IMAGING ANATOMY

Knee · Ankle · Foot

SECOND EDITION

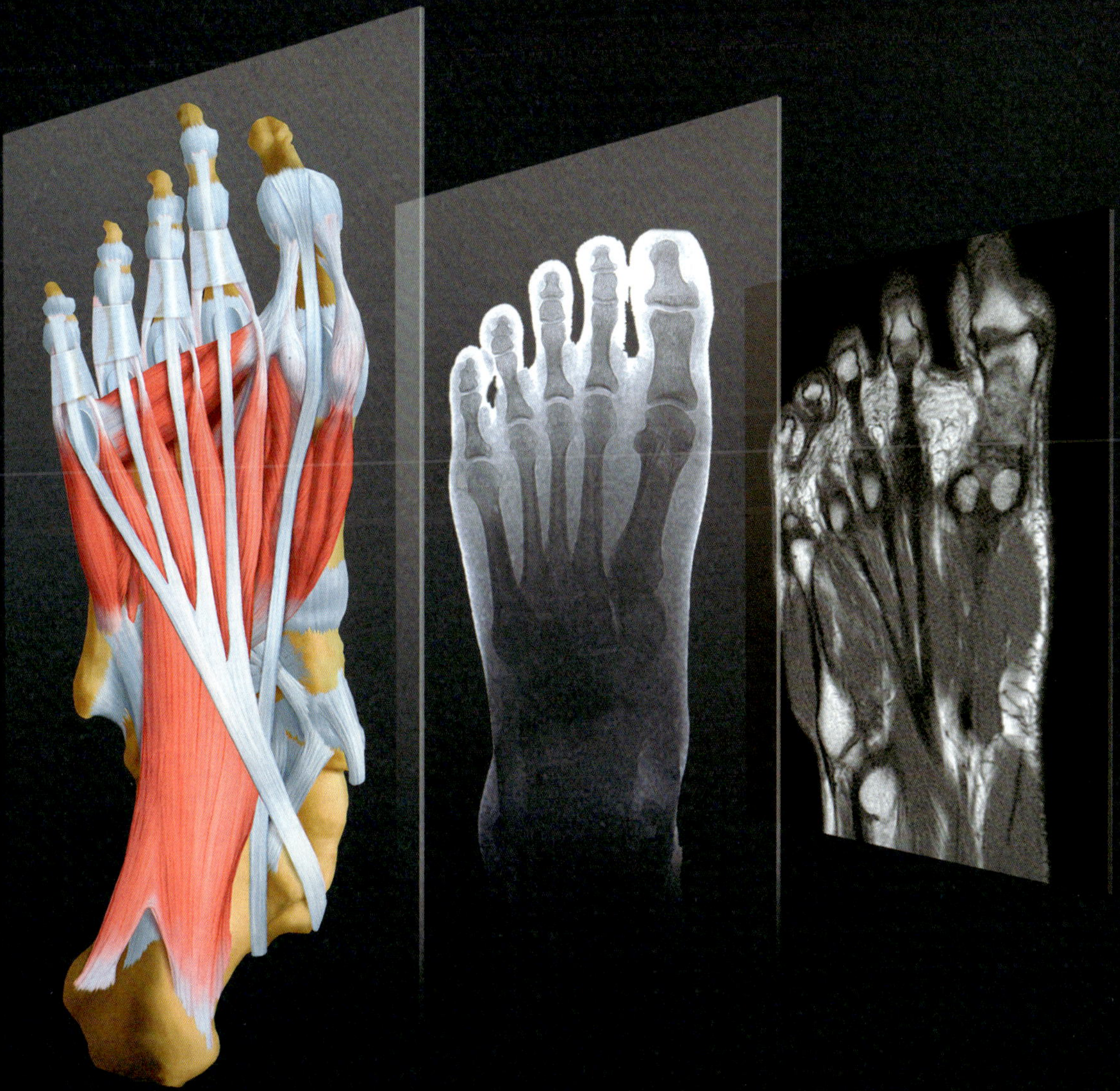

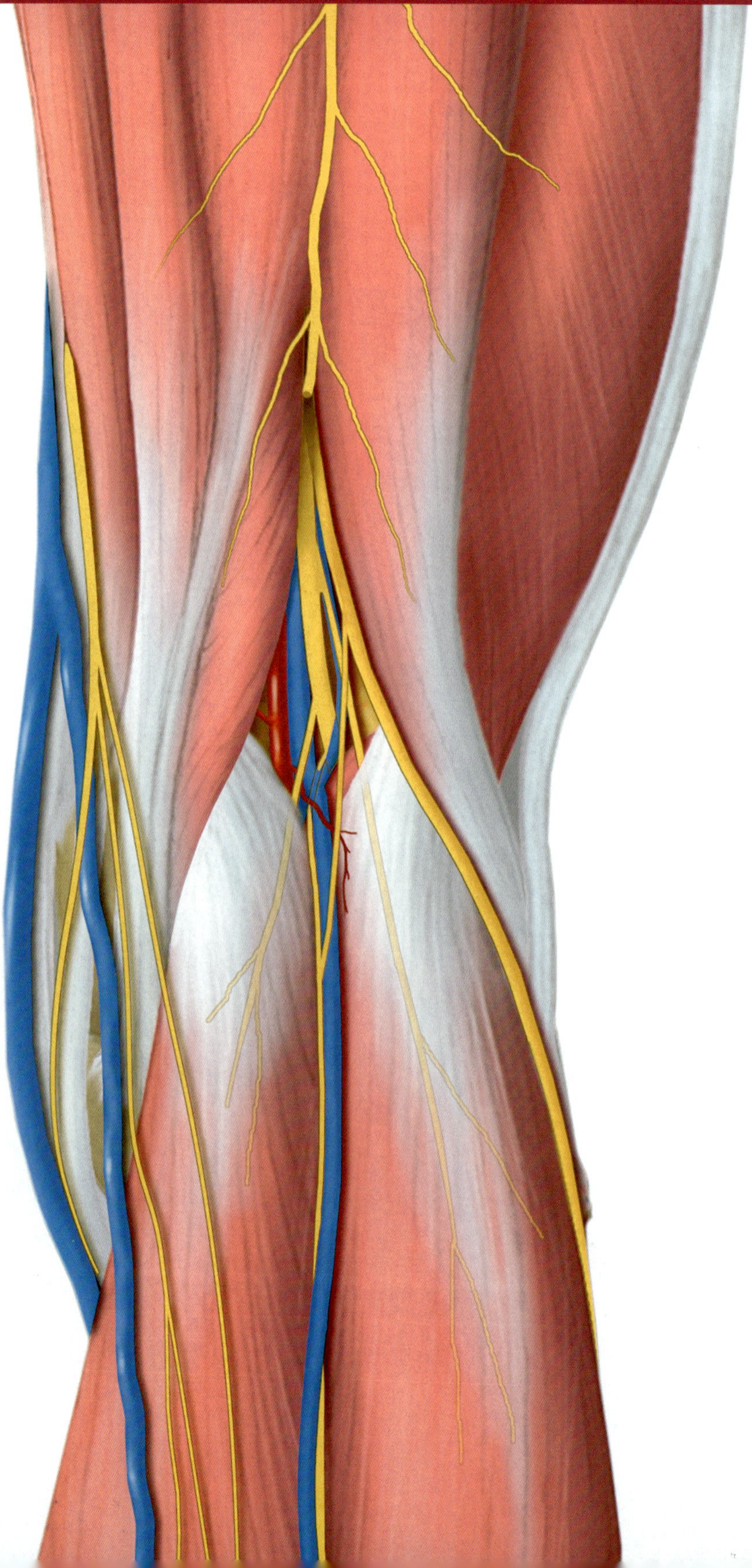

IMAGING ANATOMY

Knee · Ankle · Foot

SECOND EDITION

Julia R. Crim, MD
Chief of Musculoskeletal Radiology
Vice Chair for Clinical Affairs
Professor of Radiology
University of Missouri at Columbia
Columbia, Missouri

B.J. Manaster, MD, PhD, FACR
Emeritus Professor
Department of Radiology
University of Utah School of Medicine
Salt Lake City, Utah

Zehava Sadka Rosenberg, MD
Professor of Radiology and Orthopedic Surgery
NYU School of Medicine
NYU Langone Medical Center
New York, New York

ELSEVIER

1600 John F. Kennedy Blvd.
Ste 1800
Philadelphia, PA 19103-2899

IMAGING ANATOMY: KNEE, ANKLE, FOOT, SECOND EDITION ISBN: 978-0-323-47780-2

Notices

Knowledge and best practice in this field are constantly changing. As new research and experience broaden our understanding, changes in research methods, professional practices, or medical treatment may become necessary.

Practitioners and researchers must always rely on their own experience and knowledge in evaluating and using any information, methods, compounds, or experiments described herein. In using such information or methods they should be mindful of their own safety and the safety of others, including parties for whom they have a professional responsibility.

With respect to any drug or pharmaceutical products identified, readers are advised to check the most current information provided (i) on procedures featured or (ii) by the manufacturer of each product to be administered, to verify the recommended dose or formula, the method and duration of administration, and contraindications. It is the responsibility of practitioners, relying on their own experience and knowledge of their patients, to make diagnoses, to determine dosages and the best treatment for each individual patient, and to take all appropriate safety precautions.

To the fullest extent of the law, neither the Publisher nor the authors, contributors, or editors, assume any liability for any injury and/or damage to persons or property as a matter of products liability, negligence or otherwise, or from any use or operation of any methods, products, instructions, or ideas contained in the material herein.

Publisher Cataloging-in-Publication Data

Names: Crim, Julia R.
Title: Imaging anatomy. Knee, ankle, foot / [edited by] Julia R. Crim.
Other titles: Knee, ankle, foot.
Description: Second edition. | Salt Lake City, UT : Elsevier, Inc., [2017] | Includes bibliographical references and index.
Identifiers: ISBN 978-0-323-47780-2
Subjects: LCSH: Knee--Anatomy--Handbooks, manuals, etc. | Ankle--Anatomy--Handbooks, manuals, etc. | Foot--Anatomy--Handbooks, manuals, etc. | Knee--Imaging--Handbooks, manuals, etc. | Ankle--Imaging--Handbooks, manuals, etc. | Foot--Imaging--Handbooks, manuals, etc. | MESH: Knee--anatomy & histology--Atlases. | Ankle--anatomy & histology--Atlases. | Foot--anatomy & histology--Atlases.
Classification: LCC QM549.I43 2017 | NLM WE 17 | DDC 612'.98--dc23

International Standard Book Number: 978-0-323-47780-2

Cover Designer: Tom M. Olson, BA
Cover Art: Richard Coombs, MS

Printed in Canada by Friesens, Altona, Manitoba, Canada

Last digit is the print number: 9 8 7 6 5 4 3 2 1

Dedication

To Philip and Eleanor, in recognition of their courage, perseverance, and dedication to helping others.

JRC

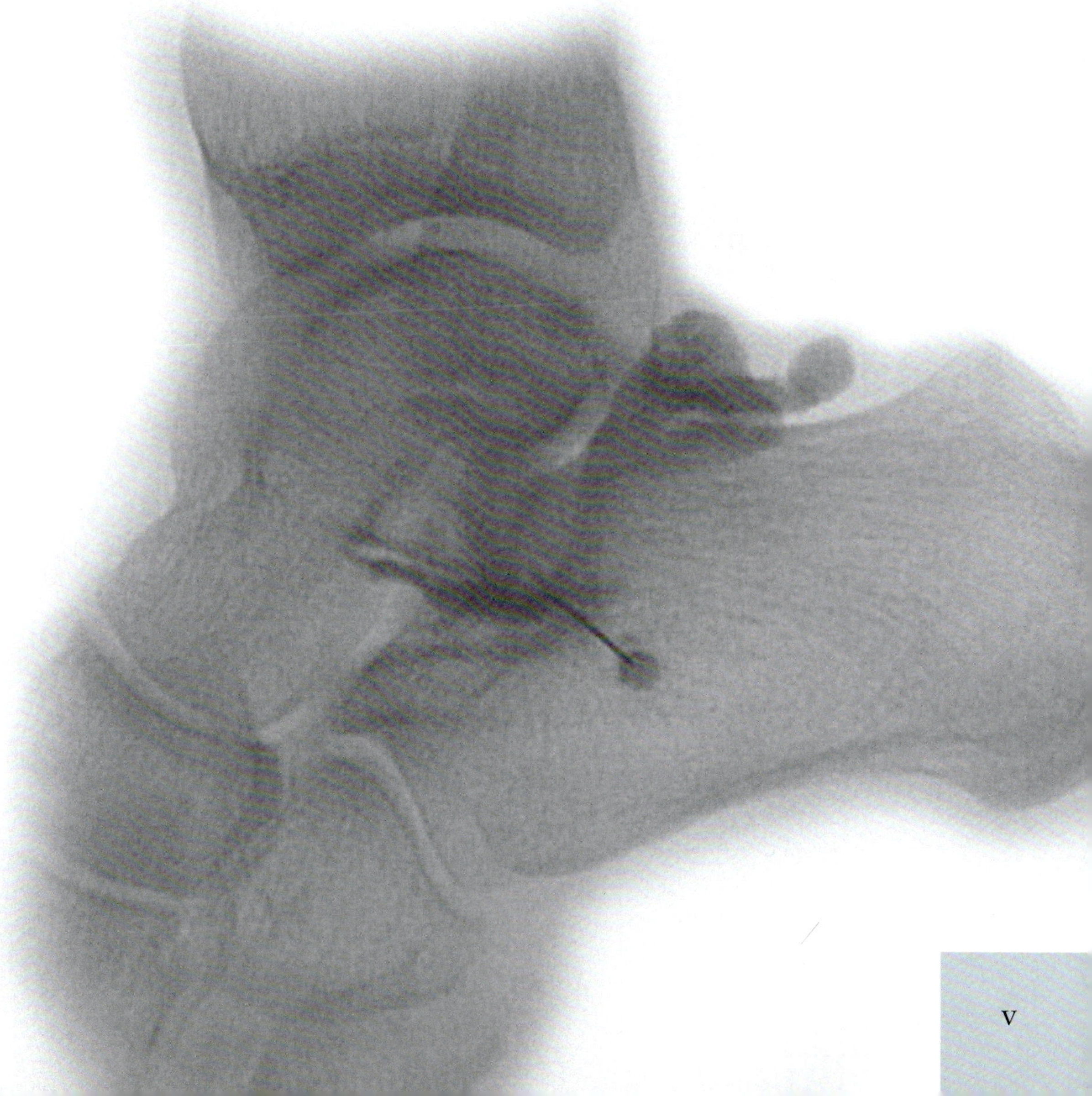

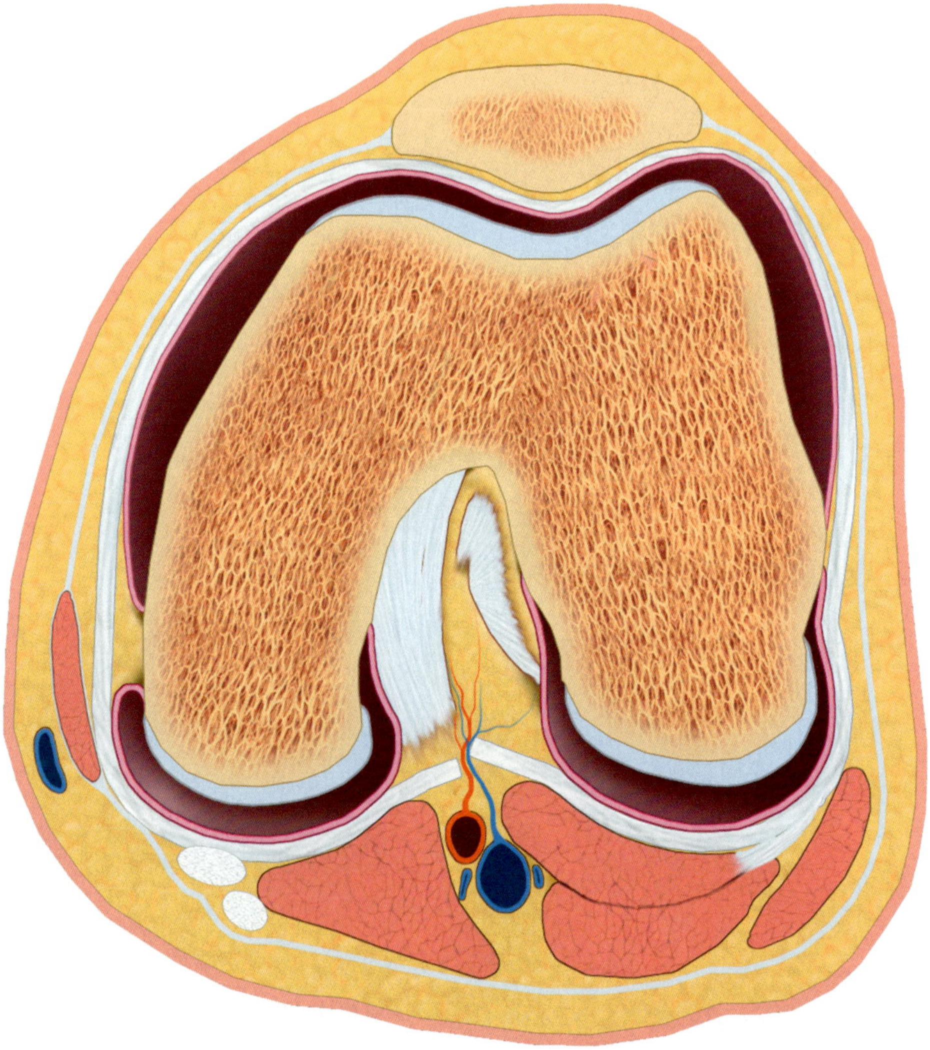

Contributing Authors

Gregory E. Antonio, MD, FRANZCR

Eric K. H. Liu, PhD, RDMS

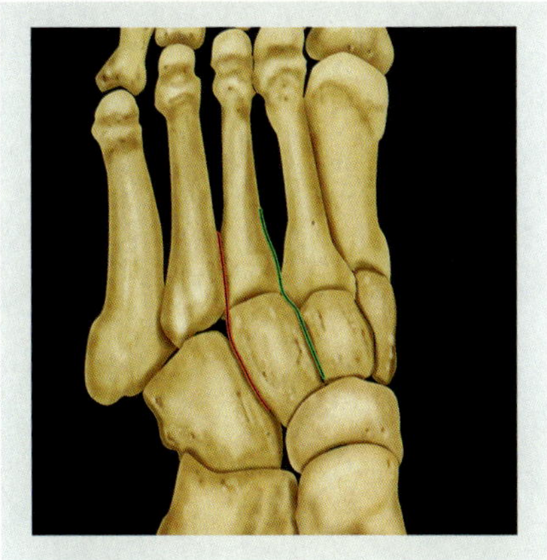

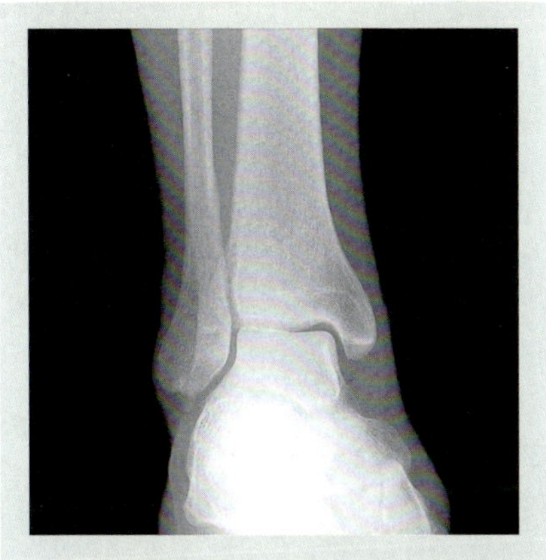

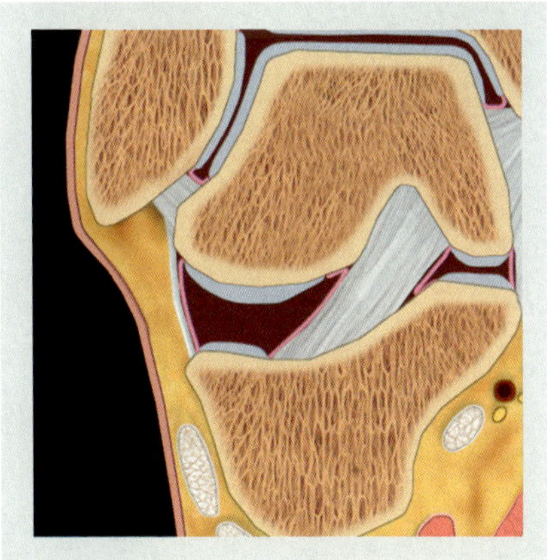

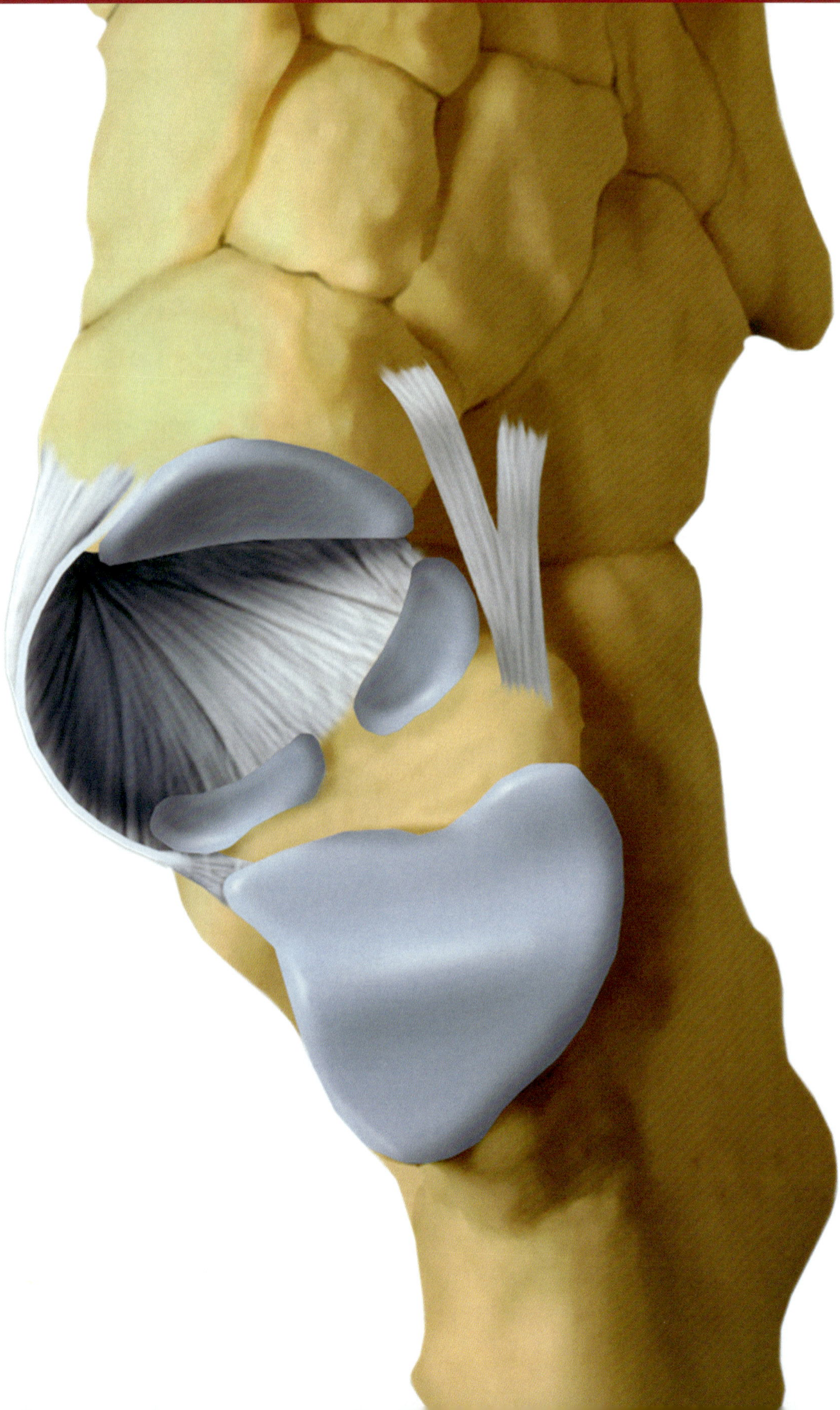

Preface

The first edition of *Imaging Anatomy: Knee, Ankle, Foot* was a successful venture, designed to serve clinicians in medical imaging and each area's related surgical and allied health specialists in sports medicine and pain management and surgeons operating on the foot and ankle. The second edition has been revised and expanded to include new information, new clinical concerns, and ultrasound imaging. Although anatomy does not change, our medical understanding of it continues to evolve, and that is reflected in our second edition.

The high-resolution CT, MR, ultrasound, and radiographic images are richly labeled. The anatomy is further elucidated by color graphics. The text is designed to give you, the busy medical professional, rapid answers to imaging anatomy questions at a level beyond what is found online or in other anatomy texts. For easy reference, *Imaging Anatomy: Knee, Ankle, Foot*, second edition is subdivided into separate sections that cover detailed normal anatomy of the knee, ankle, and foot. The joints, muscles, tendons, ligaments, nerves, and adjacent bones are discussed for each area. In addition, special sections on normal variants as well as relevant angles and measurements for the knee/leg and ankle/foot are included. Finally, needle approaches for aspiration/injection are delineated in detail.

We believe you will find that this resource for subspecialty imaging enables you to make more accurate and sophisticated diagnoses in areas of complex anatomy.

Julia R. Crim, MD
Chief of Musculoskeletal Radiology
Vice Chair for Clinical Affairs
Professor of Radiology
University of Missouri at Columbia
Columbia, Missouri

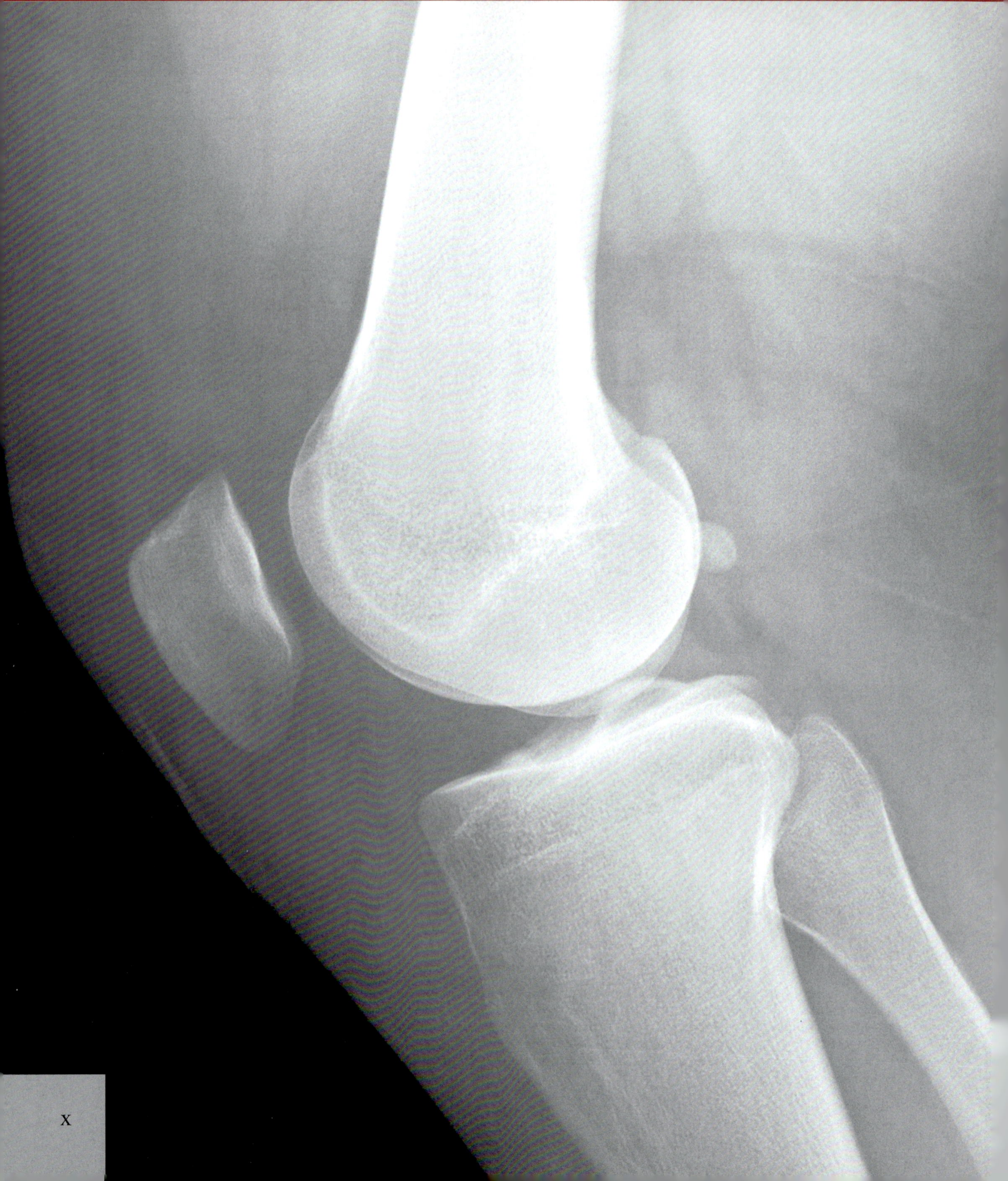

Acknowledgments

Text Editors

Nina I. Bennett, BA
Terry W. Ferrell, MS
Lisa A. Gervais, BS
Karen E. Concannon, MA, PhD
Matt W. Hoecherl, BS
Megg Morin, BA

Image Editors

Jeffrey J. Marmorstone, BS
Lisa A. M. Steadman, BS

Illustrations

Lane R. Bennion, MS
Richard Coombs, MS
Laura C. Sesto, MA

Art Direction and Design

Tom M. Olson, BA
Laura C. Sesto, MA

Lead Editor

Arthur G. Gelsinger, MA

Production Coordinators

Rebecca L. Bluth, BA
Angela M. G. Terry, BA
Emily C. Fassett, BA

ELSEVIER

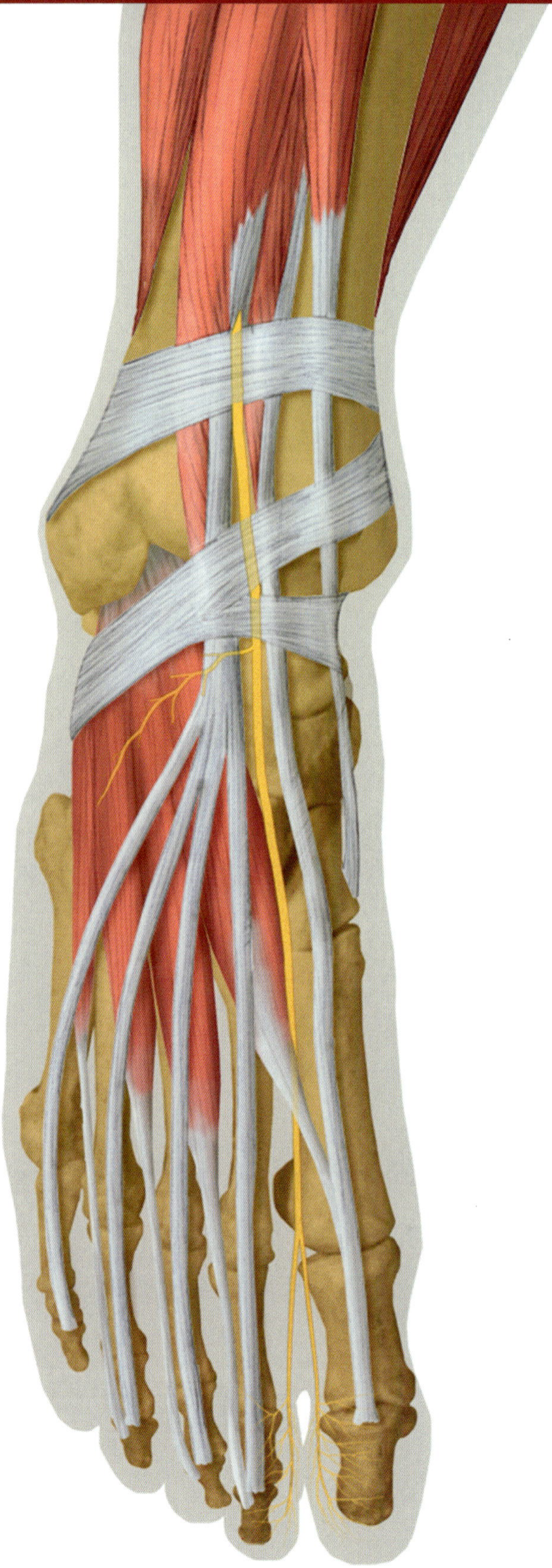

Sections

TABLE OF CONTENTS

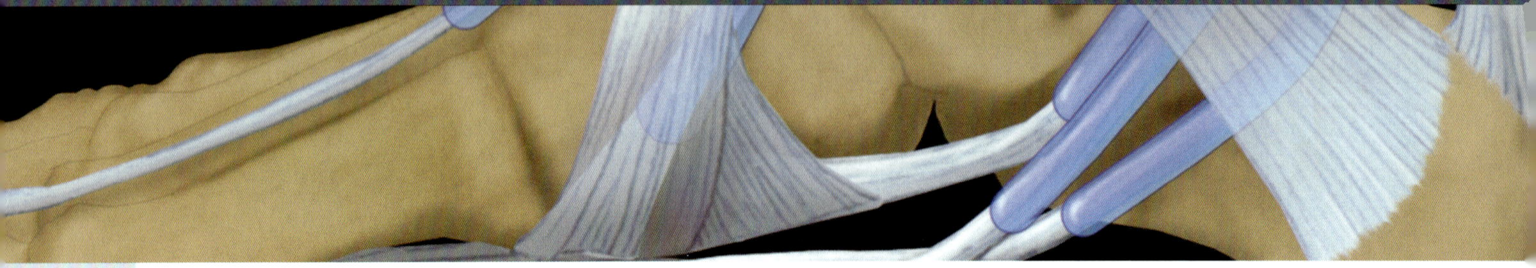

IMAGING ANATOMY

Knee · Ankle · Foot

SECOND EDITION

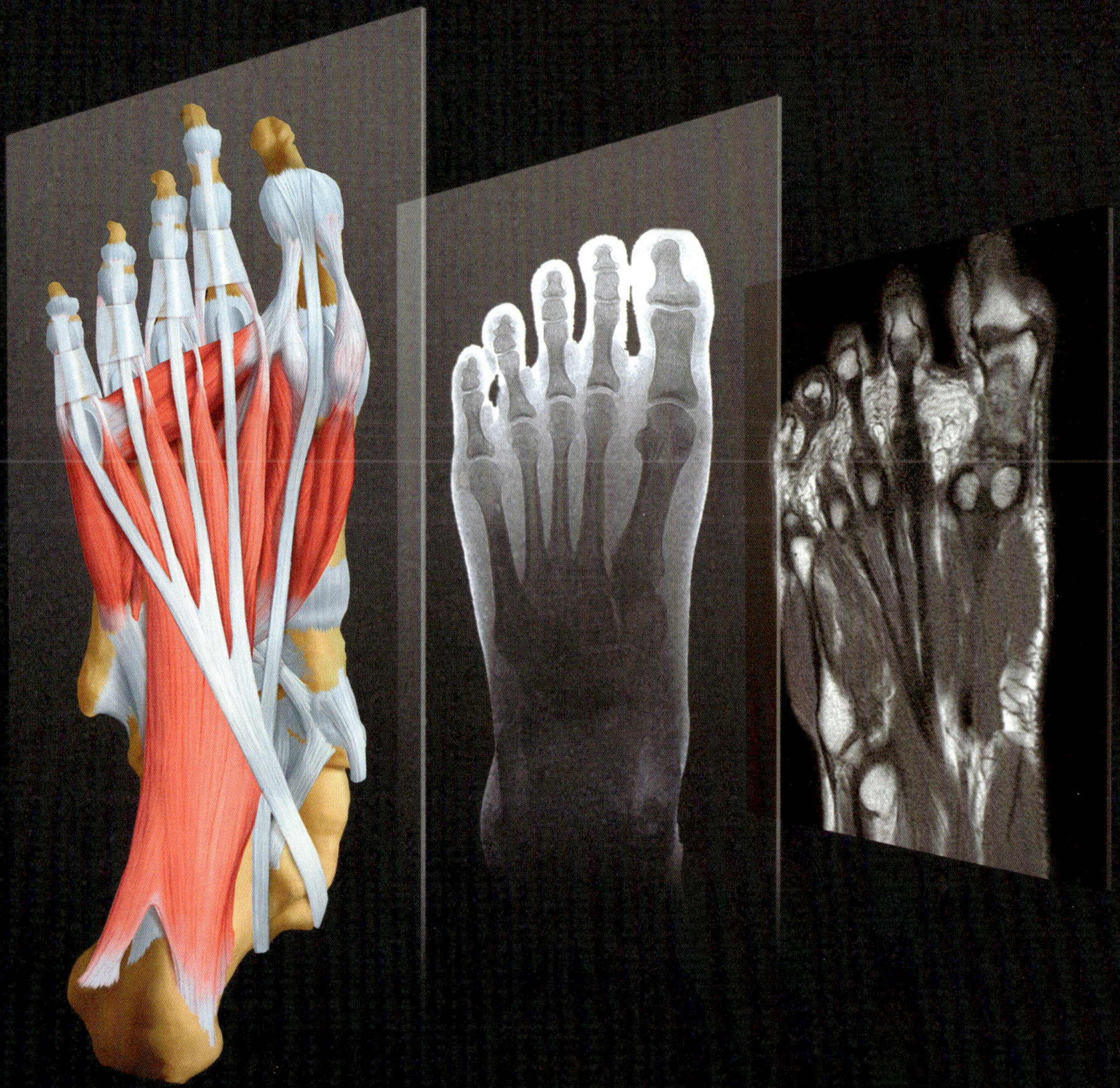

SECTION 1

Knee

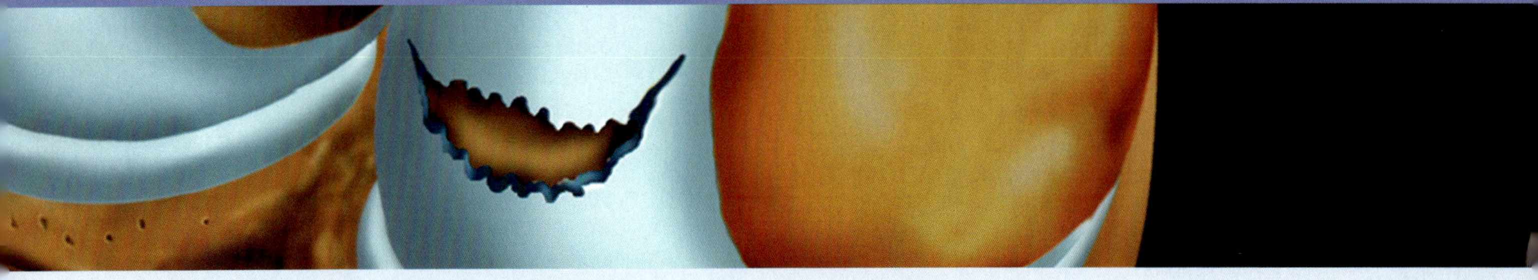

GROSS ANATOMY

Overview

- Largest and most complex joint
  - Hinge joint throughout its greatest range of motion
  - In all positions, femur in contact with tibia, with large areas of contact
  - In all positions, patella in contact with femur
  - Bones do not interlock; stability maintained by ligaments, tendons, capsule, and menisci
- **Motion** of knee and relationship of osseous structures
  - In full flexion
    - Posterior surfaces of femoral condyles articulate with posterior tibial condyles
    - Lateral facet of patella in contact with lateral femoral condyle
    - Supporting ligaments are not taut, and rotation of leg is allowed
  - During motion of extension
    - Patella slides upwards on femur, passing 1st on to its middle facet and then its lower facets
    - Femoral condyles roll forward on tibial condyles and menisci
    - Lateral femoral condyle shorter anteroposteriorly than medial and reaches full extension earlier
    - Medial femoral condyle continues to slide after lateral stops, rotates slightly medially on tibia and medial meniscus ("screwing it home"), tightens anterior cruciate ligament, collateral ligaments, and posterior capsular ligaments, turning knee into rigid pillar
  - Initiating flexion from fully extended knee
    - Requires slight medial rotation of tibia, produced by popliteus
    - "Unlocks" joint, allowing remainder of motion to take place
- **Muscles acting on knee joint: Extensors (4 parts of quadriceps femoris)**
  - Rectus femoris
    - Origin straight head: Anterior inferior iliac spine; origin reflected head: Groove immediately superior to acetabulum
    - Insertion: Patella and continuation to inferior patellar tendon
    - Action: Crosses both hip and knee joints, flexing hip and extending knee
    - Innervation: Femoral nerve
    - Vascular supply: Lateral circumflex femoral artery
  - Vastus lateralis
    - Origin: Superior portion of intertrochanteric line, anterior and inferior borders of greater trochanter, superior portion of lateral lip of linea aspera, and lateral portion of gluteal tuberosity of femur
    - Insertion: Lateral base and border of patella; also forms lateral patellar retinaculum and lateral side of quadriceps femoris tendon
    - Action: Extends knee
    - Innervation: Femoral nerve
    - Vascular supply: Lateral circumflex femoral artery
  - Vastus medialis
    - Origin: Inferior portion of intertrochanteric line, spiral line, medial lip of linea aspera, superior part of medial supracondylar ridge of femur, and medial intermuscular septum
    - Insertion: Medial base and border of patella; also forms medial patellar retinaculum and medial side of quadriceps femoris tendon
    - Action: Extends knee
    - Innervation: Femoral nerve
    - Vascular supply: Femoral artery, profunda femoris artery, and superior medial genicular branch of popliteal artery
  - Vastus intermedius
    - Origin: Superior 2/3 of anterior and lateral surfaces of femur; also from lateral intermuscular septum of thigh
    - Insertion: Lateral border of patella; also forms deep portion of quadriceps tendon
    - Action: Extends knee
    - Innervation: Femoral nerve
    - Vascular supply: Lateral circumflex femoral artery
- **Muscles acting on knee joint: Flexors**
  - Biceps femoris
    - Origin: Long head, common tendon with semitendinosus from superior medial quadrant of posterior portion of ischial tuberosity; short head, lateral lip of linea aspera, lateral supracondylar ridge of femur, and lateral intermuscular septum of thigh
    - Insertion: Primarily on fibular head; also on lateral collateral ligament and lateral tibial condyle
    - Action: Flexes knee and also rotates tibia laterally; long head also extends hip joint
    - Innervation: Long head, tibial nerve; short head, common peroneal nerve
    - Vascular supply: Perforating branches of profunda femoris artery, inferior gluteal artery, and superior muscular branches of popliteal artery
  - Sartorius
    - Origin: Anterior superior iliac spine
    - Insertion: Anteromedial tibial metaphysis near tibial tuberosity
    - Action: Crosses both hip and knee joints, flexes both hip and knee joints, rotating thigh laterally to bring limbs into position adopted by cross-legged tailor
    - Innervation: Femoral nerve
    - Vascular supply: Muscular branches of femoral artery
  - Gracilis
    - Origin: Inferior margin of pubic symphysis, inferior ramus of pubis, and adjacent ramus of ischium
    - Insertion: Medial tibial metaphysis, just posterior to sartorius
    - Action: Adducts thigh, flexes knee, and rotates flexed leg medially
    - Innervation: Anterior division of obturator nerve
    - Vascular supply: Obturator artery, medial circumflex femoral artery, and muscular branches of profunda femoris artery
  - Semitendinosus
    - Origin: From common tendon with long head of biceps femoris from superior medial quadrant of posterior portion of ischial tuberosity

- Insertion: Medial tibial metaphysis, just posterior to gracilis
- Action: Crosses both hip and knee joints, extends hip, flexes knee, medially rotates flexed leg
- Innervation: Tibial nerve
- Vascular supply: Perforating branches of profunda femoris artery, inferior gluteal artery, and superior muscular branches of popliteal artery
  - Semimembranosus
    - Origin: Superior lateral quadrant ischial tuberosity
    - Insertion: Wide insertion posterior and medial tibial condyle
    - Action: Crosses both hip and knee joints, extends hip, flexes knee, medially rotates flexed knee
    - Innervation: Tibial nerve
    - Vascular supply: Perforating branches of profunda femoris artery, inferior gluteal artery, and superior muscular branches of popliteal artery
  - Popliteus
    - Origin: Anterior part of popliteal groove on lateral surface of lateral femoral condyle
    - Insertion: Posterior surface of tibia in fan-like fashion, just superior to popliteal line
    - Action: Flexes knee and medially rotates tibia at beginning of flexion
    - Innervation: Tibial nerve
    - Vascular supply: Medial inferior genicular branch of popliteal artery and muscular branch of posterior tibial artery
- **Muscles acting on knee joint: Superficial flexors of knee**
  - Gastrocnemius
    - Origin: Medial head from posterior nonarticular surface of medial femoral condyle; lateral head from posterior edge of lateral epicondyle; heads unite to form main bulk of muscle
    - Insertion: Unites with deep tendon of soleus to form Achilles tendon, inserting on middle 1/3 of posterior calcaneal surface
    - Action: Flexes knee and plantar flexes ankle
    - Innervation: Tibial nerve
    - Vascular supply: Sural branch of popliteal artery
  - Plantaris
    - Origin: Superior and medial to lateral head of gastrocnemius origin, as well as from oblique popliteal ligament
    - Insertion: Middle 1/3 of posterior calcaneal surface, just medial to Achilles tendon
    - Action: Flexes knee and plantarflexes ankle
    - Innervation: Tibial nerve
    - Vascular supply: Sural arteries
    - Note: Absent in 7-10% of population
- **Muscles acting on knee joint: Internal rotators of leg**
  - Popliteus, gracilis, sartorius, semitendinosus, semimembranosus
- **Muscles acting on knee joint: External rotator of leg**
  - Biceps femoris
- **Extensor mechanism**
  - Quadriceps tendon and retinacula converge to inferior patellar tendon
- **Internal structures**
  - Menisci
    - Cushion lubricate and stabilize knee
  - Cruciate ligaments
    - Major stabilizing structures to anteroposterior motion
  - Medial supporting structures
    - Pes anserinus, medial collateral ligament, capsular layers, and posterior oblique ligament
  - Lateral supporting structures
    - Iliotibial band, biceps femoris, quadriceps retinaculum, fibular collateral ligament, arcuate ligament, and several small inconstant posterolateral structures
- **Nerves** of knee joint
  - **Femoral nerve** supplies
    - 3 branches, 1 to each of vasti and to anterosuperior part of joint
    - Largest is nerve to vastus medialis, which accompanies descending genicular artery
  - **Common peroneal nerve** supplies
    - Superior lateral genicular nerve descends into popliteal fossa and supplies superolateral part of joint, passing deep to biceps, through lateral intermuscular septum above femoral condyle
    - Inferior lateral genicular nerve: Small and sometimes absent; arises with superior lateral genicular nerve and curves downwards and forwards over lateral head of gastrocnemius, passing between capsule and fibular collateral ligament
    - Recurrent genicular nerve: Small twigs reaching anteroinferior part of joint
  - **Tibial nerve** supplies
    - Superior medial genicular nerve: Runs medially around femur above medial condyle, deep to adductor magnus, then through vastus medialis to superomedial part of joint
    - Middle genicular nerve: Runs forward through fibrous capsule to cruciate ligaments
    - Inferior medial genicular nerve: Largest, running along upper border of popliteus, passing forward between shaft of tibia and medial collateral ligament, curving superiorly to inferomedial part of capsule
  - **Obturator nerve**: Sends genicular branch through adductor magnus to join popliteal artery, running to posterior aspect of joint
- **Vessels** of knee joint: 8 arteries supply large anastomosis
  - **Popliteal** artery supplies 5 genicular branches
  - **Anterior tibial** artery supplies 2 recurrent branches
  - **Femoral** artery supplies descending genicular branch
  - **Lateral circumflex** artery supplies descending genicular branch

3D CT: ORIGINS AND INSERTIONS (LATERAL, ANTEROLATERAL)

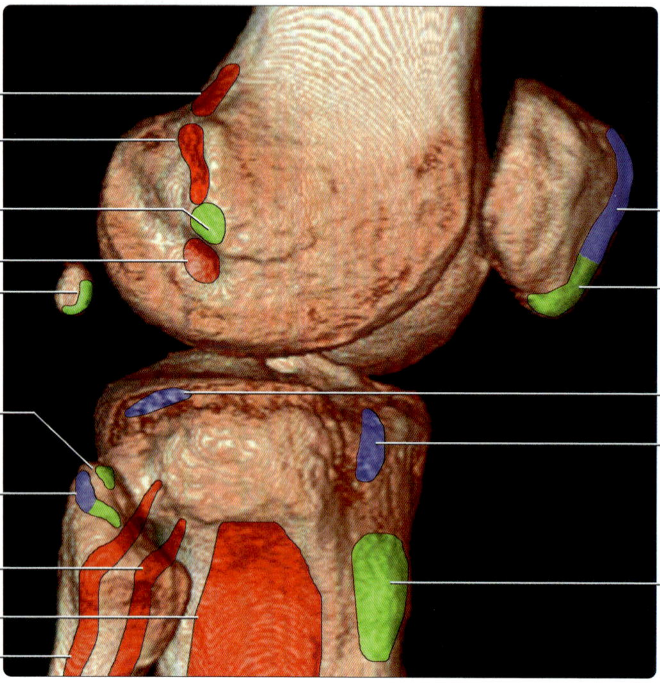

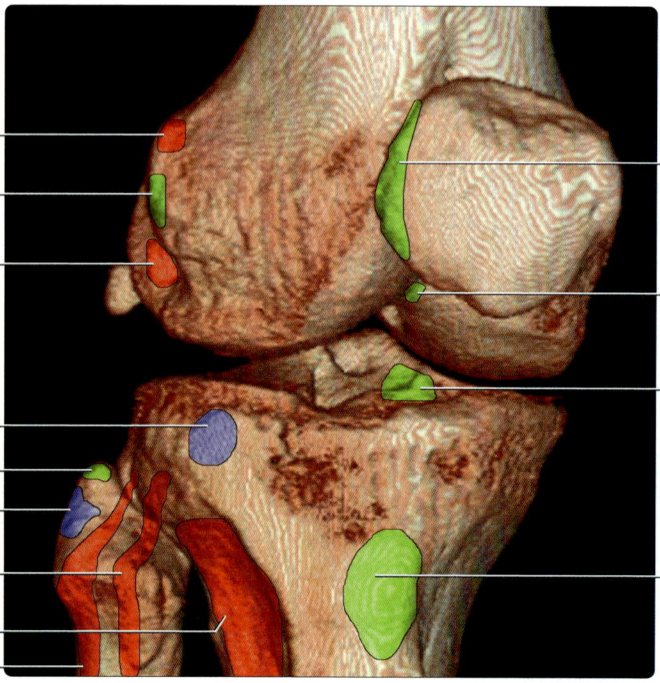

(Top) *Lateral view of the knee shows lateral stabilizing structures. Origins of anterior and lateral leg muscles are seen as well.* **(Bottom)** *This slightly anterolateral view shows the lateral stabilizers of the knee and patella. These consist primarily of the lateral collateral ligament, arcuate ligament, popliteal tendon, iliotibial band, and biceps femoris. Origins of several leg muscles are seen. The tibialis anterior, extensor digitorum longus, and peroneus longus origins extend several centimeters distally beyond the regions indicated here.*

3D CT: ORIGINS AND INSERTIONS (ANTEROMEDIAL)

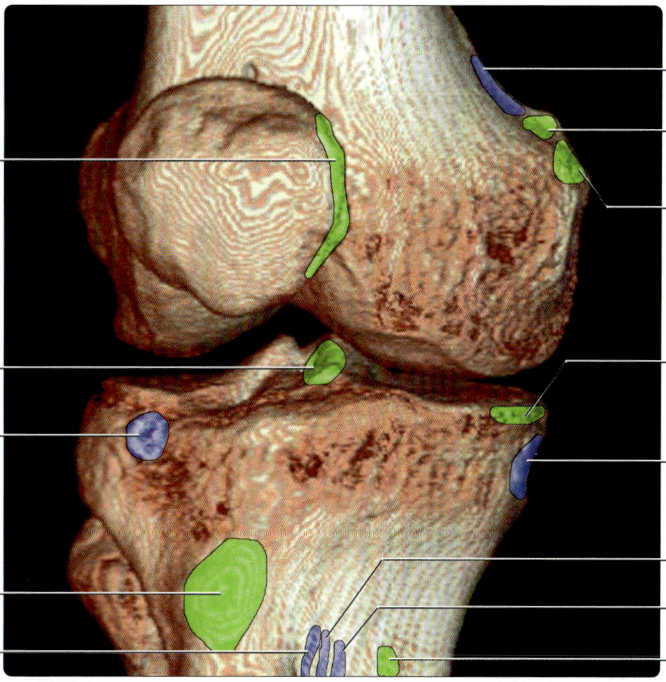

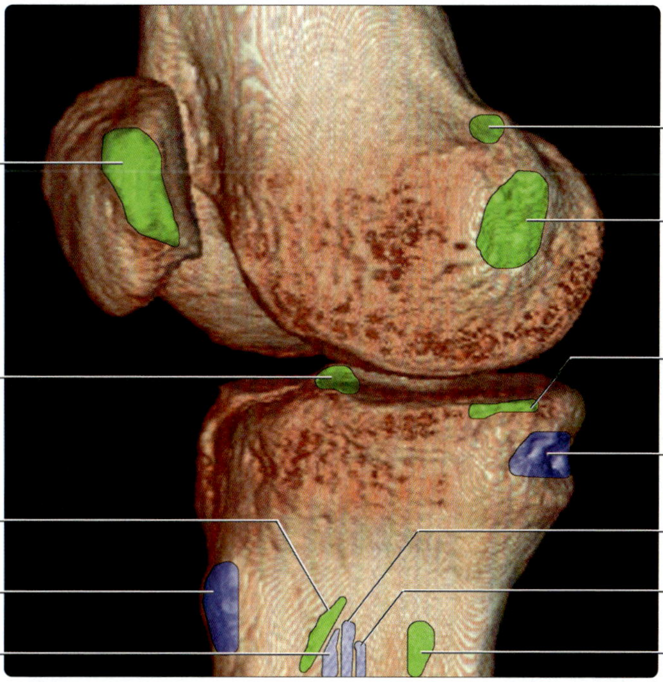

(Top) *Slightly anteromedial view shows the medial stabilizers of the knee and patella. Note that only the uppermost portion of the insertions of the pes anserinus (sartorius, gracilis, and semitendinosus), as well as superficial medial collateral ligament, are shown. These insertions actually extend several cm distally on the tibia.* **(Bottom)** *Anteromedial knee shows medial stabilizers of knee (primarily medial collateral ligament, superficial and deep fibers, secondarily pes anserinus), as well as medial stabilizers of patella (superiorly medial patellofemoral ligament, mid medial retinaculum, inferiorly patellotibial ligament).*

3D CT: ORIGINS AND INSERTIONS (MEDIAL, POSTEROMEDIAL)

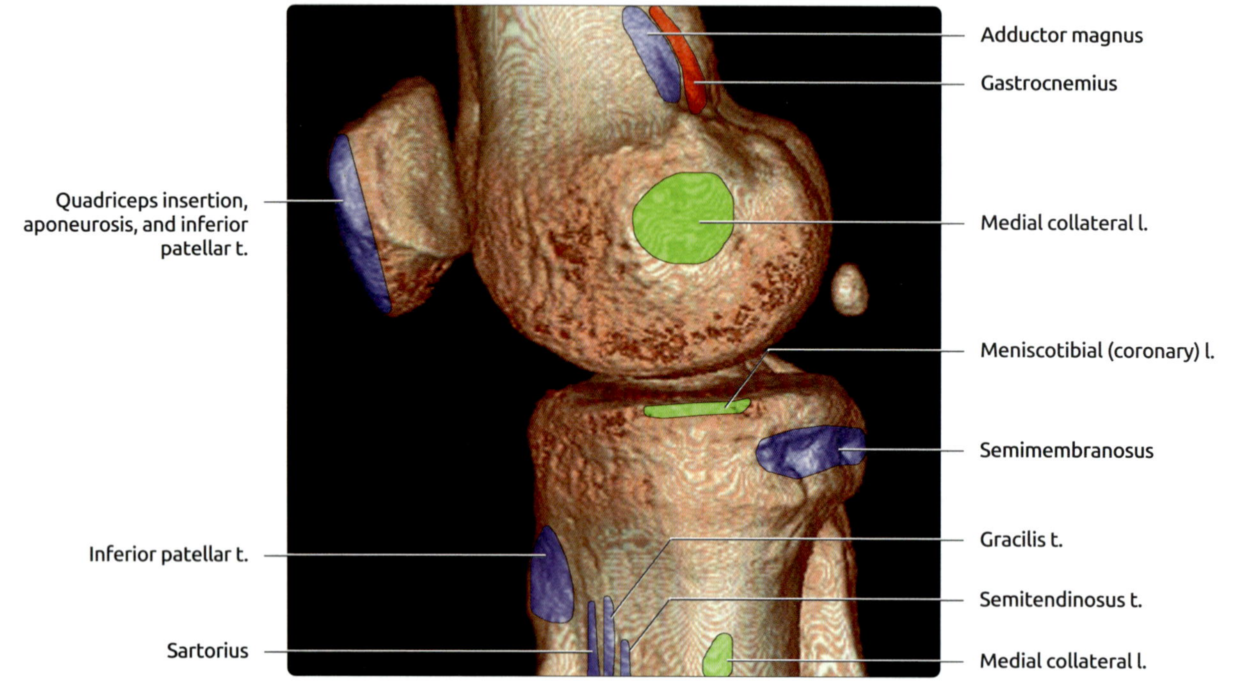

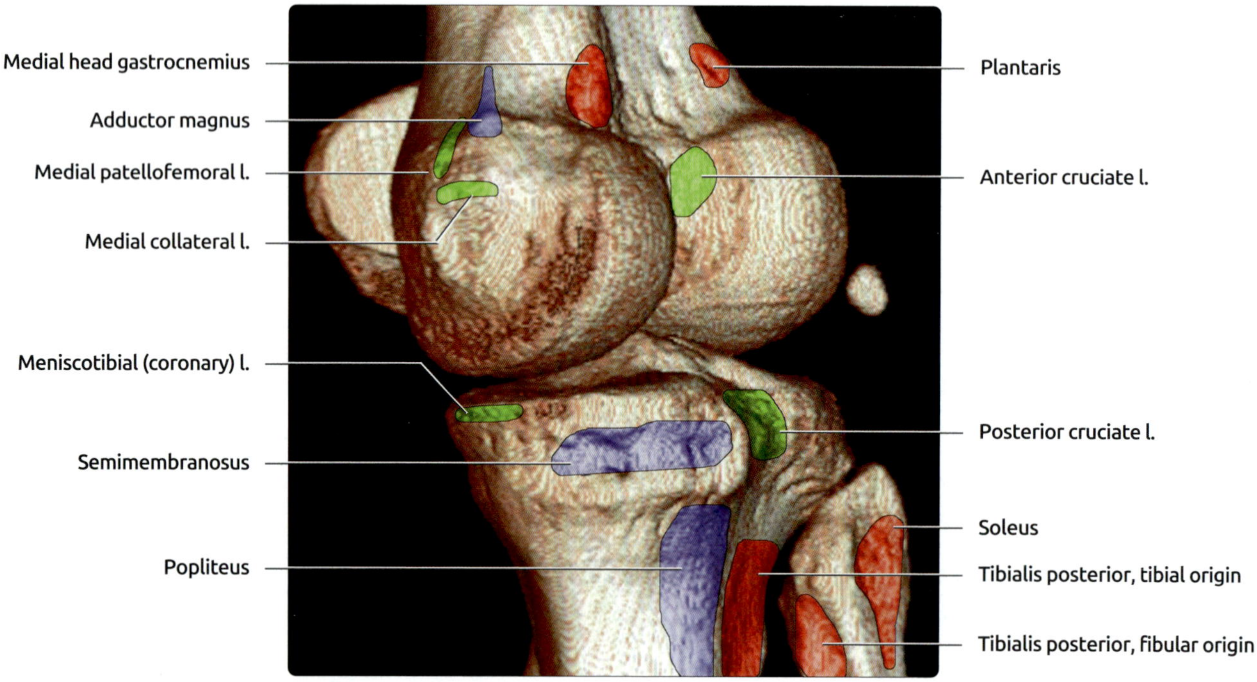

(Top) *First of 8 volume-rendered topographic CT images is shown. Image shows the medial aspect of the knee with associated muscle, tendon, and ligament origins/insertions.* **(Bottom)** *Posterior CT, oblique to medial, is shown. Note the extensive insertions of both semimembranosus and popliteus on the posteromedial tibia.*

3D CT: ORIGINS AND INSERTIONS (POSTERIOR, POSTEROLATERAL)

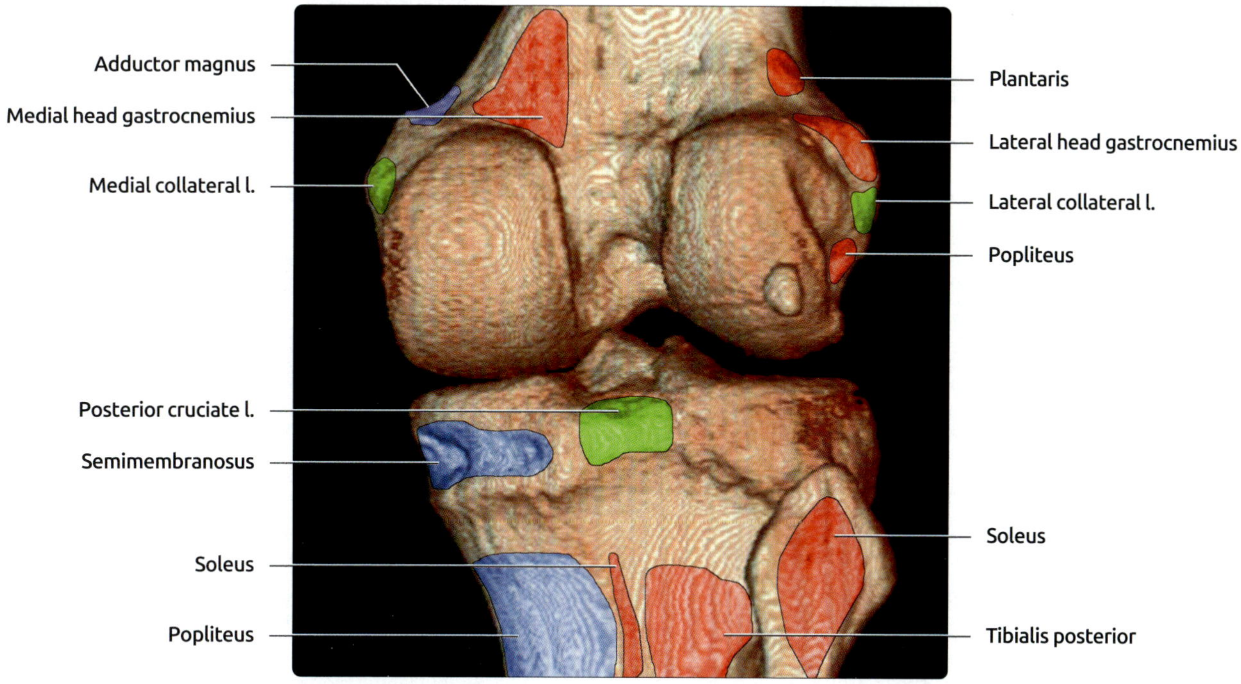

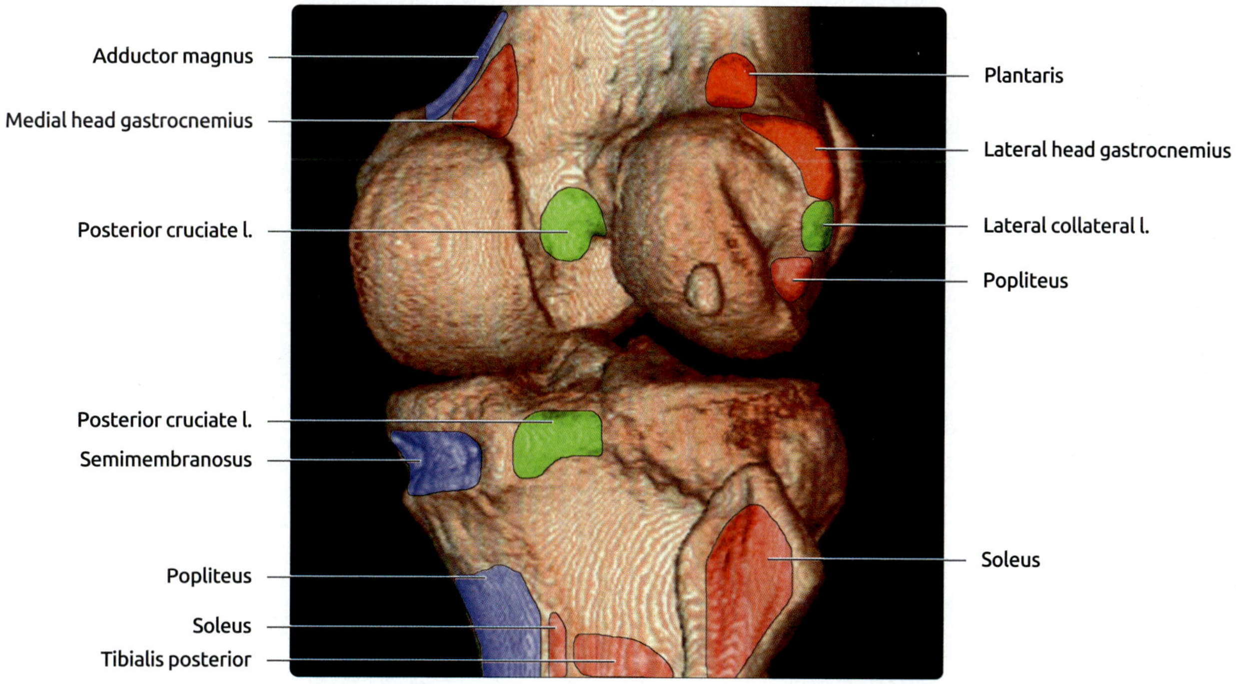

(Top) *Direct posterior view shows that the posterior cruciate ligament insertion is extraarticular on the posterior central tibia.* **(Bottom)** *Posterior (slightly oblique) view of the knee shows the attachments of the posterior structures. Note that fibular origin of the soleus is more proximal than tibial origin.*

GRAPHICS: POSTERIOR SUPERFICIAL AND DEEP MUSCLES AND NERVES

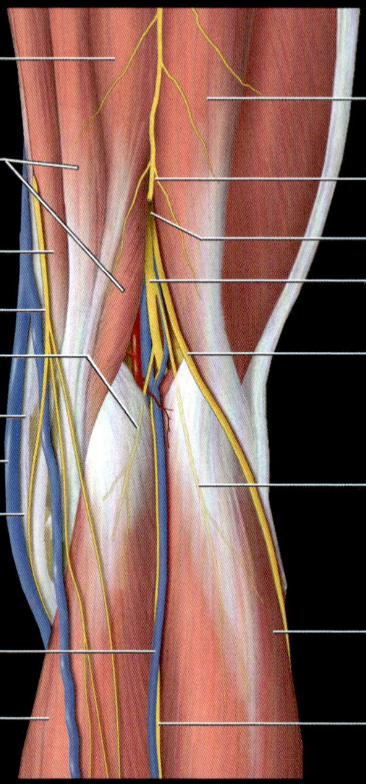

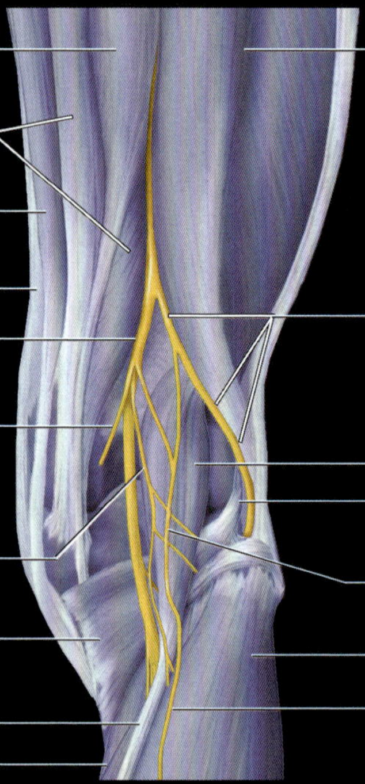

(Top) *Graphic shows the superficial posterior muscles and nerves. Note that the common peroneal nerve is part of the deeper nerve system, but travels more superficially, following the posterior biceps femoris muscle and tendon until it wraps around the fibular neck.* **(Bottom)** *Graphic shows the relationship of the common peroneal nerve to the posterior biceps femoris tendon. It also shows the tibial nerve with the numerous muscular branches. Note the plantaris muscle coursing over the popliteus (and popliteal vessels, not shown) and becoming tendinous at the level of the popliteus/soleus muscle junction. The plantaris tendon then courses downward and slightly medially between soleus and medial head gastrocnemius (not shown). The sural nerve arises from branches of both common peroneal and tibial nerves and courses down superficial to the junction of the 2 gastrocnemius heads. The tibial nerve travels downward in a deeper position, just posterior to the posterior tibial vessels.*

GRAPHICS: VESSELS AND ANASTOMOTIC NETWORK

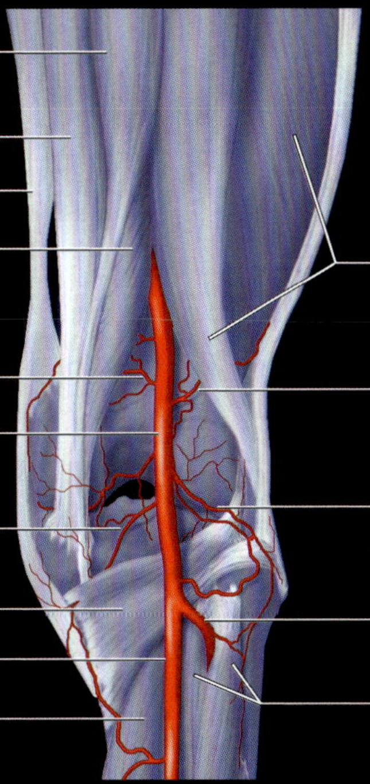

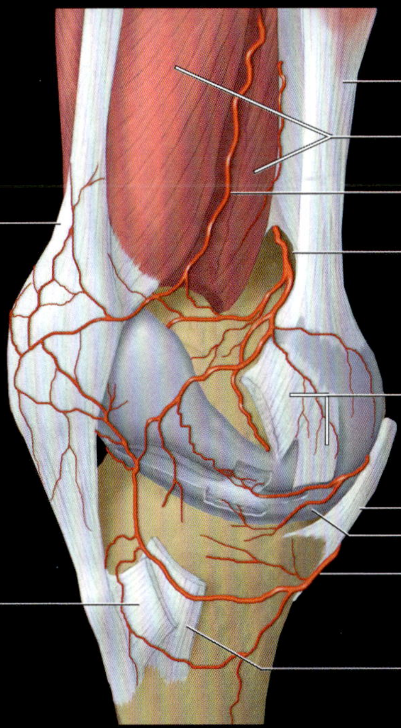

(Top) *Graphic shows the anastomoses around the knee, posteriorly. The popliteal artery is seen throughout its course, from the hiatus in adductor magnus proximally to the lower border of popliteus distally. At this point, the popliteal artery bifurcates into anterior and posterior tibial arteries. The anterior tibial is the smaller branch that extends through a slit in tibialis posterior and on through the interosseous membrane to descend along the interosseous membrane down the anterior compartment. There are 4 named geniculate branches, a superior and inferior both medially and laterally.* **(Bottom)** *Graphic of the anteromedial knee shows the rich anastomotic vascular network around the knee. There are 2 named geniculate branches of the popliteal artery in each side (superior and inferior). Additionally, there are 2 supplementary arteries. The descending geniculate artery (a branch of the femoral artery) descends superomedially. There is also an anterior recurrent branch of the anterior tibial artery that runs inferolaterally, not shown here.*

IMAGING ANATOMY

Overview

- Radiographic anatomy
  - Distal femur osseous features
    - Distal femoral metaphysis flares into medial and lateral epicondyles
    - Medial femoral condyle larger than lateral, more rounded inferiorly
    - Lateral femoral condyle has flatter contour
      - Slight concavity in anteroinferior surface at junction of patellofemoral and femorotibial articular surfaces
      - Termed terminal sulcus or lateral femoral recess
      - < 2mm depth
    - Intercondylar notch houses cruciate ligaments
      - Roof of intercondylar notch visualized as Blumensaat line on lateral radiograph
    - Anteriorly, V-shaped trochlear groove articulates with patella
  - Possible sites of avulsion from femur
    - Posterolateral intercondylar notch [anterior cruciate ligament (ACL) origin]
    - Mid medial intercondylar notch [posterior cruciate ligament (PCL) origin]
    - Medial epicondyle [medial collateral ligament (MCL) origin]
  - Proximal tibia osseous features
    - Tibial plateau refers to articular surface, condyle is bony support of plateau
    - Tibial plateaus slope about 10° inferiorly from anterior to posterior
    - Medial tibial plateau larger than lateral, has concave articular surface
    - Lateral tibial plateau has flat articular surface
    - Medial tibial condyle has squared contour posteriorly
    - Lateral tibial condyle has diagonal posterior facet for articulation with fibula
    - Tibial spines lie between tibial plateaus
      - ACL attaches to medial aspect of lateral tibial spine
    - Tibial tubercle is anterior prominence several centimeters distal to articular surface
      - Site of attachment of patellar tendon
      - Forms from separate apophysis, which may remain nonunited
  - Proximal fibula osseous features
    - Posterolaterally located relative to tibia
    - Proximal point termed fibular styloid process
  - Patellar osseous features
    - Triangular sesamoid
    - Wider at base superiorly than at apex inferiorly
    - Articular surface divided by vertical ridge into lateral and medial facets
    - Lateral facet elongated and has shallow angle
    - Medial facet short and more strongly angulated
    - Odd facet lies between medial facet, anterior margin and does not have articular cartilage
      - Variably present
    - Lower 25% nonarticular
    - Nonarticular outer surface may develop prominent enthesopathy where quadriceps tendon insertion blends into origin of inferior patellar tendon
    - Multiple vascular grooves often visible along anterior patellar surface
- Internal contents
  - **Menisci**: Cushion, lubricate, and stabilize knee
    - Composed of fibrocartilage, triangular in cross section
    - Only peripheral 1/3 is vascularized
    - Each meniscus divided into anterior horn, body, and posterior horn
    - Meniscal roots: Central portions of anterior and posterior horns, anchored to tibia
    - Transverse ligament extends between anterior horns
    - Medial meniscus: Posterior horn larger than anterior horn
    - Menisci tightly attached to medial joint capsule; small perimeniscal recesses
    - Lateral meniscus: Posterior and anterior horns equal in size
    - Loose capsular attachments of lateral meniscus allow rotational motion; large perimeniscal recesses
    - Popliteus tendon passes by body and posterior horn lateral meniscus; popliteomeniscal fascicles extend from posterior horn to popliteus sheath
  - **Cruciate ligaments**
    - Intraarticular but extrasynovial
    - ACL prevents anterior translation of tibia
    - ACL originates at posterolateral intercondylar notch, extends anteromedially, inserts at interspinous tibia and medial tibial spine
    - ACL consists of 2 bundles: Anteromedial and posterolateral
    - PCL prevents posterior translation of tibia
    - PCL originates at medial aspect of intercondylar notch, extends posterolaterally, inserts extraarticularly on posterior cortex of proximal tibia
    - PCL consists of 2 bundles: Anterolateral and posteromedial
  - **Meniscofemoral ligaments**: Extend from posterior horn lateral meniscus to medial femoral condyle adjacent to PCL origin at intercondylar notch
    - Ligament of Humphrey: Passes anterior to PCL
    - Ligament of Wrisberg: Passes posterior to PCL
  - **Medial collateral ligament**
    - Superficial portion: Thick, extends from femoral condyle to proximal tibia
    - Deep portion: Meniscofemoral (coronary) and meniscotibial ligament
    - Stabilizes to valgus stress
  - **Lateral collateral ligament complex**
    - Iliotibial band: Distal extension of tensor fascia lata, inserts on Gerdy tubercle of anterolateral tibia; anterolateral stabilizer
    - Lateral (fibular) collateral ligament (LCL): Femoral condyle to fibula
    - Anterolateral ligament: Arises immediately anterior to lateral collateral ligament, crosses obliquely and anteriorly to attach at lateral tibial condyle between Gerdy tubercle and fibular head

- Biceps femoris: Complex insertions on fibula and tibia; often forms conjoint tendon distally with fibular collateral ligament
- Posterolateral corner: LCL, biceps, popliteus; fabellofibular/arcuate/popliteofibular ligaments
- **Extensor mechanism**
  - Quadriceps tendon: Inserts on anterosuperior margin of patella
  - Patellar tendon: Continuation of quadriceps tendon, extends from anteroinferior margin of patella to tibial tubercle
  - Patella: Medial and lateral articular facets divided by median ridge (apex)
  - Hoffa fat pad: Triangle-shaped, vascularized fat pad posterior to patellar tendon
- **Hyaline cartilage surfaces**
  - Patella has thickest cartilage in body; can be up to 7 mm
  - Patella articulates with wedge-shaped trochlear groove of femur
  - Bipartite patella: Superolateral accessory ossicle, intact cartilage over junction with patella
  - Medial tibiofemoral compartment normally has thinner cartilage width than lateral compartment
  - Lateral tibiofemoral compartment has thin cartilage at lateral femoral sulcus
  - Tibial cartilage gradually thins near periphery; tibial spines, anteriorly
- **Joint capsule, recesses**
  - Suprapatellar recess: Large recess, communicates freely with remainder of joint
  - Perimeniscal recesses: Larger laterally than medially
  - Popliteus tendon sheath: Communicates with joint
  - Capsule may extend into/through origin of medial or lateral gastrocnemius
  - Popliteal cyst ("Baker cyst"): Fluid extends through weak point in capsule between semimembranosus tendon and medial head of gastrocnemius
  - Plicae: Remnants of tissue between developing compartments
  - Superior patellar plica: Curves through suprapatellar recess medial to lateral (not commonly symptomatic)
  - Infrapatellar plica: Extends from origin adjacent to ACL into Hoffa fat pad; parallels ACL
  - Medial patellar plica: Vertically oriented in medial patellofemoral recess (can result in snapping on flexion/extension and medial patellofemoral cartilage wear)

- **Extraarticular bursae**
  - Prepatellar bursa: Anterior to patella
  - Infrapatellar bursa: Within Hoffa fat pad, adjacent to tibial tubercle, deep to patellar tendon

ANATOMY IMAGING ISSUES

Imaging Approaches

- Radiographs
  - Standard includes AP standing, lateral in slight flexion, and axial patella with 20° flexion
  - Notch view often used for evaluation for arthritis
    - Tibia parallel to image detector, femur flexed 20 degrees
    - Beam from posterior to anterior centered at joint line
    - Shows joint width in posterior weight-bearing portion of joint
    - Flexion of femur causes distortion sometimes mistaken for valgus alignment
- Arthrography rarely performed today
- CT arthrogram: Useful if MR is contraindicated
  - Technique: Inject 40 cc dilute contrast of choice 50/50 with bacteriostatic saline
  - Acquire submillimeter sections; reformat
- Conventional MR arthrogram
  - Useful for postsurgical evaluation of menisci
  - Technique: Inject volume of 40 cc gadolinium diluted 1:200 in saline
- MR arthrogram usually performed using indirect technique
  - Relies on synovial excretion of gadolinium
  - Intravenous gadolinium (10-20 cc) is administered, patient exercise
  - Imaging performed 20-30 minutes after injection
  - Useful for postsurgical evaluation of menisci

Imaging Pitfalls

- Radiographic pitfalls
  - Malpositioning
    - AP radiograph: Joint line must be in center of beam or joint space cannot be accurately assessed
    - Axial patella radiograph: Flexion > 20° may reduce subluxation or tilt
  - Bipartite (multipartite) patella
    - Always upper outer quadrant
    - Osseous fragments may not appear to "match," but cartilage is continuous over osseous defect
  - Other osseous variants: Dorsal defect of patella, meniscal ossicle
- MR/CT arthrogram pitfalls
  - Positioning for oblique coronal or sagittal MR imaging
    - Incorrect alignment can either obscure or exaggerate anatomical landmarks
  - Attachment of structures to menisci can simulate tear
    - Transverse ligament: Attaches to both anterior meniscal horns
    - Meniscofemoral ligament: Attaches to posterior horn, lateral meniscus
  - Popliteus tendon sheath may mimic tear of posterior horn, lateral meniscus
  - Normal meniscal vascularity in young patients can appear hyperintense on MR
  - Anterior horn of lateral meniscus separates into fascicles at insertion, can simulate tear

FRONTAL AND SUNRISE VIEWS: KNEE

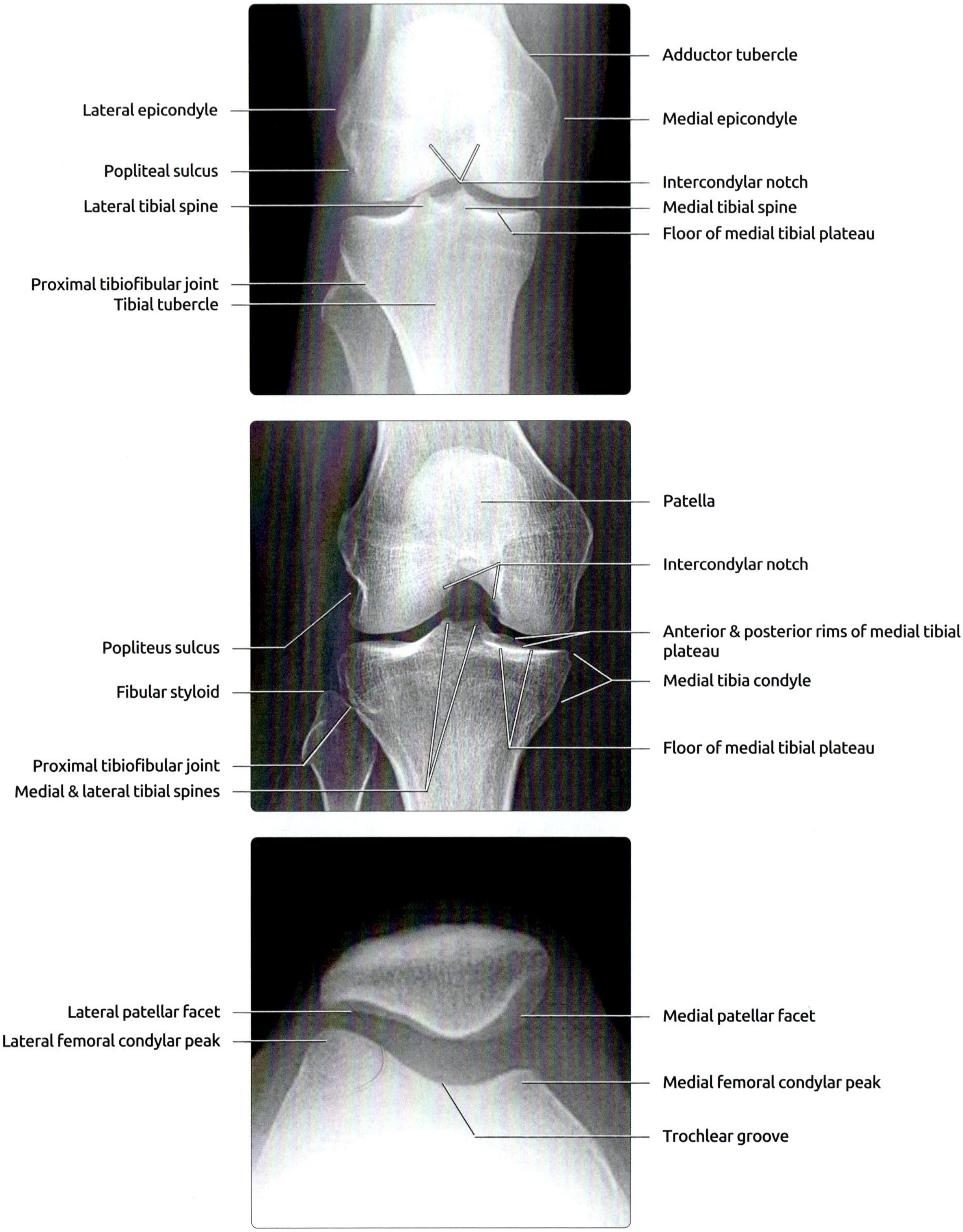

(Top) *AP radiograph of the knee shows its osseous features with the fibular head slightly posterolateral to the lateral tibial condyle.* **(Middle)** *The notch view is obtained with the beam from posterior to anterior, with the knee flexed. A more posterior portion of the femoral condyle is seen than on the AP view. The anterior and posterior rims of the medial tibial plateau should be superimposed, and the floor of the plateau forms a distinct line.* **(Bottom)** *Axial radiograph shows the knee flexed 20 degrees, allowing maximal subluxation of the patella. Note that the lateral facet of the patella is elongated and less sharply angled than the medial. There are numerous described facets of the patella, but the medial and lateral hold the greatest clinical importance.*

LATERAL VIEW: KNEE

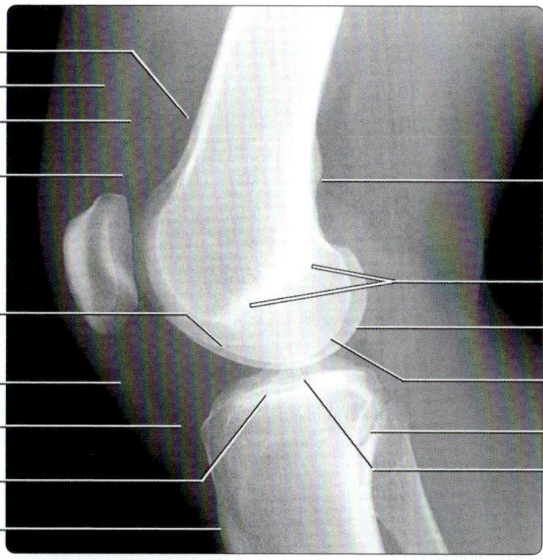

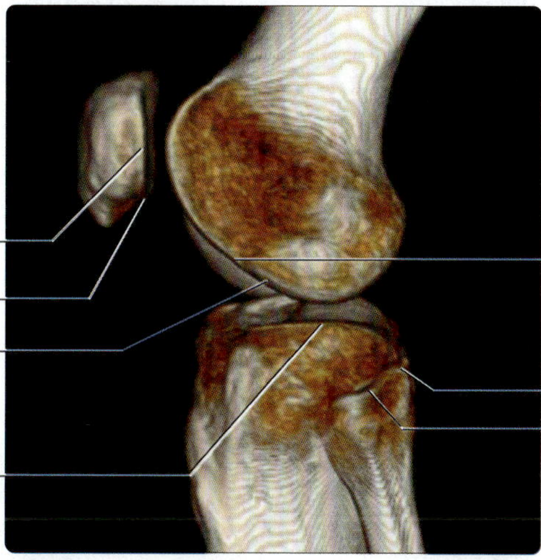

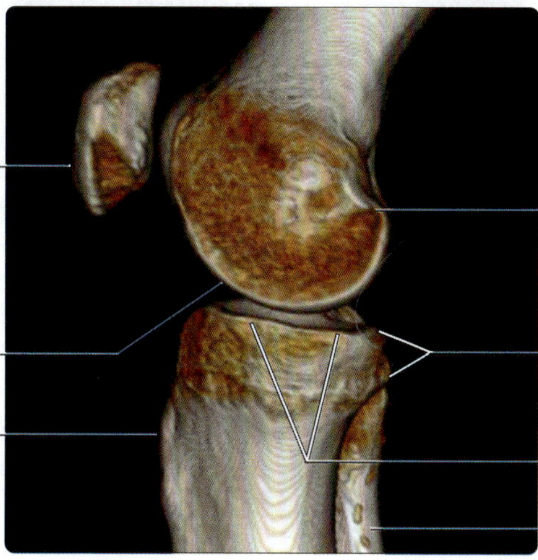

(Top) *Lateral radiograph can be difficult to interpret because of the multiple overlapping structures. Medial femoral condyle is more rounded inferiorly and larger; it corresponds to the concave medial tibial plateau. The flatter contour of the lateral femoral condyle corresponds to the flatter lateral tibial plateau.* **(Middle)** *3D CT aids in understanding the structures that are superimposed on the lateral radiograph. Here, the lateral side of the knee is shown. Note the flat contour of the lateral tibial plateau and its diagonal posterior contour articulating with the fibula.* **(Bottom)** *3D view of the medial side of the knee shows that the contour of the articular surfaces is quite different. The appearance of the femoral condyle relative to the tibial plateau has been described as a golf ball on a tee. The posterior margin of the medial tibial condyle is squared, unlike the triangular shape of the lateral tibial condyle.*

AXIAL VIEW: ARTHROGRAPHIC KNEE ANATOMY

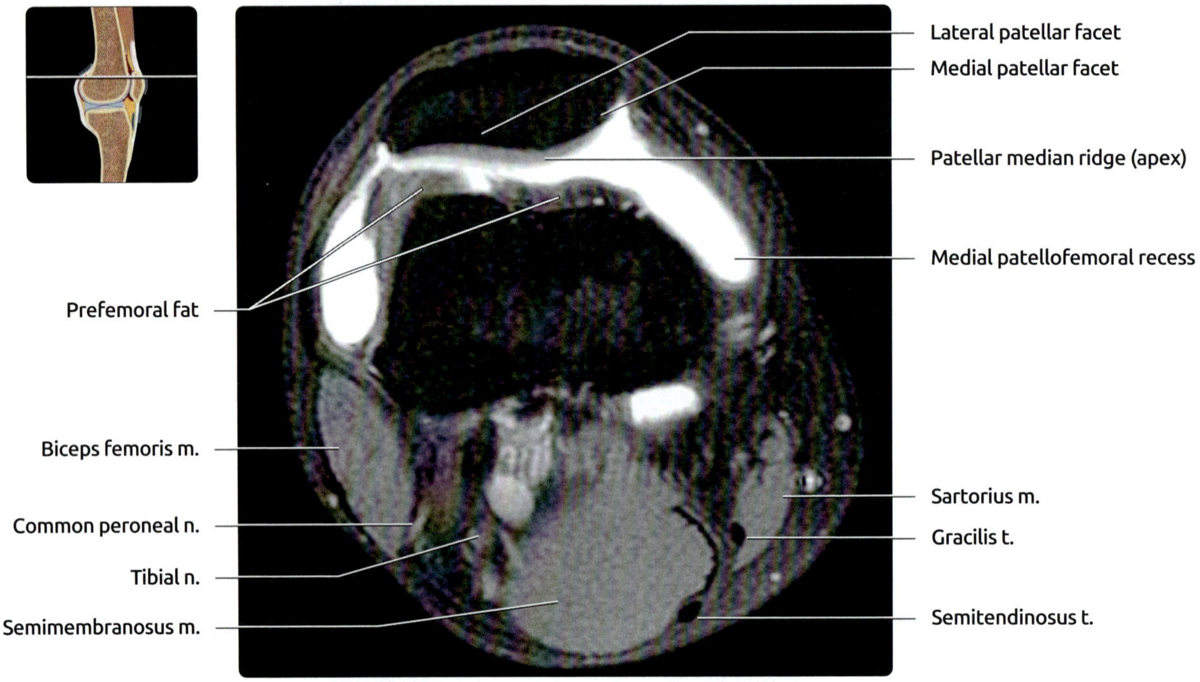

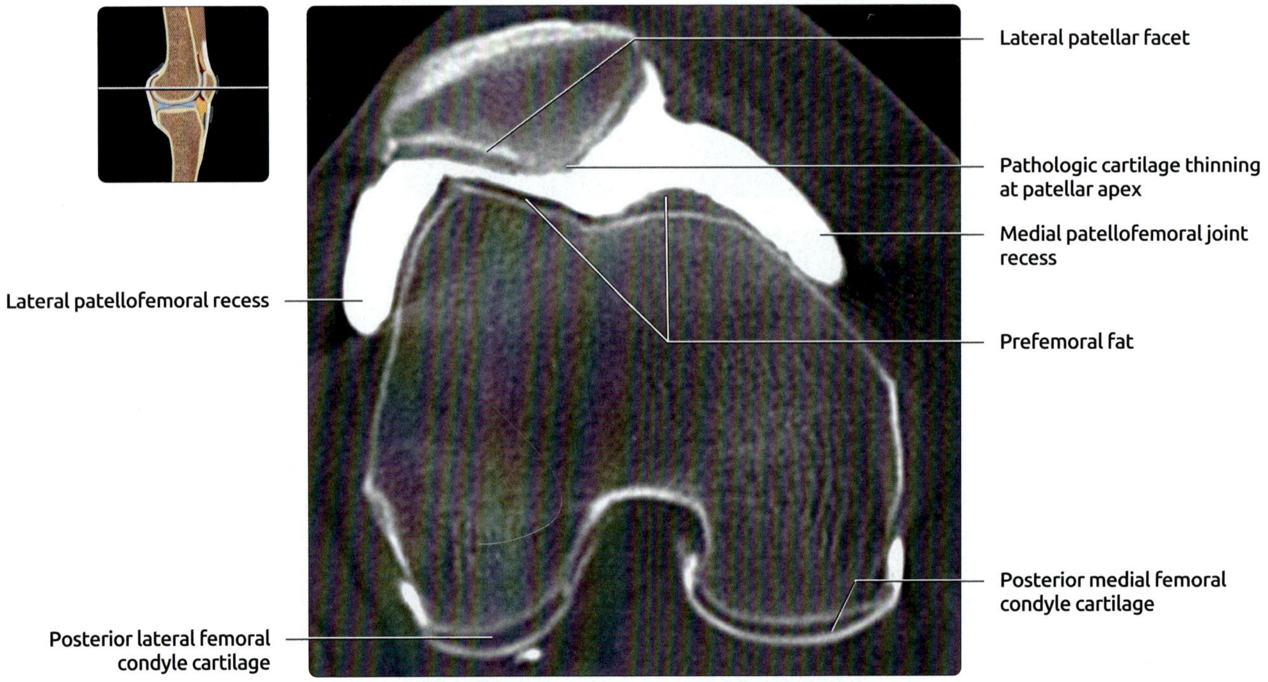

(Top) *Axial PD FS MR arthrogram through the patella shows intact cartilage. When the knee is fully extended, the patellar articular surface lies superior to the trochlear articular surface. Undulation of the prefemoral fat above the trochlea should not be confused with cartilage defects.* **(Bottom)** *Axial CT arthrogram through the femoral condyles shows contrast outlining cartilage. The patella appears slightly subluxated laterally, but this is normal in the fully extended knee. Note the capacious patellofemoral joint recesses extending around the femur. Posteriorly, the joint recesses are small.*

AXIAL VIEW: ARTHROGRAPHIC KNEE ANATOMY

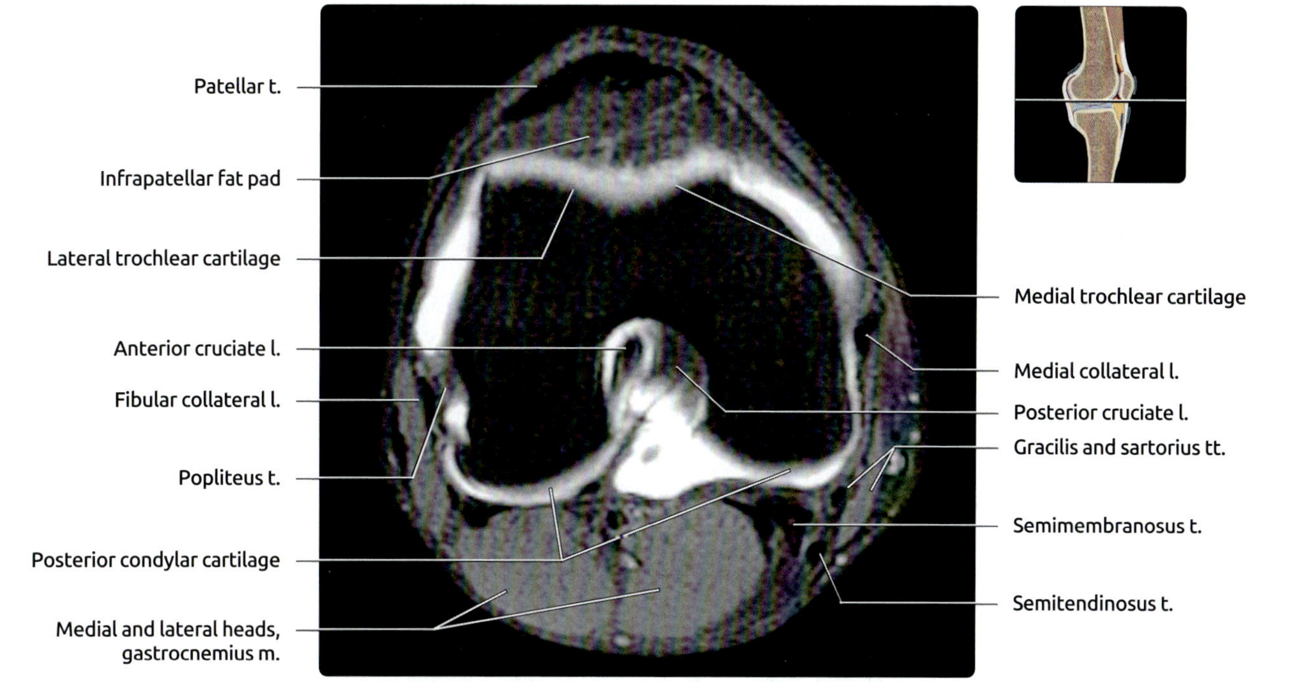

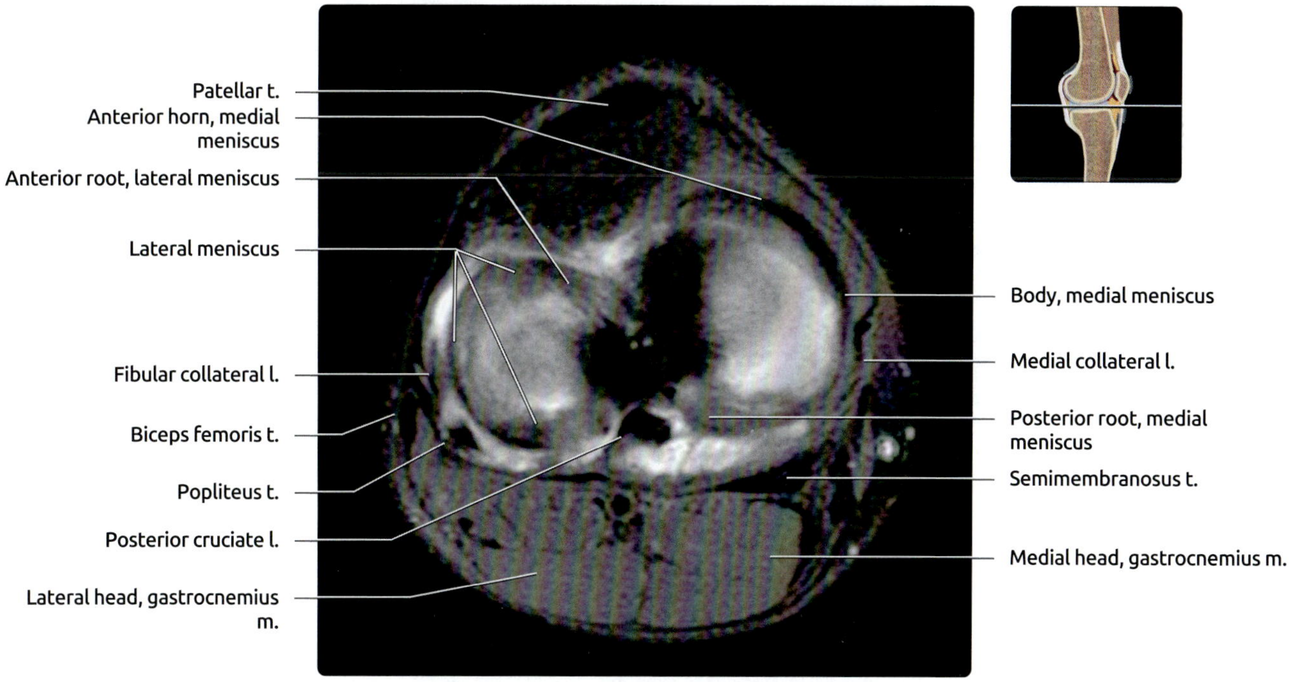

(Top) *Axial PD FS MR arthrogram through the femoral condyles shows hyaline cartilage at the trochlea (femoral surface of the patellofemoral joint) and posterior femoral condyles, as well as the anterior and posterior cruciate ligaments within the intercondylar notch.* **(Bottom)** *Axial PD FS MR arthrogram through the menisci is shown. The medial meniscus has an open C shape, while the lateral meniscus approaches a circle. The anterior root of the lateral meniscus divides into thin fascicles, which may be mistaken for a tear when seen in cross section on sagittal or coronal images.*

CORONAL VIEW: ARTHROGRAPHIC KNEE ANATOMY

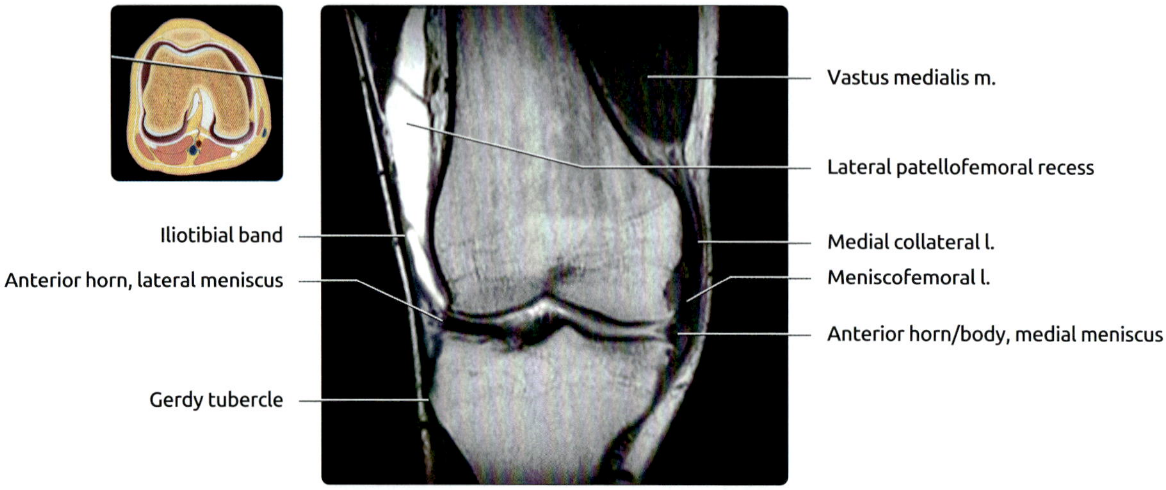

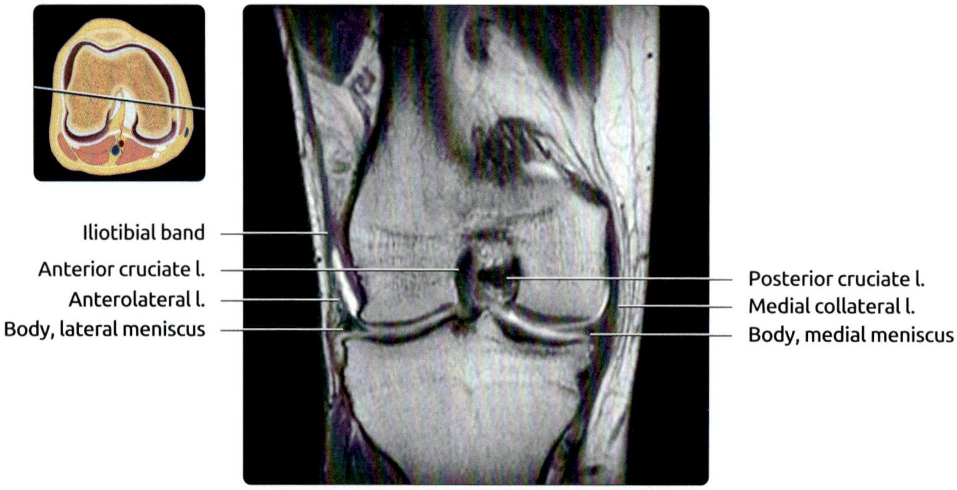

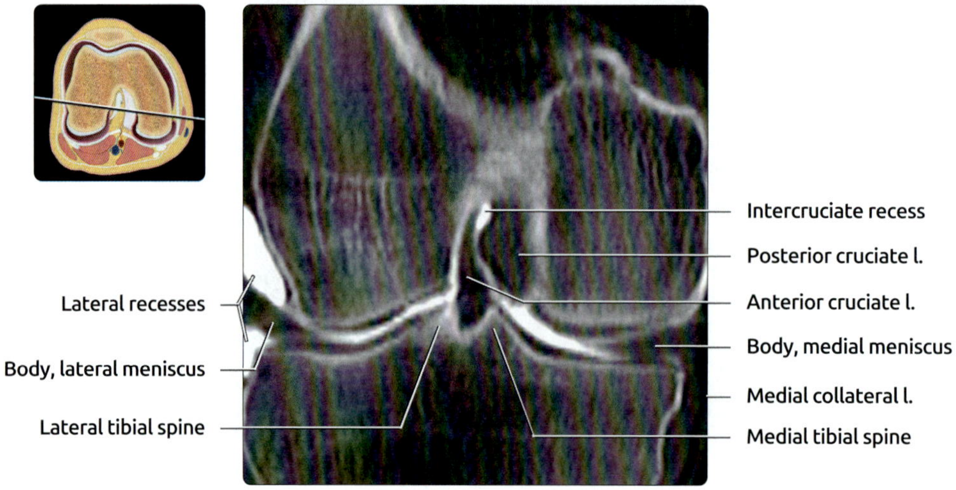

(Top) *Coronal T1WI MR arthrogram through the anterior portion of the femorotibial articulations shows the iliotibial band inserting on the tibia at Gerdy tubercle. In this example, the medial collateral ligament is thickened from prior injury.* **(Middle)** *Coronal T1WI MR arthrogram posterior to prior image shows the body of the medial and lateral meniscus, as well as the anterior and posterior cruciate ligaments within the intercondylar notch.* **(Bottom)** *Coronal CT arthrogram through the intercondylar notch, at approximately the same position as the prior MR, outlines the bodies of the menisci as well as the cruciate ligaments. Note normal capacious recesses around the lateral meniscus, compared to only minimal fluid extending above and below the medial meniscus.*

CORONAL VIEW: ARTHROGRAPHIC KNEE ANATOMY

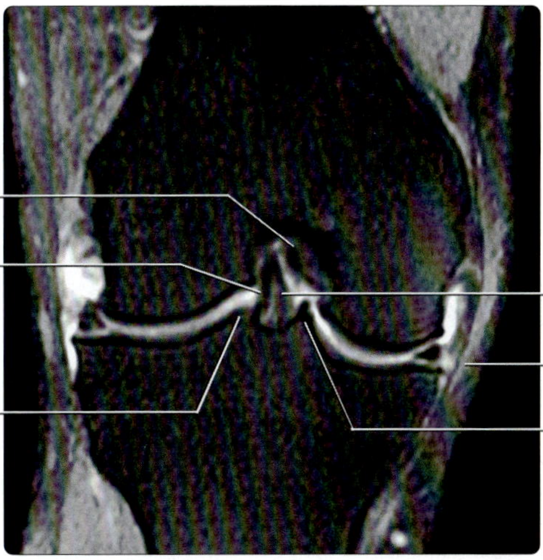

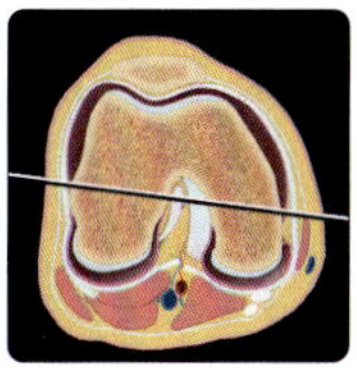

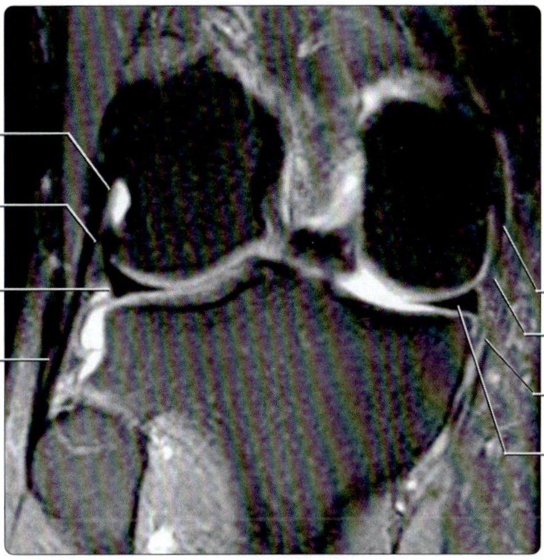

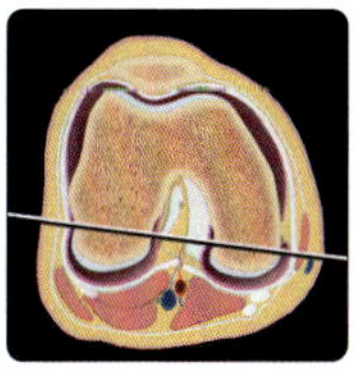

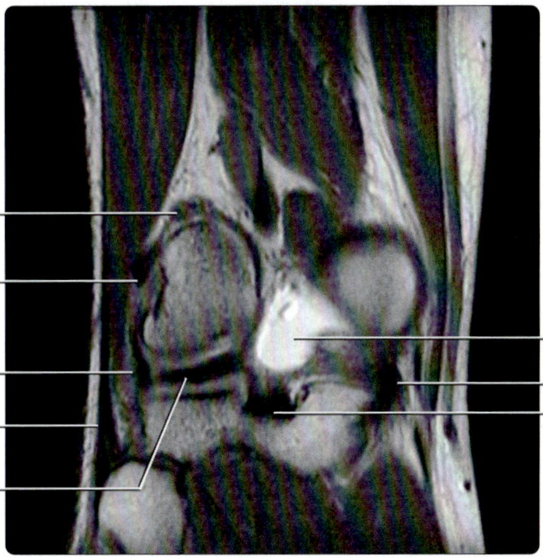

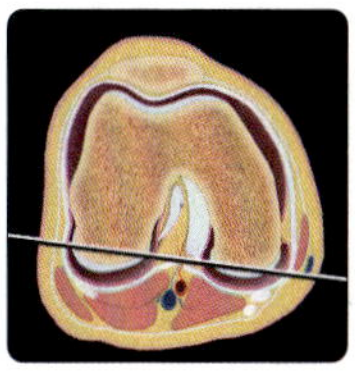

(Top) *Coronal T1WI FS MR arthrogram shows the separate bundles of the anterior cruciate ligament. The anteromedial bundle inserts on the medial tibial spine, and the posterolateral bundle inserts near the lateral tibial spine.* **(Middle)** *Coronal T1WI FS MR arthrogram shows the medial and lateral joint recesses. The medial meniscus has tight attachments to the femur and tibia (meniscofemoral and meniscotibial or coronary ligaments, respectively), resulting in small medial recesses. These meniscal-capsular ligaments comprise the deep portion of the medial collateral ligament. The lateral meniscal attachments are relatively loose, resulting in large recesses.* **(Bottom)** *Coronal T1WI MR arthrogram through the posterior joint margin shows the insertion of the posterior cruciate ligament on the posterior surface of the tibia.*

LATERAL VIEW: SAGITTAL ARTHROGRAPHIC KNEE ANATOMY

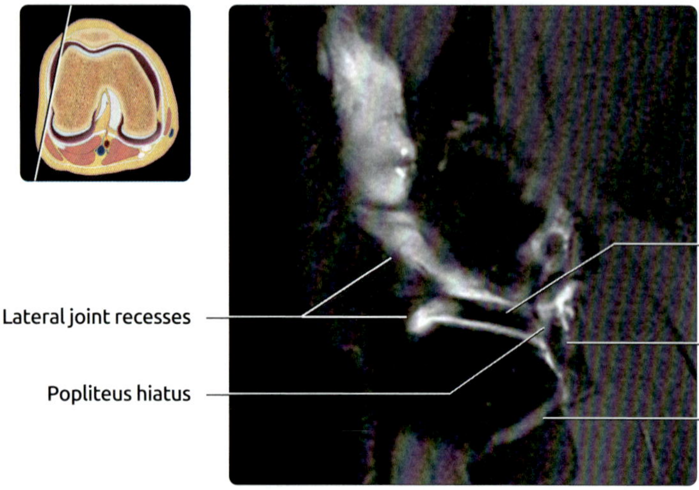

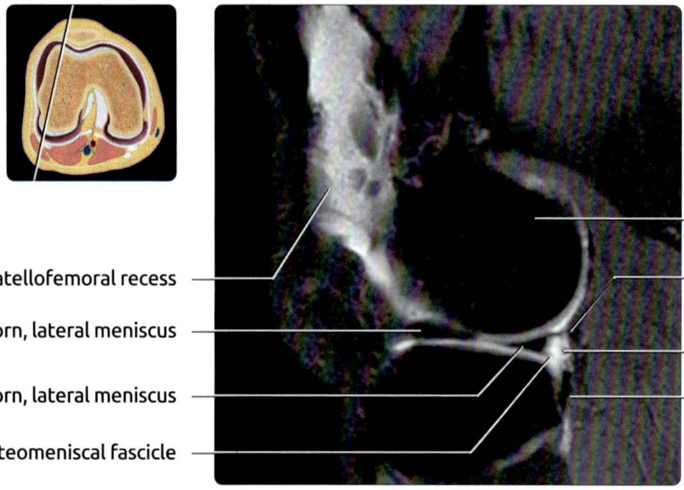

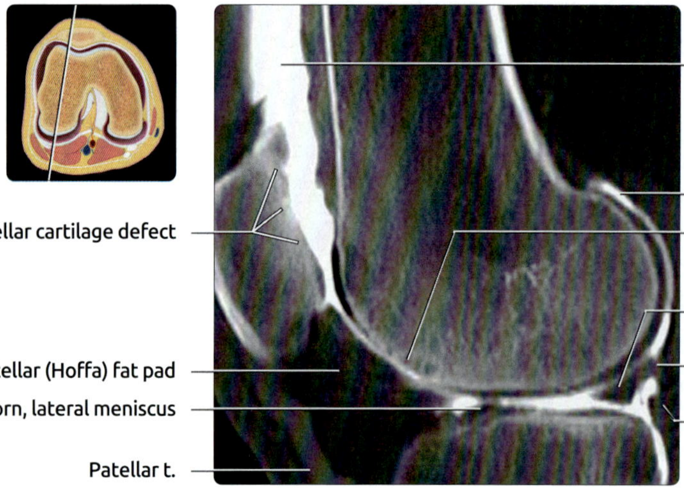

(Top) *Sagittal T1WI FS MR arthrogram through the far lateral portion of the lateral compartment shows the body of the lateral meniscus with the popliteus tendon posterior to it.* **(Middle)** *Sagittal T1WI FS MR arthrogram through the lateral portion of the lateral compartment shows the popliteus tendon passing inferiorly by the lateral meniscus. The popliteal hiatus is the opening in the capsule through which the tendon enters. Note that the inferior popliteomeniscal fascicle appears incomplete, a normal finding at the hiatus.* **(Bottom)** *Sagittal CT arthrogram through the midportion of the lateral compartment is shown. The patient has osteoarthritis, and cartilage loss is seen in multiple areas. The lateral meniscus is outlined by contrast. The superior fascicle of posterior horn is well seen, as is the popliteal tendon in its hiatus.*

SAGITTAL VIEW: MEDIAL ARTHROGRAPHIC KNEE ANATOMY

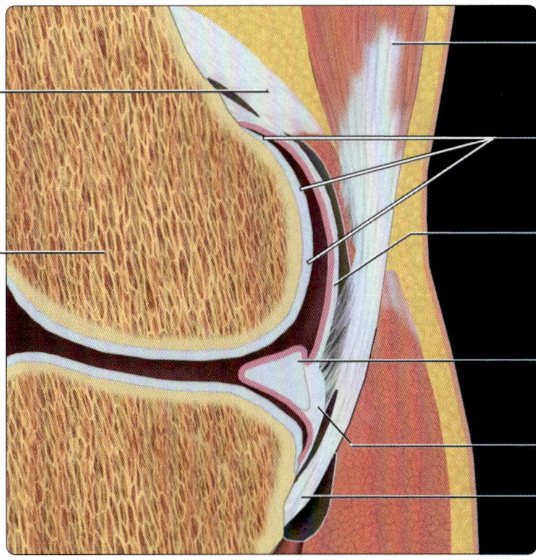

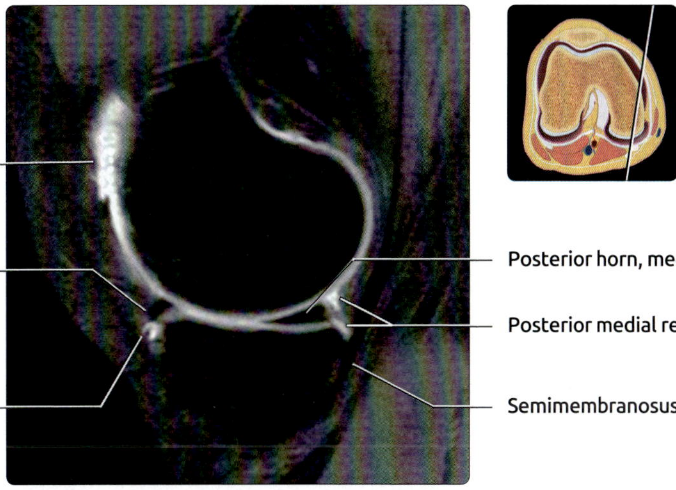

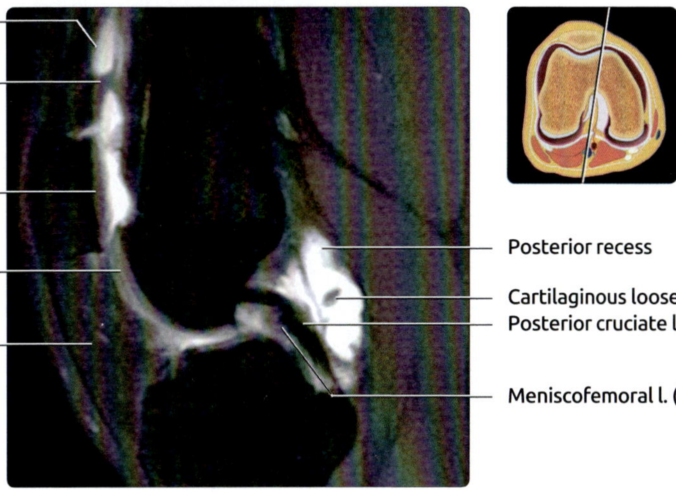

(Top) *Graphic shows a sagittal cross section through the medial compartment of the knee. The posterior oblique ligament courses along the capsular margin, reinforcing the joint against posterior tibial translation. Hyaline cartilage extends to the most superior margin of the posterior femoral condyles.* **(Middle)** *Sagittal T1WI FS MR arthrogram through the medial compartment of the joint shows contrast in small recesses around the medial meniscus. Hyaline cartilage is intermediate signal intensity on T1WI FS.* **(Bottom)** *Sagittal T1WI FS MR arthrogram through the medial portion of intercondylar notch shows the posterior cruciate ligament with anterior meniscofemoral ligament in cross section at its anterior margin. Cartilage loose body is seen posteriorly; MR arthrography is more sensitive in detection of loose bodies than noncontrast MR.*

POSTEROLATERAL CORNER STRUCTURES

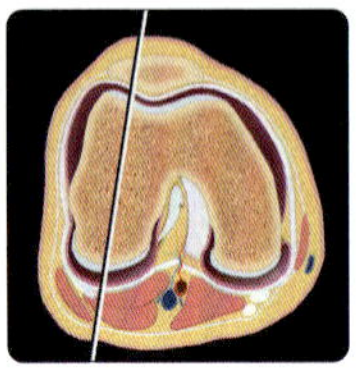

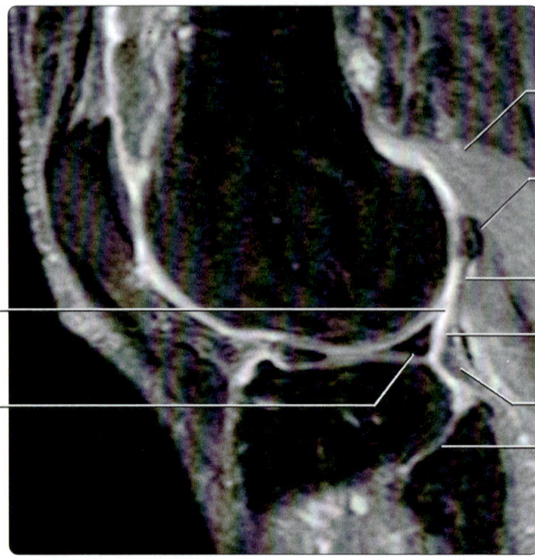

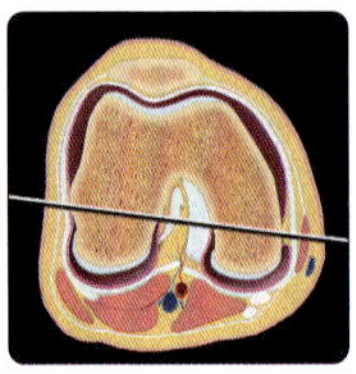

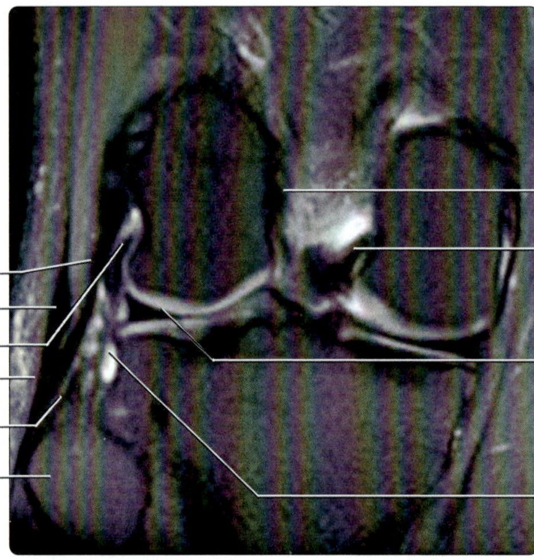

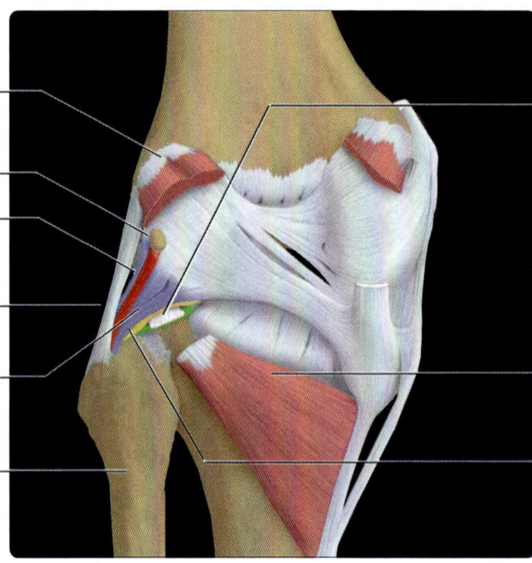

(Top) *Sagittal T1WI FS MR arthrogram through the posterolateral joint shows fabella (sesamoid in the lateral gastrocnemius) with the fabellofibular ligament extending inferiorly. This ligament (and associated fabella) is often absent.* **(Middle)** *Coronal T1WI FS MR arthrogram through the posterior joint shows posterolateral structures including the fibular collateral ligament and biceps femoris (together forming the conjoined tendon inserting on the fibula), the arcuate ligament, the popliteal-fibular ligament, and the popliteus tendon.* **(Bottom)** *Graphic of the posterior joint seen from behind shows diagrammatic representation of posterolateral joint ligaments.*

SAGITTAL VIEW: PLICAE

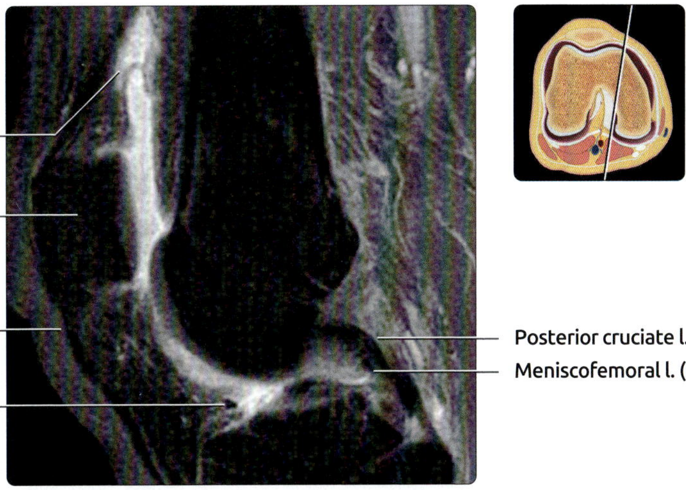

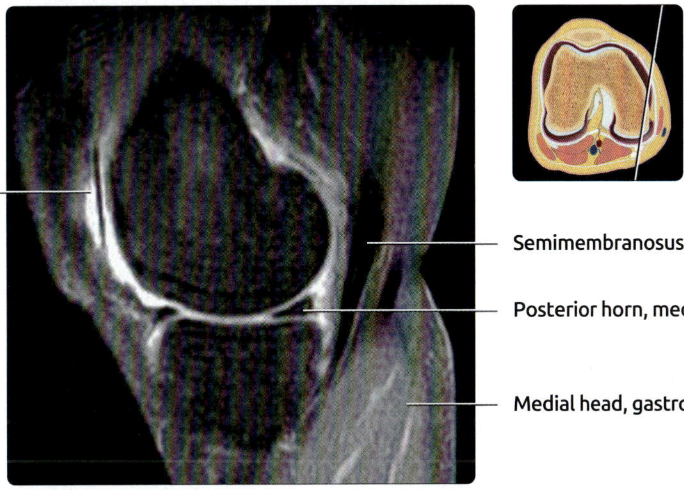

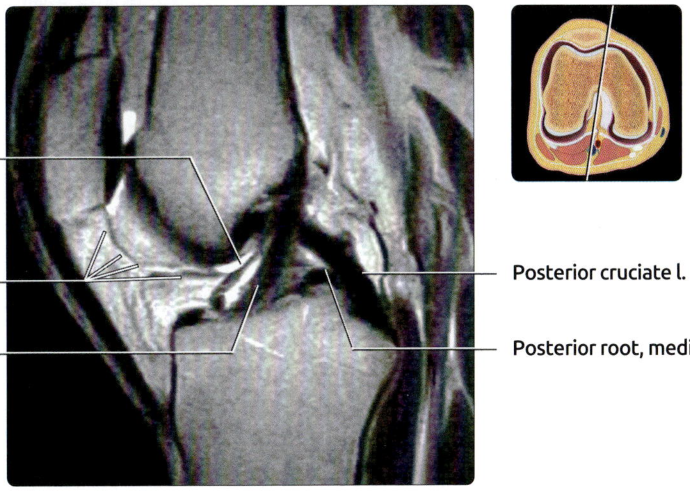

(Top) *Sagittal T1WI FS MR arthrogram shows a suprapatellar plica. A suprapatellar plica rarely can become symptomatic if it is thickened and obstructs the suprapatellar recess, leading to entrapment of fluid and synovial tissue above the plica.* **(Middle)** *Sagittal T1WI FS MR arthrogram through the medial joint shows a medial plica, which is the most common symptomatic type of plica. The plica extends vertically through the medial patellofemoral joint and can cause a snapping sensation on flexion/extension as it rubs across the femoral condyle. It may contribute to trochlear or patellar cartilage wear.* **(Bottom)** *Sagittal T1WI FS MR arthrogram shows an infrapatellar plica, which extends from Hoffa fat pad to the intercondylar notch anterior to the anterior cruciate ligament. It is not thought to cause symptoms. Fluid may dissect along the plica into Hoffa fat.*

TERMINOLOGY

Abbreviations

- Anterior cruciate ligament (ACL)
- Posterior cruciate ligament (PCL)
- Medial (tibial) collateral ligament (MCL)
- Lateral (fibular) collateral ligament (LCL)

IMAGING ANATOMY

Overview

- Multiple specific anatomic relationships must be maintained in order to assure stability and full function

Distal Femur

- **Osseous features**
  - Distal femoral metaphysis flares into medial and lateral epicondyles
  - Medial femoral condyle larger than lateral condyle, more rounded inferiorly
  - Lateral femoral condyle has flatter contour inferiorly than medial condyle
    - Shallow groove (< 2 mm deep) demarcates femoral-tibial from patellofemoral articular surface
    - Called lateral femoral condylar recess or terminal sulcus
  - Intercondylar notch accommodates cruciate ligaments; roof is seen as Blumensaat line on radiograph
  - Trochlear groove accommodates patella and is generally V-shaped, with lateral and medial articular facets corresponding to patellar facets
- **Cartilage**
  - Thicker over posterior condyles than on central weight-bearing surface
  - Focally thin at lateral femoral condylar sulcus

Proximal Tibia

- **Osseous features**
  - Medial plateau is concave; lateral plateau has straight contour
  - Posterior tilt of tibial surface: 10°
  - Tibial tubercle (apophysis) anterior and slightly lateral, several cm distal to joint
  - Gerdy tubercle anterolateral just distal to joint
  - Do not confuse terminology of tibial plateau vs. tibial condyle
    - Plateau: Horizontal articular surface
    - Condyle: Metaphyseal flare of tibia
- **Cartilage**
  - Uniformly thin

Proximal Fibula

- **Osseous features**
  - Posterolateral relative to tibia
  - Fibular styloid process

Tibiofibular Joint

- True synovial joint; subject to any arthritic process
- Connects to knee joint in 20%

Patella

- **Osseous features**
  - Triangular sesamoid in quadriceps tendon
  - Wider at base superiorly than at apex inferiorly
  - Articular surface divided by vertical ridge into lateral and medial facets
  - Lateral facet long and shallow angle
  - Medial facet short and more strongly angulated
  - Several other facets described but not of imaging importance
  - Lower 25% nonarticular
  - Nonarticular outer surface may develop prominent enthesopathy where quadriceps tendon insertion blends into origin of inferior patellar tendon
  - Bipartite (multipartite) patella: Always upper outer quadrant; osseous fragments may not appear to "match," but cartilage is continuous over defect
- **Cartilage**
  - Thickest cartilage in body (3-4 mm)
  - Uniform thickness
  - May have dorsal patellar defect or bipartite/multipartite patella as normal variant but with normal overlying cartilage

Extensor Mechanism

- Quadriceps tendon converges on patella
- Fibers of rectus femoris course over patella as quadriceps continuation
- Quadriceps continuation forms patellar tendon (a.k.a. patellar ligament) extending from patella to tibial tubercle
- Fibers of vastus lateralis and medialis contribute to lateral and medial retinacula, respectively

Internal Structures

- **Menisci**
  - Fibrocartilage cushions, which also lubricate and stabilize knee
  - Only peripheral portion vascularized
  - Attached by anterior and posterior roots to tibial surface
  - Medial attached to capsule throughout extent
  - Lateral attached to capsule at anterior horn and far posteriorly, but by fascicles to popliteus/capsule at body and posterior horn
- **Cruciate ligaments**
  - Intraarticular but extrasynovial
  - Major stabilizing structures to anteroposterior motion
  - ACL originates at posterolateral intercondylar notch, crosses anteromedially, and inserts at medial tibial spine/tibial surface
    - 2 bundles, anteromedial and posterolateral, distinct on MR
  - PCL originates at mid medial intercondylar notch, crosses posteriorly and slightly laterally, and inserts extraarticularly at posterior center of tibia below joint line
    - 2 bundles, anterolateral and posteromedial, usually not distinct on MR

Medial Supporting Structures

- Superficial (layer 1)
  - Pes anserinus: Anteromedial tibial insertion
    - Sartorius embedded in crural fascia
    - Gracilis immediately deep to sartorius
    - Semitendinosus immediately deep to gracilis

- Middle (layer 2)
  - Superficial medial collateral ligament
    - Origin is medial epicondyle; runs slightly anteromedially to insert on tibia, 5 cm distal to joint line
    - Anteriorly, longitudinal component fascia blends with layer 1
  - Posterior oblique ligament (blends with layer 3)
- Deep (layer 3)
  - Capsular layers (sometimes termed deep fibers of MCL) at mid portion of knee
    - Meniscofemoral ligament
    - Meniscotibial (coronary) ligament
  - More posteriorly, superficial MCL blends with capsular layers of MCL
  - Posterior oblique ligament arises from superficial MCL
    - Blends with posteromedial meniscus
    - Receives fibers from semimembranosus tendon
    - Envelops posterior aspect of femoral condyle, blends with oblique popliteal ligament

Lateral Supporting Structures

- Superficial (layer 1)
  - Iliotibial band (also called iliotibial tract) anteriorly, inserting on Gerdy tubercle
  - Superficial portion of biceps femoris posterolaterally, inserting on fibular styloid
- Middle (layer 2)
  - Quadriceps retinaculum anteriorly
  - Posteriorly, 2 ligamentous thickenings, which originate from lateral patella
    - Proximal terminates at lateral intermuscular septum on femur
    - Distal terminates at femoral insertion of posterolateral capsule and lateral head of gastrocnemius
- Deep (layer 3): Several thickenings in lateral part of capsule function as discrete structures
  - Lateral (fibular) collateral ligament originates from lateral femoral epicondyle, extends posterolaterally to insert on lateral fibular head
  - Anterolateral ligament
    - Originates from lateral femoral epicondyle just anterior to lateral collateral ligament (may have connecting fibers)
    - Has connecting fibers with lateral meniscus
    - Extends anteriorly and inferiorly
    - Inserts on lateral tibia posterior to Gerdy tubercle
  - Arcuate ligament originates from styloid process fibular head, interdigitates with popliteus, and inserts into posterior capsule near oblique popliteal ligament
  - Several other small and inconstant structures located posterolaterally, which are difficult to differentiate by imaging

ANATOMY IMAGING ISSUES

Imaging Recommendations

- MR
  - T1 in one plane to evaluate marrow and anatomy
  - PD (± fat saturation) is most accurate sequence to evaluate menisci
  - Fluid-sensitive sequence to evaluate location and tracking of fluid collections

Imaging Pitfalls

- Variants: Multiple osseous and soft tissue normal variants
- Loose bodies on MR: Easily missed
- Partial voluming over convex surfaces: Morphology of trochlea, femoral condyles, and patella makes them particularly difficult to evaluate in 3 standard planes

CLINICAL IMPLICATIONS

Denervation Syndromes Related to Knee Anatomy

- Tibial nerve denervation
  - Tibial nerve branches from sciatic nerve in popliteal fossa
    - Relatively protected, so compression fairly rare
    - Provides motor innervation to gastrocnemius, plantaris, popliteus, soleus, tibialis posterior, flexor digitorum longus, and flexor hallucis longus
  - Proximal tibial neuropathy symptoms
    - Sensory change on bottom of foot
    - Weakness of plantar flexor and inverter muscles
    - Weakness of intrinsic muscles of foot
  - Common causes of proximal tibial neuropathy
    - Significant fracture
    - Compression by Baker cyst
    - Nerve sheath tumor
    - Vasculitis-related neuropathy (diabetes mellitus or polyarteritis nodosa)
- Common peroneal nerve denervation
  - Most common mononeuropathy of lower extremity
  - At greatest risk for direct compression/trauma, as it winds around outer fibular neck
    - Superficial position with only subcutaneous fat and skin coverage puts nerve at risk for direct trauma
    - Nerve then pierces anterior fascia to enter anterior compartment, between tendinous origins of peroneus longus muscle; tethering may occur, making nerve susceptible to stretch injury
    - Trifurcation into recurrent articular branch, superficial peroneal nerve, and deep peroneal nerve
  - Innervation
    - Deep peroneal nerve provides innervation to extensor muscles in anterior compartment of lower leg (tibialis anterior, extensor hallucis longus, extensor digitorum longus)
    - Superficial peroneal branch innervates peroneus longus and peroneus brevis
  - Common peroneal neuropathy symptoms
    - Footdrop
    - Pain in lower lateral 2/3 of leg
  - Common causes of common peroneal neuropathy
    - Direct trauma
    - Fibular neck fracture or knee dislocation
    - Knee arthroplasty in patient with prior significant valgus deformity
    - Tight cast
    - Ganglia/mass lesions
    - Variations in distal and posterior extent of distal biceps muscle in up to 23% of population may create tunnel with entrapment of nerve

AXIAL T1 MR: RIGHT KNEE

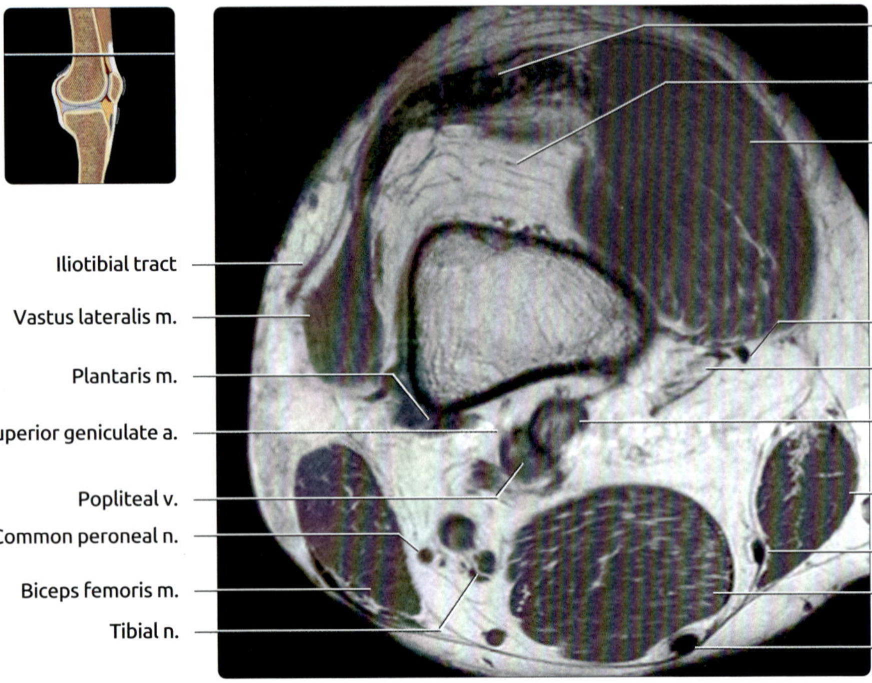

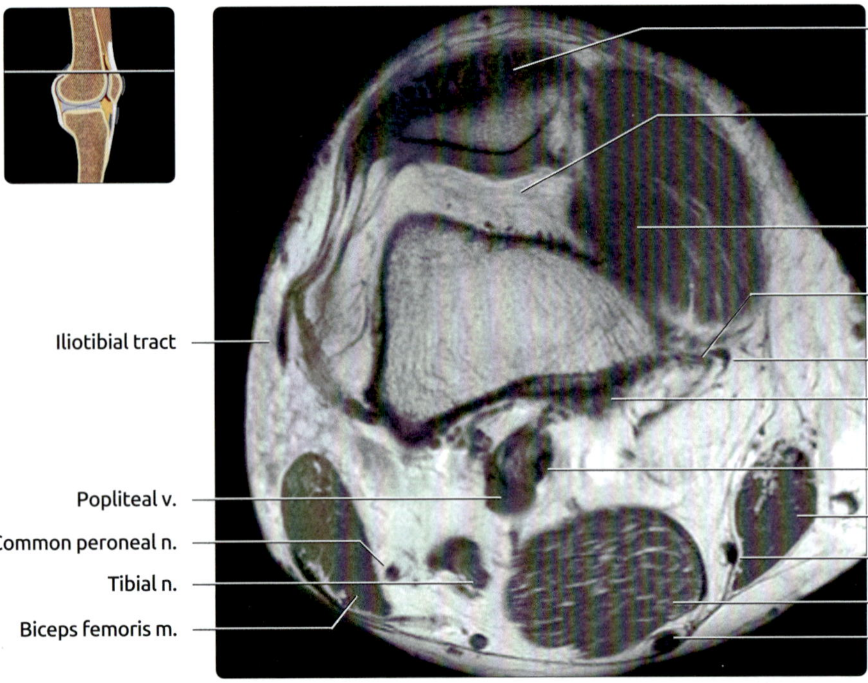

(Top) *First in a series of axial T1 MR images of the right knee shows that the cut is above the patella and at the proximal portion of the femoral metaphysis. At this level, the origin of the plantaris muscle is seen, but it is still proximal to the adductor tubercle.* **(Bottom)** *This cut is immediately above the adductor tubercle. The vastus medialis obliquus is seen, serving as medial support for the superior portion of the patella.*

AXIAL T1 MR: LEFT KNEE

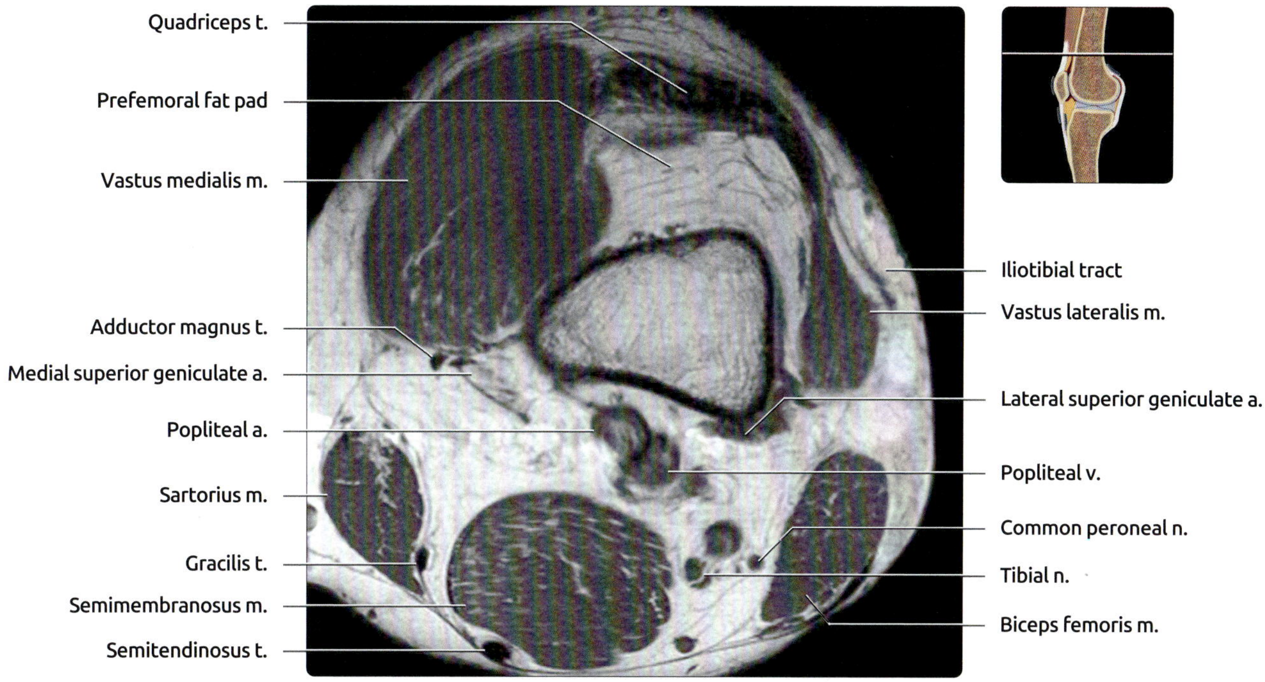

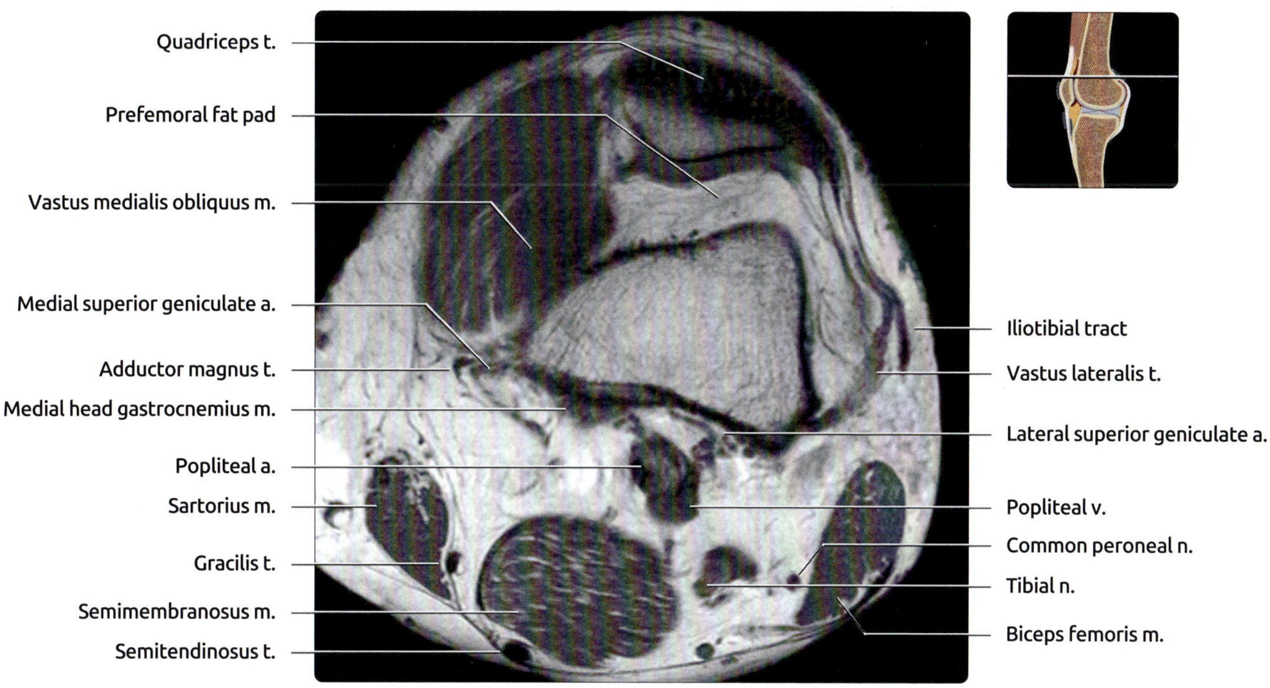

(Top) *First in a series of axial T1 MR images of the left knee shows that the cut is above the patella and at the proximal portion of the femoral metaphysis. At this level, the origin of the plantaris muscle is seen, but it is still proximal to the adductor tubercle.* **(Bottom)** *This cut is immediately above the adductor tubercle. The vastus medialis obliquus is seen, serving as medial support for the superior portion of the patella.*

AXIAL T1 MR: RIGHT KNEE

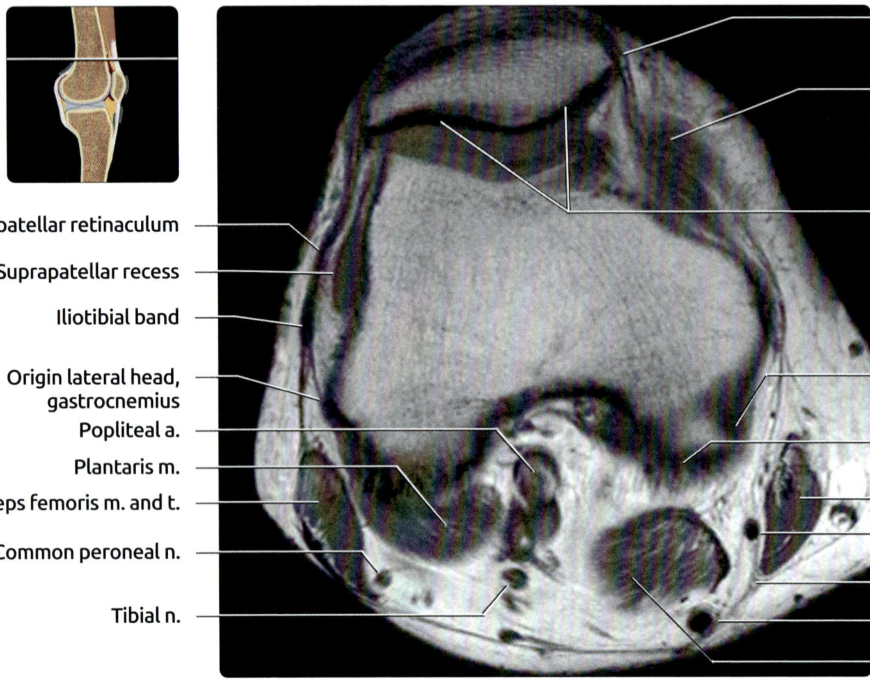

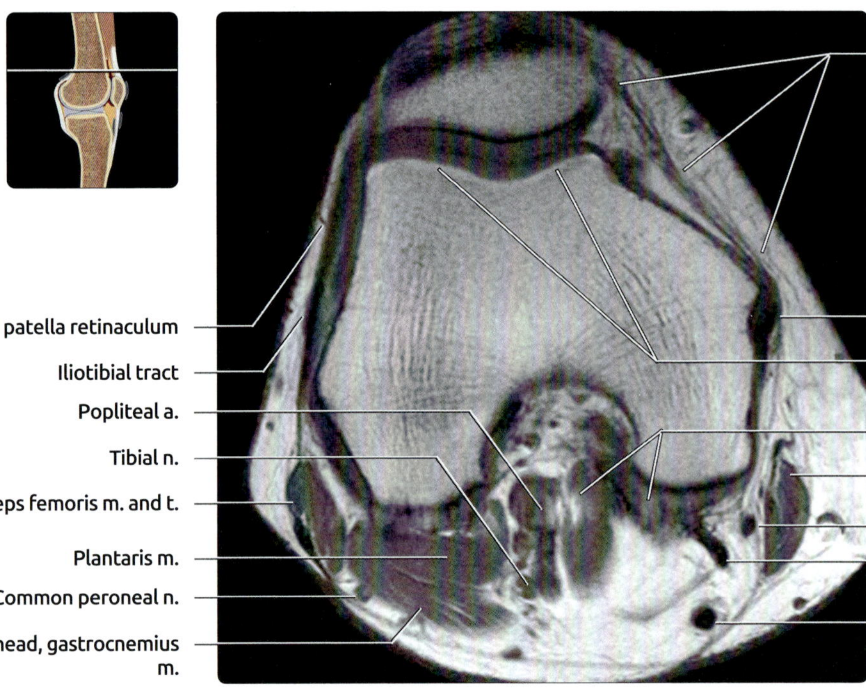

(Top) *This cut is at the level of the adductor tubercle, which serves at its superior aspect as the insertion site of the adductor magnus tendon. The superior portion of the medial patella is stabilized by the tendinous attachment of the vastus medialis obliquus. Note that the structures comprising the pes anserinus are aligning themselves.* **(Bottom)** *Slightly distal, the inferior aspect of the adductor tubercle serves as the site of origin of the medial patellofemoral ligament, which inserts on the upper 2/3 of the medial patella and is an important patellar stabilizer. It also serves as the site of origin of the superficial medial collateral ligament fibers.*

AXIAL T1 MR: LEFT KNEE

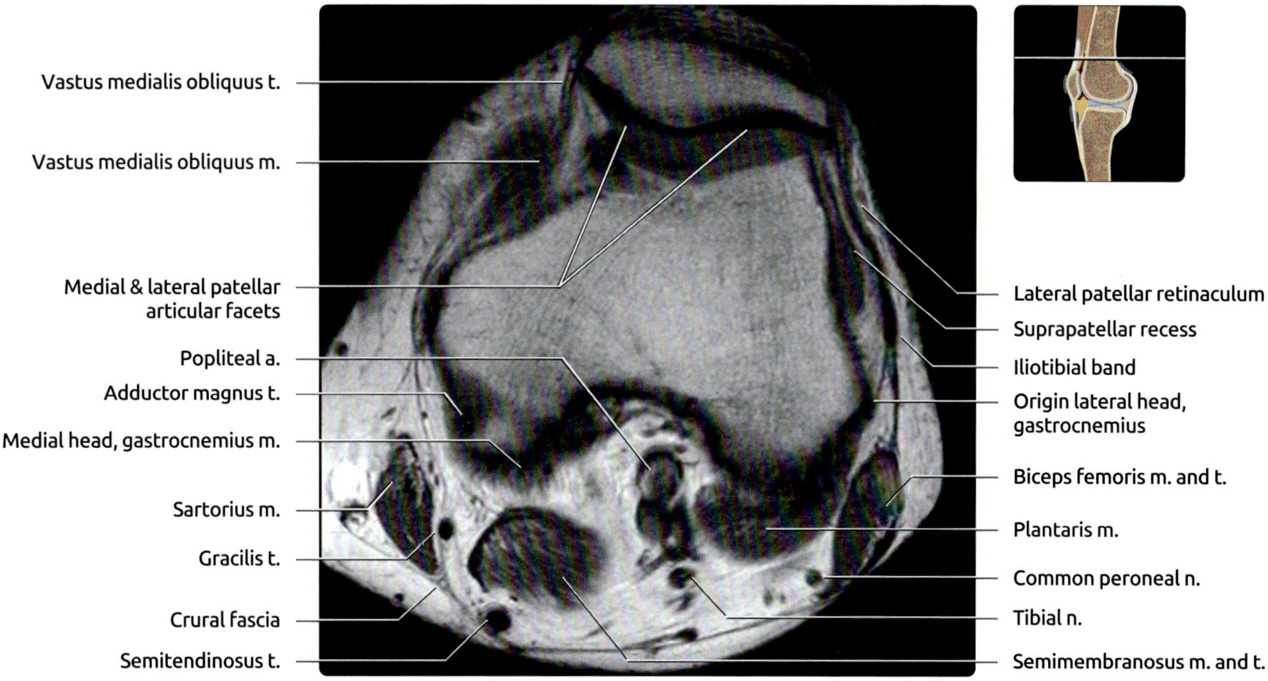

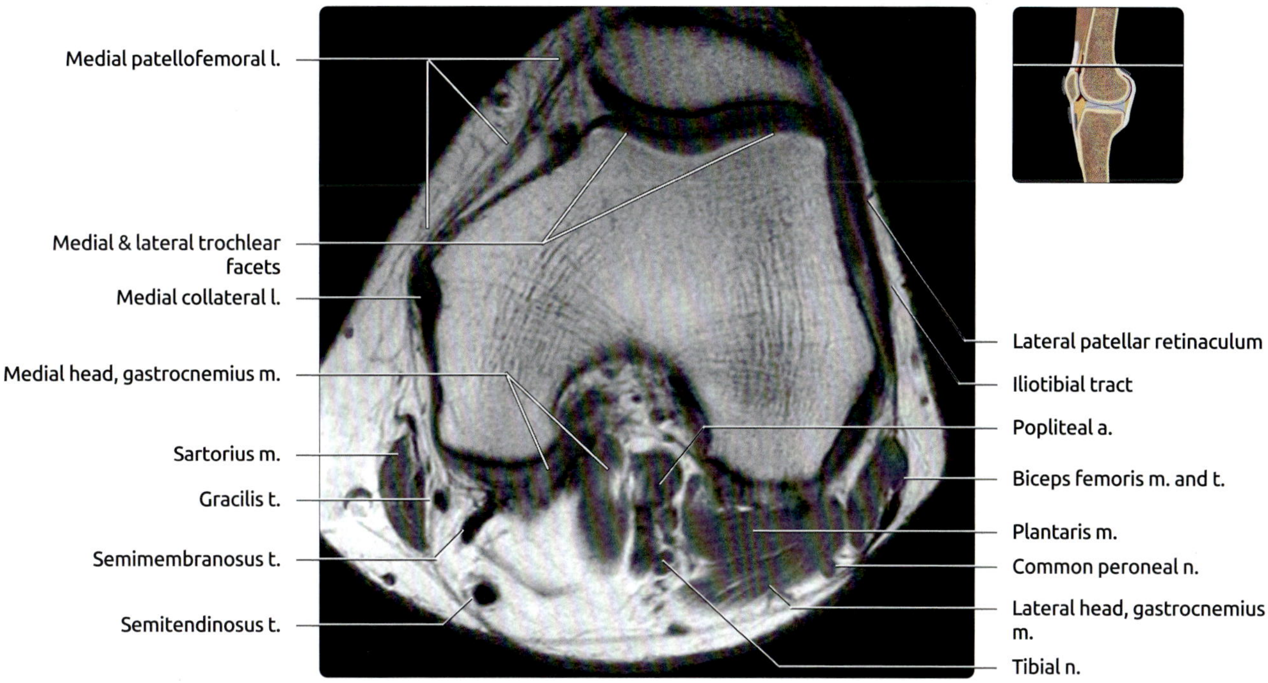

(Top) *This cut is at the level of the adductor tubercle, which serves at its superior aspect as the insertion site of the adductor magnus tendon. The superior portion of the medial patella is stabilized by the tendinous attachment of the vastus medialis obliquus. Note that the structures comprising the pes anserinus are aligning themselves.* **(Bottom)** *Slightly distal, the inferior aspect of the adductor tubercle serves as the site of origin of the medial patellofemoral ligament, which inserts on the upper 2/3 of the medial patella and is an important patellar stabilizer. It also serves as the site of origin of the superficial medial collateral ligament fibers.*

AXIAL T1 MR: RIGHT KNEE

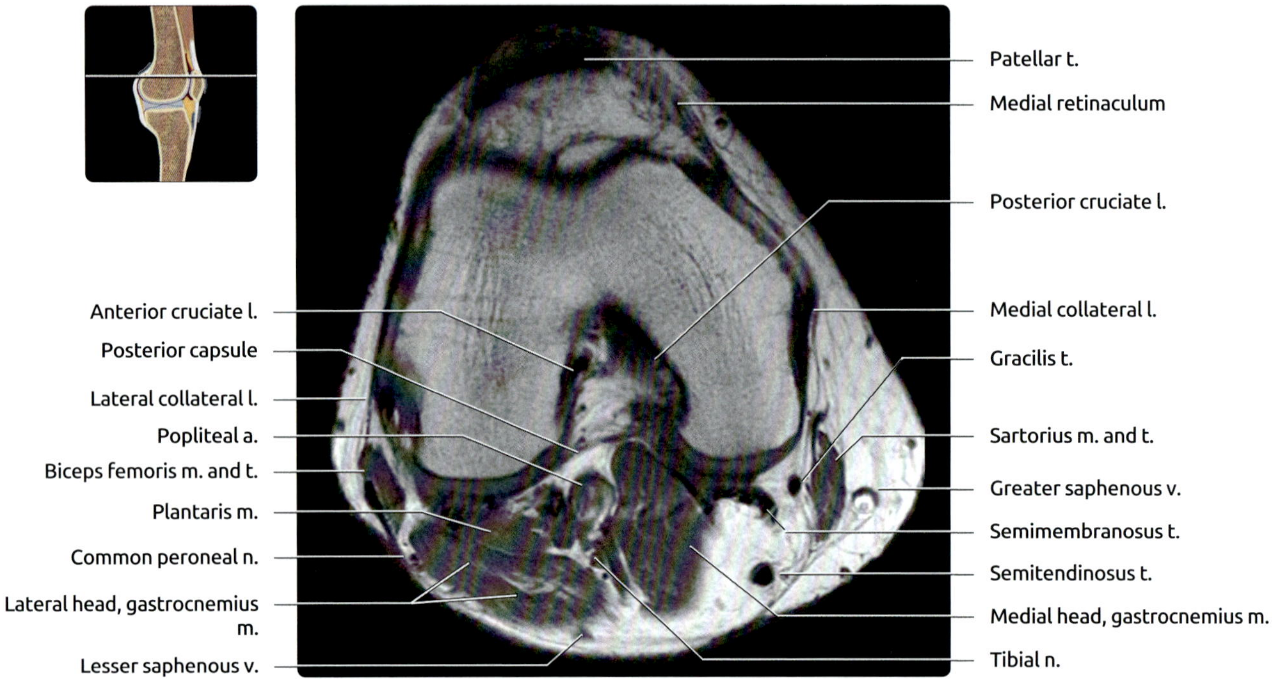

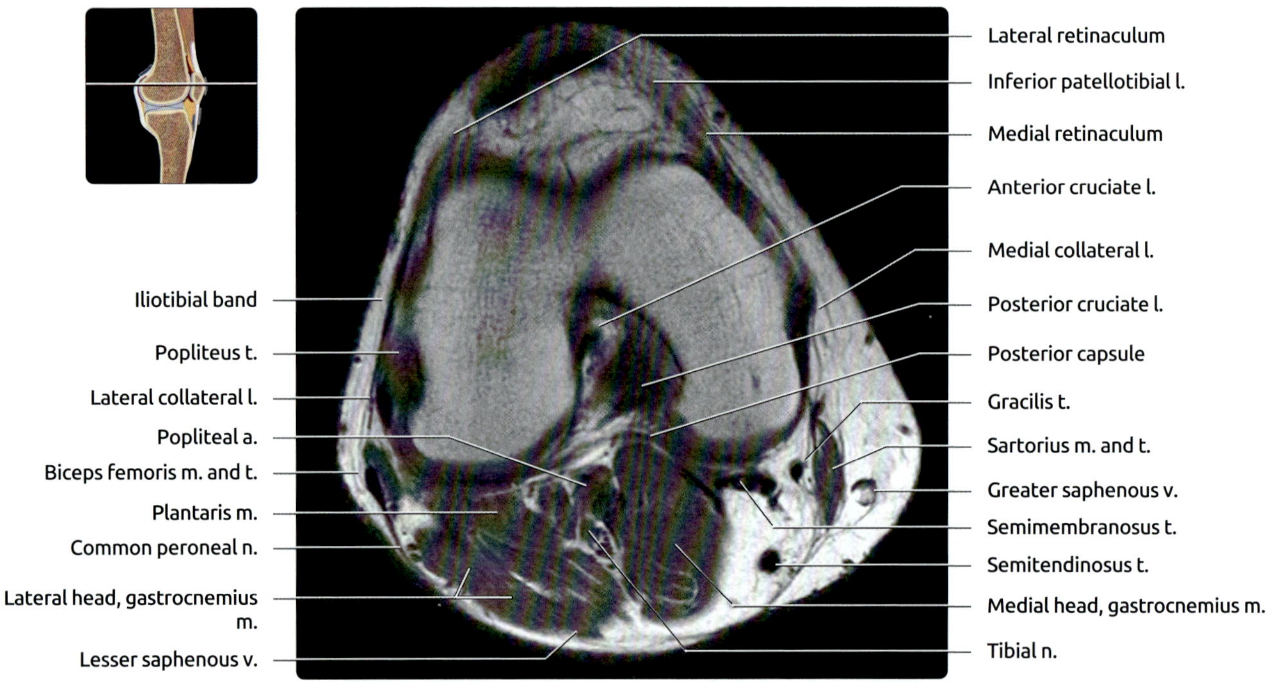

(Top) *This cut is through the intercondylar notch; origins of both the anterior and posterior cruciate ligaments are seen. The hamstrings are nearly completely tendinous, about to cross medially to the knee joint. The origins of both collateral ligaments are now seen.* (Bottom) *At the lower end of the patella, the medial support is from the inferior patellotibial ligament. The C-shaped semimembranosus tendon is distinctly different from the elements of pes anserinus (sartorius, gracilis, semitendinosus). The biceps femoris and lateral collateral ligament begin to approach one another as they extend to their insertion on the fibular head; the popliteus tendon arises from its sulcus on the lateral femoral condyle.*

AXIAL T1 MR: LEFT KNEE

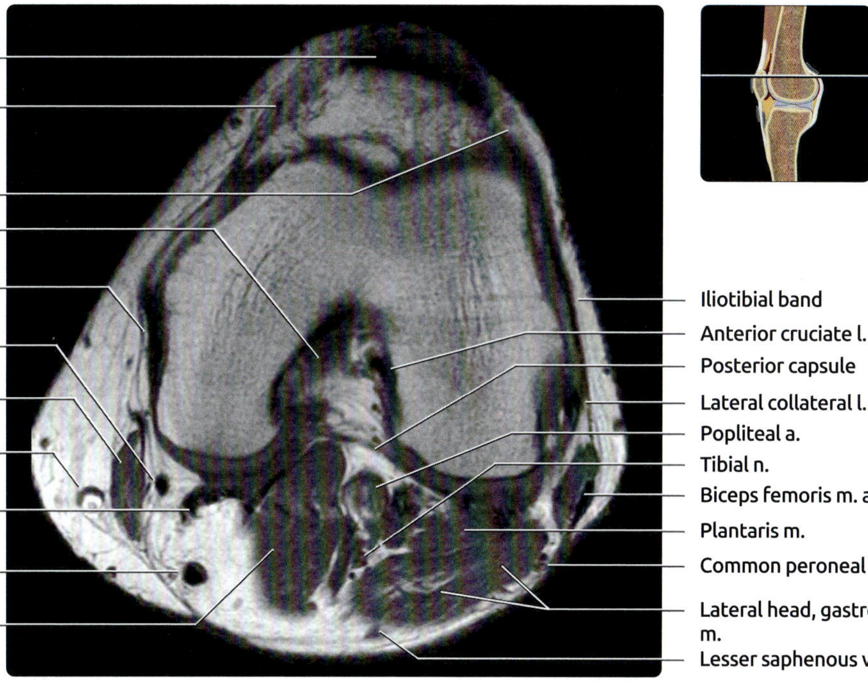

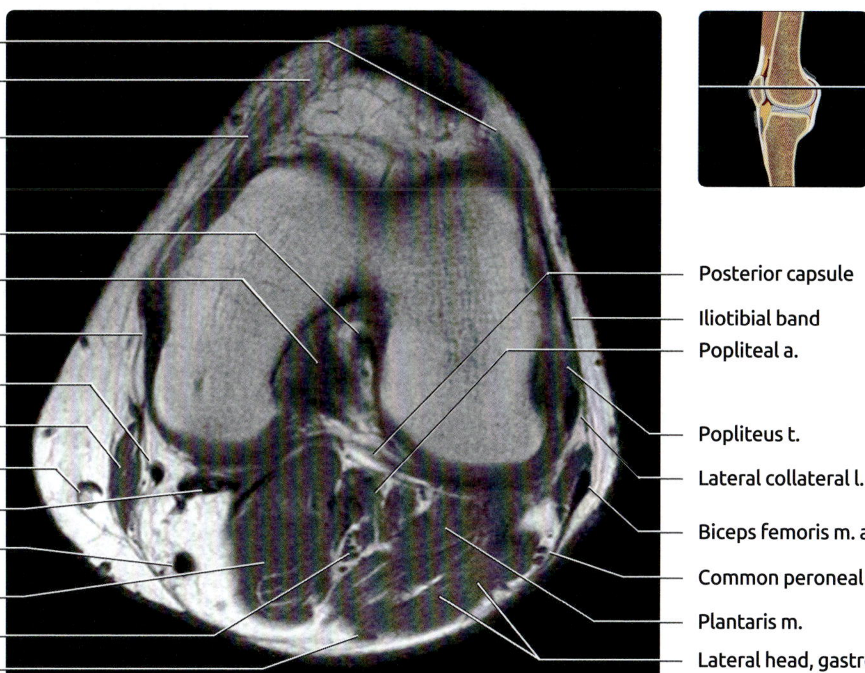

(Top) *This cut is through the intercondylar notch; origins of both the anterior and posterior cruciate ligaments are seen. The hamstrings are nearly completely tendinous, about to cross medial to the knee joint. The origins of both collateral ligaments are now seen.*
(Bottom) *At the lower end of the patella, the medial support is from the inferior patellotibial ligament. The C-shaped semimembranosus tendon is distinctly different from the elements of the pes anserinus (sartorius, gracilis, semitendinosus). The biceps femoris and lateral collateral ligament begin to approach one another as they extend to their insertion on the fibular head; the popliteus tendon arises from its sulcus on the lateral femoral condyle.*

AXIAL T1 MR: RIGHT KNEE

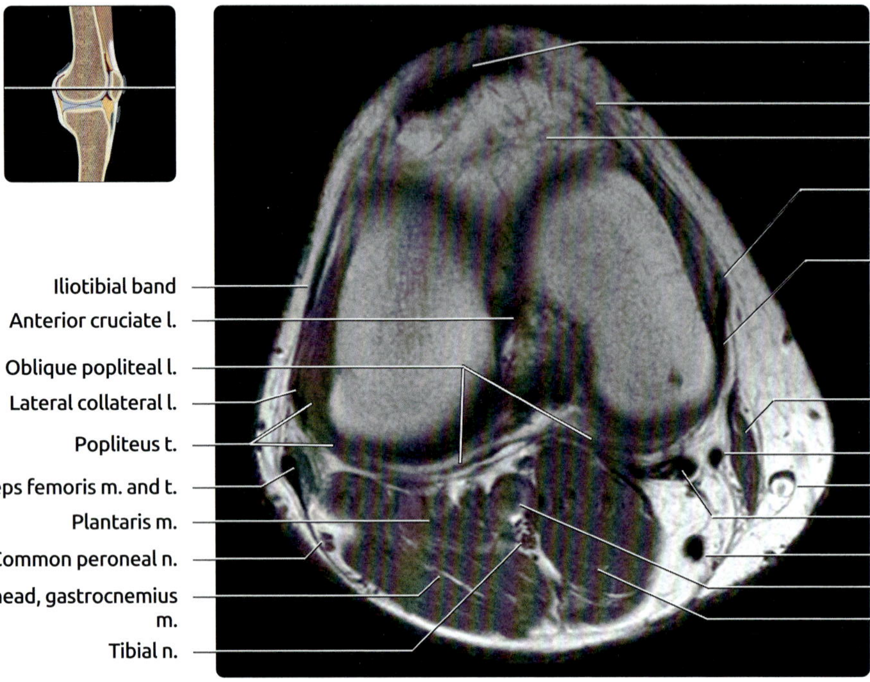

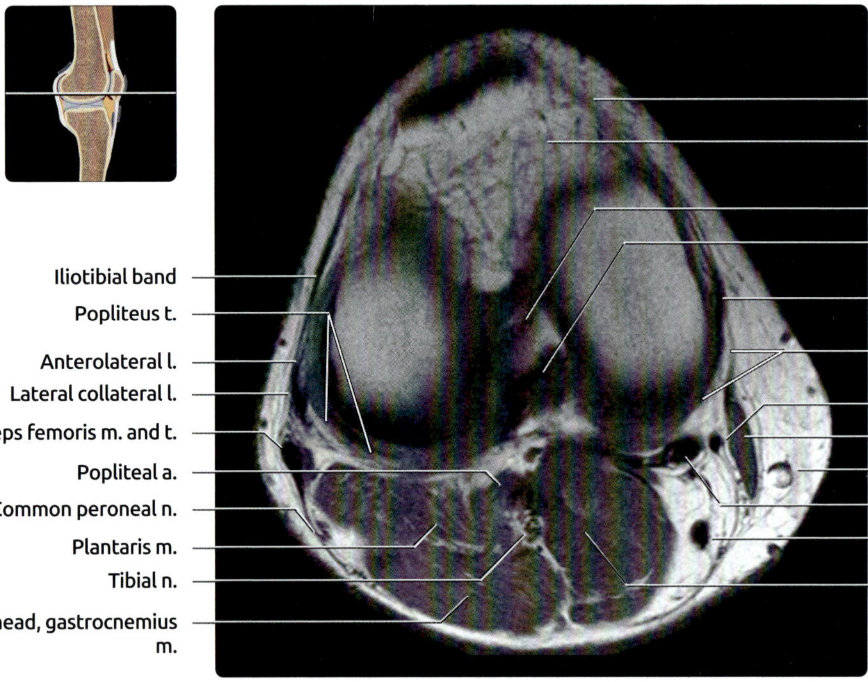

(Top) *This cut is 1.5 cm above the knee joint. The posterolateral structures now include the popliteus tendon, extending posteromedially around the lateral femoral condyle within the popliteal hiatus. Additionally, the posterior oblique ligament, arising from fibers of the medial collateral ligament, joins fibers from the semimembranosus to reinforce the posterior capsule as the oblique popliteal ligament.* **(Bottom)** *This cut is immediately above the knee joint. The posterior cruciate is approaching its insertion on the posterior tibia and the anterior cruciate spreads out toward its insertion on the plateau.*

AXIAL T1 MR: LEFT KNEE

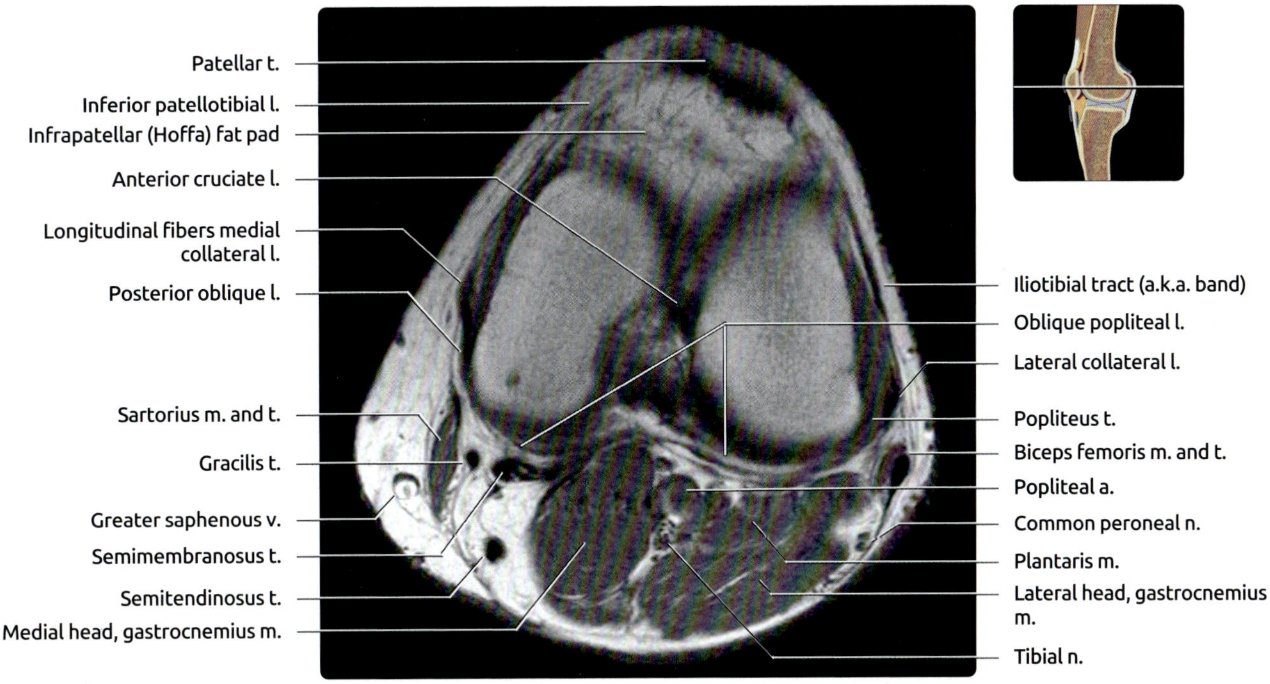

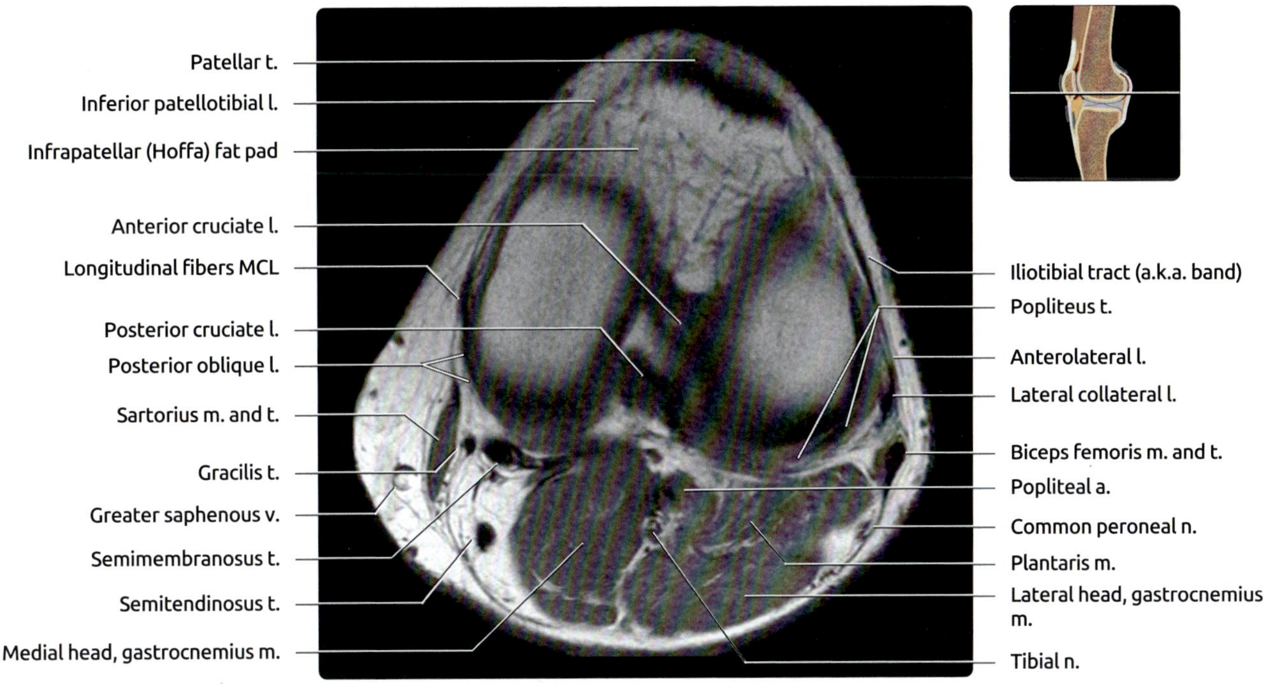

(Top) *This cut is 1.5 cm above the knee joint. The posterolateral structures now include the popliteus tendon, extending posteromedially around the lateral femoral condyle within the popliteal hiatus. Additionally, the posterior oblique ligament, arising from fibers of the medial collateral ligament, joins fibers from the semimembranosus to reinforce the posterior capsule as the oblique popliteal ligament.* **(Bottom)** *This cut is immediately above the knee joint. The posterior cruciate is approaching its insertion on the posterior tibia and the anterior cruciate spreads out toward its insertion on the plateau.*

AXIAL T1 MR: RIGHT KNEE

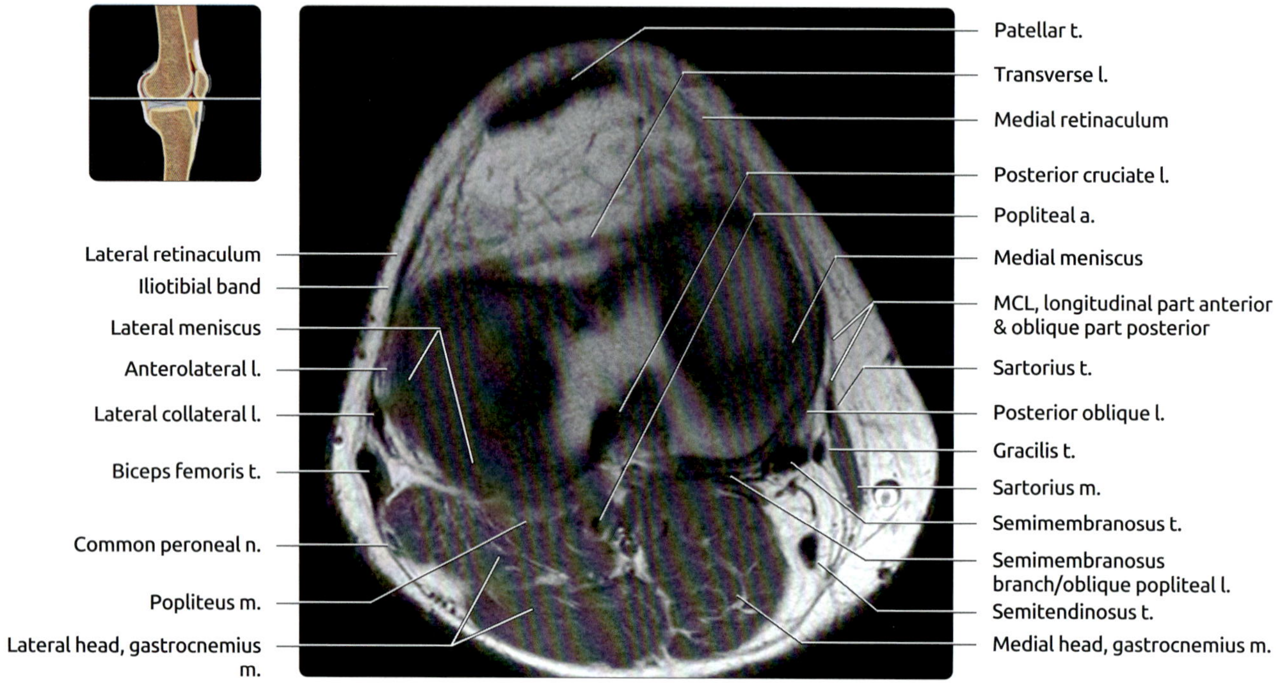

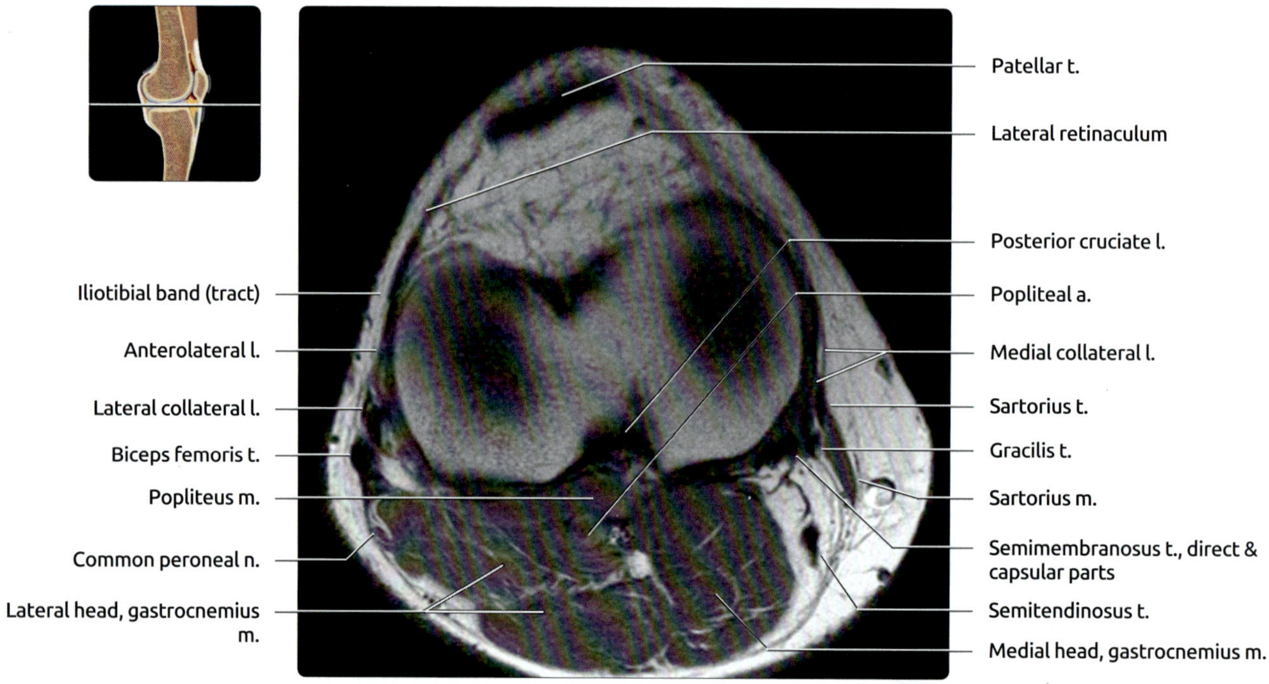

(Top) *This cut is through the knee joint. The menisci are seen, along with the transverse (anterior intermeniscal) ligament extending between the anterior horns. The anterior cruciate ligament has inserted adjacent to the tibial spines and the posterior cruciate ligament is heading posterior to its insertion on the tibia in an extraarticular position.* **(Bottom)** *This cut is immediately distal to the menisci within the joint. The semimembranosus begins to attach to the posteromedial tibia and the popliteus muscle broadens to its insertion on the posterior tibia as well.*

AXIAL T1 MR: LEFT KNEE

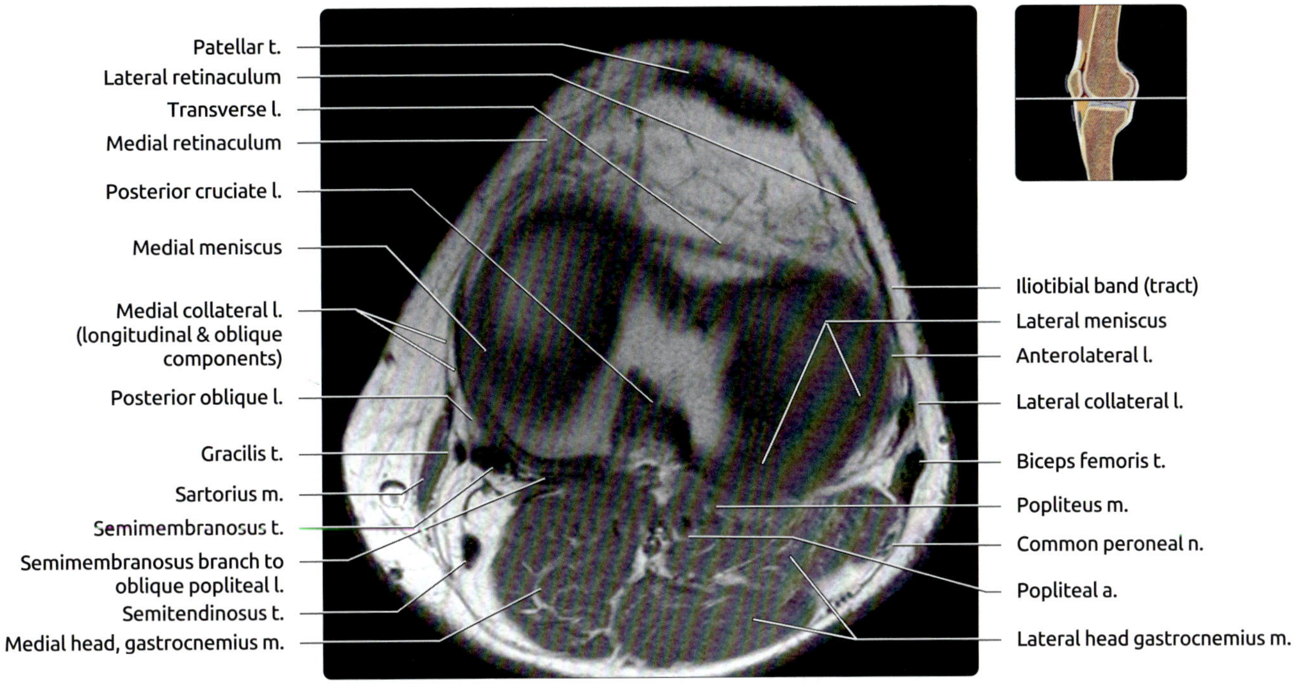

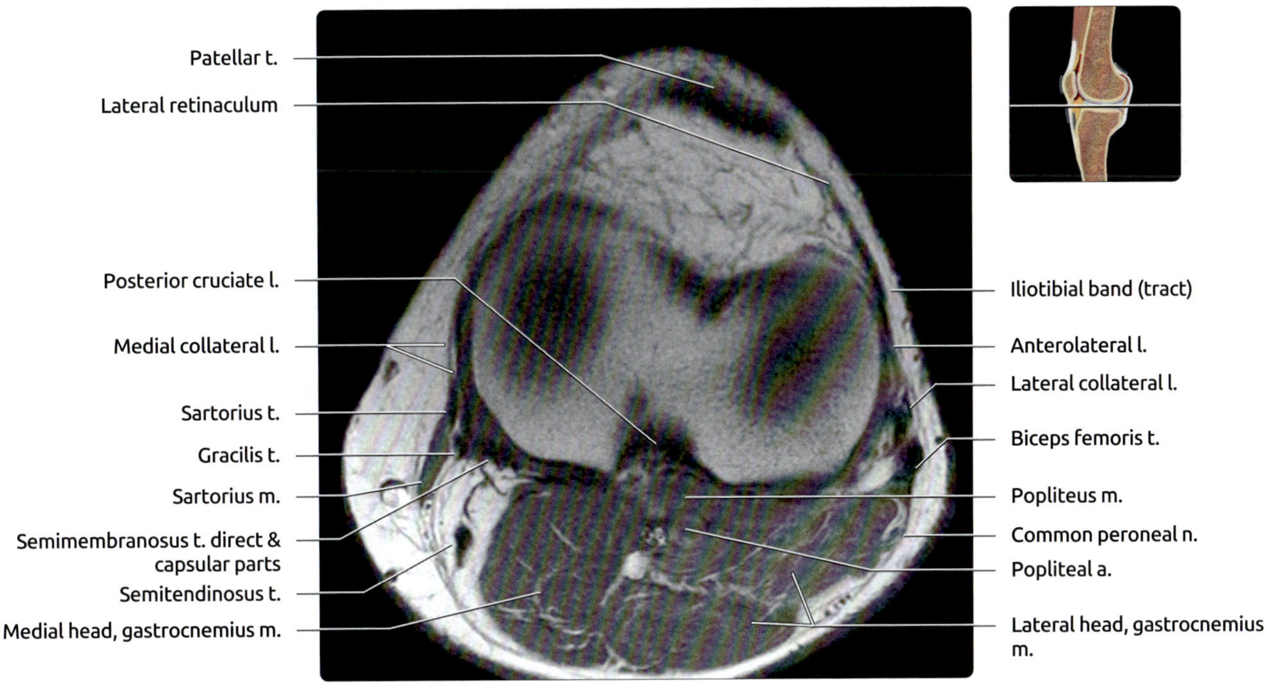

(Top) *This cut is through the knee joint. The menisci are seen, along with the transverse ligament extending between the anterior horns. The anterior cruciate ligament has inserted adjacent to the tibial spines and the posterior cruciate ligament is heading posterior to its insertion on the tibia in an extraarticular position.* **(Bottom)** *This cut is immediately distal to the menisci within the joint. The semimembranosus begins to attach to the posteromedial tibia, and the popliteus muscle broadens to its insertion on the posterior tibia as well.*

AXIAL T1 MR: RIGHT KNEE

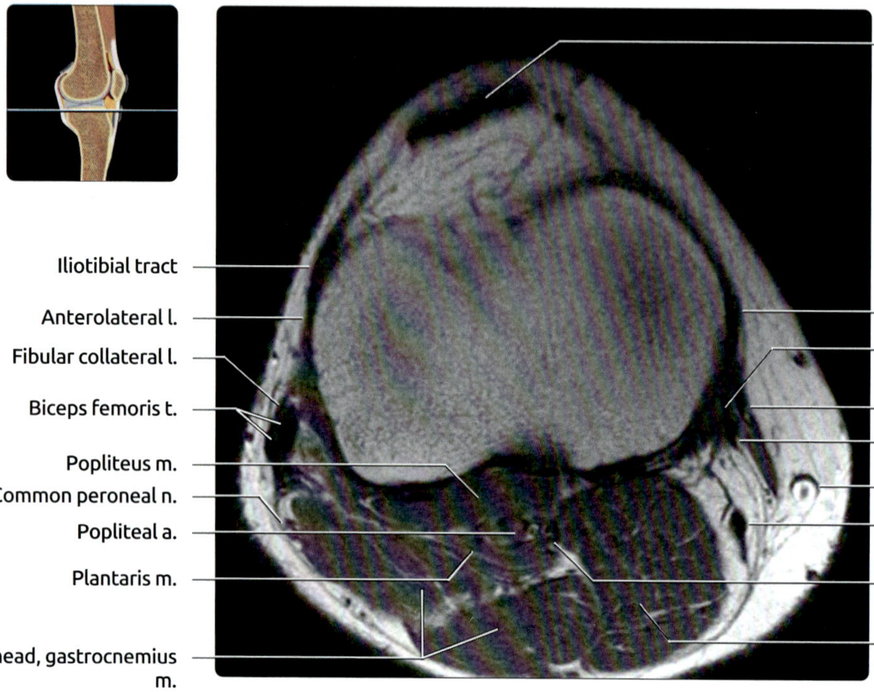

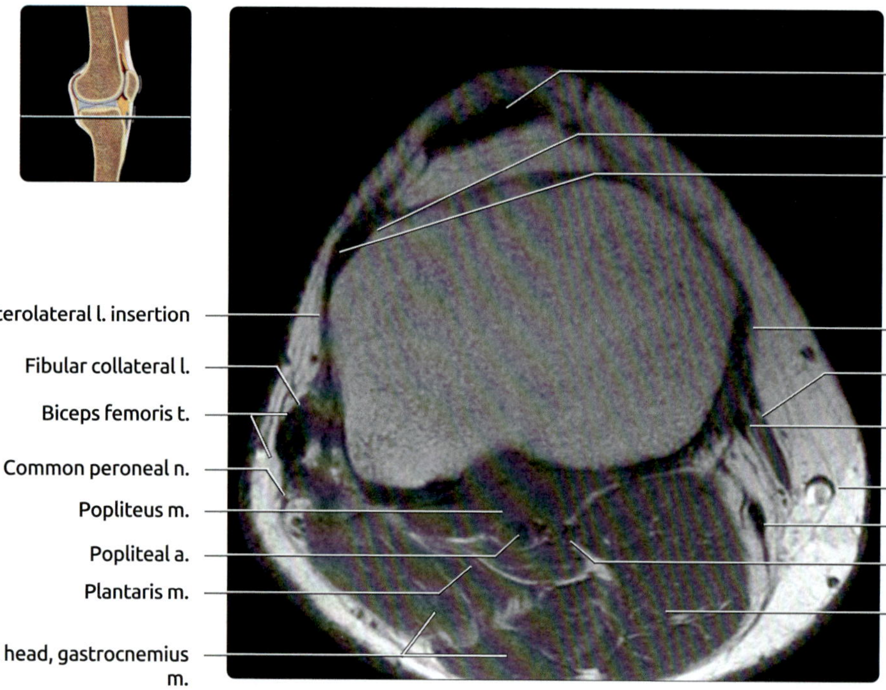

(Top) *This cut is through the tibial plateau. The tendons of pes anserinus (sartorius, gracilis, and semitendinosus) are lining up, extending toward their insertion on the anteromedial tibia. The popliteus muscle is still broad, with the tibial nerve and popliteal vessels interposed between it and the superficial muscles of the leg.* **(Bottom)** *This cut is through the lower portion of the tibial plateau, immediately proximal to the fibular head. Note the common peroneal nerve, located posterior to the biceps femoris tendon.*

AXIAL T1 MR: LEFT KNEE

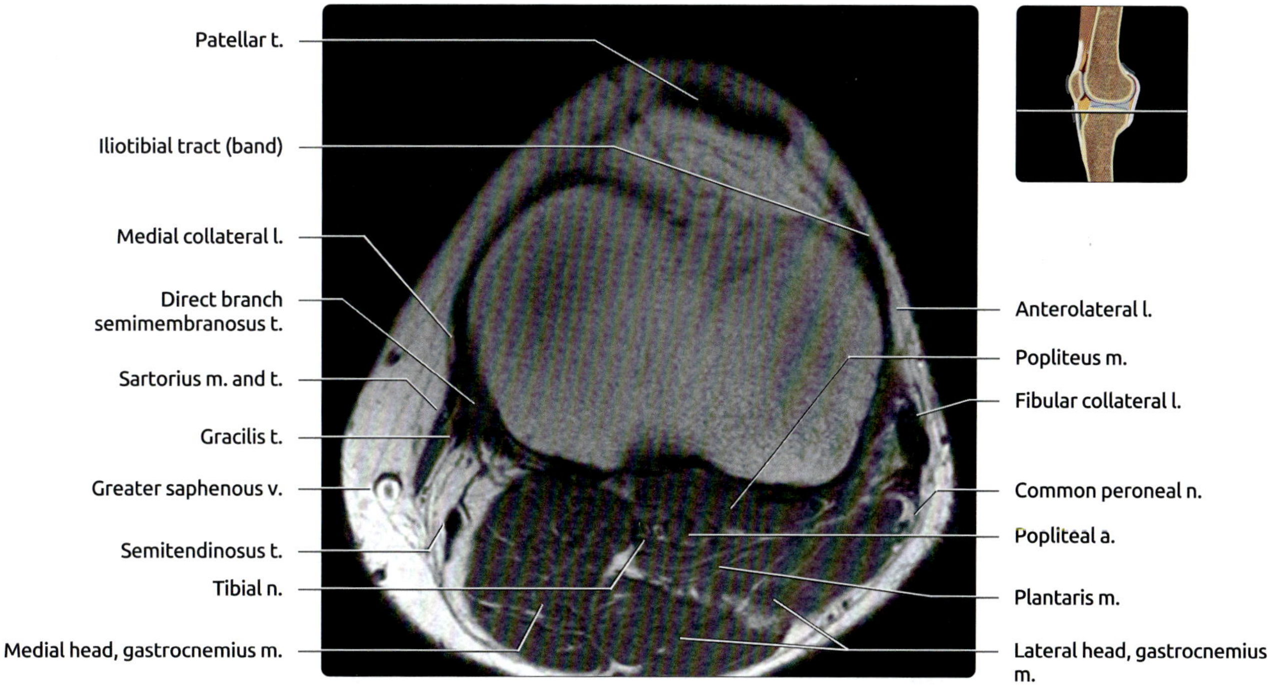

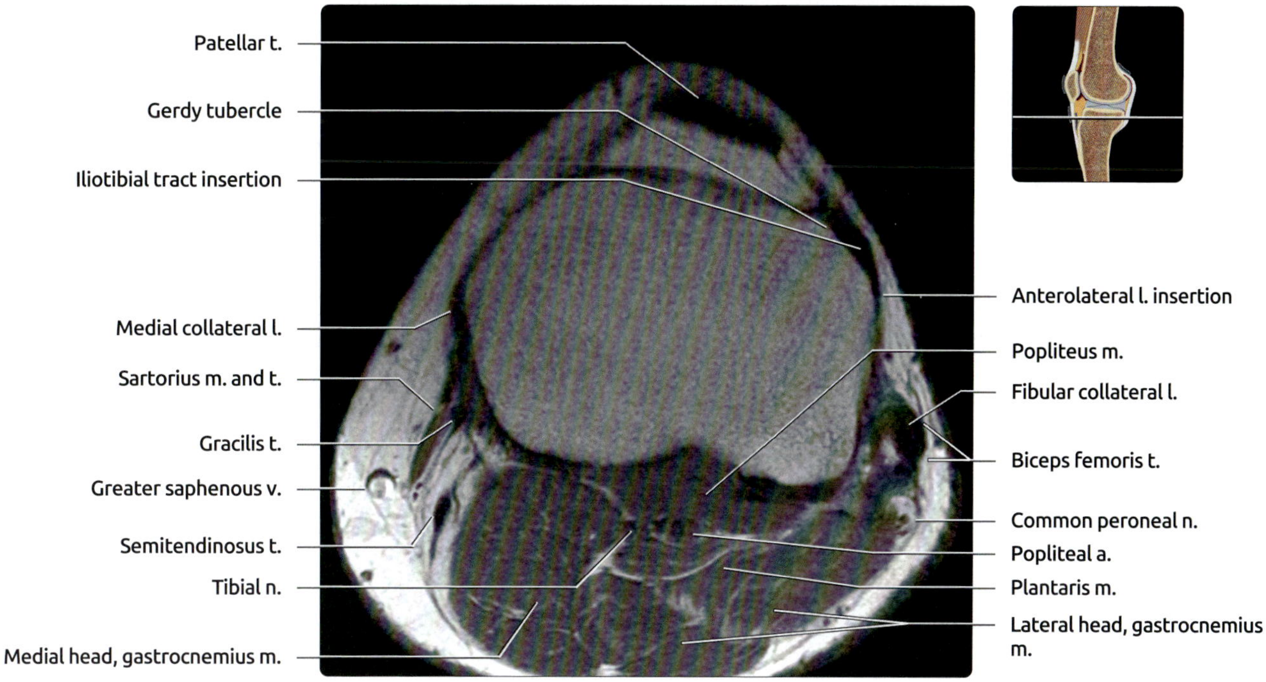

(Top) *This cut is through the tibial plateau. The tendons of the pes anserinus (sartorius, gracilis, and semitendinosus) are lining up, extending toward their insertion on the anteromedial tibia. The popliteus muscle is still broad, with the tibial nerve and popliteal vessels interposed between it and the superficial muscles of the leg.* **(Bottom)** *This cut is through the lower portion of the tibial plateau, immediately proximal to the fibular head. Note the common peroneal nerve, located posterior to the biceps femoris tendon.*

AXIAL T1 MR: RIGHT KNEE

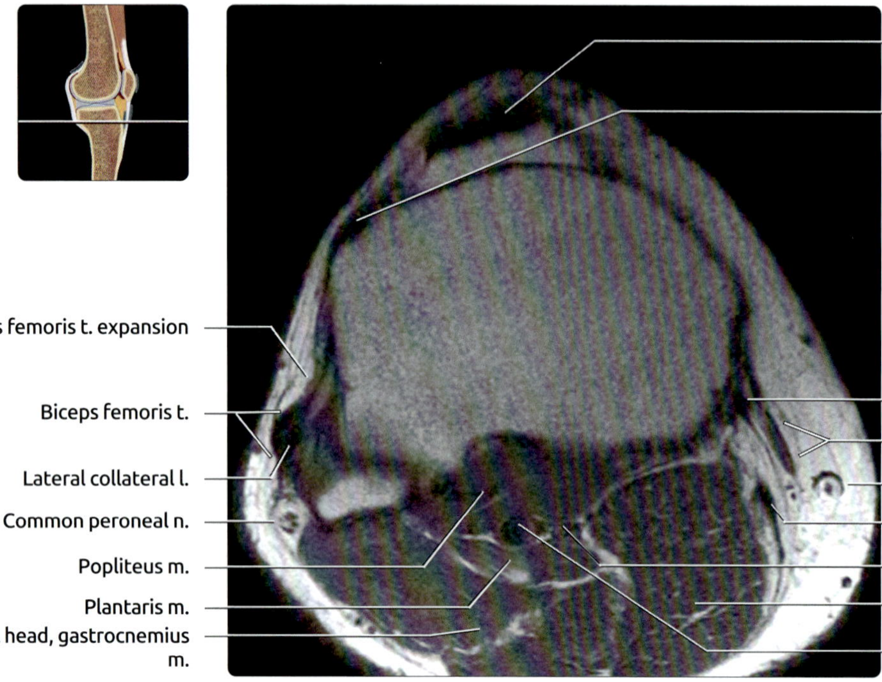

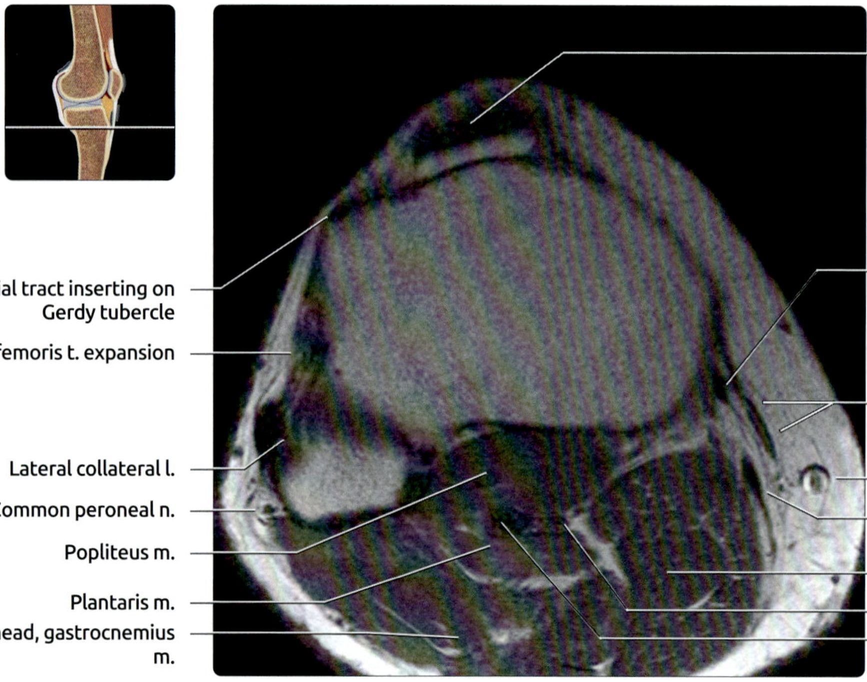

(Top) *At the level of the apex of the fibular head, the pes anserinus is wrapping around the tibial metaphysis to its insertion anteromedially. The biceps femoris tendon expands around the lateral collateral ligament as both course toward their insertion on the fibular head.* **(Bottom)** *This cut at the level of the fibular head shows the insertion of the biceps femoris and lateral collateral ligament anterolaterally on the head. The short head of the biceps femoris has a thin anterior expansion that extends to the anterolateral tibia.*

AXIAL T1 MR: LEFT KNEE

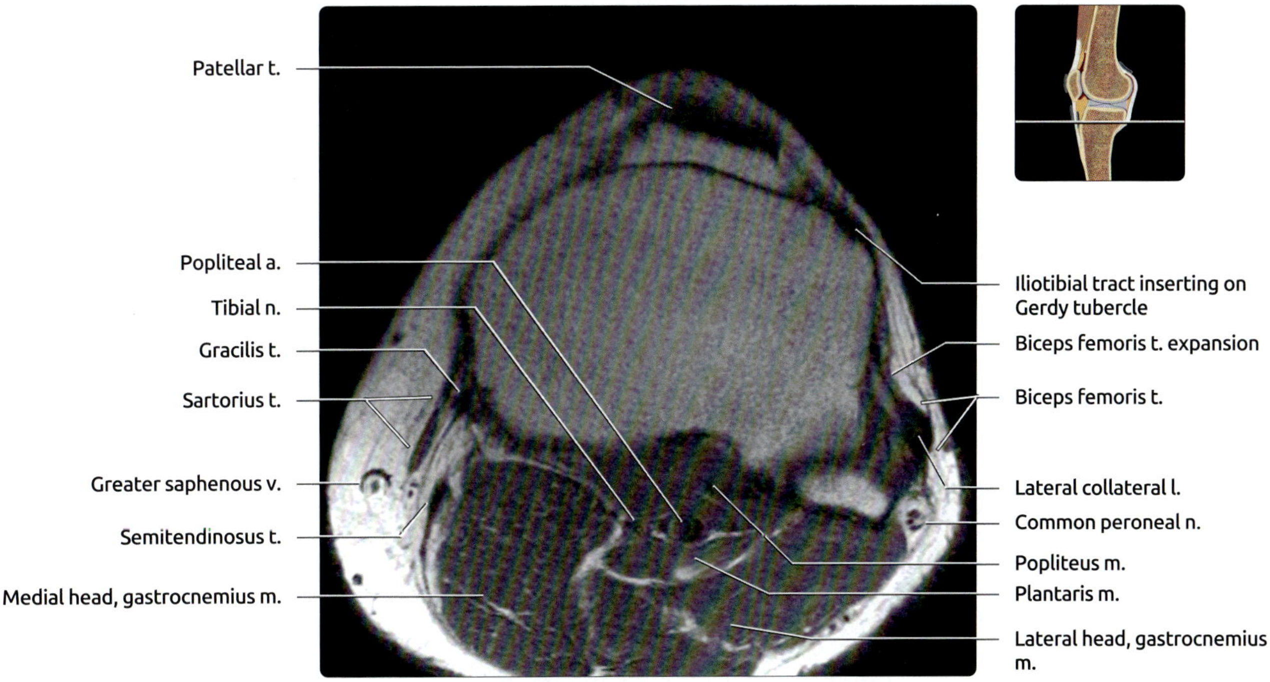

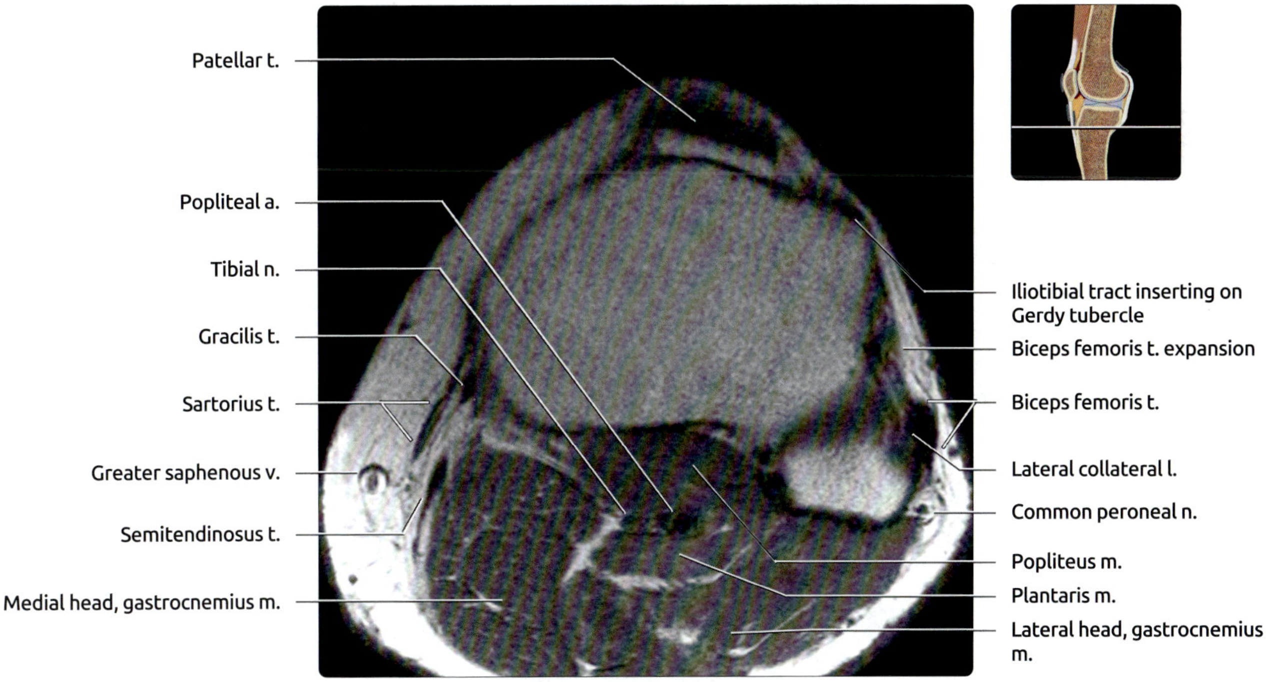

(Top) *At the level of the apex of the fibular head, the pes anserinus is wrapping around the tibial metaphysis to its insertion anteromedially. The biceps femoris tendon expands around the lateral collateral ligament as both course toward their insertion on the fibular head.* **(Bottom)** *This cut is at the level of the fibular head and shows the insertion of the biceps femoris and lateral collateral ligament anterolaterally on the head. The short head of the biceps femoris has a thin anterior expansion that extends to the anterolateral tibia.*

CORONAL T1 MR: RIGHT KNEE

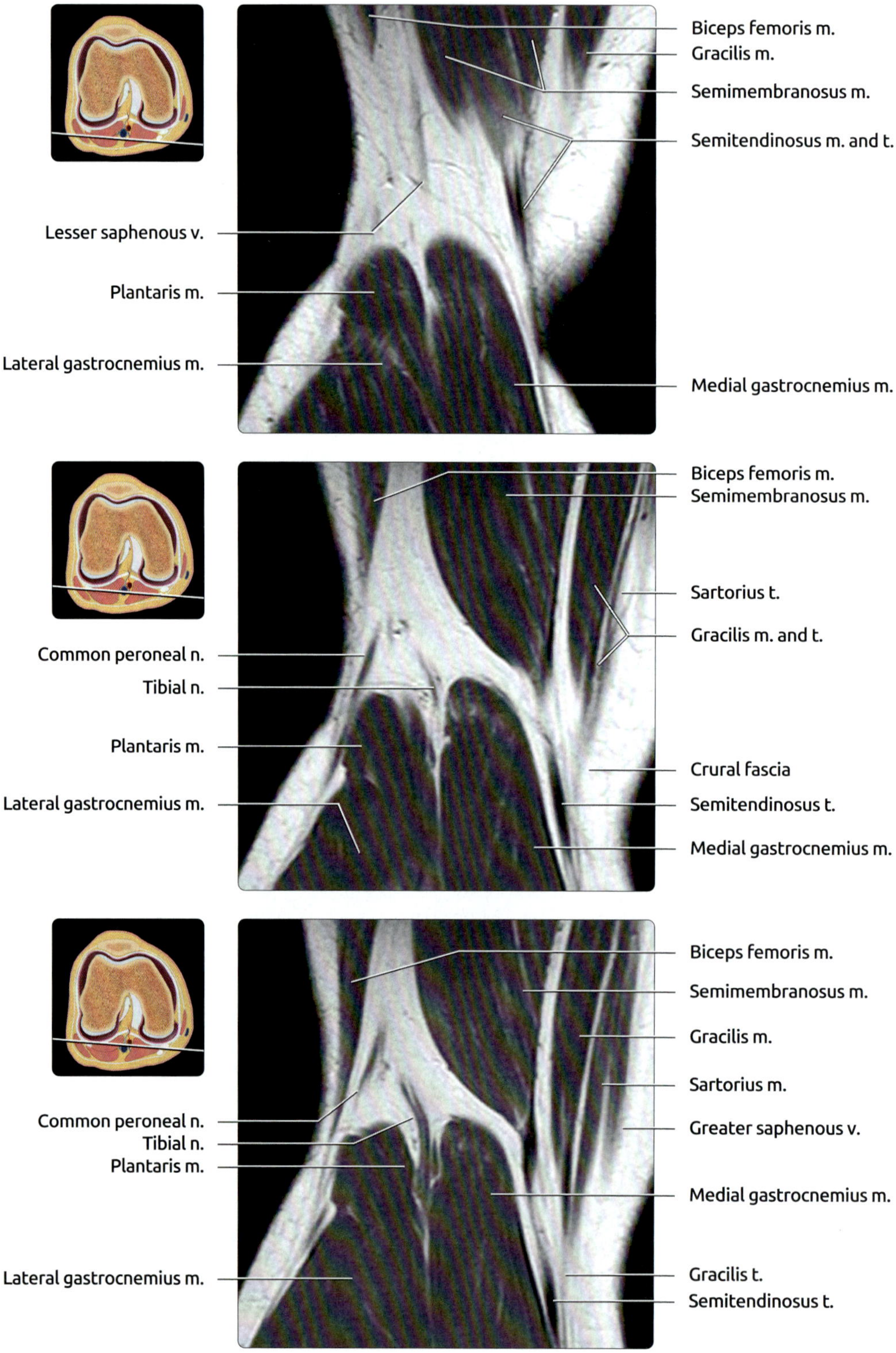

(Top) *First in a series of coronal posterior T1 MR images of the right knee, displayed from posterior to anterior, shows the semitendinosus muscle as well as tendon. This image is posterior enough to also see the lesser saphenous vein. More distally in the leg, the sural nerve accompanies this structure.* **(Middle)** *Slightly more anterior, the courses of the common peroneal and tibial nerves can be seen. The semitendinosus tendon is distinctly seen as the posterior portion of the pes anserinus.* **(Bottom)** *In this slightly more anterior cut, the course of the common peroneal nerve is seen following the posterior biceps femoris tendon. The elements of the pes anserinus are distinctly seen, with the gracilis and sartorius muscles in this plane posterior to their tendons (seen in slightly more anterior cuts). The semitendinosus tendon, the most posterior of the 3 elements of the pes, is seen in this section; however, its muscle fibers are in a more posterior section.*

CORONAL T1 MR: LEFT KNEE

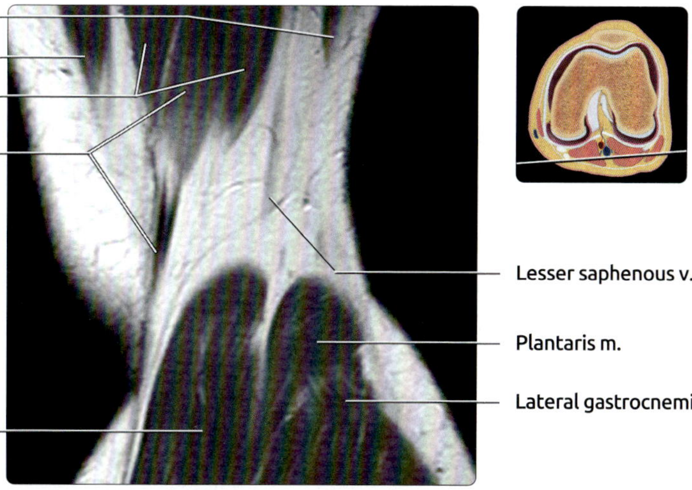

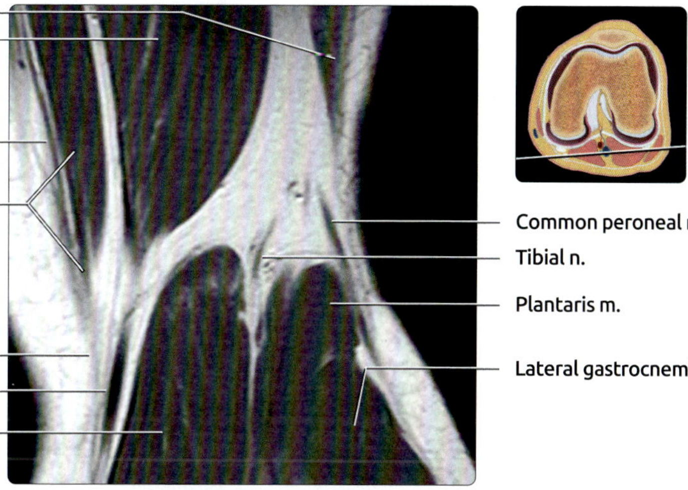

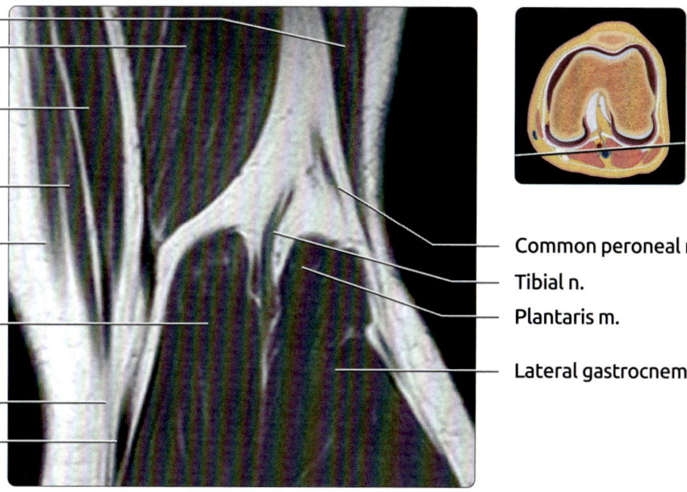

(Top) *First in a series of posterior coronal T1 MR images of the left knee, displayed from posterior to anterior, shows the semitendinosus muscle and tendon. The images are posterior enough to also see the lesser saphenous vein. More distally in the leg, the sural nerve accompanies this structure.* **(Middle)** *Slightly more anterior, the courses of the common peroneal and tibial nerves can be seen. The semitendinosus tendon is distinctly seen as the posterior portion of the pes anserinus.* **(Bottom)** *In this slightly more anterior cut, the course of the common peroneal nerve is seen following the posterior biceps femoris tendon. The elements of the pes anserinus are distinctly seen, with the gracilis and sartorius muscles in this plane posterior to their tendons (seen in slightly more anterior cuts). The semitendinosus tendon, the most posterior of the 3 elements of the pes, is seen in this section; however, its muscle fibers are in a more posterior section.*

CORONAL T1 MR: RIGHT KNEE

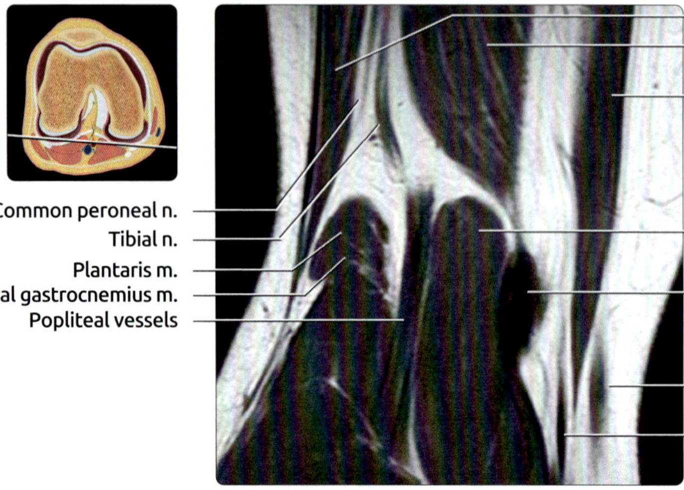

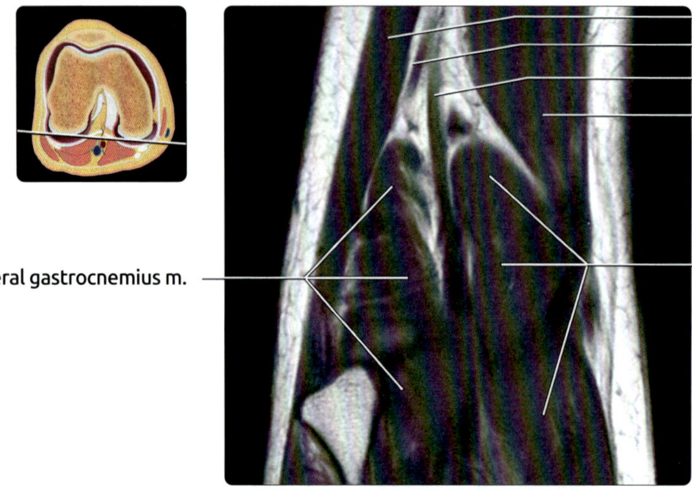

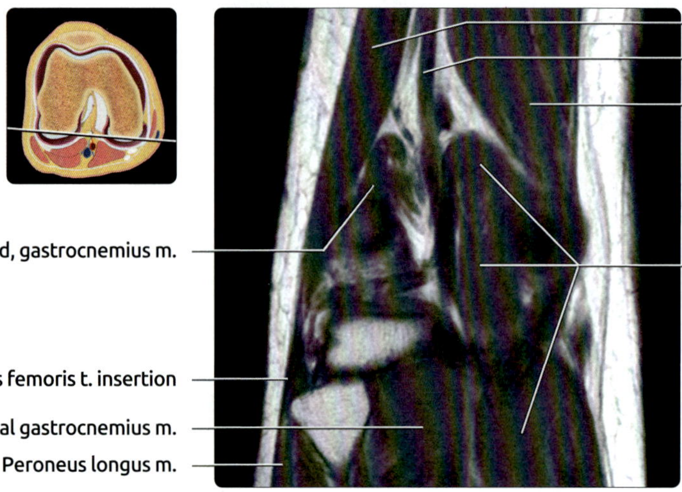

(Top) *In the most anterior cut of this series, the division of the tibial and common peroneal nerves can be seen as well as the separate components of the pes anserinus.* **(Middle)** *First in a series of coronal T1 MR images of the right knee is shown. This series is in a slightly different obliquity than the prior series, allowing slightly different combinations of structures to be seen in a single cut. The series is shown from posterior to anterior. The tibial nerve and common peroneal nerve are seen in this cut, as they lie more posterior than the popliteal vessels.* **(Bottom)** *In this slightly more anterior image, the gastrocnemius muscles predominate in the posterior portion of the lower knee; the deeper muscles are smaller at this point. Laterally, the origin of the peroneus longus muscle is seen at the fibula.*

CORONAL T1 MR: LEFT KNEE

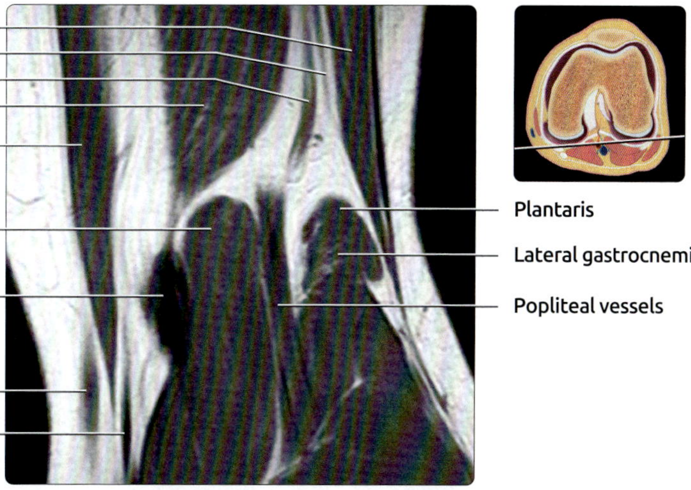

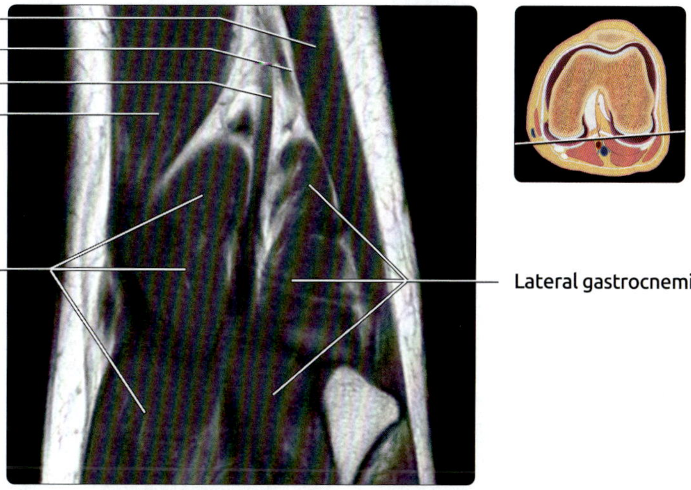

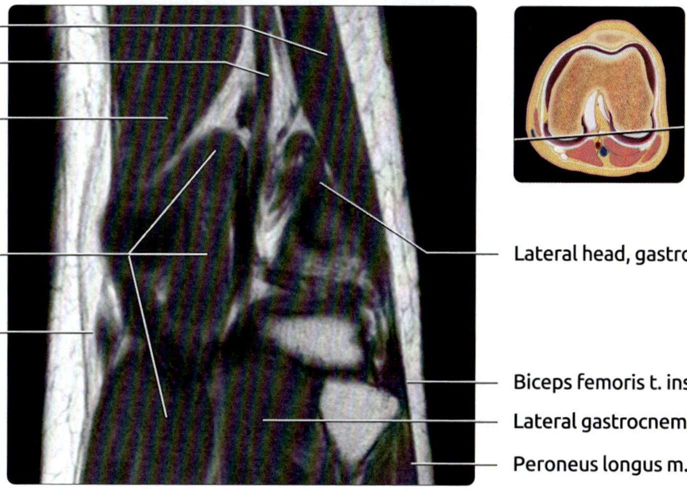

(Top) *In this most anterior cut of this series, we see the division of the tibial and common peroneal nerves as well as the separate components of the pes anserinus.* **(Middle)** *First in a series of T1 MR images of the left knee, shown from posterior to anterior, shows a slightly different obliquity than the prior series, allowing slightly different combinations of structures to be seen in a single cut. The tibial nerve and common peroneal nerve are seen in this cut, as they lie more posterior than the popliteal vessels.* **(Bottom)** *In this slightly more anterior image, the gastrocnemius muscles predominate in the posterior portion of the lower knee; the deeper muscles are smaller at this point. Laterally, the origin of the peroneus longus muscle is seen at the fibula.*

CORONAL T1 MR: RIGHT KNEE

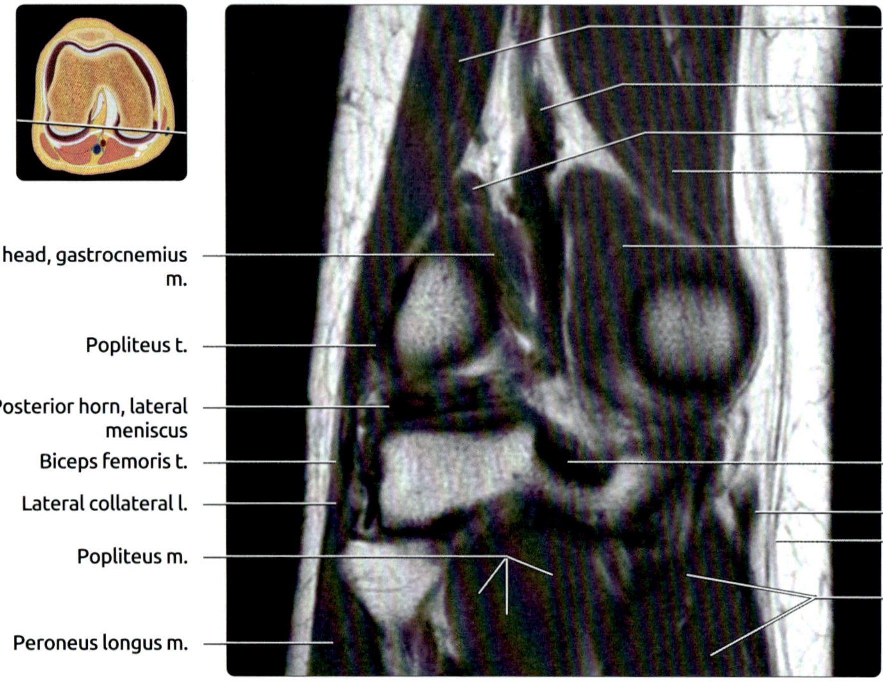

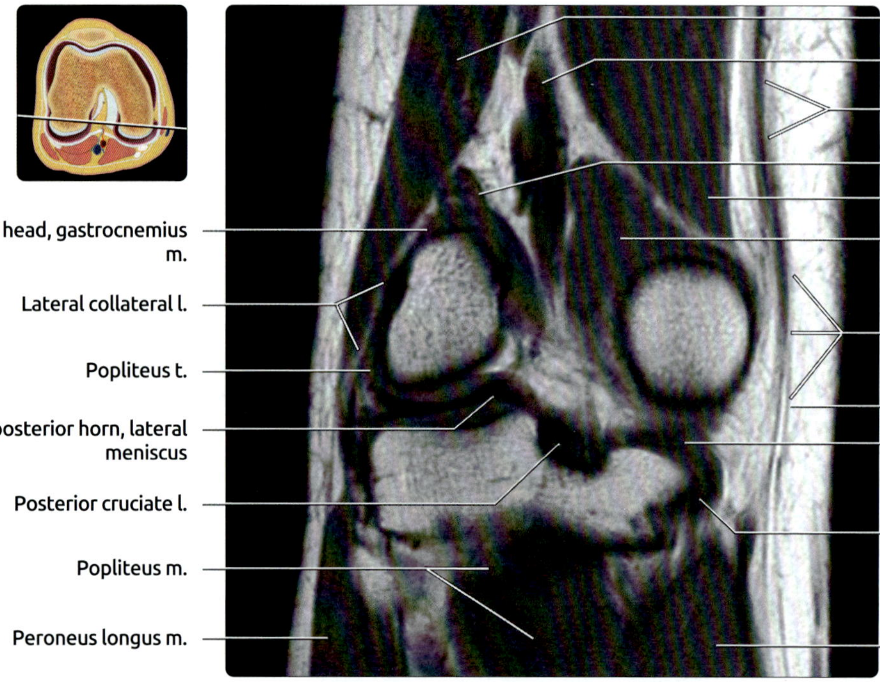

(Top) *Slightly more anterior and deep to the majority of the gastrocnemius muscle mass, the popliteus tendon is seen arising from its notch on the lateral femoral condyle, extending posteriorly and inferiorly to the popliteal hiatus. The individual structures in the posterolateral corner are generally better seen on fluid-sensitive sequences because of the fluid in the popliteal hiatus.* **(Bottom)** *The lateral collateral ligament can now be seen arising from lateral femoral condyle, coursing toward its insertion, along with the biceps femoris, on the fibular styloid process.*

CORONAL T1 MR: LEFT KNEE

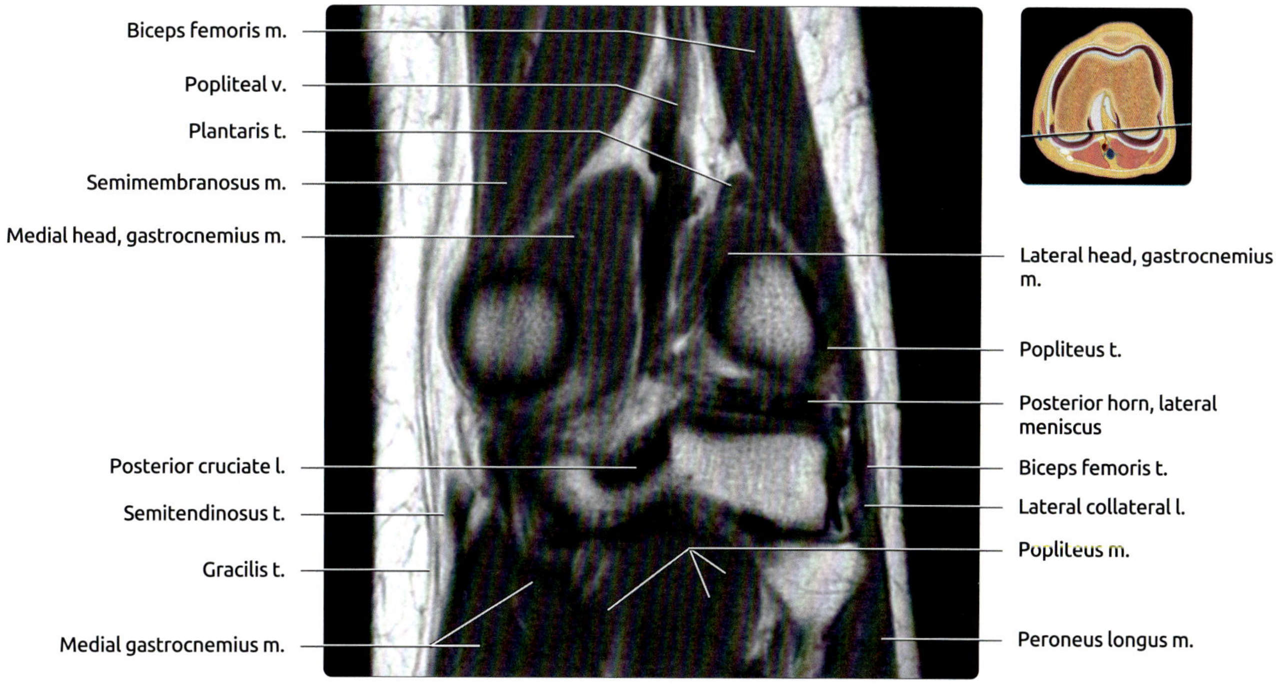

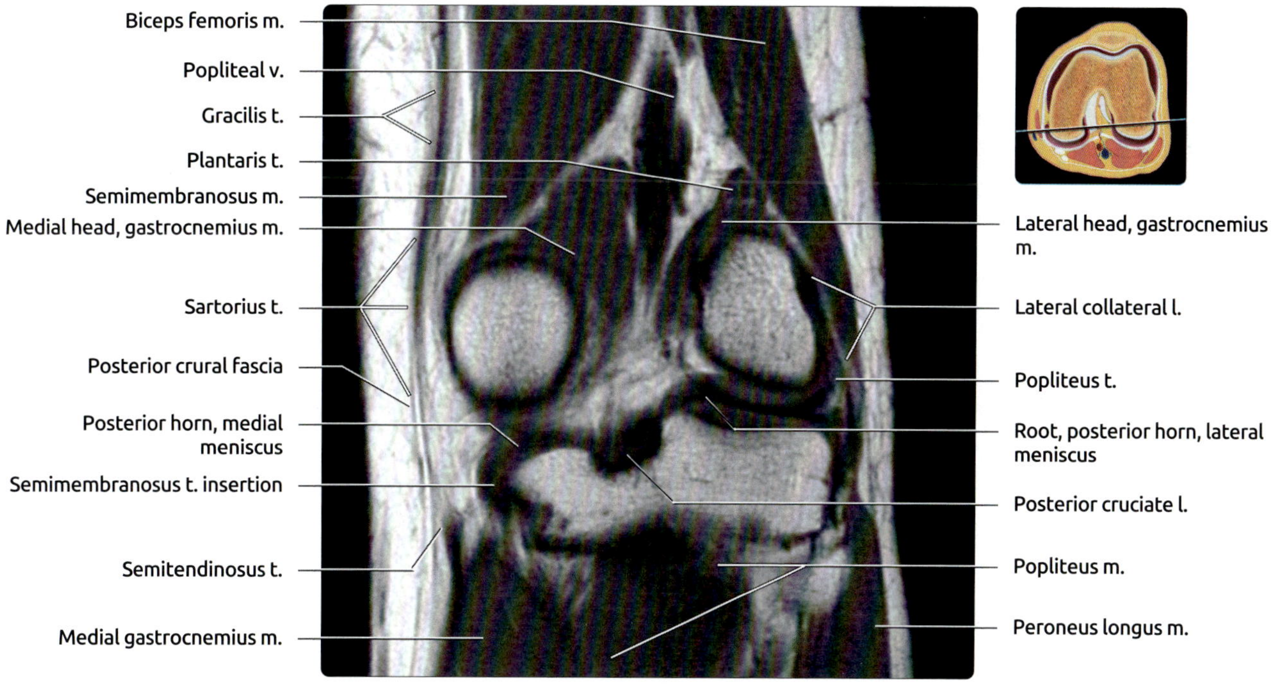

(Top) *Slightly more anterior and deep to the majority of the gastrocnemius muscle mass, the popliteus tendon is seen arising from its notch on the lateral femoral condyle, extending posteriorly and inferiorly to the popliteal hiatus. The individual structures in the posterolateral corner are generally better seen on fluid-sensitive sequences because of the fluid in the popliteal hiatus.* **(Bottom)** *The lateral collateral ligament can now be seen arising from lateral femoral condyle, coursing toward its insertion, along with the biceps femoris, on the fibular styloid process.*

CORONAL T1 MR: RIGHT KNEE

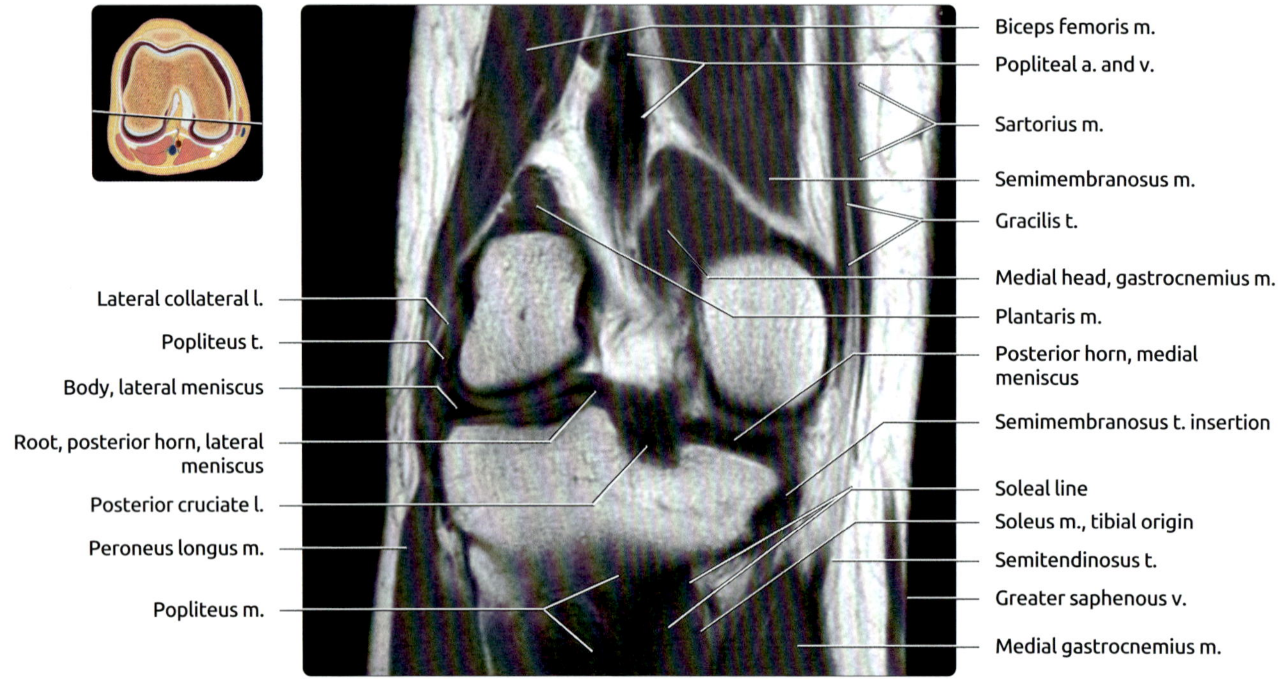

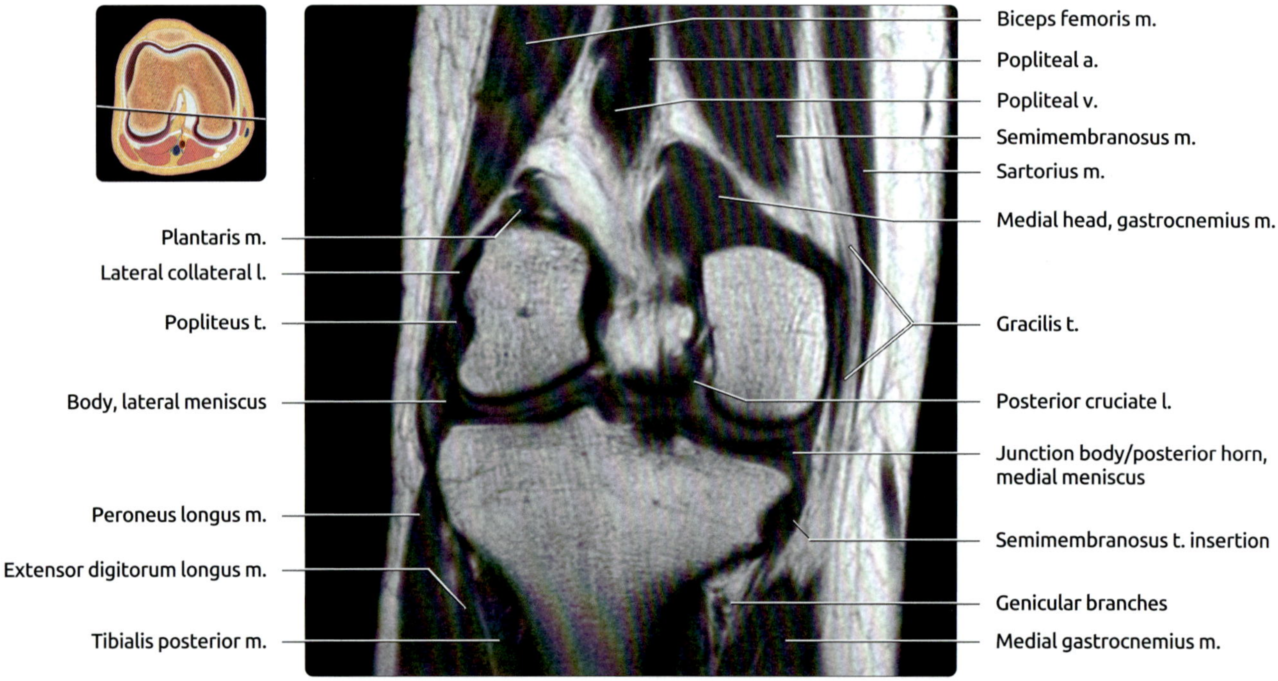

(Top) *More anteriorly, note the large expanse of insertion of the popliteus muscle on the posterior tibia. The medial soleus origin arises at its distal edge, along the soleal line. The fibular origin of the soleus occurs more proximally.* **(Bottom)** *Coronal T1WI MR shows the posterior portion of the knee joint, which is more complex than the anterior. The gastrocnemius and posterior vessels are still seen as well as the hamstring muscles. Inferolaterally, the muscles can be confusing on coronal imaging since in a single plane such as this, muscles from the lateral compartment (peroneus), anterior compartment (extensor digitorum longus), and posterior compartment (tibialis posterior) can be seen. This is because the cut extends obliquely across the interosseous membrane between the tibia and fibula.*

CORONAL T1 MR: LEFT KNEE

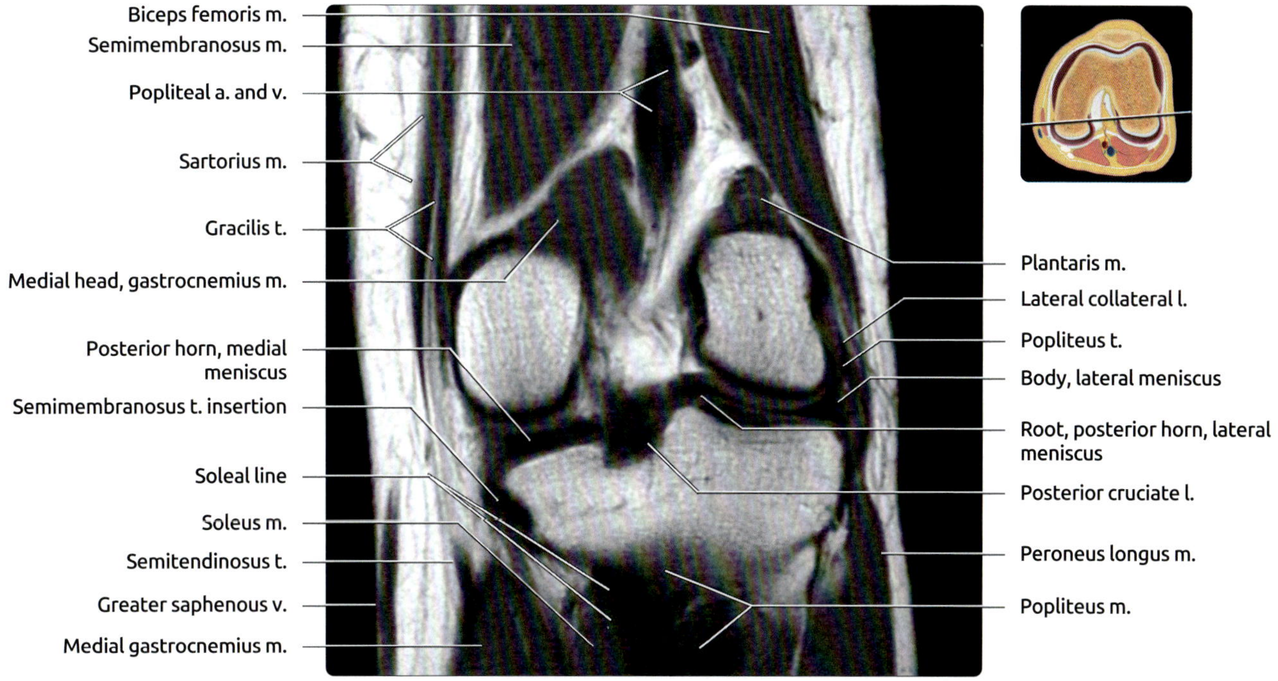

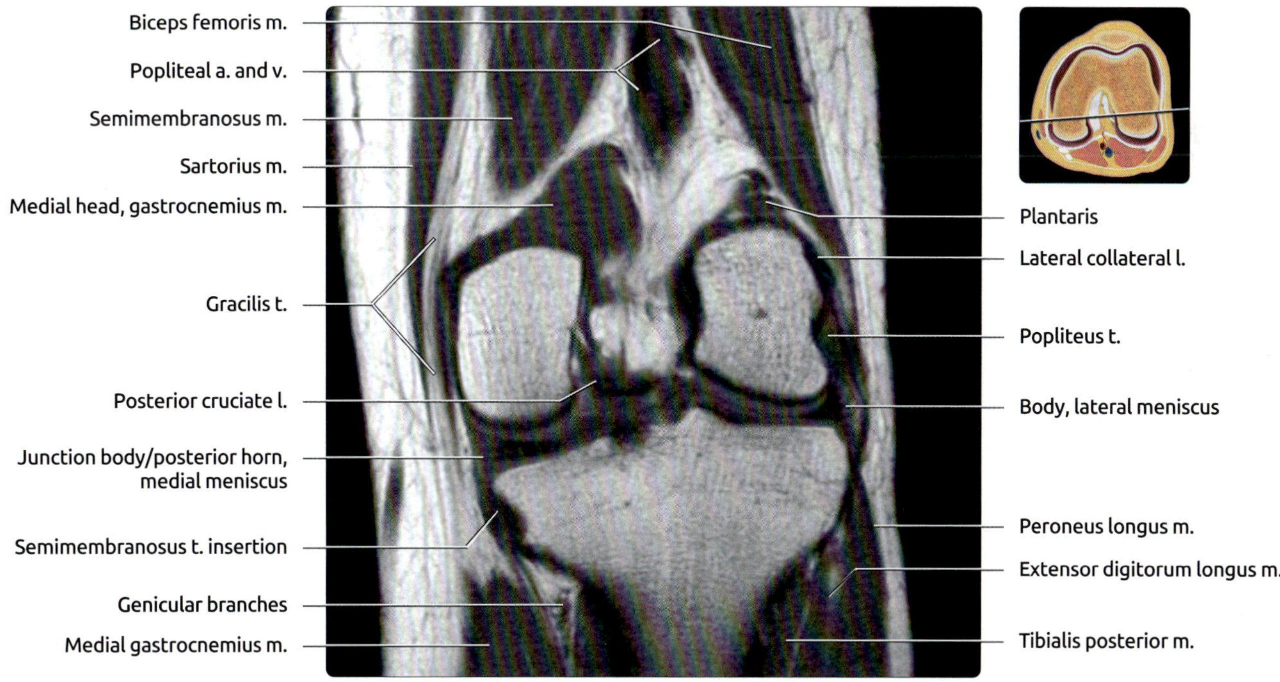

(Top) *More anteriorly, note the large expanse of insertion of the popliteus muscle on the posterior tibia. The medial soleus origin arises at its distal edge, along the soleal line. The fibular origin of the soleus occurs more proximally.* **(Bottom)** *Coronal T1WI MR shows the posterior portion of the knee joint, which is more complex than the anterior. The gastrocnemius and posterior vessels are still seen as well as the hamstring muscles. Inferolaterally, the muscles can be confusing on coronal imaging since in a single plane such as this, muscles from the lateral compartment (peroneus), anterior compartment (extensor digitorum longus), and posterior compartment (tibialis posterior) can be seen. This is because the cut extends obliquely across the interosseous membrane between tibia and fibula.*

CORONAL T1 MR: RIGHT KNEE

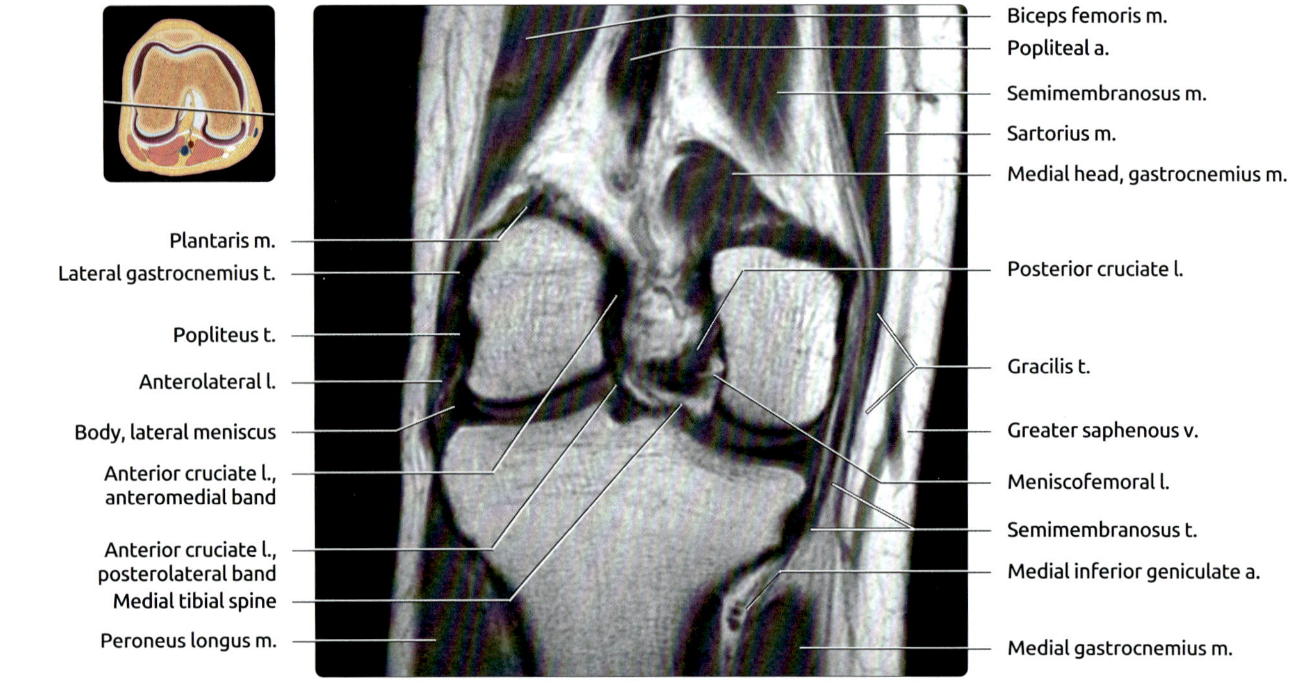

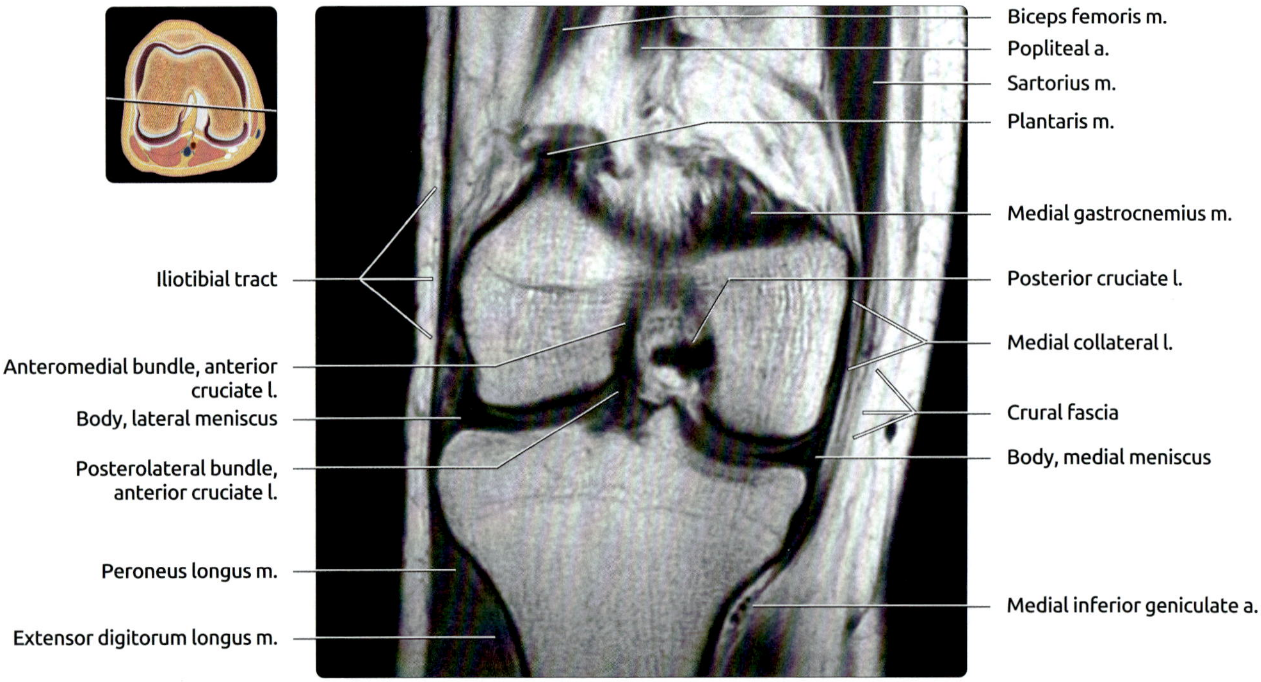

(Top) *As the images become more anterior, the last elements of the pes anserinus can be seen. The sartorius and gracilis are shown in this image located more anteriorly at the joint line than the 3rd element of the pes and semitendinosus. The most posterior fibers of the anterior cruciate ligament are seen as well.* **(Bottom)** *More anteriorly within the notch, the anterior cruciate ligament is seen in its oblique route from the lateral femoral condyle to the insertion adjacent to the medial spines. The posterolateral bundle attaches to the femoral condyle inferior to the attachment of the anteromedial bundle.*

CORONAL T1 MR: LEFT KNEE

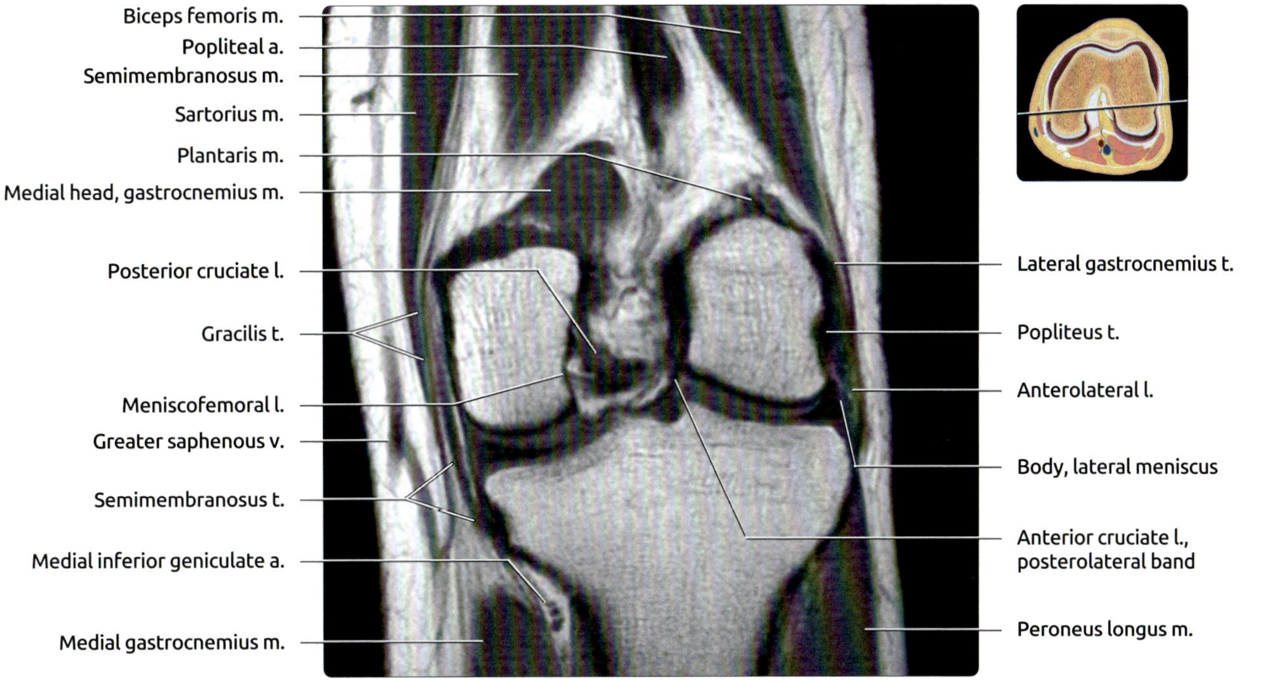

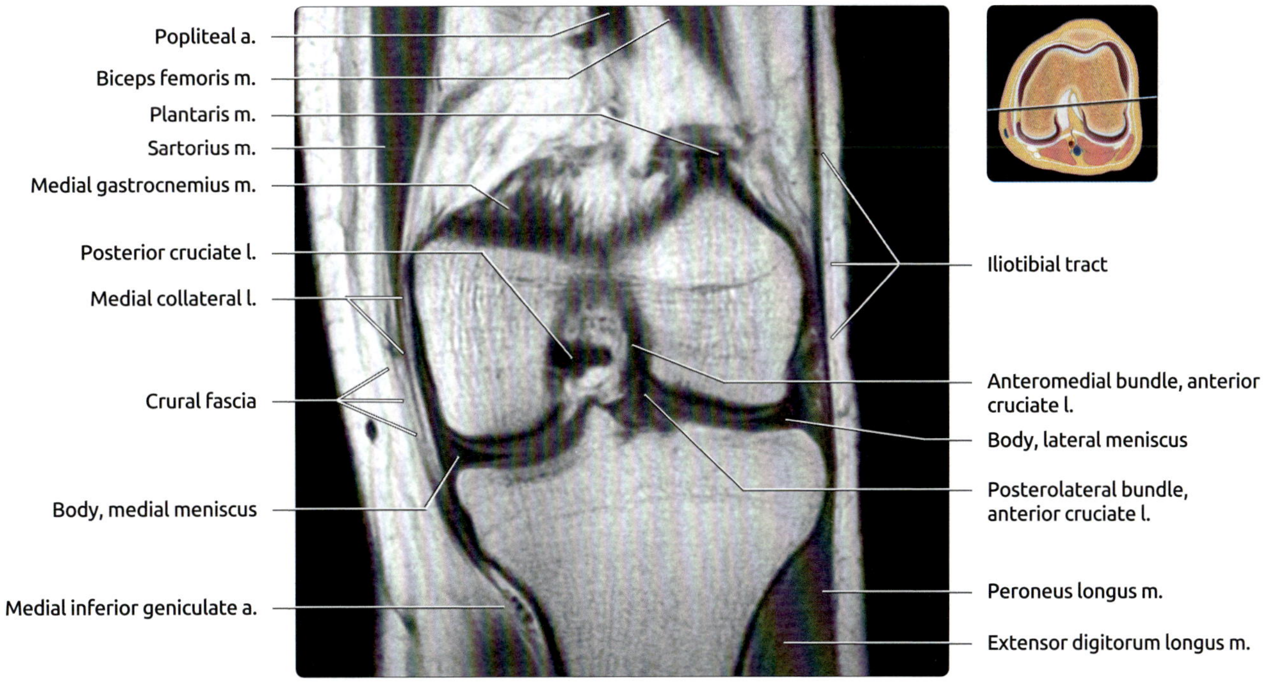

(Top) *As the images become more anterior, the last elements of the pes anserinus can be seen. The sartorius and gracilis are shown in this image located more anteriorly at the joint line than the 3rd element of the pes and semitendinosus. The most posterior fibers of the anterior cruciate ligament are seen as well.* **(Bottom)** *More anteriorly within the notch, the anterior cruciate ligament is seen in its oblique route from the lateral femoral condyle to the insertion adjacent to the medial spines. The posterolateral bundle attaches to the femoral condyle inferior to the attachment of the anteromedial bundle.*

CORONAL T1 MR: RIGHT KNEE

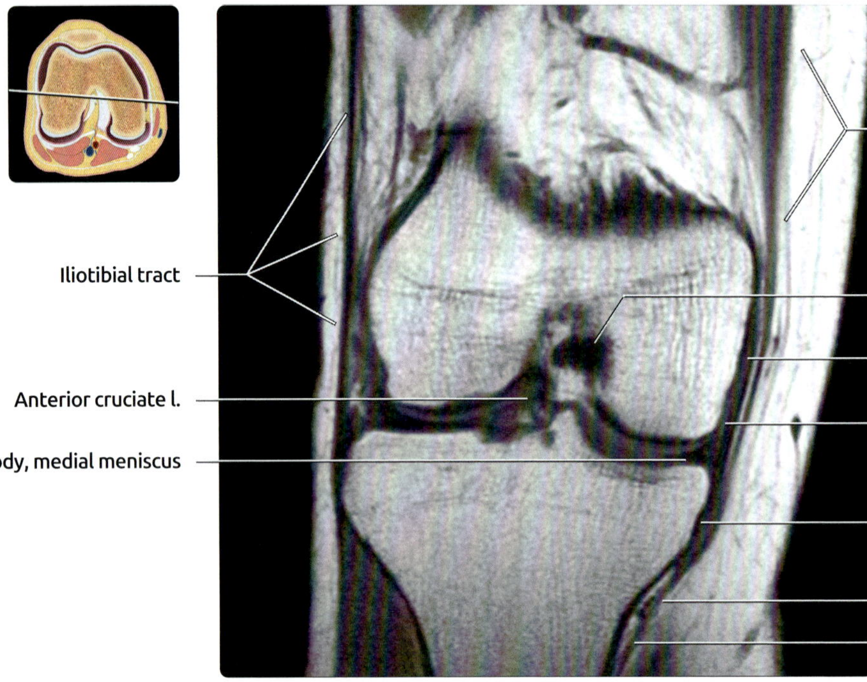

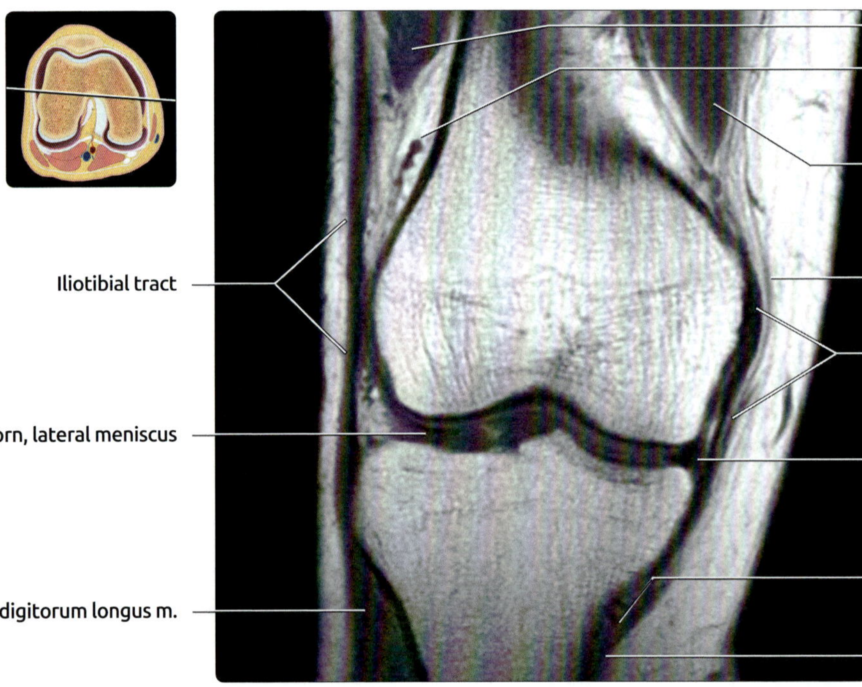

(Top) *Note the length of the medial collateral ligament in this image. The origin is intimately associated with the origin of the medial patellofemoral ligament, immediately distal to the adductor tubercle. The insertion is about 5 cm distal to the knee joint and is usually not entirely included in standard knee MR exams. The medial inferior geniculate arterial branches are seen in cross section between the superficial medial collateral ligament and the tibial cortex.* **(Bottom)** *The anterior cut is through the anterior midportion of the joint. Because these are T1 images, there is little contrast between the hyaline cartilage and menisci.*

CORONAL T1 MR: LEFT KNEE

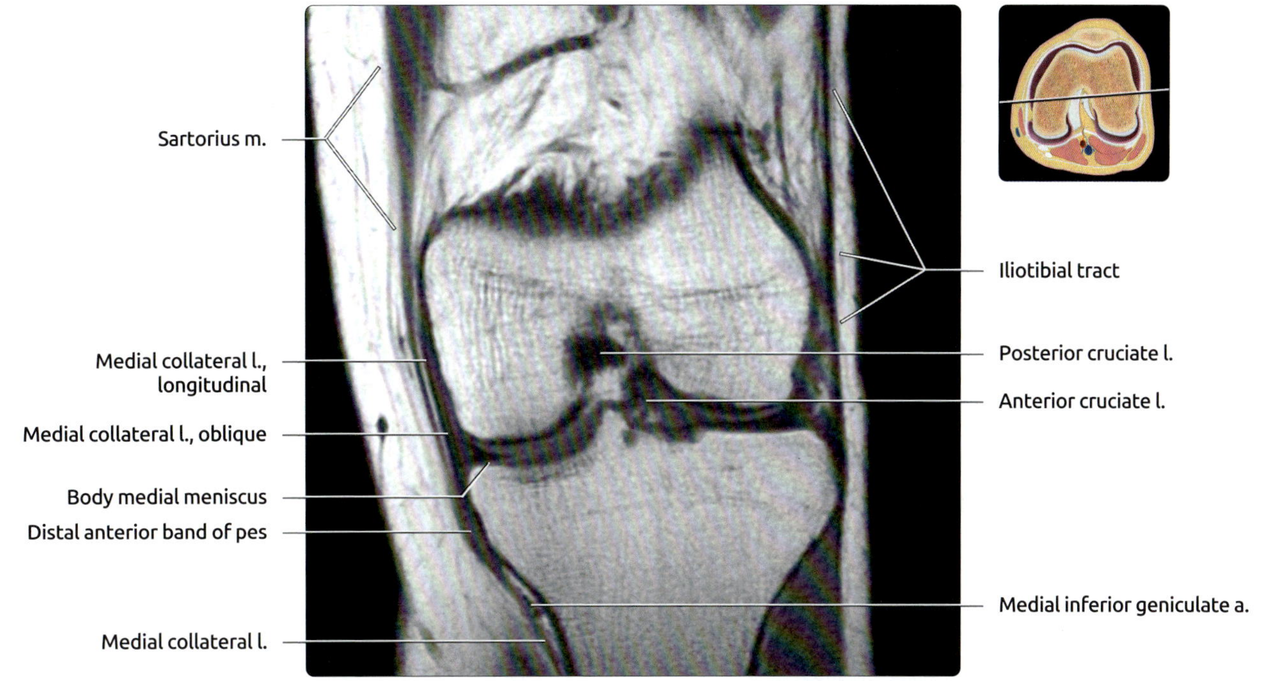

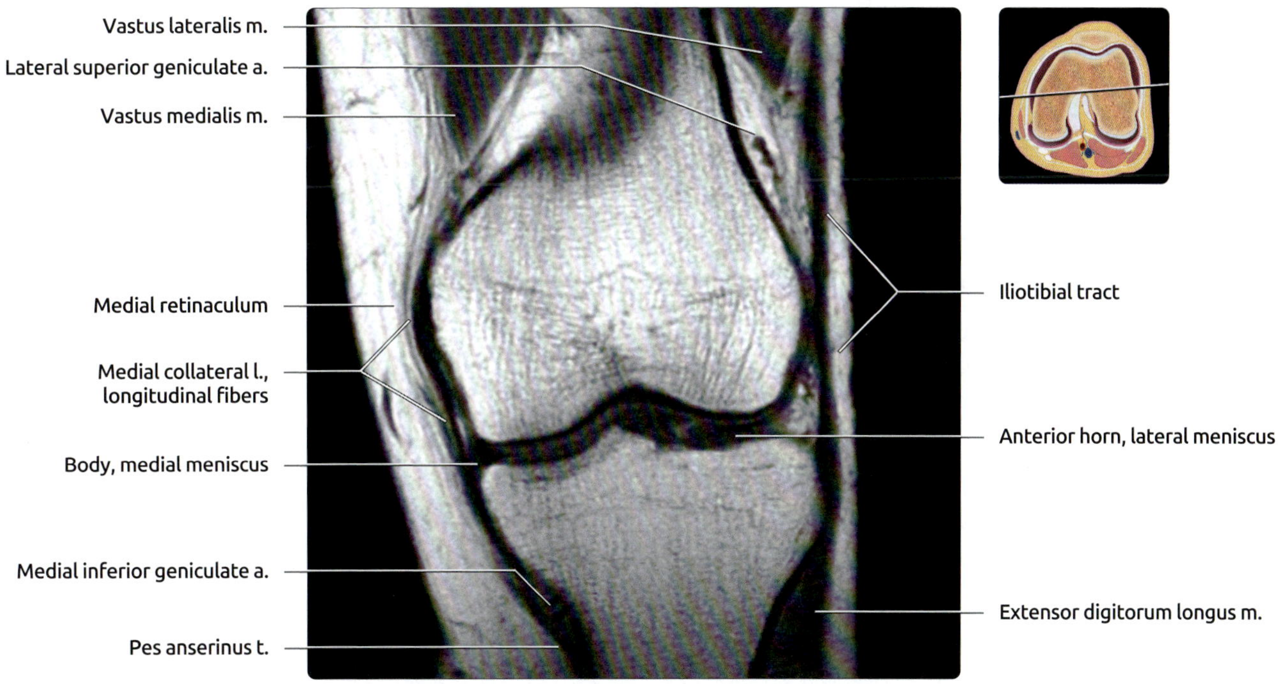

(Top) *Note the length of the medial collateral ligament in this image. The origin is intimately associated with the origin of the medial patellofemoral ligament, immediately distal to the adductor tubercle. The insertion is about 5 cm distal to the knee joint and is usually not entirely included in standard knee MR exams. The medial inferior geniculate arterial branches are seen in cross section between the superficial medial collateral ligament and the tibial cortex.* **(Bottom)** *The anterior cut is through the anterior midportion of the joint. Because these are T1 images, there is little contrast between the hyaline cartilage and menisci.*

CORONAL T1 MR: RIGHT KNEE

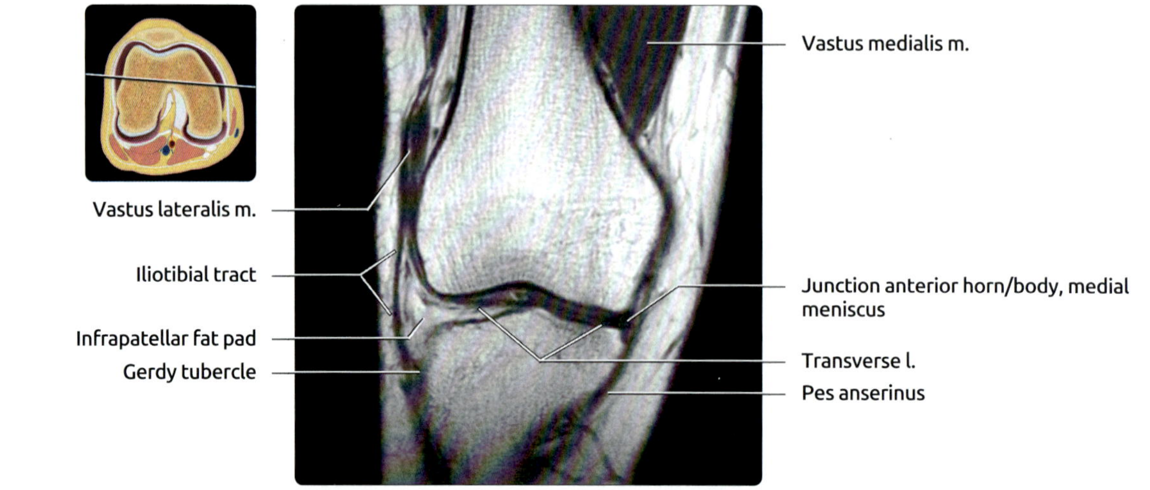

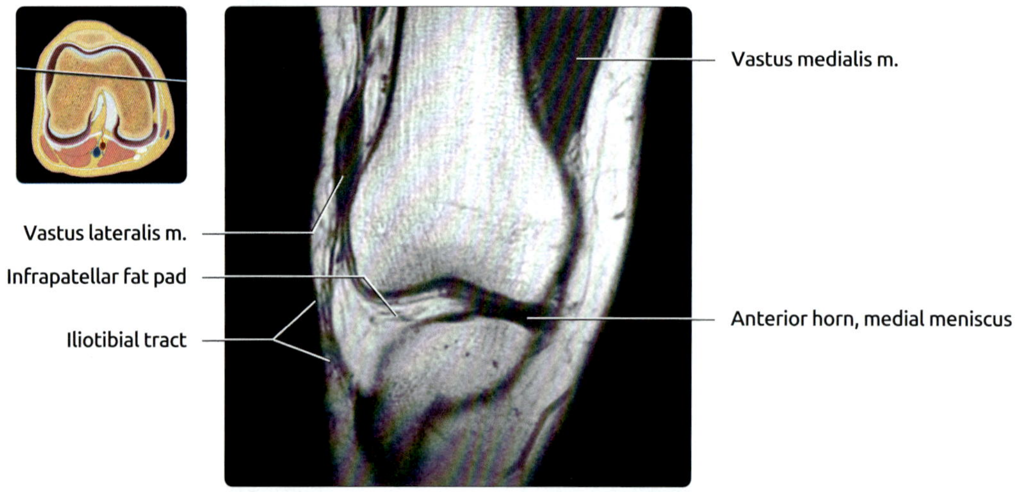

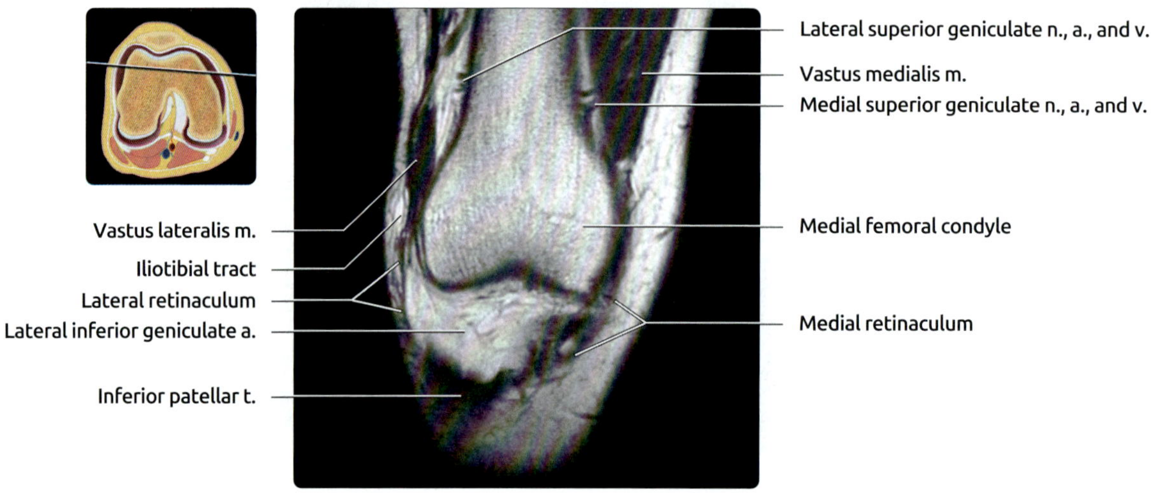

(Top) *In this far anterior image, the transverse ligament is seen crossing the anterior joint from the anterior horn medial meniscus toward the anterior horn lateral meniscus. The iliotibial tract is seen inserting on the Gerdy tubercle.* **(Middle)** *In this far anterior cut through the joint space, note that because of the slightly oblique angle at which coronal knee MR images are obtained, the anterior horn of the medial meniscus is visualized in the far anterior coronal cuts without any portion of the lateral meniscus.* **(Bottom)** *Coronal cut through the anterior femoral shaft shows that the joint is fairly featureless, consisting mostly of fat pads and anastomosing vascular structures.*

CORONAL T1 MR: LEFT KNEE

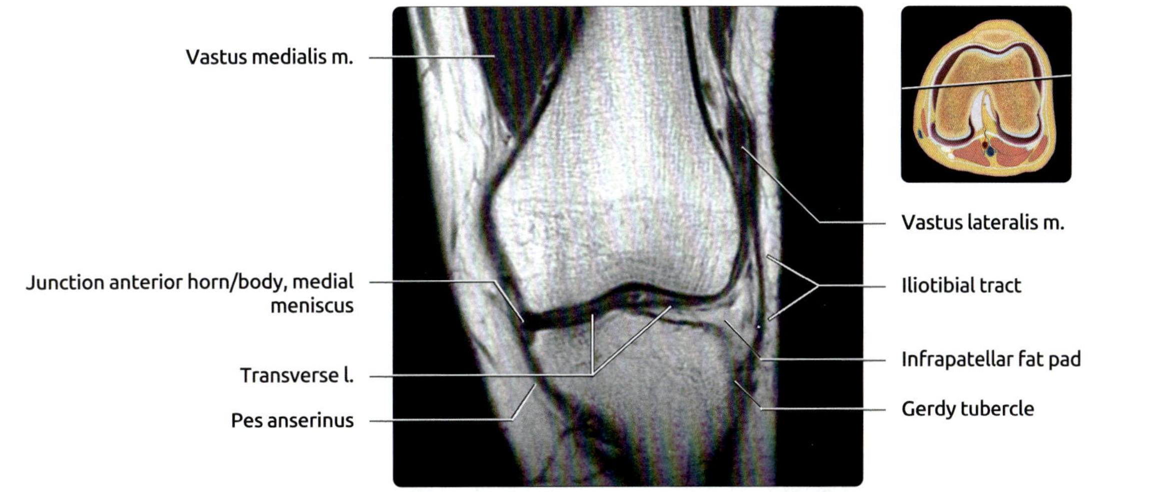

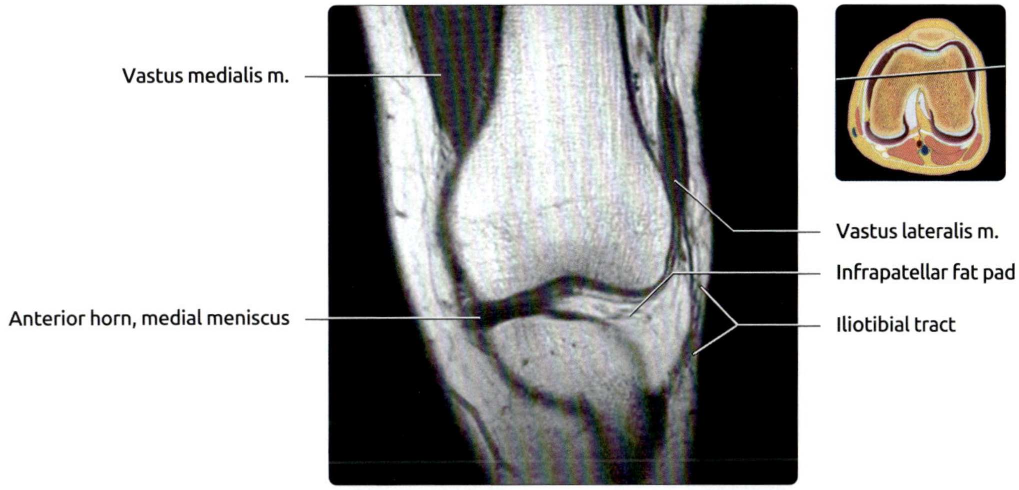

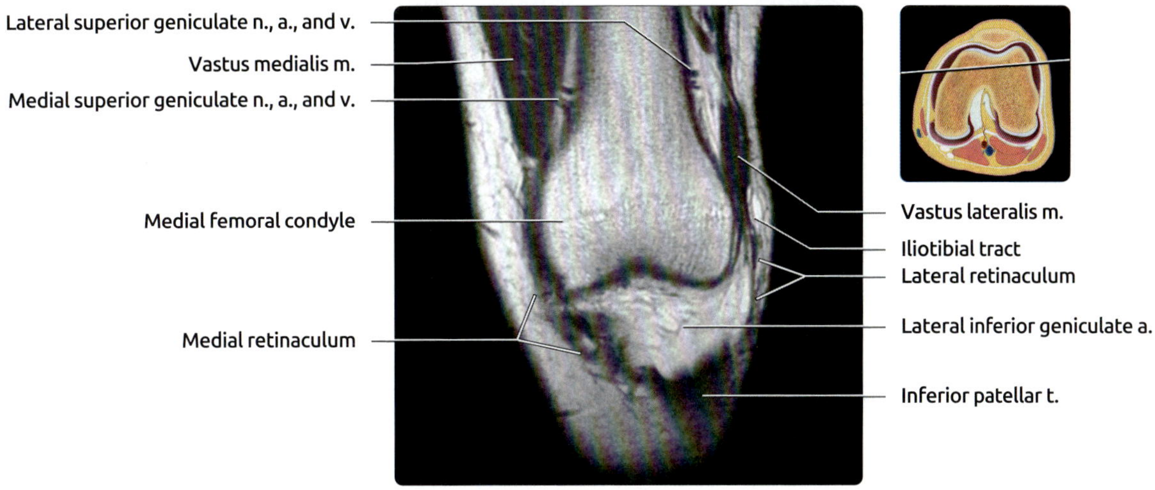

(Top) *In this far anterior image, the transverse ligament is seen crossing the anterior joint from the anterior horn of the medial meniscus toward the anterior horn of the lateral meniscus. The iliotibial tract is seen inserting on the Gerdy tubercle.* **(Middle)** *In this far anterior cut through the joint space, note that because of the slightly oblique angle at which the coronal knee MR images are obtained, the anterior horn of the medial meniscus is visualized in far anterior coronal cuts without any portion of the lateral meniscus.* **(Bottom)** *Coronal cut through the anterior femoral shaft shows that the joint is fairly featureless, consisting mostly of fat pads and anastomosing vascular structures.*

CORONAL T1 MR: RIGHT KNEE

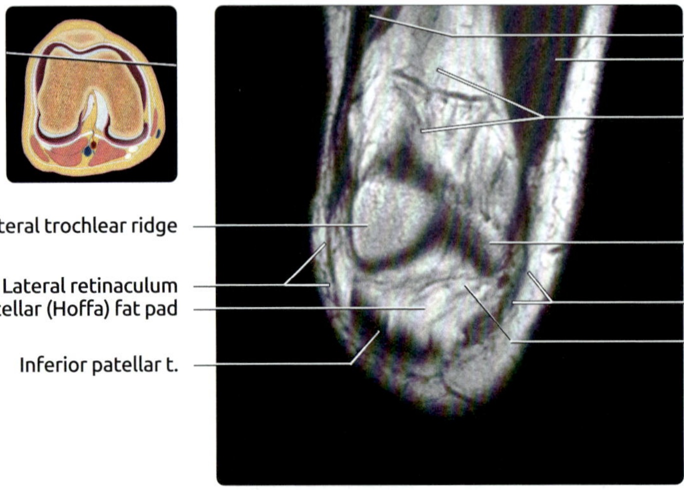

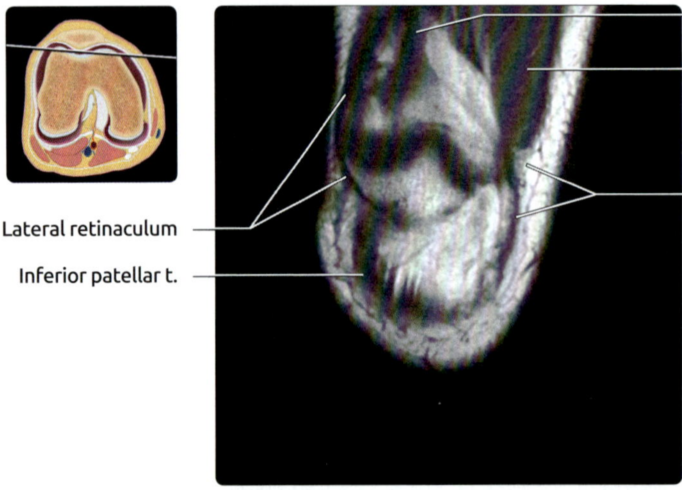

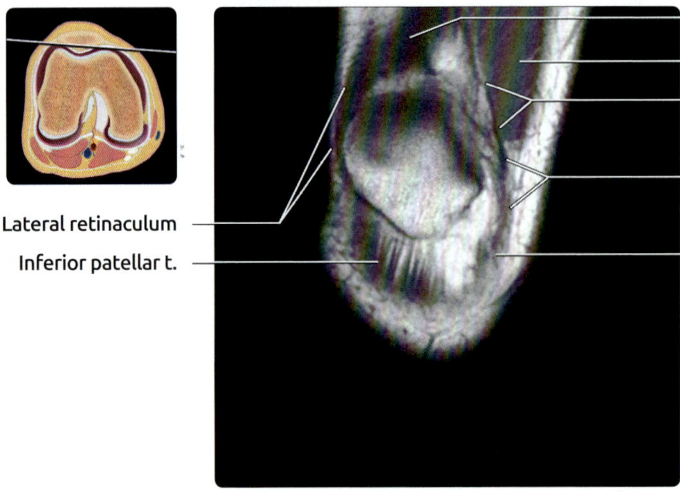

(Top) *The cut is through the anterior femoral condyles. Fat pads, both prefemoral and infrapatellar, predominate in the anterior joint. The retinacula are seen as well. Note the multiple geniculate and collateral arteries supplying the knee joint.* **(Middle)** *This is a coronal cut through the posterior patella. Note the large size of the vastus medialis. This can help identify the medial side of the knee on coronal or axial planes.* **(Bottom)** *This anterior-most image of the series shows the medial and lateral supporting structures of the patella as well as the quadriceps and inferior patellar tendons. Both the quadriceps and inferior patellar tendons are fairly broad, as are the medial and lateral retinacula, effectively surrounding the patella.*

CORONAL T1 MR: LEFT KNEE

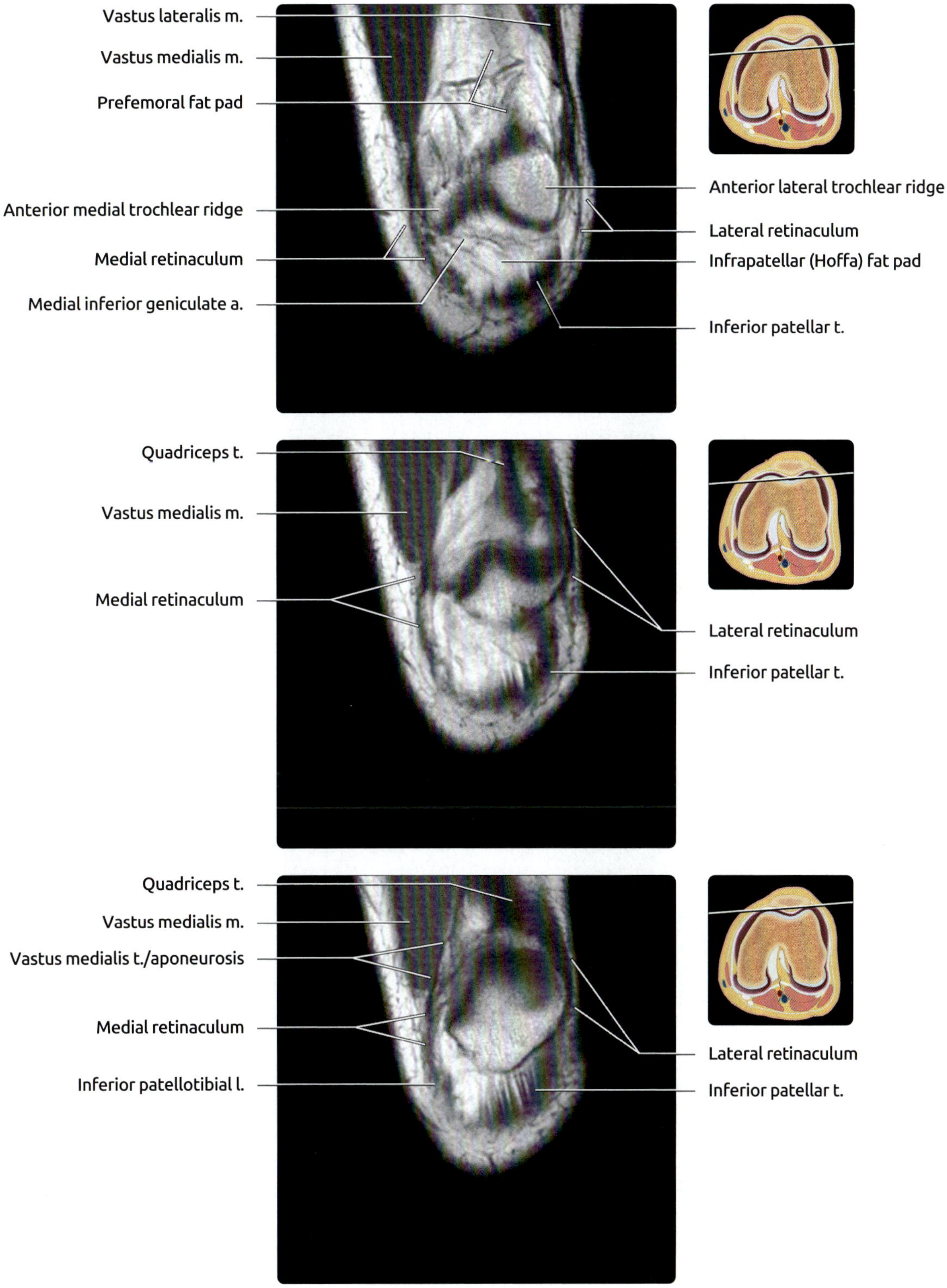

(Top) *This cut is through the anterior femoral condyles. Fat pads, both prefemoral and infrapatellar, predominate in the anterior joint. The retinacula are seen as well. Note the multiple geniculate and collateral arteries supplying the knee joint.* **(Middle)** *This is a coronal cut through posterior patella. Note the large size of the vastus medialis. This can help identify the medial side of the knee on coronal or axial planes.* **(Bottom)** *This anterior-most image of the series shows the medial and lateral supporting structures of the patella as well as the quadriceps and inferior patellar tendons. Both the quadriceps and inferior patellar tendons are fairly broad, as are the medial and lateral retinacula, effectively surrounding the patella.*

SAGITTAL T1 MR: LEFT KNEE

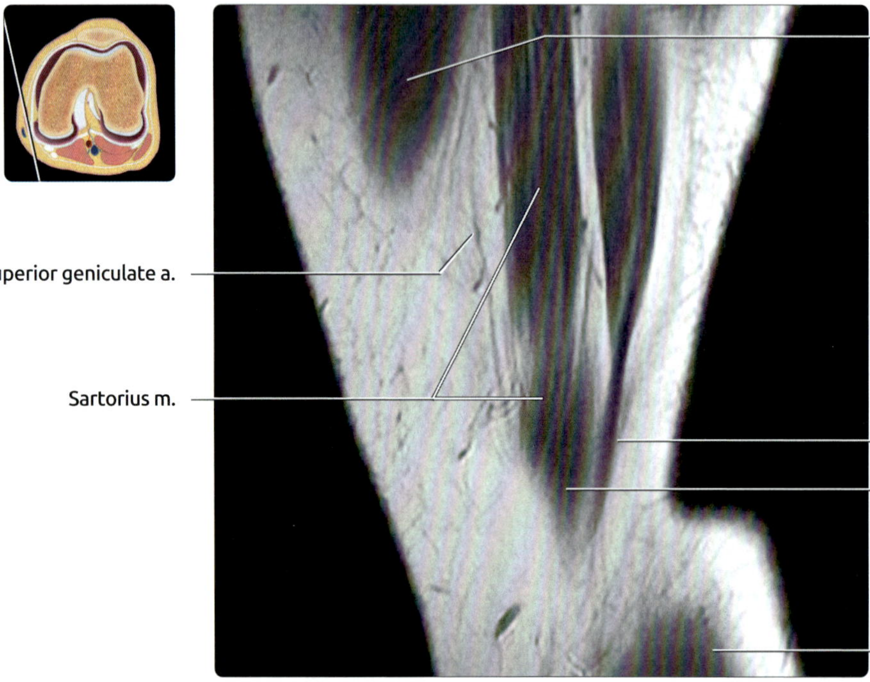

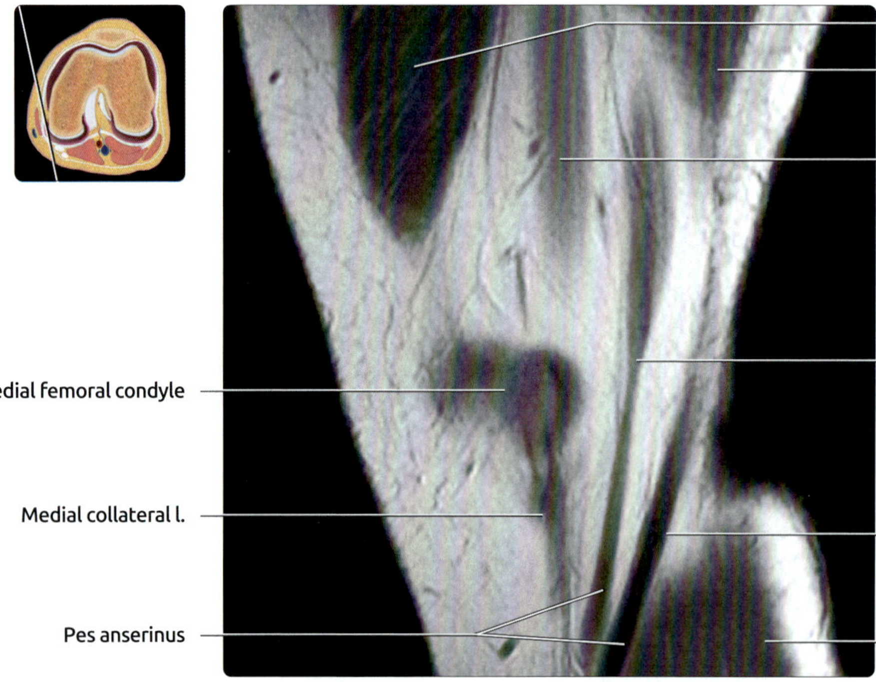

(Top) *First of 20 sagittal T1 MR images of the knee shows a far medial cut. Note the sartorius muscle and tendon, with the gracilis muscle and tendon extending immediately posterior to it.* **(Bottom)** *This cut is barely through the medial femoral condyle, and only a small portion of the sartorius is seen. The gracilis and semitendinosus tendons are seen extending posteriorly, forming with the sartorius and the 3 tendons of the pes anserinus.*

SAGITTAL T1 MR: RIGHT KNEE

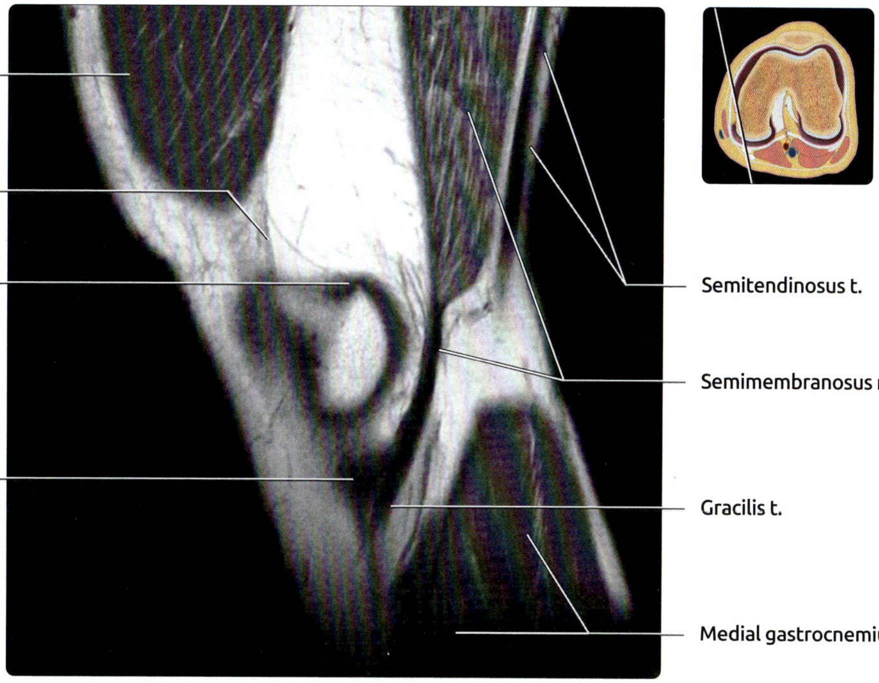

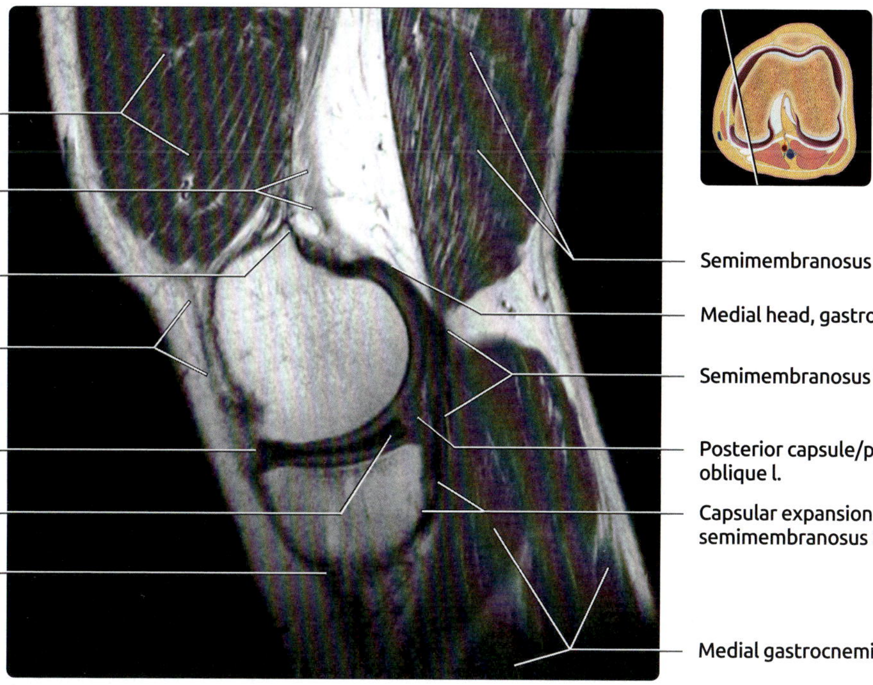

(Top) *This is a medial cut through the femoral condyle. Note the large semimembranosus tendon with its extensive insertion along the posteromedial tibia.* **(Bottom)** *This cut goes through the medial compartment, near the central edge of the body of the medial meniscus. This is still a slightly bowtie configuration of the meniscus.*

SAGITTAL T1 MR: LEFT KNEE

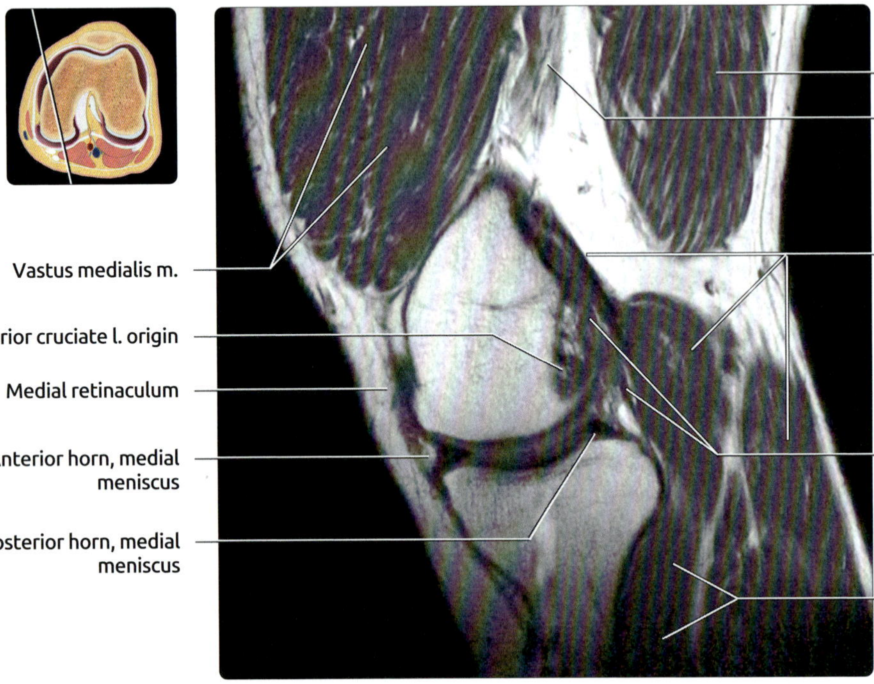

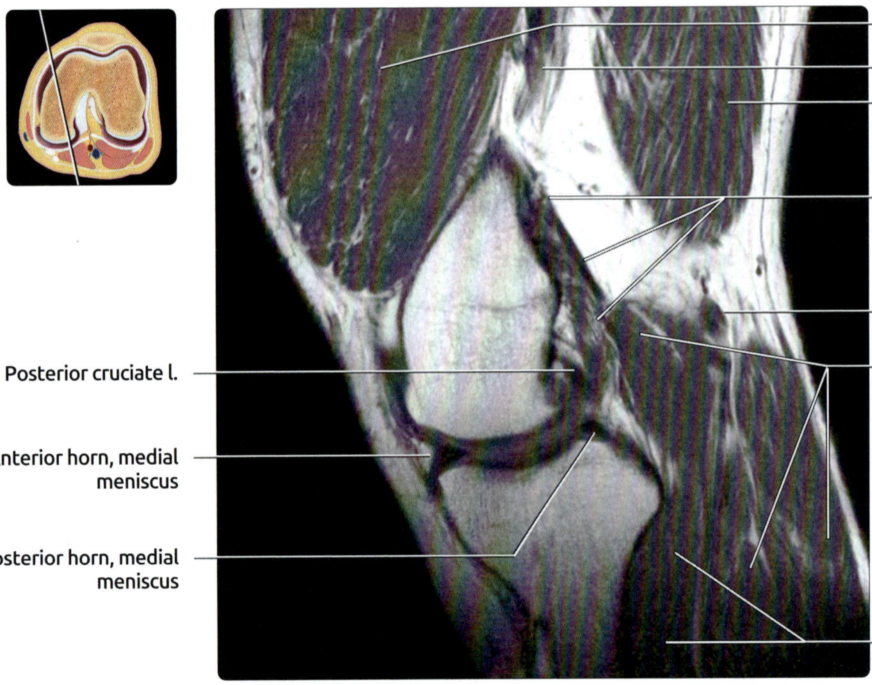

(Top) *This cut is through the medial compartment, approaching the intercondylar notch. The posterior aspect of the medial femoral condyle is only partially seen. The oblique popliteal ligament contributes to the posterior capsule at this point.* **(Bottom)** *This cut is at the medial-most aspect of the intercondylar notch, where the origin of the posterior cruciate ligament is 1st seen. Note that by this point, the oblique popliteal ligament contributes more fully to the posterior joint capsule.*

SAGITTAL T1 MR: RIGHT KNEE

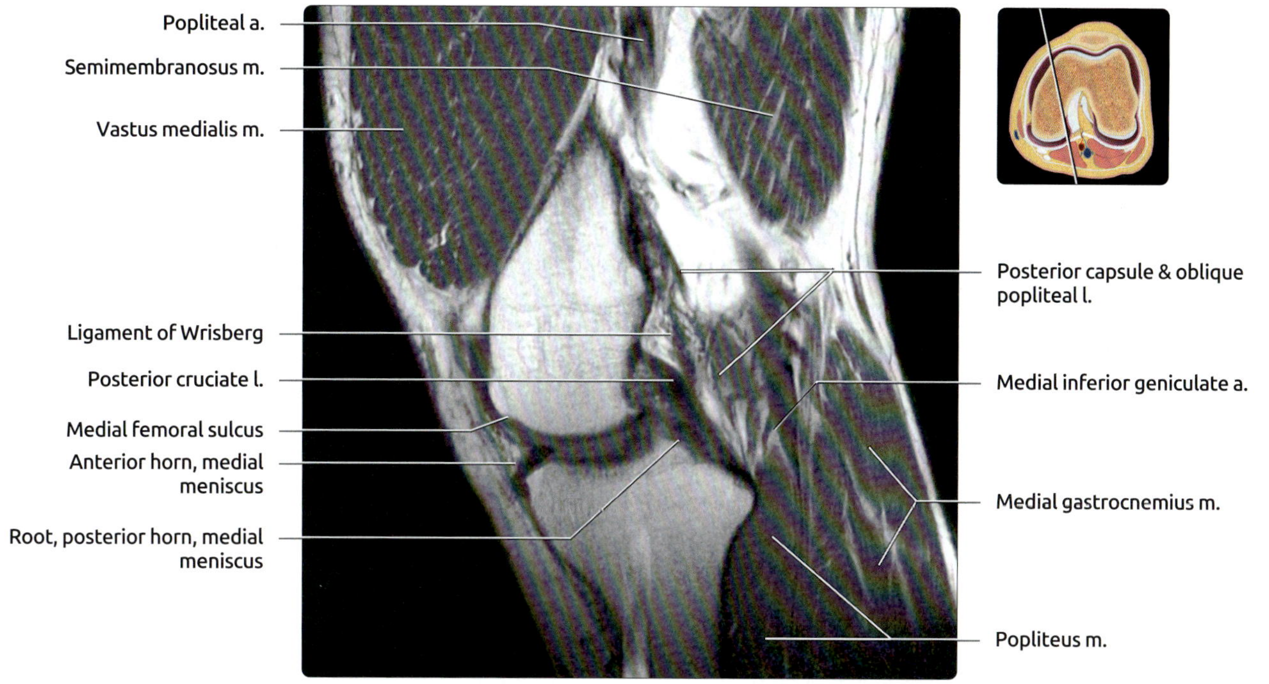

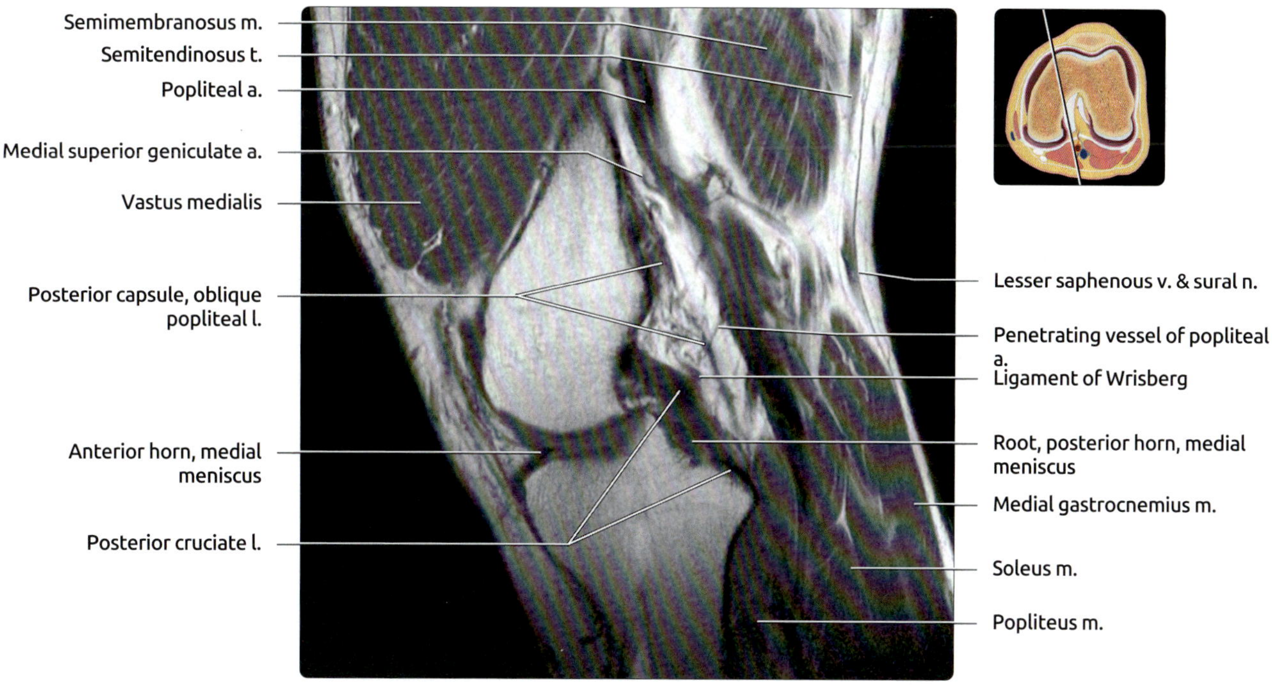

(Top) *This cut is through the medial aspect of the intercondylar notch. The medial femoral sulcus divides the femorotibial from the patellofemoral articulations. It is less prominent than the lateral terminal sulcus.* **(Bottom)** *The mid intercondylar notch is shown. Note that at the posterior intercondylar notch, the posterior capsule is penetrated by vessels from the popliteal artery. The capsule is therefore incomplete posteriorly.*

SAGITTAL T1 MR: LEFT KNEE

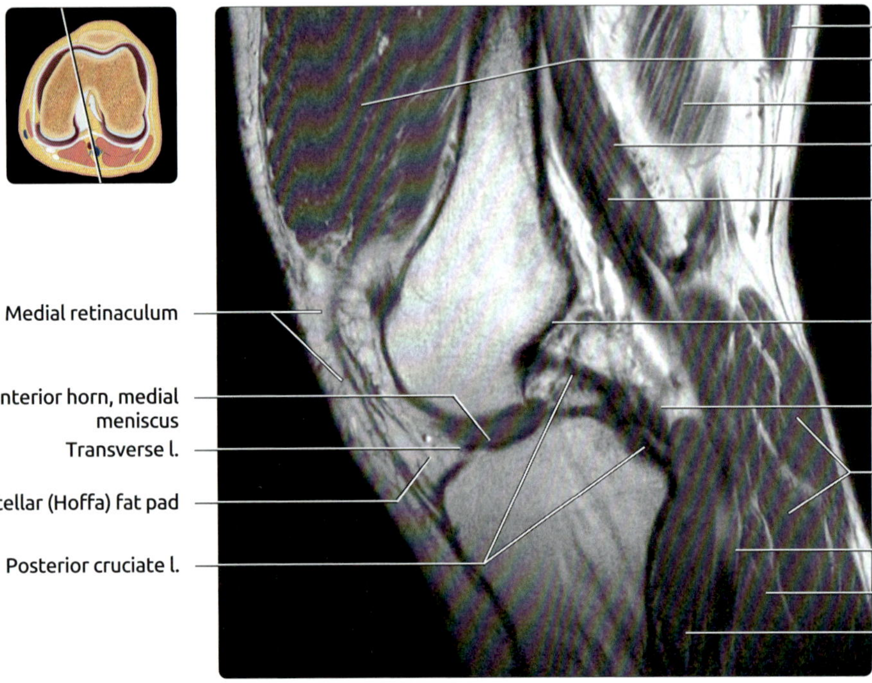

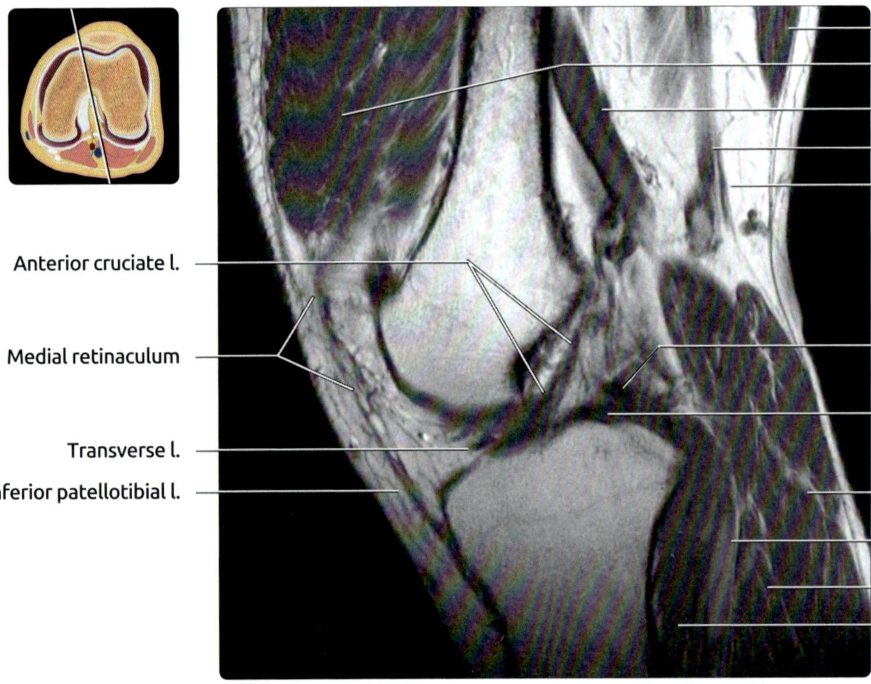

(Top) *This cut is at the mid intercondylar notch, transitioning from the posterior to anterior cruciate ligament. The posterior capsule is still incomplete due to penetrating vessels.* **(Bottom)** *Slightly laterally within the intercondylar notch, the anterior cruciate ligament is most fully seen. Note the pathway of the ligament of Wrisberg (posterior meniscofemoral ligament), arising from the medial aspect of the intercondylar notch, traversing posterior and superior to the posterior cruciate ligament, and inserting on the superior aspect of the root of the posterior horn of the lateral meniscus.*

SAGITTAL T1 MR: RIGHT KNEE

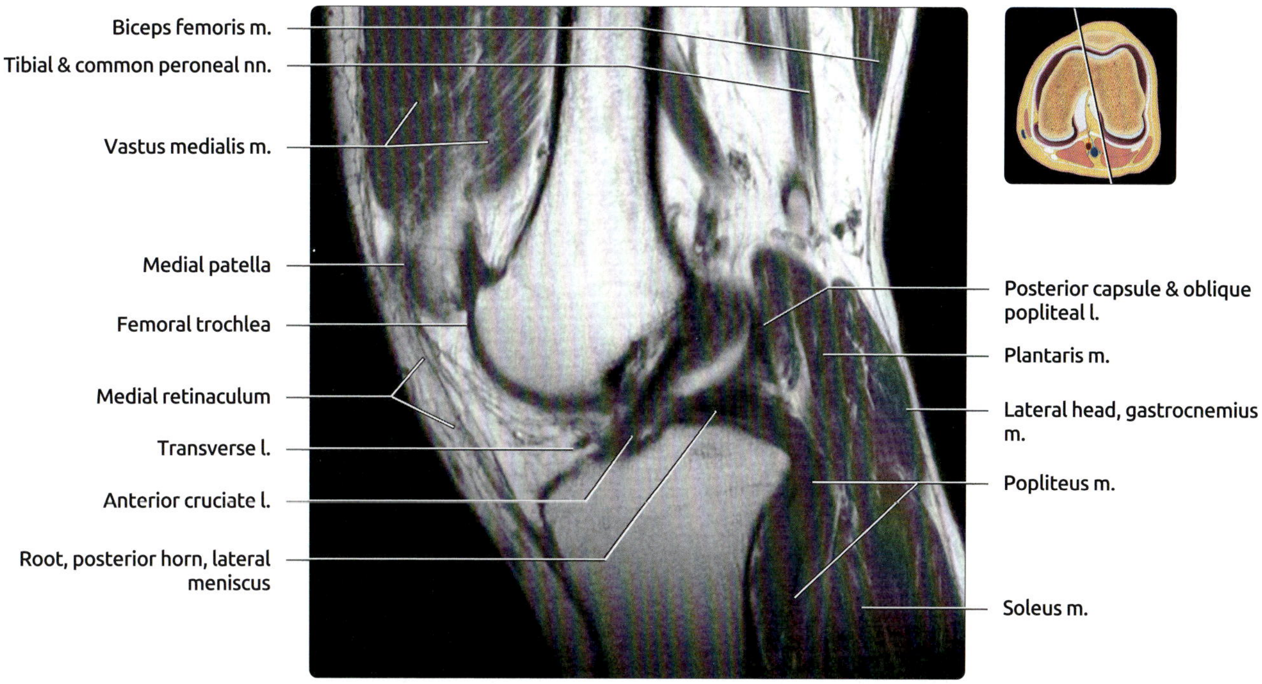

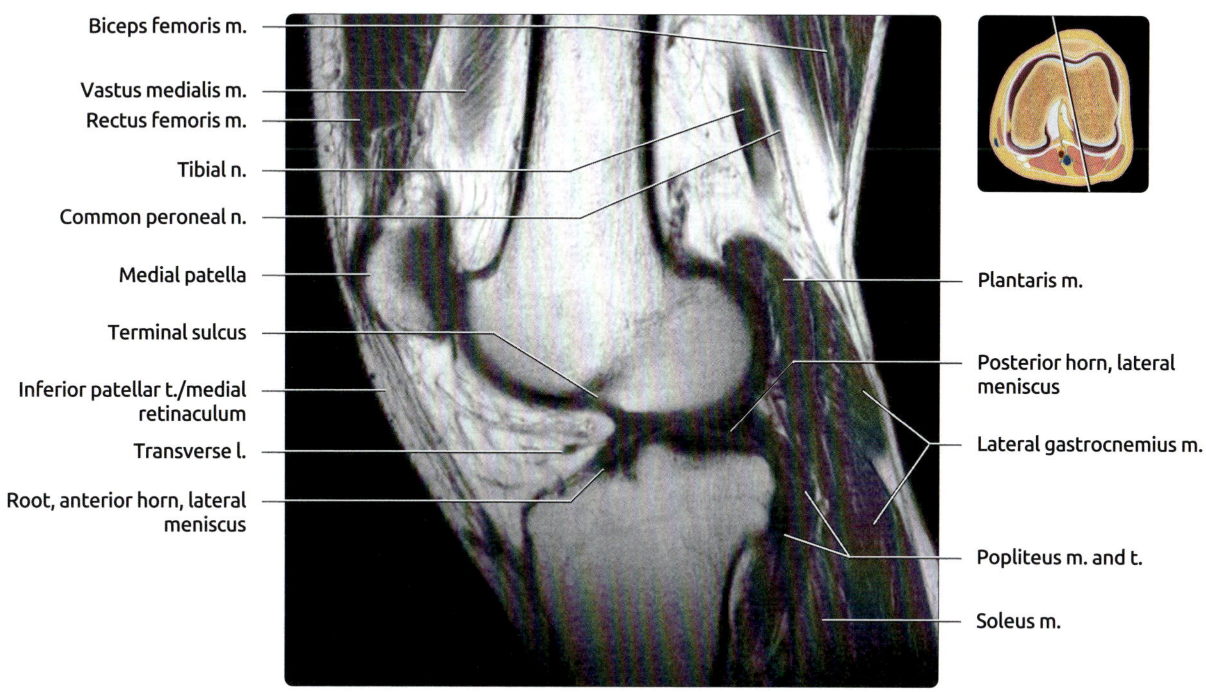

(Top) *This image is in the lateral position within the intercondylar notch where there is partial voluming of the anterior cruciate/lateral femoral condyle at the ACL insertion. Note the transverse ligament, seen in cross section, extending across in front of the anterior cruciate ligament toward the root of the anterior horn lateral meniscus. The anterior horn is not yet seen.* **(Bottom)** *This cut shows the beginning of the lateral compartment, immediately adjacent to the intercondylar notch. Note the musculotendinous junction of the popliteus.*

SAGITTAL T1 MR: LEFT KNEE

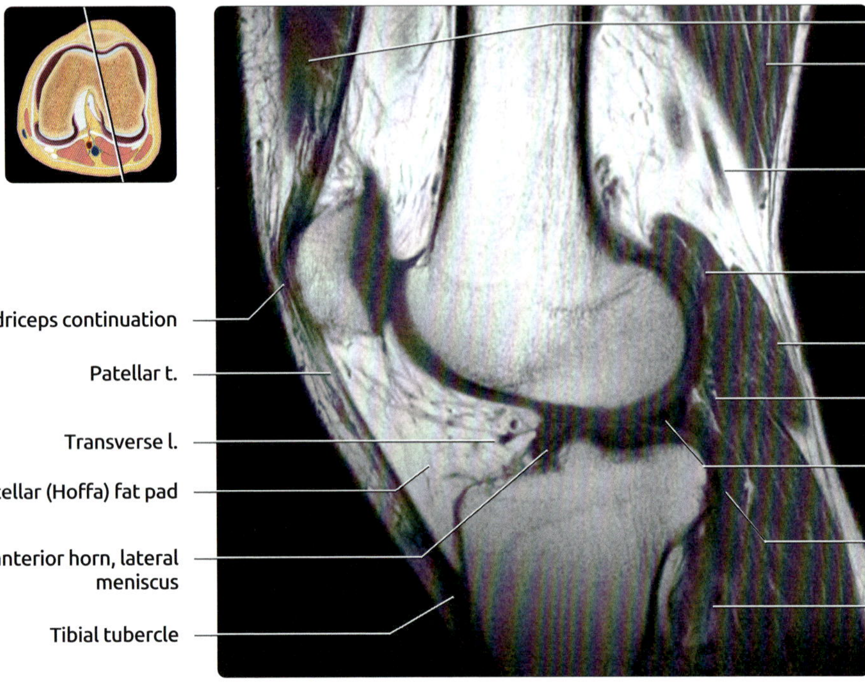

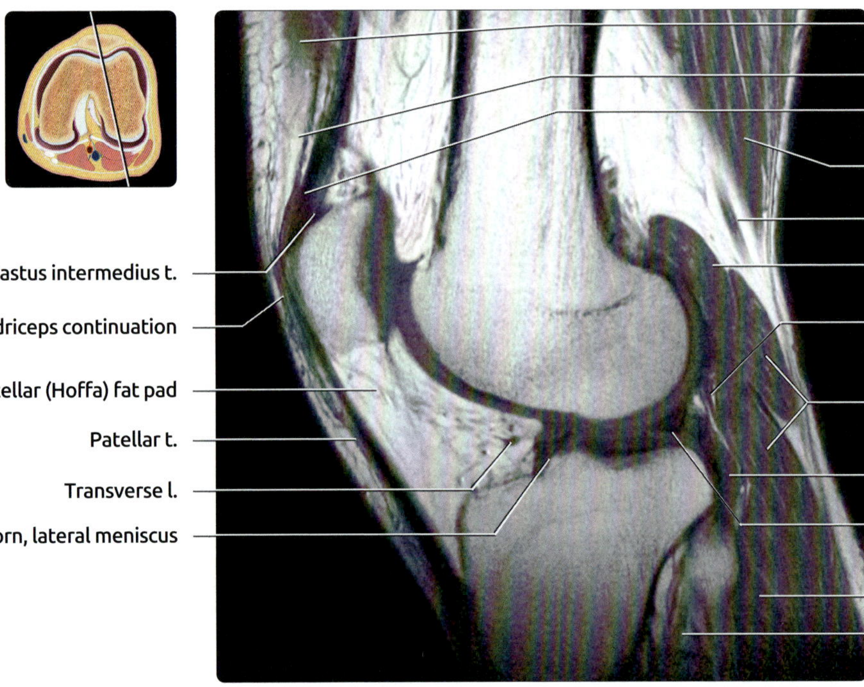

(Top) *The lateral compartment is shown. Note the path of the common peroneal nerve, anteromedial to the bulk of the biceps femoris muscle. The plantaris muscle is seen, arising on the lateral femoral condyle, just medial to the lateral head of the gastrocnemius. Quadriceps continuation is the aponeurosis along the anterior margin of the patella, providing continuity between the rectus femoris tendon and the patellar tendon.* **(Bottom)** *Because of the obliquity with which sagittal images are obtained, the extensor complex is seen in the more lateral sagittal images. The trilaminate nature of the quadriceps tendon is demonstrated here. The transverse ligament has not yet contacted the anterior horn of the lateral meniscus. Note the popliteus tendon. Although it is within the popliteal hiatus, it is difficult to distinguish from fluid in the hiatus as well as the lateral meniscus. This region is better imaged with fluid-sensitive sequences.*

SAGITTAL T1 MR: RIGHT KNEE

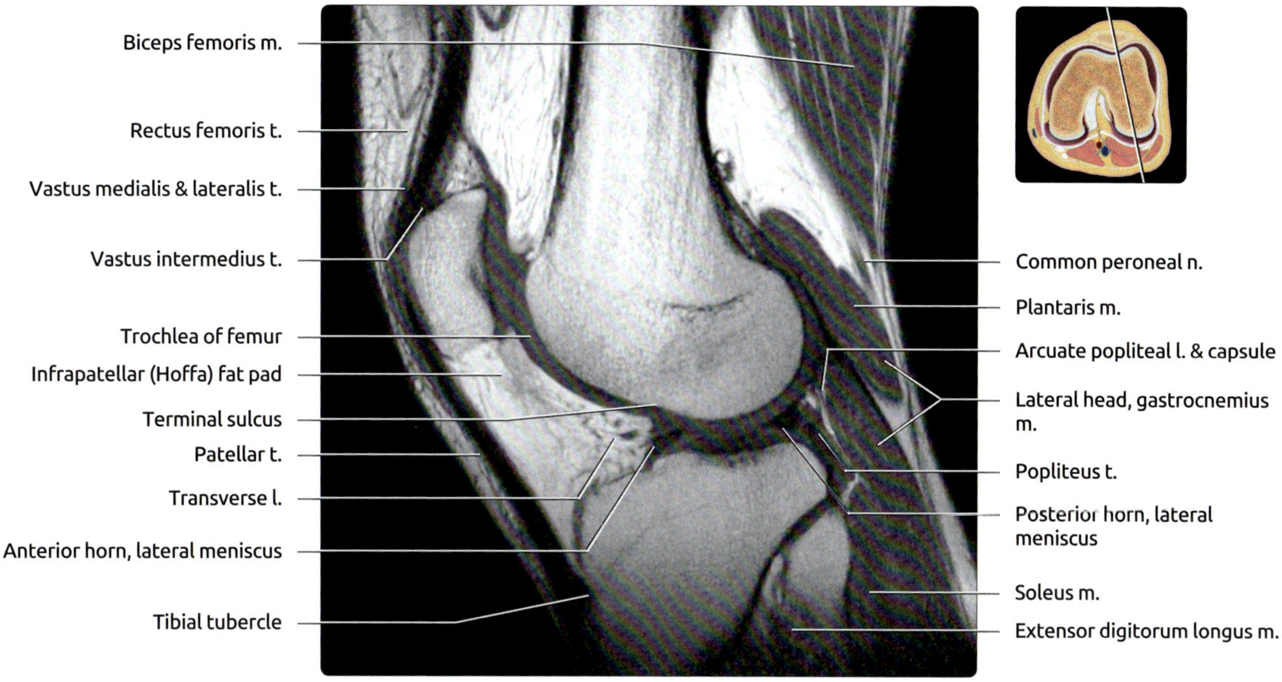

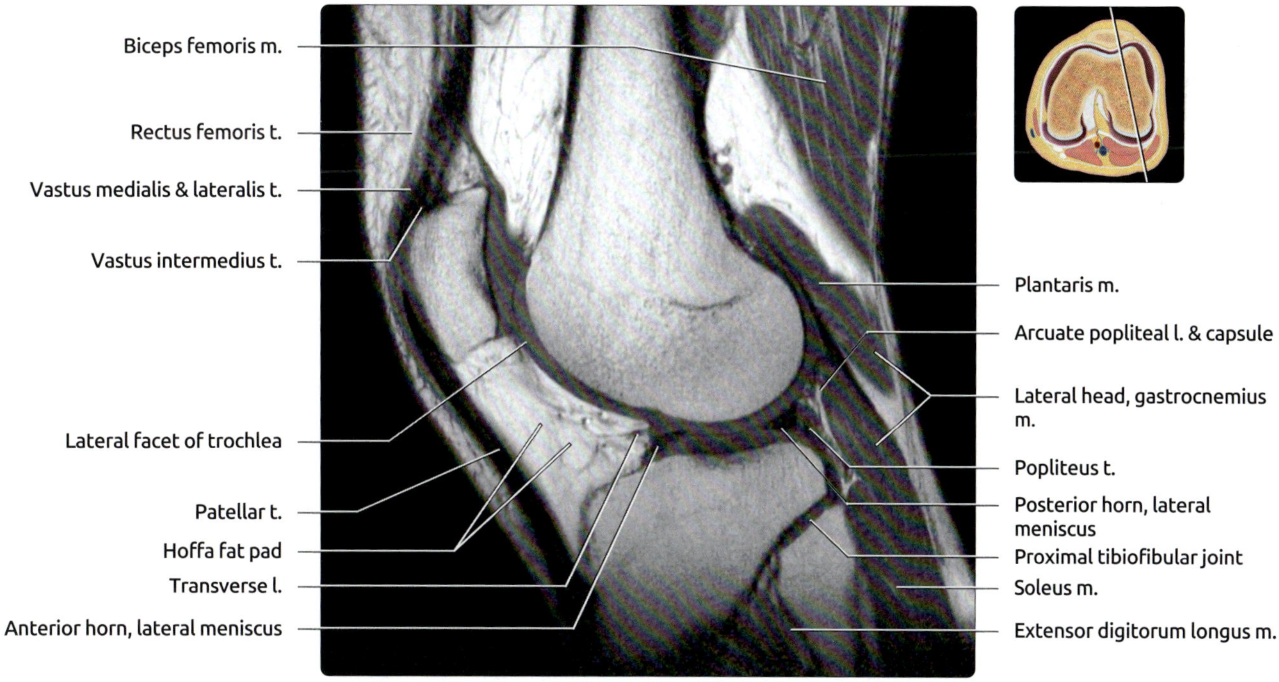

(Top) *In the lateral portion of the knee joint, the popliteus tendon is seen within the popliteal hiatus, adjacent to the lateral meniscus. It is connected to the posterior horn lateral meniscus by the popliteomeniscal ligaments. The terminal sulcus (a.k.a. lateral femoral condylar recess) is the demarcation between the portion of the femur articulating with the tibia and the portion articulating with the patella.* **(Bottom)** *As shown here, the transverse ligament approaches its insertion site on the anterior horn of the lateral meniscus, which is composed of multiple parallel fascicles. When viewed in cross section, as in this image, it is important not to mistake the normal fascicles for a meniscal tear.*

SAGITTAL T1 MR: LEFT KNEE

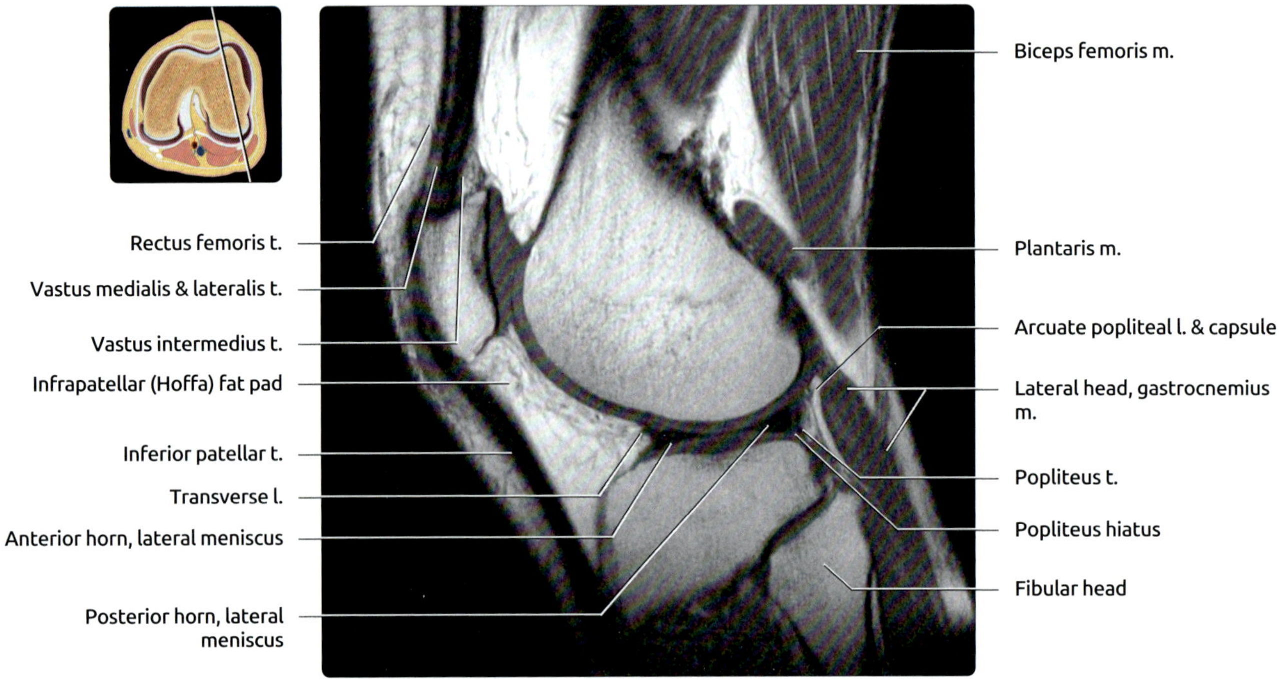

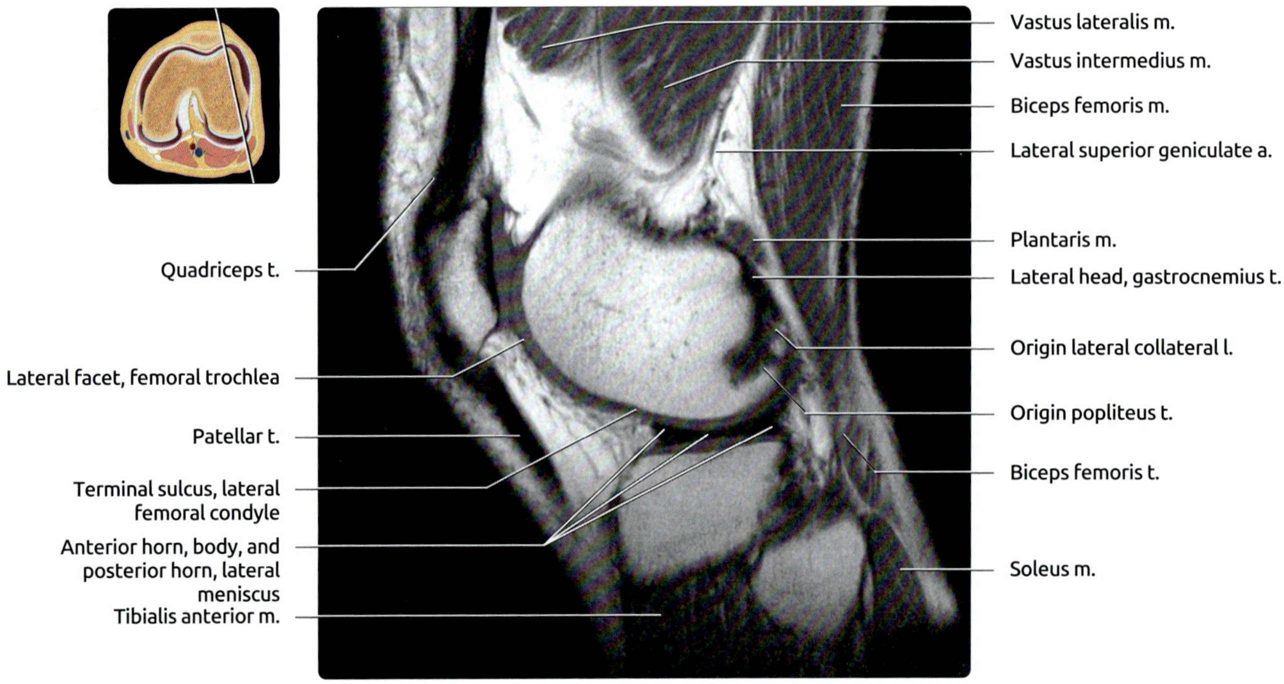

(Top) *The popliteus tendon approaches the posterior horn of the lateral meniscus on this image, and it is important not to mistake the small amount of fluid in the popliteus hiatus for a meniscal tear.* **(Bottom)** *At the lateral aspect of the lateral femoral condyle, one sees the origin of the lateral head of the gastrocnemius from the lateral femoral epicondyle as well as the lateral collateral ligament and the popliteal tendon.*

SAGITTAL T1 MR: RIGHT KNEE

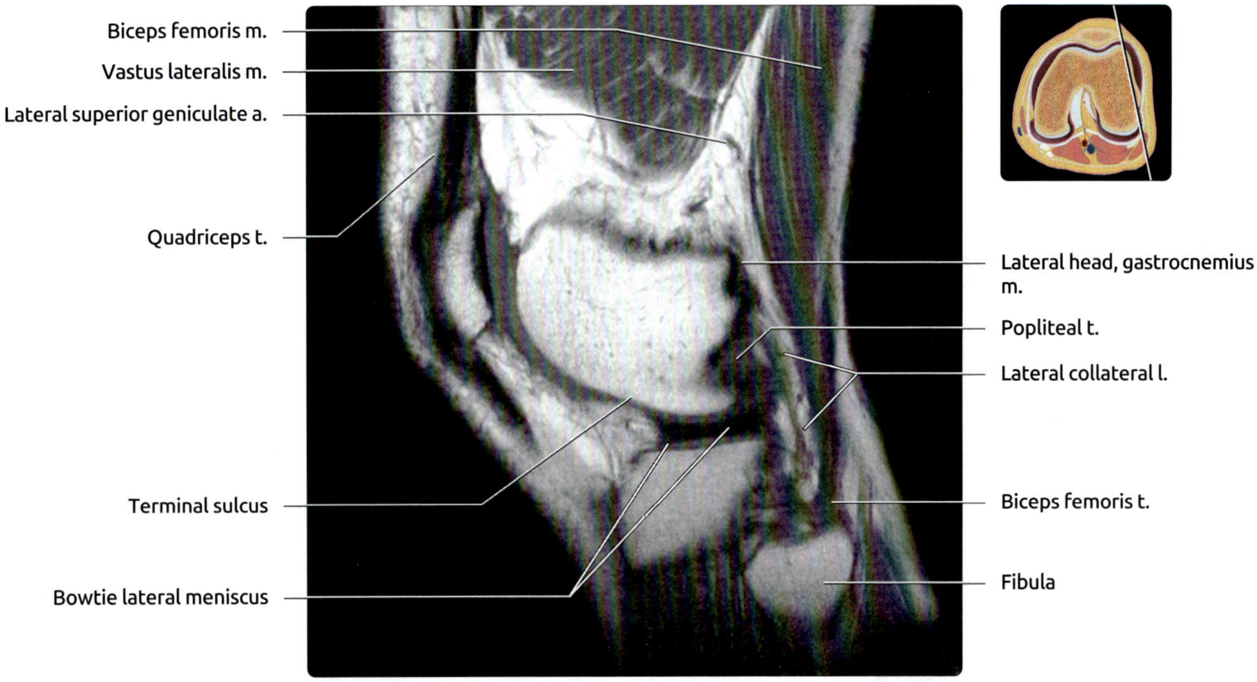

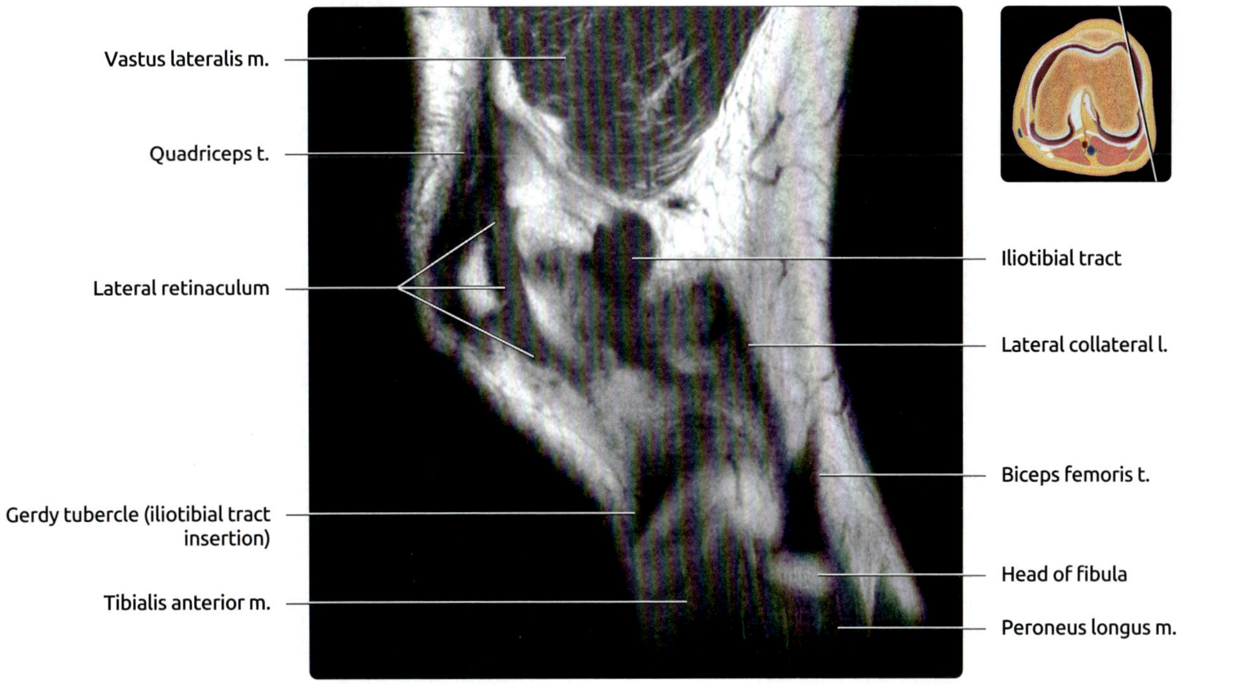

(Top) *This is the lateral-most portion of the joint in which the bowtie configuration of the meniscus is seen. The lateral collateral ligament is also seen extending posteroinferiorly toward its insertion on the fibular head, adjacent to the insertion of the biceps femoris tendon.* **(Bottom)** *Far lateral in the knee, the lateral collateral ligament and biceps femoris tendon insert adjacent to one another on the head of the fibula. Only portions of other lateral stabilizing structures (iliotibial tract, lateral retinaculum) are seen on this image.*

ARTHROSCOPIC PHOTOGRAPHS

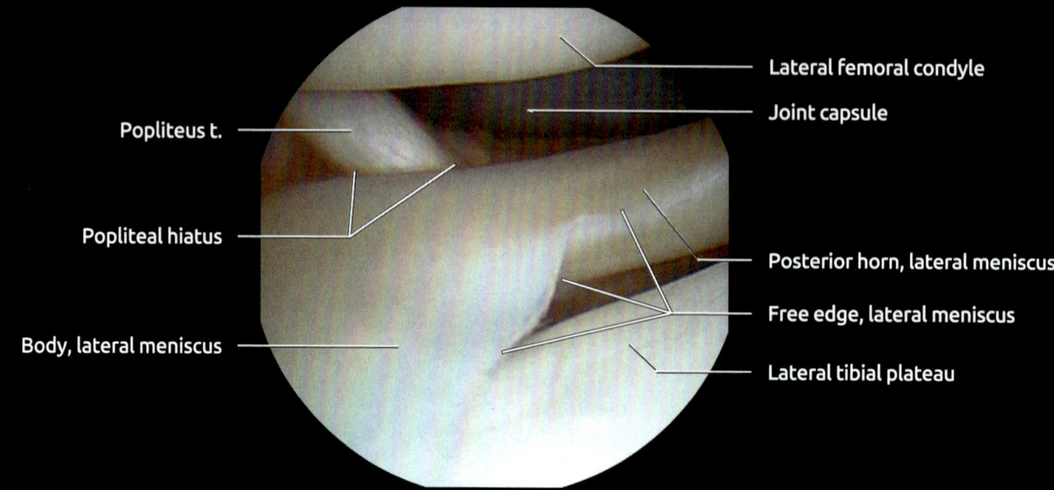

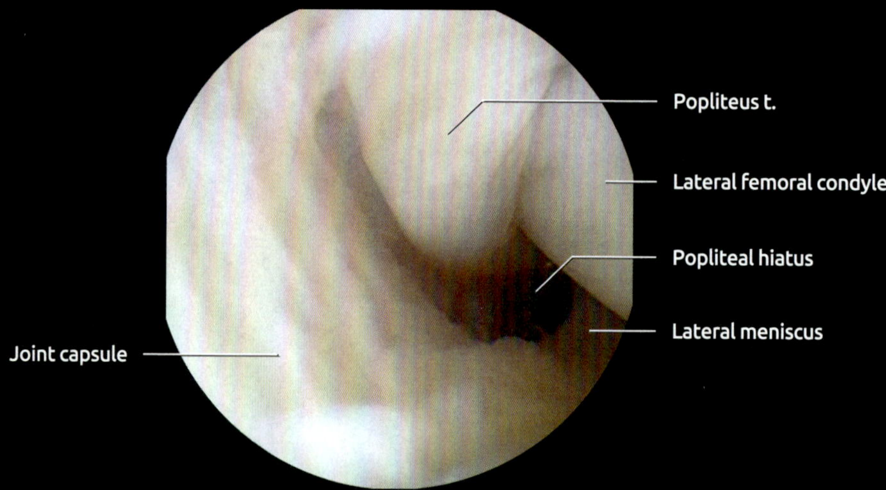

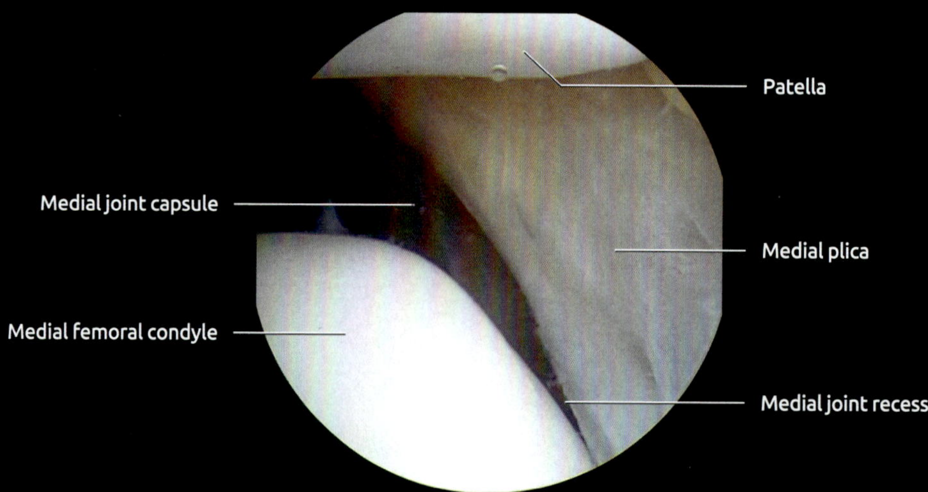

(Top) *First in a series of 6 arthroscopic photographs of the knee is shown. The arthroscope is positioned anteriorly, with a view of the posterior portion of the lateral compartment. Structures are separated by fluid injected for the arthroscopy.* **(Middle)** *Arthroscopic photograph of the posterolateral gutter shows the popliteus tendon is curving around the condyle through the popliteal hiatus toward its insertion on the popliteal groove of the femur (not shown).* **(Bottom)** *After evaluating the lateral recess, the arthroscope is moved into the medial recess and proximally into the suprapatellar pouch. A normal suprapatellar plica is seen in 80-90% of knees. The suprapatellar plica may cross the suprapatellar pouch to the lateral sidewall and, rarely, may compartmentalize the suprapatellar pouch. The patellofemoral joint is inspected.*

ARTHROSCOPIC PHOTOGRAPHS

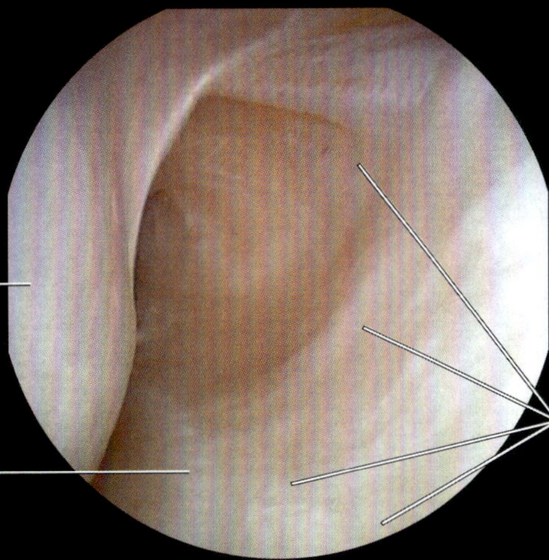

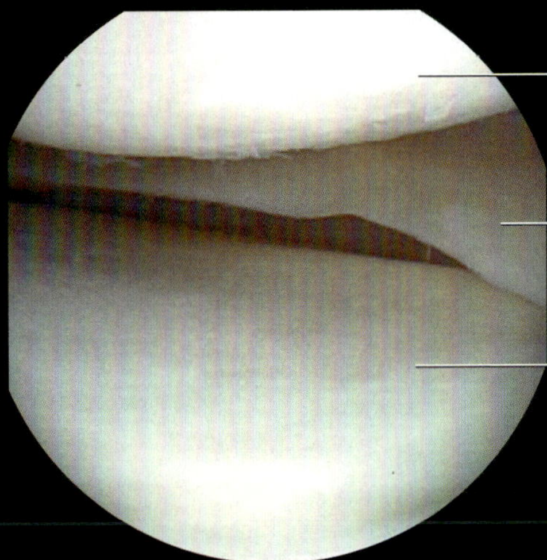

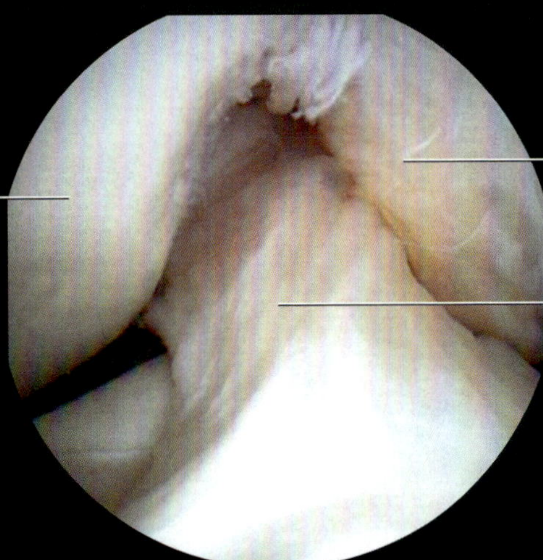

(Top) *The arthroscope is positioned in the medial gutter of the knee, showing the deep surface of the medial joint capsule and its attachments to the femur and tibia.* **(Middle)** *The medial tibial plateau is slightly concave. Normal cartilage has a smooth, glistening surface. The medial femoral condyle in this patient shows mild cartilage fibrillation, while tibial cartilage is normal.* **(Bottom)** *In this image, the anterior and posterior cruciate ligaments are probed. There is a smooth synovial covering overlying the ligaments.*

3D RECONSTRUCTION CT: ORIGINS & INSERTIONS

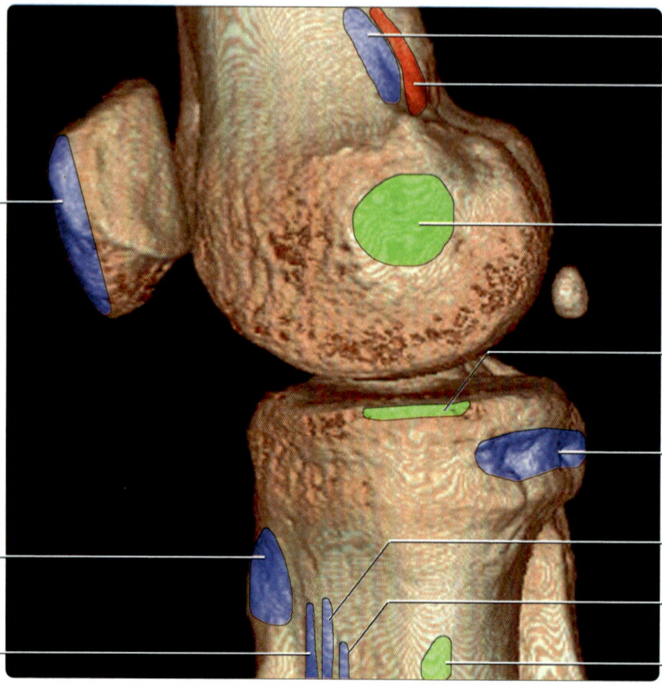

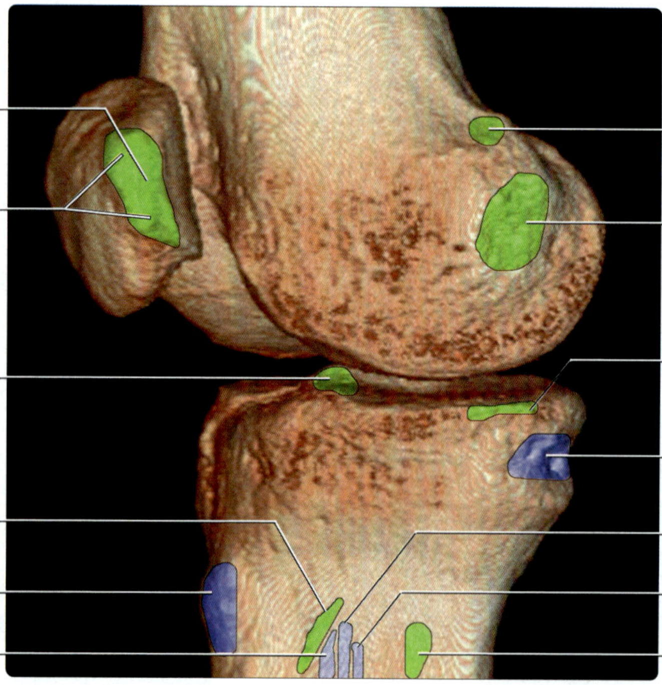

(Top) *First of 8 volume-rendered topographic CT images shows the medial aspect of the knee, with associated muscle, tendon, and ligament origins/insertions. The quadriceps tendon has an aponeurotic sheath along the anterior border of the patella called the quadriceps continuation. This in turn gives rise to the patellar tendon (a.k.a. patellar ligament).* **(Bottom)** *This image of the anteromedial knee shows medial stabilizers of the knee (primarily medial collateral ligament, superficial and deep fibers, secondarily pes anserinus), as well as medial stabilizers of the patella. The medial patellofemoral ligament is a thickening in the medial patellar retinaculum, extending from the midpole of the patella to the medial femoral condyle, immediately superior to the origin of the medial collateral ligament.*

3D RECONSTRUCTION CT: ORIGINS & INSERTIONS

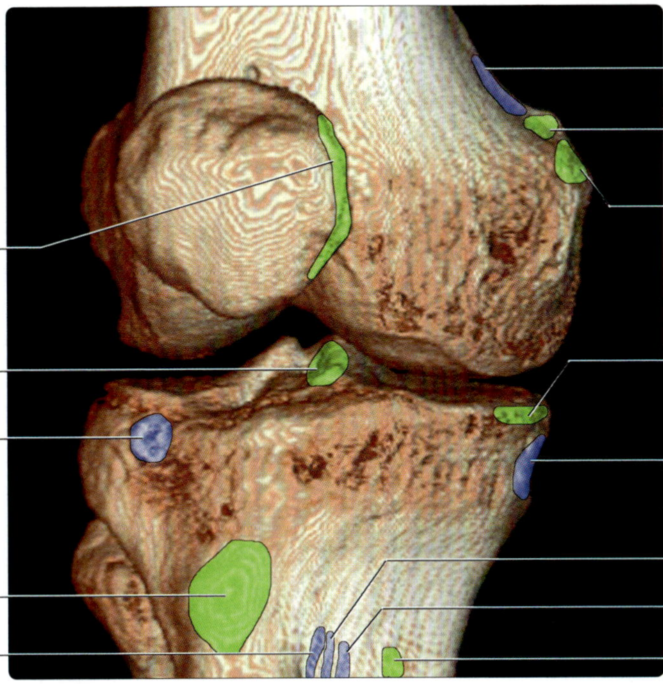

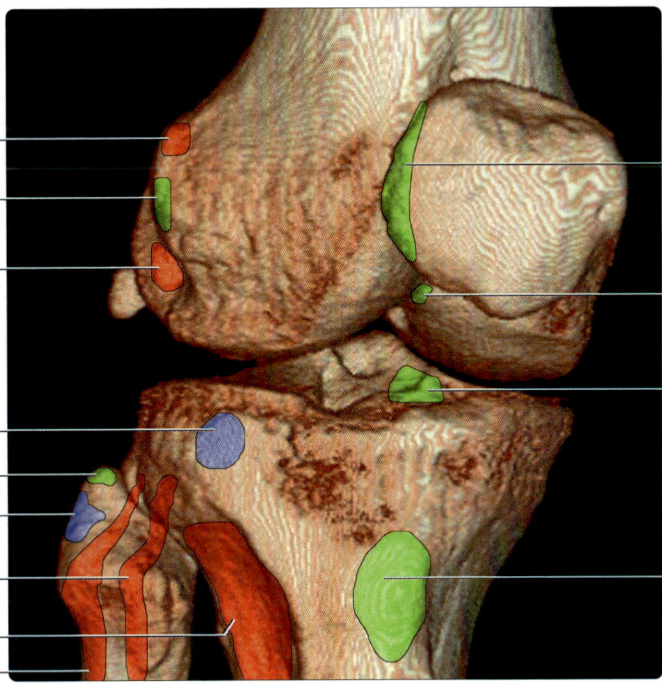

(Top) *A slightly anteromedial view shows the medial stabilizers of the knee and patella. Note that only the uppermost portion of the insertions of the pes anserinus (sartorius, gracilis, and semitendinosus) as well as superficial medial collateral ligament are shown; these insertions actually extend several cm distally on the tibia.* **(Bottom)** *A slightly anterolateral view shows the lateral stabilizers of the knee and patella. These consist primarily of lateral collateral ligament, arcuate ligament, popliteal tendon, iliotibial band, and biceps femoris. Origins of several leg muscles are seen; the tibialis anterior, extensor digitorum longus, and peroneus longus origins extend several cm distally beyond the regions indicated here.*

3D RECONSTRUCTION CT: ORIGINS & INSERTIONS

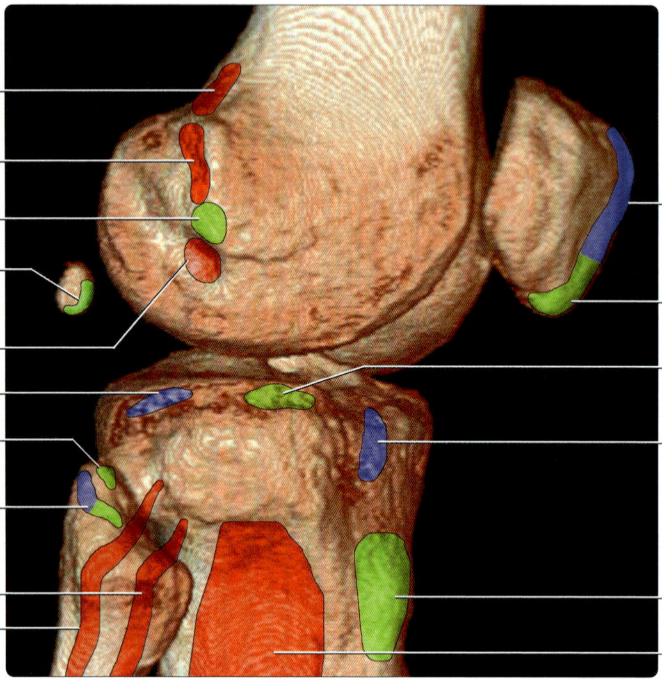

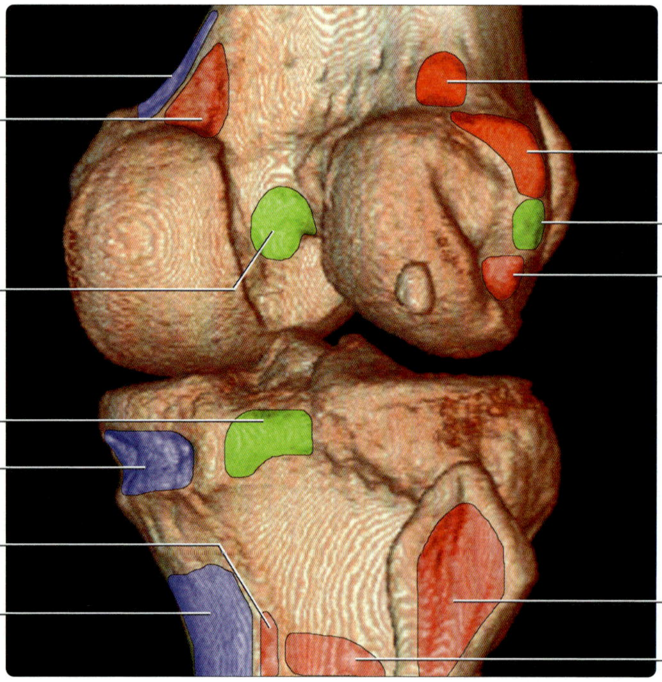

(Top) *A lateral view of the knee shows muscle and ligament attachments.* **(Bottom)** *A posterior (slightly oblique) view of the knee shows the attachments of the posterior structures. Note that the fibular origin of the soleus is more proximal than the tibial origin.*

3D RECONSTRUCTION CT: ORIGINS & INSERTIONS

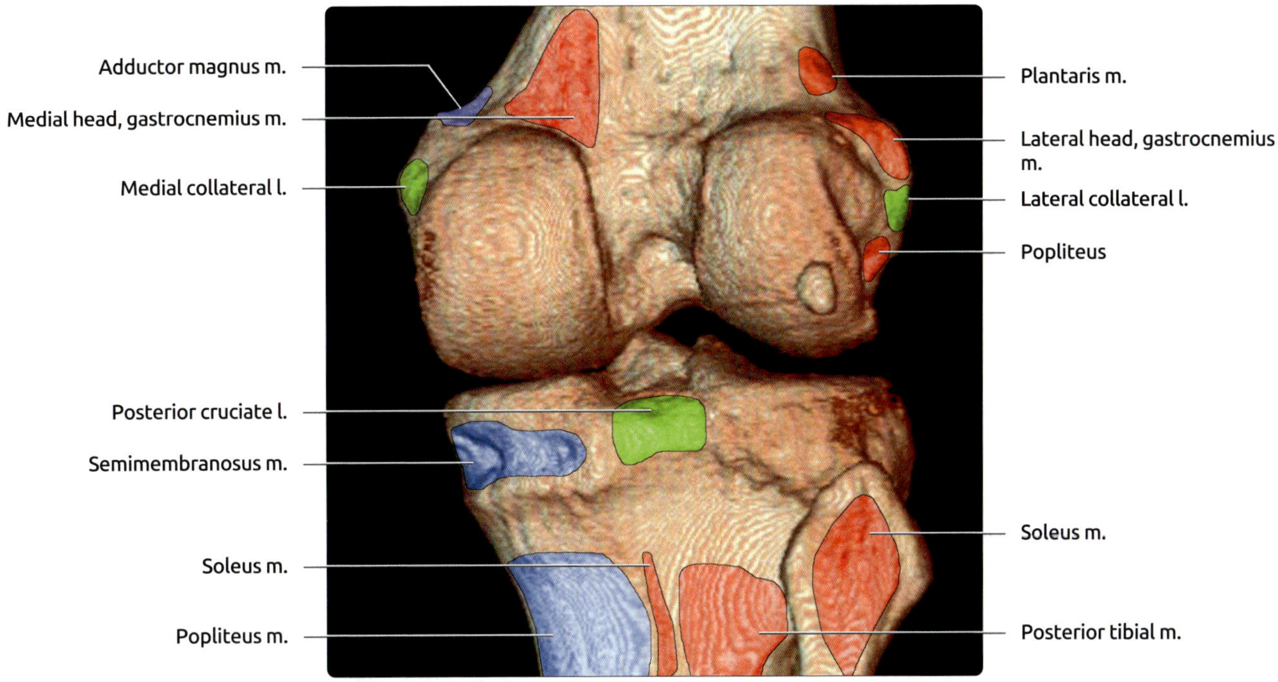

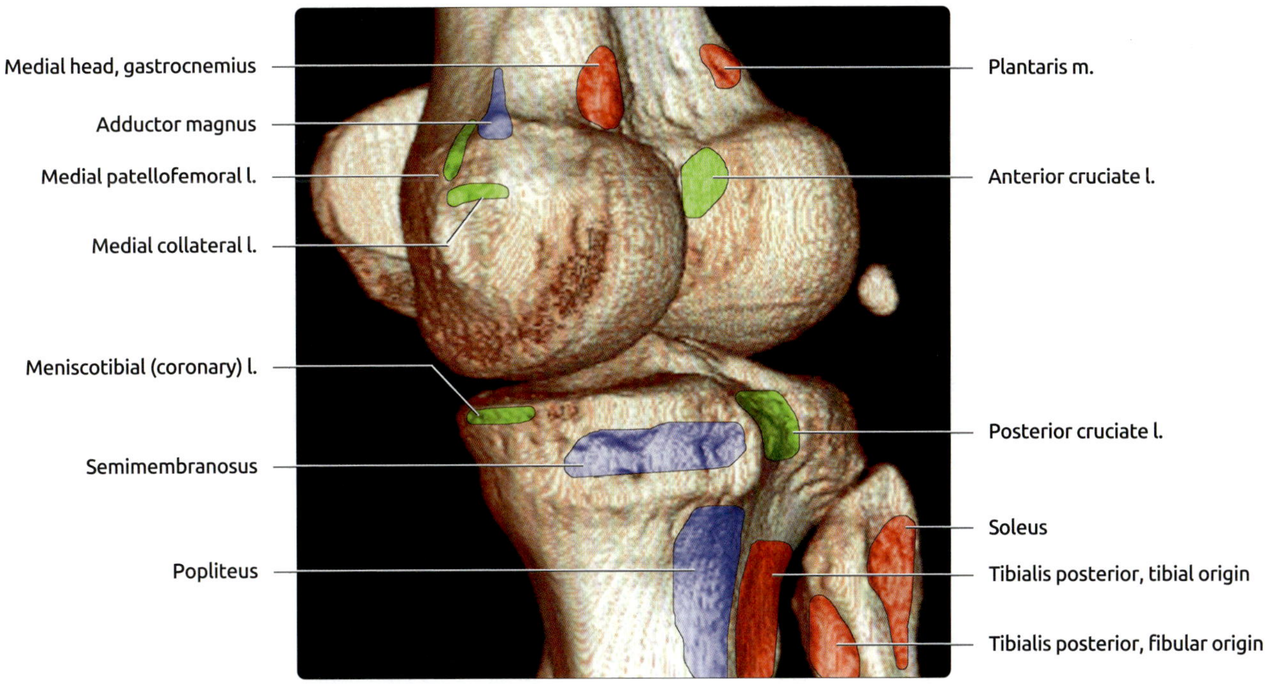

(Top) *In this direct posterior view, note that posterior cruciate ligament attachment is extraarticular, on the posterior central tibia.* **(Bottom)** *On this posterior (oblique to medial) view, note the extensive insertions of both the semimembranosus tendon and popliteus vein on the posteromedial tibia.*

IMAGING ANATOMY

Overview

- Extensor mechanism: Quadriceps muscle and tendon, patella, patellar tendon, and patellar retinacula

Quadriceps

- **Muscles**: Rectus femoris, vastus lateralis, vastus medialis, vastus intermedius
- **Quadriceps tendon**
  - Trilaminar configuration (generally): Fascia of component muscles with interposed fat
    - Superficial (anterior on sagittal): Rectus femoris
    - Middle: Vastus lateralis and vastus medialis
    - Deep (posterior on sagittal): Vastus intermedius
  - May appear as 2 or 4 layers: Medial and lateral components of middle layer merge in different combinations or remain discrete
  - Tendon inserts on nonarticular (anterior) patella

Patellar Tendon

- Mainly composed of rectus femoris fibers that course over patella forming prepatellar quadriceps seam of fibrocartilage connecting to inferior patellar tendon
- Extends from inferior pole of patella to tibial tuberosity
- Length ~ 5 cm
  - Length ~ equal to height of patella
  - Variation by > 20% of craniocaudal length of patella results in patella alta or baja
- 3 cm wide superiorly to 2 cm inferiorly; 5-6 mm thick

Medial Retinaculum Complex

- Medial stabilizer of patellofemoral joint
- Extends from patella to vastus medialis
- Medial retinacular complex divided into superior, mid, and inferior portions that blend into one another
  - **Superior: Vastus medialis obliquus (VMO) and medial patellofemoral ligament (MPFL)**
    - VMO: Muscular slip of vastus medialis; arises either from adductor magnus tendon or from adductor tubercle
    - VMO inserts at superior medial border of patella
    - VMO aponeurosis tightly adherent to underlying MPFL
    - MPFL: Arises from adductor tubercle adjacent to medial collateral ligament (MCL) origin and inserts at medial border of patella
  - **Midportion**: Thin fibers of superficial MCL fascia
  - **Inferior**
    - Patellotibial ligament arises from tibia at level of insertion of gracilis and semitendinosus and inserts on inferior aspect patella and patellar tendon
    - Medial patellomeniscal ligament lies deep to patellotibial ligament

Lateral Retinaculum

- Lateral stabilizer of patellofemoral joint
- Extends from patella to vastus lateralis
- 3 layers
  - **I (superficial)**: Iliotibial tract (band) and its anterior expansion, supplemented posteriorly by superficial portion of biceps femoris and its anterior expansion
  - **II (mid)**: Retinaculum of quadriceps (vastus lateralis)
  - **III (deep)**: Lateral part of joint capsule

Anterior Fat Pads

- Each interposed between joint capsule externally and synovium-lined joint cavity (intracapsular but extrasynovial)
- Suprapatellar bursa outlined by anterior (quadriceps) and posterior (prefemoral) suprapatellar fat pads
- Infrapatellar (Hoffa fat pad)
  - Bordered by
    - Inferior pole patella (superior)
    - Joint capsule and patellar tendon (anterior)
    - Proximal tibia and deep infrapatellar bursa (inferior)
    - Synovial-lined joint capsule (posterior)
  - Can be tethered posteriorly at apex by infrapatellar plica
  - Attached to anterior horns of menisci inferiorly and to tibial periosteum
  - Transverse ligament courses within fat pad
  - Interface between posterior aspect of fat pad and joint space consists of several synovial recesses
  - Anastomotic vessels course through fat pad, seen in cross section on sagittal images

Plica

- Synovial folds; persistent embryonic remnants
- **Superior** (suprapatellar, superomedial): Common
  - Medial suprapatellar pouch, 2 cm superior to patella
  - Seen as fold or (rarely) complete septum
  - Runs obliquely downward from synovium at anterior aspect of femoral metaphysis to posterior aspect of quadriceps tendon
  - Inserts above patella; best seen on sagittal
- **Medial** (plica synovialis, patellar shelf, medial intraarticular band)
  - Arises from medial wall of synovial pouch or under medial retinaculum and extends obliquely downward to insert on synovium covering infrapatellar fat pad
  - Inserts on synovium covering infrapatellar fat pad, at medial edge of patella; seen on sagittal or axial
  - If large, can impinge on medial facet of trochlea or under medial facet of patella
- **Inferior** (infrapatellar plica/fold/septum, ligamentum mucosa): Common
  - Extends from Hoffa fat pad in intercondylar notch, paralleling and anterior to anterior cruciate ligament; best seen on sagittal
  - May be split or fenestrated; dimensions vary
- **Lateral**: Rare
  - Originates from lateral wall superior to popliteal hiatus and extends to infrapatellar fat pad
  - Oblique coronal orientation; 1-2 cm lateral to patella
- Size and morphologic features of given plica do not reliably indicate whether it is clinically significant

SELECTED REFERENCES

1. Wangwinyuvirat M et al: Prepatellar quadriceps continuation: MRI of cadavers with gross anatomic and histologic correlation. AJR Am J Roentgenol. 192(3):W111-6, 2009

GRAPHIC & MR: EXTENSOR TENDON

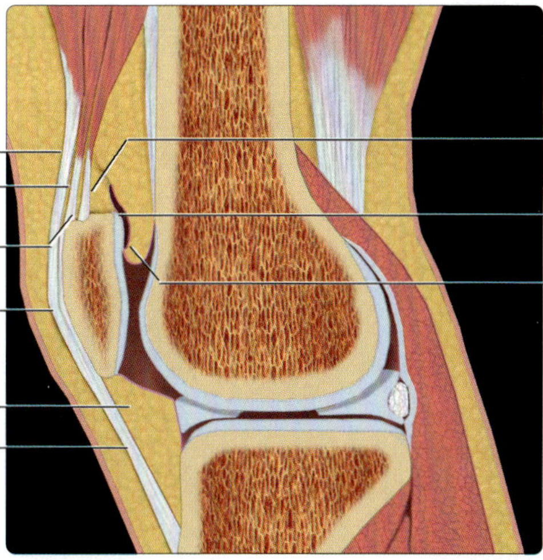

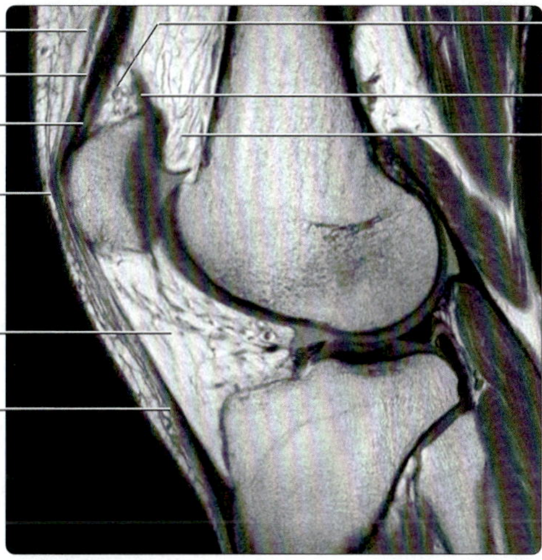

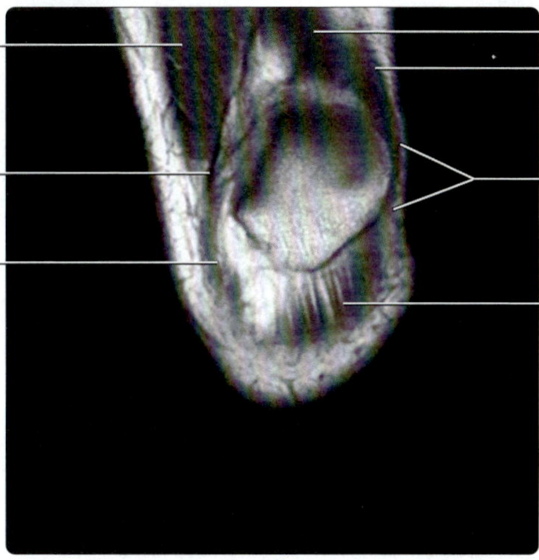

(Top) *Graphic shows trilaminar configuration of the quadriceps tendon. The superficial portion is rectus femoris, the middle portion is the aponeurosis of the vastus medialis and lateralis, and the deep portion is the vastus intermedius tendon.* **(Middle)** *Sagittal PD MR shows the trilaminate character of the extensor tendon. The suprapatellar bursa is not distended. The surrounding fat pads are well demonstrated. The infrapatellar fat pad, with anastomosing joint vessels coursing through it, is also seen.* **(Bottom)** *Anterior coronal T1WI MR shows components of patellar attachments. The quadriceps and inferior patellar tendons attach superiorly and inferiorly, respectively. The lateral retinaculum attaches along the entire lateral edge of patella. The vastus medialis obliquus (VMO), medial patellofemoral, and inferior patellotibial ligaments contribute to medial retinaculum from superior to inferior.*

GRAPHIC & MR: PATELLAR STABILIZERS

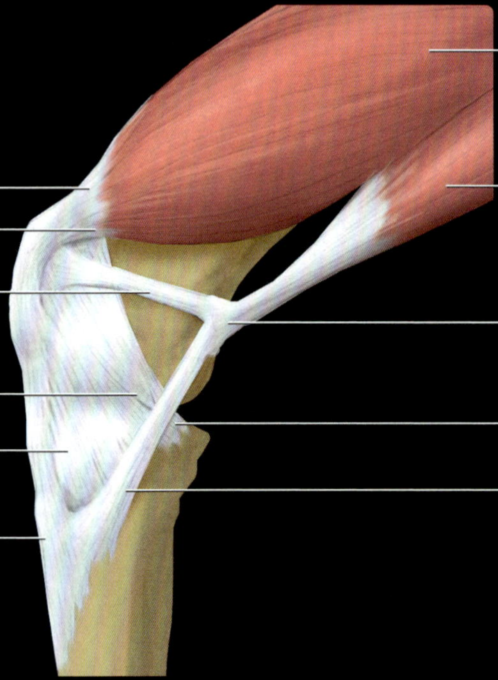

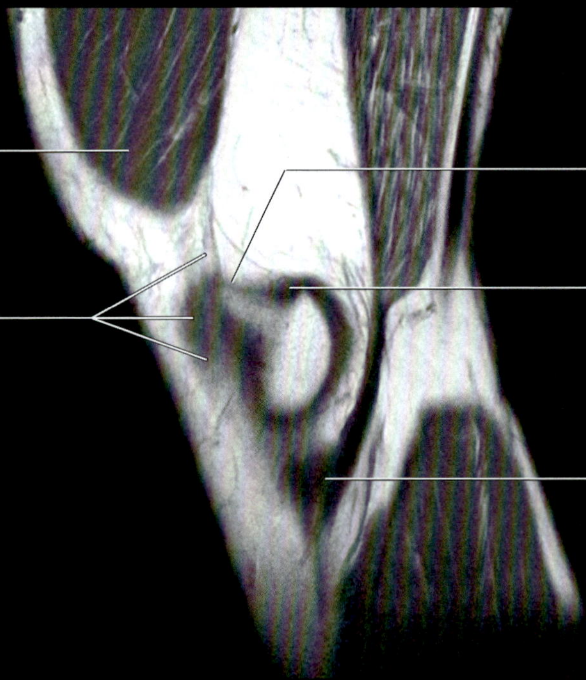

(Top) *Graphic shows medial patellar stabilizers. The VMO arises from the adductor magnus tendon. The medial patellofemoral ligament (MPFL) arises from the adductor tubercle; both insert along superior 1/3 of the medial patella. The patellotibial ligament originates on the tibia at the level of insertion of the pes anserinus; it inserts on inferior 2/3 of the patella and on the patellar tendon. The medial patellomeniscal ligament is deep in relation to the patellotibial ligament. Fibers from superficial medial collateral ligament also contribute to medial retinaculum.* **(Bottom)** *Sagittal PD MR shows that the individual components of the medial retinaculum are rarely seen in this plane. The semimembranosus contributes thin fibers to the superficial medial collateral ligament, which in turn contributes to the medial retinaculum. The fibers labeled medial retinaculum are contributed from the VMO, MPFL, patellotibial ligament, and patellomeniscal ligament.*

SAGITTAL MR: PATELLAR STABILIZERS

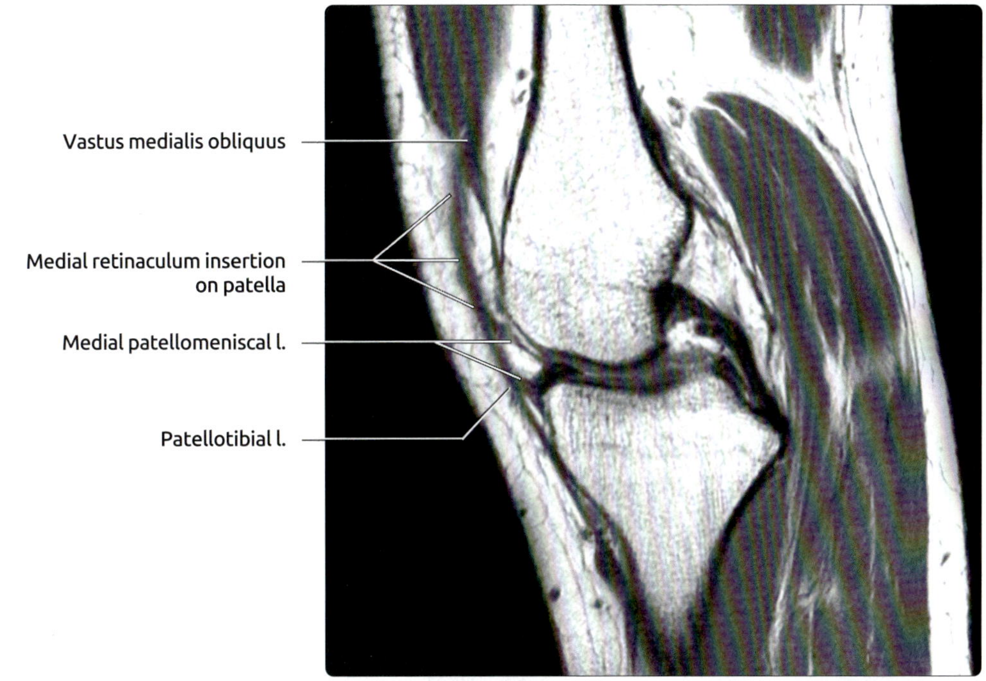

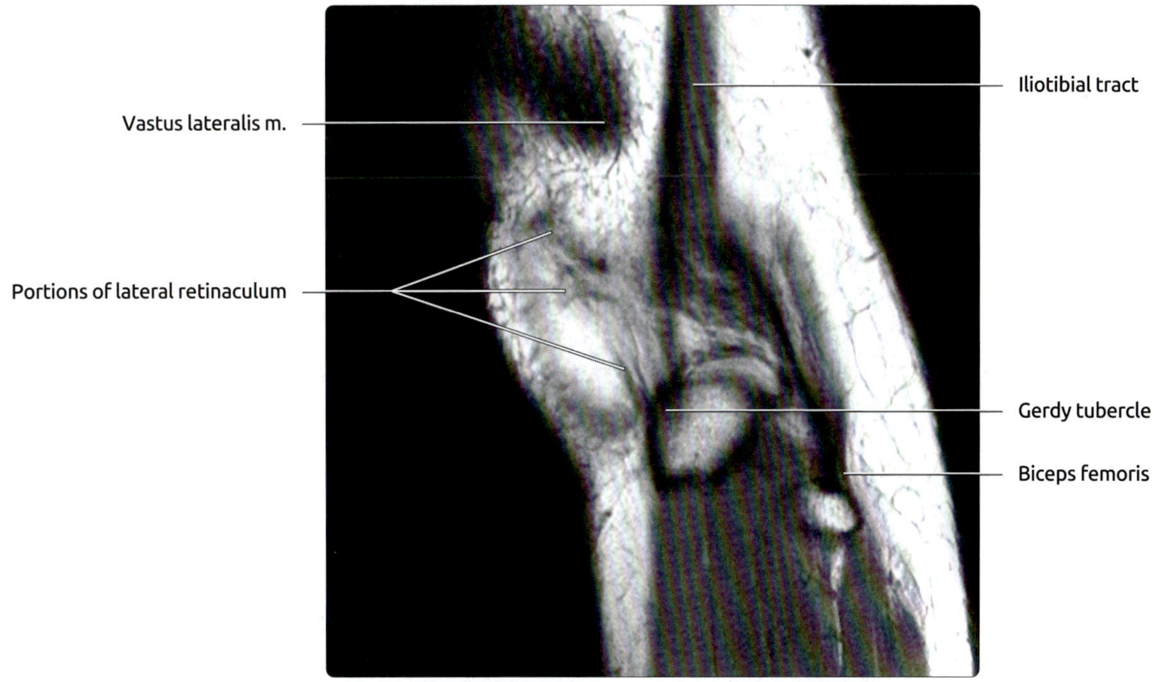

(Top) *Sagittal PD MR through the medial portion of the intercondylar notch shows various portions of the medial retinaculum, including the VMO, medial patellomeniscal ligament, and patellotibial ligament. These, along with the MPFL, blend together to form the medial retinaculum.* **(Bottom)** *Sagittal PD MR, far lateral, shows portions of the lateral retinaculum. Contributions come from the vastus lateralis, anterior expansion iliotibial tract, anterior expansion superficial biceps femoris, and joint capsule.*

AXIAL MR: PATELLAR STABILIZERS

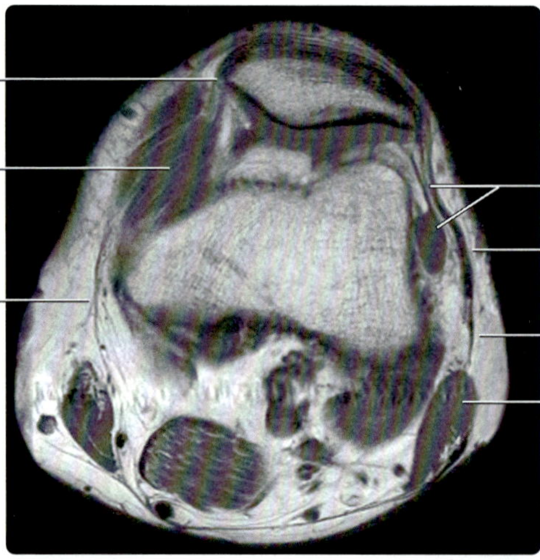

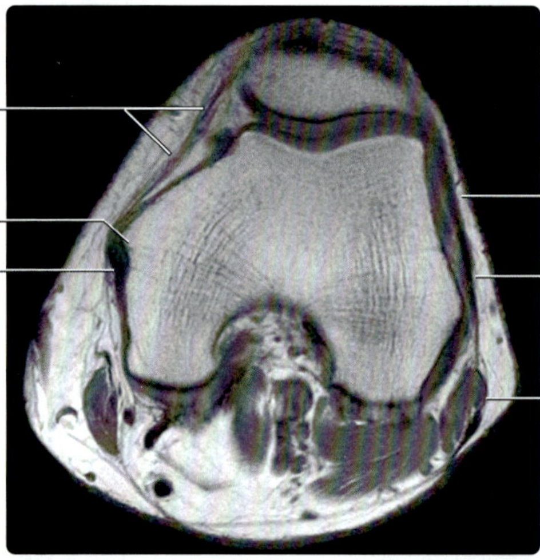

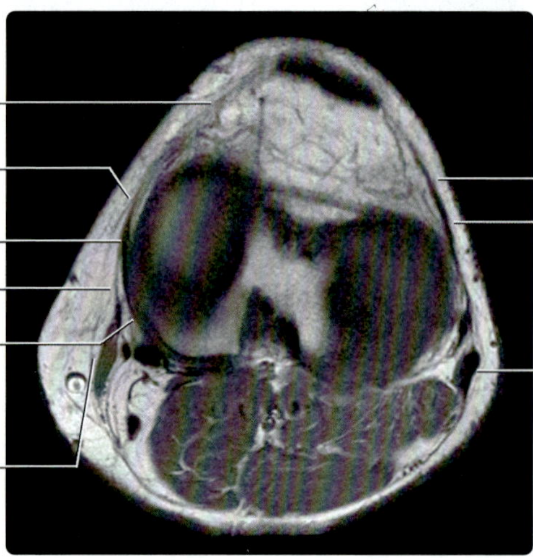

(Top) *First of 3 axial PD MR images, located just above the adductor tubercle, shows the VMO contributing to the superior portion of the medial retinaculum. The lateral retinaculum receives fibers from the anterior expansions of both the iliotibial tract and the biceps femoris.* **(Middle)** *At the level of the adductor tubercle, the superficial fibers of the medial collateral ligament and the MPFL are seen at their origin. The MPFL extends to the patella as the superior portion of the medial retinaculum at this level.* **(Bottom)** *At the level of the joint line, the medial retinaculum receives a contribution from the merged fibers of the superficial medial collateral ligament fascia and its overlying crura. The patellotibial ligament is also a major contributor at this level.*

MR: PLICA

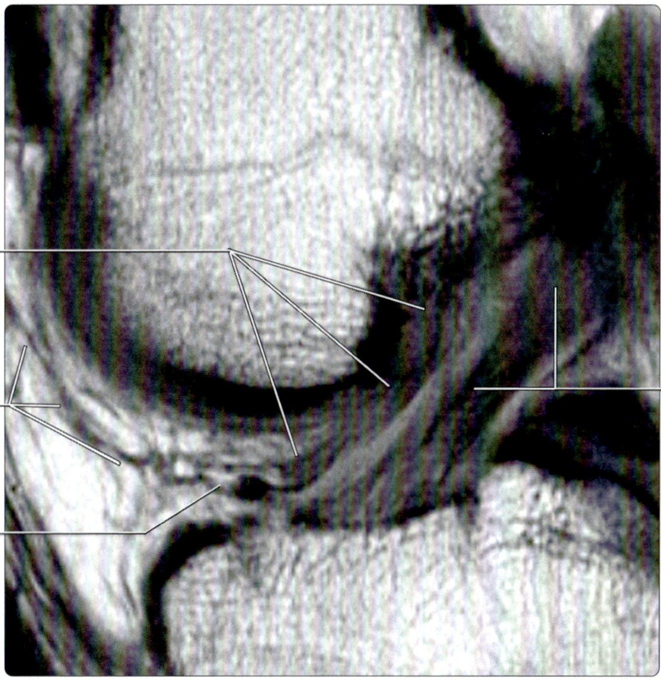

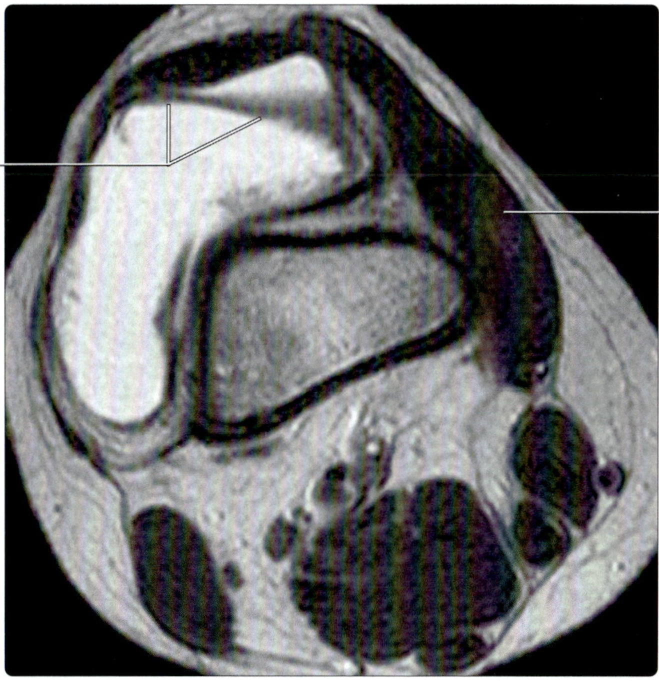

(Top) *Sagittal PD MR through the intercondylar notch shows a typical inferior (infrapatellar) plica. This normal variant extends from the inferior pole of the patella, through the Hoffa fat pad, parallels the anterior cruciate ligament, and attaches to the femoral condyle at the intercondylar notch. It may simulate a meniscocruciate ligament, but the anterior sites of origin are distinctly different.* **(Bottom)** *Axial T2WI MR at the level of the distal femur shows a synovial fold extending across the medial side of the suprapatellar pouch. This is a common form of plica, seen particularly well because of the large effusion. It is termed the superior, or suprapatellar, plica.*

SAGITTAL MR: PLICA

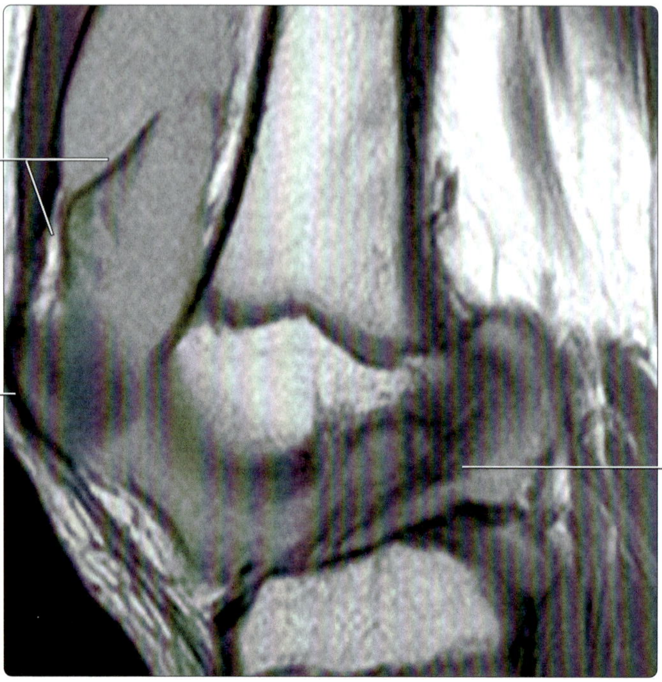

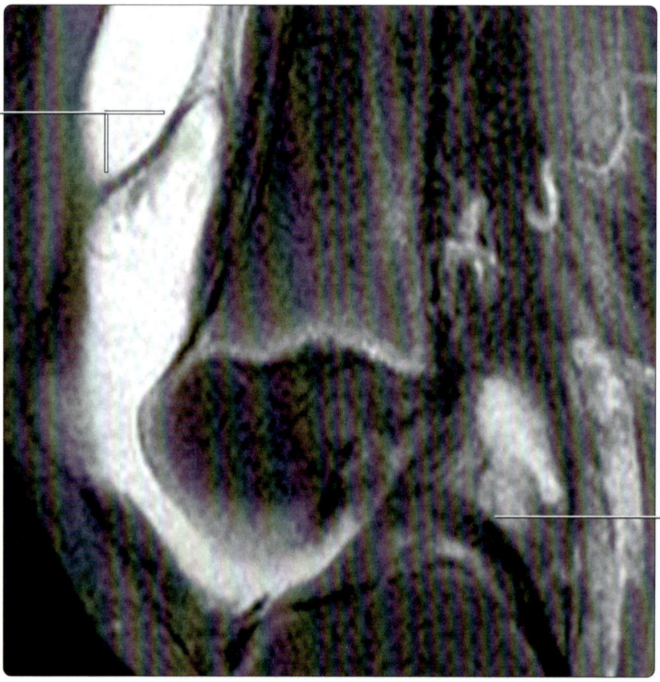

(Top) *Sagittal PD MR through the intercondylar notch of the same patient shows a superior (suprapatellar) plica. The plica extends from just superior to the patella, medially through the suprapatellar pouch.* **(Bottom)** *Sagittal PD FS MR shows the plica extending further superomedially. This is a common variant, which does not have clinical consequences. Note the posterior cruciate ligament.*

AXIAL MR: PLICA

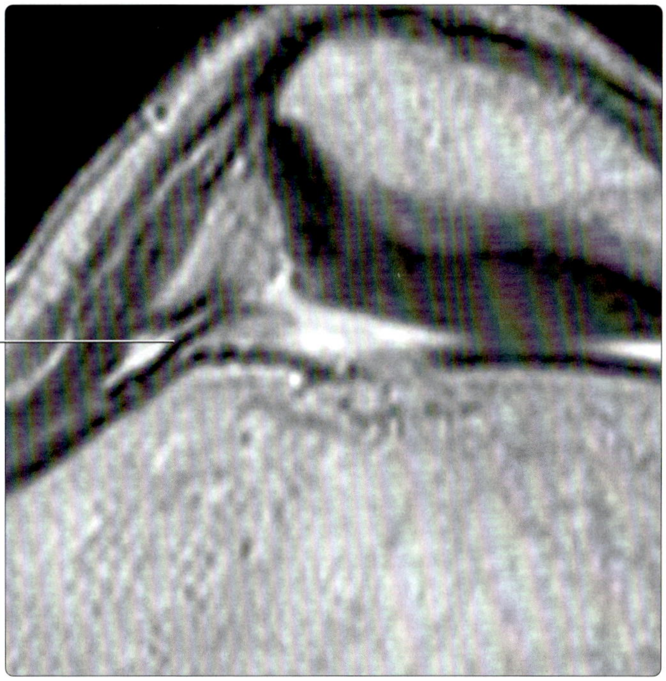

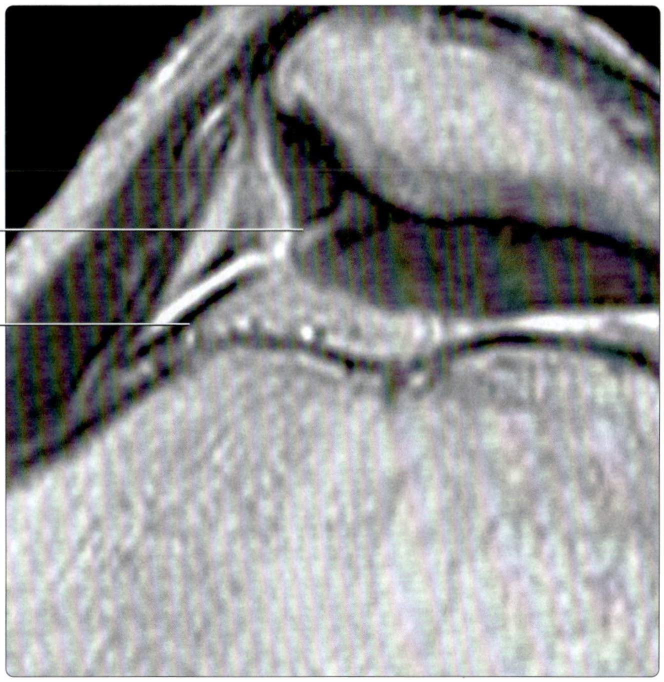

(Top) *First of 2 axial T2 MR images through the midpatella shows a medial plica extending over the medial facet of the trochlea and under the medial facet of the patella.* **(Bottom)** *Slightly distal image shows the medial plica, with signal abnormality, approaching the medial facet of the patella, which also shows signal abnormality. The medial plica is more likely to result in symptomatic damage (either at the medial patellar facet or medial trochlea) than the other plicae.*

TERMINOLOGY

Abbreviations

- Anterior/posterior cruciate ligament (ACL/PCL)
- Lateral/medial meniscus (LM/MM)
- Medial collateral ligament (MCL)

IMAGING ANATOMY

Overview

- Menisci evaluated by morphology, signal, and attachments
- Triangular shape tapers from height of 3-5 mm peripherally to sharp, thin, central (free) edge
- Normally specific and predictable size/shape
- Anterior and posterior root attachments to tibia are key for meniscal stability
- Central 2/3 is avascular (white zone); outer 1/3 is vascularized (red zone)
    - Vascularity is more prominent in children
- Avascular portion is low signal intensity on all sequences
- Vascularized portion shows central high signal extending to periphery
- Crucial to distribution of weight across knee joint
- Improve congruity of femoral condyle to tibial plateau
- Contribute to knee stability via bumper effect

Morphology

- **LM**
    - Tightly curved shape with close proximity of anterior, posterior roots
    - Posterior, anterior horns same size in cross section
    - Anterior horn divides into separate fascicles near root
        - Fluid between fascicles should not be mistaken for tear
    - Normal recess: Peripheral, inferior at anterior horn
- **MM**
    - Open, C-shape
    - Posterior horn is larger than anterior horn in cross section
    - Normal recess: Peripheral, superior at posterior horn

Meniscal Attachments

- **Osseous attachments: Both menisci are firmly attached to tibia at their roots**
    - **LM roots**
        - Anterior horn attaches immediately lateral to origin of ACL
        - Posterior horn attaches just posterior to ACL and anterior to PCL as PCL extends behind tibial plateau to its insertion on posterior tibia
        - Root of posterior horn LM also is anterior to root of posterior horn MM
    - **MM roots**
        - Root anterior horn MM anterior to origin of ACL
        - Root posterior horn MM immediately anterior to PCL but posterior to root of posterior horn LM
- **Capsular attachments**
    - **LM entirely attached to joint capsule only in anterior and far posterior portions**, with attachment being interrupted at body and much of posterior horn by popliteal hiatus
        - After origination from lateral femoral condyle, popliteus tendon penetrates capsule and takes intraarticular course
        - Intraarticularly, popliteus tendon extends distally in posteromedial direction
        - Popliteus tendon separates LM from its capsular insertion along body & majority of posterior horn
        - Superior and inferior fascicles serve as attachments between LM and popliteal tendon and, in turn, capsule
        - Inferior popliteomeniscal fascicle extends from lateral edge of body of meniscus to inferior portion of popliteus paratenon, forming floor of popliteal hiatus
        - Inferior fascicle complete at level of body of LM, but not posterior horn
        - Superior popliteomeniscal fascicle extends from body/posterior horn LM to superior portion popliteal paratenon and on to capsule, forming ceiling of popliteal hiatus
        - Superior fascicle incomplete at body, but complete at body/posterior horn LM
    - **MM entirely attached to joint capsule**, with exception of small interruption at MCL
        - MM serves as origin of meniscofemoral ligament portion of deep fibers of MCL; this ligament either inserts on adjacent femur or superficial MCL
        - MM also serves as origin of meniscotibial ligament (coronary ligament) portion of deep fibers of the MCL, which inserts on the adjacent tibia
        - Fibrofatty tissue as well as MCL bursa separate MM and deep fibers of MCL from superficial MCL

Meniscal Variants

- **Discoid meniscus**
    - Widened body of meniscus
    - May be medial or lateral
    - Predisposes to tear
- **Transverse ligament**: Connects menisci anteriorly
    - Oblique insertion on LM anterior horn may simulate tear; may be absent
- **Meniscofemoral ligaments**: Extend from posterior medial femoral condyle to posterior horn LM
    - At insertion on LM, may simulate tear
    - Ligament of Wrisberg passes posterior to PCL
    - Ligament of Humphrey passes anterior to PCL
- **Oblique menisco-meniscal ligaments**: Cross from anterior horn of one meniscus to posterior horn of other meniscus, passing between ACL and PCL
- **Meniscal "flounce"**: Buckling of portion of meniscus, perhaps related to femorotibial subluxation

GRAPHICS: MEDIAL MENISCUS

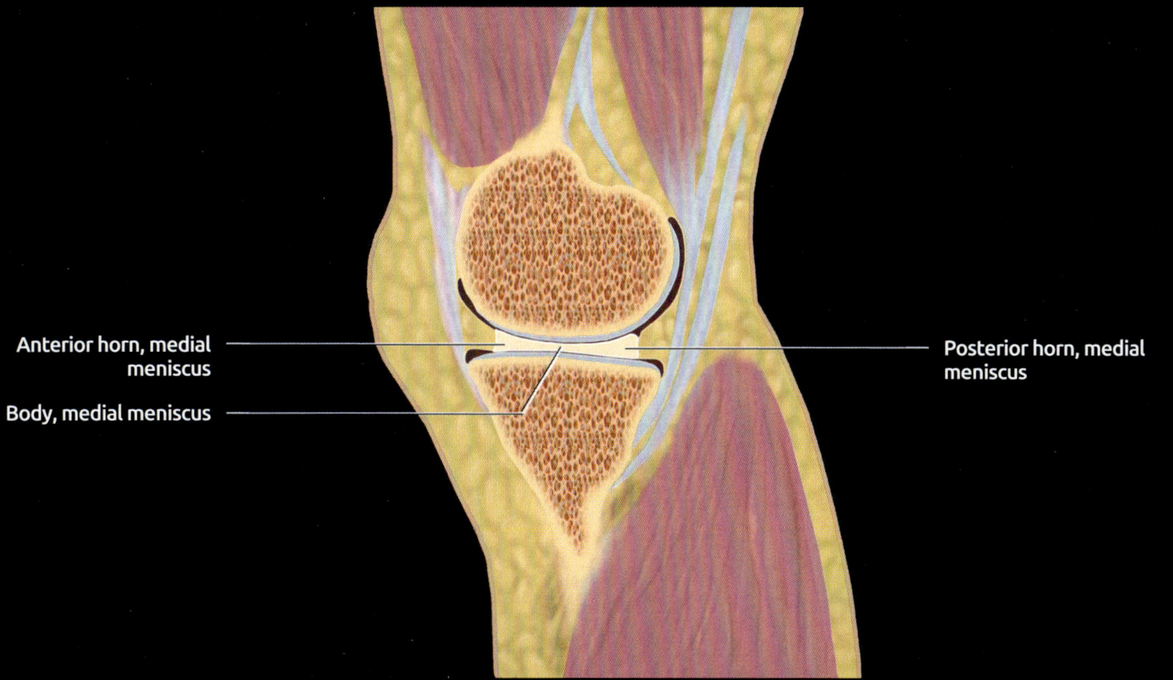

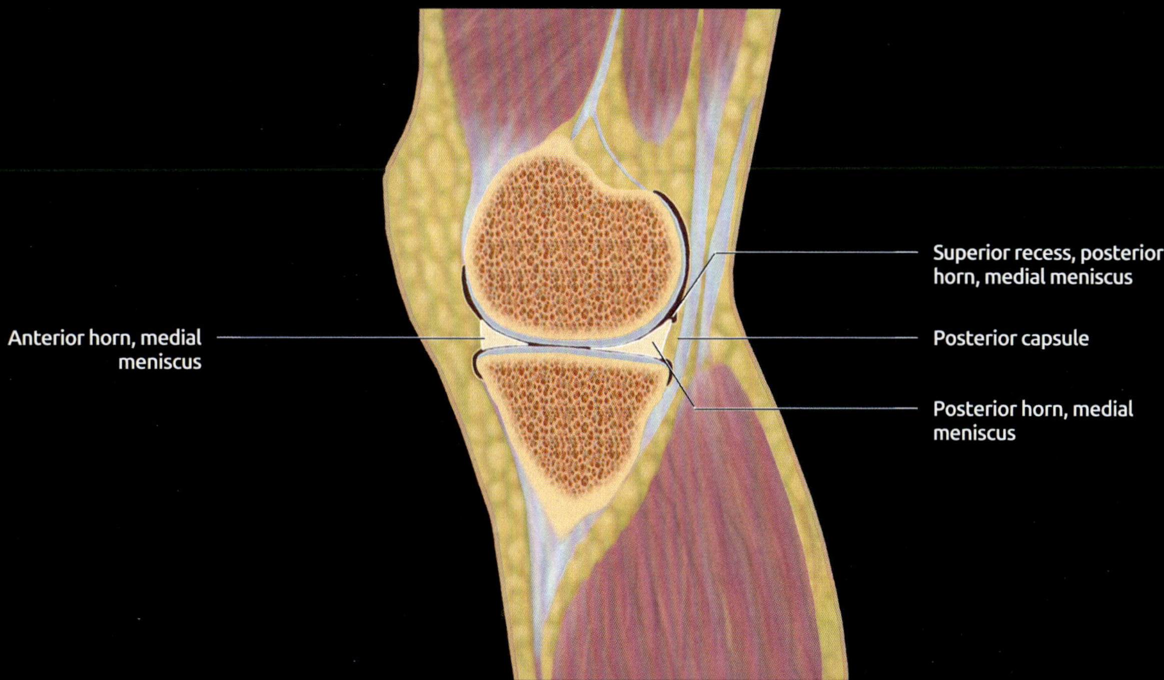

(Top) *Sagittal cut through the medial-most aspect of the medial meniscus shows the bowtie configuration. This appearance is due to the cut extending across the full thickness of both the anterior and posterior horns but across only the thinner mid portion of the body.* **(Bottom)** *Sagittal cut through the mid portion of the medial meniscus shows the triangular anterior and posterior horns. The posterior horn of the medial meniscus is normally elongated and larger than the anterior horn. There may be a superior recess at the meniscocapsular junction of the posterior horn.*

SAGITTAL PD MR: MEDIAL MENISCUS

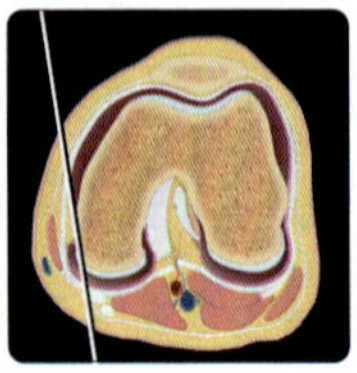

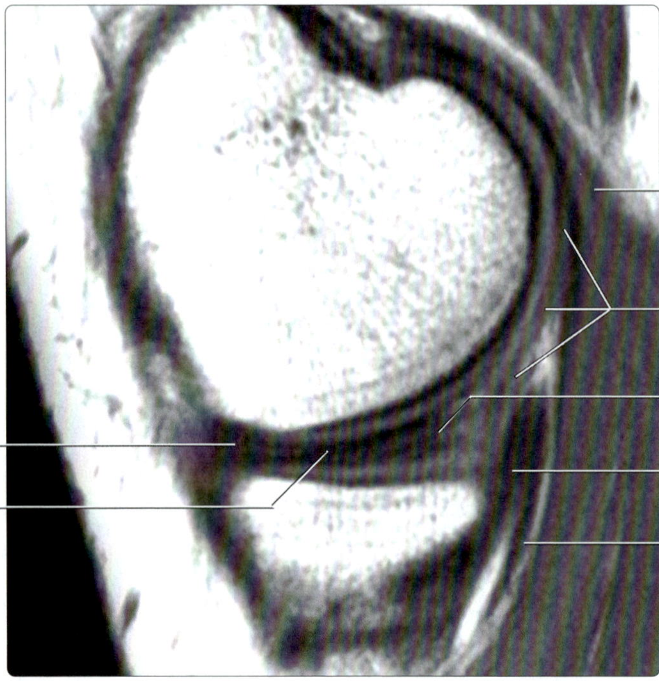

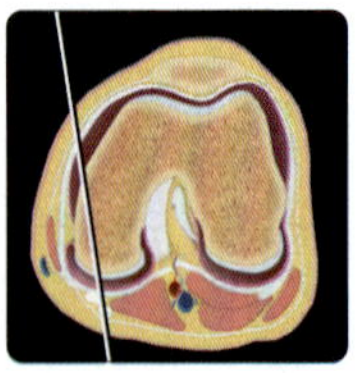

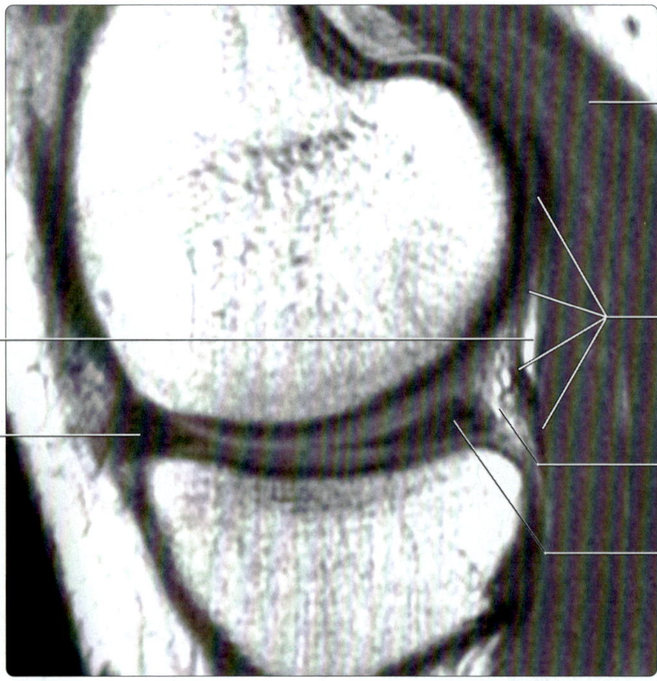

(Top) *First of 8 sagittal PD MR images through the medial meniscus is shown. Far medial (peripheral) sagittal cut through the medial meniscus shows the bowtie configuration encompassing portions of the anterior horn, body, and posterior horn of the medial meniscus.* **(Bottom)** *Midline sagittal cut through the medial meniscus shows the differential size and shape of the anterior and posterior horns. This image and the previous image show the low-signal meniscus blending indistinctly into the gray vascular portion of the meniscus, which in turn blends into the capsule.*

SAGITTAL PD MR: MEDIAL MENISCUS

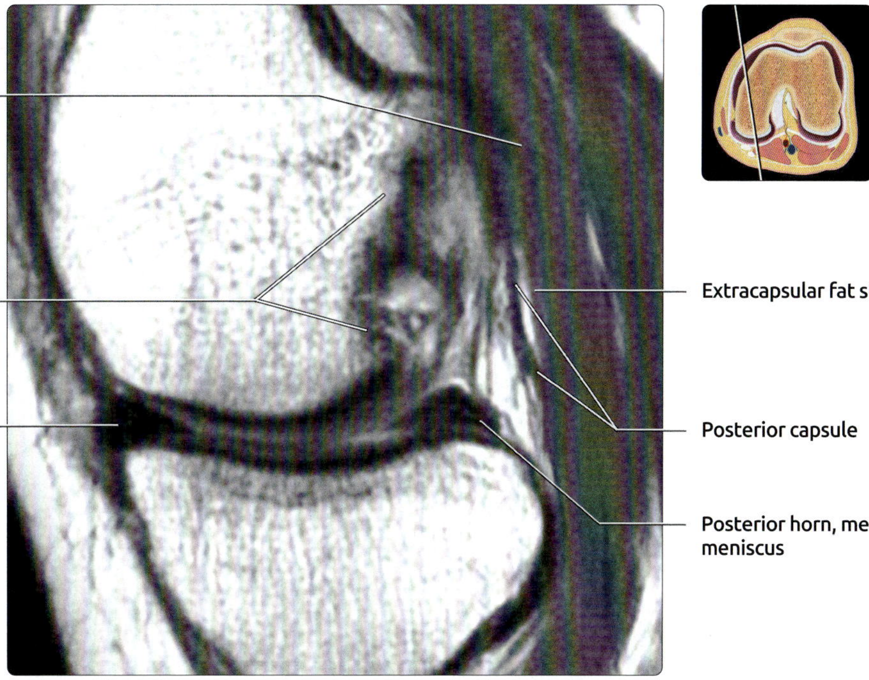

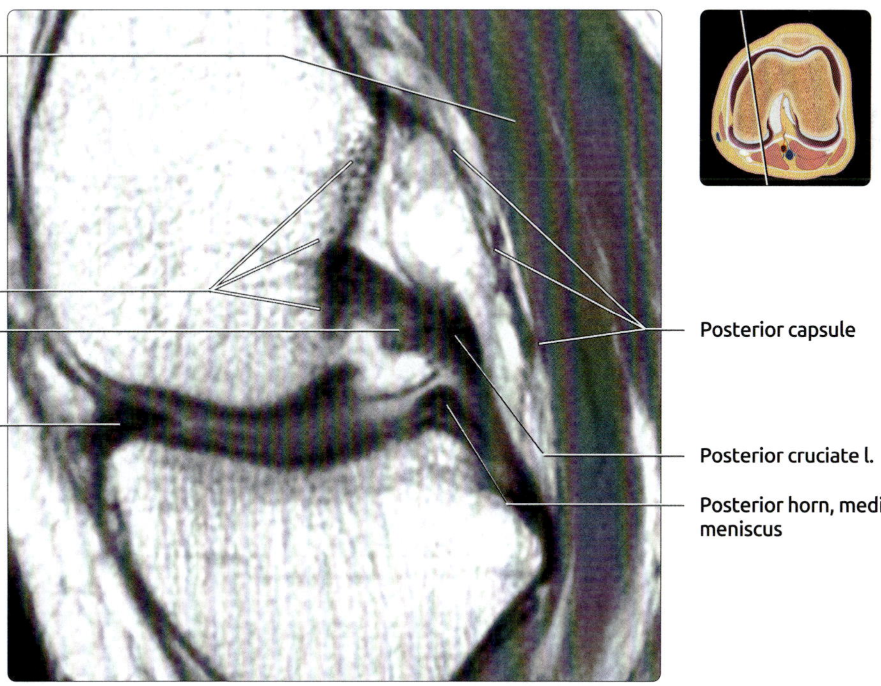

(Top) *Sagittal PD MR shows a cut through the medial meniscus, approaching the intercondylar notch. The anterior and posterior horns retain their differential size and shape.* **(Bottom)** *Sagittal PD MR shows the medial meniscus as it enters the medial portion of the intercondylar notch. The posterior cruciate ligament is seen, arising from the mid portion of Blumensaat line along the medial femoral condyle. The anteroinferior meniscofemoral ligament (of Humphrey) is seen in cross section beneath the posterior cruciate ligament. The posterior horn of the medial meniscus is beginning to change its shape as it approaches its root attachment to the tibial plateau. Because of the obliquity at which the knee is scanned for the sagittal images, the anterior horn is not yet approaching its root, but retains its triangular shape.*

SAGITTAL PD MR: MEDIAL MENISCUS

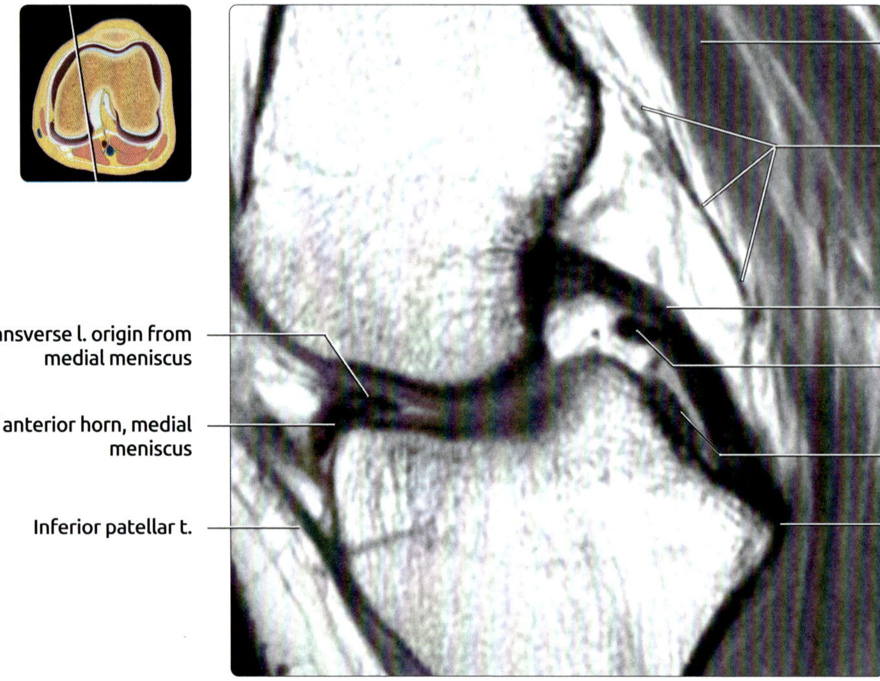

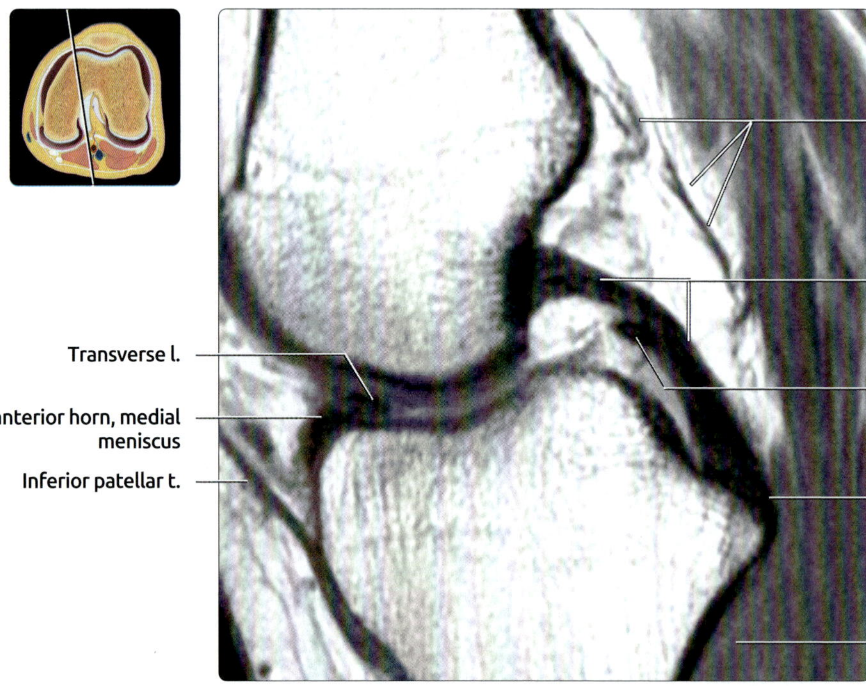

(Top) *Sagittal PD MR shows the roots of both the anterior and posterior horns of the medial meniscus. The root of the posterior horn of the medial meniscus terminates immediately in front of the posterior cruciate insertion on the tibia.* **(Bottom)** *Adjacent image shows the anterior horn of the medial meniscus terminating in its root; the transverse ligament arises at this point. Both the transverse and meniscofemoral ligaments are seen in cross section.*

SAGITTAL PD MR: MEDIAL MENISCUS

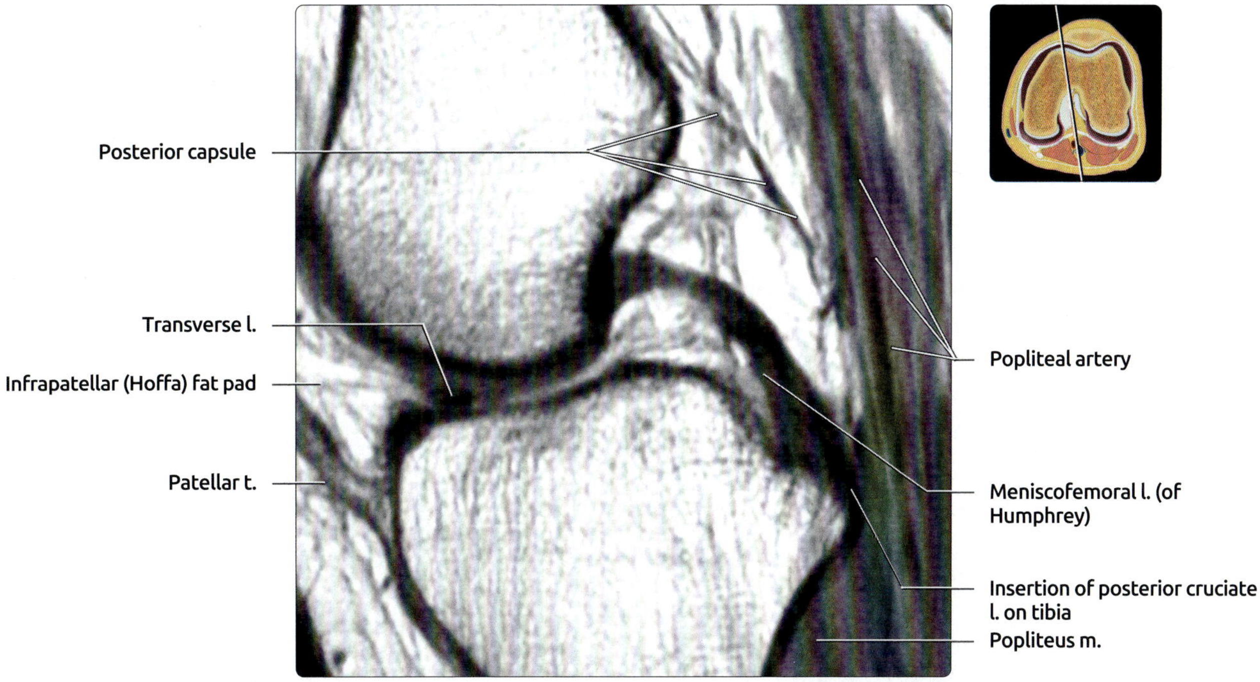

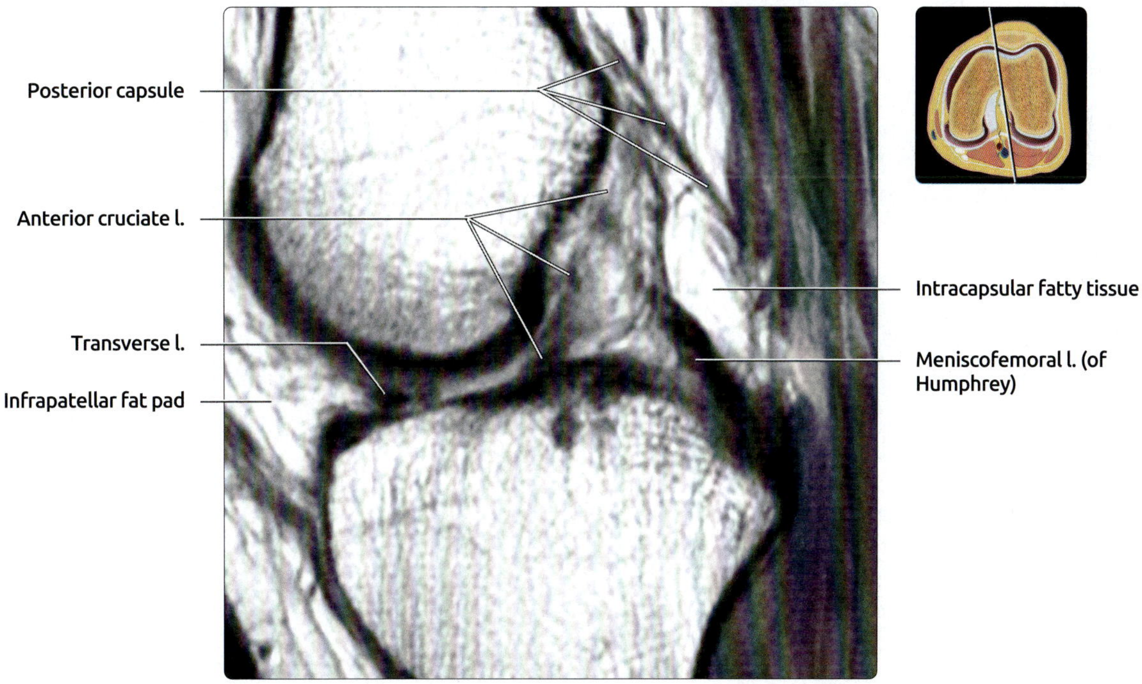

(Top) *Sagittal PD MR shows no menisci; the meniscofemoral ligament is beginning to elongate and parallel the posterior cruciate ligament. Note that the posterior capsule is interrupted, allowing neurovascular structures to enter the joint.* **(Bottom)** *Sagittal PD MR between the cruciate ligaments shows the transverse ligament in cross section, continuing across the anterior joint space. The meniscofemoral ligament elongates towards its insertion on the posterior horn of the lateral meniscus; the latter structure is not seen until the next cut toward the lateral side.*

GRAPHICS: MENISCAL ROOTS & MORPHOLOGY

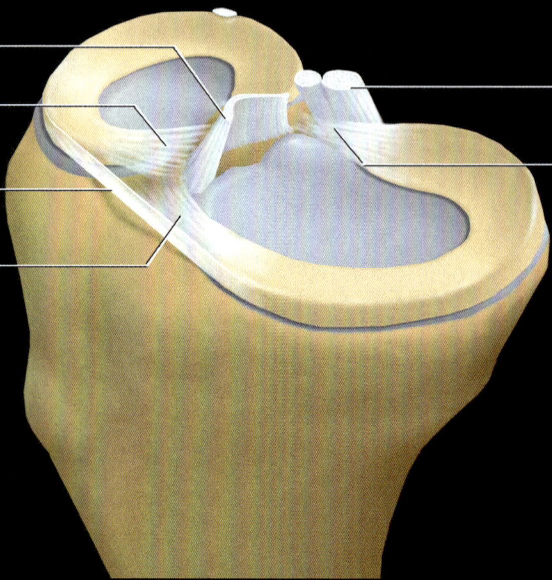

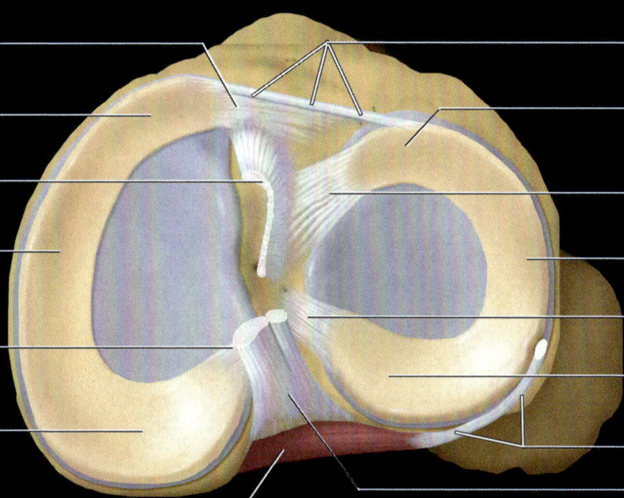

(Top) *Oblique axial graphic shows the tibial surface of the knee joint in an external oblique position. It highlights the semilunar medial meniscus, with its anterior and posterior roots located anterior to the ACL and PCL, respectively. The transverse ligament is seen coursing between the anterior horns of the medial and lateral menisci.* **(Bottom)** *Axial graphic through the joint line shows the semilunar medial meniscus with its wider C-shape compared to the more circular lateral meniscus. The position of the meniscal roots is seen relative to one another as well as to the anterior cruciate ligament (ACL) and posterior cruciate ligament (PCL). The transverse ligament and popliteal tendon are shown in relation to the menisci. Note also the different sizes of the various parts of the menisci.*

AXIAL PD FS MR: MENISCI

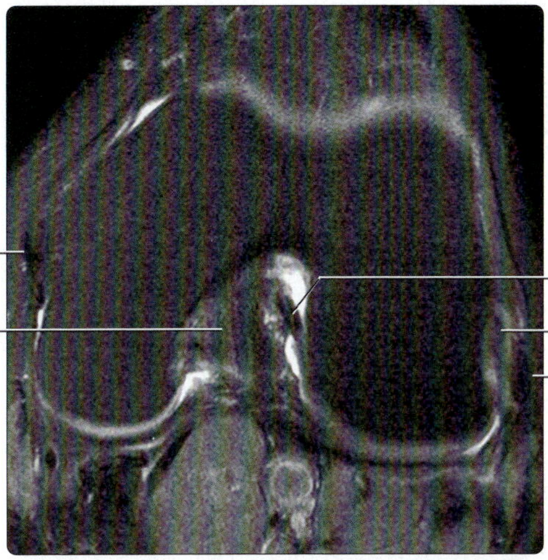

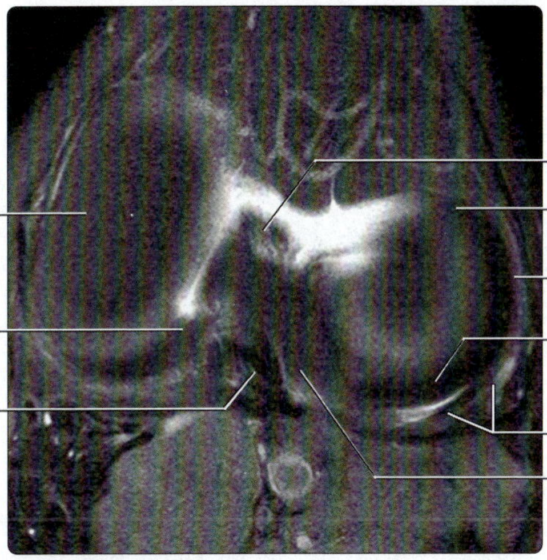

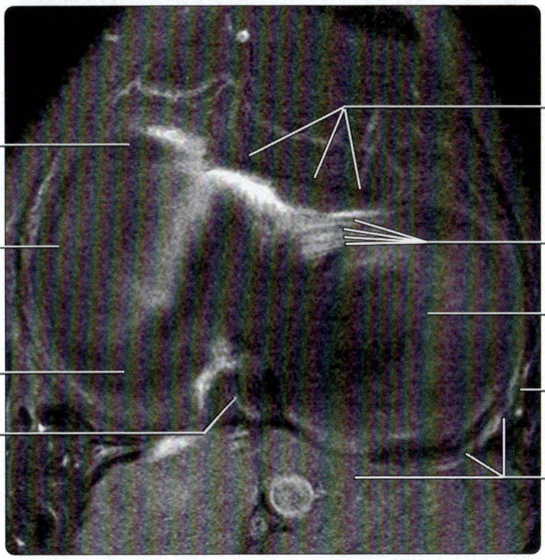

(Top) *First of 3 axial PD FS MR images through the knee joint line, located immediately above it, is shown. The cruciate ligaments as well as the origins of the medial and lateral collateral ligaments are seen.* **(Middle)** *Axial PD FS MR through the knee joint line shows parts of the menisci as well as the course of the popliteal tendon through the popliteal hiatus.* **(Bottom)** *Axial PD FS MR through the tibial plateau at the joint line shows parts of the menisci and their roots. The division of the anterior horn of the lateral meniscus into separate fascicles at its root is well seen. It is easy to understand how these separate fascicles, seen in cross section on sagittal images, can mimic tear. The transverse meniscal ligament bridges between the 2 anterior horns.*

GRAPHICS: POPLITEAL TENDON, HIATUS, & FASCICLES

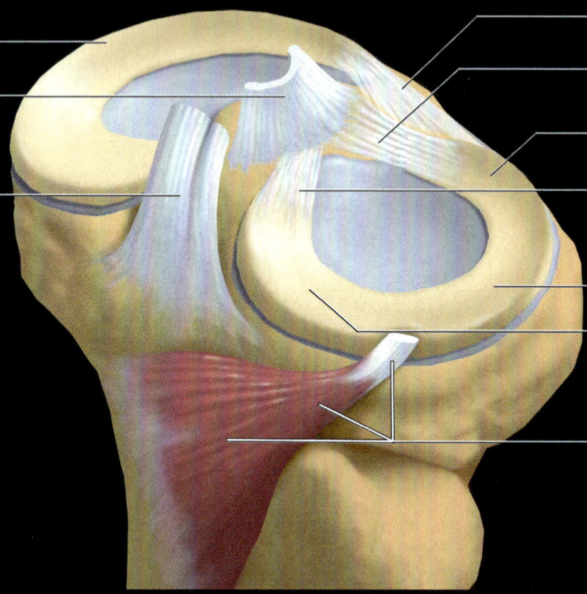

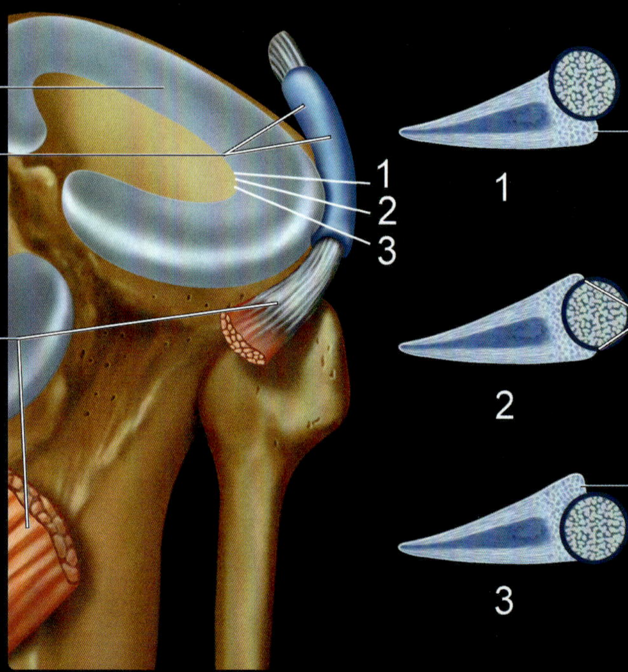

(Top) *Posterolateral oblique view of the knee joint line shows the radius of the lateral meniscus is tightly curved, and its roots are in close proximity. The popliteal tendon is shown curving around the lateral meniscus.* **(Bottom)** *Oblique axial graphic shows the course of the popliteal tendon through the knee joint. After the popliteal tendon originates from the lateral femoral condyle, it enters the joint space, interrupting the capsular attachment of the body of the lateral meniscus. It travels posteriorly and downward, curving around the body and posterior horns of the lateral meniscus. It is bathed in synovial fluid within this space (termed the popliteal hiatus). Note the inferior fascicle, which forms the floor of the hiatus at the body of the lateral meniscus, and the superior fascicle, which forms the roof of the hiatus at the lateral meniscus body/posterior horn. Different combinations of the superior and inferior fascicles are visualized as the popliteal tendon proceeds through the hiatus from the level of the body to the posterior horn of the lateral meniscus.*

GRAPHICS: LATERAL MENISCUS

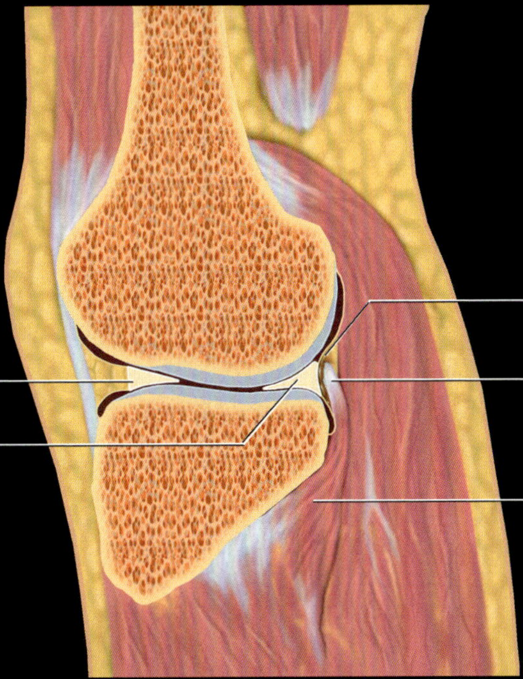

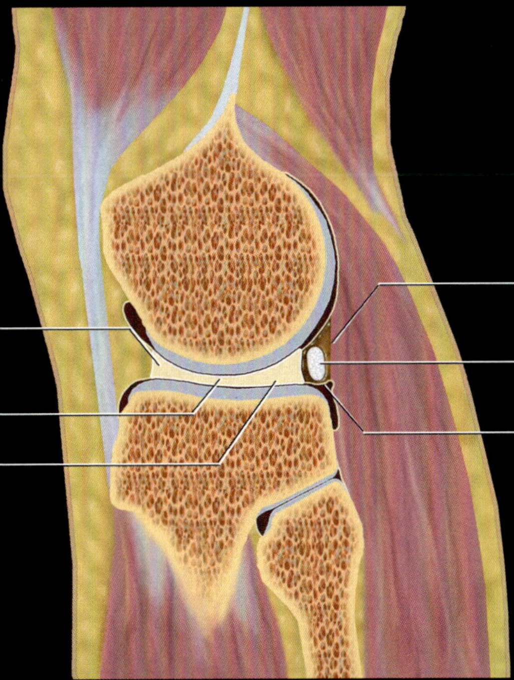

(Top) *In the mid portion of the lateral compartment, the anterior and posterior horns of the lateral meniscus are nearly equal in size and shape. The popliteal tendon extends into the popliteus muscle. The superior fascicle can be seen extending from the superior portion of the posterior horn to the superior edge of the popliteal tendon (paratenon), continuing to the capsule and forming the roof of the popliteal hiatus. The inferior fascicle is not continuous at this level since it is interrupted by passage of the popliteal tendon inferolaterally through the hiatus.* **(Bottom)** *Sagittal graphic located far laterally in the joint shows the bowtie configuration of the anterior horn, body, and posterior horn of the lateral meniscus. The popliteal tendon is seen in the hiatus; at this junction of body and posterior horn of the lateral meniscus, the inferior fascicle can be seen extending from the meniscus toward (but not connecting to) the popliteal tendon. It forms the floor of the popliteal hiatus. At this site, the superior fascicle is interrupted by the popliteal tendon.*

SAGITTAL PD MR: LATERAL MENISCUS

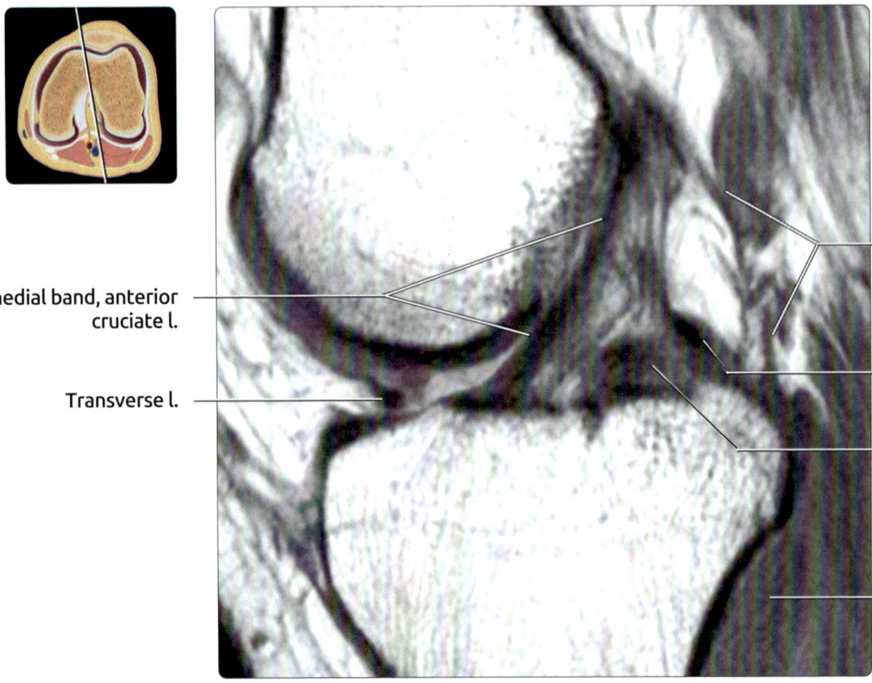

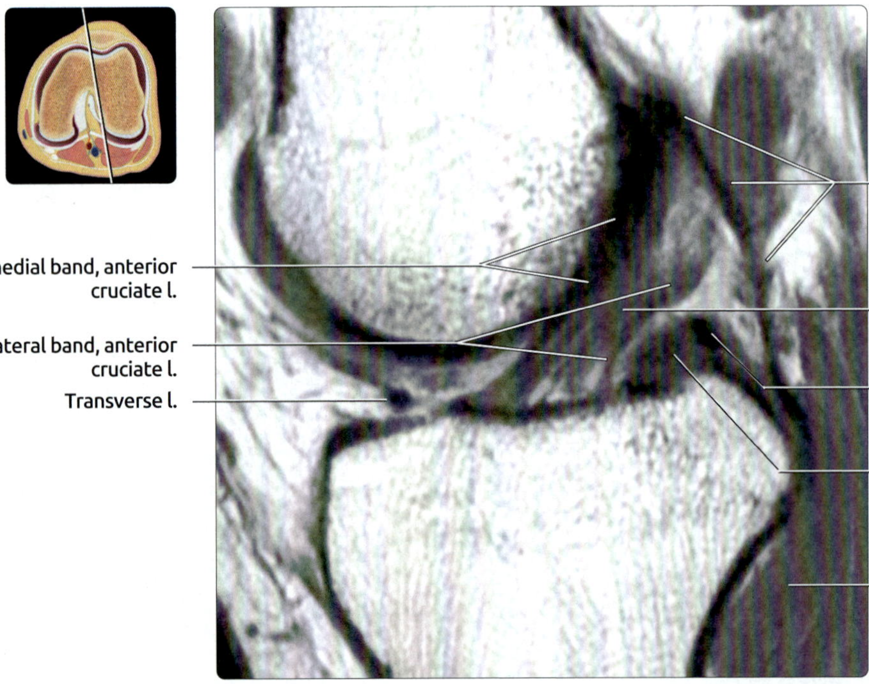

(Top) *First of 8 sagittal PD MR images through the lateral compartment shows the mid portion of the intercondylar notch. Note the meniscofemoral ligament approaching the posterior horn of the lateral meniscus.* **(Bottom)** *At the lateral aspect of intercondylar notch, the meniscofemoral ligament joins the posterior horn if the lateral meniscus near its root. This attachment may be misinterpreted as a torn meniscus. Note that, due to the obliquity with which sagittal sequences are routinely obtained, it is not uncommon to see the transverse ligament anteriorly as well as the root of the posterior horn for several cuts before the root of the anterior horn of the lateral meniscus is seen. The root of the lateral meniscal anterior horn arises lateral to the origin of the anterior cruciate ligament from the tibia; therefore, one should not expect to see it in these images.*

SAGITTAL PD MR: LATERAL MENISCUS

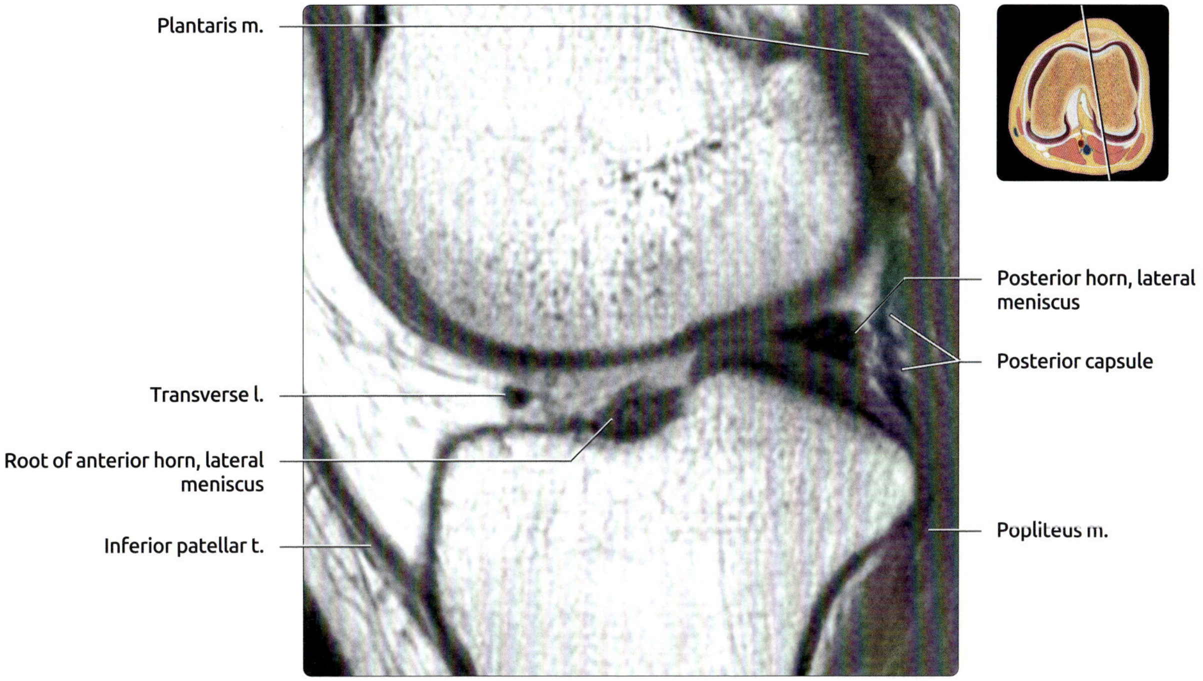

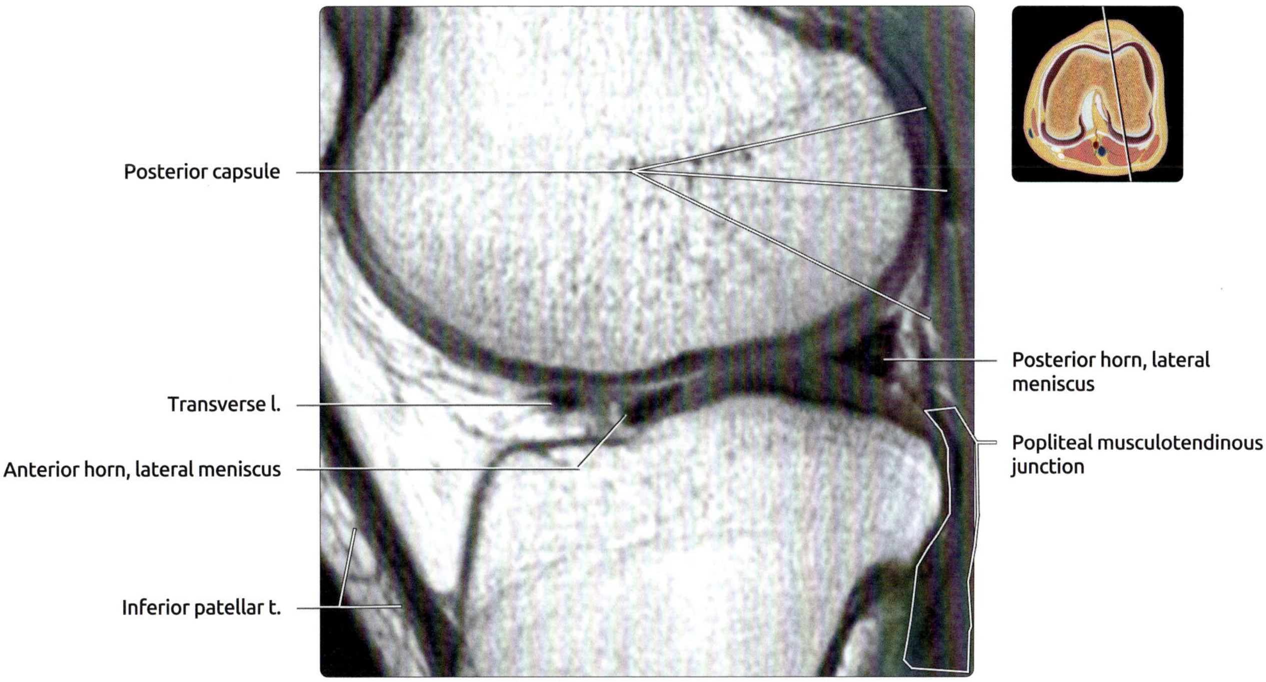

(Top) *In the lateral compartment, adjacent to the intercondylar notch, the root of the anterior horn of the lateral meniscus is seen with the transverse ligament approaching it. The anterior root has a stippled appearance on sagittal images, because the individual fascicles of the root are seen in cross section.* **(Bottom)** *In this adjacent, slightly more lateral image, the transverse ligament more closely approaches the anterior horn of the lateral meniscus. In these cuts, the popliteus muscle (top) and popliteal musculotendinous junction (bottom) are extraarticular. This far posterior region is the only portion of the lateral meniscus which directly attaches to the posterior capsule and is not interrupted by the popliteal hiatus.*

SAGITTAL PD MR: LATERAL MENISCUS

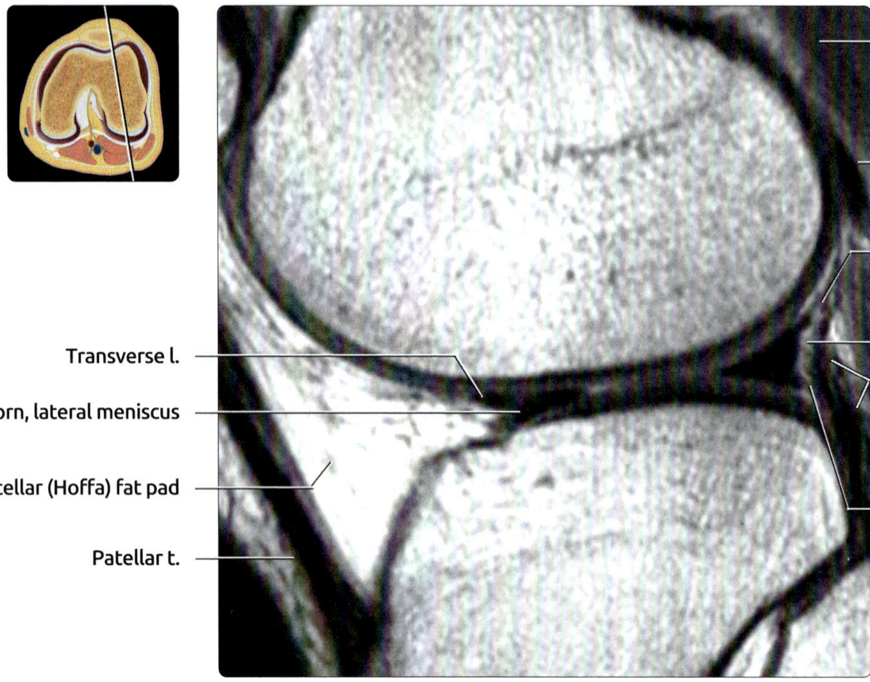

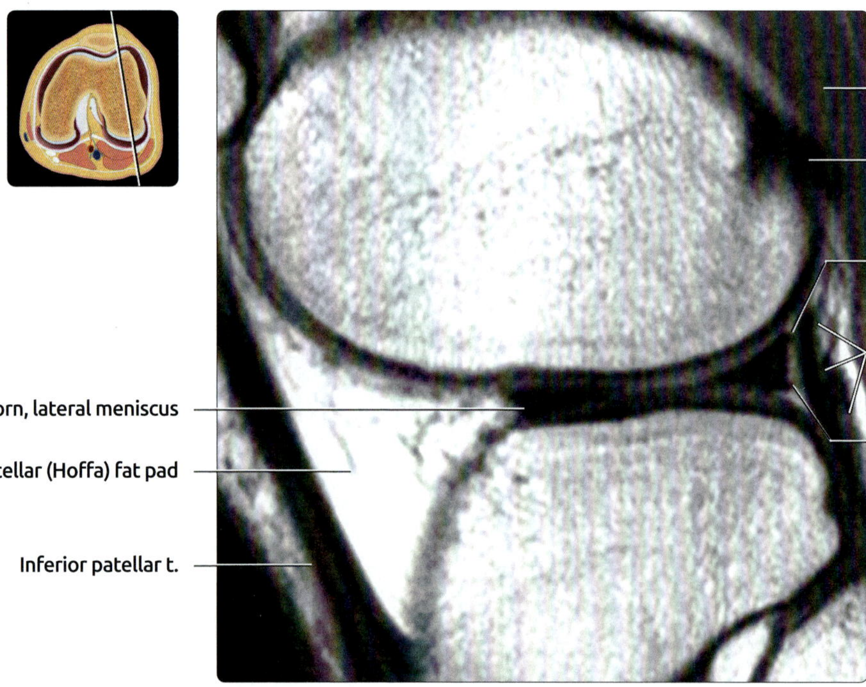

(Top) *Sagittal PD MR through the lateral compartment shows the transverse ligament joining the anterior horn of the lateral meniscus. Posteriorly, the popliteal tendon is seen within the popliteal hiatus. This structure is intraarticular but extrasynovial. The superior fascicle extends from the superior aspect of the posterior horn of the lateral meniscus to the paratenon of the popliteal tendon and on to the capsule, forming the roof of the popliteal hiatus. The inferior fascicle extends from the inferior aspect of the posterior horn of the lateral meniscus toward the popliteal tendon but is interrupted by the tendon's passage into the extraarticular position of the musculotendinous junction.* **(Bottom)** *This adjacent, more lateral cut shows a similar relationship of the fascicles, with the superior extending to the popliteal tendon and capsule, and the inferior fascicle being interrupted.*

SAGITTAL PD MR: LATERAL MENISCUS

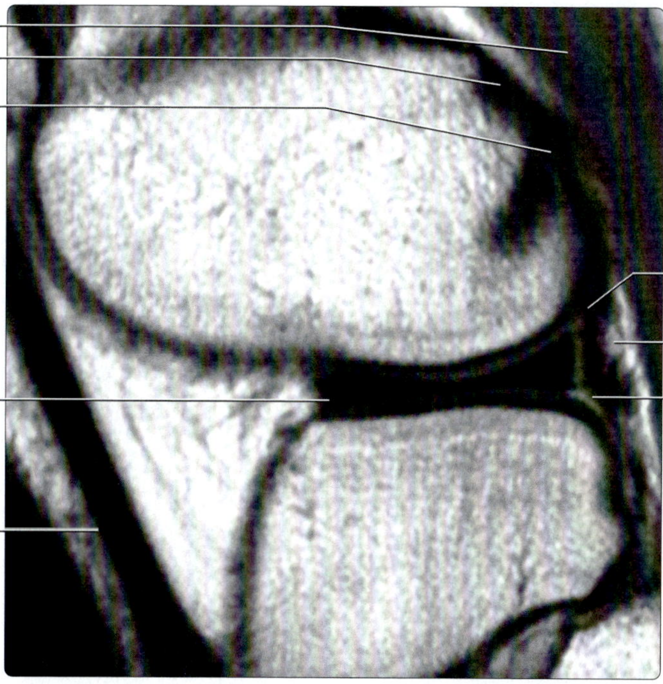

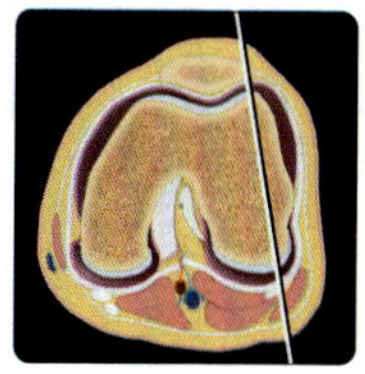

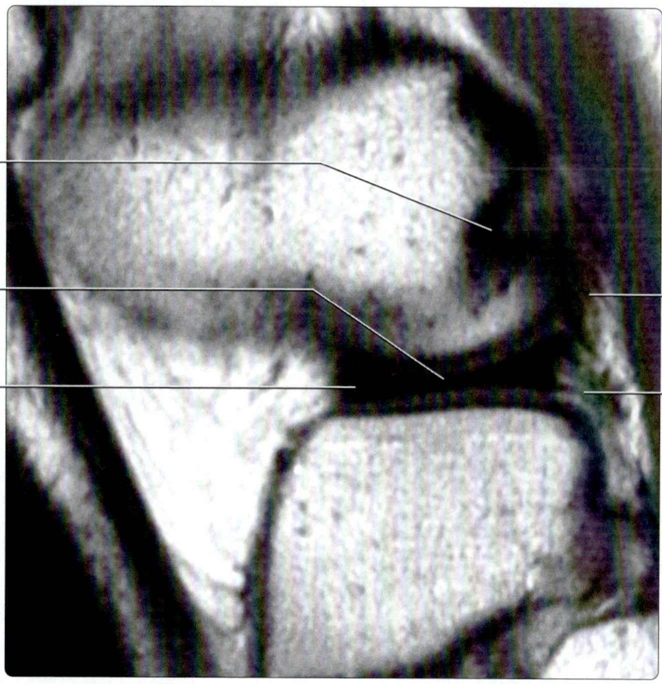

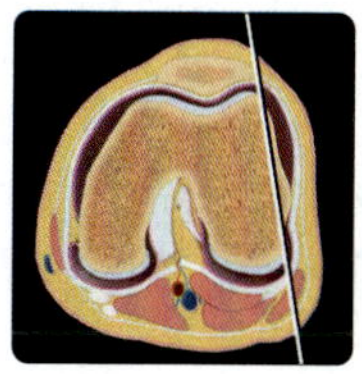

(Top) *Sagittal PD MR through the lateral compartment shows the beginning of the bowtie configuration of the meniscus. The popliteal tendon is within the hiatus, outlined superiorly by the superior popliteomeniscal fascicle and inferiorly by the inferior popliteomeniscal fascicle.* **(Bottom)** *Farther laterally, the lateral meniscus has a bowtie configuration with a thin central body flaring into the anterior and posterior horns. The origin of the popliteus tendon (located just anteriorly and inferiorly to the origin of the lateral collateral ligament on the lateral femoral condyle) is seen. A portion of the popliteal tendon is seen coursing towards its intraarticular position in the popliteal hiatus. The superior popliteomeniscal fascicle has not yet formed as the popliteal tendon passes the superior portion of the posterior horn, but the inferior popliteomeniscal fascicle clearly forms the floor of the hiatus.*

GRAPHICS: CORONAL MENISCI

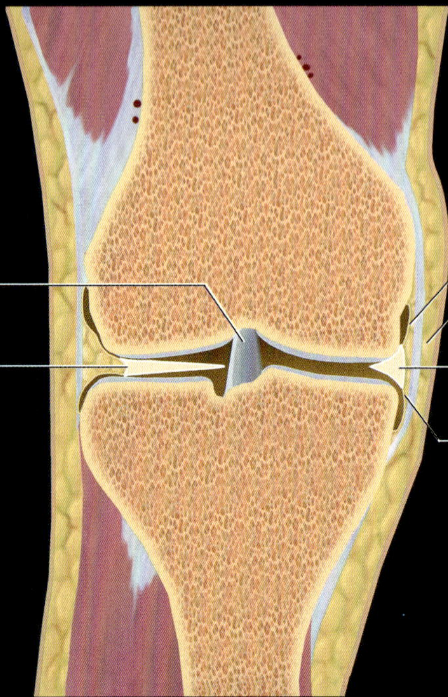

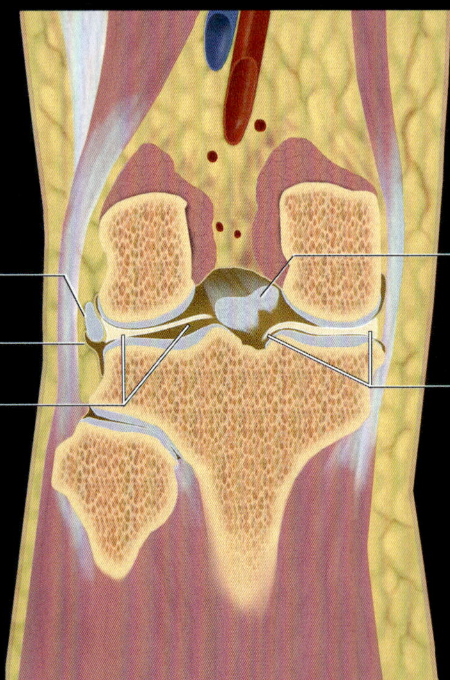

(Top) *Coronal graphic through the anterior/mid knee joint shows the anterior horn near the root of the lateral meniscus. The same cut shows the body of the medial meniscus, which is short and shaped as an equilateral triangle. The deep fibers of the medial collateral ligament arise from the body of the medial meniscus; the meniscofemoral ligament inserts either on the femoral condyle or the superficial medial collateral ligament while the meniscotibial (coronary) ligament inserts on the tibia.* **(Bottom)** *Coronal graphic more posteriorly shows the posterior root of the medial meniscus. Note that it curves around the central margin of the medial tibial plateau, in a characteristic comma shape. The posterior root of the lateral meniscus will insert slightly anterior to this, and forms a similar curve around the central margin of the lateral tibial plateau.*

CORONAL T2 FS MR: MENISCI

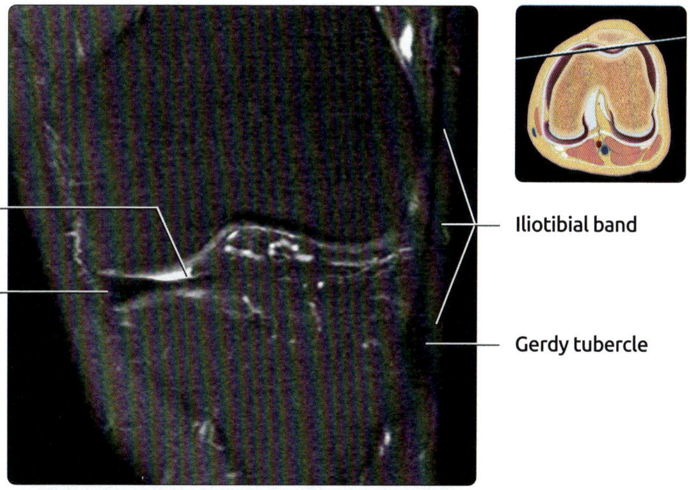

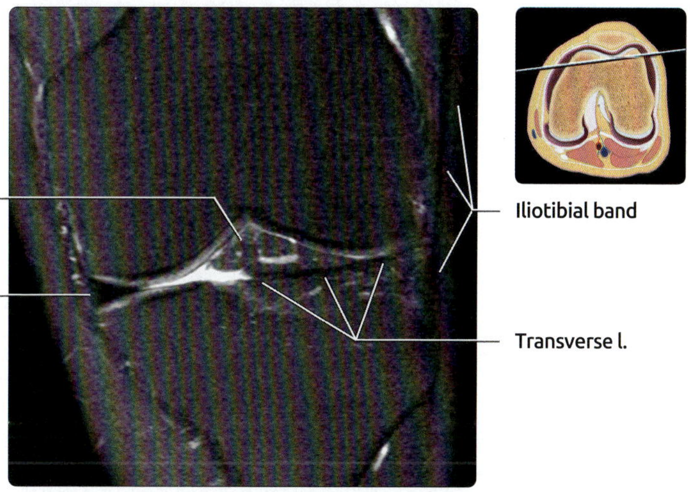

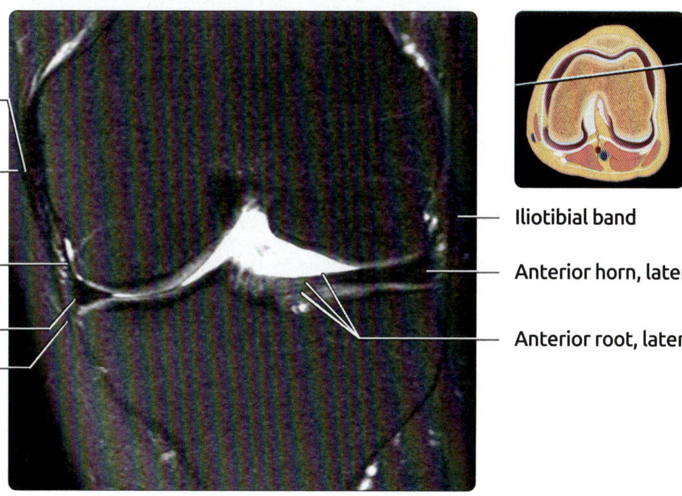

(Top) *First of 9 coronal T2 FS MR images, anterior to posterior, is shown. Anterior cut shows that the anterior horn of medial meniscus is located anterior to the anterior horn of lateral meniscus. This appearance is due to the obliquity of the image. Transverse ligament extends from the anterior horn of medial meniscus toward the anterior horn of lateral meniscus.* **(Middle)** *Transverse ligament extends toward anterior horn of the lateral meniscus, which itself is not yet visible due to the obliquity of the image.* **(Bottom)** *The root of the anterior horn of lateral meniscus is several mm posterior to that of medial meniscus. Note its division into distinct fascicles. By this cut, medial meniscus is transforming from anterior horn to body. In mid portion of knee, there is separation between layer 2 and 3 of medial supporting structures (superficial & deep fibers of medial collateral ligament, respectively). Deep fibers consist of meniscofemoral ligament, extending from body of meniscus to superficial medial collateral ligament, and meniscotibial (coronary) ligament.*

CORONAL T2 FS MR: MENISCI

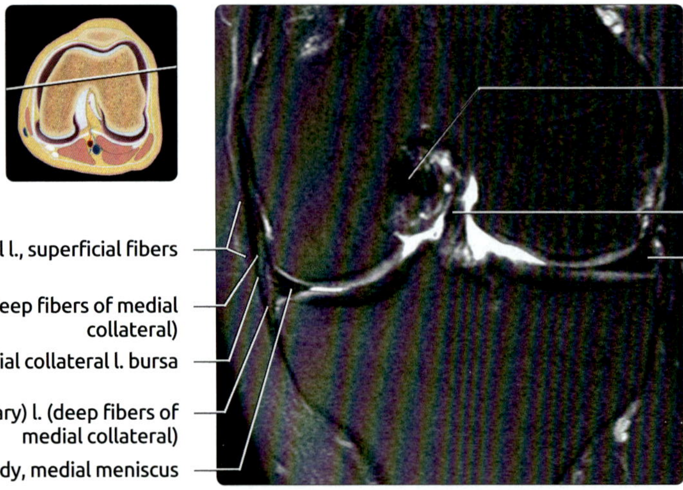

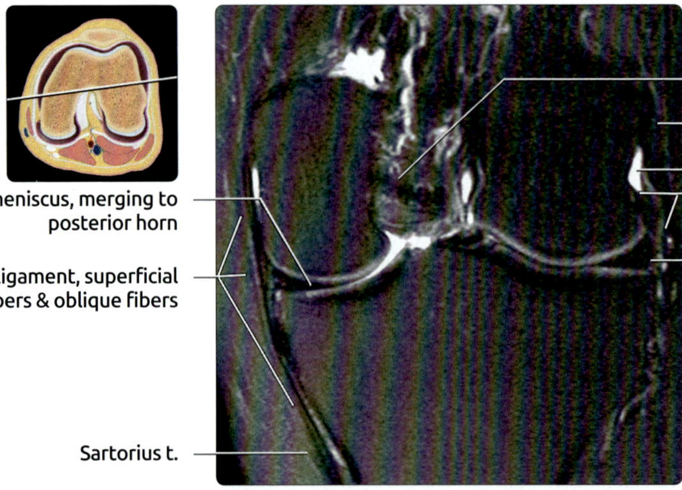

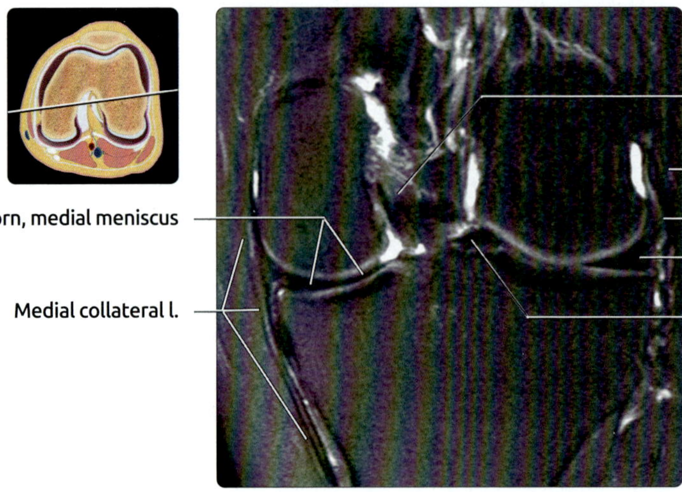

(Top) *Coronal cut through the mid joint shows the body of the medial meniscus to be the smallest, approaching an equilateral triangle in shape. The anterior cruciate ligament is reliably seen in this mid cut, as are both the deep and superficial layers of the medial collateral ligament.* **(Middle)** *In a cut that is slightly more posterior, note the deep and superficial layers of the medial collateral ligament merge together. On the lateral side, the popliteal tendon is seen at its origin, extending towards the joint line. The body of the lateral meniscus is still firmly attached to the capsule.* **(Bottom)** *Even more posteriorly, the medial meniscus is transforming to its posterior horn. On the lateral side, the popliteal tendon is seen entering the joint superiorly to the body of the lateral meniscus, at the beginning of the popliteal hiatus.*

CORONAL T2 FS MR: MENISCI

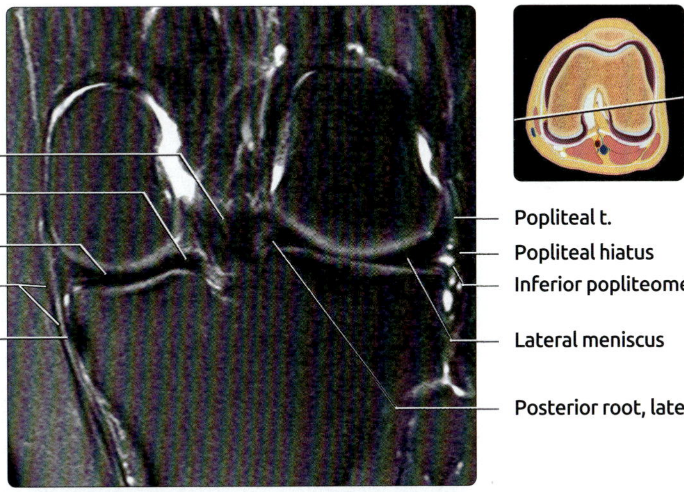

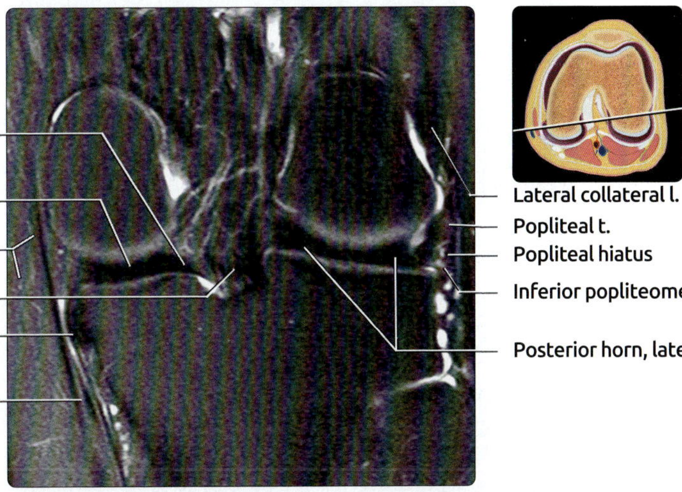

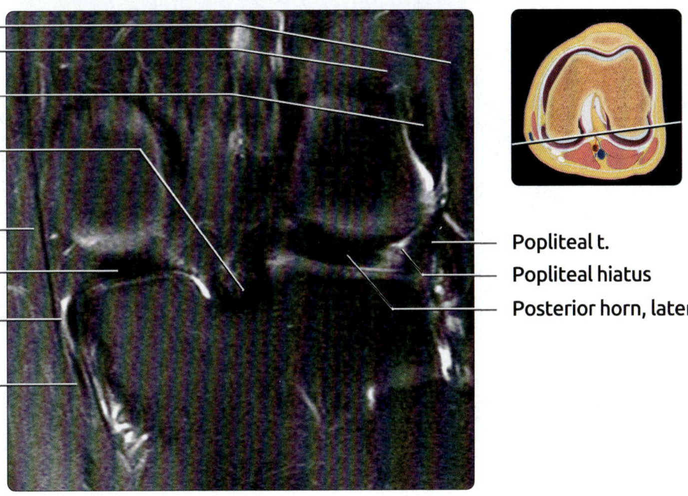

(Top) *Both posterior roots are visible on this image, curving around the central margin of their respective tibial plateaus to lie adjacent to the posterior cruciate ligament. Medially, the medial collateral ligament has merged with the capsule. Laterally, the popliteal tendon enters the articular space by way of the popliteal hiatus.* **(Middle)** *The popliteal hiatus becomes more prominent as the tendon extends posteriorly and downward. The inferior popliteomeniscal fascicle forms the floor of the popliteal hiatus at this point.* **(Bottom)** *At the posterior extent of the intraarticular portion of the knee joint, the popliteal tendon crosses in its downward and posterior course to its musculotendinous junction. The hiatus is prominent here, and must not be mistaken for a tear in the posterior horn of the lateral meniscus. Both posterior horns are seen this far posteriorly, beyond their roots (which are located more anteriorly).*

VARIANT: DISCOID MENISCUS

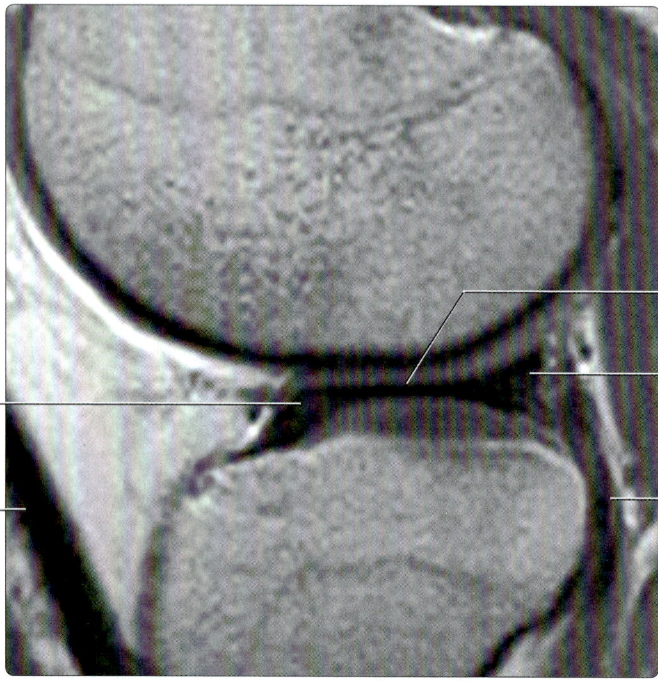

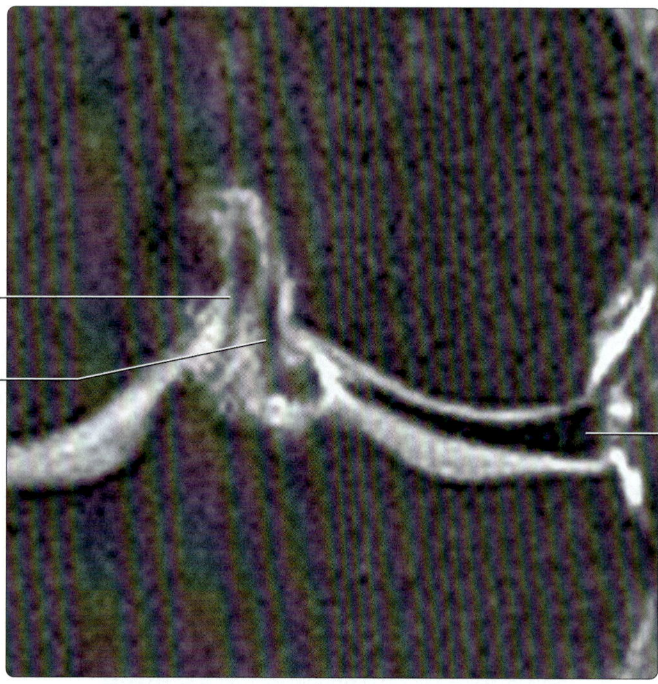

(Top) *Sagittal image of the mid portion of the lateral compartment shows a discoid lateral meniscus. Note that the meniscus is seen with all 3 portions (anterior horn, body, and posterior horn). This bowtie appearance should be seen only in the outer portion of the joint. The fact that the fibula is not seen, as well as that the popliteus musculotendinous junction (rather than just the popliteus tendon) and patellar tendon are both in this image, indicates that the location is far too interior in the joint for a normal body of meniscus to be seen. Thus, the body of the meniscus is too large, indicating the discoid variant.* **(Bottom)** *Coronal image through the mid portion of the joint (as indicated by the morphology and presence of the ACL) shows the body of the lateral meniscus to be too large, confirming that it is discoid.*

ARTHROGRAM: DISTENDED JOINT SHOWING POSTERIOR MENISCAL ATTACHMENTS

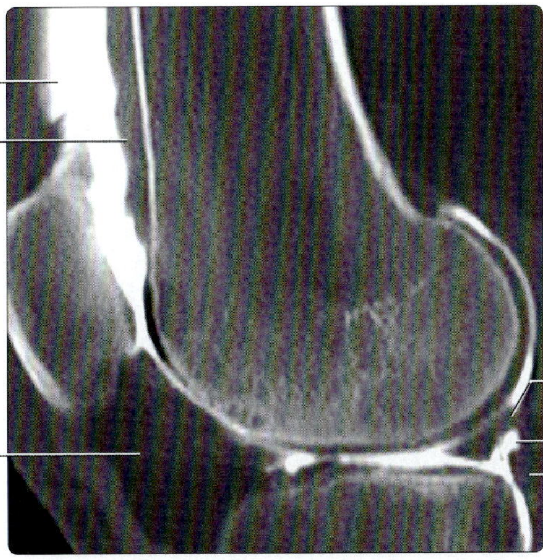

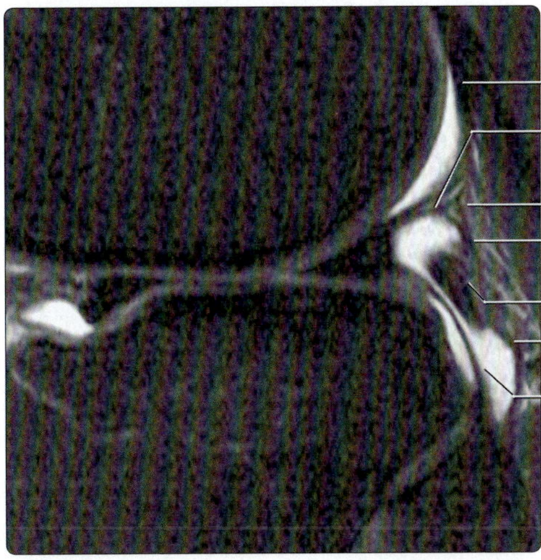

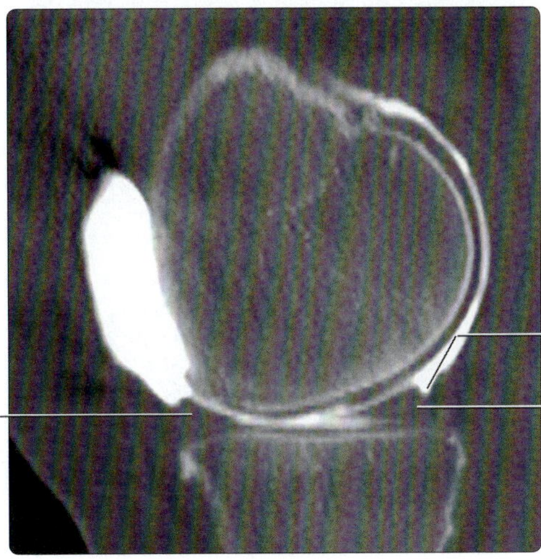

(Top) *Reformatted sagittal PD MR shows the lateral compartment. Note that, with distension of the joint by contrast, continuum of the joint fluid with the popliteal hiatus is readily seen. The superior popliteomeniscal fascicle, extending between the posterior horn of the lateral meniscus and the popliteal paratenon, is outlined by fluid.* **(Middle)** *MR arthrogram shows distended popliteal hiatus and outlines both the superior and inferior meniscopopliteal fascicles (struts) as well as the popliteal tendon. The popliteofibular and arcuate ligaments are seen well.* **(Bottom)** *Reformatted sagittal CT arthrogram through the medial compartment shows the superior recess of the posterior horn of the medial meniscus. This should not be mistaken for a peripheral meniscal tear or meniscocapsular separation. Note that cartilage width varies over the femoral condyle (thicker posteriorly).*

MENISCOFEMORAL LIGAMENT

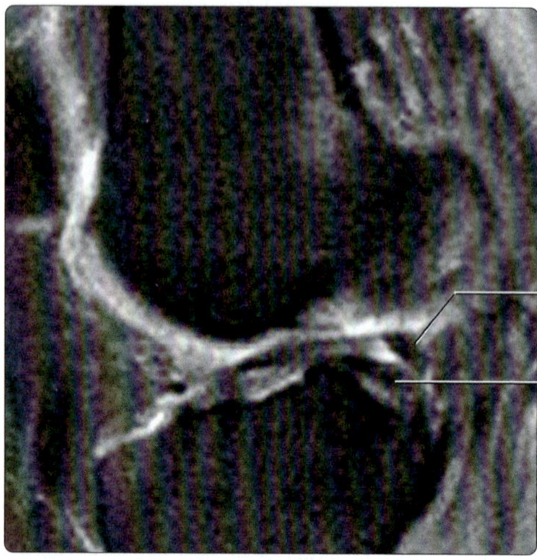

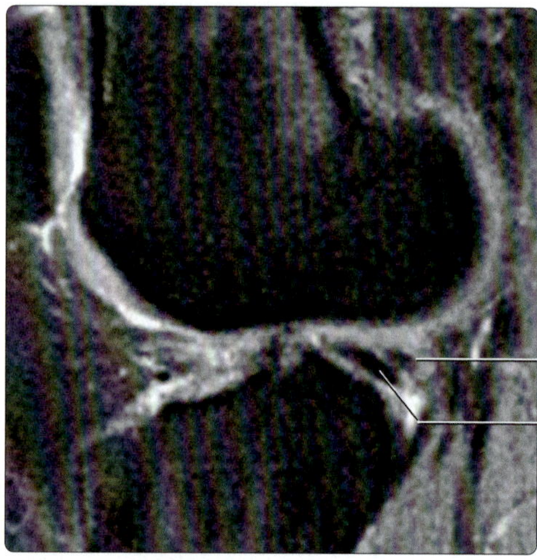

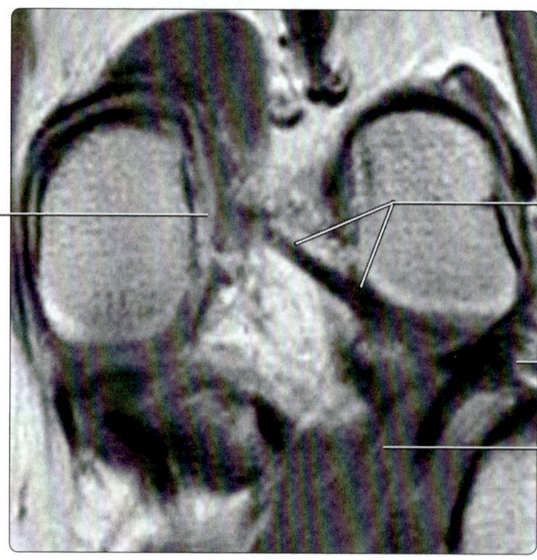

(Top) *First of 3 images depicting the meniscofemoral ligament of Wrisberg is shown. This sagittal image is slightly lateral to the intercondylar notch and the root of the posterior horn of lateral meniscus. The meniscofemoral ligament is distinctly separate from the meniscus.* **(Middle)** *Approaching the intercondylar notch and the root of posterior horn of the lateral meniscus, the meniscofemoral ligament more closely approaches the lateral meniscus to merge with it. It is at this point that a tear of the posterior horn could be mistakenly diagnosed.* **(Bottom)** *Coronal image located posteriorly in the joint shows the meniscofemoral ligament of Wrisberg over nearly its entire extent, originating at the medial femoral condyle in the intertrochanteric notch and merging with the posterior horn of the lateral meniscus.*

VARIANTS: LARGE TRANSVERSE LIGAMENT & MENISCOCRUCIATE LIGAMENT

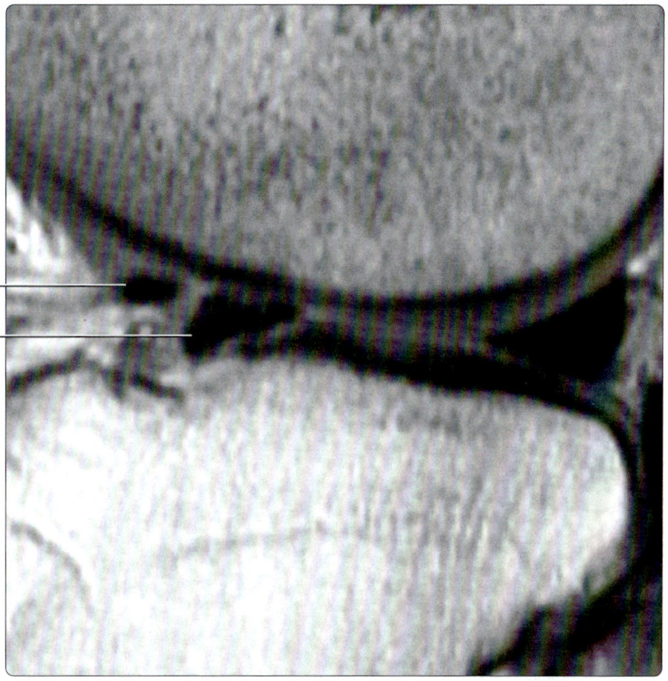

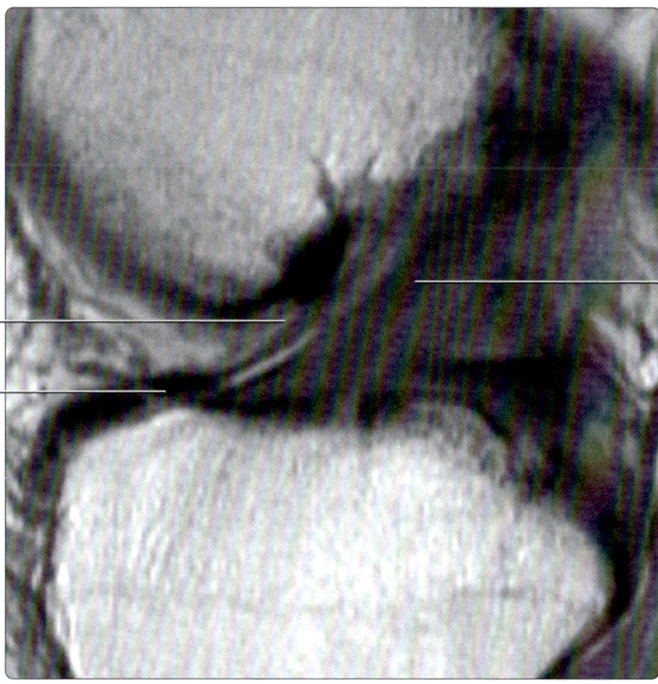

(Top) *First of 2 sagittal PD MR images near the intercondylar notch, lateral to medial, shows a large transverse ligament. This ligament connects the 2 anterior meniscal horns and is seen in cross section on sagittal images. It could possibly be confused for a meniscal tear as it merges with the lateral meniscus, closer to the notch. The ligament is generally smaller than this, or may be absent.* **(Bottom)** *Sagittal PD MR through the lateral portion of the intercondylar notch shows a discrete structure that parallels the anterior cruciate ligament and extends from the root of the anterior horn of the lateral meniscus to the lateral femoral condyle. This represents the normal variant, anterior lateral meniscocruciate ligament. It is distinguished from the infrapatellar plica (which can also parallel the ACL in the same manner) by its site of origin at the meniscus rather than the patella.*

VARIANT: MENISCOCRUCIATE LIGAMENT

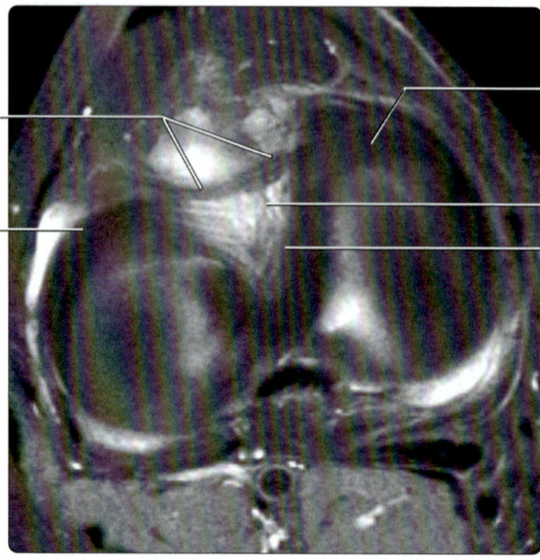

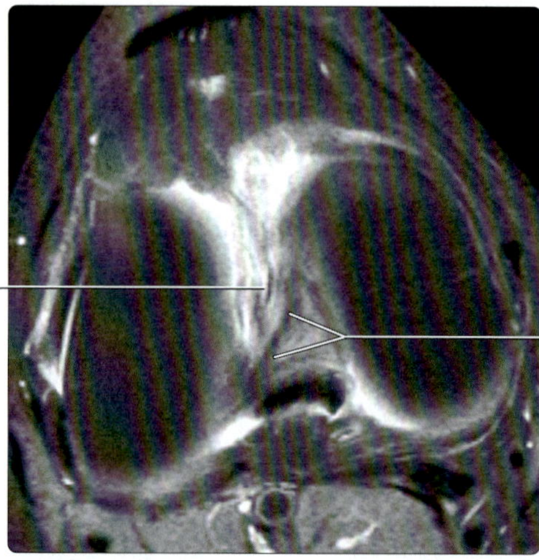

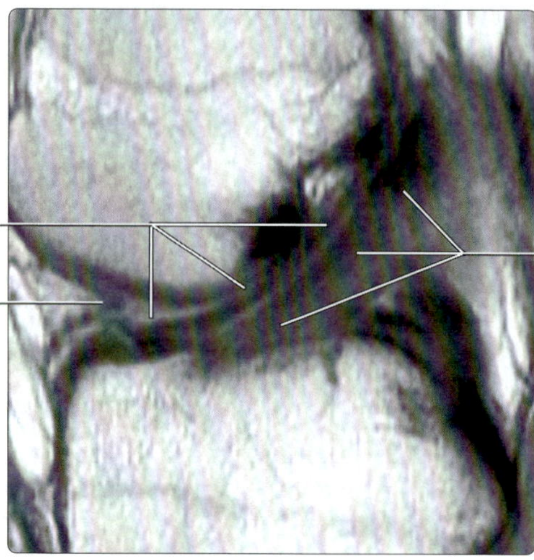

(Top) *First of 2 axial PD FS MR images at the level of the joint line shows a slightly tethered transverse ligament with an anterior meniscocruciate ligament arising from it. Note that the ligament is anterior to the anterior cruciate ligament.* **(Middle)** *Axial PD FS MR, slightly higher than the previous image, shows the intercondylar notch. The anterior meniscocruciate ligament parallels the anterior cruciate ligament throughout the notch.* **(Bottom)** *Sagittal PD MR shows the length of the anterior meniscocruciate ligament, paralleling the anterior cruciate ligament. This normal variant should not be mistaken for an intrasubstance tear of the anterior cruciate. Note that the apex of the Hoffa fat pad is free of this ligament (not attached as in an infrapatellar plica).*

VARIANT: MENISCOCRUCIATE FASCICLES

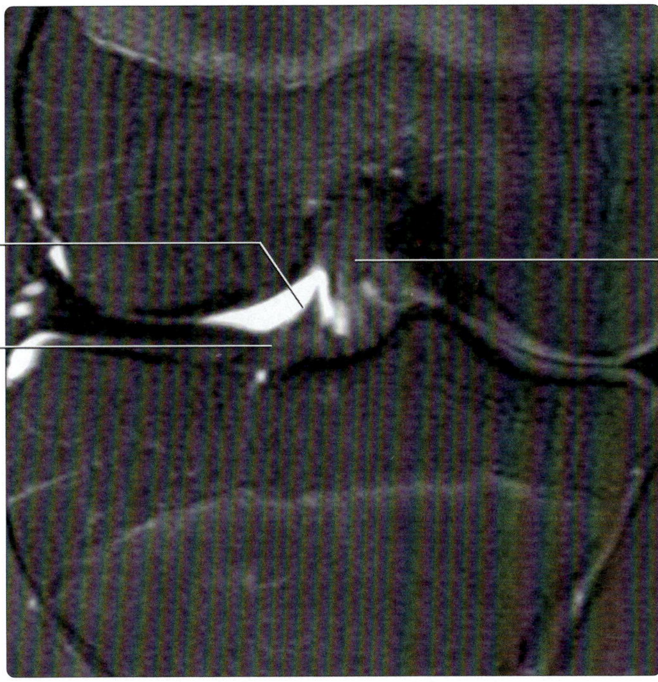

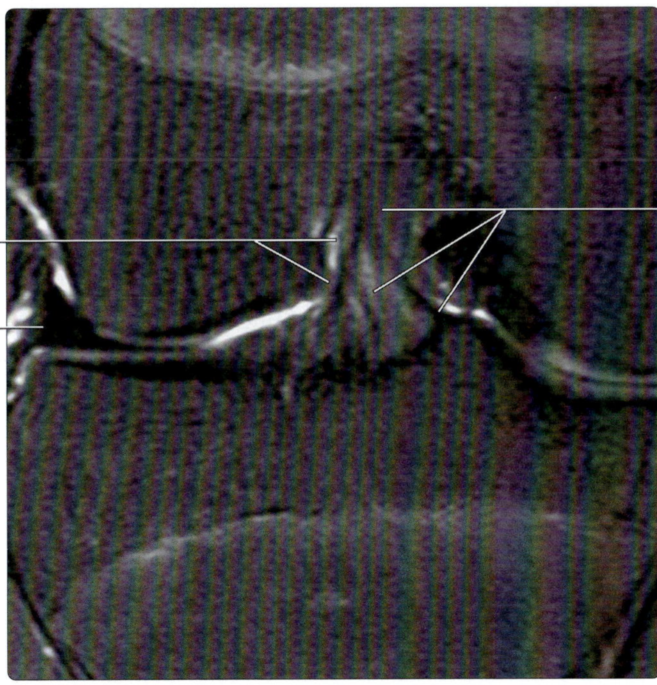

(Top) *First of 2 coronal PD FS MR images in the anterior portion of the joint is shown. The transverse ligament in this patient was absent (more anterior cut not shown). The fibers of the anterior horn of the lateral meniscus, which normally blend into the transverse ligament, instead form discrete lateral meniscal fascicles, which ascend toward the ACL.* **(Bottom)** *Coronal PD FS MR, slightly posterior to the previous image, shows the lateral meniscal fascicles ascending to intersect the anterior cruciate ligament. These fibers clearly are not part of the ACL since they ascend at a different angle. This normal variant should not be mistaken for pathology such as a disrupted ACL or a meniscal fragment from a bucket handle tear.*

VARIANT: MENISCOMENISCAL LIGAMENT

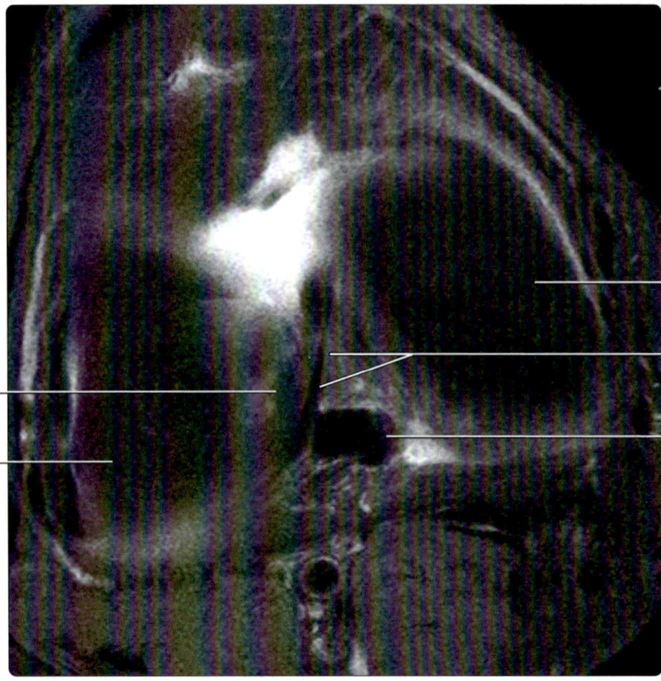

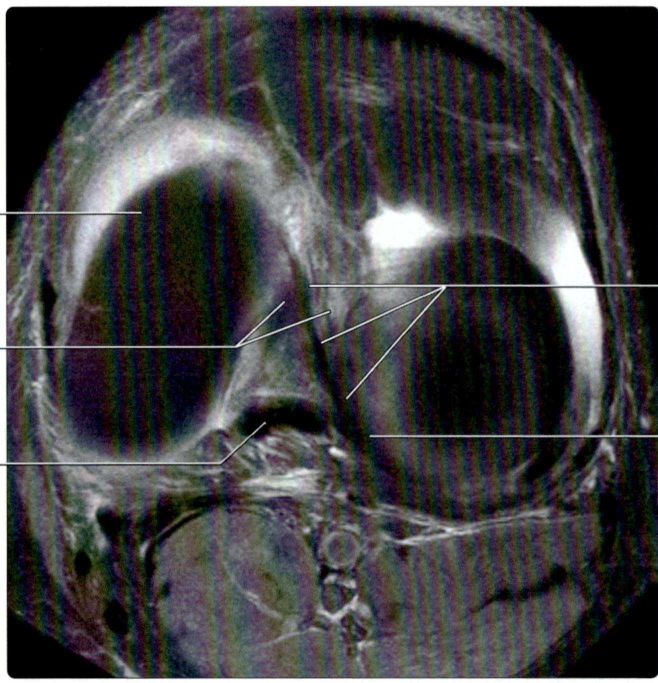

(Top) *Axial image, just above the joint line, shows the normal variant medial oblique meniscomeniscal ligament. It arises from the anterior horn of the medial meniscus and inserts on the posterior horn of the lateral meniscus, threading its way between the ACL and PCL.* **(Bottom)** *First of 3 PD FS MR images through the joint line shows a normal variant, the medial oblique meniscomeniscal ligament. The ligament extends from the anterior horn of the medial meniscus across the intercondylar notch to insert on the posterior horn of the lateral meniscus. At this level of the menisci, the variant ligament appears to split the ACL at its insertion on the tibia. It normally extends between the ACL and PCL. The mirror image variant, lateral meniscomeniscal ligament, extends from the anterior horn of the lateral meniscus to the posterior horn of the medial meniscus (not shown here).*

VARIANT: MENISCOMENISCAL LIGAMENT

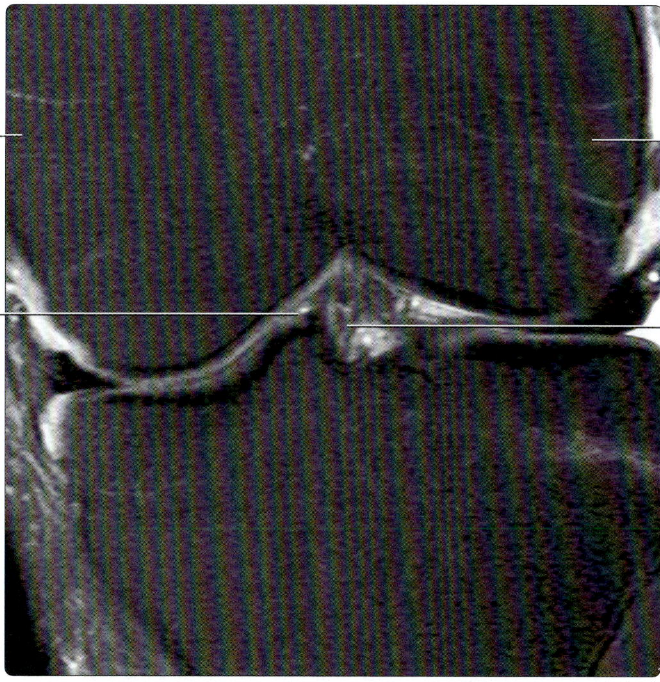

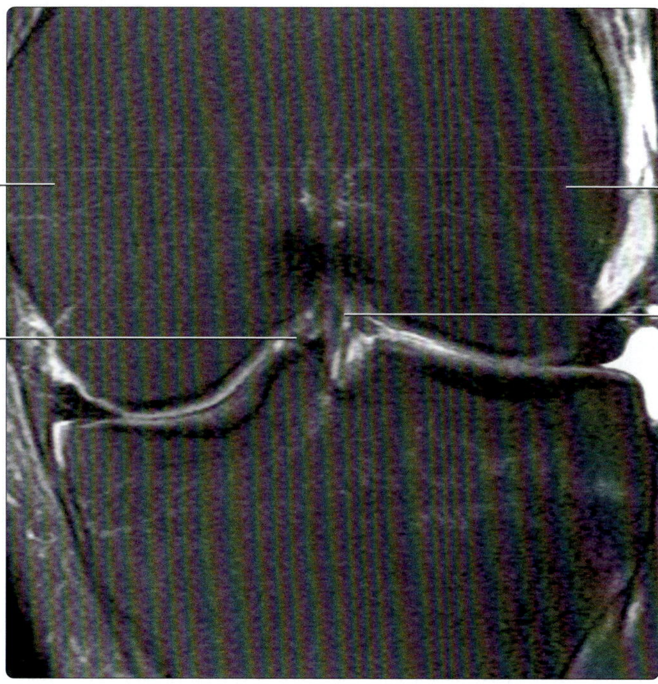

(Top) *At the anterior portion of mid joint, the tiny medial meniscomeniscal ligament is seen in cross section, adjacent to the anterior cruciate ligament. This is the same patient as shown on the immediate previous axial image.* **(Bottom)** *3 mm posterior, the meniscomeniscal ligament is shown giving the appearance of a loose body or fragment adjacent to the ACL. The location and low signal of this normal variant ligament may be misdiagnosed as a meniscal fragment or bucket handle fragment. It is important to correlate it with the appearance on either axial or sagittal images, where the ligament will be seen as a longitudinal structure placed between the ACL and PCL and angling obliquely across the notch between the 2 menisci.*

TERMINOLOGY

Abbreviations

- Anterior cruciate ligament (ACL)
- Posterior cruciate ligament (PCL)

IMAGING ANATOMY

Overview

- Cruciate ligaments are in **extrasynovial but intracapsular** location
  - Fatty tissue lies between cruciates
  - Synovial membrane surrounds anterior, medial, and lateral portions of cruciates but is reflected posteriorly from PCL to adjoining parts of joint capsule

ACL

- **Multiple separate fascicles**, which spiral laterally from femur to tibia (fibers rotate externally 90°); fatty tissue is seen between fibers
  - Continuum of fibers allows variable tension, with some taut throughout knee range of motion
  - **Anteromedial bundle**: Tight in flexion, lax in extension
  - **Posterolateral bundle**: Tight in extension, lax in flexion
- **Origin of ACL**: Posteriorly from lateral femoral condyle at intercondylar notch (seen on radiograph as junction of posterior femoral cortex and Blumensaat line)
- **Insertion of ACL**: Anteromedial tibial spine and adjacent plateau; bundles fan out at tibial attachment, forming "foot"
- **Function**
  - Primary restraint to anterior tibial translation
  - Major secondary restraint to internal rotation; minor secondary restraint to external rotation
  - Minor secondary restraint to varus/valgus at full extension
- **MR imaging**: Seen well in all 3 planes, low signal with fat interspersed between bundles
- Blood supply: Middle geniculate artery (pierces posterior capsule from popliteal); lesser supply from fat pad (inferior medial and lateral geniculates)
- Nerve: Posterior articular (branch of posterior tibial)

PCL

- **Appears as single round ligament** but consists of 2 major parts; rotates 90° from anteroposterior alignment at femoral origin to medial-lateral alignment at insertion on posterior tibia
  - **Anterolateral bundle**: Bulk of ligament, taut in flexion, lax in extension
  - **Posteromedial (oblique) bundle**: Taut in extension, lax in flexion
- **Origin of PCL**: Mid portion of medial femoral condyle at intercondylar notch
- **Insertion of PCL**: Mid posterior tibia, 1 cm below joint line, where it blends in with posterior capsule
- **Function**: Primary restraint against posterior translation
- **Meniscofemoral ligaments**
  - Both arise from posterior horn lateral meniscus and insert on medial femoral condyle; at least 1 present 70% of time
  - **Posterior (Wrisberg)** lies posterior to PCL
  - **Anterior (Humphrey)** lies anterior to PCL; intact ligament of Humphrey may mimic intact PCL in setting of complete PCL tear
  - May play role in secondary restraint to posterior instability; may stabilize lateral meniscus during flexion
- **MR imaging**: Seen well in all 3 planes, solid low signal throughout
- Blood supply: Middle geniculate artery proximal and middle 1/3; geniculate and popliteal artery base; capsular vessels through entire length

Posterior Capsule

- **Complex fibrous structure**: Augmented by extensions of adjacent tendons
- **Incomplete**: Pierced centrally by neurovascular structures
- **Proximal attachment**: Vertical fibers attached to posterior margins of femoral condyles and intercondylar fossae
- **Distal attachment** is to posterior margins of tibial condyles and intercondylar areas
- **Tendons/ligaments**: Attach to posterior capsule to provide reinforcement
  - **Proximally** (medially and laterally): Tendinous heads of gastrocnemius
  - **Posteromedial corner**: Semimembranosus and posterior oblique ligament
  - **Posterolateral corner**: Arcuate ligament and iliotibial tract
  - **Posterior central**: Oblique popliteal ligament

Spaces Within Cruciate/Posterior Capsule

- Synovial membrane surrounds anterior, medial, and lateral portions of cruciates but is reflected posteriorly from PCL to adjoining parts of joint capsule
- Results in potential space (**PCL bursa or recess**)
  - Seen only when fluid filled; best on coronal and sagittal planes
  - Seen posterior to PCL and adjacent to lateral aspect of medial femoral condyle
  - No contact between PCL recess and proximal 1/3 of PCL (fat is interposed)
  - Communicates with medial (femorotibial) compartment of knee
  - Does not communicate with lateral compartment
  - If ligament of Wrisberg is present, it lies posterosuperior to PCL recess
- **Intercruciate recess**
  - Localized potential fluid collection between ACL and PCL; best seen on sagittal and axial planes
  - Communicates with either lateral or medial (femorotibial) compartments

SELECTED REFERENCES

1. De Maeseneer M et al: Normal anatomy and pathology of the posterior capsular area of the knee: findings in cadaveric specimens and in patients. AJR Am J Roentgenol. 182(4):955-62, 2004
2. Delgado GJ et al: Tennis leg: clinical US study of 141 patients and anatomic investigation of four cadavers with MR imaging and US. Radiology 224(1):112-9, 2002

SAGITTAL MR: CRUCIATE LIGAMENTS

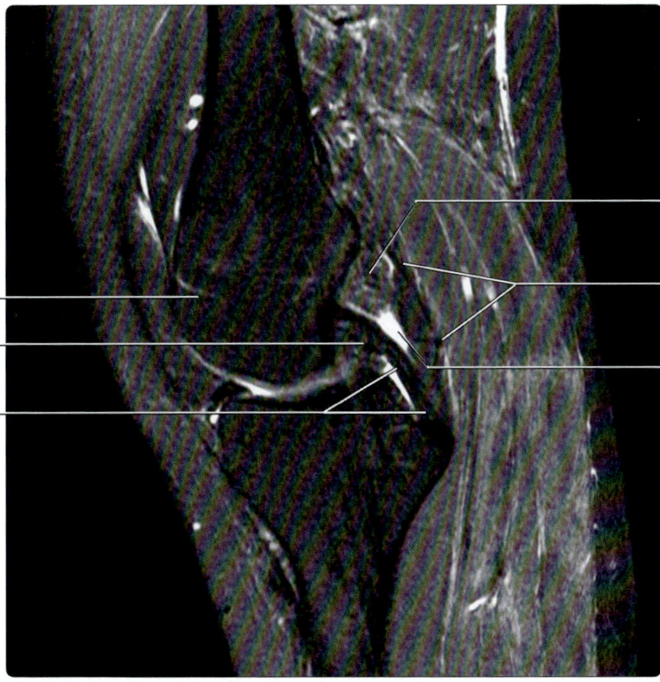

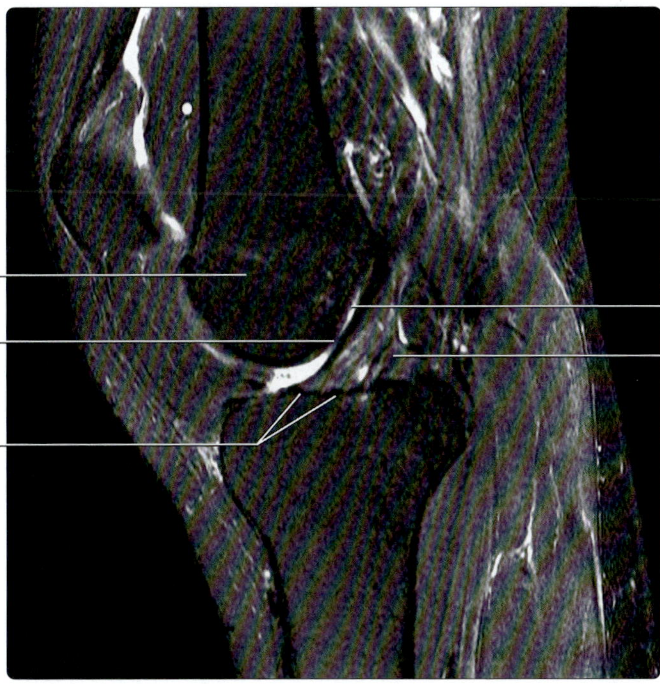

(Top) *First of 2 sagittal T2 FS MR images through the intercondylar notch in the more medial portion of the notch shows the origin of the posterior cruciate ligament (PCL) from the anterior portion of the medial notch, as well as the insertion posteriorly on the tibia, 1 cm below the joint line. The PCL appears as a thick single band, usually in at least 2 adjacent images. There is fat located immediately posterior to the proximal portion of the PCL. More distally, the posterior joint recess abuts the PCL. The posterior capsule lies behind this fat and the recess. In this case, the meniscofemoral ligament of Humphrey is present; the ligament of Wrisberg is absent.* **(Bottom)** *This image is located slightly laterally to the previous image, within the intercondylar notch. The anterior cruciate ligament (ACL) arises from the posterior lateral femoral condyle within the notch; the broad insertion on the tibial plateau is seen.*

CORONAL MR: CRUCIATE LIGAMENTS

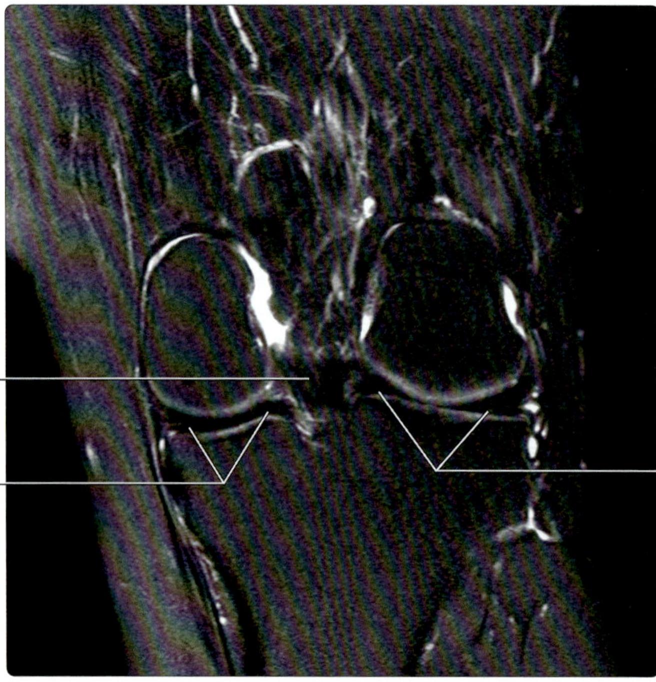

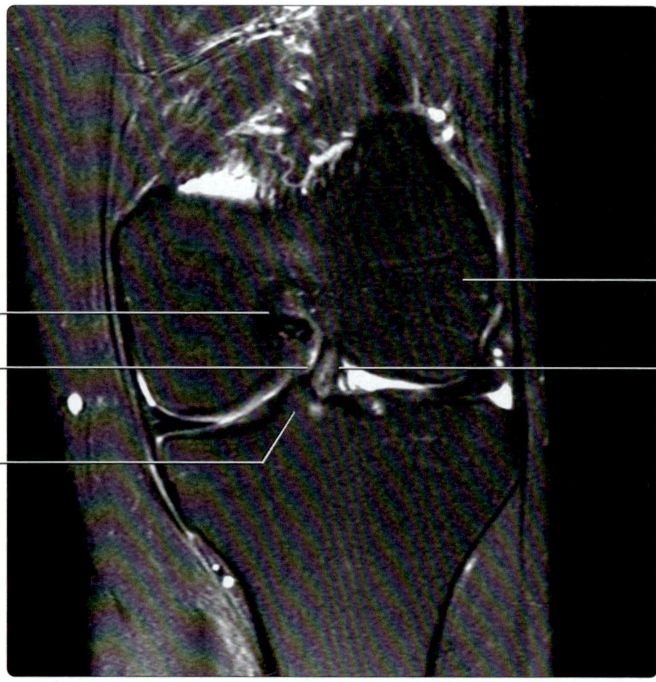

(Top) *First of 2 coronal T2 FS MR images shows the cruciate ligaments. This more posterior image shows the PCL approaching its insertion on the posterior aspect of the tibial plateau. No portion of the anterior cruciate is seen. Note that while we expect to see the ACL as a complete band on coronal images located more anteriorly, the PCL is incompletely seen on coronal images.* **(Bottom)** *This more anterior image also shows the cruciate ligaments. The anteromedial bundle and posterolateral bundle of the ACL are seen arising from the lateral femoral condyle and inserting on the tibial plateau adjacent to the medial tibial spine. Both are seen on the same cut because of the obliquity at which coronal images are obtained. Because the leg is in extension, the posterolateral bundle is taut.*

AXIAL MR: CRUCIATE LIGAMENTS

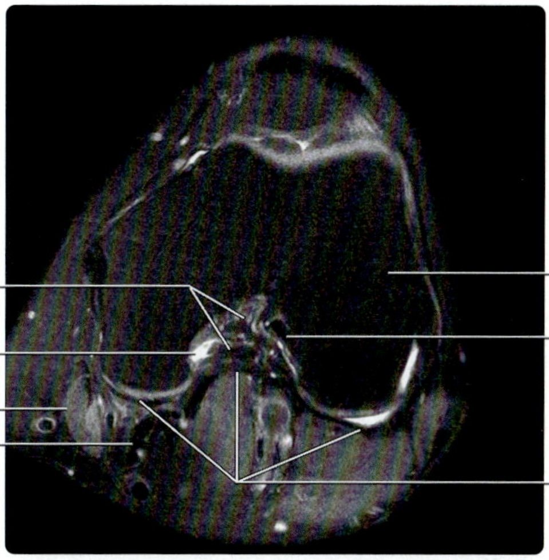

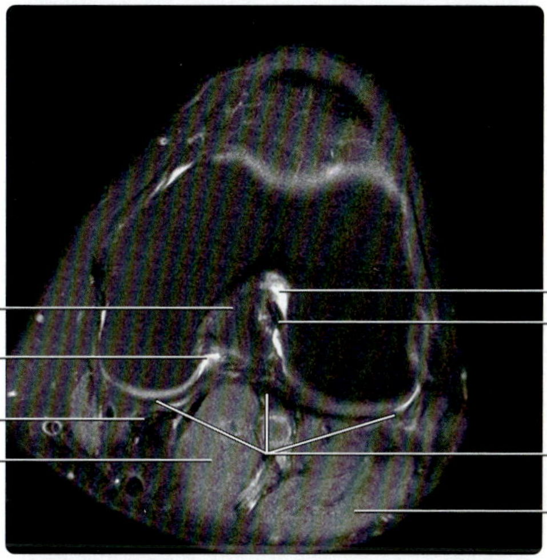

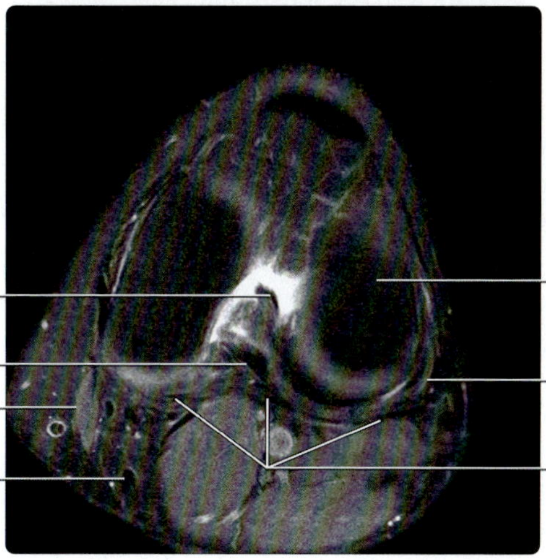

(Top) *First of 3 axial T2 FS MR images through the upper portion of the intercondylar notch shows the cruciate ligaments within the intercondylar notch. In the upper portion of the notch, the ACL is seen arising from the posterior aspect of the lateral femoral condyle within the notch. The remainder of the notch is filled with fat and is a potential space (posterior cruciate bursa).* **(Middle)** *Axial cut through the mid portion of the intercondylar notch is shown. The ACL extends obliquely toward its insertion on the tibial plateau. The origin of PCL is seen at the anterior medial femoral condyle within the notch. Fluid-filled recesses are seen anterior to the ACL and posteromedial to the PCL.* **(Bottom)** *The inferior portion of the intercondylar notch shows the ACL as it approaches insertion on the tibial plateau. The PCL is still within the capsule but beginning to blend with it as it approaches insertion on the posterior tibia. The cruciates are well seen axially.*

VARIANTS: MENISCOMENISCAL LIGAMENT AND INFRAPATELLAR PLICA

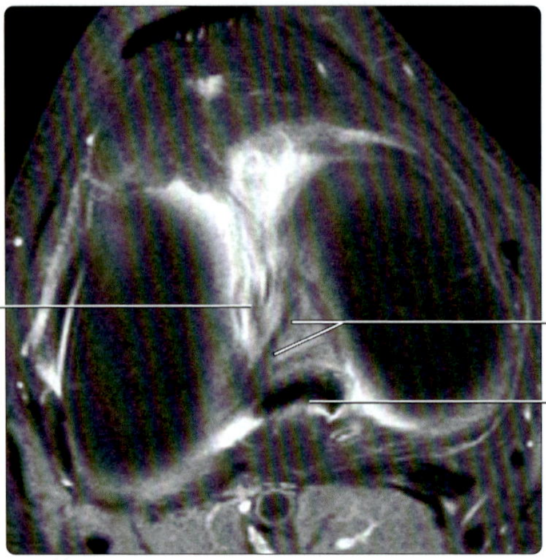

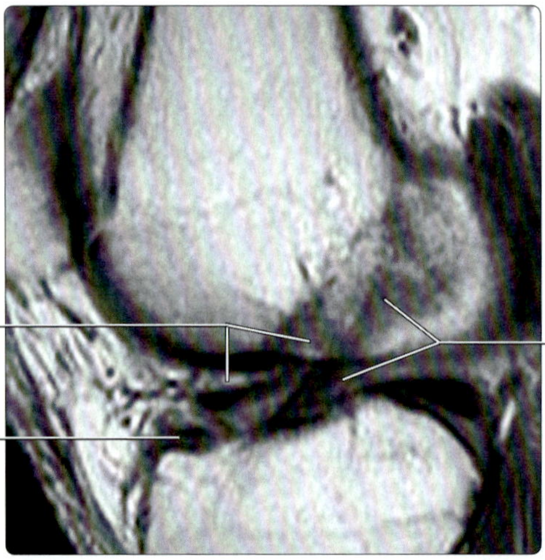

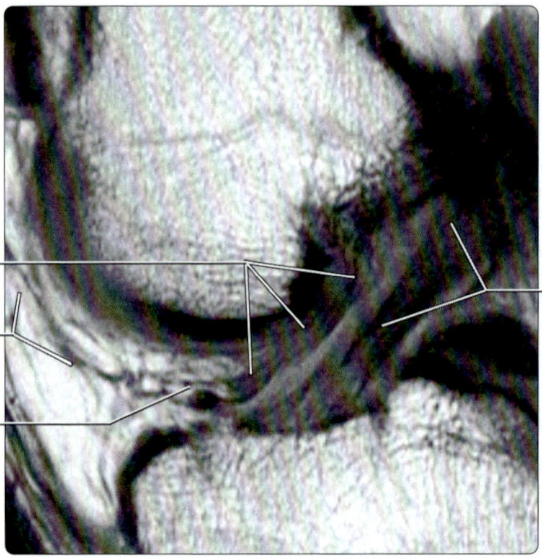

(Top) *Axial PD FS MR through the femoral condyles shows an oblique meniscomeniscal ligament. This uncommon variant connects the anterior horn of one meniscus with the posterior horn of the contralateral meniscus. It runs between the anterior and posterior cruciate ligaments.* **(Middle)** *Sagittal PD MR through the intercondylar notch shows the variant infrapatellar plica. This plica arises from the patella, extends across the Hoffa fat pad and along the anterior surface of the anterior cruciate ligament. It should not be mistaken for a longitudinal split in the ACL.* **(Bottom)** *Sagittal PD MR through the intercondylar notch shows an infrapatellar plica. The plica is seen extending through the Hoffa fat pad, paralleling the curvature of the femoral condyle, and then paralleling the anterior cruciate ligament.*

VARIANT: MENISCOCRUCIATE LIGAMENT

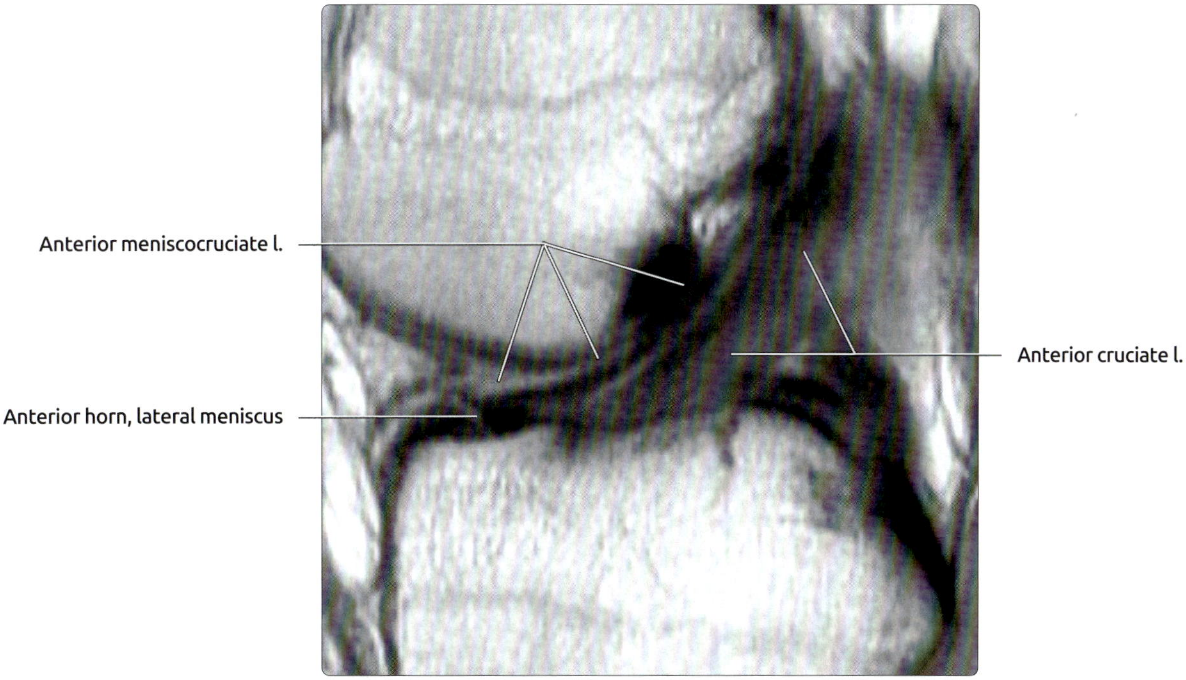

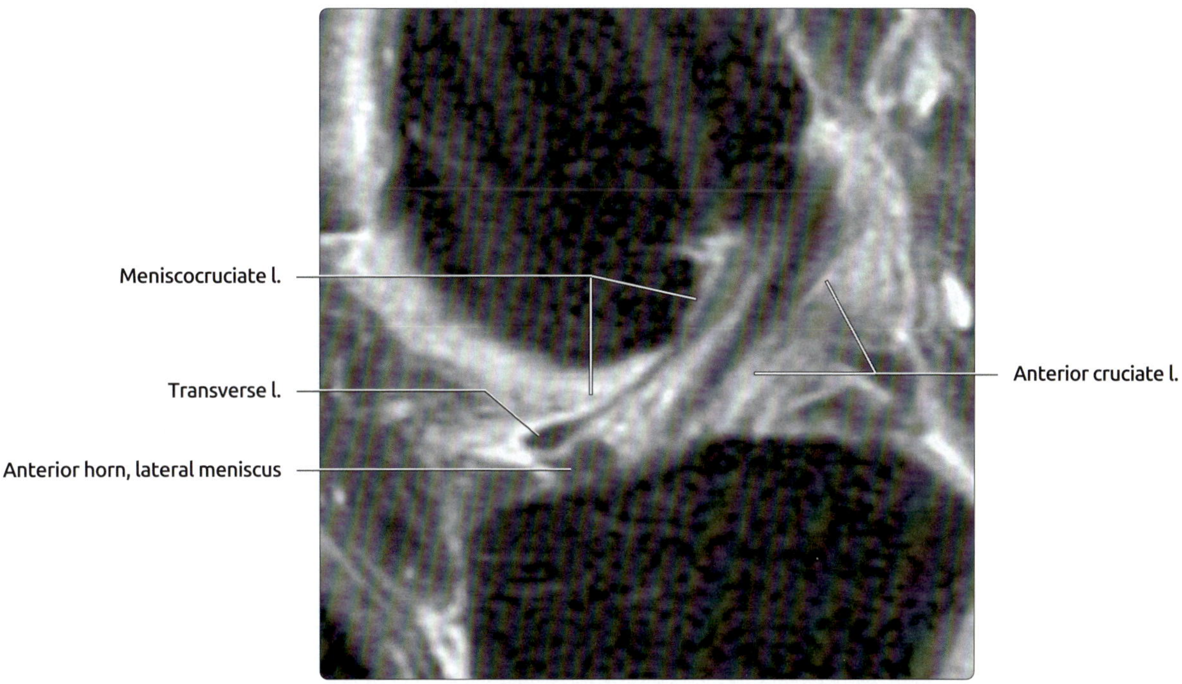

(Top) *Sagittal PD MR through the intercondylar notch shows a meniscocruciate ligament. The ligament arises from the anterior horn medial meniscus and extends along the anterior surface of the ACL to the femoral condyle. It could possibly be mistaken for a longitudinal tear in the anterior cruciate.* **(Bottom)** *Sagittal PD FS MR shows another variant meniscocruciate ligament. This ligament is arising from the transverse ligament; as it extends parallel to and anterior to the ACL it could simulate a longitudinal or partial tear in this cruciate.*

VARIANT: MENISCAL FASCICLE

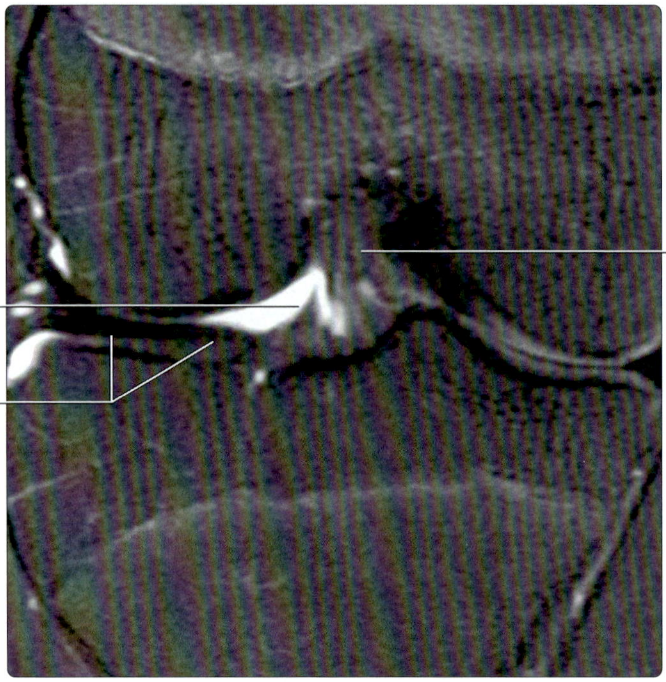

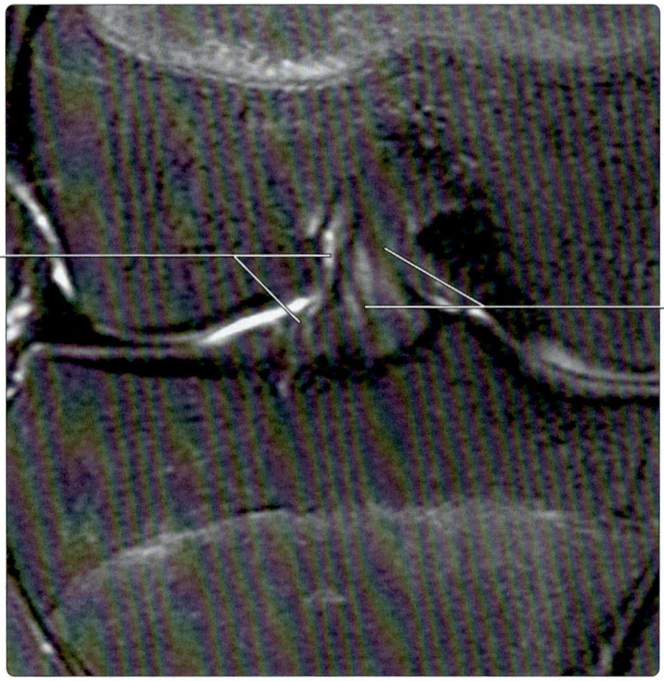

(Top) *First of 2 coronal PD FS MR images shows a variant anterior meniscal fascicle extending to the ACL. The fascicle arises from the anterior horn lateral meniscus and its root. It then extends upward to merge with the synovium over the ACL. In this anterior slice, the fascicle appears as a separate fiber. The anterior cruciate is in its normal position, extending from the lateral femoral condyle to its insertion adjacent to the medial tibial spine.* **(Bottom)** *Coronal image located slightly posterior to the previous image shows the meniscal fascicle extending from inferolateral to superomedial, an opposite angulation relative to the anterior cruciate. This is a potentially confusing appearance and should not be confused with cruciate pathology.*

MR: MENISCOFEMORAL LIGAMENT OF WRISBERG

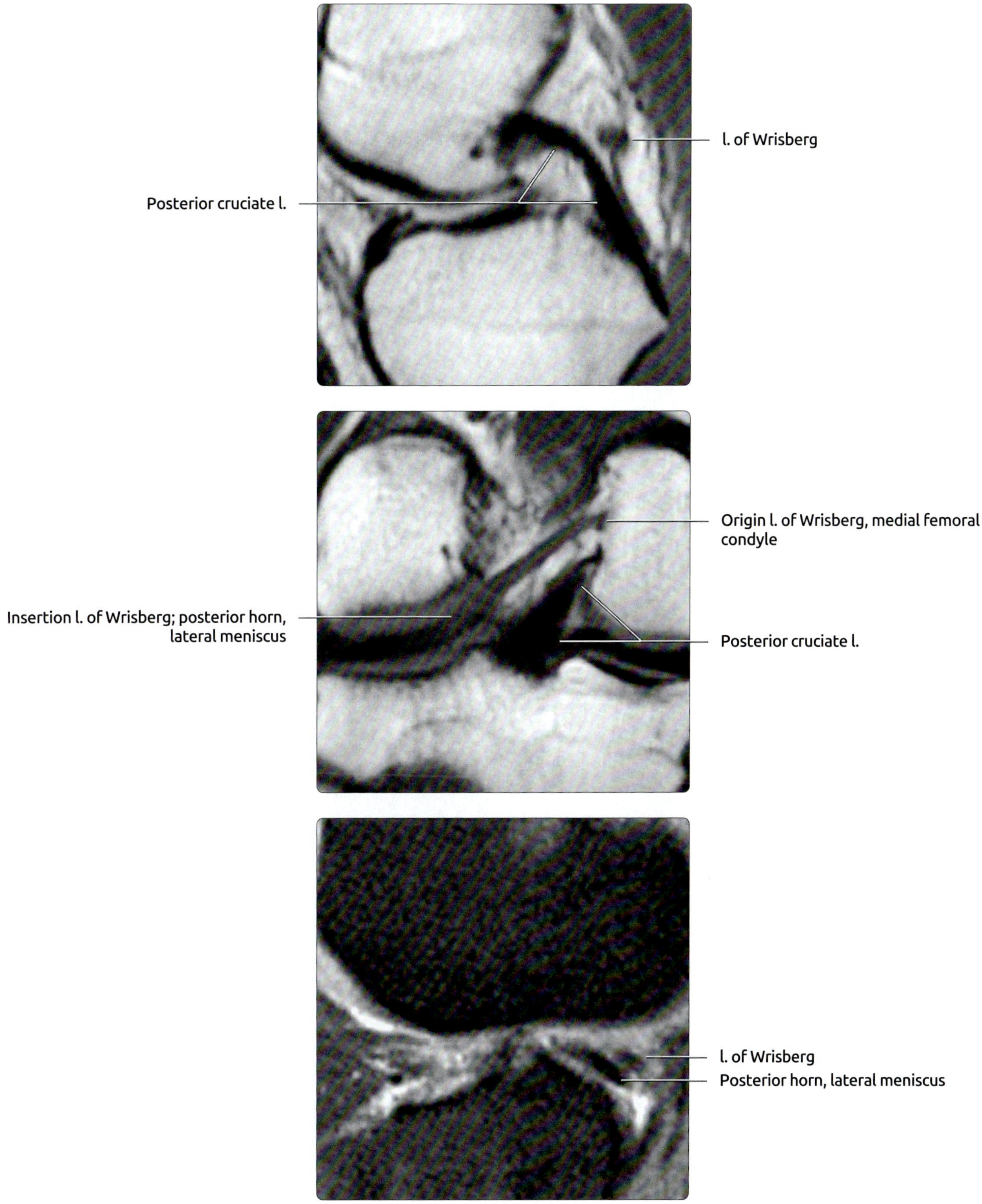

(Top) *First of 3 images of the PCL and associated posterior meniscofemoral ligament (Wrisberg) through the posterior cruciate shows the ligament of Wrisberg in cross section as it extends from the medial femoral condyle toward the posterior horn lateral meniscus.* **(Middle)** *Coronal PD MR located posteriorly in the joint shows the ligament of Wrisberg paralleling the PCL in its path from the medial femoral condyle to the posterior horn lateral meniscus.* **(Bottom)** *Sagittal PD FS MR shows the lateral compartment immediately adjacent to the intercondylar notch at the root of posterior horn lateral meniscus. The ligament of Wrisberg inserts at this point; just prior to the insertion, this appearance could give a false impression of a meniscal tear.*

MR: MENISCOFEMORAL LIGAMENT OF HUMPHREY

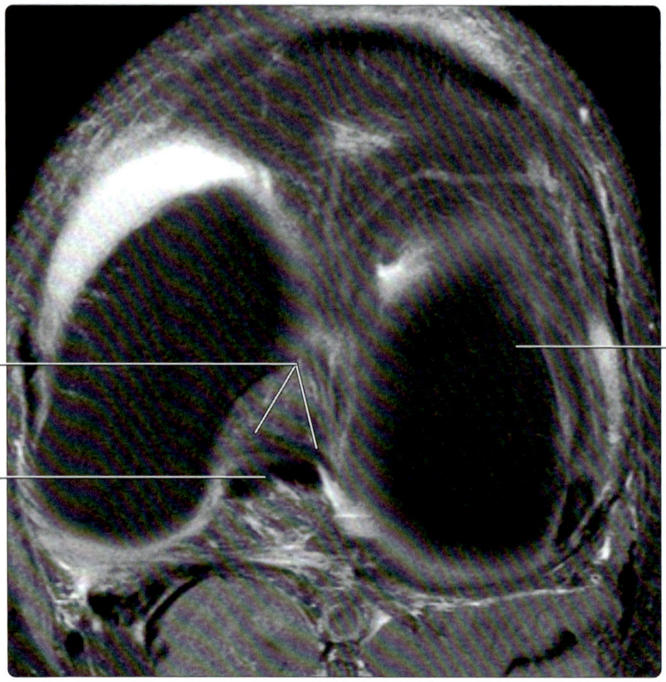

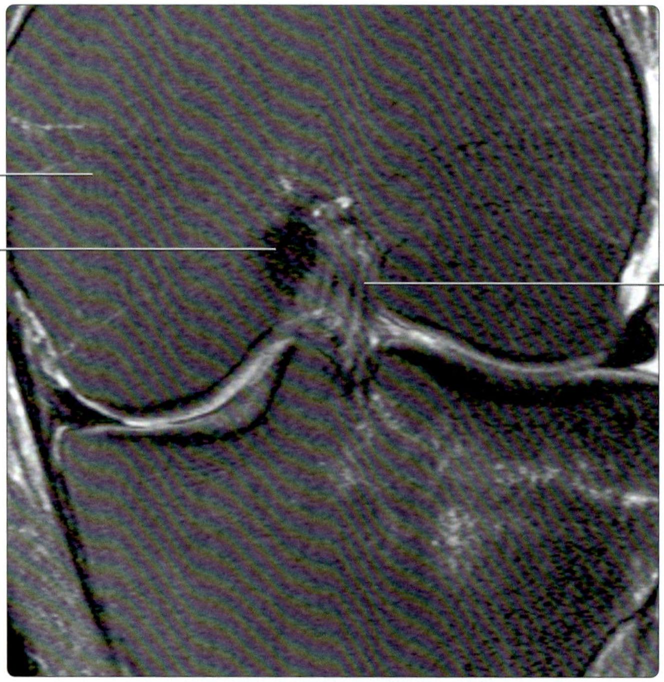

(Top) *Axial PD FS MR through the femoral condyles and intercondylar notch is shown. The meniscofemoral ligament of Humphrey extends from the medial femoral condyle across in front of the PCL toward its insertion on the posterior horn lateral meniscus.*
(Bottom) *First of 3 coronal PD FS MR images shows the ACL extending from the lateral femoral condyle toward the tibial spine. At the same level, there is a ligamentous structure arising from the medial femoral condyle. This is located slightly anterior to the origin of the PCL and is the meniscofemoral ligament of Humphrey.*

MR: MENISCOFEMORAL LIGAMENT OF HUMPHREY

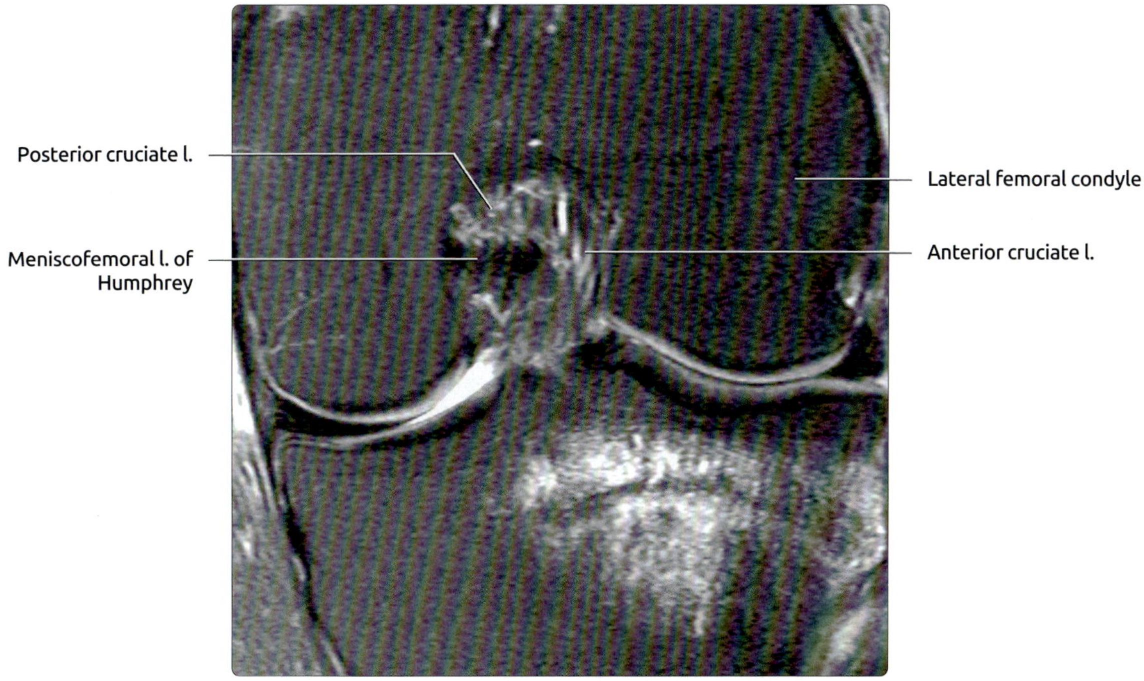

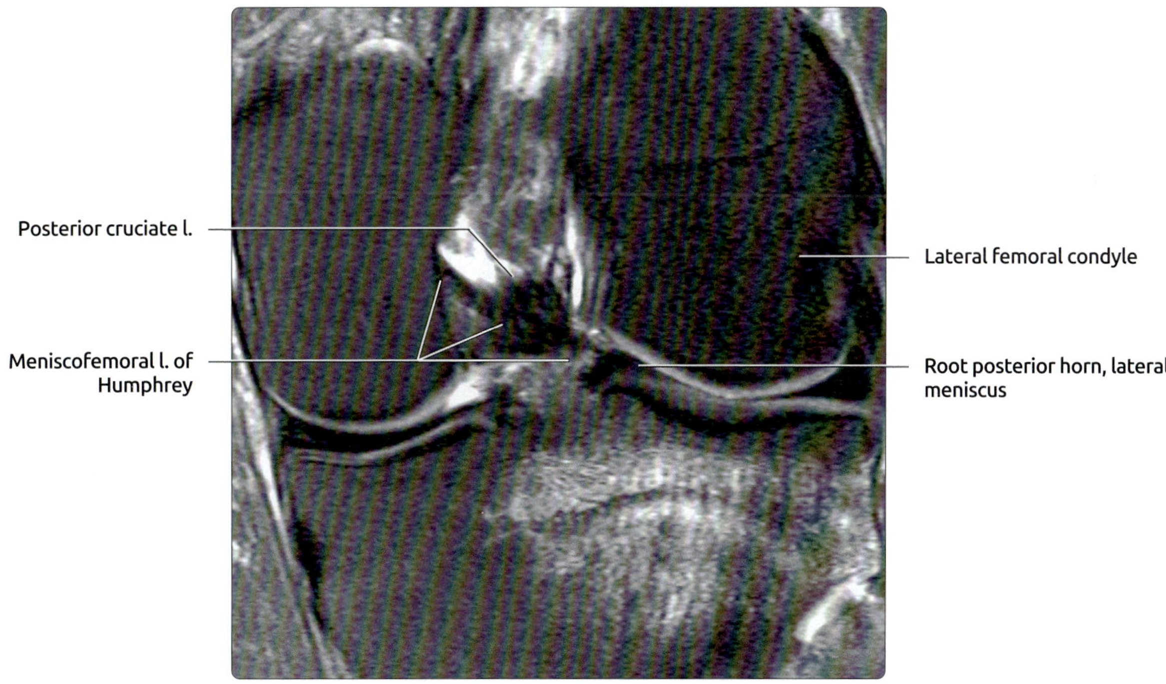

(Top) *Coronal PD FS MR located slightly posterior to the previous image is shown. The intercondylar notch is quite full, containing the normally positioned ACL as well as the origin of PCL. The origin of the meniscofemoral ligament of Humphrey is noted immediately anterior and inferior to that of posterior cruciate.* **(Bottom)** *Coronal image located further posteriorly shows the meniscofemoral ligament of Humphrey crossing from the medial femoral condyle to insert on the root of the posterior horn lateral meniscus. It crosses directly in front of the PCL. It is somewhat unusual to see it in its entirety on a single coronal image. Bone bruise on the lateral tibial plateau is incidentally seen in this example.*

MR: MENISCOFEMORAL LIGAMENT OF HUMPHREY

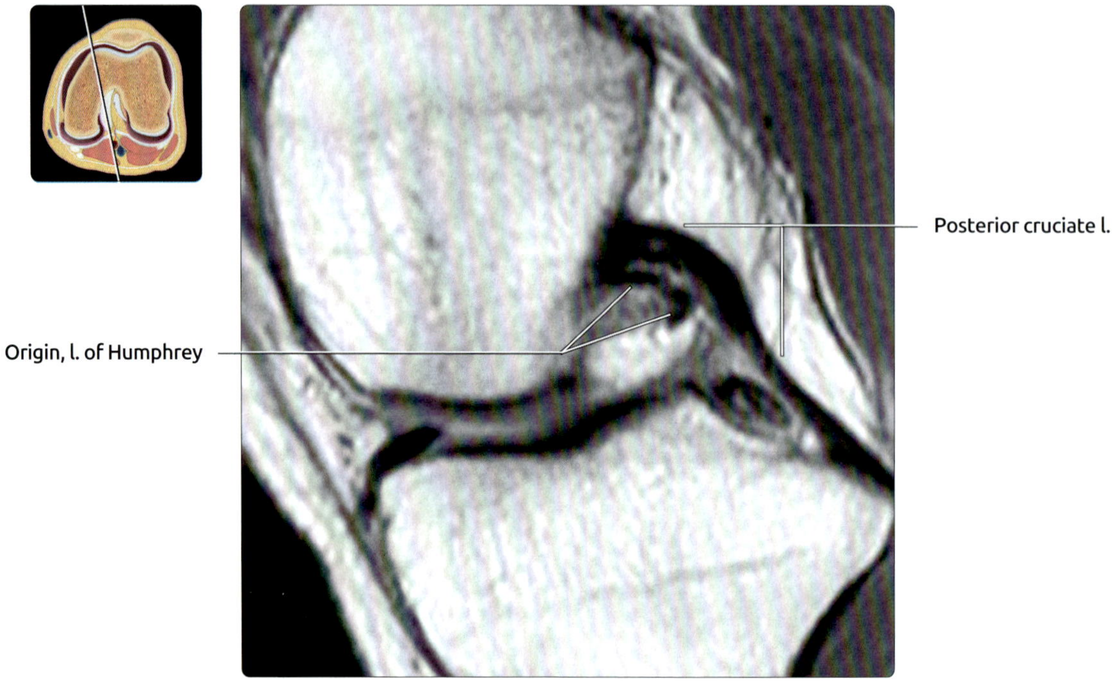

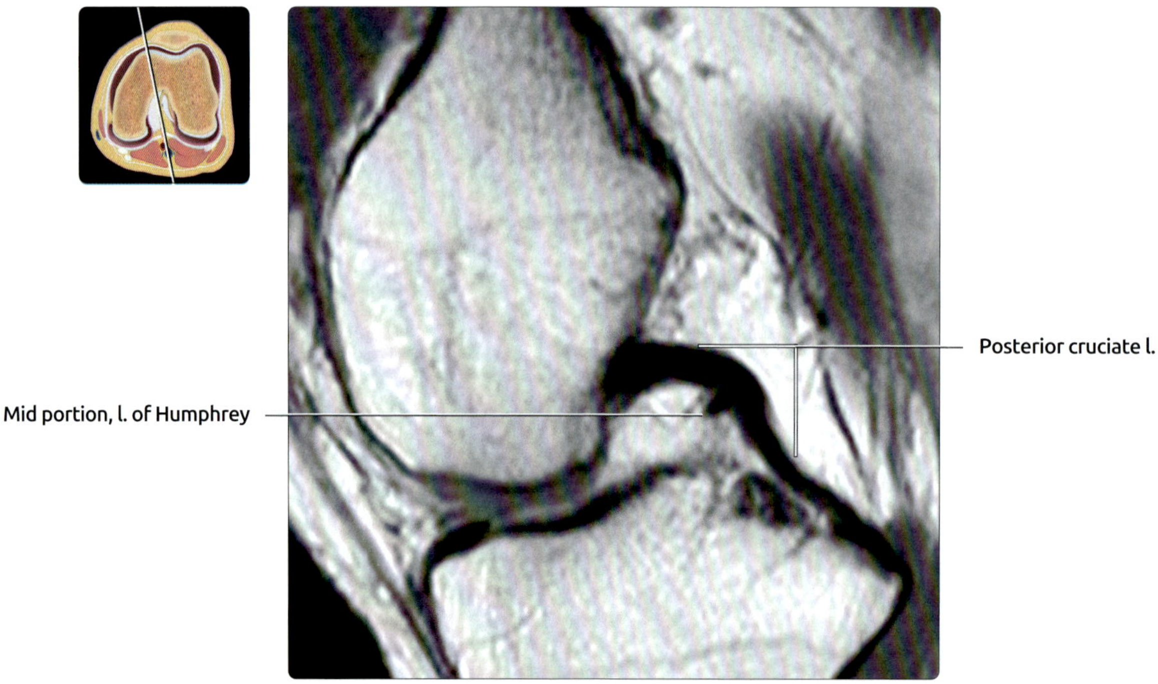

(Top) *First of 4 sagittal PD MR images shows the meniscofemoral ligament of Humphrey. Image is medial within the intercondylar notch, at the level of the PCL. The ligament of Humphrey is seen originating from the medial intercondylar notch, immediately inferior and anterior to the PCL.* **(Bottom)** *Sagittal PD MR, minimally lateral to the previous image, shows the ligament of Humphrey in cross section, immediately inferior to the PCL.*

MR: MENISCOFEMORAL LIGAMENT OF HUMPHREY

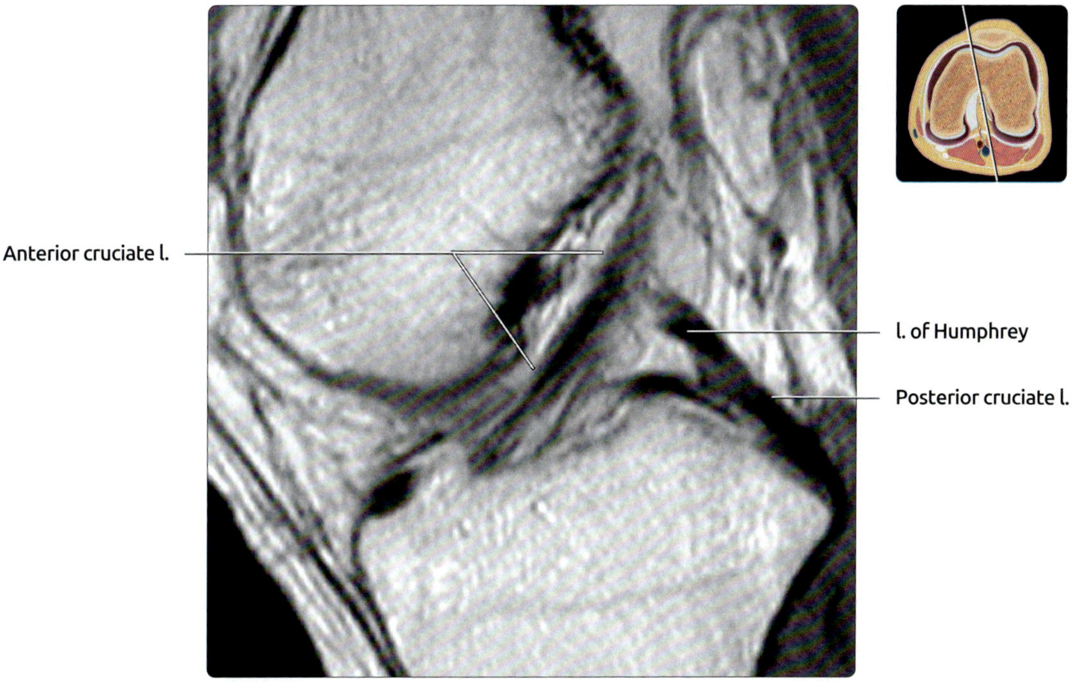

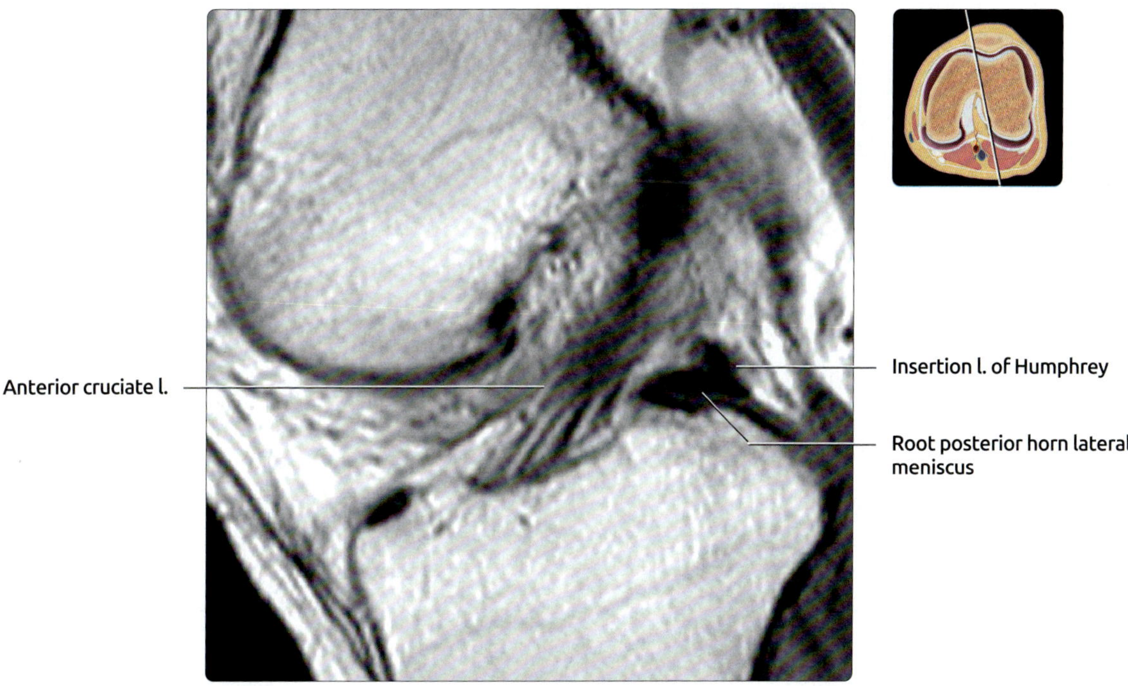

(Top) *This image is further lateral within the intercondylar notch compared with the previous 2 images. Fibers of both the ACL and PCL are seen. The ligament of Humphrey is still located anteroinferior to the posterior cruciate, extending toward the root of the posterior horn lateral meniscus.* **(Bottom)** *Further lateral within the intercondylar notch, this image shows the termination of the ligament of Humphrey as it inserts on the posterior horn of the lateral meniscus at its root. This insertion may be mistaken for a loose body, meniscal fragment, or other abnormality if it is not correctly identified.*

GRAPHIC & MR: POSTERIOR CAPSULE

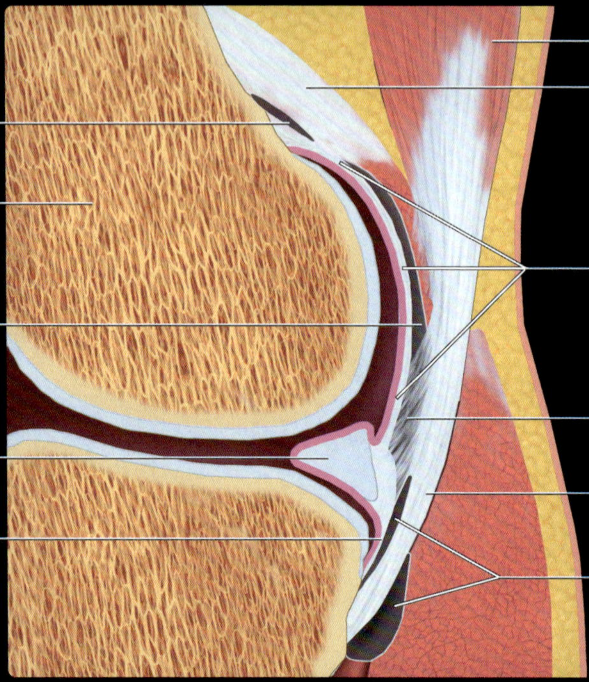

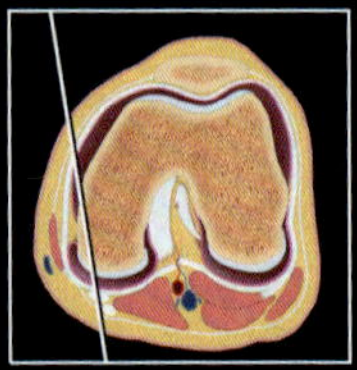

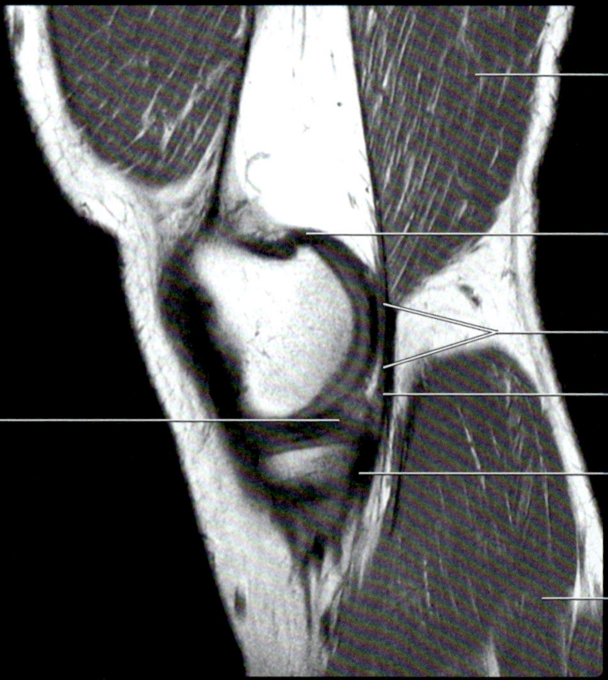

(Top) *Graphic shows the far medial portion of the posterior capsule. The capsule proper is complete, and the posterior horn of the meniscus attaches to it. Superiorly, the capsule attaches to the cortex of the posterior femoral condyle and then fuses with fibers of the medial gastrocnemius. A portion of the distal semimembranosus tendon contributes fibers to the oblique popliteal ligament; these continue as the posterior oblique ligament, contributing to the posterior capsule. Possible fluid collections in this area include the retrocondylar bursa superiorly, the subgastrocnemius bursa, and deep/superficial bursae on either side of semimembranosus tendon as it inserts on tibia.* **(Bottom)** *Sagittal PD MR, located far medially, shows the contribution made by the semimembranosus tendon to the posterior capsule. Note that the posterior horn medial meniscus blends directly into the posterior capsule.*

GRAPHIC & MR: POSTERIOR CAPSULE

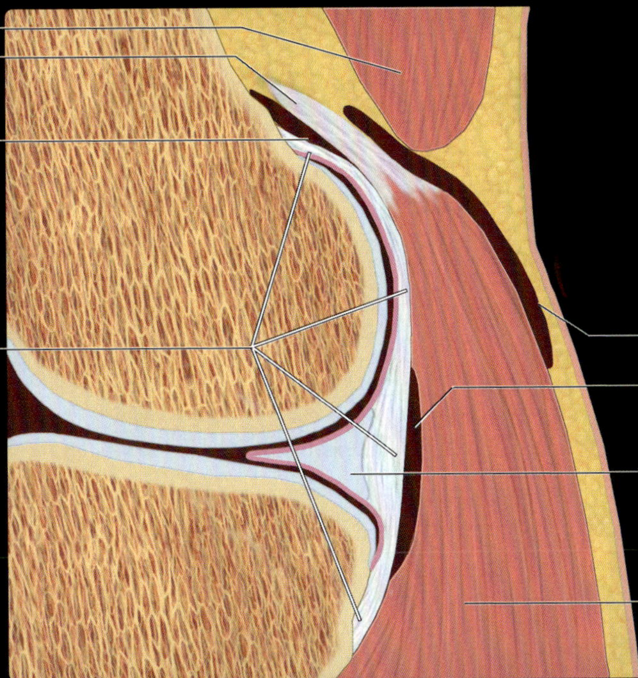

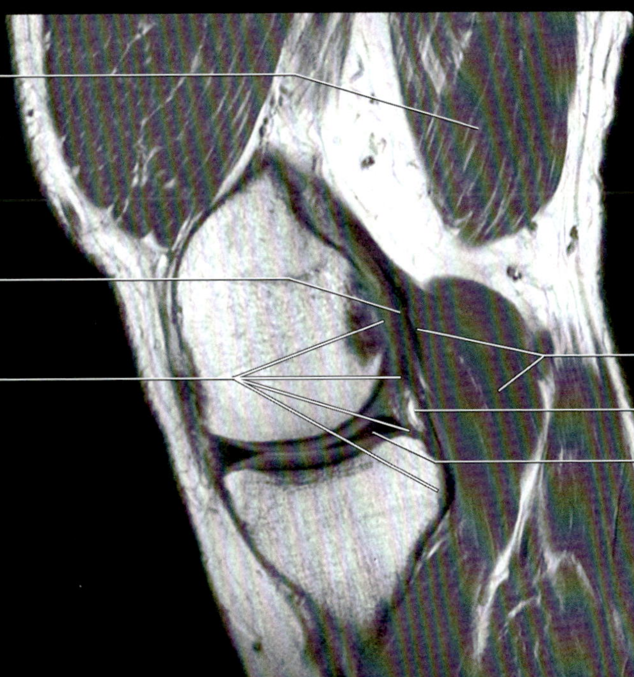

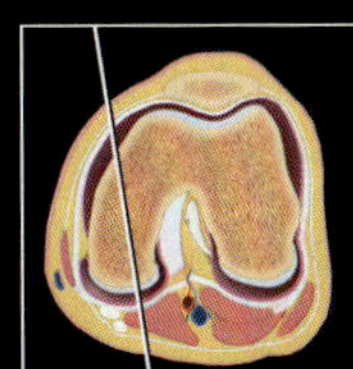

(Top) *Sagittal graphic medially in the joint is shown. The capsule is fused superiorly with the gastrocnemius tendon. A Baker (popliteal) cyst is shown at the gastrocnemius-semimembranosus bursa. The posterior horn medial meniscus is attached to the posterior capsule, reinforced by the oblique popliteal ligament. A small subgastrocnemius bursa is between the capsule and gastrocnemius muscle; another bursa is more superior between the joint capsule and gastrocnemius tendon, the retrocondylar bursa.* **(Bottom)** *Sagittal image shows the posterior capsule to be inseparable from the medial gastrocnemius tendon, proximally. Behind the meniscal attachment to the capsule, however, there is a subgastrocnemius bursa separating the capsule and gastrocnemius muscle. This case does not show a Baker (popliteal) cyst, but if it were present, it would lie between the semimembranosus and gastrocnemius muscle bellies.*

GRAPHIC & MR: POSTERIOR CAPSULE

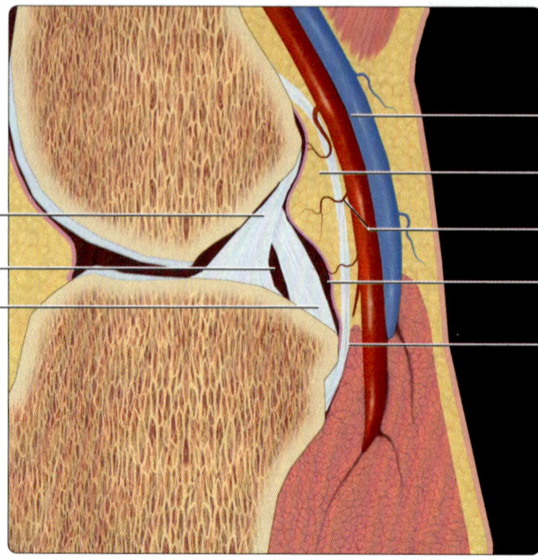

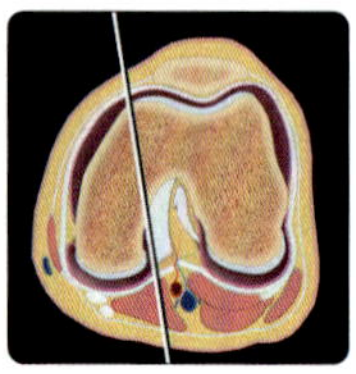

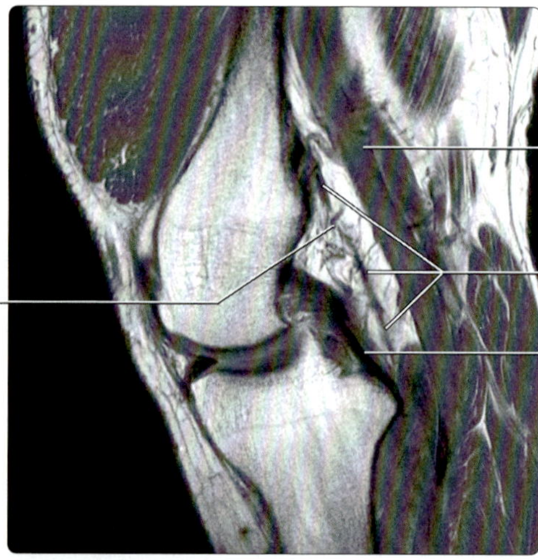

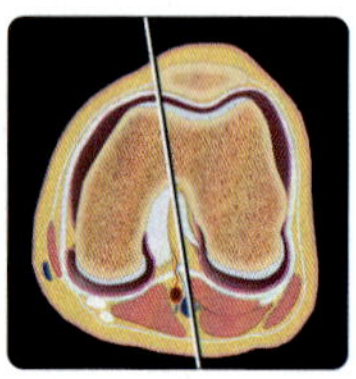

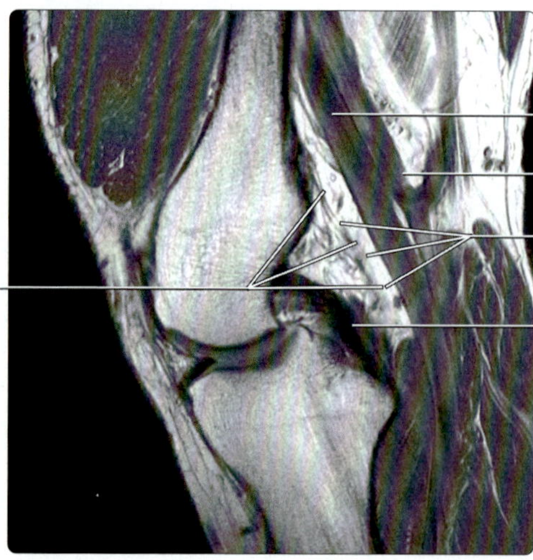

(Top) *Graphic at the level of the cruciate ligaments is shown. The capsule, strengthened by the oblique popliteal ligament, extends from the posterior margin of the femoral condyles to the intercondylar fossa at the tibia. It is incomplete, with several small perforations at its mid portion for vessels extending from the popliteal vessels to the joint. The posterior cruciate recess is found between the capsule and the lower 2/3 of the PCL. There may be a small amount of fluid in the intercruciate recess.* **(Middle)** *Sagittal image through the posterior cruciate shows posterior capsule with only a small perforation for a vessel; the majority of the capsule appears complete.* **(Bottom)** *Immediately adjacent, this slightly lateral sagittal image shows several more perforations in posterior capsule for vessels. The capsule is incomplete at this point but is surrounded both anteriorly and posteriorly by fat.*

GRAPHIC & MR: POSTERIOR CAPSULE

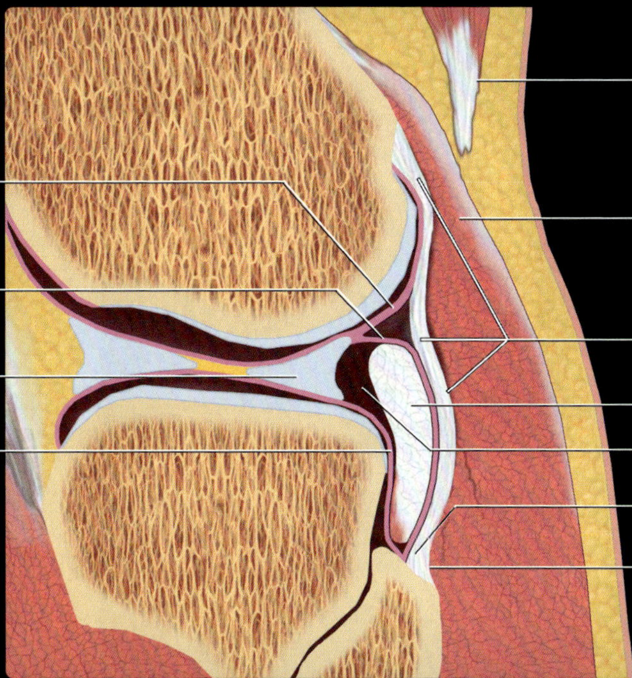

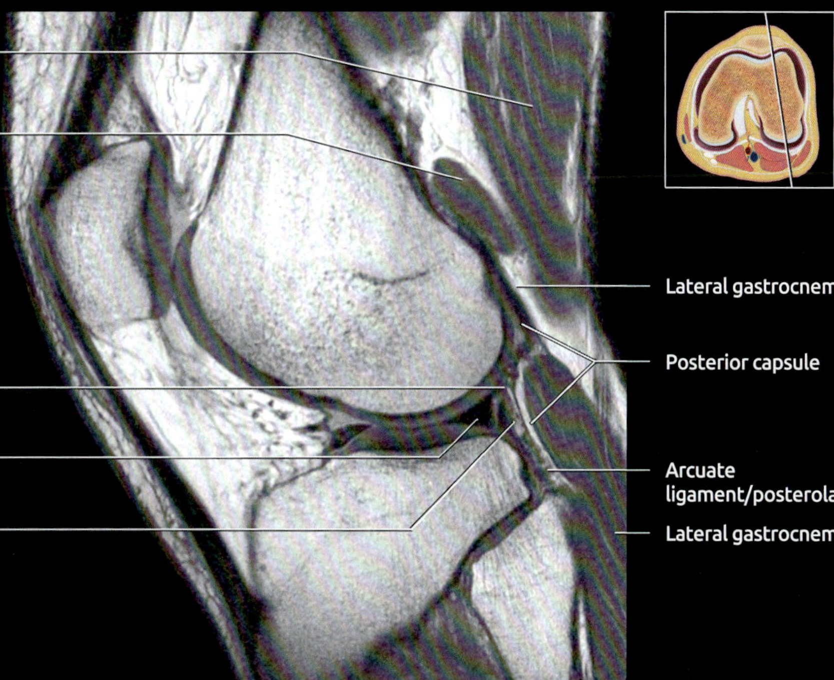

(Top) *Graphic of the lateral part of posterior capsule shows that it is intimately attached to the lateral gastrocnemius muscle. The popliteus tendon is intraarticular, but extrasynovial, and is attached to the capsule. Fibers from the posterolateral corner and arcuate ligament originating from the fibular head contribute to the lateral portion of the posterior capsule.* **(Bottom)** *Sagittal MR shows the gastrocnemius tendon contributing to the posterior capsule as well as the arcuate ligament (and fibers from other posterolateral structures). The popliteus tendon and superior fascicle (popliteomeniscal ligament) attach to the capsule as well.*

GRAPHIC & MR: SPACES WITHIN POSTERIOR CAPSULE REGION

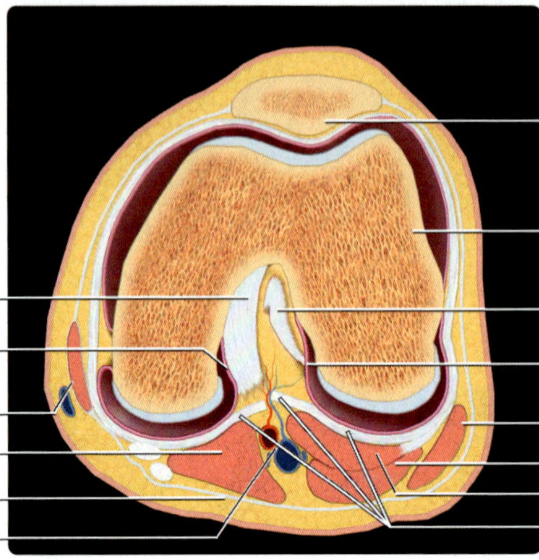

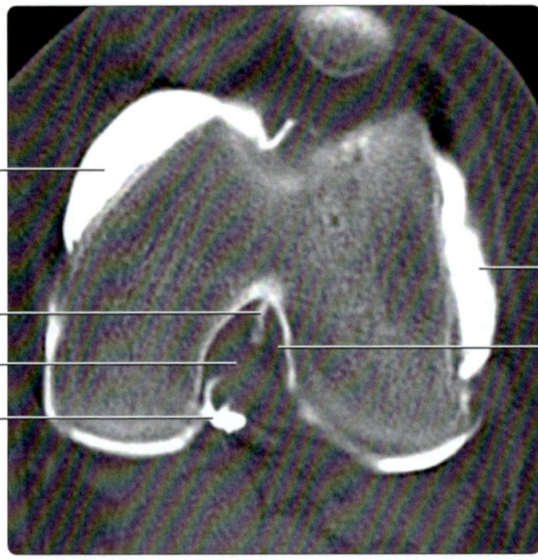

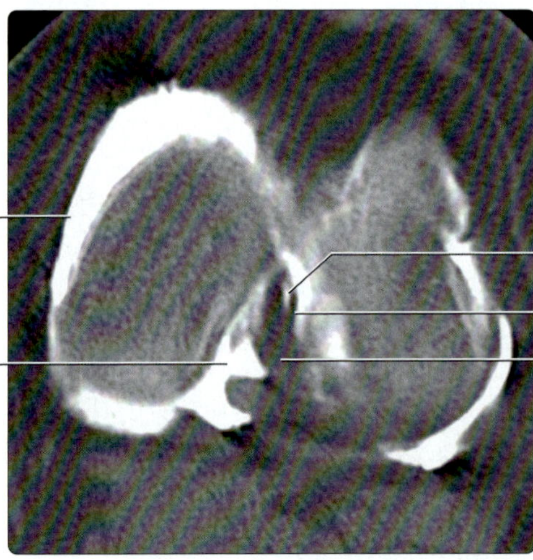

(Top) *Graphic shows the relationships of the posterior capsule. The most superficial layer is the crural fascia, which envelops the sartorius and otherwise confines all the structures. The posterior capsule (white) is continuous with the synovium (pink, next to purple synovial fluid) both posteromedially and posterolaterally. However, at the intercondylar area, the synovium separates from the capsule and covers the cruciate ligaments. It is this feature that allows us to outline the cruciates with injected fluid; they are intraarticular but extrasynovial. Thus, at this intercondylar area, the posterior capsule has no synovial covering. The capsule continues across the posterior aspect of the joint, anterior to the popliteal vessels, and is interrupted by perforating vessels.* **(Middle)** *CT arthrogram shows fluid-filled spaces.* **(Bottom)** *Here, the spaces are seen more distally.*

CORONAL MR: SPACES WITHIN POSTERIOR CAPSULE REGION

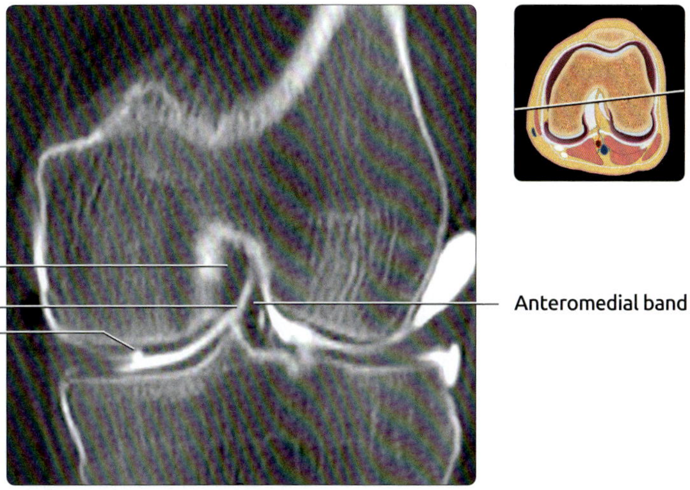

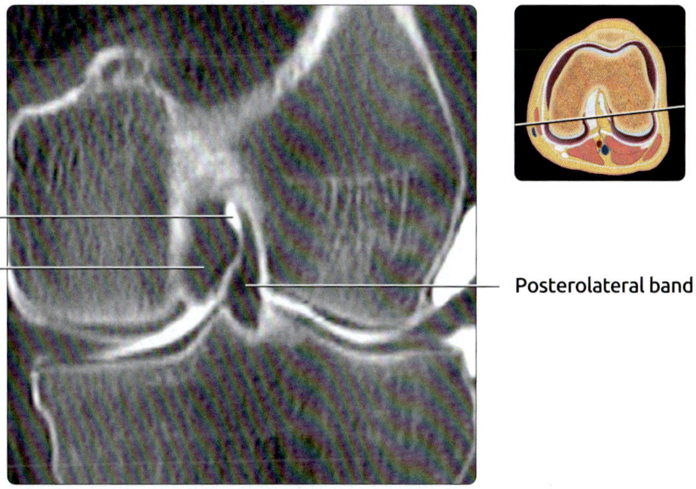

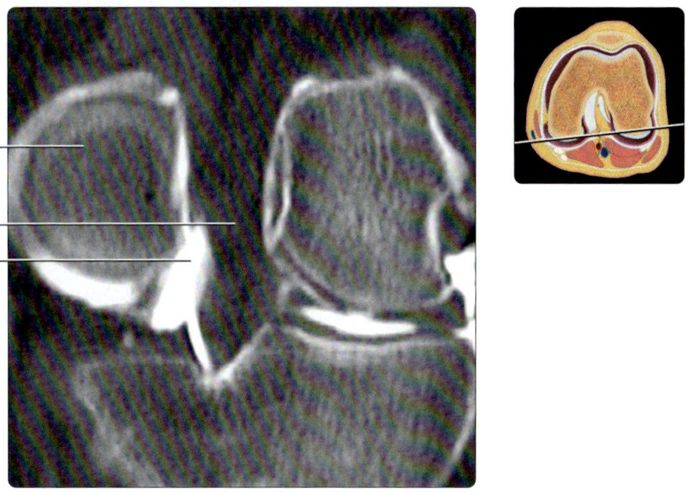

(Top) *First of 3 coronal reformatted images from CT arthrogram is shown. With joint distension, the synovial-lined surfaces of the cruciate ligaments are outlined. In this more anterior cut, the anteromedial band of the ACL is primarily seen; only the origin of the PCL is seen at the medial femoral condylar portion of the notch. There is an intercruciate recess that fills with joint distension. Incidental note is made of a focal cartilage defect in the medial femoral weight-bearing surface.* **(Middle)** *Slightly more posteriorly, both the posterolateral band of the ACL and a larger portion of the PCL are seen. The menisci are well outlined, and the intercruciate recess is again noted.* **(Bottom)** *More posteriorly, the PCL is seen approaching its posterior tibial insertion. The posterior cruciate recess contacts the distal 2/3 of the PCL and flows into the medial (not lateral) compartment of the knee.*

TERMINOLOGY

Abbreviations

- Medial (tibial) collateral ligament (MCL)
- Vastus medialis obliquus (VMO)
- Medial patellofemoral ligament (MPFL)

IMAGING ANATOMY

Overview

- Medial capsuloligamentous complex has **3 layers** that vary from anterior to mid to posterior; highly complex, with layers merging at different sites
- Primary stabilizers of femorotibial joint in valgus motion; secondary stabilizers to rotation
- Primary stabilizer against lateral subluxation/dislocation of patella

Superficial Layer (Layer 1)

- Primarily consists of **crural fascia**
- Anteriorly and superiorly, this crural fascia is continuous with fascia overlying vastus medialis
- **Sartorius** muscle/tendon enveloped by this fascia and is part of superficial layer
- Semimembranosus, semitendinosus, and gracilis are immediately deep to sartorius and superficial fascia
- Tendons of semitendinosus and gracilis blend with fascia of layer 1 and fibers of MCL as they insert distally on tibia
  - This means semitendinosus and gracilis cross just superficial to MCL (layer 2) and are between layers 1 and 2
  - Sartorius, semitendinosus, and gracilis together form pes anserinus at their insertion on anteromedial tibia, ~ 5 cm below joint line
    - Sartorius crosses medial knee joint anterior to gracilis, which in turn is anterior to semitendinosus
    - Sartorius has broadest and most anterior insertion on tibia
    - Gracilis inserts directly adjacent to sartorius, with semitendinosus directly posterior and slightly inferior to gracilis

Middle Layer (Layer 2)

- **Anteriorly**, superficial (longitudinal) fibers of MCL (layer 2) merge with crural fascia (layer 1)
- **Mid knee**: Superficial fibers of MCL form layer 2
  - Vertical fibers
  - 12 cm long
  - 1-2 cm wide
  - 2-4 mm thick
  - Origin: Medial epicondyle
  - Courses slightly anteriorly to insert on tibia ~ 5 cm below joint line
  - Layer of fat containing medial inferior genicular artery lies between superficial MCL and tibia
- **Posteriorly**, continuation of MCL is posterior oblique ligament
  - Oblique fibers extend from layer 2 posteriorly and fuse with layer 3
  - Attaches closely to posteromedial portion of meniscus; this conjoined structure is termed posterior oblique ligament

Semimembranosus

- Complex insertion, involving both middle and deep layers
- Main portion inserts on posteromedial tibial plateau
- Other attachments
  - Tibia beneath MCL
  - Posteromedial capsule
  - Oblique popliteal ligament
  - Superficial fibers of MCL

Deep Layer (Layer 3)

- **Anterior**
  - Continuous with capsule along suprapatellar recess
  - Patellomeniscal ligament extends anteriorly from meniscus to patella margin
- **Mid knee**: Capsular layer, sometimes termed deep fibers of MCL
  - Capsule thickens to form these 2 ligaments
  - **Meniscofemoral**
    - 1-2 cm long
    - Extends from outer superior aspect of body of medial meniscus obliquely and cephalad
    - Attaches to either superficial MCL or femur
  - **Meniscotibial (coronary ligament**)
    - Short (1 cm)
    - Extends from outer inferior aspect of body of medial meniscus to tibia just distal to joint line
    - Slightly more posterior than meniscofemoral
  - Capsular layers fuse posteriorly with oblique fibers of superficial MCL (no fat interposed) to form posterior oblique ligament
- **Posteriorly**, primarily capsule but receives fibers from
  - Semimembranosus
  - Oblique fibers of superficial MCL (in form of **posterior oblique ligament)**
  - **Oblique popliteal ligament**
    - Receives fibers from semimembranosus, superficial MCL (posterior oblique ligament), and synovial sheath
    - Envelops posterior aspect of femoral condyle to become posterior structure

Bursae

- Variable amounts of fat between layers 1, 2, and 3
- May see small bursa (MCL bursa) between superficial and deep layers of MCL
  - Requires fluid (distension) to be seen on MR
  - Bursa can extend to distal extent of superficial MCL, though usually is smaller, lying just over body of meniscus and deep fibers of MCL
  - Delineated anteriorly by anterior margin of superficial MCL
  - Delineated posteriorly by merger of superficial and deep fibers of MCL
- Another bursa separates semimembranosus tendon from posterior capsule

Medial Stabilizers of Patella

- Loosely termed medial retinaculum
  - Extends from vastus medialis superiorly to tibia inferiorly
  - Inserts along medial edge of patella
- Highly complex, with **3 layers**, which differ in superior, mid, and inferior portions

- Layer 1 is most superficial, just deep to subcutaneous tissues
    - Deep crural fascia
    - Anterosuperiorly, continuous with fascia overlying vastus medialis
  - **Layer 2** is just deep to layer 1 and just superficial to layer 3 (joint capsule)
  - Within layers 2 and 3, condensations of fibers form ligaments of **medial retinacular complex**
  - Within layer 2, medial retinacular complex ligaments form inverted triangle in sagittal plane, with central split, which defines 3 separate ligaments
    - MPFL: Superior aspect of triangle
    - Superficial MCL: Posterior aspect of triangle
    - Patellotibial ligament: Anteroinferior aspect of triangle
  - **Layer 3**: Joint capsule
- **Superior portion** of medial patellar stabilizers
  - **VMO**
    - Inferior portion of vastus medialis
    - Acts as dynamic stabilizer, neutralizing lateralizing forces on patella exerted by vastus lateralis during quadriceps contraction
    - Arises from adductor magnus tendon, medial intermuscular septum, or adductor tubercle
    - Merges with MPFL and inserts on superior 2/3 of medial patella
  - **MPFL**
    - Major ligamentous restraint preventing lateral patellar subluxation (50-60% total restraining force)
    - Origin is variable: Adductor tubercle, medial epicondyle, or superficial MCL
    - Runs forward and slightly inferiorly, just deep to VMO, fuses with aponeurosis of VMO
    - Inserts on superior 2/3 of medial patella; seen as distinct structure at insertion
    - 4.5-6.0 cm in length
    - < 0.5 cm thick
    - Width: 1-2 cm at femur, 2-3 cm at patella
    - Merges with layer 2 (medial retinaculum) inferiorly
- **Mid portion** of medial patellar stabilizers
  - Superficial MCL (layer 2), fuses with crural fascia (layer 1) to form medial retinaculum (proper) anteriorly
  - Merges with VMO fascia anteriorly
  - Inserts into medial margin of patella
- **Inferior portion** of medial patellar stabilizers
  - Patellotibial ligament
    - Originates on tibia at level of insertion of gracilis and semitendinosus
    - Joins layer 1 and extends obliquely proximally to insert on inferior aspect of patella and on patellar tendon
  - Medial patellomeniscal ligament
    - Deep in relation to patellotibial ligament (anatomically in layer 3)

Posteromedial Capsule

- **Medial side of posterior capsule**: Fibers from several structures merge with and contribute to capsule
  - Fibers from distal semimembranosus tendon, forming oblique popliteal ligament
  - Fibers from superficial MCL, forming posterior oblique ligament, which also contribute to oblique popliteal ligament
  - Capsule attaches to posterior femoral cortex a few cm above level of most superior aspect of cartilage
  - Capsule attaches inferiorly to tibia 1-2 cm below joint line
  - Bursa separates capsule and semimembranosus tendon
  - Little more toward center of knee, semimembranosus is replaced by medial gastrocnemius
  - Superiorly, capsule joins gastrocnemius tendon
- **Midportion of posterior capsule**
  - Capsule is incomplete posteriorly
  - Therefore, intraarticular space is not completely separate from extraarticular fat
  - Popliteal artery and vein course behind capsule
    - Perforating vessels extend from these through posterior capsule
    - Perforating nerves accompany vessels

ANATOMY IMAGING ISSUES

Imaging Recommendations

- Superficial MCL: Coronal and axial
- Capsular layers (deep MCL): Coronal
- MPFL and VMO best seen on axials immediately inferior to adductor tubercle
  - MPFL seen at its origin in 80%
  - MPFL seen at patellar insertion in 100%
- Medial retinaculum seen just inferior to MPFL/VMO, also on axials
  - Medial retinaculum seen at midsubstance and patellar insertion in 100%
- Patellotibial and medial patellomeniscal meniscal ligaments seen at level of knee joint, on axials
- Oblique popliteal ligament envelops posterior aspect of femoral condyle, best seen on axials
  - Seen 100% on axial MR

SELECTED REFERENCES

1. Elias DA et al: Acute lateral patellar dislocation at MR imaging: injury patterns of medial patellar soft-tissue restraints and osteochondral injuries of the inferomedial patella. Radiology. 225(3):736-43, 2002
2. De Maeseneer M et al: Three layers of the medial capsular and supporting structures of the knee: MR imaging-anatomic correlation. Radiographics. 20 Spec No:S83-9, 2000
3. Spritzer CE et al: Medial retinacular complex injury in acute patellar dislocation: MR findings and surgical implications. AJR Am J Roentgenol. 168(1):117-22, 1997

SAGITTAL GRAPHIC & MR: PES ANSERINUS

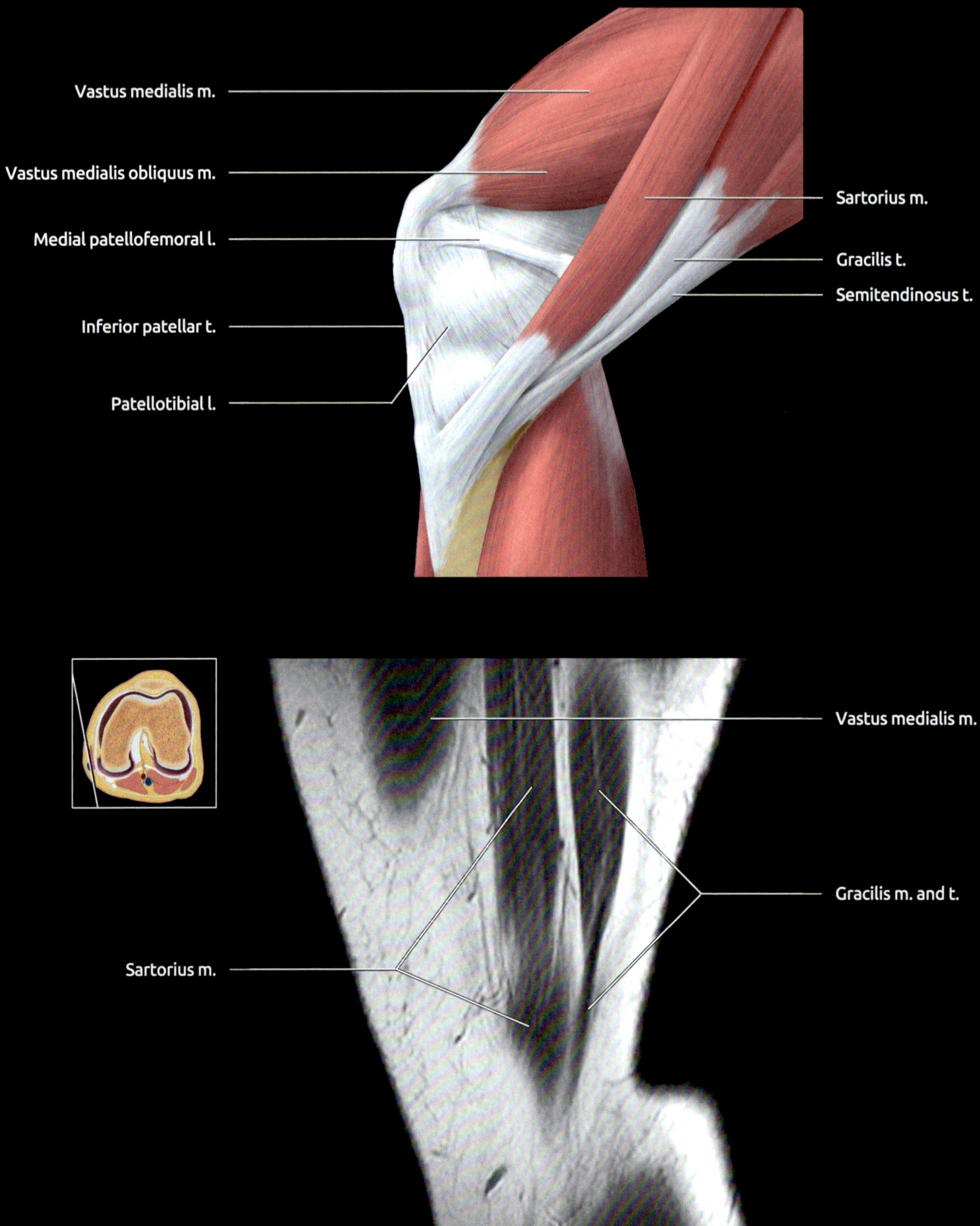

(Top) *Graphic shows the anteromedial attachment of the pes anserinus tendons. The sartorius is the most anterior and superficial. The gracilis inserts directly adjacent and deep to the sartorius, and the semitendinosus inserts directly posterior and slightly inferior to the gracilis. These tendons and their crural fascia comprise the superficial layer of the medial capsuloligamentous complex.* **(Bottom)** *First of 4 sagittal T1 MR images, starting far medially, shows the components of the pes anserinus. The sartorius has a straight course above the knee joint, directly medial to the knee. The sartorius is invested by the crural fascia to form layer 1 of the medial capsuloligamentous complex. The gracilis maintains its position slightly posterior and deep to sartorius.*

SAGITTAL MR: PES ANSERINUS

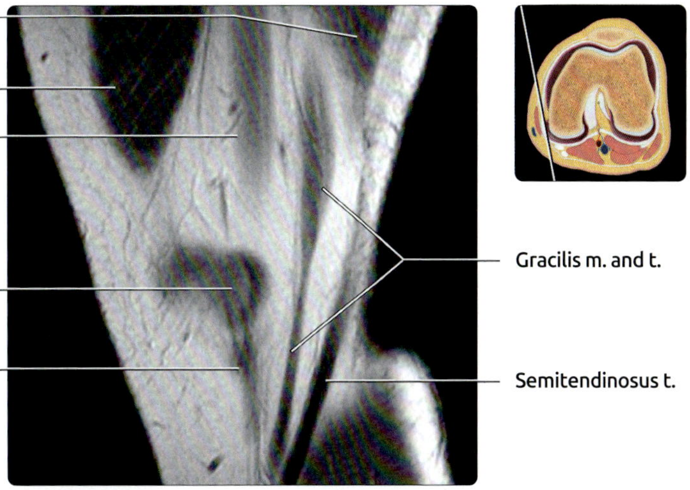

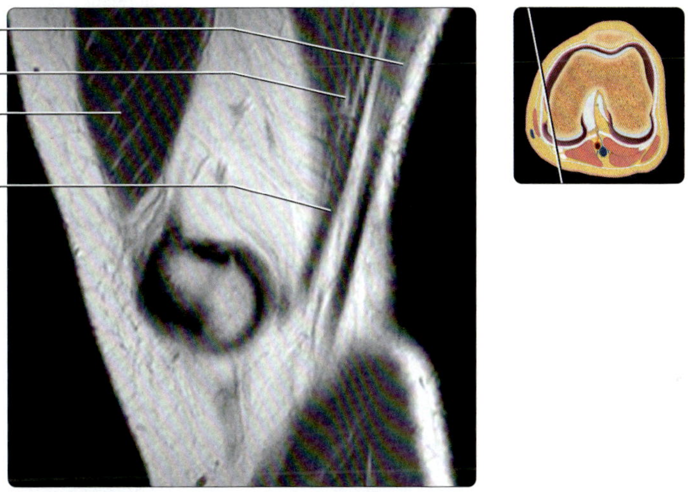

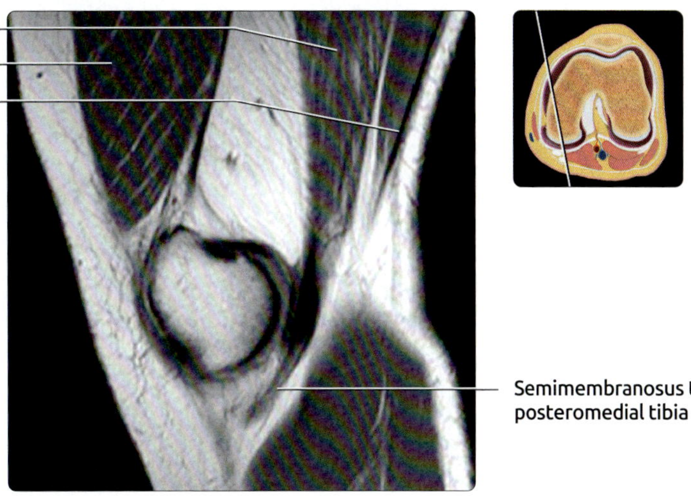

(Top) *Slightly more lateral cut (toward the intercondylar notch) shows a remnant of the sartorius. The gracilis tendon is immediately posterior and deep to the sartorius. The semitendinosus tendon follows even more posteriorly and medially. The medial collateral ligament (MCL) is barely seen arising from the medial femoral condyle.* **(Middle)** *More laterally, the semimembranosus muscle and tendon are seen, with the semitendinosus muscle and tendon remaining behind them. While the semitendinosus continues its course, following the gracilis toward its anteromedial tibial insertion, the semimembranosus inserts at the proximal tibia posteriorly and medially.* **(Bottom)** *Approaching the tibia with a more lateral section, the semimembranosus is seen to broaden at its tendinous insertion on the posterior as well as medial tibia, immediately below the joint line. The slips from the semimembranosus to the MCL and posterior capsule via the posterior oblique ligament are not seen as separate structures here.*

CORONAL MR: PES ANSERINUS

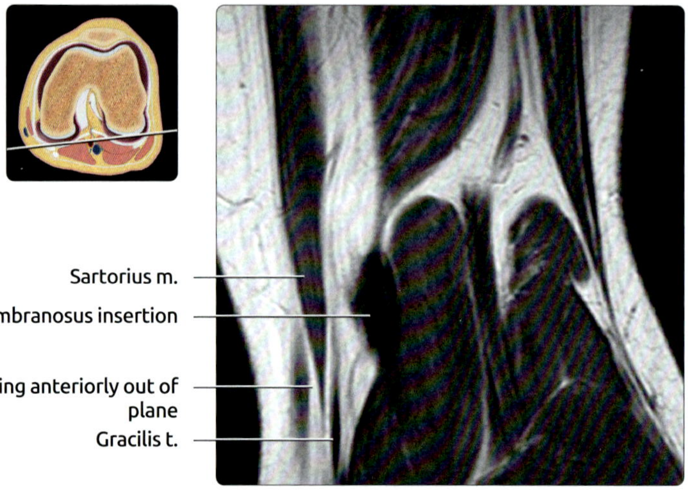

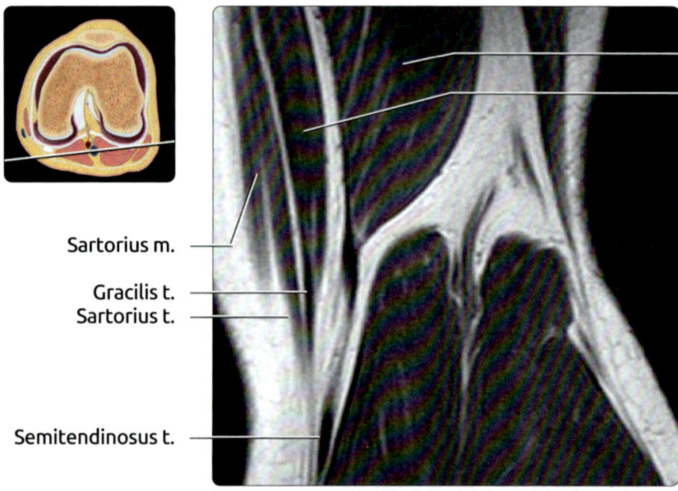

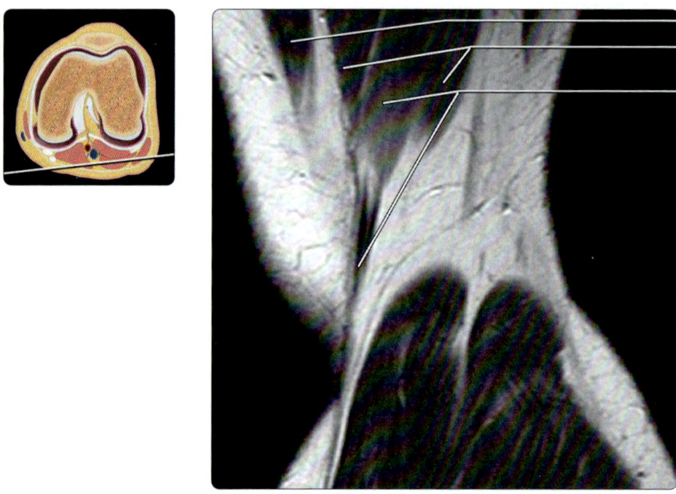

(Top) *First of 3 coronal T1 MR images through the posterior portion of the joint shows the medial-lateral relationships of the tendons comprising the pes anserinus. At the level of the popliteal vessels, just posterior to the tibia, the semimembranosus spreads out into its insertion, which is wide at the posterior as well as the posteromedial tibia. The sartorius muscle is seen at this level, with its tendon curving anteriorly out of the plane. A portion of the gracilis tendon is seen parallel and deep to the sartorius tendon.* **(Middle)** *Shown slightly more posteriorly, a remnant of the sartorius muscle and tendon is seen, but the gracilis muscle and tendon are more completely seen. A very small portion of the semitendinosus tendon is seen distally, behind and medial to the gracilis. The semitendinosus muscle is more proximal and posterior and out of plane.* **(Bottom)** *Even more posteriorly, the semitendinosus muscle and tendon are shown posterior to the muscle belly of the semimembranosus.*

AXIAL MR: PES ANSERINUS

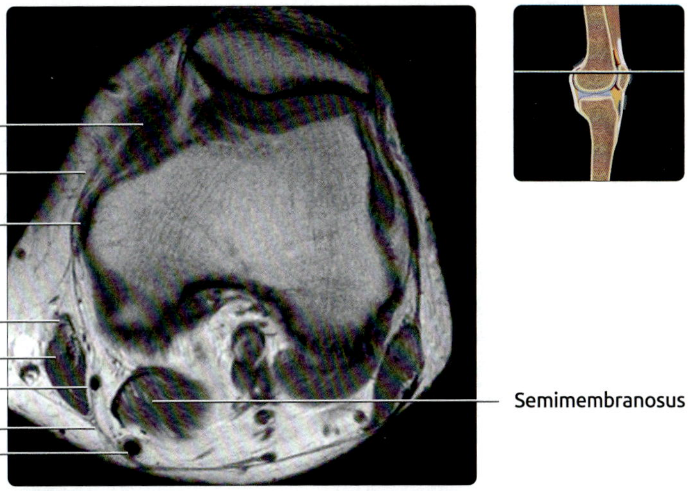

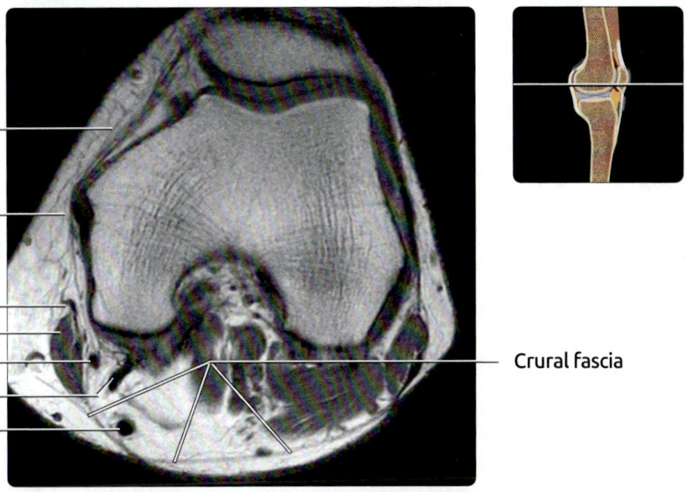

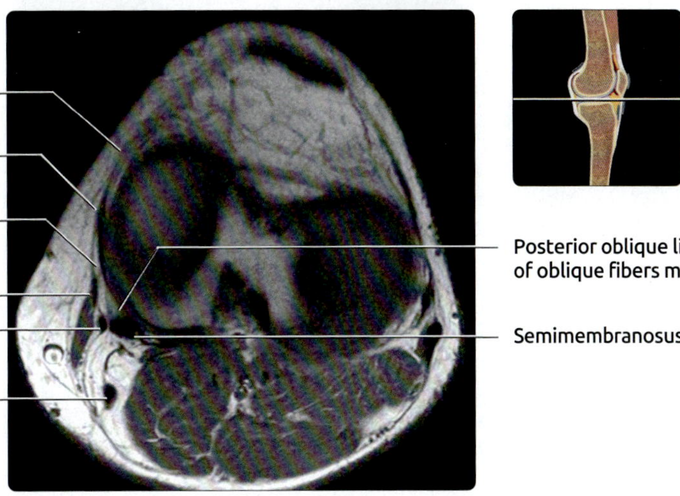

(Top) *First of 3 axial T1 MR images shows the anatomy of the pes anserinus. The sartorius is the most superficial. It is invested by the crural fascia to form layer 1. The gracilis tendon is medial to the sartorius and follows its tendon in a slightly posterior position. The semitendinosus is posterior to the semimembranosus and distinctly posterior and lateral (toward the intercondylar notch) relative to the gracilis tendon.* **(Middle)** *Superficial MCL arises distal to the adductor tubercle and forms layer 2.* **(Bottom)** *At the level of the joint line, the elements of the pes anserinus line up in order of their insertion (sartorius, gracilis, semitendinosus) on the anteromedial tibia. Anteriorly, layers 1 (sartorius) and 2 (superficial MCL) merge to contribute to the medial retinaculum. The gracilis and semitendinosus lie between layers 1 and 2. Posteriorly, layers 2 and 3 (superficial and deep MCL, respectively) merge to form the posterior oblique ligament, contributing to the capsule.*

GRAPHIC: POSTEROMEDIAL STRUCTURES

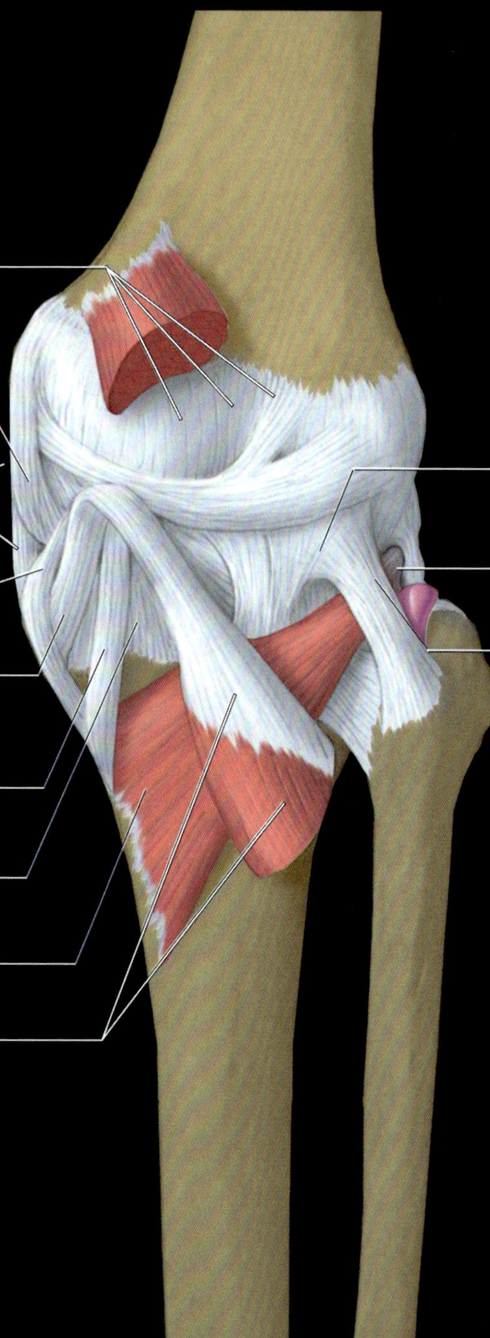

The semimembranosus tendon has a complex insertion, both at the posteromedial tibia and more anteriorly at the medial tibia. The semimembranosus also provides slips to the posterior aspect of the MCL, as well as providing an expansion to the oblique popliteal ligament. The posterior oblique ligament arises from several arms of the superficial MCL, both superiorly and inferiorly, as well as from the posterior aspect of the deep MCL (therefore, both layers 2 and 3 contribute to it). The posterior oblique ligament then extends from its posteromedial position to contribute to the oblique popliteal ligament, which in turn strengthens the posterior capsule. On the lateral side, fibers from the arcuate ligament blend into and contribute to the oblique popliteal ligament as well.

MR: POSTEROMEDIAL STRUCTURES: SEMIMEMBRANOSUS

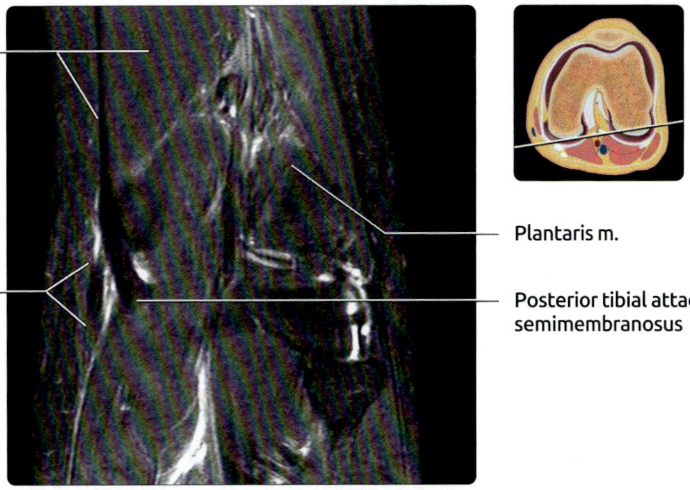

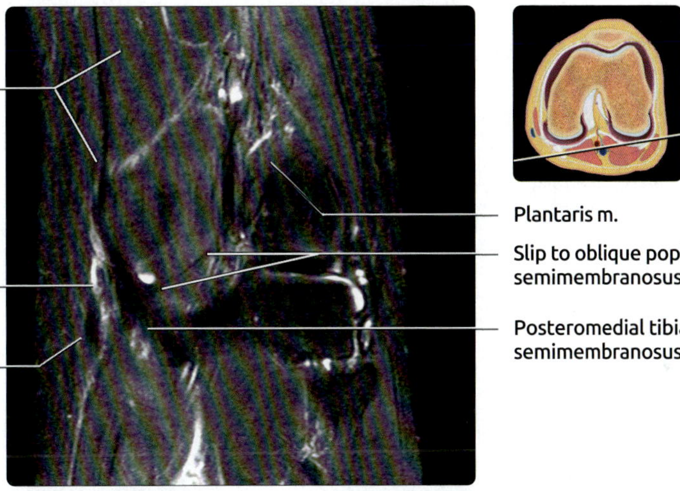

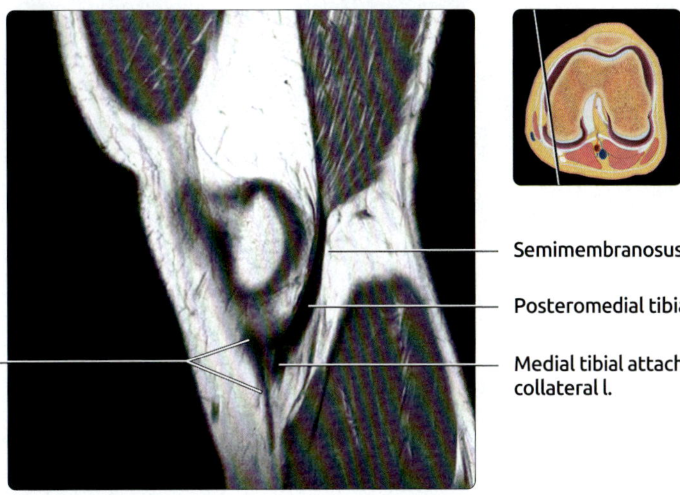

(Top) *First of 2 posterior coronal T2 FS images shows semimembranosus insertion at the posteromedial tibia.* **(Middle)** *Slightly more anterior cut shows the multiple slips of the semimembranosus. These include insertions at the posteromedial tibia and another more directly medially. Additionally, there are slips extending from the semimembranosus to the oblique popliteal and MCLs.* **(Bottom)** *Sagittal PD MR shows the semimembranosus insertion on the posteromedial tibia, along with its slip extending to the MCL.*

GRAPHIC & MR: MEDIAL CAPSULOLIGAMENTOUS COMPLEX

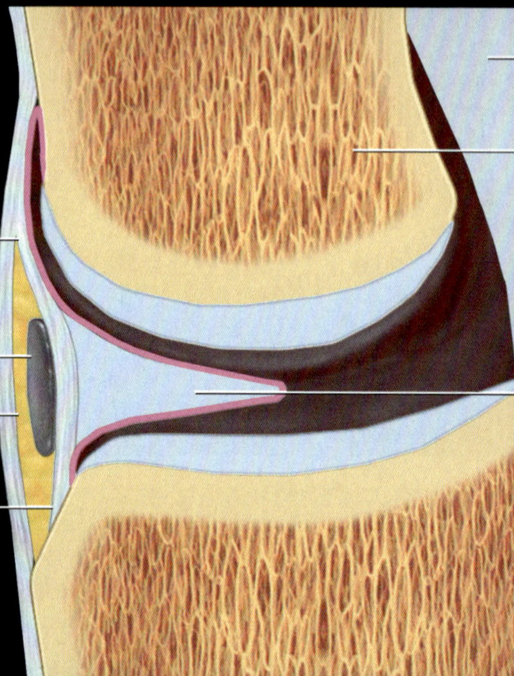

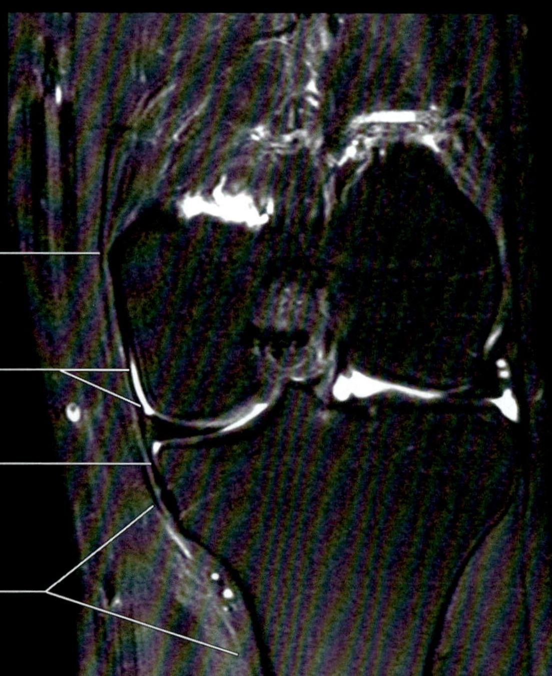

(Top) *Coronal graphic at midjoint shows the relationship of the deep and superficial fibers of the MCL. Superficial fibers extend from adjacent to the adductor tubercle to approximately 5 cm distal to the joint line. Deep fibers are much shorter: The meniscotibial (coronary) ligament extends from the meniscus to the tibia adjacent to the joint line, and the meniscofemoral ligament extends from the meniscus to either the femur or superficial MCL. A variable amount of fat and a small bursa may be seen between deep and superficial fibers.* **(Bottom)** *Coronal MR shows the deep medial collateral fibers outlined by joint fluid. The meniscofemoral ligament inserts on the femur in this case; it may also normally insert on the superficial MCL at the same level above the joint. The short coronary (meniscotibial) ligament is seen. The superficial MCL is only faintly seen due to the fat saturation. There is no bursal fluid present to separate the deep and superficial layers of the MCL.*

GRAPHIC & MR: MEDIAL CAPSULOLIGAMENTOUS COMPLEX

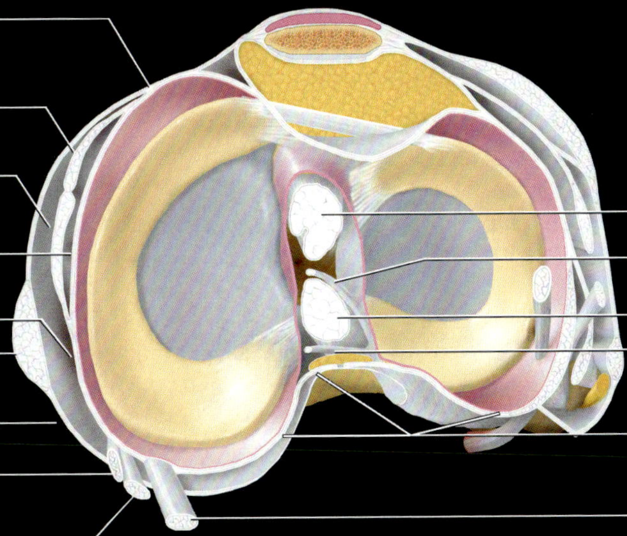

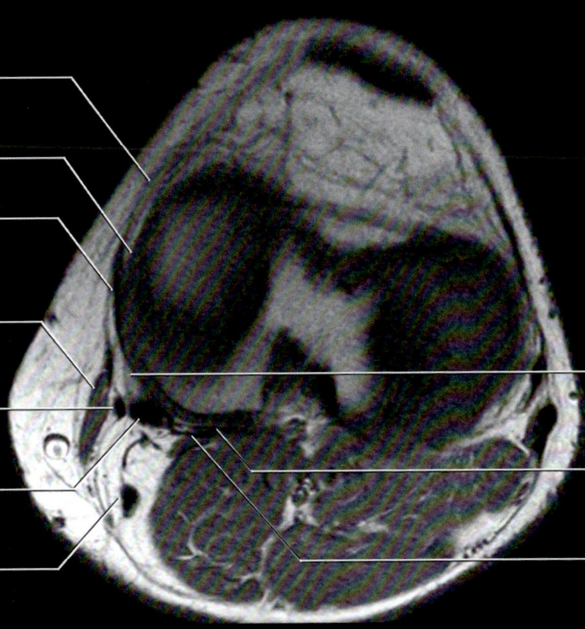

(Top) *Graphic shows 3 layers of medial capsuloligamentous complex. Layer 1 consists of the crural fascia, which envelops the sartorius. The superficial fibers of MCL form layer 2. Layers 1 and 2 merge anteriorly to contribute to medial retinaculum. The gracilis and semitendinosus lie between layers 1 and 2. Posteriorly, the superficial MCL fibers (layer 2) fuse with deep MCL fibers (layer 3) to form the posterior oblique ligament; this ligament contributes to the posterior capsule at its posteromedial aspect.* **(Bottom)** *Axial T1 MR shows some of the complexity of the posteromedial structures, including the elements of the pes anserinus as well as the various attachments and slips of the semimembranosus tendon. Note the slip from the semimembranosus extending to the posterior oblique ligament and posterior capsule.*

TERMINOLOGY

Abbreviations

- Iliotibial (IT) tract
- Lateral (fibular) collateral ligament (LCL)

IMAGING ANATOMY

Overview

- Combination of muscles, tendons, and ligaments that contribute to lateral stability of knee

Muscles Contributing to Lateral Stability

- **IT tract**
  - **Origin**: Strong band of deep fascia composed of fusion of aponeurotic coverings of tensor fascia lata, gluteus maximus, gluteus minimus
  - **Main insertion**
    - Gerdy tubercle (anterolateral tibia near plateau)
  - Additional insertions
    - Above knee, IT tract fibers insert on
      - Supracondylar tubercle of lateral femoral condyle
      - Intermuscular septum
    - Small attachments to patella and patellar ligament
  - **Function**
    - Extends, abducts, and laterally rotates hip
- **Biceps femoris**
  - Long head joined by short head above knee
  - **Insertions**
    - Long head: 2 major tendinous components
      - Direct arm inserts on fibular head
      - Anterior arm inserts just anterior to direct arm on fibular head and continues distally as anterior aponeurosis that extends anterolaterally around leg
    - Short head: 2 tendinous components
      - Direct arm inserts on fibular head anterior to styloid process and medial to long head biceps
      - Anterior arm passes medial to LCL and inserts into superolateral edge of lateral tibial condyle inferior to anterolateral ligament
  - **Function**
    - Both heads flex knee
    - Long head also aids hip extension
    - Slight lateral rotation when knee semiflexed
- **Popliteus**
  - Tendinous attachment at **popliteal sulcus** of lateral femoral condyle
    - Inferior and deep to origin of LCL
  - Extends posteromedially through **popliteal hiatus** (runs deep to fabellofibular and arcuate ligaments)
  - **Superior popliteomeniscal fascicle** extends from posterior horn lateral meniscus to paratenon tissues of popliteus tendon
    - Superior popliteomeniscal fascicle and arcuate ligament form **roof of popliteal hiatus**
  - **Inferior popliteomeniscal fascicle** extends from posterior horn lateral meniscus to paratenon tissues of popliteus tendon
    - Inferior popliteomeniscal fascicle forms **floor of popliteal hiatus**
  - Superior and inferior fascicles join and insert on fibular styloid as **popliteofibular ligament**
  - **Popliteus muscle** has wide attachment to posteromedial aspect of proximal tibial metaphysis
  - **Function**
    - Assists with flexion of knee
    - Internally rotates tibia on femur (at initiation of flexion of knee)
    - Protects posterior horn lateral meniscus by withdrawing it from joint space during flexion and rotation
    - Stabilizes posterolateral corner from rotatory instability

Lateral Support System: Consists of 3 Layers

- **Layer 1 (superficial)**
  - Anteriorly, IT tract
  - Posterolaterally, superficial portion of biceps
- **Layer 2 (middle)**
  - Anteriorly, lateral retinaculum
  - 2 ligamentous thickenings originate from lateral patella
    - Proximal: Terminates at lateral intermuscular septum
    - Distal: Terminates at femoral insertion of posterolateral capsule and lateral head of gastrocnemius tendon
- **Layer 3 (deep)**
  - Forms lateral part of capsule
  - Contains several thickenings that function as discrete structures
    - Anterolateral ligament
      - Originates on femur immediately anterior to LCL
      - Extends anteroinferiorly, inserts on tibia midway between Gerdy tubercle and fibular head
      - Firm attachment to lateral meniscus
    - Lateral (fibular) collateral ligament
    - Arcuate complex, including arcuate, popliteofibular, fabellofibular, and coronary (meniscotibial) ligaments

Posterolateral Corner Structures: Superficial and Deep Layers

- All insert on fibular head and provide posterolateral support
- Not all are seen with equal reliability on imaging
- **Superficial posterolateral corner structures: Biceps femoris and LCL**
  - Biceps femoris insertions
    - Fibula: Proximal, medial, and distal insertions
      - Inserts both anterior and posterior to lateral collateral ligament
    - Tibia: Inserts immediately inferior to anterolateral ligament
    - Soft tissue: Several tendinous and fascial insertional components, including portion that inserts on posterior edge of IT tract
  - LCL
    - Proximal attachment at distal femur just proximal and posterior to lateral epicondyle
    - Proximal attachment is slightly proximal and anterior to sulcus for origin of popliteus tendon
    - LCL extends posterolaterally to insert on upper facet of fibular head

- Anterolateral to attachment of fabellofibular and arcuate ligaments
- **Deep posterolateral corner structures**
  - Posterolateral reinforcements of fibrous capsule, including fabellofibular, arcuate, oblique popliteal, and popliteofibular ligaments
  - **Fabellofibular ligament**
    - Originates at fabella (or proximal to it)
    - Inserts at lateral aspect of apex of fibular head (styloid process)
    - Inserts just anterolateral to insertion of popliteofibular ligament on fibular head
    - Fabellofibular ligament may be dominant when arcuate is diminutive
  - **Arcuate ligament**
    - Y-shaped
    - Arises from fibular styloid process, just deep to fabellofibular ligament
    - Lateral limb courses straight upward along lateral knee capsule to reach lateral femoral condyle
    - Medial limb crosses over posterior surface of popliteal tendon and attaches to posterior knee capsule
      - Medial limb, along with superior popliteomeniscal fascicle, forms bowed roof of popliteal hiatus
      - At insertion on posterior knee capsule, medial limb arcuate merges with fibers from oblique popliteal ligament
    - Arcuate may be dominant when fabellofibular is absent (or may contain fibers of fabellofibular ligament)
    - Inferior lateral geniculate artery passes anterior relative to arcuate
  - **Oblique popliteal ligament**
    - Arises medially from slips of semimembranosus and medial tibial condyle, courses superolaterally
    - Joins arcuate ligament posterolaterally at its femoral insertion (margin of intercondylar fossa and posterior surface of lateral femoral condyle)
  - **Popliteofibular ligament**
    - Arises from confluence of superior and inferior popliteomeniscal fascicles
    - Inserts on fibular head
    - Popliteofibular ligament may be dominant, with neither arcuate or fabellofibular ligaments present

ANATOMY IMAGING ISSUES

Imaging Recommendations

- Crucial posterolateral structures seen on axial and routine oblique sagittal imaging
- **Coronal oblique** suggested to increase probability of visualizing posterolateral structures
  - Prescribed off sagittal image
  - Obliquity runs anterosuperior to posteroinferior, generally parallel to popliteal tendon as seen on sagittals

Imaging Sweet Spots

- Structures are variably seen on MR
  - Following statistics are based on 1.5T imaging
- Biceps seen well in all 3 planes; 100%
  - Individual components may be seen separately on axials near fibular attachment
    - Short head biceps, direct arm 70%
    - Long head biceps, direct and anterior arms 70%
- LCL seen well in all 3 planes; 100%
- Superior popliteomeniscal fascicle seen best on sagittal fluid sensitive sequence, at level of posterior horn lateral meniscus; 100%
- Inferior popliteomeniscal fascicle seen best on coronal fluid sensitive sequence, at level of body lateral meniscus; 100%
- Arcuate ligament
  - In cadaver study, at least 1 limb seen in 70% on sagittal or coronal MR
    - Lateral limb arcuate seen 57% (better when fabella absent)
    - Medial limb arcuate seen 57% (better when fabella present)
  - Coronal oblique MR may increase likelihood
- Fabellofibular ligament rarely seen as separate entity (coronal or sagittal)
- Popliteofibular ligament
  - In cadaver study, seen 57% using coronal oblique (38% with standard planes)
- Oblique popliteal ligament 100%, axial

CLINICAL IMPLICATIONS

Clinical Importance

- Posterolateral structures act primarily as static constraints to varus angulation and external rotation of knee
- Secondary restraint against posterior translation of tibia

Biomechanical Selective Cutting Study

- Major structures preventing posterolateral instability are LCL and popliteus tendon
- Popliteofibular ligament also important in providing static stability
- Surgery primarily focuses on restoring these ligaments
- Identifying popliteofibular on MR is variable (even with coronal oblique)
  - Limitation in assessing posterolateral corner injuries

Avulsion Fractures at Posterolateral Corner

- **Arcuate sign**
  - Thin sliver avulsion at posterosuperior portion of fibular styloid
  - Site of (near) common insertion of fabellofibular, popliteofibular, and arcuate ligaments
  - Marrow edema may also indicate injury at this site
  - Posterior cruciate ligament injury is often associated
- **Anterolateral fibular head avulsion** (distal to fibular styloid)
  - LCL/biceps avulsion

SELECTED REFERENCES

1. Porrino J Jr et al: The anterolateral ligament of the knee: MRI appearance, association with the Segond fracture, and historical perspective. AJR Am J Roentgenol. 204(2):367-73, 2015
2. Jadhav SP et al: Comprehensive review of the anatomy, function, and imaging of the popliteus and associated pathologic conditions. Radiographics. 34(2):496-513, 2014

GRAPHICS: POSTEROLATERAL STRUCTURES

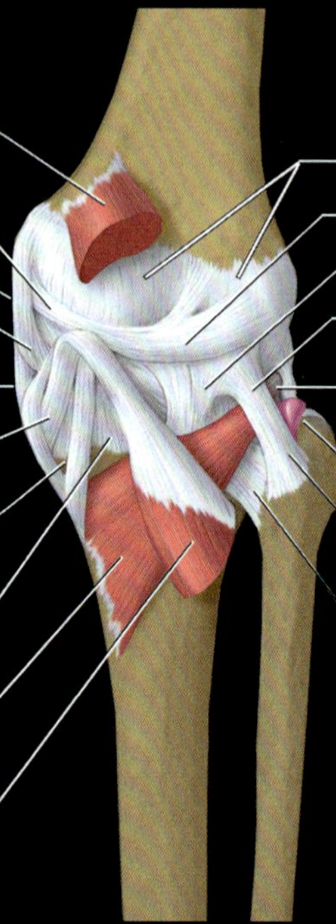

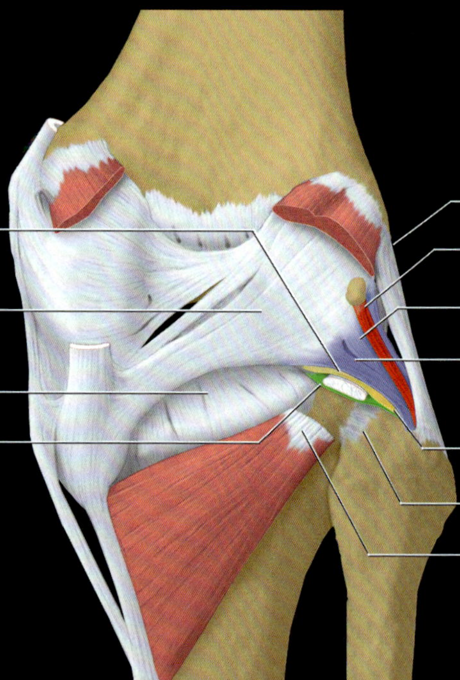

(Top) *Graphic shows the posterior stabilizing structures of the knee. The arcuate ligament arises from the posterior fibular head; both the lateral and medial branches contribute to the oblique popliteal ligament, which strengthens the posterior capsule. The posterior oblique ligament, originating from posterior fibers of medial collateral ligament (MCL), blends posteriorly into the capsule and the oblique popliteal ligament.* **(Bottom)** *Graphic with popliteus tendon cut shows its complex attachments. The superior fascicle extends from the posterior horn meniscus over the popliteus tendon to attach to its paratenon and capsule. Medial (oblique) arcuate joins this to form the roof of popliteal hiatus. Inferior fascicle forms the floor of hiatus; the convergence of the superior and inferior fascicles attach on the fibula forms the popliteofibular ligament.*

GRAPHICS & MR: POSTEROLATERAL CORNER

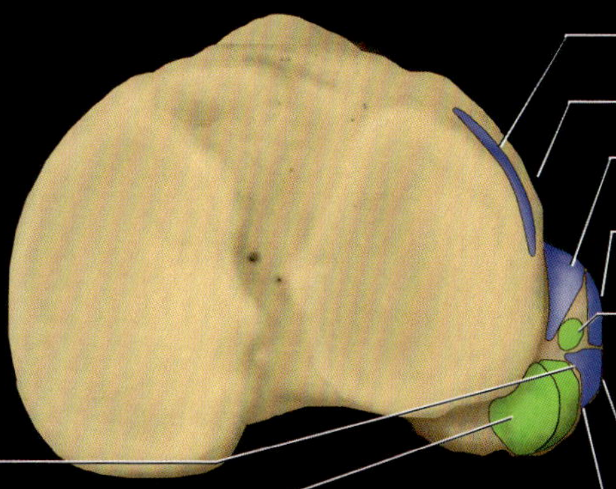

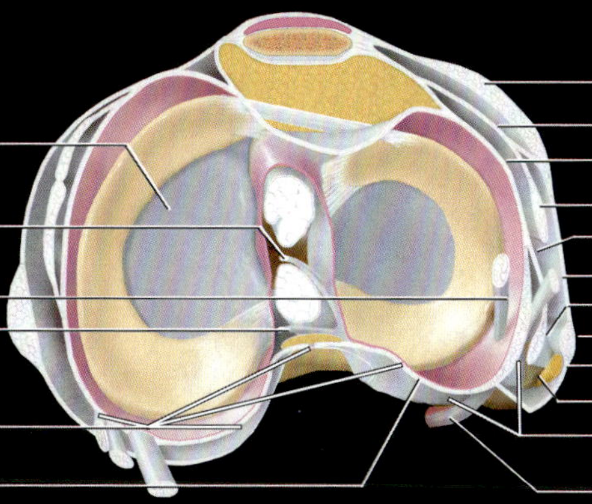

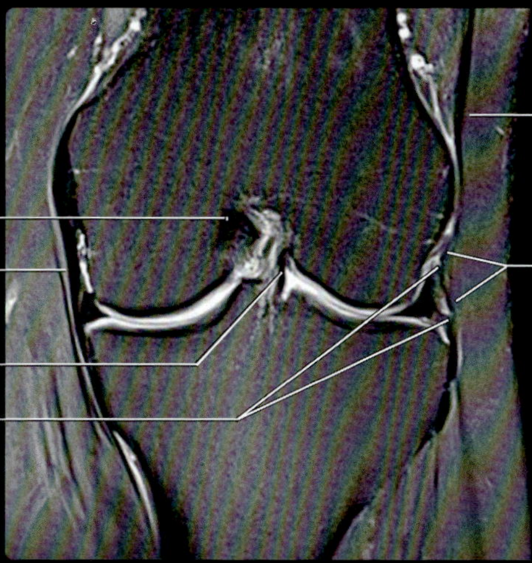

(Top) *Axial graphic shows the insertion sites of posterolateral structures on the proximal fibula. Note that the 2 heads of the short head biceps femoris insert most anteriorly, with the lateral collateral ligament (LCL) and 2 heads of the long head biceps femoris directly posterior to them. The arcuate, fabellofibular, and popliteofibular ligaments insert more posteriorly at the apex of the fibular head (fibular styloid process).* **(Middle)** *Axial graphic shows the lateral capsuloligamentous complex. Superficial posterolateral structures include long and short heads biceps femoris and LCLs. Deep posterolateral structures include the fabellofibular, arcuate, oblique popliteal, and popliteofibular ligaments. The posterior fibers of the anterolateral ligament blend with the LCL.* **(Bottom)** *Coronal PD FS MR shows the anterolateral ligament attaching to the tibia posterior to the attachment of the iliotibial band. Its attachments to the body of the lateral meniscus are well seen.*

AXIAL MR: POSTEROLATERAL CORNER

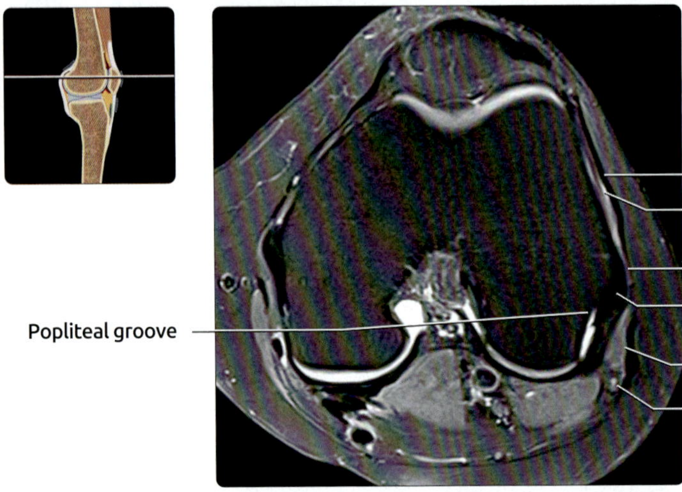

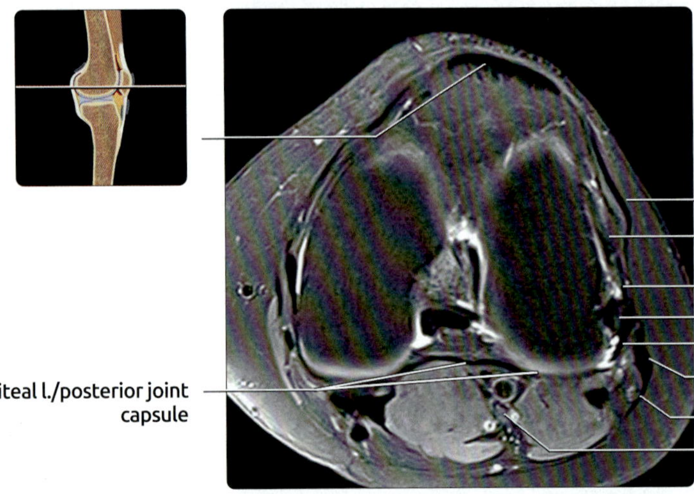

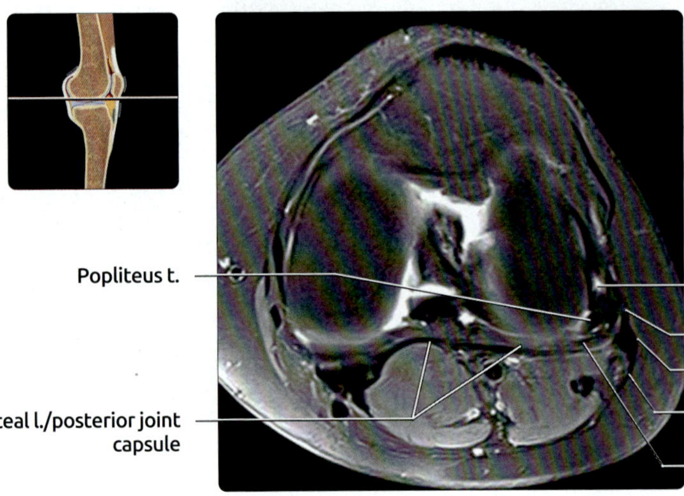

(Top) *First of 6 axial PD FS MR images demonstrating the structures of the posterolateral corner of the knee is shown. The LCL and anterolateral ligament are seen arising at the superior margin of the popliteal groove of the femur.* **(Middle)** *The popliteus tendon is seen at its insertion on the popliteal groove. The LCL is immediately superficial to it, coursing posteriorly, laterally, and inferiorly. The anterolateral ligament diverges from the LCL, coursing anteriorly and inferiorly, close to the lateral margin of the femoral condyle.* **(Bottom)** *The arcuate ligament is seen superficial to the popliteus tendon. The LCL is approaching the biceps femoris tendon.*

AXIAL MR: POSTEROLATERAL STRUCTURES

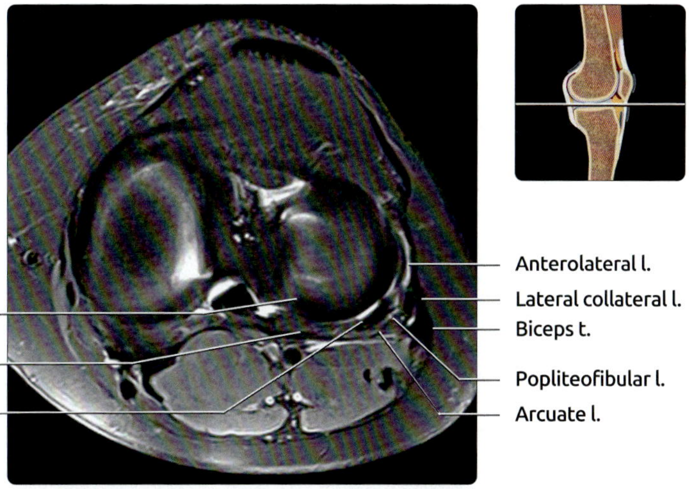

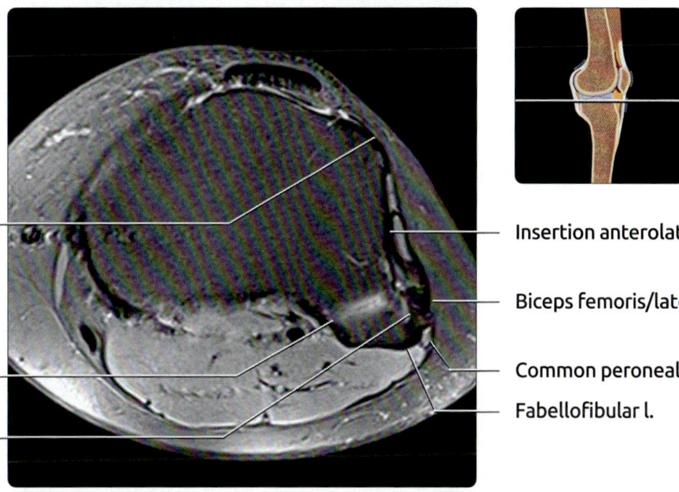

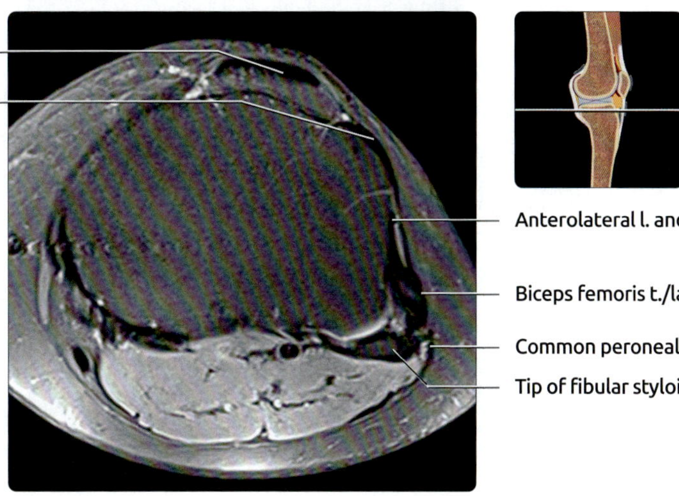

(Top) *The popliteofibular ligament extends from the popliteus tendon just distal to the meniscopopliteal fascicles and inserts posteriorly on the tip of the fibula.* **(Middle)** *The LCL and the fibular fibers of the biceps femoris are seen inserting along the lateral margin of the fibular styloid.* **(Bottom)** *The conjoint biceps femoris tendon and LCL are seen just proximal to their attachment to the fibula. The anterolateral ligament blends with anterior fibers of the biceps femoris attaching to the tibia.*

CORONAL & SAGITTAL MR: POSTEROLATERAL STRUCTURES: FABELLOFIBULAR LIGAMENT

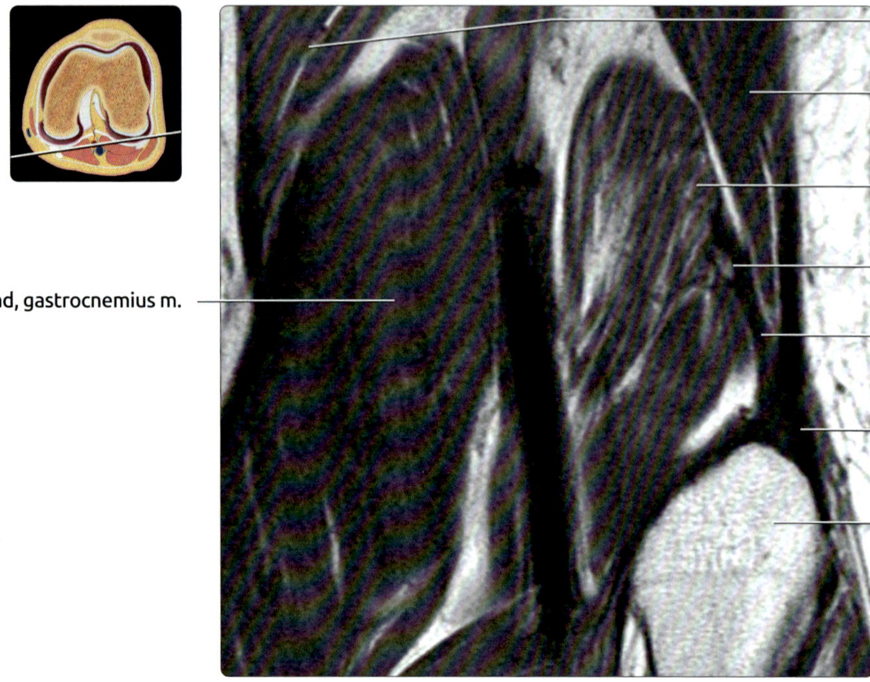

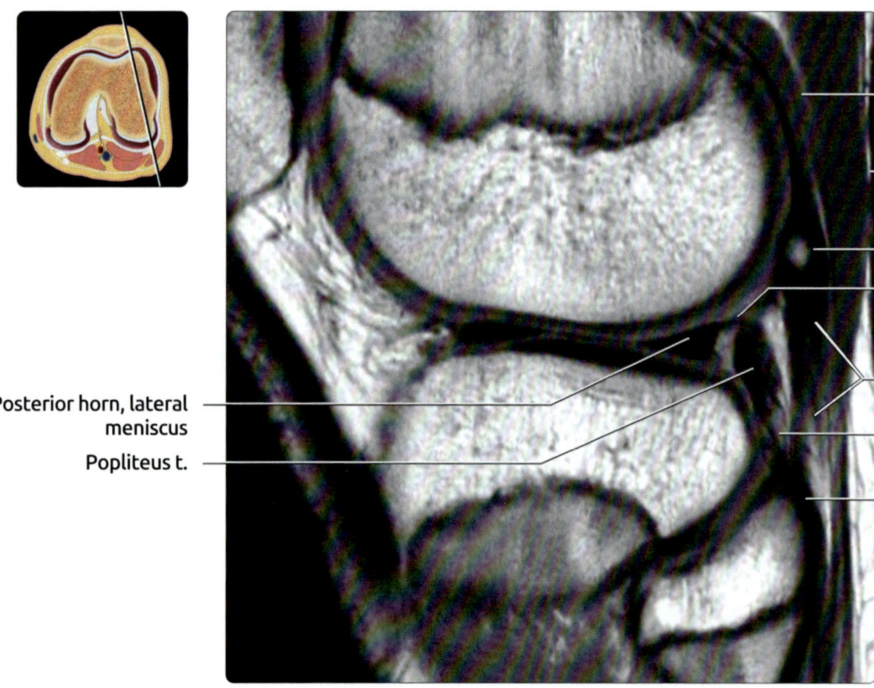

(Top) *This far posterior coronal cut shows a fabella within the lateral head of the gastrocnemius. There is a prominent fabellofibular ligament, extending from the fabella to the posterior aspect of the head of the fibula, immediately posteromedial to the long head biceps tendon insertion. This ligament is hypertrophied; it is not usually seen this well.* **(Bottom)** *Sagittal cut located laterally shows the hypertrophied fabellofibular ligament in the same patient. The fabella is distinctly seen with the fabellofibular ligament investing it and extending to the apex of fibular styloid. The popliteus tendon is within the popliteal hiatus; the superior fascicle extends from the posterior horn lateral meniscus to the superior paratenon of popliteus. The thin popliteofibular ligament is seen extending from the fibular head to the popliteus as well.*

SAGITTAL MR: POSTEROLATERAL STRUCTURES: BICEPS FEMORIS, FABELLOFIBULAR, ARCUATE

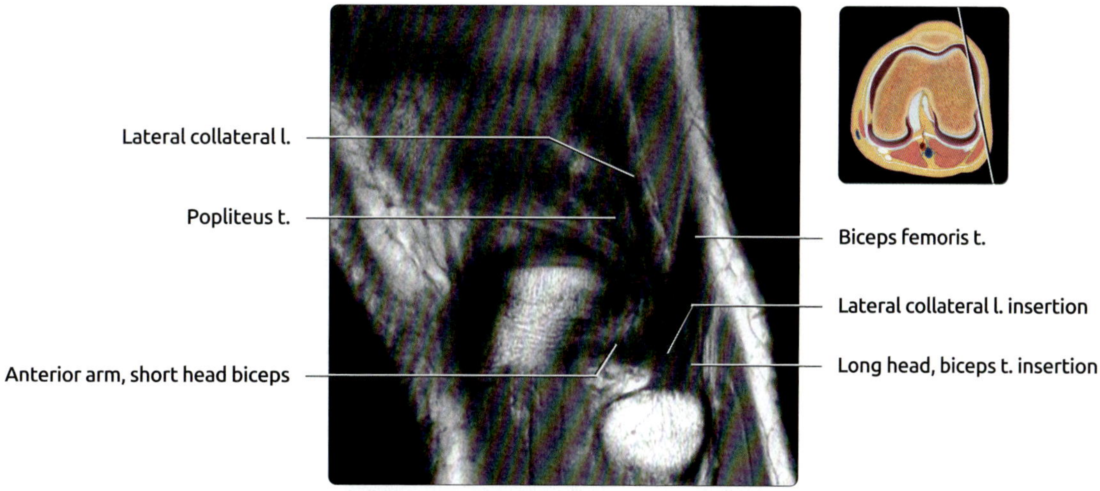

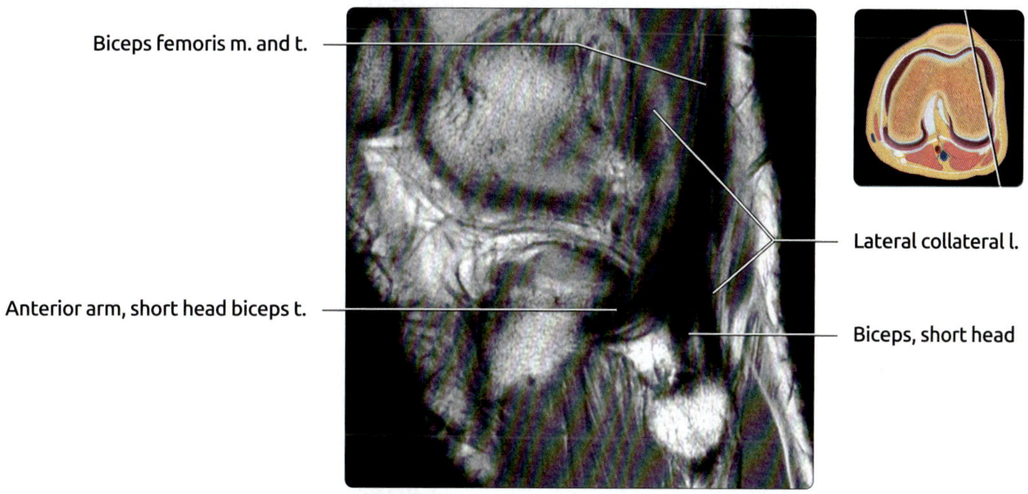

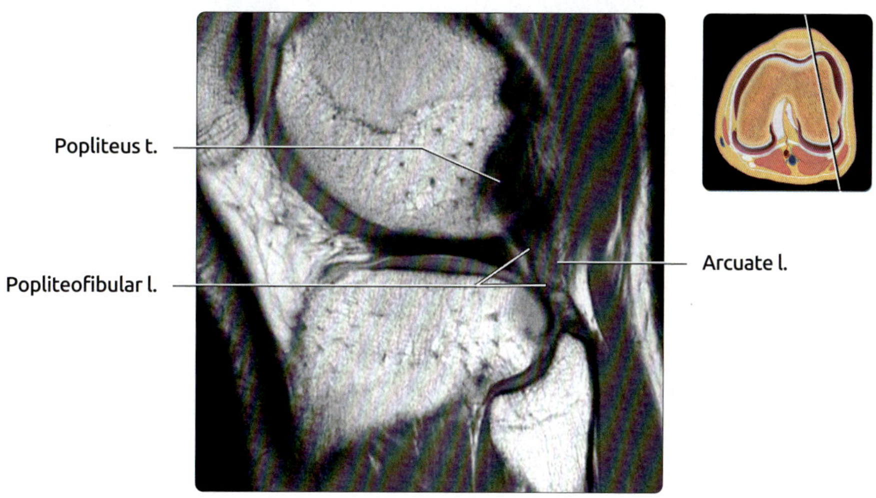

(Top) *First of 3 sagittal T1 MR images, far lateral, shows the complex set of insertions of long and short heads of biceps femoris. Although they are not often discerned as separate on MR imaging, the long head of biceps has 2 insertions on the posterolateral portion of fibular head. The short head of biceps has 1 insertion on the fibular head immediately anterior to the long head and a 2nd broad insertion on anterolateral tibia. The LCL inserts immediately medial to long head biceps.* **(Middle)** *Slightly medial, one sees partial voluming of the LCL. Short head of biceps is still seen inserting on the anterolateral tibia with a branch inserting on fibular head.* **(Bottom)** *Image at the level of the bow tie of the meniscus shows the popliteus tendon extending to hiatus, the popliteofibular ligament extending from the paratenon to fibula, and posteriorly, the arcuate ligament.*

SAGITTAL PD MR: POPLITEUS TENDON

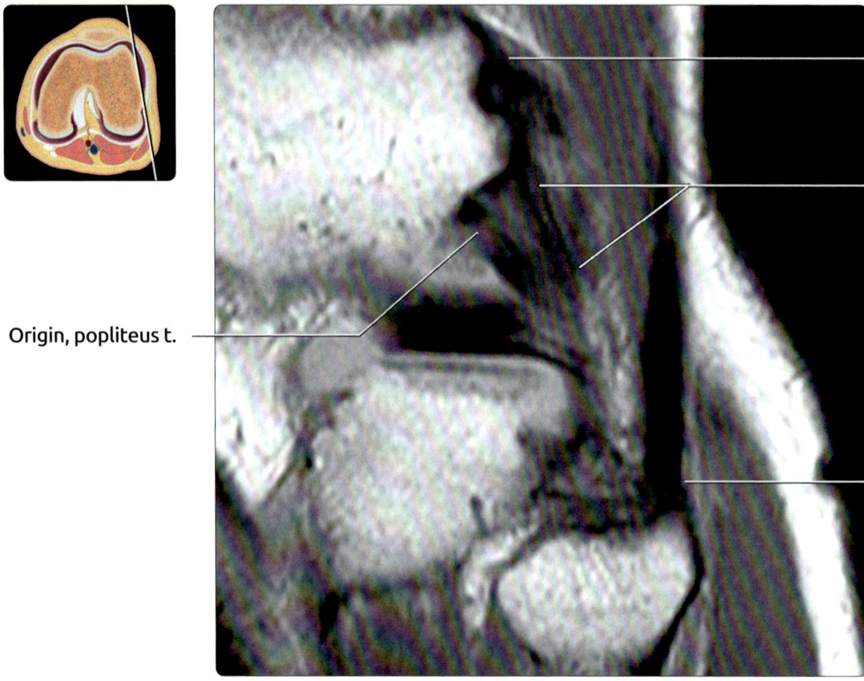

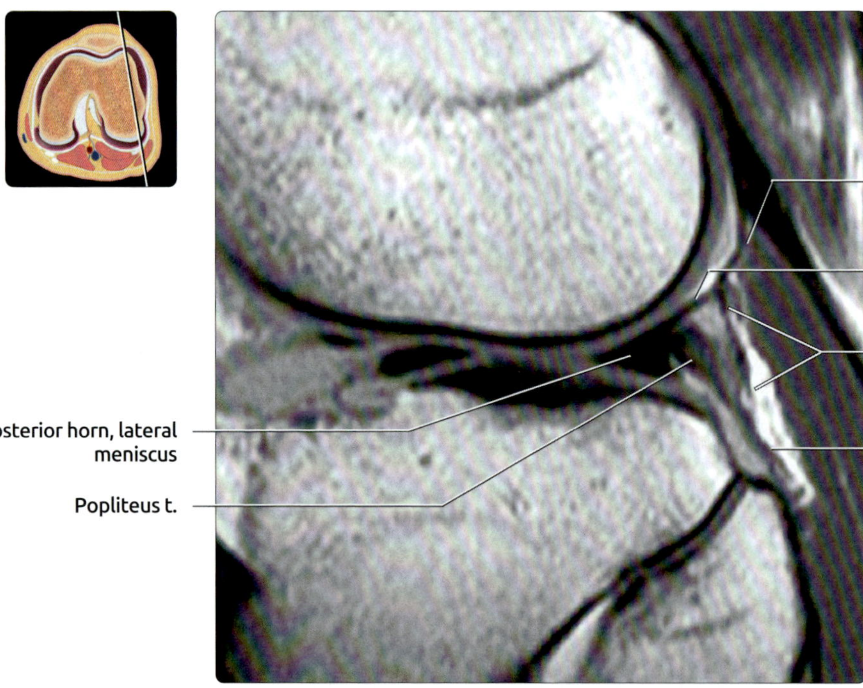

(Top) *First of 5 sagittal PD MR images following the course of the popliteus tendon is shown. In this far lateral image, the biceps femoris is seen inserting on the fibular head. A hint of origin of the popliteus tendon in its sulcus in the lateral femoral condyle is seen, along with the origin of the LCL.* **(Bottom)** *Slightly medially, the popliteus tendon enters the joint and its hiatus. The lateral (oblique) head of the arcuate ligament is seen arising along with the popliteofibular ligament from the fibular styloid; the arcuate ligament continues toward the oblique popliteal ligament and capsule of the joint.*

SAGITTAL PD MR: POPLITEUS TENDON

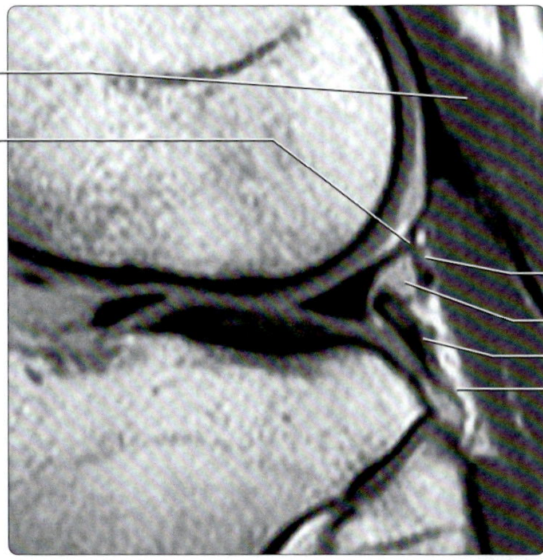

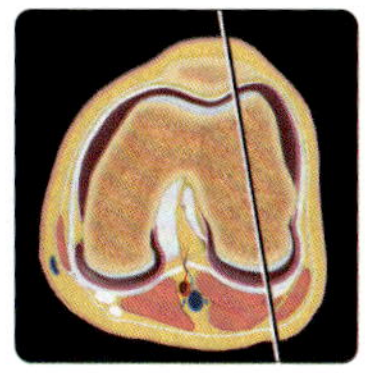

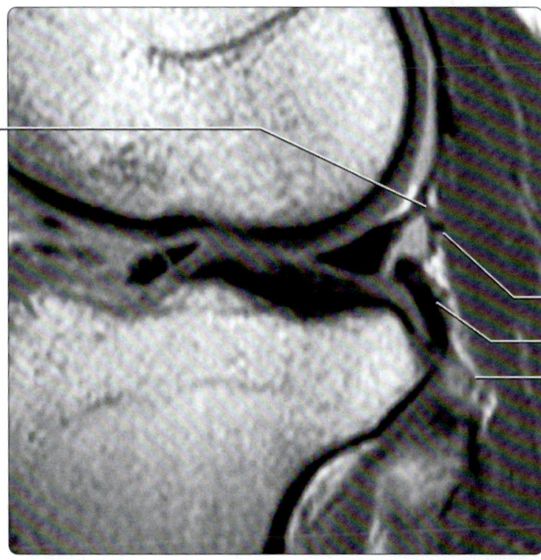

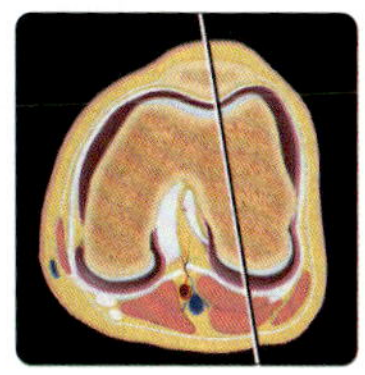

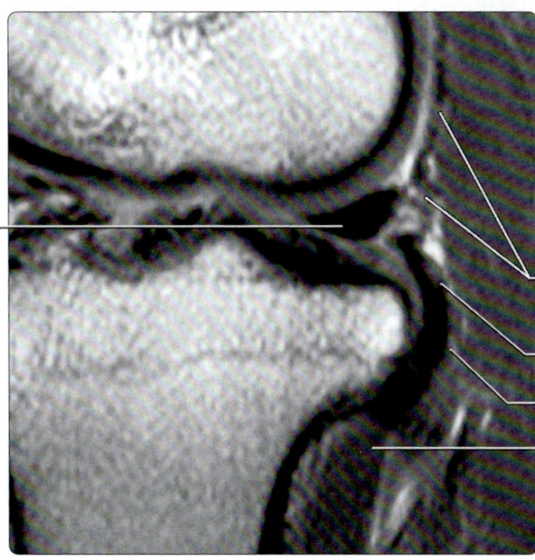

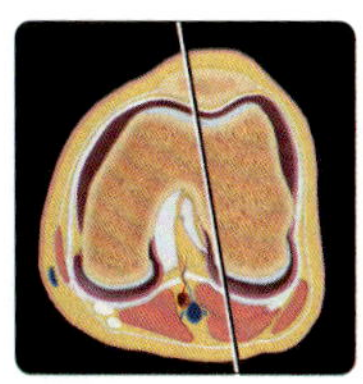

(Top) *Slightly more medially, the popliteus elongates downward; the popliteofibular ligament merges with its paratenon. By this point, the medial branch of the arcuate ligament has joined the superior fascicle to form the roof of the popliteal hiatus.* **(Middle)** *The popliteus tendon approaches its musculotendinous junction. Note the arched roof of the popliteal hiatus formed by the superior fascicle and the medial branch of the arcuate ligament.* **(Bottom)** *Approaching, but not yet in the intercondylar notch, the popliteus tendon is seen at its musculotendinous junction. The muscle can be seen extending distally toward its insertion on the posterior tibia. By this point, the posterior horn of the lateral meniscus has rejoined the posterior capsule.*

CORONAL MR: POSTEROLATERAL STRUCTURES

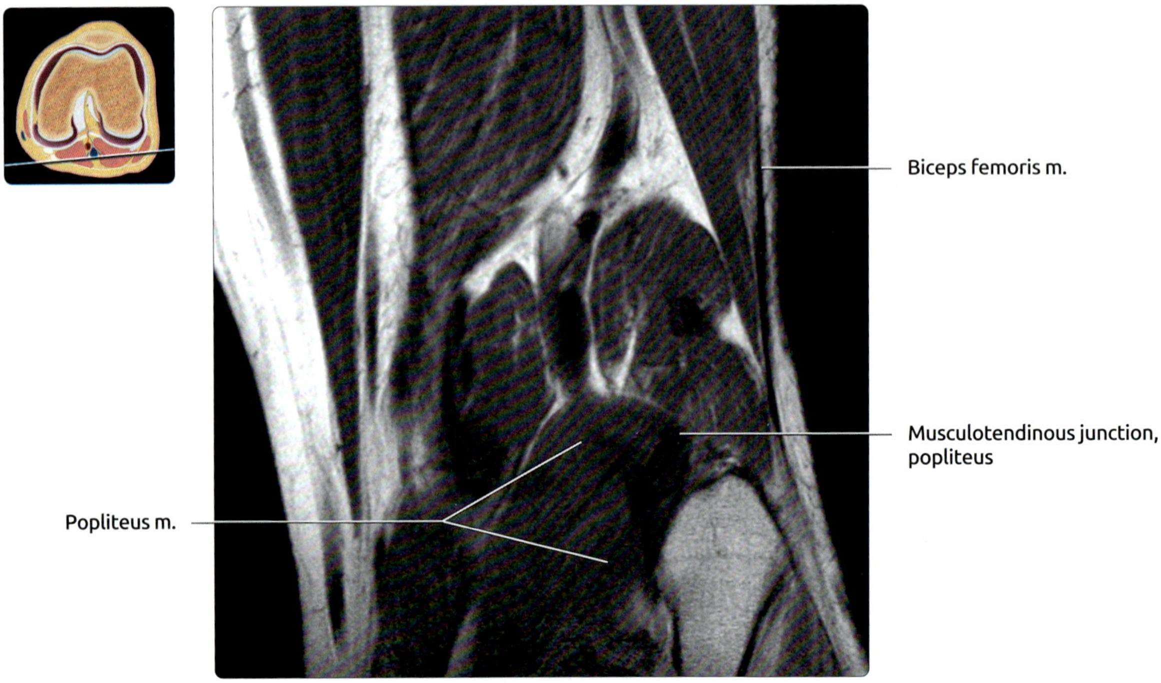

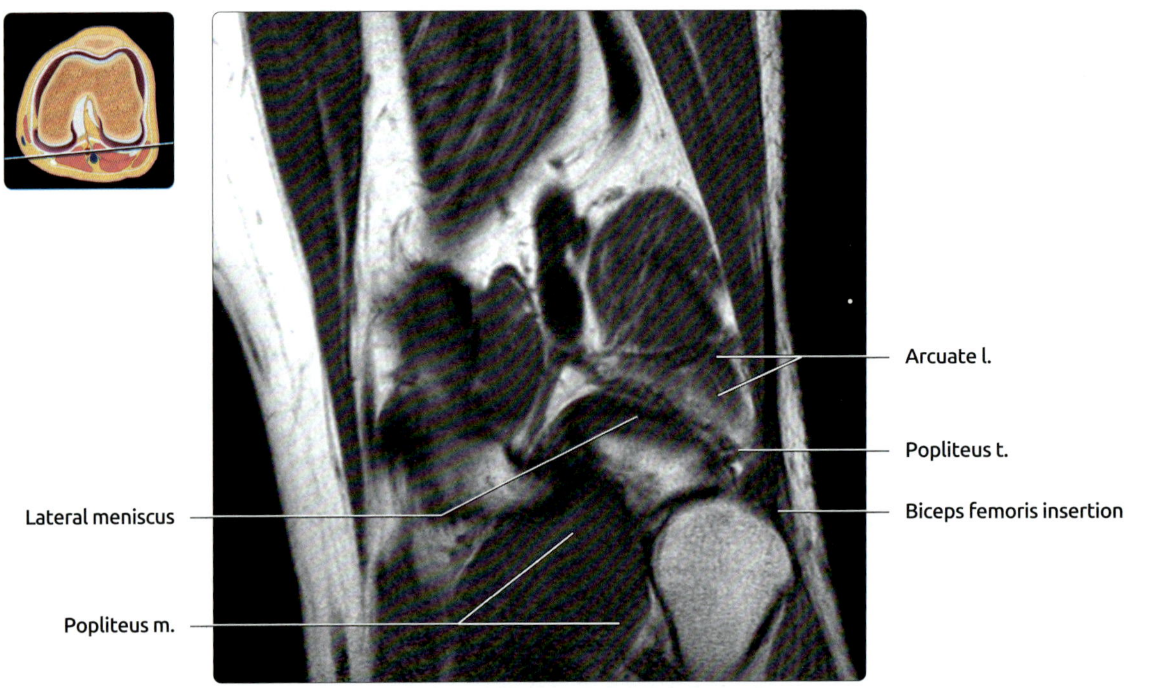

(Top) *First of 2 coronal T1 MR images, far posterior, shows structures in the posteriormost aspect of posterolateral corner. The musculotendinous junction of the popliteus is seen, extending into the popliteus muscle.* **(Bottom)** *Slightly more anteriorly, the long head of biceps femoris inserts on the outer aspect of the fibular head. A corner of the popliteus tendon is seen extending around the posterolateral tibia toward its musculotendinous junction. Arcuate ligament is seen joining the posterior capsule.*

CORONAL MR: POSTEROLATERAL STRUCTURES

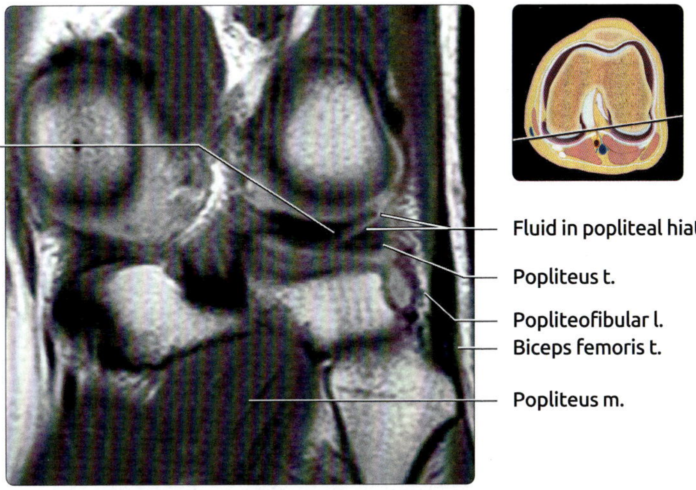

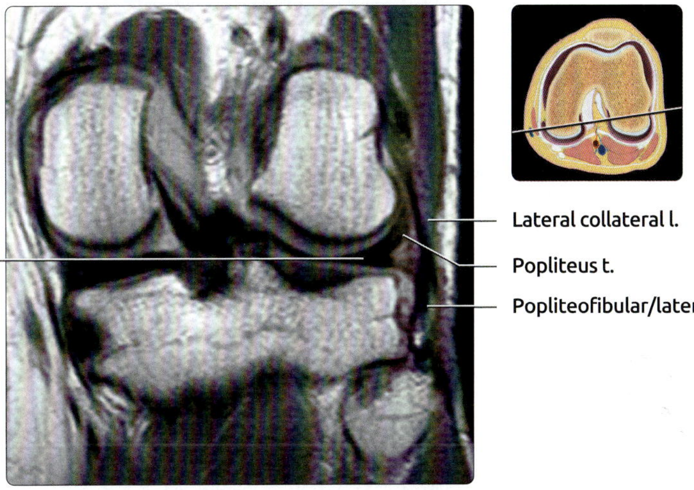

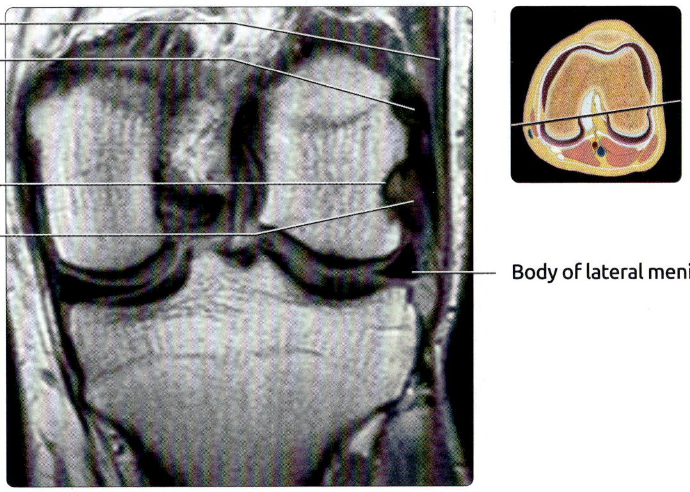

(Top) *First of 3 coronal PD MR images following the popliteus tendon is shown, outlined here by fluid within the popliteal hiatus. This more posterior view of the 3 shows the popliteus muscle, as well as the popliteus tendon as it traverses the hiatus, with fluid separating the tendon from the posterior horn, lateral meniscus. Biceps femoris tendon inserts laterally on the fibular head.* **(Middle)** *Slightly more anteriorly, the midportion of the LCL is seen extending toward its insertion on the lateral femoral head. Popliteus tendon is just entering the hiatus at the level of junction of the posterior horn/body of lateral meniscus.* **(Bottom)** *At a midcoronal cut, the origins of both the LCL and popliteus tendon are seen. At this point, the body of the lateral meniscus is directly attached to capsule since the popliteus has not yet entered the hiatus.*

CORONAL OBLIQUE T1 MR: POSTEROLATERAL STRUCTURES

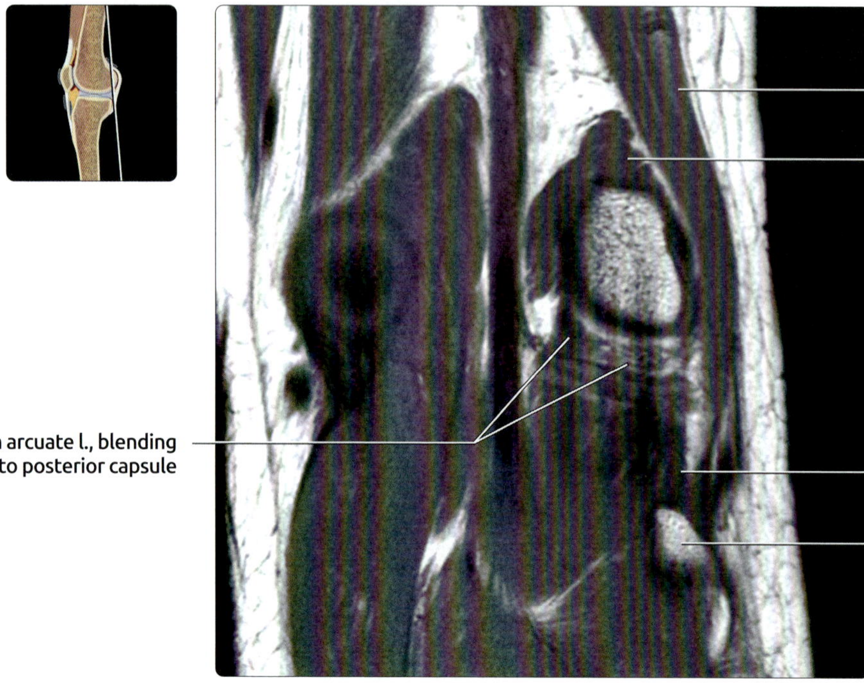

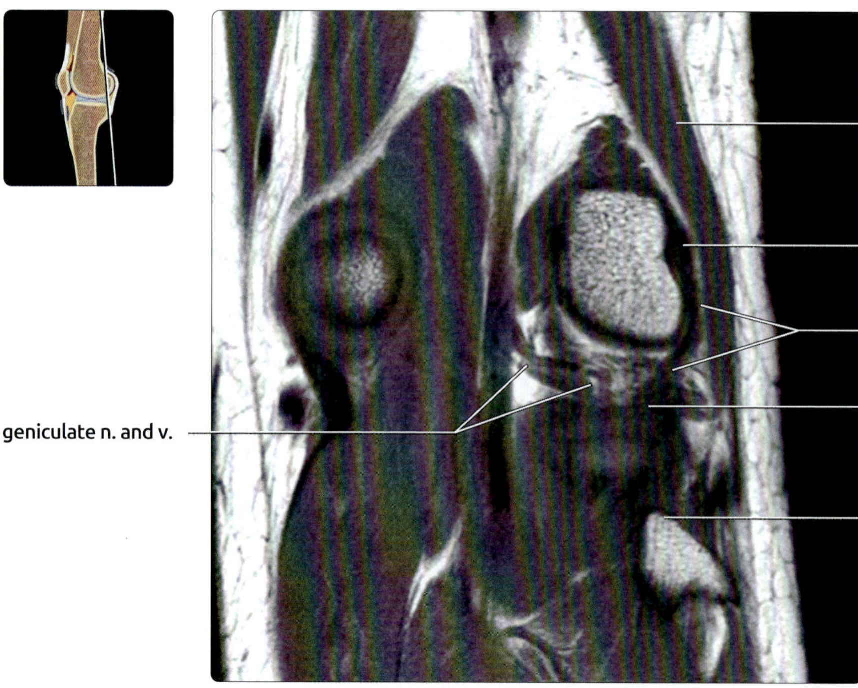

(Top) *First of 4 coronal oblique T1 MR images of posterolateral structures is shown. The images are prescribed off a sagittal, angling from anterosuperior to posteroinferior, following the popliteus tendon. Thus, in this image, we see more of the lateral femoral condyle than fibula. It allows visualization of oblique posterior structures, such as the fabellofibular ligament and arcuate ligament. This image is too far posterior to include much popliteus tendon.* **(Bottom)** *Slightly anterior to the previous image, this lays the popliteus tendon out such that it is seen from its origin to the musculotendinous junction. The fibular origin of the popliteofibular ligament is seen with fibers stretching up to meet the popliteal paratenon. Portions of the arcuate ligament may be present but are not well seen. Since we are at the apex of the fibula, the biceps has not yet inserted.*

CORONAL OBLIQUE T1 MR: POSTEROLATERAL

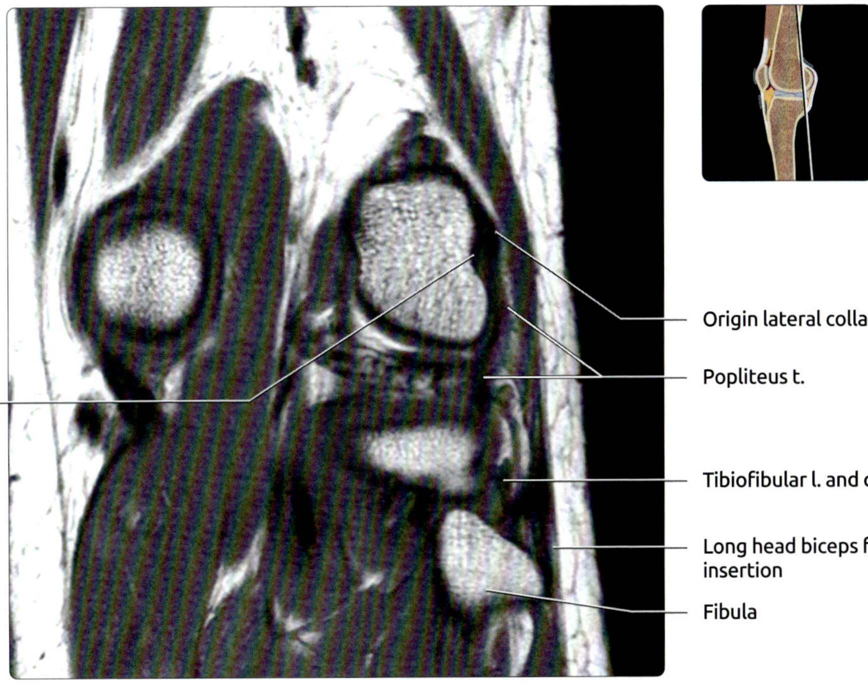

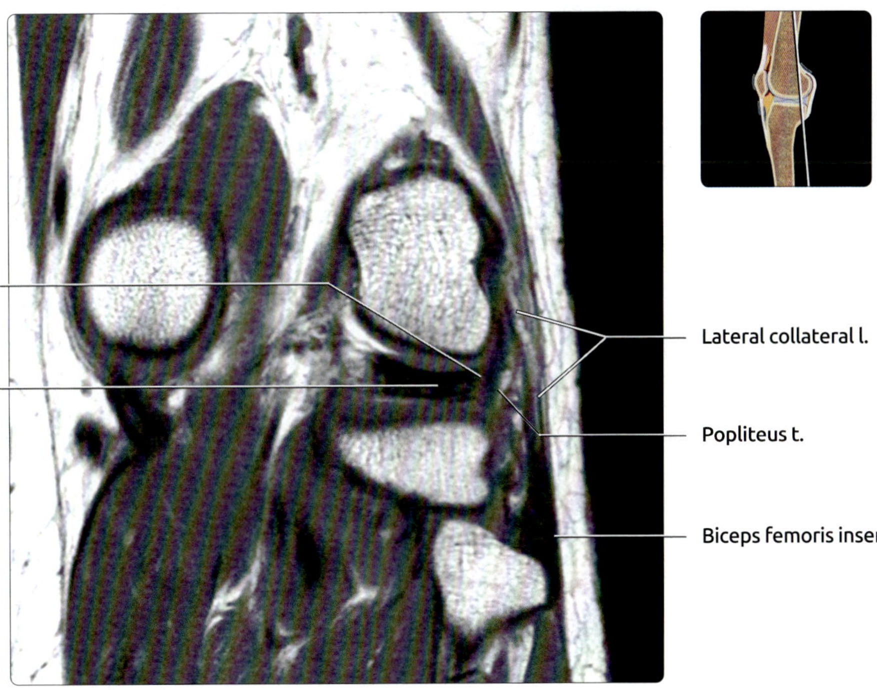

(Top) *Slightly anterior MR continues to show more of the origin of the popliteus tendon. The origin of the LCL is seen, and the long head of the biceps femoris inserts on the midportion of the fibula laterally.* **(Bottom)** *More anteriorly, the popliteus tendon is seen separated from the posterior horn of the lateral meniscus by fluid in the popliteal hiatus. The biceps more fully inserts on the fibula, with the LCL inserting immediately medial to it.*

GROSS ANATOMY

Overview

- Largest and most complex joint
  - Hinge joint throughout its greatest range of motion
  - Bones do not interlock; stability is maintained by ligaments, tendons, capsule, and menisci
- **Extensors of knee**
  - Quadriceps: 4 muscles form common tendon, inserting on patella & patellar retinacula
    - Rectus femoris, vastus medialis, vastus intermedius, vastus lateralis
  - Semimembranosus: Inserts on posterior aspect of medial tibial condyle
- **Flexors of knee**
  - Pes anserinus: Conjoined tendon of sartorius, gracilis, semitendinosus
    - Inserts on anteromedial tibia
    - Immediately distal and anterior to insertion of medial collateral ligament (MCL)
  - Biceps femoris inserts on fibular head and tibia
  - Popliteus: Originates on posterior surface of proximal tibia, inserts on popliteal groove

IMAGING ANATOMY

Extensor Mechanism

- Quadriceps tendon inserts on patella
- Quadriceps continuation is aponeurosis of quadriceps along anterior patella, continuous with patellar tendon
- Patellar tendon (a.k.a. patellar ligament) extends from inferior pole of patella to tibial tubercle

Retinacula

- Medial, lateral retinacula extend from patella to femur
- Condensation of medial retinaculum is known as medial patellofemoral ligament
  - Extends from midpole of patella to medial femoral condyle, immediately superior to origin of MCL
- Fibers of vastus lateralis and medialis contribute to lateral and medial retinacula, respectively

Fat Pads

- Suprapatellar: Anterior and posterior to suprapatellar bursa
- Infrapatellar (Hoffa fat pad): Inferior to patella and between patellar ligament and anterior knee joint
- Posterior: Around joint margin extending into intercondylar region

Medial Supporting Structures

- Superficial (layer 1)
  - Pes anserinus
    - Sartorius, gracilis, semitendinosus tendons
    - Sartorius embedded in crural fascia
    - Gracilis immediately deep to sartorius
    - Insert on anteromedial tibia, immediately anterior to MCL insertion
- Middle (layer 2)
  - Superficial MCL
    - Anteriorly, longitudinal component fascia blends with layer 1
    - Posteriorly, oblique component blends with layer 3 as posterior oblique ligament
    - 2 tibial insertions: 1st on condyle, 2nd on proximal metadiaphysis
- Deep (layer 3)
  - Meniscofemoral ligament
  - Meniscotibial ligament
  - Posterior oblique ligament
    - Posterior to MCL
    - Blends with posteromedial meniscus
    - Receives fibers from semimembranosus tendon
    - Envelops posterior aspect of femoral condyle

Lateral Supporting Structures

- Iliotibial band
  - Inserts on Gerdy tubercle
- Posterolateral corner complex
  - Lateral (fibular) collateral ligament originates from lateral femoral epicondyle, inserts on lateral margin of fibular head
  - Popliteus tendon inserts on popliteal groove of femur
  - Biceps femoris tendon inserts on fibula, tibia
  - Arcuate ligament originates from styloid process of fibular head, inserts into posterior capsule
  - Other ligaments are variable and small, not well seen by ultrasound

Internal Structures

- **Menisci**: Cushion and stabilize knee
  - Fibrocartilage
  - Only peripheral portion visualized by ultrasound
- **Cruciate ligaments**: Stabilize to anteroposterior motion, twisting
  - Not well visualized by ultrasound

Synovial Recesses of Knee Joint

- Suprapatellar, medial patellar, lateral patellar
- Increase in synovial fluid 1st accumulates in either medial or lateral recess and then suprapatellar recess
- Small amount of fluid in knee joint is normal but should not get more than small amount
- Synovial proliferation can also be best assessed at medial and lateral recesses
- Baker cyst is distension of gastrocnemius-semimembraneous bursa
- Usually has very small communication to knee joint
  - Fluid may not be able to reenter knee (1-way valve)

ANATOMY IMAGING ISSUES

Imaging Approaches

- Ultrasound
  - Good at assessing extracapsular structures and their abnormalities but limited evauation of internal structures of knee
  - Ideal for assessing extraarticular abnormalities, e.g., tendinosis, ligament disruptions, bursitis, masses, etc.

GRAPHICS: EXTENSOR MECHANISM

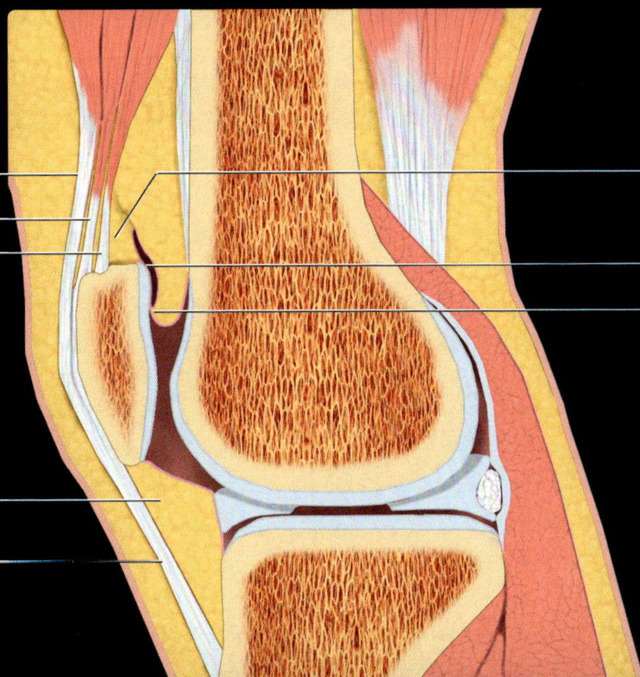

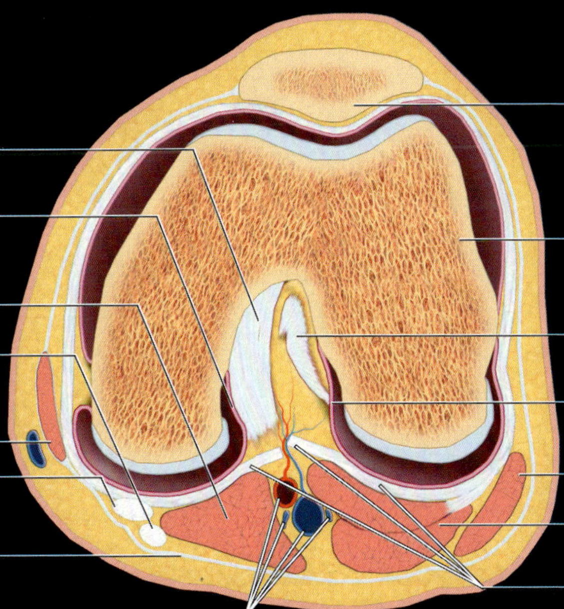

(Top) *Graphic shows trilaminar configuration of the quadriceps tendon. The superficial portion is the rectus femoris, the middle portion is the aponeurosis of the vastus medialis and lateralis, and the deep portion is the vastus intermedius tendon.* **(Bottom)** *Graphic shows the relationships of the posterior capsule and overlying structures. The most superficial layer is the crural fascia, which envelops the sartorius and otherwise confines all of the structures. The posterior capsule (white) is continuous with the synovium (pink thin line) both posteromedially and posterolaterally. Superficial to the capsule are the plantaris and gastrocnemius muscles, hamstring muscle and tendons, and the popliteal vessels.*

PANORAMIC: EXTENSOR MECHANISM

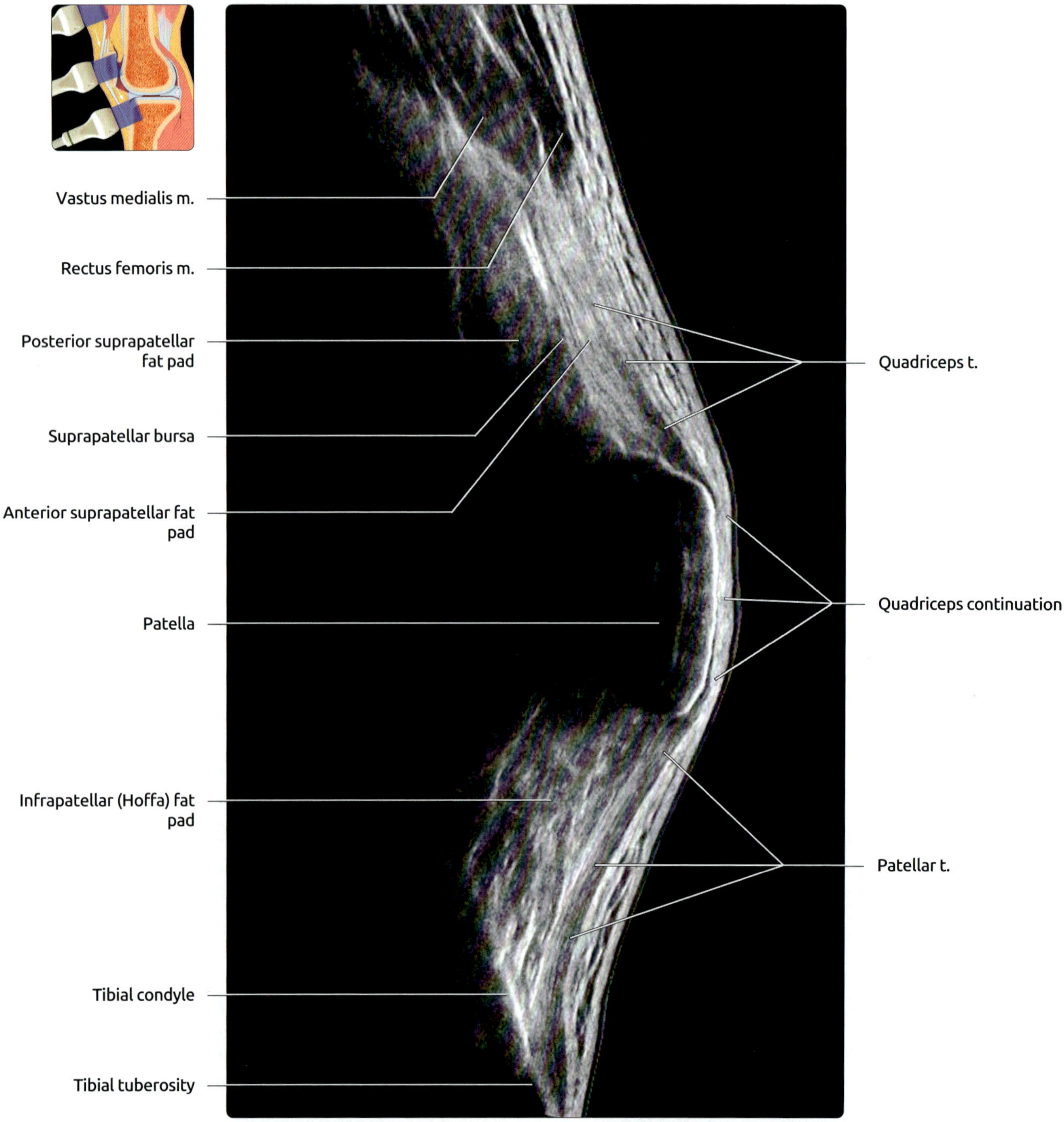

Sagittal panoramic scan of the anterior knee shows the main components of the extensor mechanism: Quadriceps muscles and tendon, patella, and patellar tendon. The scan performed here is with the knee in extension. More focused views of individual components of the anterior knee can be performed with the knee in flexion (with a pillow to support the popliteal region). Flexion increases the tension of the extensor mechanism, thus straightening the tendons. This will help highlight abnormalities in terms of tendon alignment and continuity. However, the amount of suprapatellar fluid may be decreased (due to displacement) in flexion, and assessment of the suprapatellar region in extension may be more sensitive in this respect.

SAGITTAL & TRANSVERSE US: EXTENSOR MECHANISM

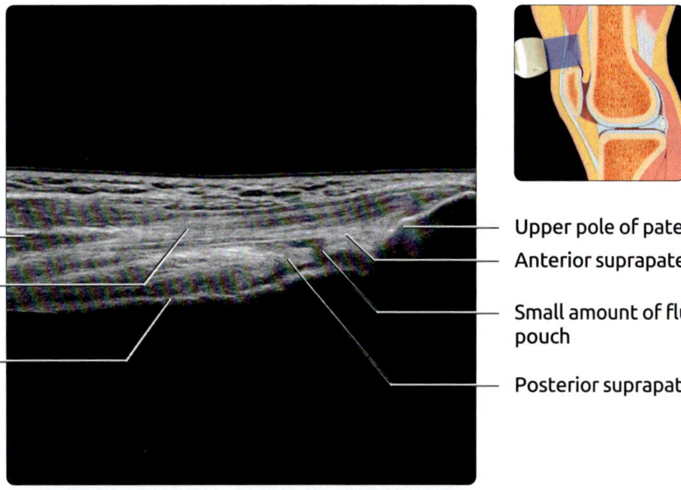

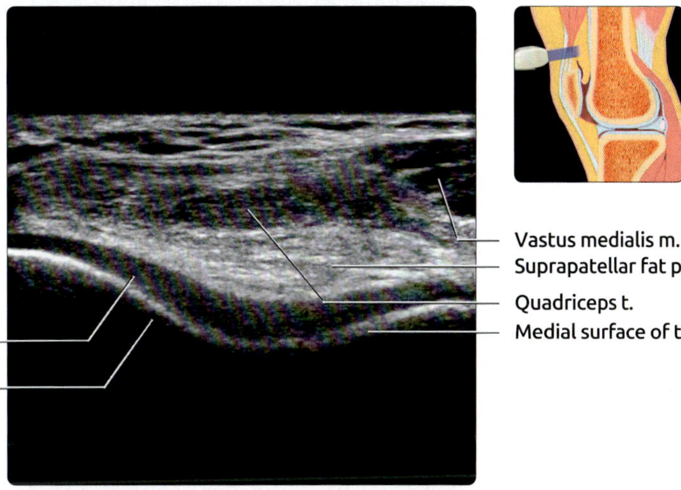

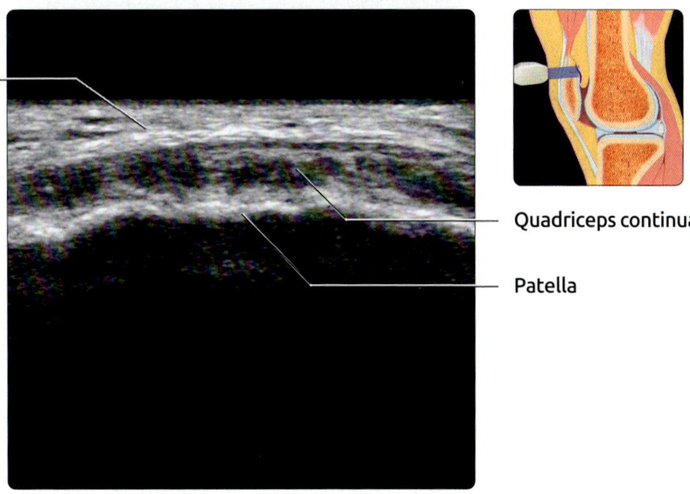

(Top) *Sagittal scan shows the quadriceps tendon. The quadriceps tendon is the direct continuation of the rectus femoris with contributions medially and laterally from the vastus medialis and the vastus lateralis, respectively, and posteriorly from vastus intermedius. The tendon inserts on the superoanterior surface of the patella. In this scan, the suprapatellar pouch can be seen. It may normally contain a small amount of fluid (several millimeters thick).* **(Middle)** *Transverse scan shows quadriceps tendon with the knee flexed. The central position of the quadriceps tendon can be appreciated here, receiving contributions from the vastus muscles. The articular cartilage of the trochlear groove can also be seen with the patella out of the way during flexion.* **(Bottom)** *Transverse scan of the anterior surface of the patella shows the quadriceps continuation, an aponeurosis along the anterior margin of the patella, continuous with both the quadriceps tendon and the patellar tendon.*

SAGITTAL US: EXTENSOR MECHANISM

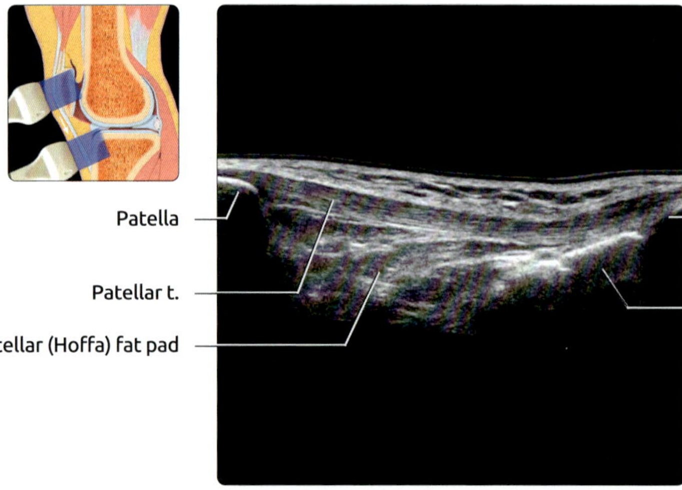

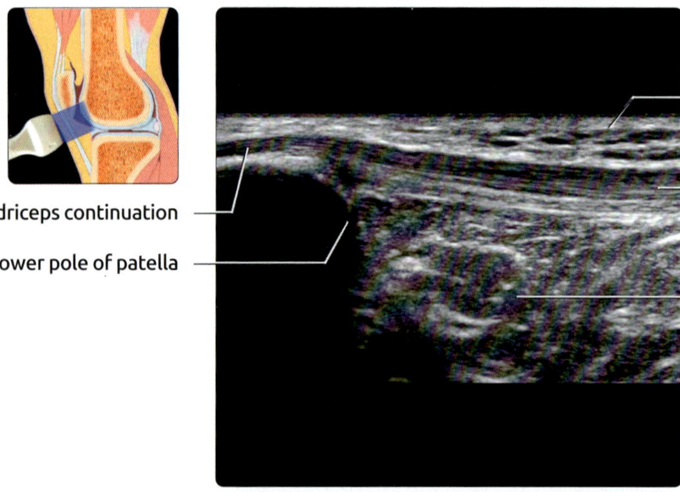

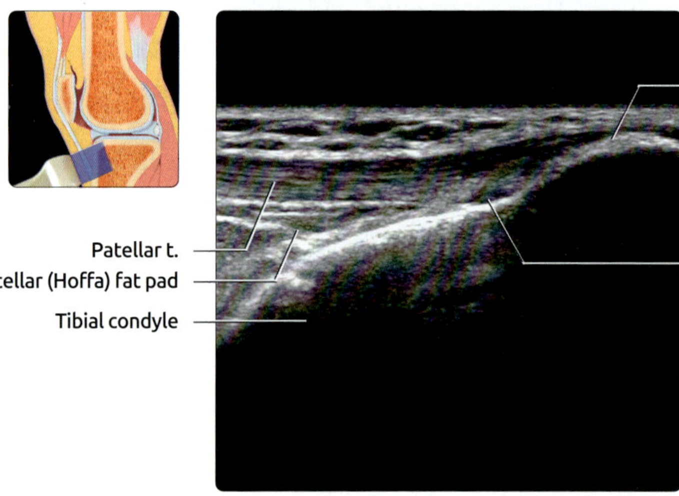

(Top) *Sagittal panoramic view shows the patellar tendon. Most of the fibers of the tendon are continuations of quadriceps tendon fibers.* **(Middle)** *Focused sagittal view of the apex of the patella shows quadriceps continuation on the anterior surface of the patella, continuing distally as the patellar tendon. Also seen here are fibers originating from the apex of the patella itself.* **(Bottom)** *Focused sagittal scan shows the tibial tuberosity. The distal fibers of the patellar tendon are separated from the anterior surface of the tibial condyle by the infrapatellar bursa. A small amount of fluid (2-3 mm thick) may be normally present in this bursa.*

TRANSVERSE US: EXTENSOR MECHANISM

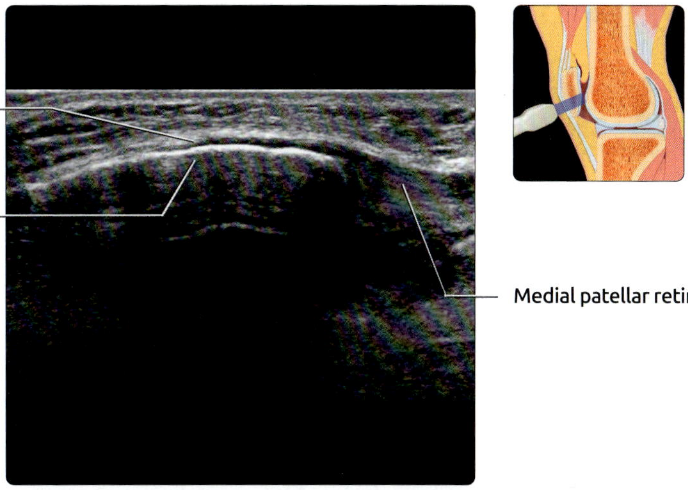

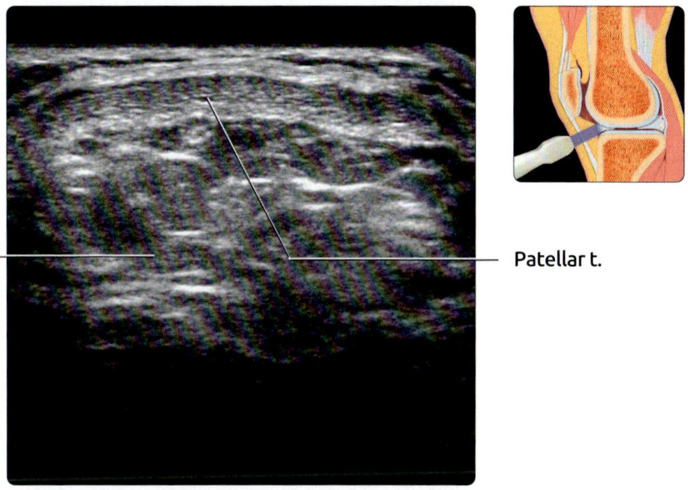

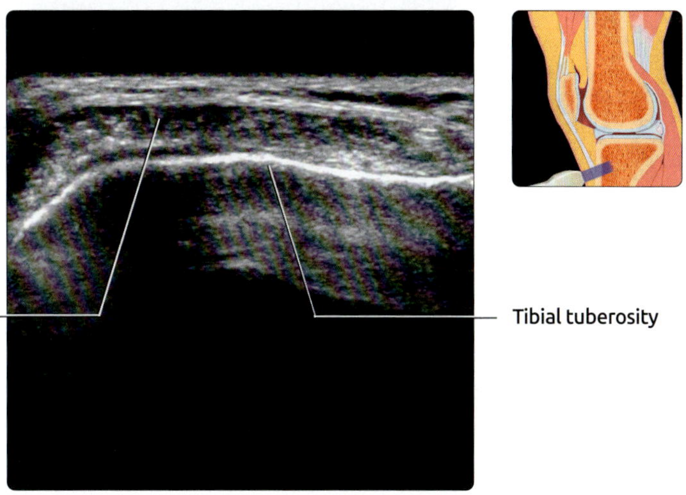

(Top) *Series of 3 transverse scans through the patellar tendon is shown. Proximally, fibers from the quadriceps tendon continue over the anterior patellar surface to contribute to the patellar tendon. On both sides, fibers from the medial and lateral patellar retinaculum also insert onto the patella and blend with the patellar tendon fibers.* **(Middle)** *At the midsubstance of the patellar tendon, the tendon assumes a flattened appearance. The fibers within the tendon can be seen as tiny hyperechoic dots. A disruption to the uniformity of these dots or a change in thickness (focal or general) of the patellar tendon suggests tendinosis.* **(Bottom)** *More inferiorly, a transverse scan shows the patellar tendon inserting onto the tibial tuberosity. The patellar tendon paratenon is seen as a thin echogenic line on the anterior surface and side walls of the tendon. It becomes thickened in patellar paratenonitis. This is an infrequently encountered condition.*

TRANSVERSE & SAGITTAL US: EXTENSOR MECHANISM

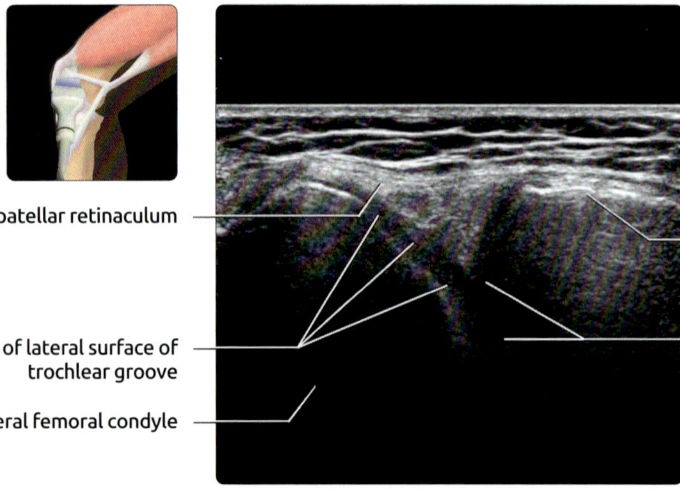

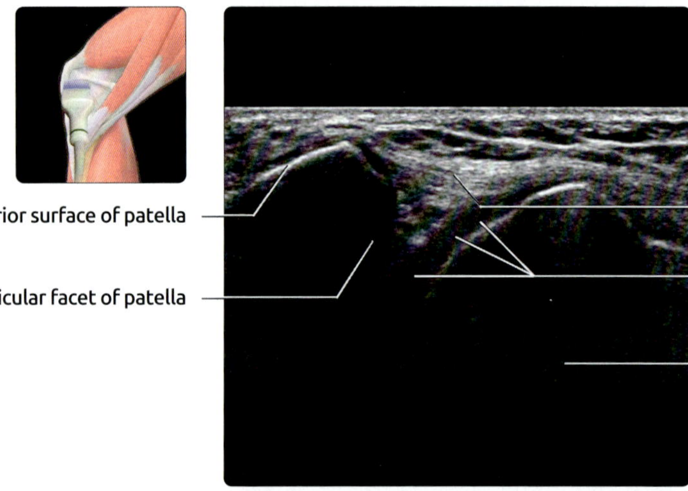

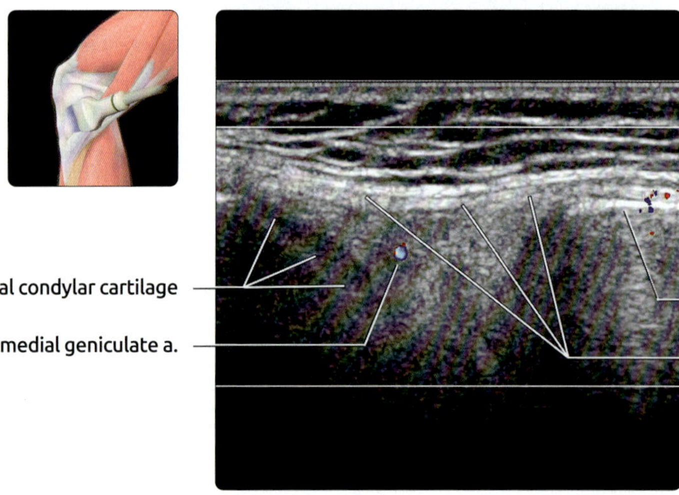

(Top) *Transverse scan at the lateral margin of the patella shows the articulation between the lateral patella and the lateral surface of the trochlear groove. This articular plane is steeper (closer to sagittal) than the medial side for mechanical advantage. As a result of the obliquity of the course of the patellar tendon with respect to the tibial axis, the patella is prone to lateral dislocation or subluxation. The steeper lateral articular plane helps prevents this.* **(Middle)** *Transverse scan at the medial margin of the patella shows the articulation between the patella and the medial surface of the trochlear groove, showing the medial patellofemoral ligament as a thick structure.* **(Bottom)** *Sagittal color Doppler scan of the medial infrapatellar region shows the patellar retinaculum inserting onto the tibia. At this level, the retinaculum has fanned out, becoming much thinner.*

GRAPHICS: MEDIAL KNEE

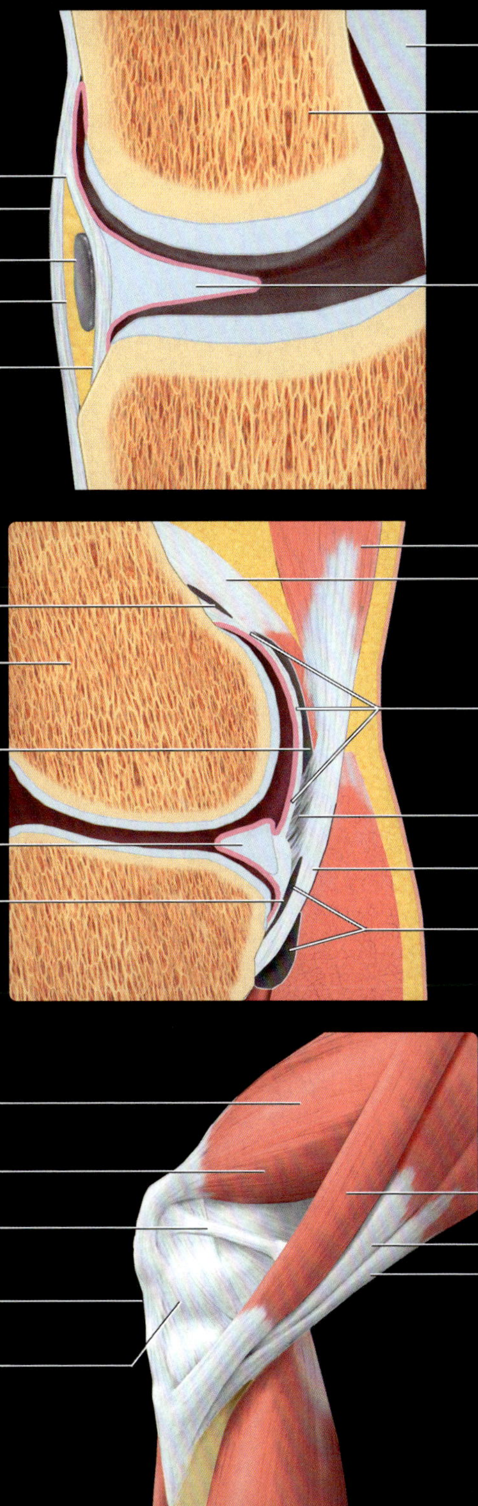

(Top) *Coronal graphic at midjoint shows superficial fibers extending from adductor tubercle to ~ 5 cm below the joint line. Deep fibers are shorter. The meniscotibial (coronary) ligament extends from the meniscus to the tibia adjacent to the joint line & the meniscofemoral ligament extends from the meniscus to the femur or superficial medial collateral ligament (MCL).* **(Middle)** *Sagittal graphic shows the far medial portion of posterior capsule. Superiorly, the capsule attaches to the cortex of the posterior femoral condyle and fuses with fibers of the medial gastrocnemius.* **(Bottom)** *Graphic shows the anteromedial attachment of pes anserinus tendons. The sartorius is the most anterior and superficial. The gracilis inserts directly adjacent and deep to the sartorius, and the semitendinosus inserts directly posterior and inferior to the gracilis. These tendons and their crural fascia comprise the superficial layer of the medial capsuloligamentous complex.*

CORONAL, TRANSVERSE, & SAGITTAL US: MEDIAL KNEE

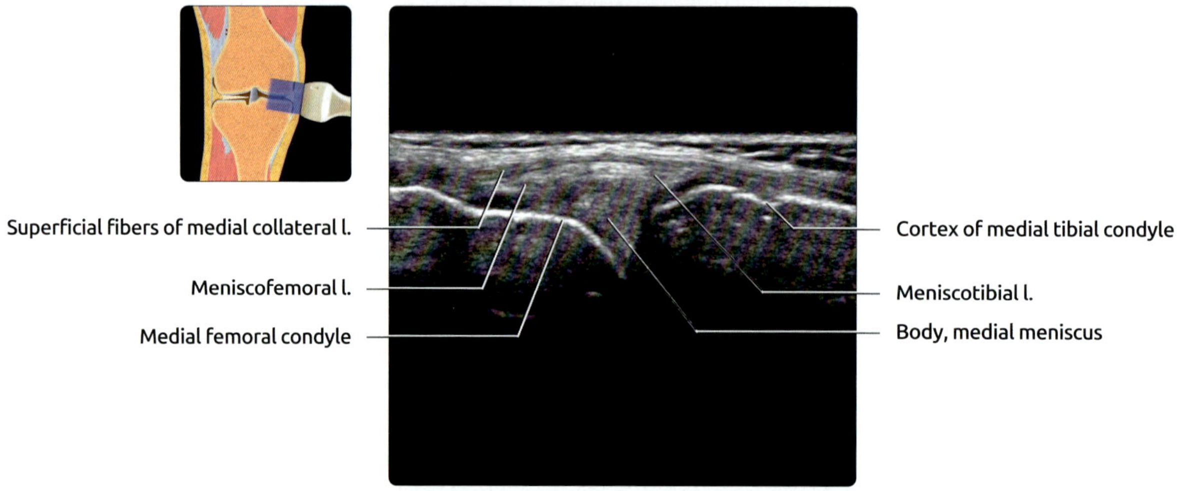

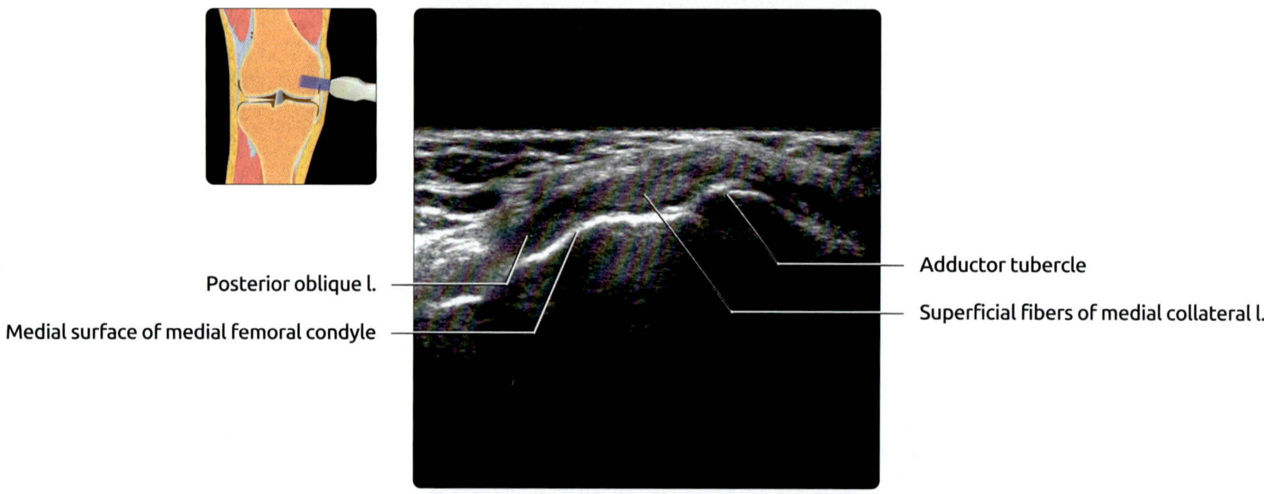

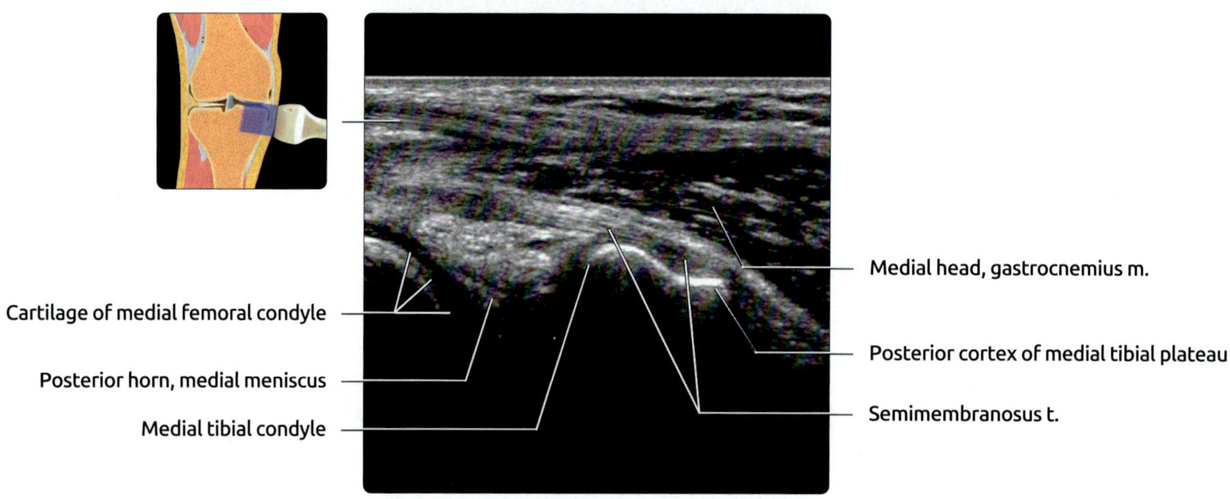

(Top) *Coronal scan shows the medial joint line. The MCL is composed of 2 layers: Superficial and deep. The superficial fibers run from the medial femoral condyle to the tibial condyle 5 cm below the joint line. The deep layer consists of the meniscofemoral (femoral condyle to body of meniscus) and meniscotibial (body of meniscus to tibia just distal to joint line).* **(Middle)** *Transverse scan shows the medial condylar region. The superficial fibers of the MCL arise just distal to the adductor tubercle. The popliteal oblique ligament arises adjacent to this and runs posterior to the posterior joint capsule.* **(Bottom)** *Sagittal scan shows the posteromedial joint line. The semimembranosus tendon inserts onto the posterior surface of the medial tibial condyle, just below the joint margin. Only the outer part of the meniscus is visible.*

GRAPHICS: LATERAL KNEE

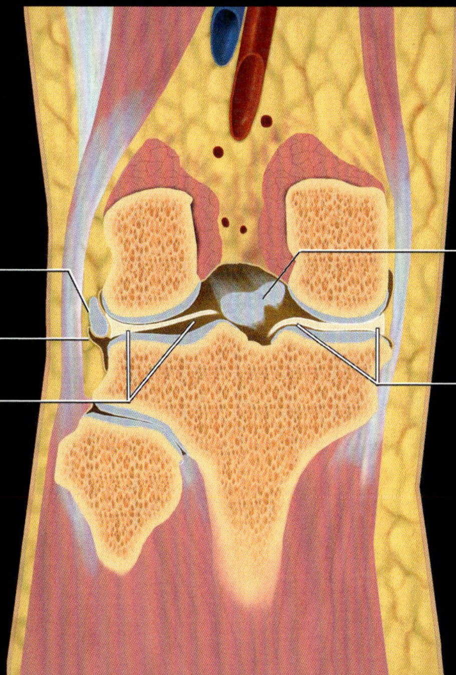

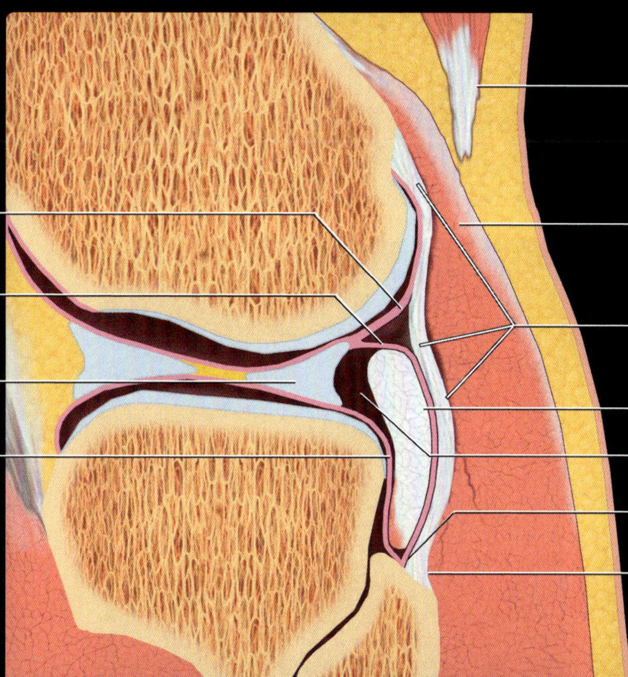

(Top) *Coronal graphic shows the roots of the posterior horns of both the medial and lateral menisci. The popliteus tendon courses through the hiatus adjacent to the body/posterior horn of the lateral meniscus.* **(Bottom)** *Sagittal graphic of lateral part of posterior capsule shows that it is intimately attached to the lateral gastrocnemius muscle. The popliteus tendon is intraarticular but extrasynovial and is attached to the capsule. Fibers from the posterolateral corner and arcuate ligament originating from the fibular head contribute to the lateral portion of the posterior capsule.*

SAGITTAL & TRANSVERSE US: LATERAL KNEE

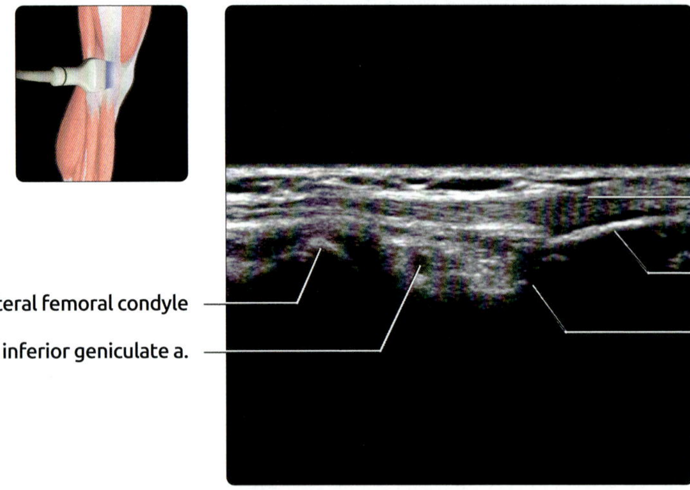

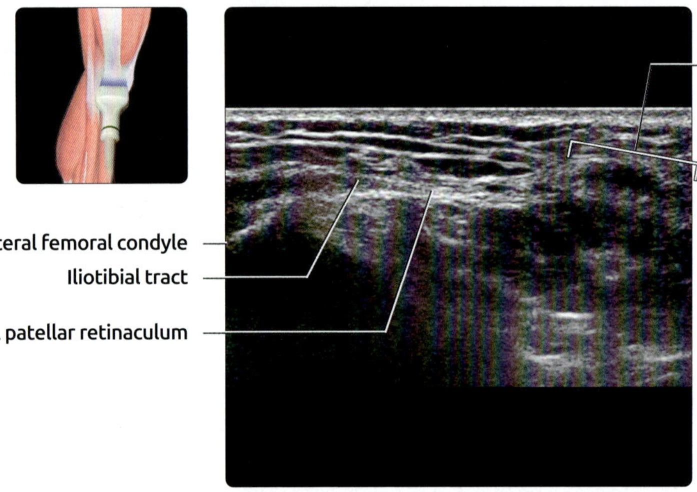

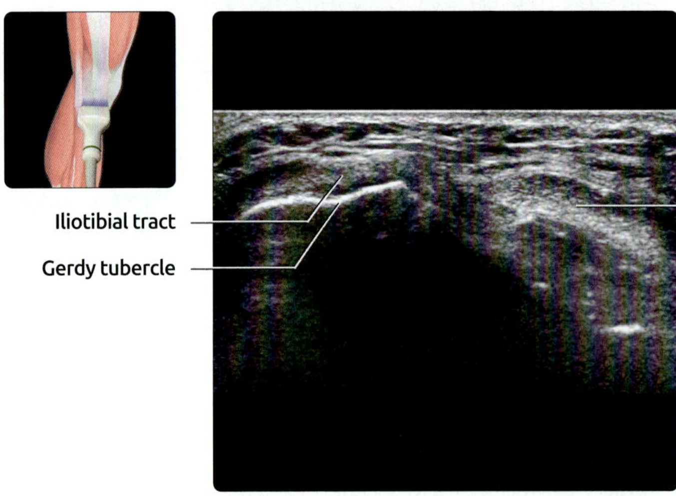

(Top) *Oblique sagittal scan shows the lateral aspect of the joint line using Gerdy tubercle as a landmark. The iliotibial tract is shown here, passing over the edge of the lateral femoral condyle [where it is subject to impingement (iliotibial tract syndrome)] before inserting on the Gerdy tubercle on the anterior surface of the lateral tibial condyle.* **(Middle)** *Transverse scan of the anterolateral knee at the level of the femoral condyle shows that the iliotibial tract and the patellar tendon are connected by fibers of the lateral patellar retinaculum.* **(Bottom)** *More inferiorly, the 2 tendons have moved closer to each other. This transverse scan shows insertion of the iliotibial tract onto the Gerdy tubercle. The patellar tendon is also approaching its tibial insertion.*

CORONAL US: LATERAL KNEE

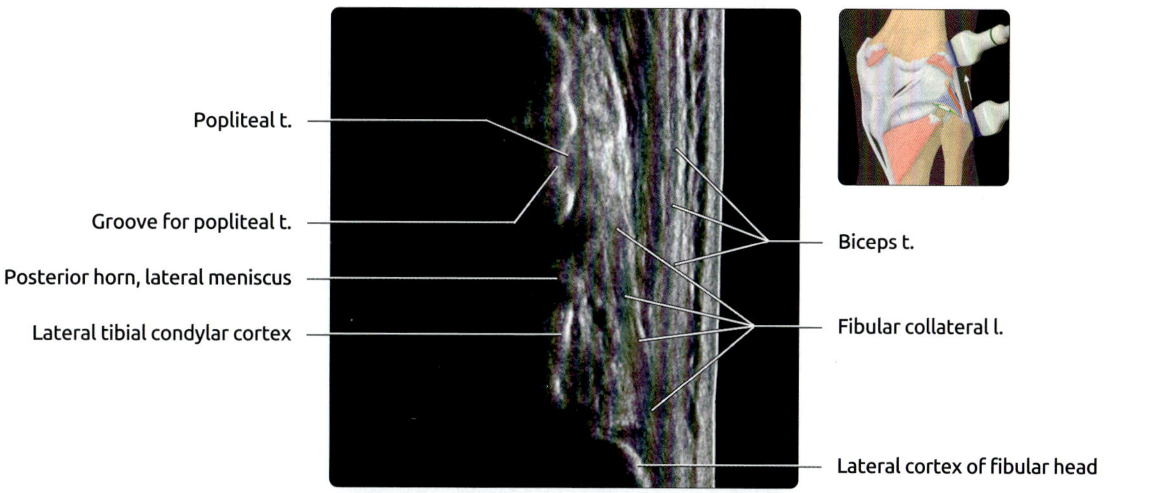

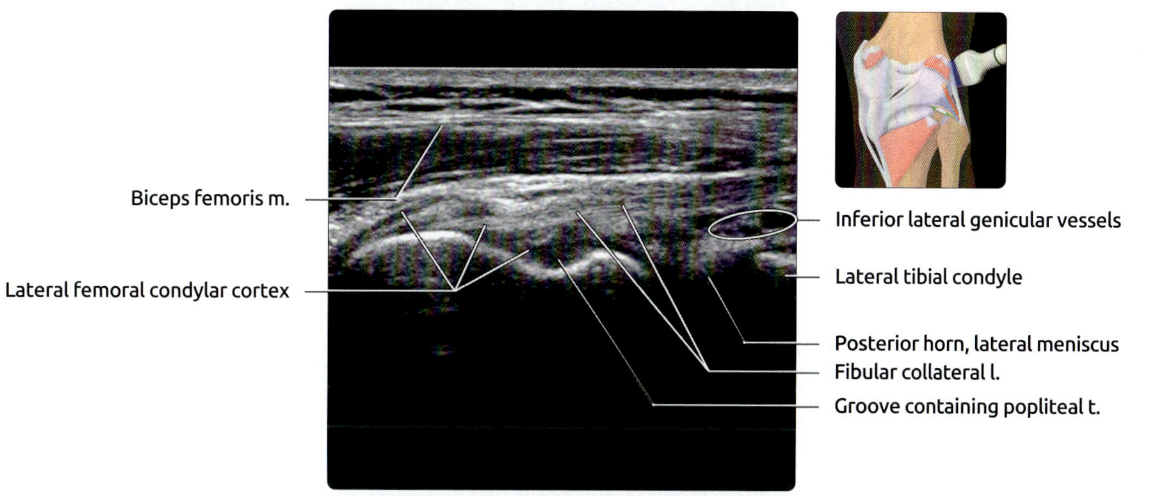

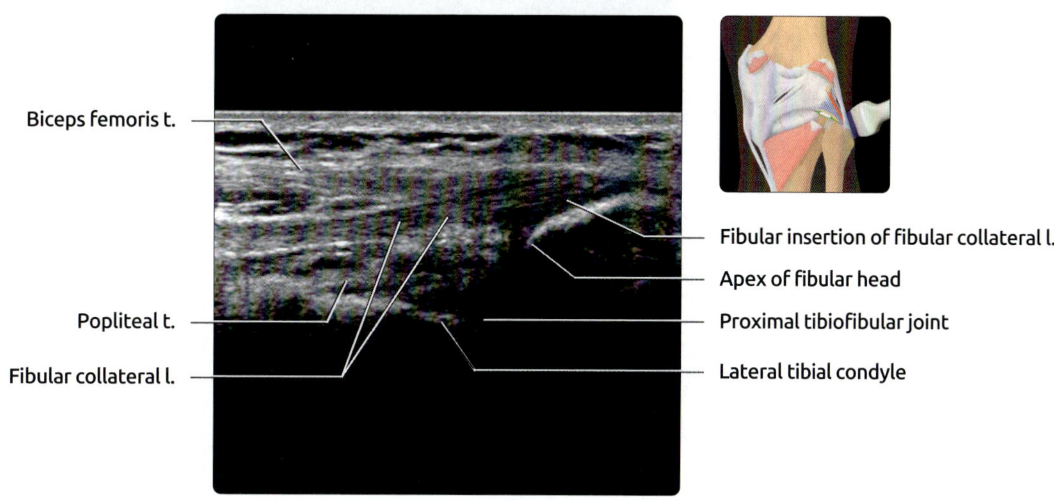

(Top) *Coronal panoramic scan shows the lateral collateral complex. The biceps femoris muscle is the dominant muscle on this side of the knee. Its long head originates from the ischial tuberosity and its short head from the femoral shaft. The tendon has insertions on the fibula and lateral margin of the tibia.* **(Middle)** *Coronal scan of the lateral femoral condyle shows the insertion of the fibular collateral ligament. Just under this insertion is the groove for the popliteal tendon. The fibular collateral ligament is cord-like compared to the superficial component of the lateral collateral ligament, which is a flatter strap.* **(Bottom)** *The fibular collateral ligament inserts onto the lateral wall of the head of the fibula. The tendon of the biceps femoris inserts at and around the apex of the fibular head.*

PANORAMIC: POSTERIOR KNEE

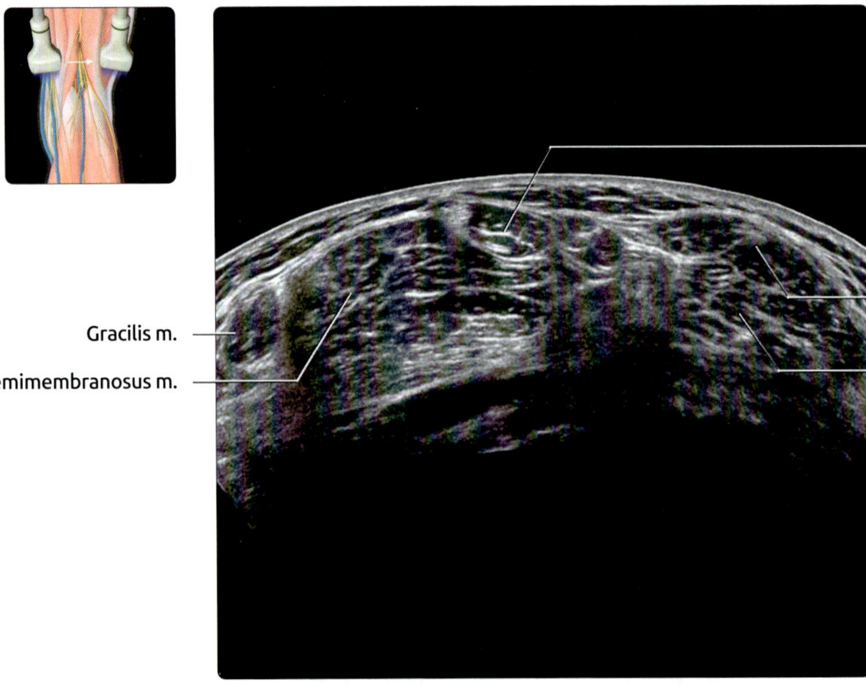

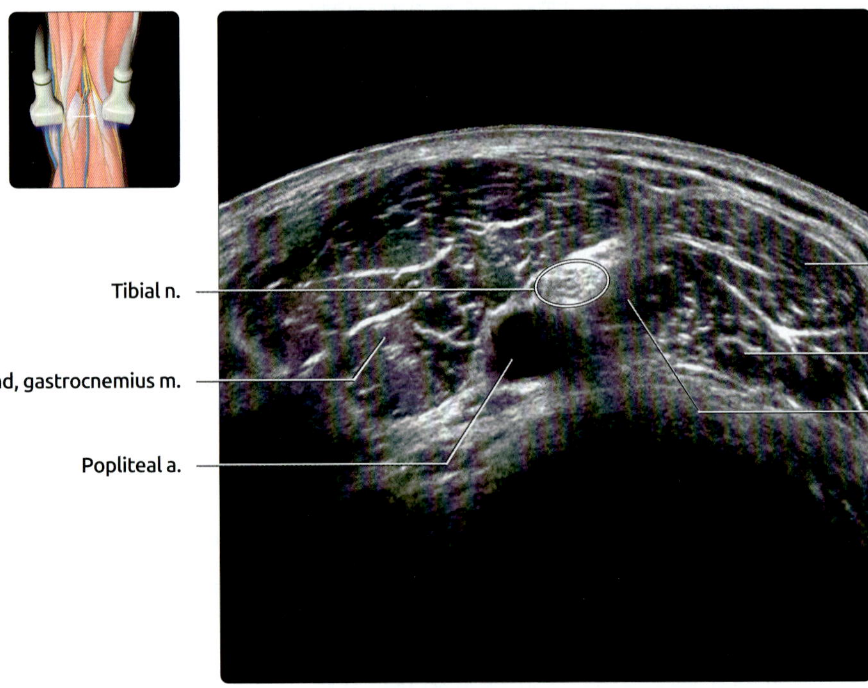

(Top) *Panoramic transverse scan of the posterior knee shows the upper popliteal fossa. At this level, the hamstring muscles form the superior boundaries (medial and lateral) of the popliteal fossa. The semimembranosus and semitendinosus muscles form the medial margin while the biceps femoris muscle forms the lateral margin.* **(Bottom)** *Panoramic view of the posterior knee shows the lower aspect of the popliteal fossa. At this level, the boundaries of the popliteal fossa are the heads of the gastrocnemius muscle, the lateral head of gastrocnemius being the lateral margin and the medial head the medial margin. The popliteal vessels are a continuation of the superficial femoral vessels after they have emerged through the adductor hiatus.*

SAGITTAL US: POSTERIOR KNEE

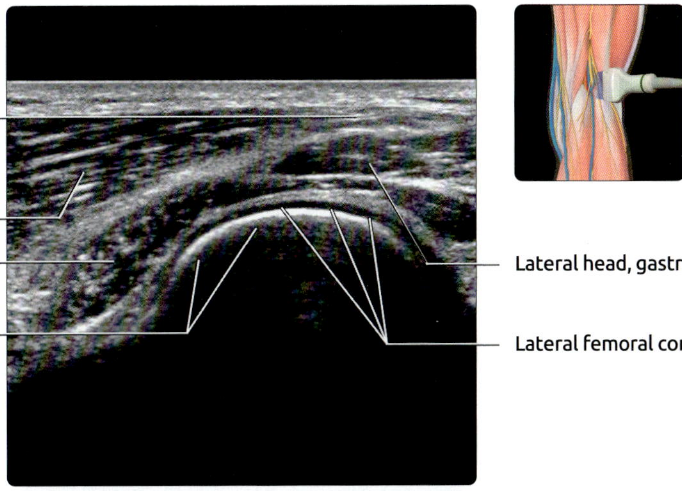

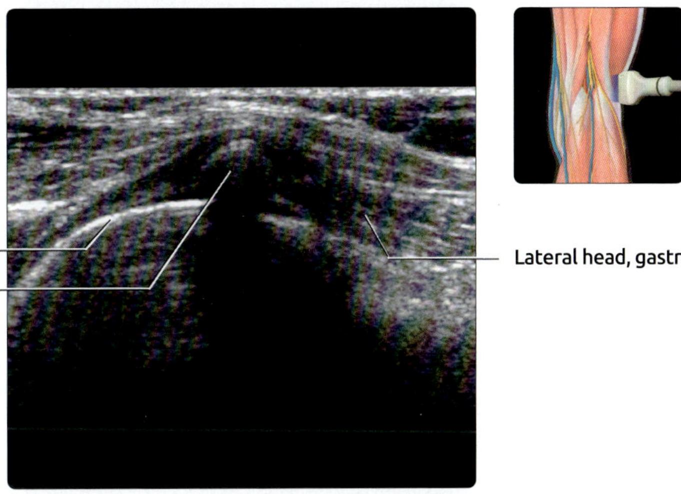

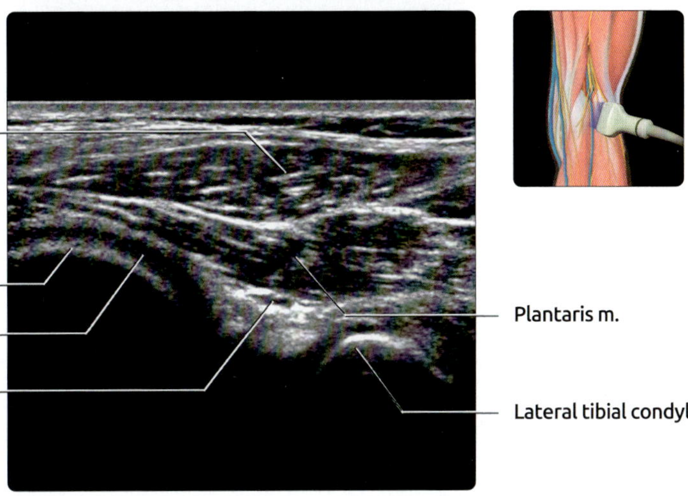

(Top) *Sagittal scan shows the lateral femoral condyle. The plantaris muscle originates slightly more superior and medial to the lateral head of the gastrocnemius. The plantaris runs inferomedially across the thigh to lie on the medial side of the Achilles tendon. More superficially, the bicipital tendon runs laterally toward its fibular head insertion.* **(Middle)** *A more lateral sagittal view shows the sesamoid bone within the lateral head of the gastrocnemius muscle, the fabella.* **(Bottom)** *A more inferior oblique scan shows both the plantaris and lateral heads of the gastrocnemius muscle running over the posterior surface of the knee joint. Further distally, the plantaris muscle becomes a thin tendon and is difficult to discern until it reaches the medial side of the Achilles tendon in the distal calf.*

TRANSVERSE & CORONAL US: POSTERIOR KNEE

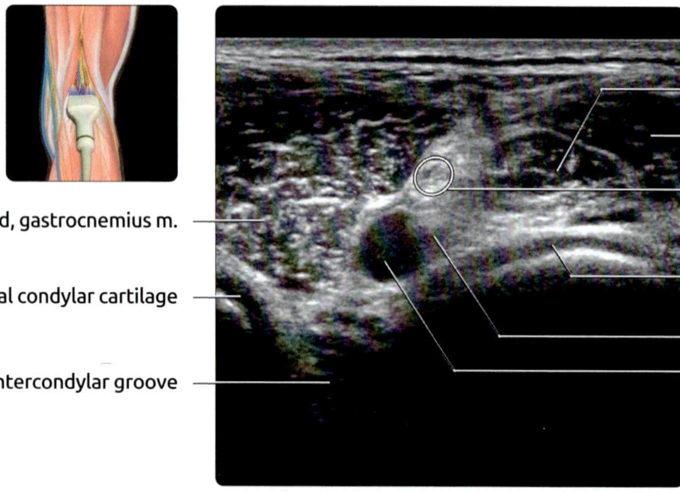

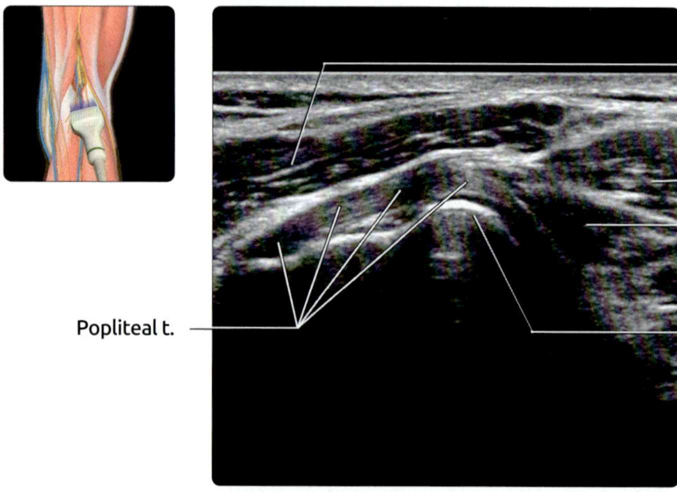

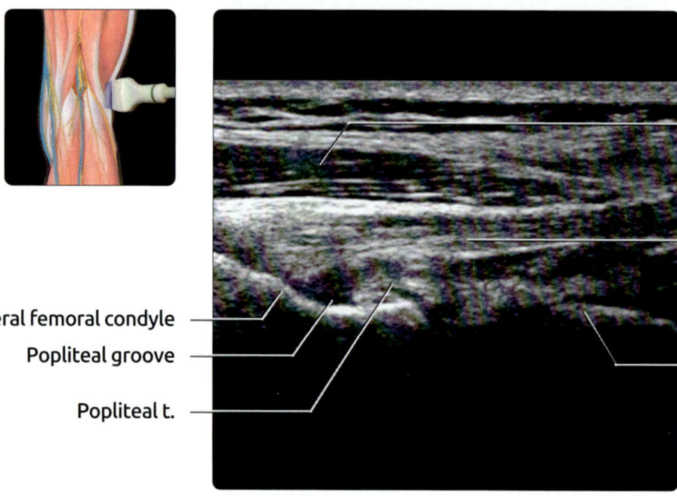

(Top) *Transverse scan shows the posterolateral aspect of the knee joint at the level of the inferior popliteal fossa. The sciatic nerve is the largest nerve in the body. In cross section, nerve fibrils are seen as hypoechoic dots separated by hyperechoic perineurium.* **(Middle)** *Scanning more laterally and inferiorly, the popliteal muscle and its tendon can be demonstrated. The popliteal tendon originates from the proximal posterior tibial surface and runs superolaterally under the lateral head of the gastrocnemius muscle to insert onto the lateral cortex of the lateral femoral condyle.* **(Bottom)** *Coronal scan shows the popliteal groove on the lateral femoral condyle and the popliteal tendon entering this groove as it heads toward its insertion.*

TRANSVERSE US: POSTERIOR KNEE

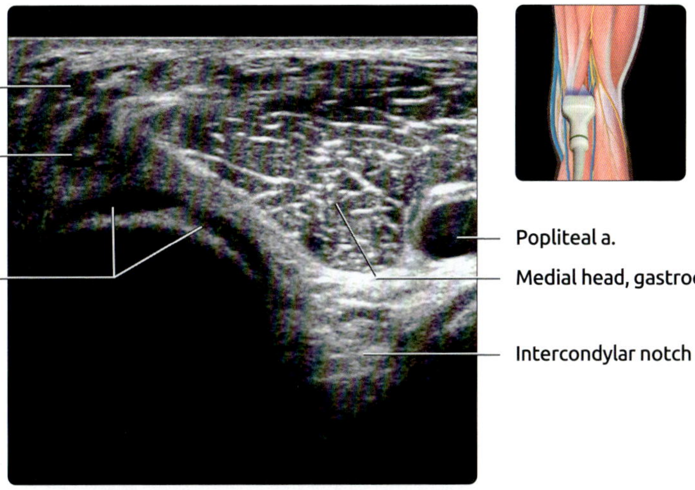

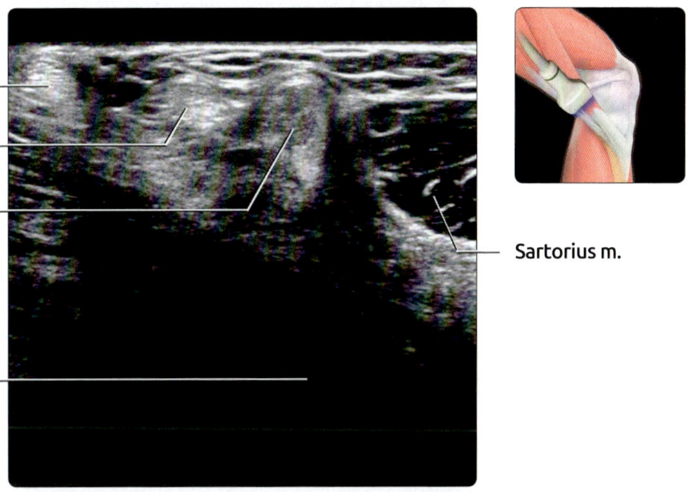

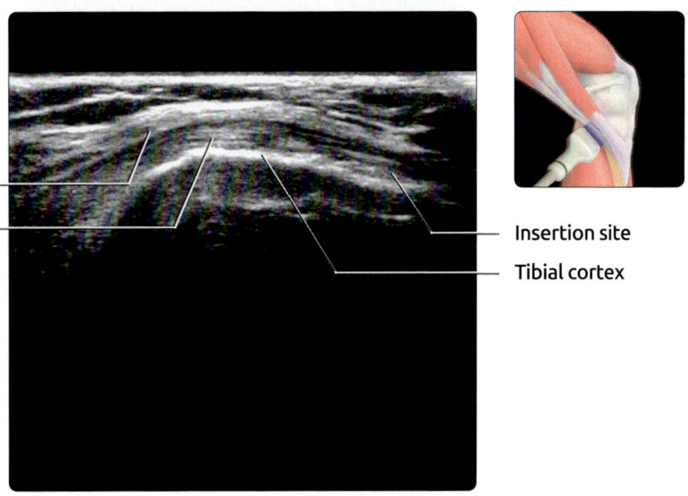

(Top) *Transverse scan shows the posteromedial knee at the level of the femoral condyles. The semimembranosus tendon can be seen running medial to the medial head of the gastrocnemius muscle and deep to the semitendinosus tendon. The semimembranosus tendon will continue inferiorly to its posterior tibial insertion, whereas the semitendinosus will be joined by others to insert on the anteromedial surface of the tibia.* **(Middle)** *More superiorly, transverse scan of the posteromedial aspect of the supracondylar region shows the medial tendons and muscles. Three of these, the sartorius, gracilis, and semitendinosus, will continue together inferiorly and insert adjacent to each other as the pes anserine on the anteromedial aspect of the proximal tibial shaft.* **(Bottom)** *Oblique transverse scan along the course of the pes anserine tendons shows their insertion on the anteromedial tibial cortex.*

SECTION 2

Leg

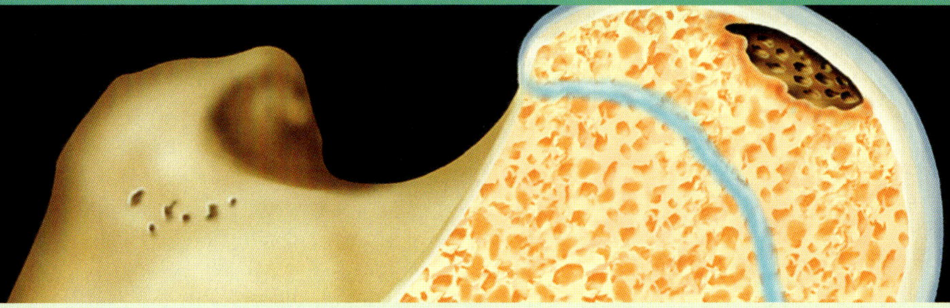

GROSS ANATOMY

Osseous Anatomy

- **Tibia**
  - Proximal tibiofibular joint
    - Head of fibula and lateral condyle tibia joined by fibrous capsule
    - May communicate with knee joint
    - Posterolaterally located
    - Synovial; at risk for any articular process
  - Anterolateral tibia: Origin of anterior muscles of leg
  - Anterior border (shin): Sharp ridge running from tibial tuberosity proximally to anterior margin of medial malleolus
  - Medial tibial surface
    - Wide and flat
    - Proximally, covered by pes anserinus
    - Remainder is subcutaneous
  - Medial border of tibia: Saphenous nerve and great saphenous vein run along it
  - Posterior tibia: Origin of deep posterior muscles of leg
  - Lateral border of tibia: Ridge for attachment of interosseous membrane
  - Medial malleolus: 2 colliculi, anterior longer than posterior
  - Distal tibiofibular joint
    - Fibula articulates with tibia at fibular notch; joined by interosseous ligament
    - Strengthened by anterior and posterior tibiofibular ligaments
    - Posterolaterally located
- **Fibula**
  - Anterior fibula
    - Origin of lateral muscles of leg
  - Medial fibula
    - Origin of deep posterior muscles of leg
  - Posterolateral fibula
    - Origin of posterior muscles of leg
  - Lateral malleolus: 1 cm longer than medial malleolus

Interosseous Membrane

- Stretches across interval between tibia and fibula
- Greatly extends surface for origin of muscles
- Strong, oblique fibers run downward and laterally from tibia to fibula
- In upper part, below lateral condyle of tibia, there is an opening for passage of anterior tibial vessels
- Distally, opening allows passage of perforating branch of peroneal artery
- Tibialis posterior and flexor hallucis longus partially originate from back of membrane
- Tibialis anterior, long extensors of toes, and peroneus tertius partially originate from front of membrane

Retinacula

- Superior extensor retinaculum
  - Strong, broad band
  - Stretches across front of leg from tibia to fibula, immediately above ankle joint
  - Ends attached to anterior borders of tibia and fibula
  - Long extensors, peroneus tertius, anterior tibial vessels, and deep peroneal nerve pass behind retinaculum
  - Medial part of retinaculum splits to enclose tendon of tibialis anterior, forming sling for muscle
- Inferior extensor retinaculum: Distal to ankle joint except for attachment of 1 band to anterior part of medial malleolus
- Superior peroneal retinaculum
  - Thickened deep fascia securing peroneal tendons to back of lateral malleolus, peroneus longus superficial to brevis
  - Retinaculum attached to back of lateral malleolus and to lateral retrotrochlear tubercle of calcaneus
- Flexor retinaculum: Extends from posterior corner of medial malleolus medially and inferiorly

Muscles of Leg

- Compartments separated by deep fascia, which give partial origin to several muscles
- **Posterior compartment: Superficial muscles**
  - **Gastrocnemius**
    - Origin: Medial from posterior femoral metaphysis; lateral from posterior edge of lateral epicondyle
    - Heads separated from posterior capsule by bursa
    - 2 heads unite to form main bulk of muscle
    - Join in thin aponeurotic tendon near mid leg
    - Joins soleus aponeurosis to form Achilles tendon; concave in cross section; musculotendinous junction 5 cm above calcaneal insertion
    - Nerve supply: Tibial nerve
    - Action: Plantar flexor of ankle and flexor of knee
  - **Plantaris**
    - Origin: Superior and medial to lateral head of gastrocnemius origin, as well as from oblique popliteal ligament
    - Continues deep to lateral head gastrocnemius
    - Myotendinous junction at level of origin of soleus (muscle is 5-10 cm long)
    - Tendon then lies between medial head of gastrocnemius and soleus
    - Follows medial side of Achilles to insert either anteromedially on Achilles or on calcaneus
    - Plantaris absent 7-10%
    - Nerve supply: Tibial nerve
    - Action: Acts with gastrocnemius
  - **Soleus**
    - Origin
      - ☐ Extensive origin from back of fibular head and upper 1/3 of posterior surface of shaft of fibula, soleal line and middle 1/3 of medial border of tibia, and tendinous arch joining these across popliteal vessels
    - Flat, thick, powerful muscle ends in strong tendon
    - Joins with tendon of gastrocnemius to form Achilles tendon
    - Nerve supply: Tibial nerve
    - Action: Stabilizes ankle in standing, plantarflexes ankle
    - Accessory soleus (rare variant)
      - ☐ Arises from anterior surface of soleus or from fibula and soleal line of tibia

- Inserts into Achilles or onto calcaneus anteromedially to Achilles
- **Posterior compartment: Deep muscles**
  - **Popliteus**
    - Origin: Tendon from popliteal groove of lateral femoral condyle
    - Passes through popliteal hiatus posteriorly and medially, pierces posterior capsule of knee
    - Muscle fibers directed medially & downward to insert on posterior surface of tibia above soleal line
    - Nerve supply: Tibial nerve
    - Action: Flexes knee and medially rotates leg at onset of flexion (unlocking extension "screwing home" mechanism)
  - **Posterior tibial (tibialis posterior)**
    - Origin: Interosseous membrane and adjoining parts of posterior surfaces of tibia and fibula
    - Superior end bifid; anterior tibial vessels pass forward between the 2 attachments
    - Distally it inclines medially, under flexor digitorum longus
    - Grooves and curves around medial malleolus
    - Nerve supply: Tibial nerve
    - Action: Plantarflexes and inverts foot
  - **Flexor digitorum longus**
    - Origin: Posterior surface of tibia, below popliteus, and medial to vertical ridge
    - Crosses superficial to distal part of tibialis posterior
    - Tendon grooves lower end of tibia lateral to that of tibialis posterior, passes around medial malleolus to foot
    - Nerve supply: Tibial nerve
    - Action: Flexes interphalangeal and metatarsophalangeal joints of lateral 4 toes; plantarflexes and inverts foot
  - **Flexor hallucis longus**
    - Origin: Posterior surface of fibula, below origin of soleus
    - Passes medially, descends down posterior to mid tibia
    - Associated with os trigonum posterior to talus
    - Tendon occupies deep groove on posterior surface of talus, passes around medial malleolus, to great toe
    - Nerve supply: Tibial nerves
    - Action: Flexes interphalangeal and metatarsophalangeal joints of great toe; plantar flexes foot
- **Lateral compartment**
  - Peroneals separated from extensors by anterior intermuscular septum and from posterior muscles by posterior septum
  - **Peroneus longus**
    - Origin upper 2/3 lateral surface of fibula and intermuscular septa and adjacent muscular fascia
    - Becomes tendinous a few cm above lateral malleolus
    - Curves forward behind lateral malleolus, posterior to peroneus brevis
    - Nerve supply: Superficial peroneal
    - Action: Everts foot and secondarily plantarflexes foot
  - **Peroneus brevis**
    - Origin lower 2/3 lateral surface of fibula and intermuscular septa and adjacent muscular fascia
    - Muscle is medial to peroneus longus at origin but overlaps peroneus longus in middle 1/3
    - Tendon curves forward behind lateral malleolus, in front of peroneus longus tendon
    - Nerve supply: Superficial peroneal
    - Action: Everts foot and secondarily plantarflexes foot
  - Synovial sheath for peroneals begins 5 cm above tip of lateral malleolus and envelopes both tendons; divides into 2 sheaths at level of calcaneus
  - Peroneus tertius (see anterior compartment)
  - **Peroneus quartus**
    - Accessory muscle with prevalence of 10%; originates from distal leg, frequently from peroneal muscles, with variable insertion sites at foot; at level of malleolus, located medial or posterior to both peroneal tendons
  - **Peroneus digiti minimi**
    - Accessory with prevalence of 15-36%; extends from peroneus brevis muscle around medial malleolus to foot; tiny tendinous slip
- **Anterior compartment**
  - **Anterior tibial (tibialis anterior)**
    - Origin upper 1/2 of lateral surface of tibia and interosseous membrane
    - Tendon originates in distal 1/3; passes through retinacula
    - Nerve supply: Deep peroneal and recurrent genicular
    - Action: Dorsiflexor and invertor of foot
  - **Extensor digitorum longus**
    - Origin from upper 3/4 anterior surface fibula
    - Descends behind extensor retinacula to ankle
    - Nerve supply: Deep peroneal
    - Action: Extends IP and MTP joints of lateral 4 toes, dorsiflexes foot
  - **Peroneus tertius**
    - Small, not always present
    - Origin: Continuous with extensor digitorum longus, arising from distal 1/4 of anterior surface of fibula and interosseous membrane
    - Inserts into dorsal surface base 5th metatarsal
    - Nerve supply: Deep peroneal
    - Action: Dorsiflexes ankle and everts foot
  - **Extensor hallucis**
    - Thin muscle hidden between tibialis anterior and extensor digitorum longus
    - Origin: Middle 2/4 of anterior surface of fibula and interosseous membrane
    - Tendon passes deep to retinacula to great toe
    - Nerve supply: Deep peroneal
    - Action: Extends phalanges of great toe and dorsiflexes foot

Vessels of Leg

- **Popliteal artery**
  - Ends at distal border of popliteus in 2 branches: Anterior and posterior tibial arteries
  - Paired venae comitantes of anterior and posterior tibial arteries join to form popliteal vein
- **Anterior tibial artery**
  - Smaller of 2 terminal branches of popliteal
  - Origin in back of leg, at distal border of popliteus muscle

- Passes through upper part of interosseous membrane
- Straight course down front of leg → dorsalis pedis
- Muscular branches along length
- Malleolar branches ramify over malleoli; lateral branch anastomoses with perforating branch of peroneal artery

- **Posterior tibial artery**
  - Larger of 2 terminal branches of popliteal
  - Main blood supply to foot
  - Passes downward and slightly medially along with tibial nerve to end in space between medial malleolus and calcaneus
  - Divides into lateral and medial plantar arteries
  - Branches
    - Circumflex fibular (may arise from anterior tibial), runs laterally around neck of fibula
    - Nutrient artery to tibia
    - Muscular branches
    - **Peroneal artery**: Largest branch of posterior tibial artery; runs obliquely downward and laterally beneath soleus to fibula, along which it descends deep to flexor hallucis longus
- **Great saphenous vein**
  - Begins at medial border of foot
  - Ascends in front of medial malleolus
  - Passes obliquely upward and backwards across medial surface of distal 1/3 of tibia
  - Passes vertically upward along medial border of tibia to posterior part of medial side of knee
- **Small saphenous vein**
  - Extends behind lateral malleolus, ascends lateral to Achilles
  - At midline of calf in lower popliteal region, pierces popliteal fascia and terminates in popliteal vein

Nerves of Leg

- **Common peroneal**
  - Smaller of 2 terminal divisions of sciatic nerve
  - Arises mid thigh, runs downward laterally along medial border of biceps femoris
  - Crosses plantaris and lateral head of gastrocnemius, passes posterior and superficial to head of fibula
  - This location at fibular head/neck puts peroneal nerve at risk in multiple clinical situations
    - Fibular neck fracture may result in foot drop
    - Total knee replacement in patient who had been in chronic valgus may damage nerve when knee is realigned
  - Ends between lateral side of neck of fibula and peroneus longus by dividing into 2 terminal branches
  - **Deep peroneal nerve**: 1st of 2 terminal branches
    - Arises lateral to neck of fibula, under peroneus longus
    - Pierces anterior intermuscular septum and extensor digitorum longus to enter anterior compartment
    - Extends down to ankle between tibialis anterior and long extensors
    - Near ankle, crossed by extensor hallucis and passes to ankle midway between malleoli
    - Muscular branches to anterior compartment and articular twig to ankle joint
    - Medial terminal branch to dorsum of foot
    - Lateral terminal branch to lateral dorsum of ankle
  - **Superficial peroneal nerve**: 2nd of 2 terminal branches
    - Descends in substance of peroneus longus until it reaches peroneus brevis
    - Passes obliquely over anterior border of brevis and descends in groove between peroneus brevis and extensor digitorum longus
    - In distal 1/3 of leg, pierces deep fascia and divides into medial and lateral branches to foot
- **Tibial nerve**
  - Descends under fascial septum that separates deep and superficial posterior muscle compartments
  - In upper 2/3, lies on fascia of tibialis posterior and on flexor digitorum longus
  - In lower 1/3, located midway between Achilles tendon and medial border of tibia
  - Crosses posterior surfaces of tibia and ankle joint
  - Posterior tibial vessels run with it, crossing in front of it from lateral to medial side
  - At ankle, under flexor retinaculum, divides into lateral and medial plantar nerves
- **Saphenous nerve**
  - Longest branch of femoral nerve, arising 2 cm below inguinal ligament and descending via adductor canal
  - Passes posterior to sartorius, descends posteromedial to knee where it pierces deep fascia
  - In leg, accompanies great saphenous vein
- **Sural nerve**
  - Arises in popliteal fossa from tibial nerve
  - Descends between 2 heads of gastrocnemius
  - Pierces deep fascia midway between knee and ankle
  - Accompanies small saphenous vein to lateral foot border

IMAGING ANATOMY

Anatomy Relationships

- Critical variant: 3rd head of gastrocnemius
  - Muscular anomalies of gastrocnemius are numerous
  - 2% show anomalous 3rd head of gastrocnemius
    - Originate from posterior distal femoral metaphysis either medially or at mid portion
    - Courses laterally to join lateral head of gastrocnemius
    - Popliteal vessels located between 3rd head and medial head of gastrocnemius
  - These anomalies have potential for causing popliteal compression, and should be sought (axial images), but may be asymptomatic
- Critical variant: Hypertrophy of short head biceps
  - May cause encroachment on fat surrounding common peroneal nerve
- Abnormalities which may cause peroneal neuropathy
  - Hypertrophied short head biceps
  - Distal extension of long head of biceps
  - Prominent lateral head of gastrocnemius
  - Diabetics may accumulate excess fat around peroneal nerve at fibular neck

GRAPHICS: MUSCLE ATTACHMENTS

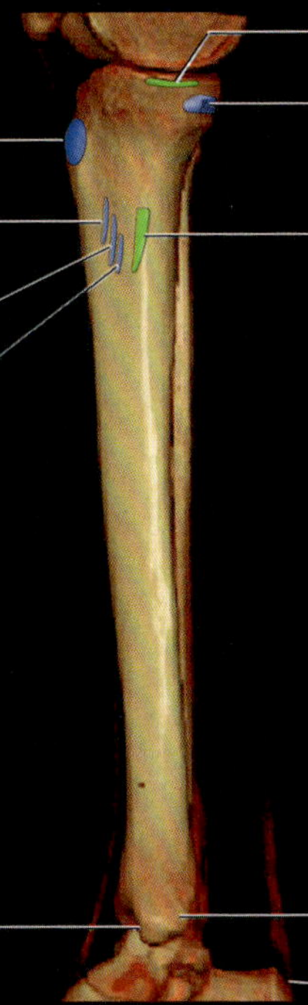

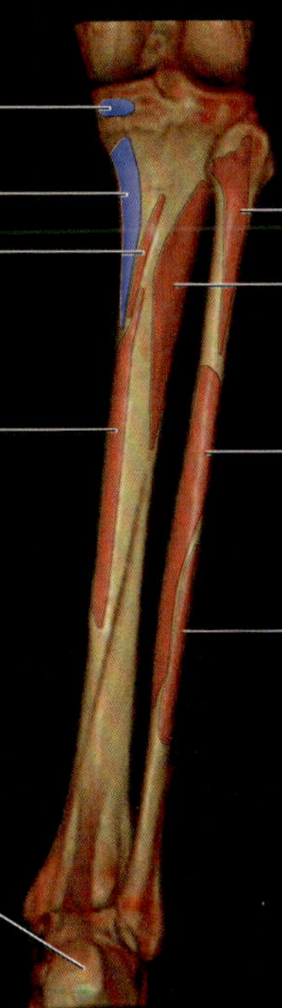

(Top) *Graphic of the medial leg is shown. Other than insertions of the pes anserinus and medial collateral ligament proximally, the medial tibial surface is subcutaneous. Note the attachment of the Achilles tendon is not at the posterosuperior margin of the calcaneus, but more inferiorly. Above its insertion, it is separated from the posterior process of the calcaneus by the pre-Achilles bursa.* **(Bottom)** *Posterior graphic of the leg is shown. Note the large surface area that serves as origin of muscles from the tibia and fibula. The interosseous septum extends across this surface area and is also a site of muscle origin.*

GRAPHICS: MUSCLE ATTACHMENTS

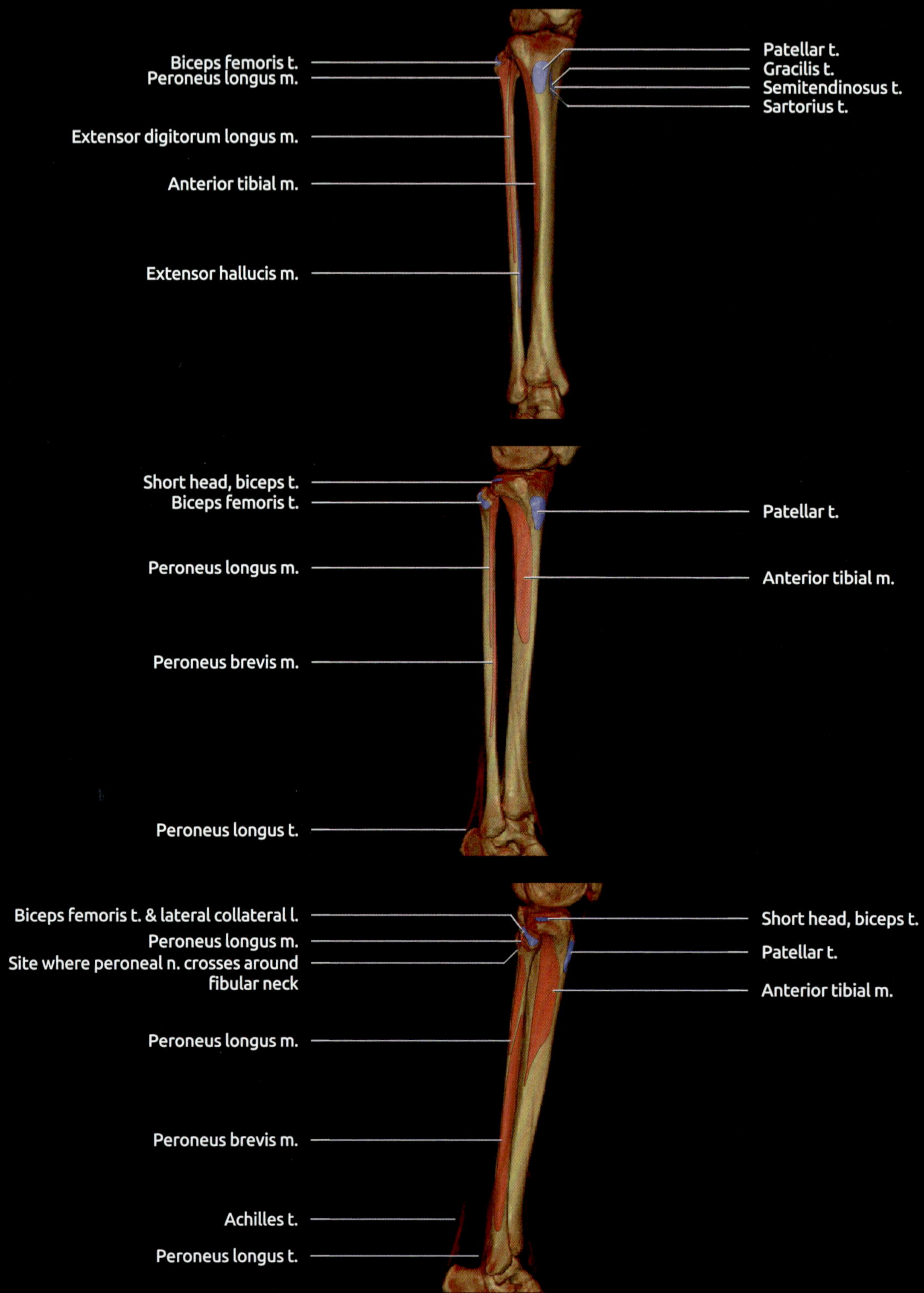

(Top) *Anterior view of the leg shows the extensive origins of the anterior tibial muscle from the anterolateral aspect of the tibia and the long origins of the peroneus longus, extensor hallucis, and extensor digitorum longus muscles from the fibula. These muscles also all have extensive origin from the interosseous membrane.* **(Middle)** *Anterior view of leg, internally rotated, shows the extensive origins of tibialis anterior, peroneus longus, and peroneus brevis.* **(Bottom)** *Lateral view of the leg is shown. Note that the peroneus longus is shown as having 2 separate origins, so that the site of passage of the common peroneal nerve around the neck of the fibula is seen. Also note that there is some overlap of sites of origin of the peroneus longus and brevis from the anterolateral fibula, with peroneus longus originating in the upper 2/3 and brevis in the lower 2/3 of the bone.*

STANDARD RADIOGRAPHS OF LEG

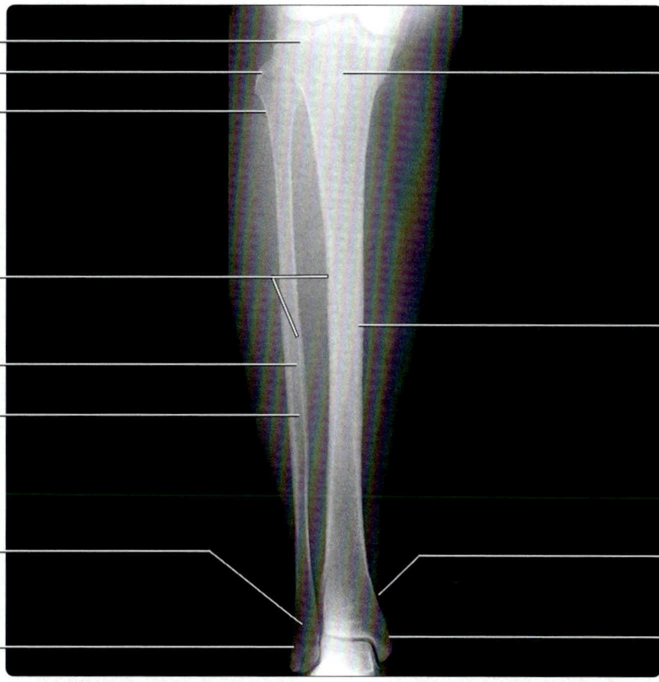

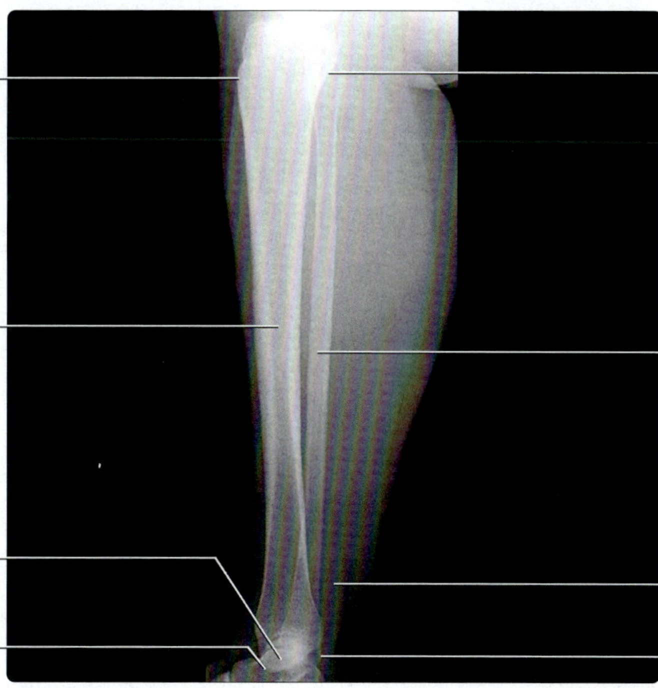

(Top) *Anteroposterior radiograph shows the leg. Note that the fibula is slightly posterolateral to the tibia, and that there is expected overlap at both the proximal and distal tibiofibular joints. The interosseous borders of both long bones are often irregular; this relates to the insertion of the strong interosseous membrane and is not abnormal periosteal reaction. The lateral malleolus extends 1 cm farther distal than the medial malleolus.* **(Bottom)** *Lateral radiograph shows the leg. As on the anteroposterior view, there is overlap of the bones at both the proximal and distal tibiofibular joints. At the ankle, both the colliculi of the medial malleolus can be seen, along with the slightly longer lateral malleolus. The flexor hallucis longus muscle forms a distinct convex shadow posterior to the tibia.*

GRAPHICS: POSTERIOR SUPERFICIAL MUSCLES

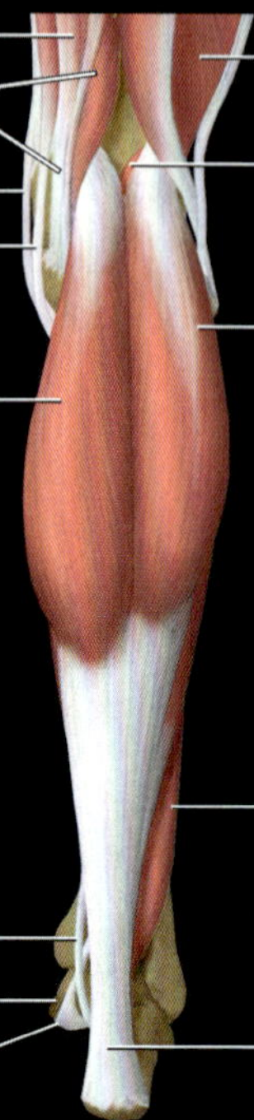

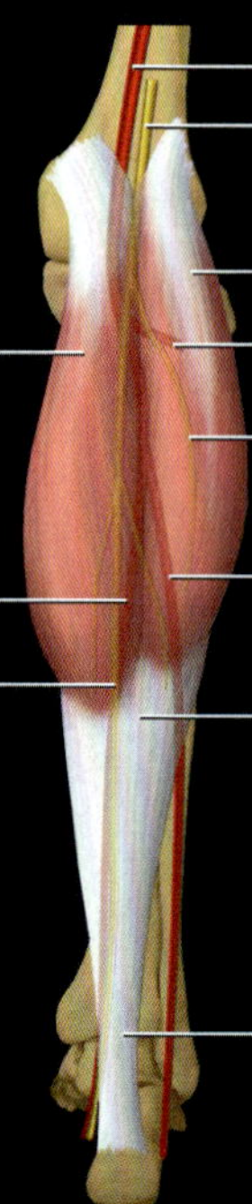

(Top) *Posterior view shows superficial muscles and tendons of the leg. The gastrocnemius muscles are bulky in the proximal 1/2 of the leg and taper to an aponeurosis that blends with the soleus more distally to become the Achilles tendon.* **(Bottom)** *Posterior view shows the gastrocnemius muscles, with the plantaris and proximal muscles removed. The medial head arises from the posterior femoral metaphysis, and the lateral head arises from the posterior edge of the lateral epicondyle (just lateral to the origin of plantaris muscle). The 2 heads unite to form the main bulk of muscle that extends as far as mid leg. The muscles then form a thin aponeurotic tendon at mid leg and extend distally. After the soleus joins the aponeurotic tendon of the gastrocnemius at the distal leg (~ 10 cm proximal to the calcaneus), the strong Achilles continues to its attachment at the posterior tuberosity of the calcaneus.*

GRAPHICS: SOLEUS, PLANTARIS, NEUROVASCULAR STRUCTURES

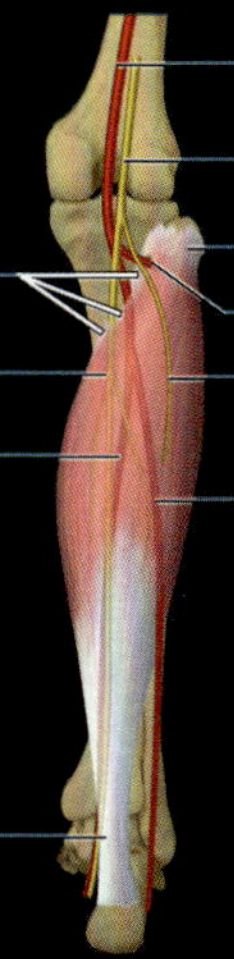

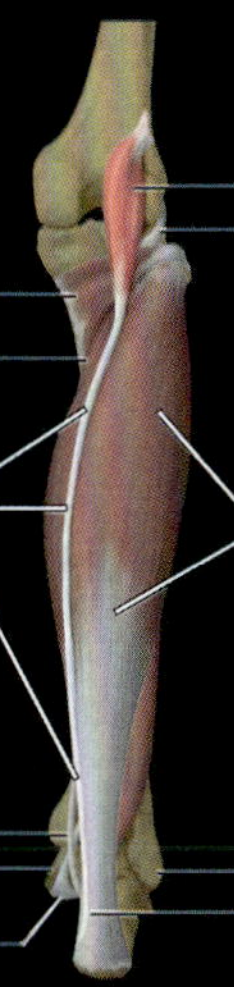

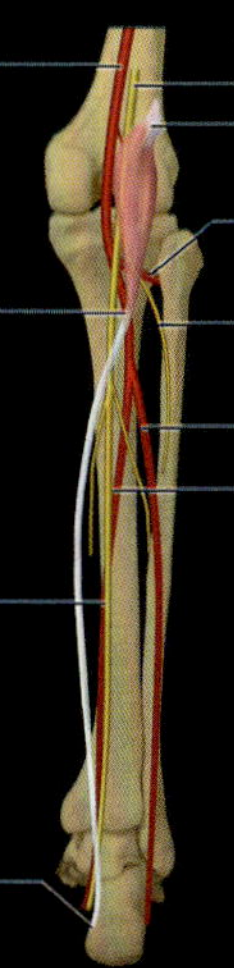

(Top) *Posterior view of the soleus shows its extensive lateral origin from the back of the fibular head and the upper 1/3 of its shaft. The medial portion originates from the medial border of the tibia and the soleal line on the posterior tibia. There is a thick tendinous arch joining the medial and lateral origins of the soleus across the popliteal vessels. Distal to this arch, the neurovascular bundle lies deep to the soleus.* **(Middle)** *Graphic shows the course of the plantaris muscle and tendon. The origin of the plantaris is superficial, adjacent to the origin of the lateral gastrocnemius. The muscle is fleshy over a short distance. The tendon then continues to course distally, located between the soleus (anterior to plantaris) and medial gastrocnemius (posterior to plantaris). The plantaris tendon moves slightly medially over this course. It becomes superficial once the soleus joins the Achilles tendon, and inserts either on the Achilles or the calcaneus, medial to the Achilles.* **(Bottom)** *Graphic shows a posterior view of the plantaris with all other muscle structures deleted.*

GRAPHIC AND MR: POPLITEUS

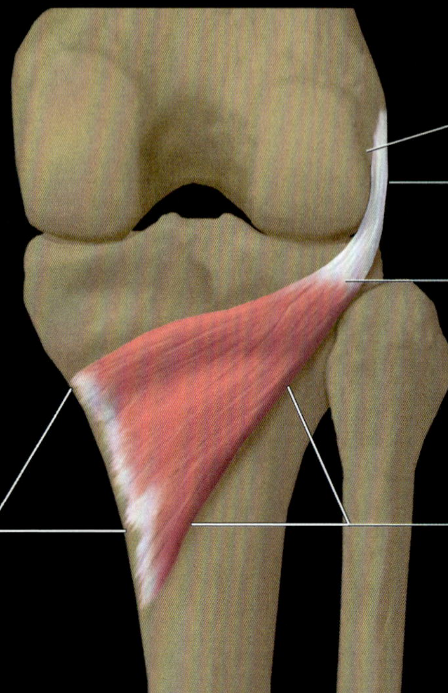

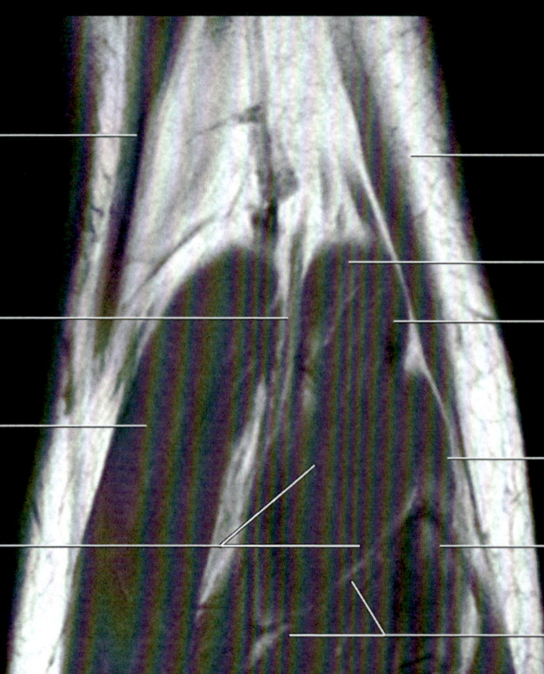

(Top) *Graphic shows the complicated path of the popliteus tendon and muscle. It can be viewed as originating on the tibia and inserting on the femur, or vice versa. The popliteus tendon attaches to the sulcus at the lateral femoral condyle, passes through the popliteal hiatus and then expands to the musculotendinous junction. The muscle broadens over a large area of the proximal posterior tibia and attaches at the posteromedial tibia, immediately proximal to the tibial origin of the tibial head of the soleus.* **(Bottom)** *Posterior coronal T1WI MR shows the large popliteus muscle, which is found deep to the popliteal vessels and gastrocnemius muscles. Note that in this example the popliteus muscle fibers are oriented superolateral to inferomedial, as opposed to the portion of gastrocnemius seen, which runs superoinferior. The proximal aspect of the tibial head of the soleus is located at the distal aspect of the popliteus insertion on the tibia.*

GRAPHICS: POSTERIOR DEEP MUSCLES OF LEG

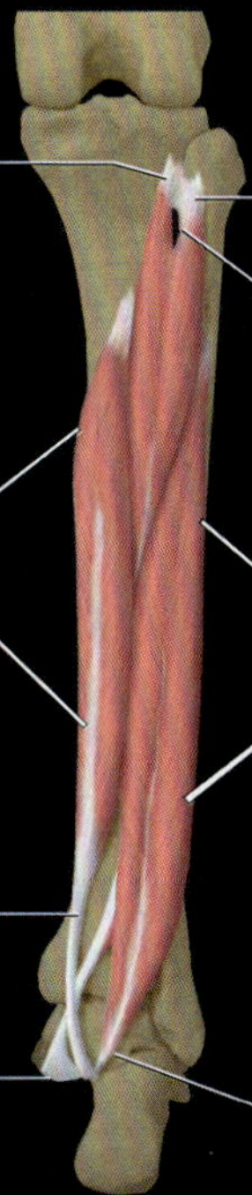

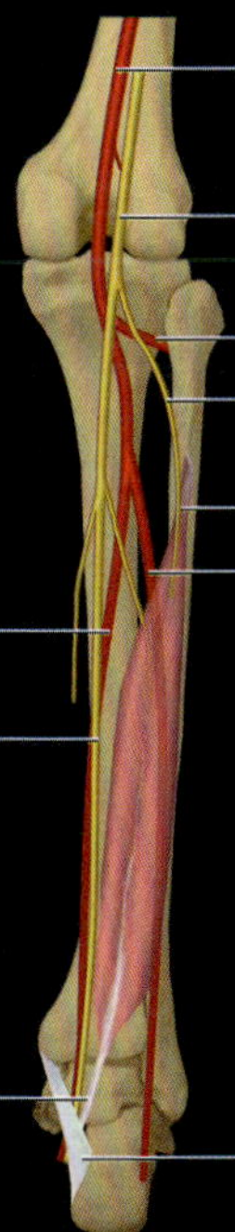

(Top) *Graphic shows the deep muscles of the leg. Flexor hallucis longus is the largest of the muscles; its muscular portion extends far distal to the others, becoming tendinous at the level of the talus. The posterior tibial muscle originates from the interosseous membrane and adjoining parts of the posterior surfaces of the tibia and fibula; in the distal leg its tendon crosses anterior to the tendon of flexor digitorum longus, so that it is the most medial of the 3 tendons coursing around the medial malleolus.* **(Bottom)** *Graphic shows the flexor hallucis longus muscle, which originates from the posterior surface of the fibula, below the origin of the soleus. It passes medially and descends distally posterior to the peroneal artery. It passes through 3 fibroosseous tunnels. The 1st is between the medial and lateral talar tubercles on the posterior talus. The 2nd is in a groove under the sustentaculum tali. The 3rd is between the medial and lateral sesamoids of the great toe to its insertion on the base of the distal phalanx.*

GRAPHICS: FLEXOR DIGITORUM LONGUS & TIBIALIS POSTERIOR

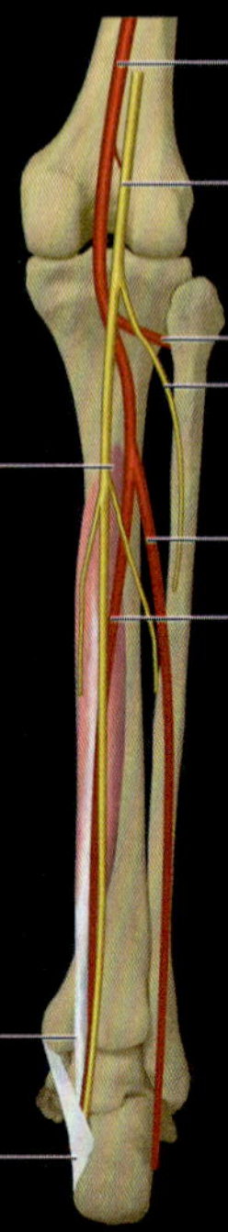

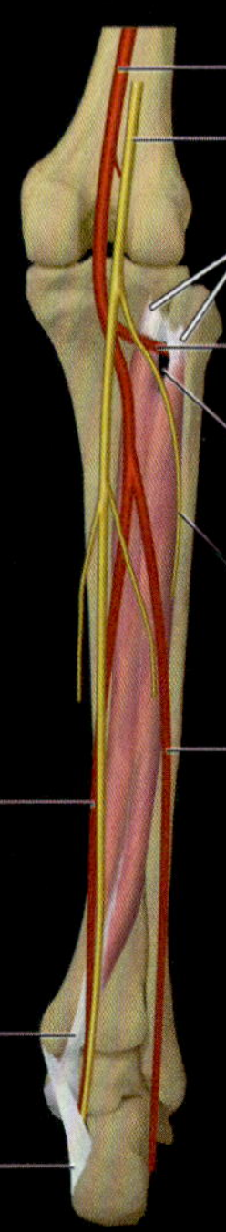

(Top) *Graphic of the flexor digitorum longus shows the origin at the posterior surface of the tibia, below the popliteus. It crosses superficial to the distal part of the tibialis posterior to become tendinous at the level of the distal leg. The tendon passes in a groove at the lower end of the tibia, lateral to the tibialis posterior tendon, and passes around the medial malleolus. It crosses the flexor hallucis longus tendon at the master knot of Henry and proceeds to its insertions on the bases of digits 2-5.* **(Bottom)** *Graphic of the posterior tibial (tibialis posterior) muscle shows its origin from adjacent areas of the posterior fibula, tibia, and interosseous membrane. Distally, the muscle inclines medially, beneath the flexor digitorum longus. The tendon passes in a groove around the medial malleolus, medial to the tendon of flexor digitorum longus. There are multiple sites of insertion, including the navicular tuberosity, cuneiforms, sustentaculum tali, and bases of the 2nd through 4th metatarsals.*

GRAPHICS: ANTERIOR LEG MUSCLES

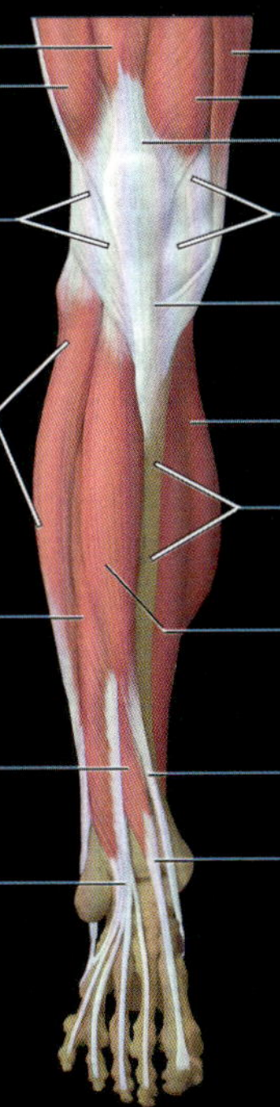

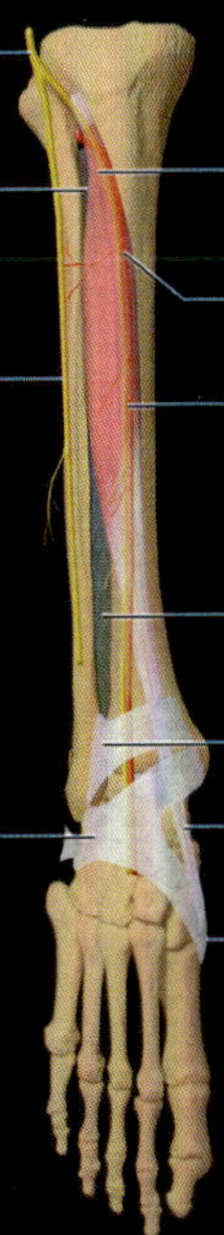

(Top) *Graphic shows the anterior leg muscles. Note that nearly the entire anteromedial tibia is bare of muscle; it is thus poorly vascularized, resulting in slow fracture healing. The anterior tibial (tibialis anterior) has an extensive origin from both tibia and interosseous membrane and is the most substantial muscle of the anterior compartment. The extensor digitorum originates from the fibula. The extensor hallucis longus originates between the tibialis anterior and extensor digitorum, from the fibula and interosseous membrane. These 3 muscles retain the same orientation as they become tendinous, anterior to the ankle.* **(Bottom)** *Graphic of the tibialis anterior shows its origin from the upper half of the lateral surface of the tibia and the interosseous membrane. The tendon originates at the distal 1/3 and passes beneath the flexor retinacula. The tibialis anterior is the most medial and largest tendon in the anterior compartment. It inserts on the medial and plantar surface of the medial cuneiform and the base of the 1st metatarsal.*

GRAPHICS: EXTENSOR DIGITORUM MUSCLE & EXTENSOR HALLUCIS LONGUS

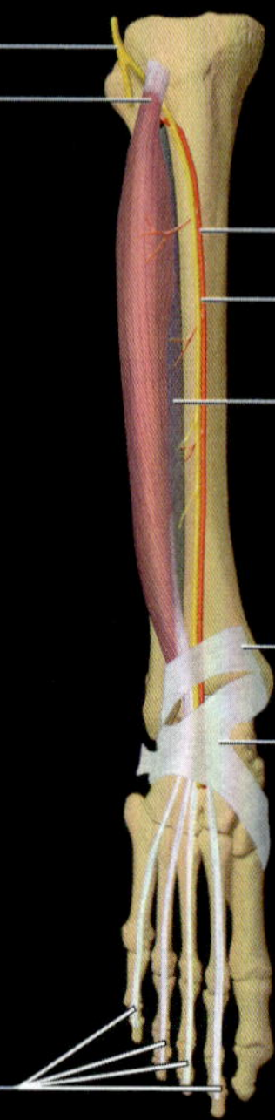

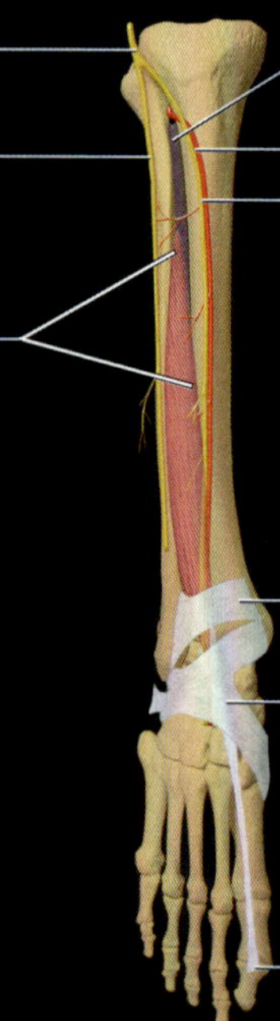

(Top) *Graphic of the extensor digitorum longus shows the origin from the lateral aspect of the tibial condyle, the anteromedial aspect of the proximal fibula and the interosseous membrane. It passes beneath the extensor retinacula where it divides into 4 slips. These slips receive tendinous contributions from the extensor digitorum brevis, the lumbricals, and the interosseous muscles. Each slip accepts slips from the extensor digitorum brevis, which insert at the base of middle phalanges, with the tendon continuing to its terminal insertion on the bases of distal phalanges 2-5.* **(Bottom)** *Graphic shows the extensor hallucis longus, with anterior tibial, flexor digitorum longus, and lateral compartment muscles peeled away. The extensor hallucis longus originates from the anterior aspect of the mid fibula (over its middle 2/4) and the adjacent interosseous membrane. It passes beneath the extensor retinacula to insert on the dorsal base of the distal phalanx of the great toe.*

GRAPHICS: PERONEUS TERTIUS AND LATERAL LEG MUSCLES

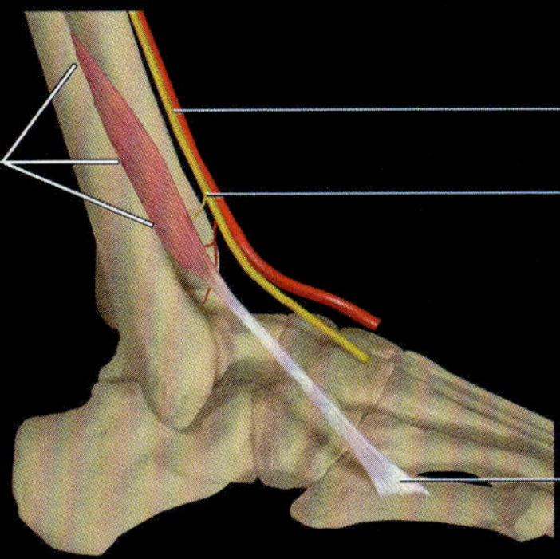

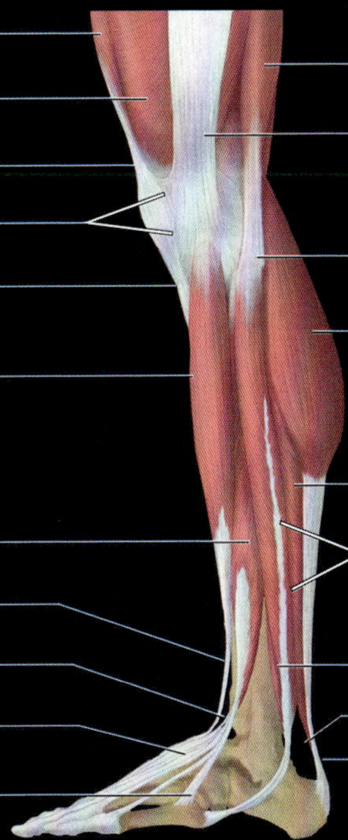

(Top) *Graphic shows the peroneus tertius, with all other extensors and lateral compartment muscles peeled away. The peroneus tertius is a variably present lateral slip of the extensor digitorum longus. Its origin is along the anterior aspect of the distal fibula. It inserts on the dorsal aspect of the proximal shaft of the 5th metatarsal.* **(Bottom)** *Graphic of the lateral leg shows the anterior compartment (extensors), lateral compartment (peroneals), and superficial muscles of the posterior compartment.*

GRAPHICS: PERONEUS LONGUS & PERONEUS BREVIS MUSCLES

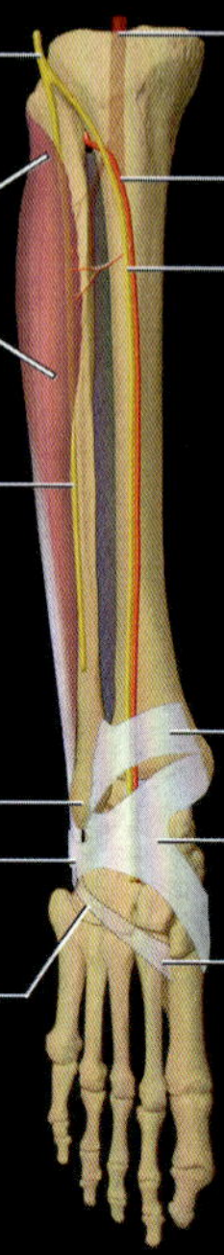

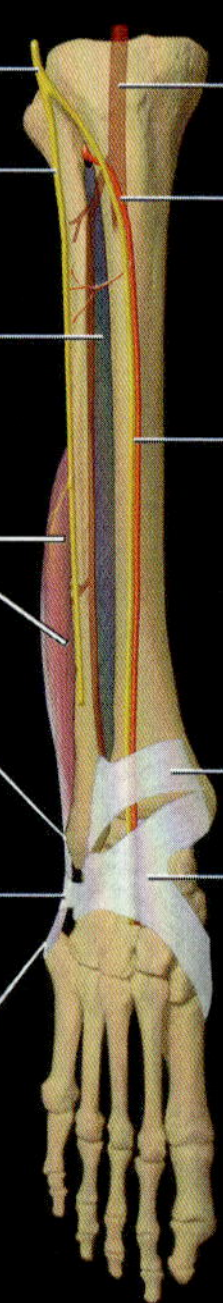

(Top) *Graphic of the peroneus longus (PL) shows its origin from the upper 2/3 of the lateral fibula and the adjacent intermuscular septa/fascia. It extends distally and becomes tendinous a few centimeters above the lateral malleolus. It curves forward around the lateral malleolus, posterolateral to the peroneus brevis (PB) tendon within the retrofibular groove. It passes deep to the superior retinaculum, then crosses the lateral calcaneus behind the peroneal tubercle, deep to the inferior peroneal retinaculum, and curves under the cuboid to insert on the bases of the medial cuneiform and 1st metatarsal.* **(Bottom)** *Graphic of the peroneus brevis shows its origin from the inferior 2/3 of the lateral aspect of the fibula and the adjacent intermuscular septa/fascia. It lies medial to the peroneus longus at its origin, overlaps the PL in its middle 1/3, then lies anteromedial to the peroneus longus in the retrofibular groove, deep to the superior peroneal retinaculum. It descends anterior to the calcaneal peroneal tubercle to insert at the base of the 5th metatarsal.*

GRAPHICS: LEG VESSELS & NERVES

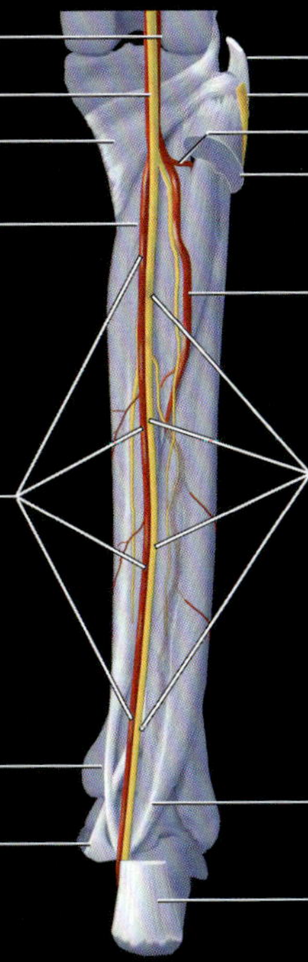

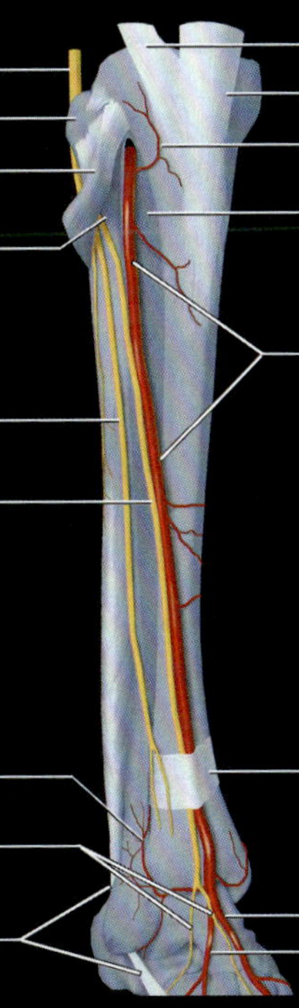

(Top) *Graphic shows the anterior tibial artery passing through a slit in the tibialis posterior muscle and interosseous membrane to the anterior compartment. The posterior tibial artery passes downward and slightly medially, adjacent to the tibial nerve. The largest branch of the posterior tibial artery is the peroneal, which runs obliquely downward and laterally beneath the soleus to the fibula. The common peroneal nerve follows posterior to the biceps and around the lateral fibular neck. The tibial nerve descends between the deep and superficial posterior leg muscles, paralleling the posterior tibial artery.* **(Bottom)** *Graphic of the anterior leg shows the anterior tibial artery perforating the interosseous septum proximally and descending along this membrane down the front of the leg to terminate as the dorsalis pedis. The common peroneal nerve is seen extending through the peroneal tunnel, branching into deep and superficial components. The deep peroneal nerve parallels the anterior tibial artery and terminates in medial and lateral branches.*

IMAGING ANATOMY

Anatomy Relationships

- **Tibial borders**
  - Anterolateral tibia: Origin of anterior muscles of leg
  - Anterior border (shin): Sharp ridge running from tibial tuberosity proximally to anterior margin of medial malleolus
  - Medial tibial surface
    - Wide and flat
    - Proximally, covered by pes anserinus
    - Remainder is subcutaneous
  - Medial border of tibia: Saphenous nerve and great saphenous vein run along it
  - Posterior tibia: Origin of deep posterior muscles of leg
  - Lateral border of tibia: Ridge for attachment of interosseous membrane
- **Relationships of tibia and fibula**
  - Tibia and fibula are connected by synovial joint superiorly, interosseous membrane along their lengths, and syndesmosis inferiorly
  - Proximal tibiofibular joint
    - Synovial joint
    - Obliquely oriented
    - Usually does not connect to knee joint
  - Interosseous membrane
    - Extends from fibular neck to ankle
    - Thickened above ankle to form interosseous ligament
    - Chronic stress often creates mild periosteal reaction along its attachments to fibia, fibula
    - In upper part, below lateral condyle of tibia, there is an opening for passage of anterior tibial vessels
    - Distally, opening allows passage of perforating branch of peroneal artery
    - Site of attachment for multiple muscles
  - Distal tibiofibular syndesmosis
    - Holds tibia & fibula tightly to create stable mortise configuration of ankle
    - Posterolaterally located
    - Composed of interosseous ligament, anterior and posterior inferior tibiofibular ligaments
- **Fibular borders**
  - Anterior fibula: Origin of lateral muscles of leg
  - Medial fibula: Origin of deep posterior muscles of leg
  - Posterolateral fibula: Origin of posterior muscles of leg
- **Muscle compartments**
  - **Posterior compartment**
    - Divided into superficial and deep compartments
    - Superficial posterior compartment: Gastrocnemius, plantaris, and soleus
      - All innervated by tibial nerve
      - Rare variant: Accessory soleus
    - Deep posterior compartment: Popliteus, posterior tibial (tibialis posterior), flexor digitorum longus
      - All innervated by tibial nerve
  - Lateral compartment: Peroneus longus & brevis
    - Both innervated by superficial peroneal nerve
    - Uncommon variant: Peroneus quartus
  - **Anterior compartment**: Anterior tibial (tibialis anterior), extensor hallucis longus, extensor digitorum longus
    - All innervated by deep peroneal nerve
    - Anterior tibial also innervated by recurrent genicular nerve

Patient Positioning

- Leg usually somewhat obliquely positioned in scanner, knee more anterior and lateral than ankle
- Coronal, sagittal images should be angled with plane of tibia
- Axial images should be perpendicular to tibia

Structures Optimally Seen in Axial Plane

- Muscle compartments and individual muscles
- Nerves (very difficult to trace on sagittal, coronal planes)
- Blood vessels

Structures Optimally Seen in Coronal Plane

- Tibial, fibular morphology and bone marrow
- Proximal tibiofibular joint

Structures Optimally Seen in Sagittal Plane

- Gastrocnemius, soleus muscles
- Achilles tendon

Anatomy imaging issues

- **Imaging recommendations**
  - Axial PD often shows muscles more sharply than axial T1
  - Coronal T1 ideal for evaluating marrow
  - Fluid-sensitive sequences with fat suppression in at least 2 planes should always be obtained
- **Imaging pitfalls**
  - Accessory muscles often overlooked, can cause compression, pain, exertional compartment syndrome
    - Clinically can be mistaken for mass
  - Be sure to include plantaris tendon in search pattern; tear is easily missed because of small size
  - Critical variant: 3rd head of gastrocnemius
    - Muscular anomalies of gastrocnemius are numerous
    - 2% show anomalous 3rd head of gastrocnemius
      - Originate from posterior distal femoral metaphysis either medially or at mid portion
      - Courses laterally to join lateral head of gastrocnemius
      - Popliteal vessels located between 3rd head and medial head of gastrocnemius
    - These anomalies have potential for causing popliteal compression, and should be sought (axial images), but may be asymptomatic
  - Critical variant: Hypertrophy of short head biceps
    - May cause encroachment on fat surrounding common peroneal nerve
  - Anatomic variants which may cause peroneal neuropathy
    - Hypertrophied short head biceps
    - Distal extension of long head of biceps
    - Prominent lateral head of gastrocnemius

STANDARD RADIOGRAPHS: LEG

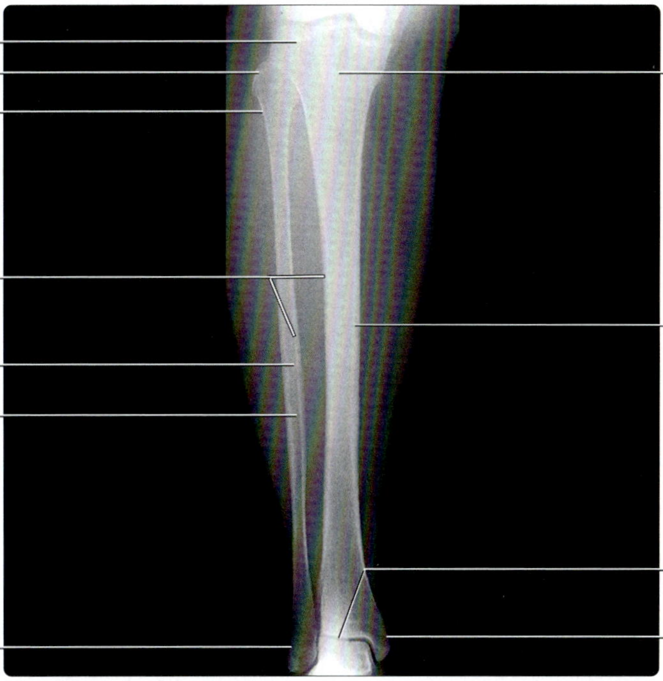

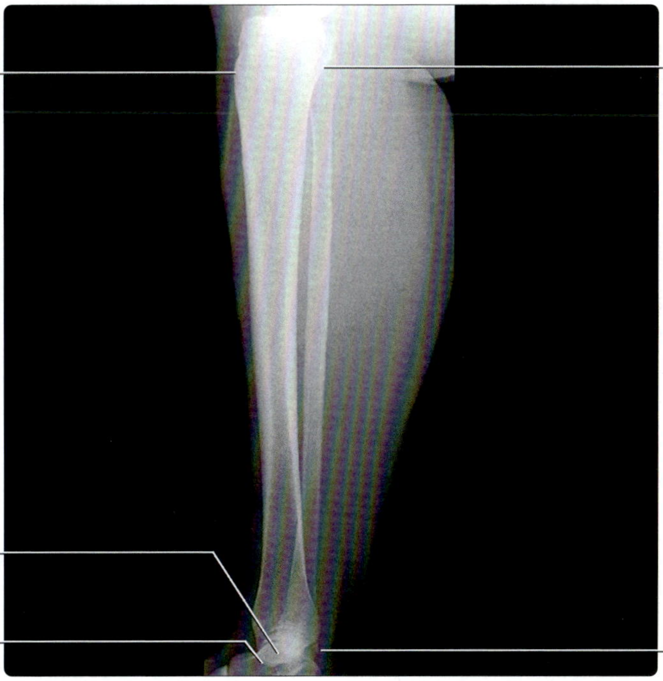

(Top) *Anteroposterior radiograph of the leg is shown. Note that the fibula is slightly posterolateral to the tibia, and there is expected overlap at both the proximal and distal tibiofibular joints. The interosseous borders of both long bones are often irregular; this relates to the insertion of the strong interosseous membrane and is not periosteal reaction. The lateral malleolus extends 1 cm farther distal than the medial malleolus.* **(Bottom)** *Lateral radiograph of the leg is shown. As on the anteroposterior view, there is overlap of the bones at both the proximal and distal tibiofibular joints. At the ankle, both the colliculi of the medial malleolus can be seen, along with the slightly longer lateral malleolus.*

AXIAL T1 MR: RIGHT LEG

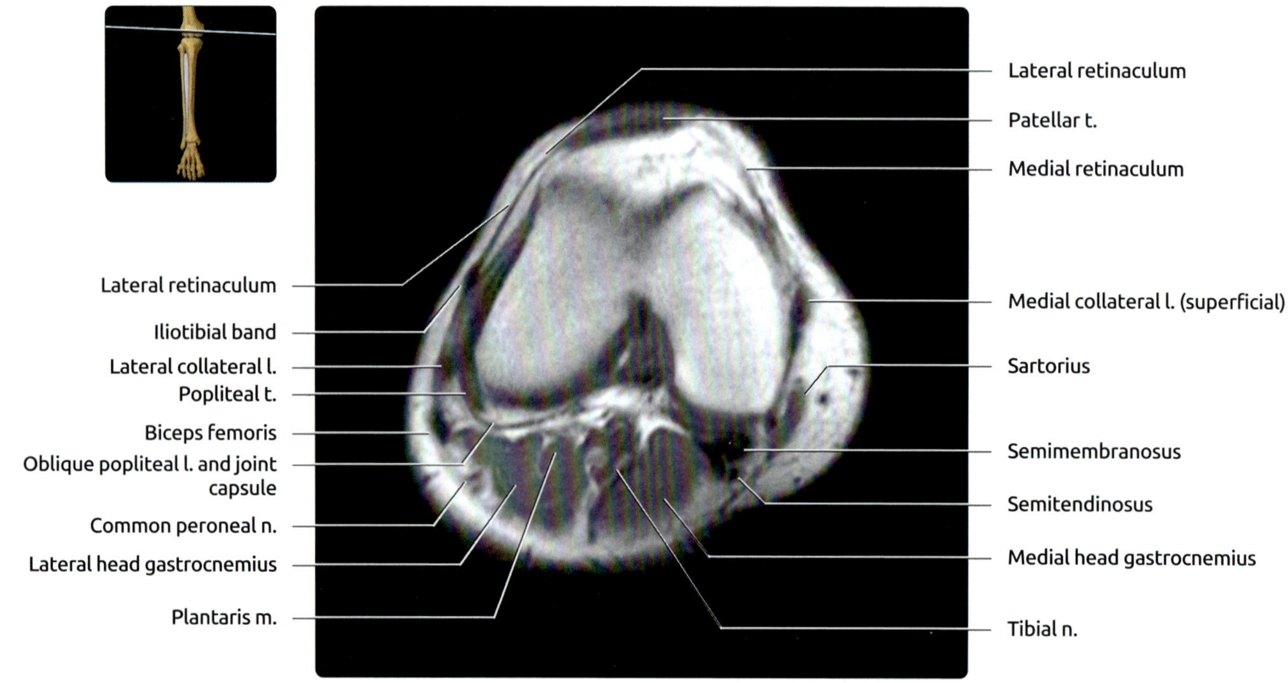

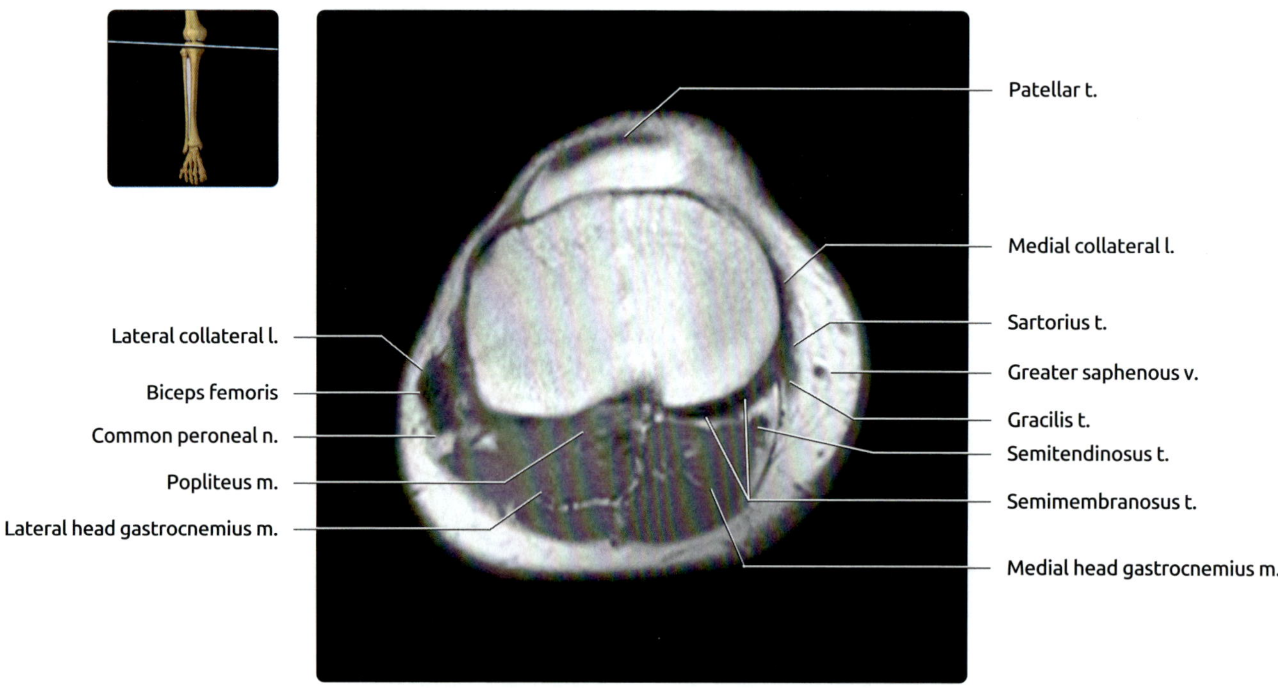

(Top) *First in a series of axial T1 MR images of the right leg is shown just above the knee joint, included for continuity of structures. The gastrocnemius and plantaris originate in the distal femur, cross the knee joint, and insert at the calcaneus.* **(Bottom)** *Axial T1WI MR shows the right leg just below the knee joint. The semimembranosus is shown inserting on the posterior tibia. The 3 tendons of the pes anserinus (sartorius, gracilis, and semitendinosus) are approaching their insertion on the tibia.*

AXIAL T1 MR: LEFT LEG

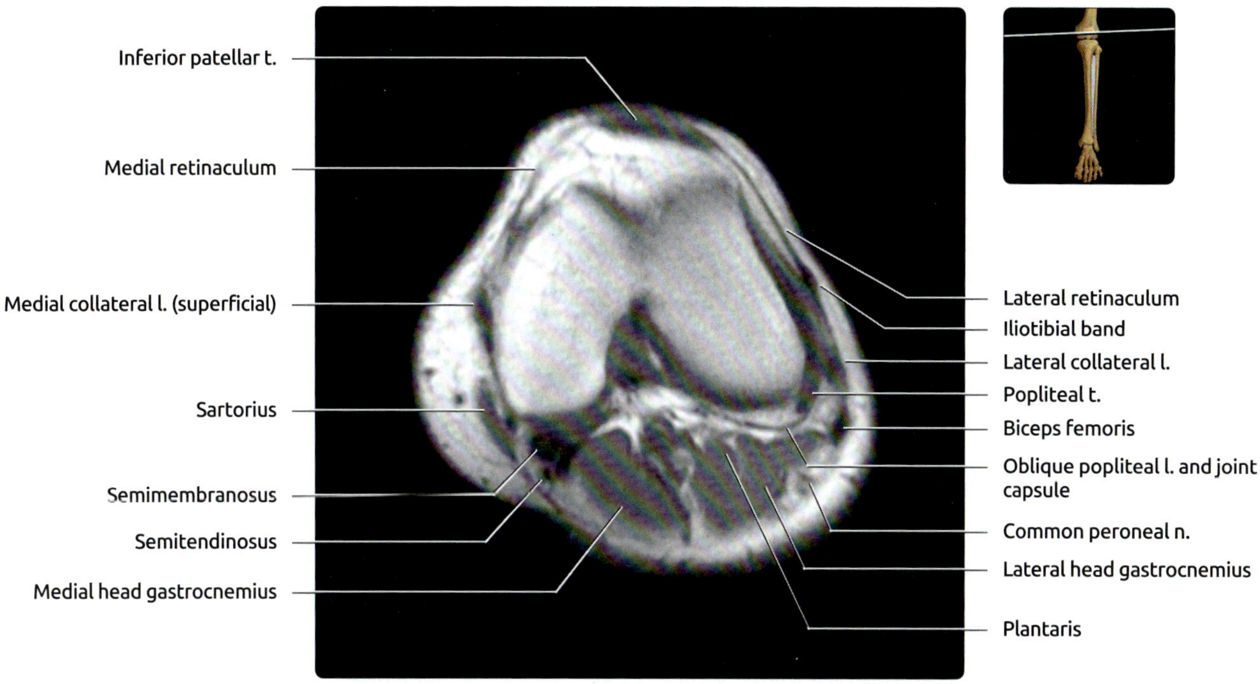

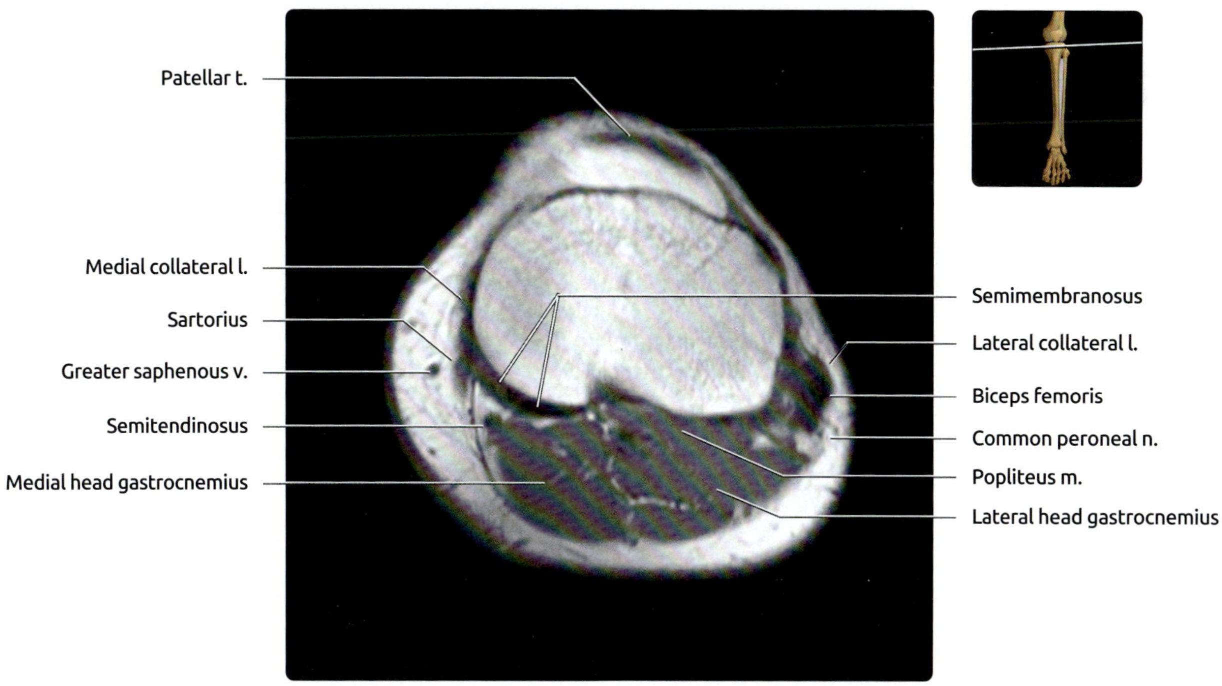

(Top) *First in series of axial T1 MR images of the left leg is shown just above the knee joint, included for continuity of structures. The gastrocnemius and plantaris originate in the distal femur, cross the knee joint, and insert at the calcaneus.* **(Bottom)** *Axial T1WI MR shows the left leg just below the knee joint. The semimembranosus is shown inserting on the posterior tibia. The 3 tendons of the pes anserinus (sartorius, gracilis, and semitendinosus) are approaching their insertion on the tibia.*

AXIAL T1 MR: RIGHT LEG

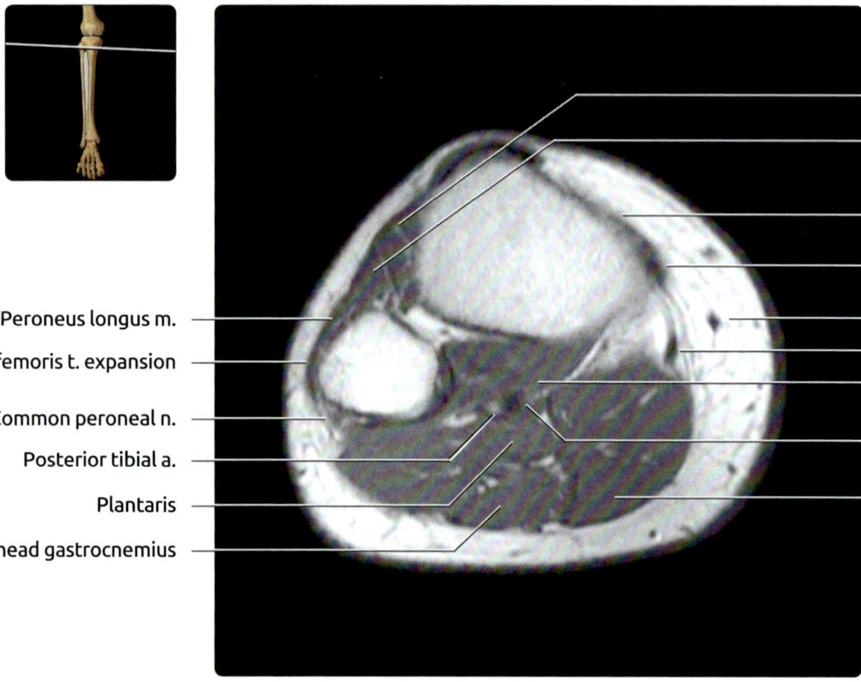

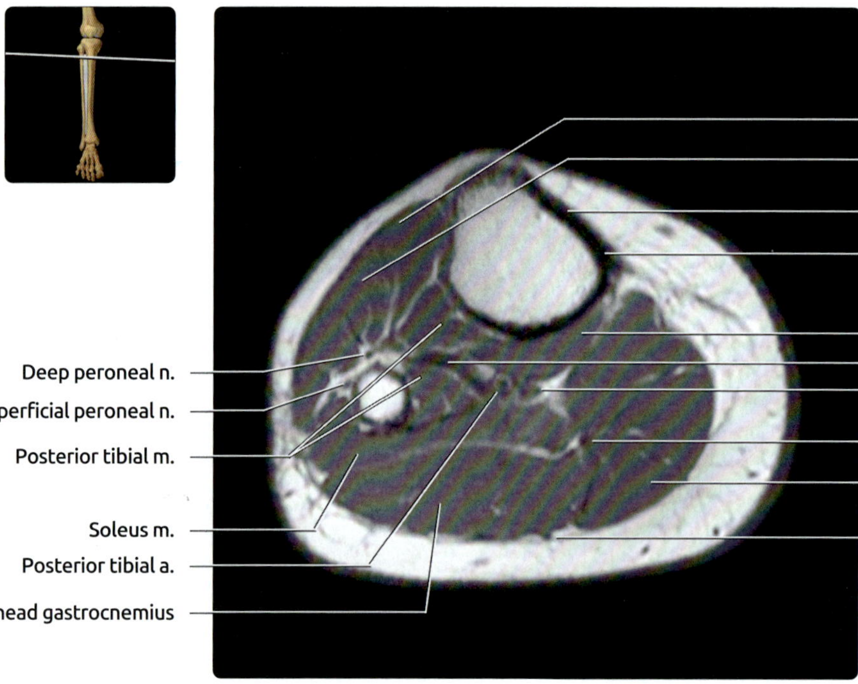

(Top) *Axial T1WI MR shows the right leg at the proximal tibiofibular joint. Note that the plantaris is still muscular, lying in front of the lateral head of the gastrocnemius.* **(Bottom)** *Axial T1WI MR shows the right leg at the proximal metaphysis. By this point, the soleus has arisen from the fibula; the section is too proximal to see the tibial origin of the soleus, since the popliteal muscle is still present. The plantaris is now tendinous, lying between the soleus and the medial head of gastrocnemius. At this level, the posterior tibial (tibialis posterior) is seen arising as a bifid structure from both tibia and fibula; the anterior tibial vessels are seen coursing forward toward the anterior compartment, between these 2 attachments.*

AXIAL T1 MR: LEFT LEG

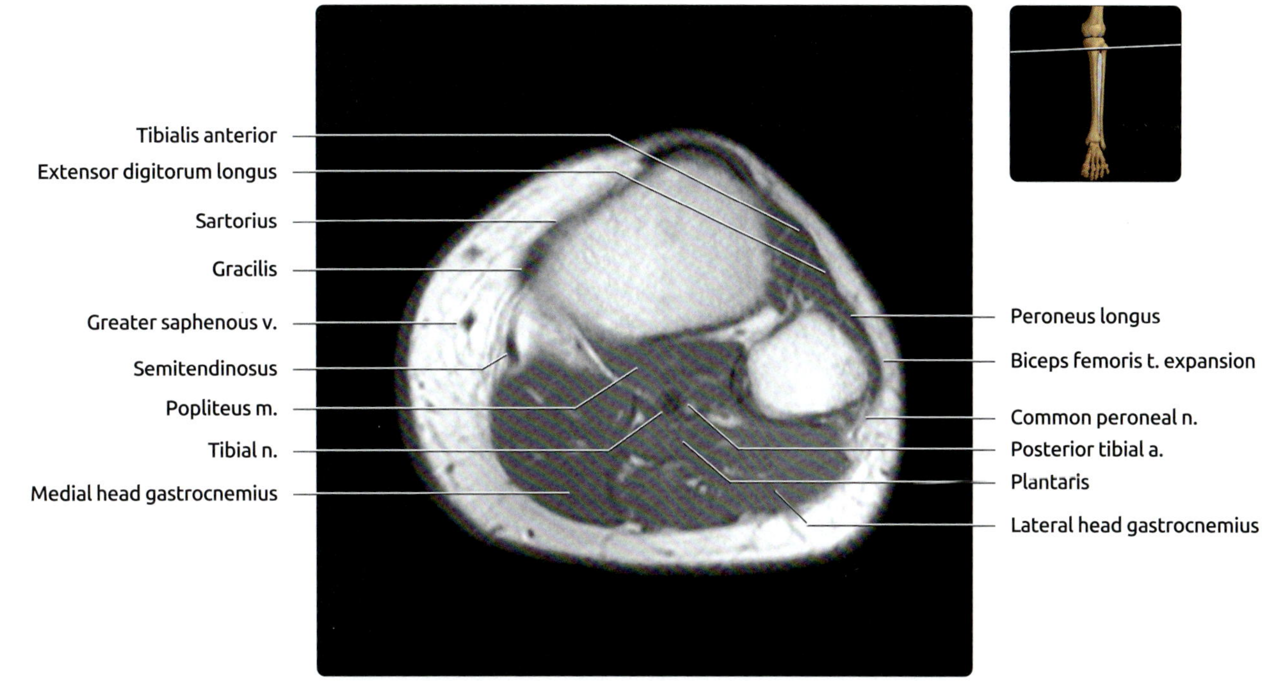

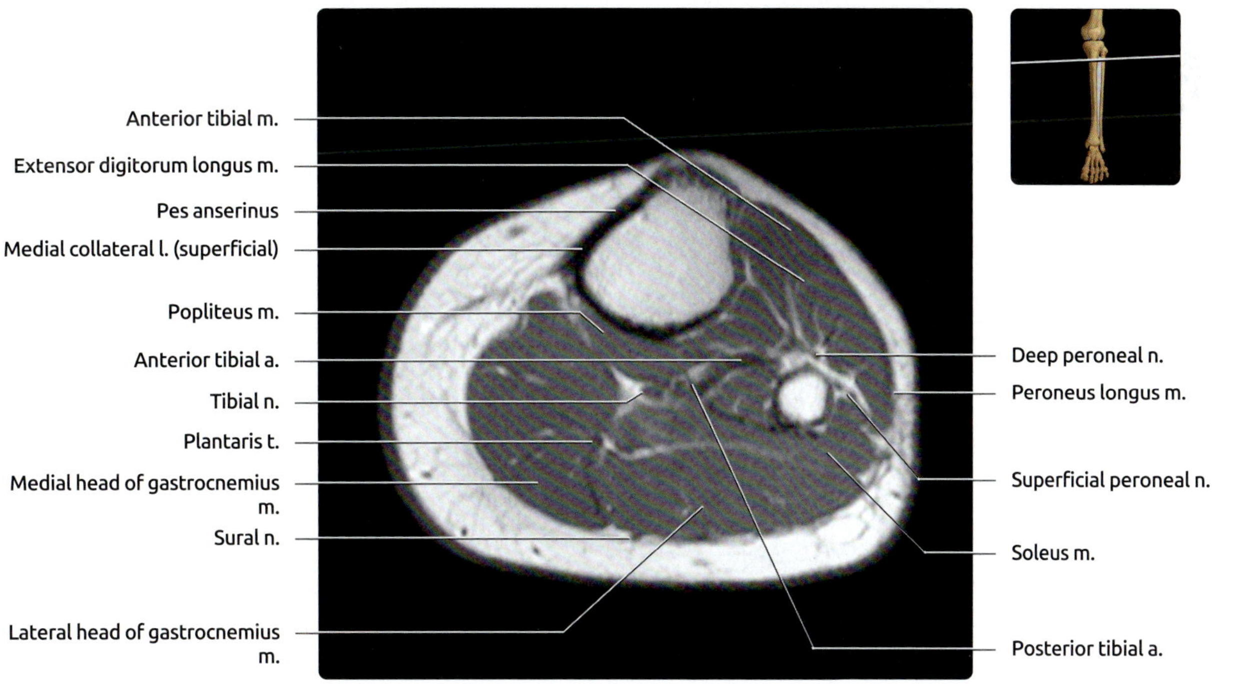

(Top) *Axial T1WI MR shows the left leg at the proximal tibiofemoral joint. Note that the plantaris is still muscular, lying in front of the lateral head of the gastrocnemius.* **(Bottom)** *Axial T1WI MR shows the left leg at the proximal metaphysis. By this point, the soleus has arisen from the fibula; the section is too proximal to see the tibial origin of the soleus, since the popliteal muscle is still present. The plantaris is now tendinous, lying between the soleus and the medial head of gastrocnemius. At this level, the posterior tibial (tibialis posterior) is seen arising as a bifid structure from both tibia and fibula; the anterior tibial vessels are seen coursing forward towards the anterior compartment, between these 2 attachments.*

AXIAL T1 MR: RIGHT LEG

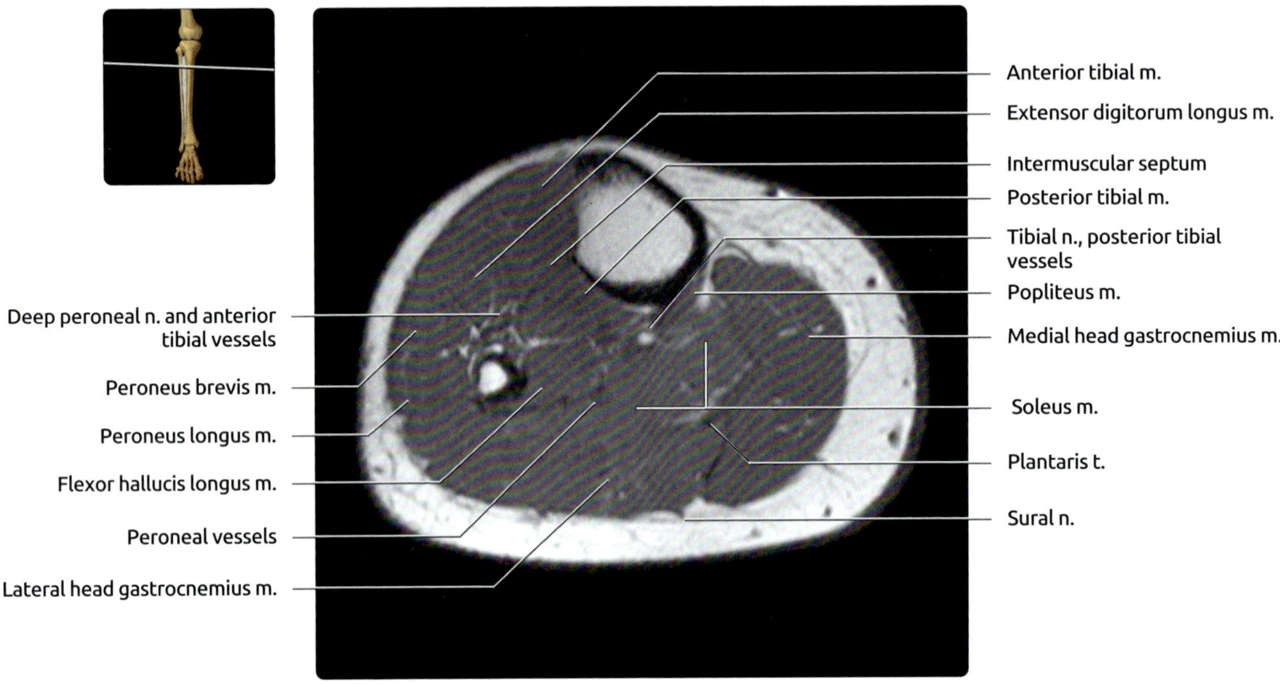

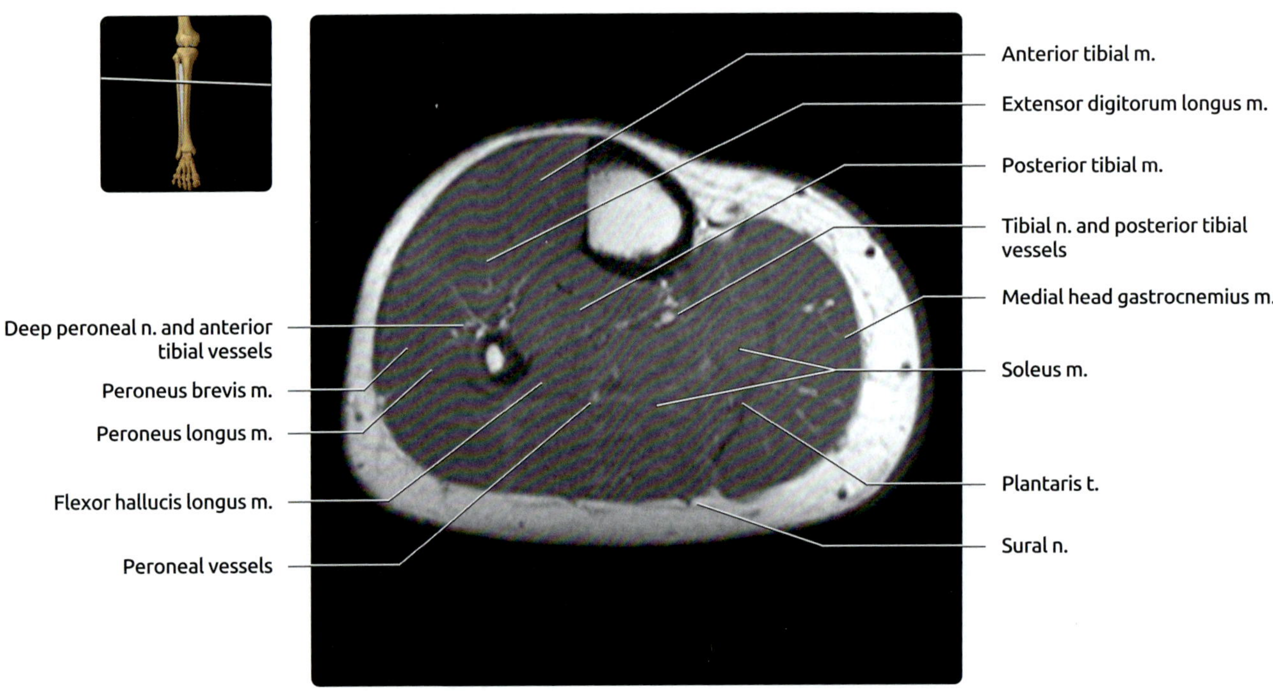

(Top) *Axial T1WI MR shows the right leg at the proximal diaphysis. Note that by this point, the peroneus brevis and flexor hallucis begin to originate from the fibula. There remains a slip of popliteus at the posterior tibia. The major vessels of the leg have trifurcated.* **(Bottom)** *Axial T1WI MR shows the right leg, slightly distal. Note that the popliteus insertion on the tibia has ended, and the soleus gains its tibial origin. The lateral head of gastrocnemius has become entirely tendinous.*

AXIAL T1 MR: LEFT LEG

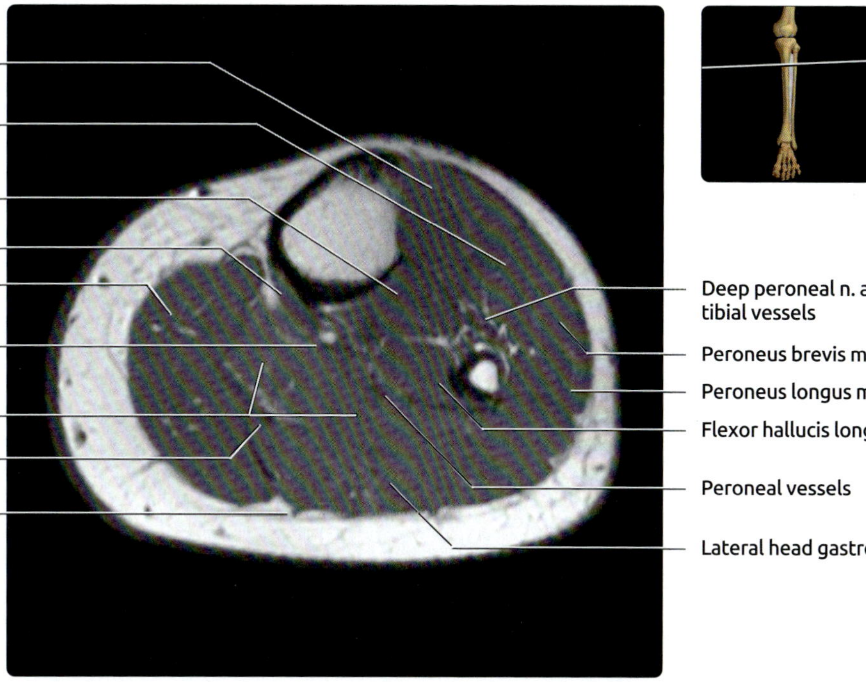

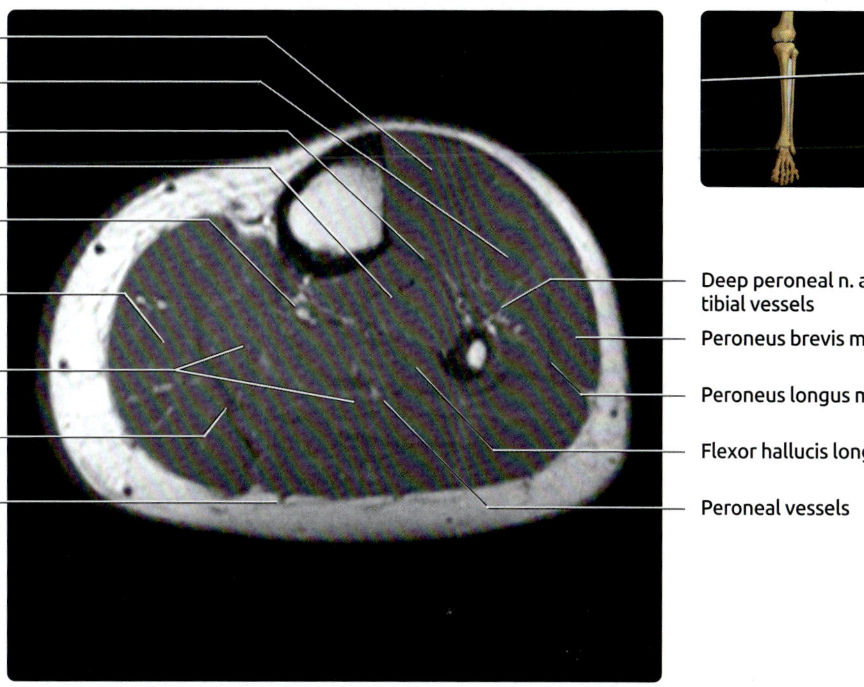

(Top) *Axial T1WI MR shows the left leg at the proximal diaphysis. Note that by this point the peroneus brevis and flexor hallucis begin to originate from the fibula. There remains a slip of popliteus at the posterior tibia. The major vessels of the leg have trifurcated.* **(Bottom)** *Axial T1WI MR shows the left leg, slightly distal. Note that the popliteus insertion on the tibia has ended and the soleus gains its tibial origin. The lateral head of the gastrocnemius has become entirely tendinous.*

AXIAL T1 MR: RIGHT LEG

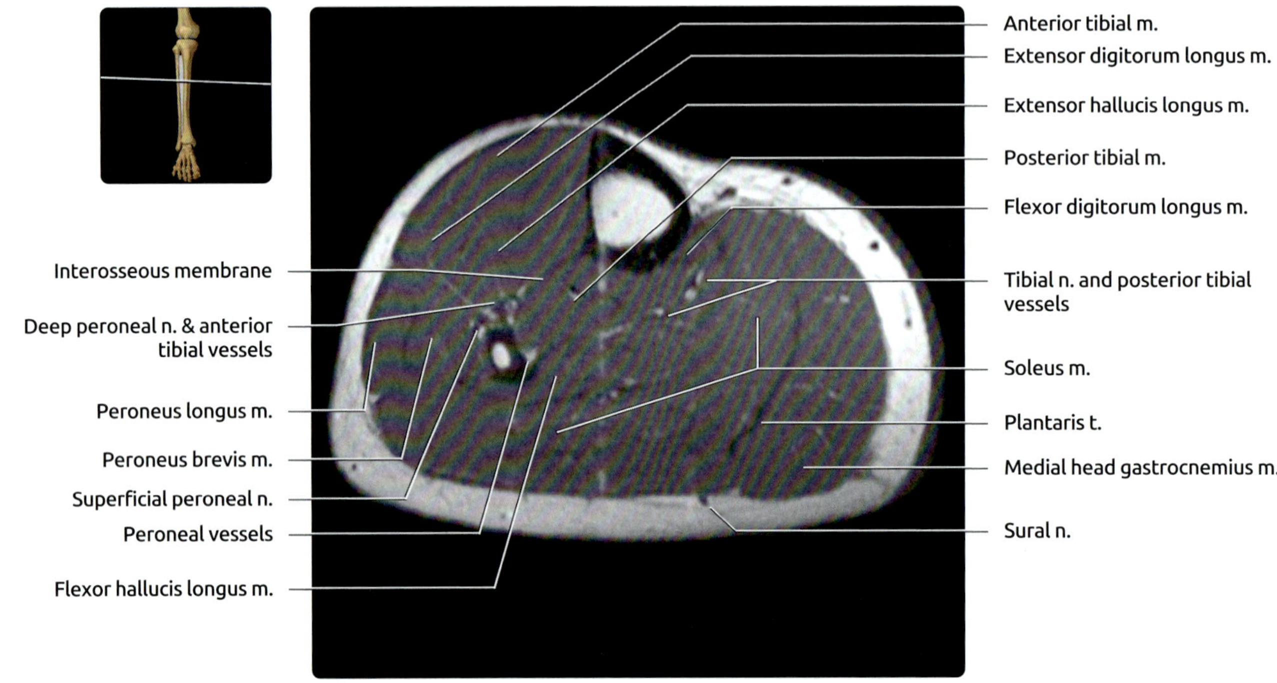

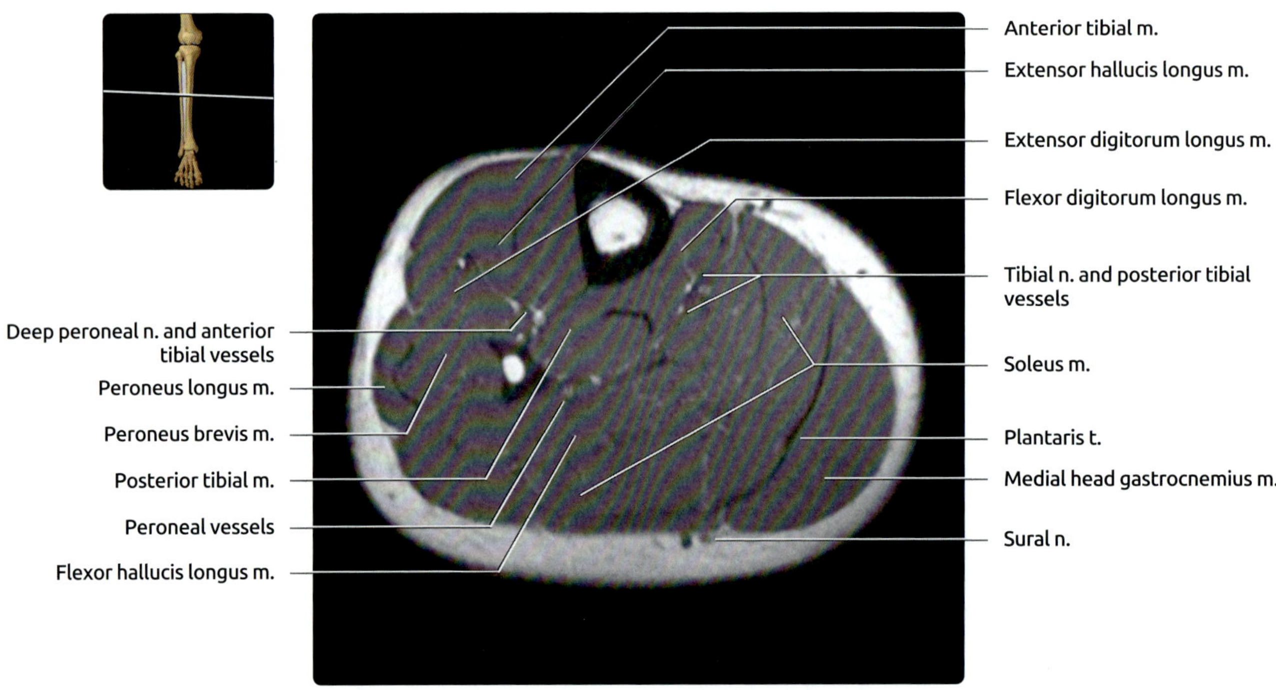

(Top) *Axial T1WI MR shows the right leg at the junction of proximal and middle thirds. At this point, the extensor hallucis longus makes its appearance, arising from the anterior fibula and interosseous membrane. Flexor digitorum longus is now also seen arising from the posterior tibia. The lateral head of the gastrocnemius has become tendinous with the soleus making up the bulk of the posterior muscles.* **(Bottom)** *Slightly distal axial T1WI MR shows the right leg. At this point, the extensor hallucis longus is located between the anterior tibial and extensor digitorum longus and is not easily distinguished from them. Similarly, the peroneal muscle/tendons are not easily distinguished because of poorly visualized fat planes in the leg. Note also that the plantaris tendon still lies between the medial head of the gastrocnemius and the soleus but is tracking medially.*

AXIAL T1 MR: LEFT LEG

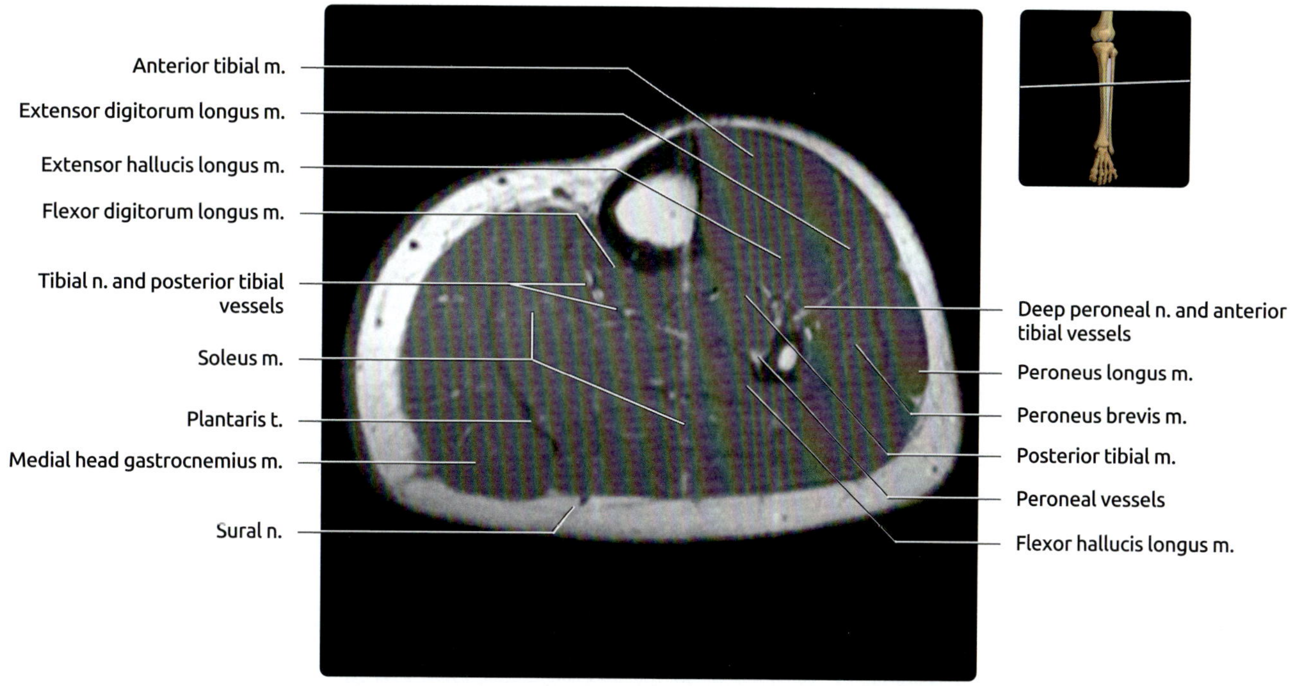

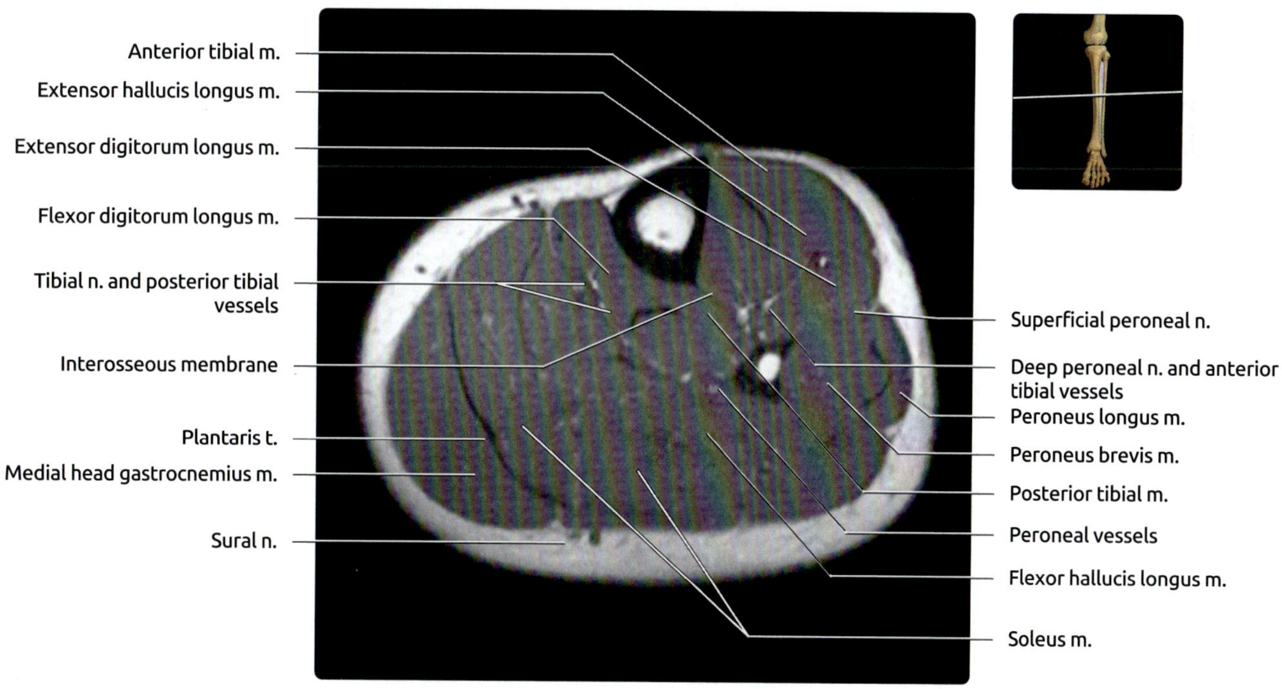

(Top) *Axial T1WI MR shows the left leg at the junction of proximal and middle thirds. At this point, the extensor hallucis longus makes its appearance, arising from the anterior fibula and interosseous membrane. The flexor digitorum longus is now also seen arising from the posterior tibia. The lateral head of the gastrocnemius has become tendinous with the soleus making up the bulk of the posterior muscles.* **(Bottom)** *Slightly distal axial T1WI MR shows the left leg. At this point, the extensor hallucis longus is located between the anterior tibial and extensor digitorum longus and is not easily distinguished from them. Similarly, the peroneal muscle/tendons are not easily distinguished because of poorly visualized fat planes in the leg. Note also that the plantaris tendon still lies between the medial head of gastrocnemius and soleus but is tracking medially.*

AXIAL T1 MR: RIGHT LEG

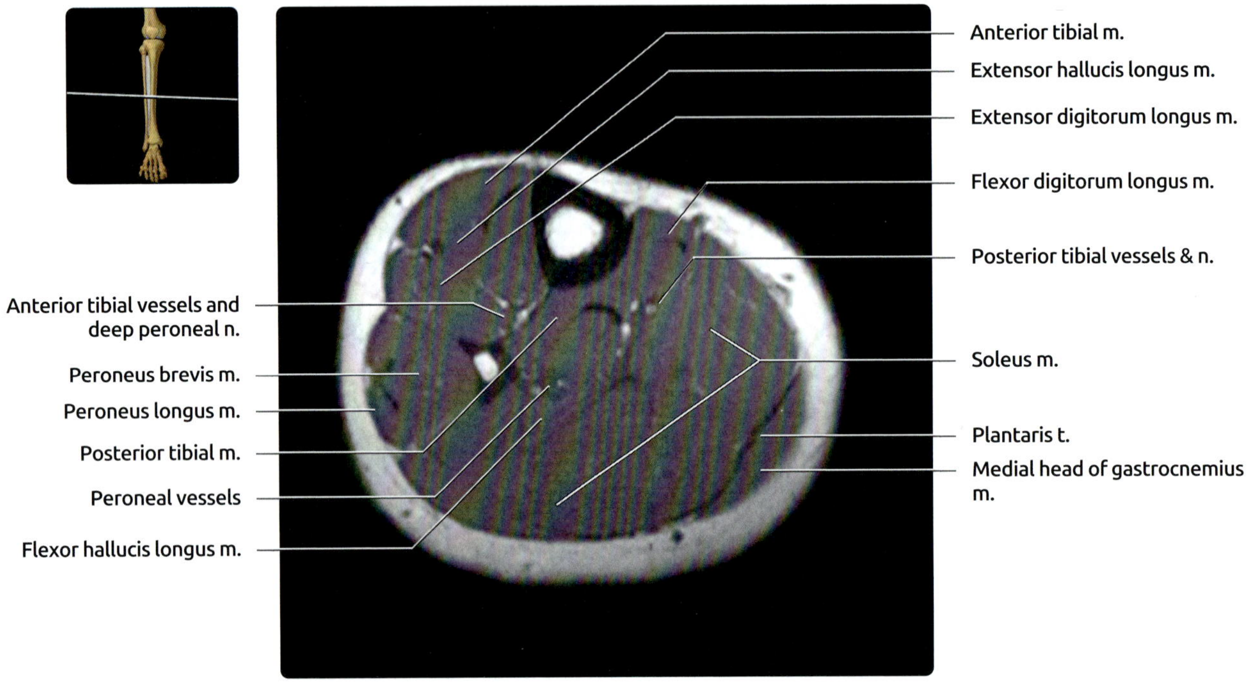

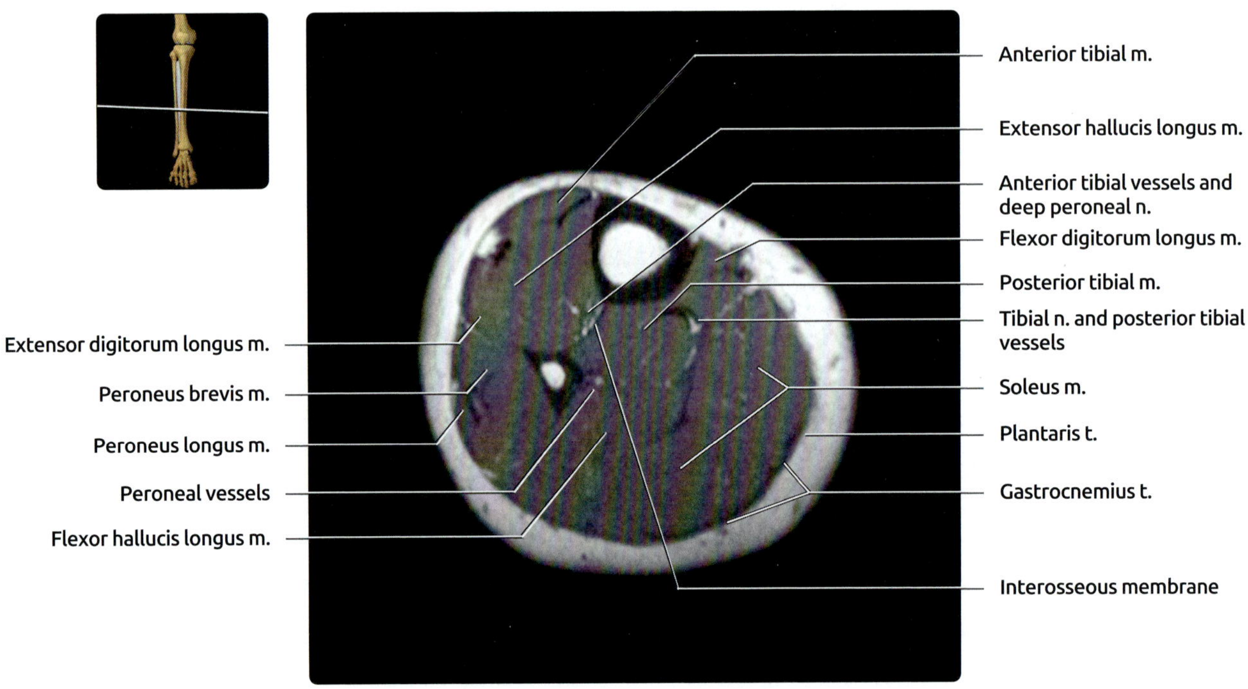

(Top) *Axial T1WI MR shows the right leg at the middiaphysis. At this point in the midleg the gastrocnemius muscle has become nearly completely tendinous.* **(Bottom)** *Slightly distal axial T1WI MR shows the right leg. The gastrocnemius forms an aponeurosis on which the soleus inserts. The plantaris tendon lies subcutaneously adjacent to the medial aspect of the gastrocnemius tendon.*

AXIAL T1 MR: LEFT LEG

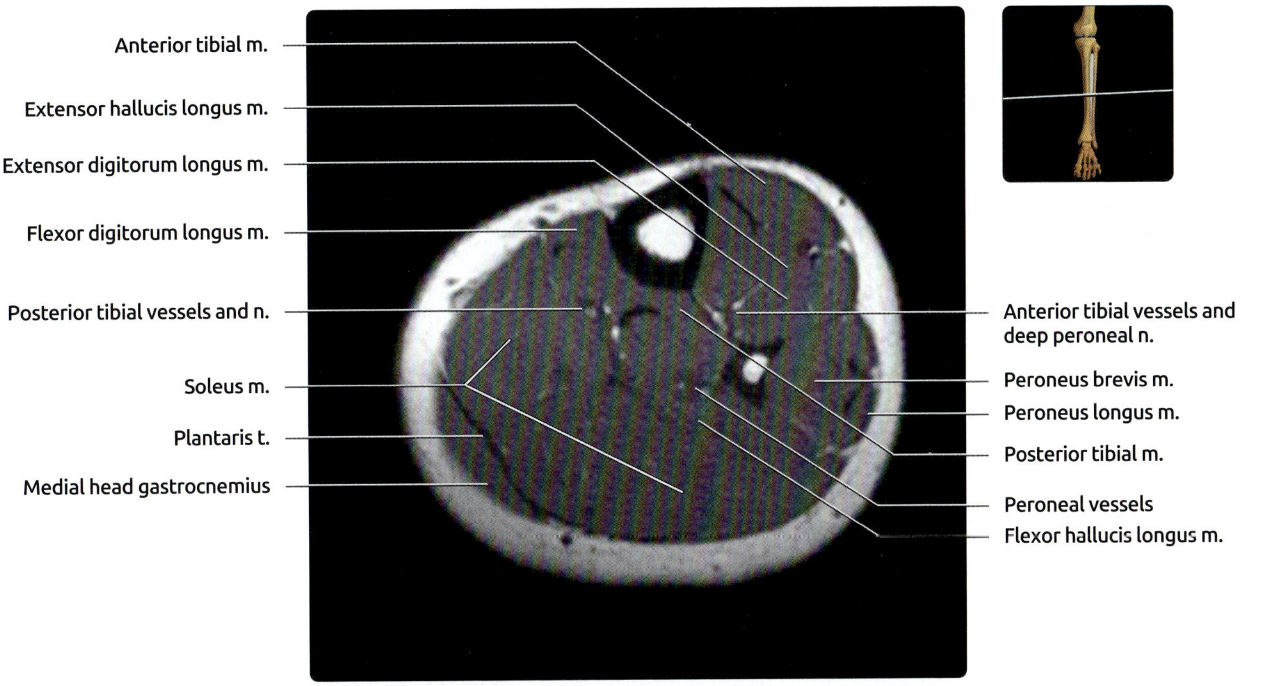

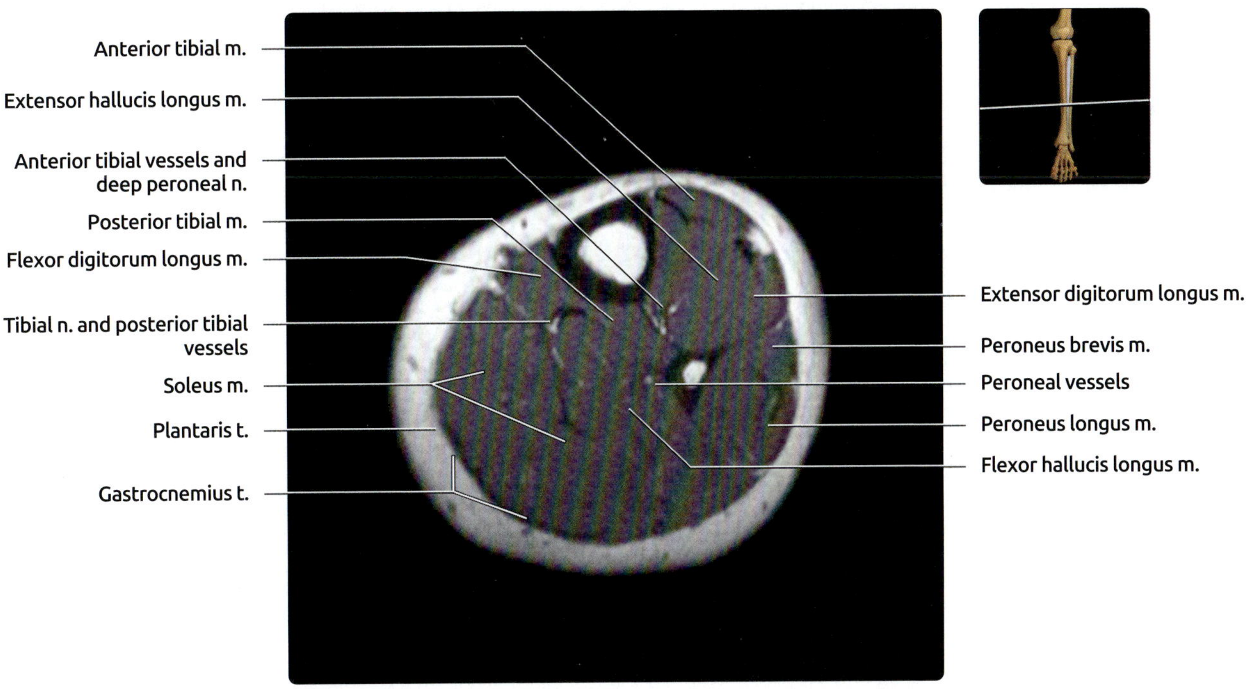

(Top) *Axial T1WI MR shows the left leg at the middiaphysis. At this point in the midleg the gastrocnemius muscle has become nearly completely tendinous.* **(Bottom)** *Slightly distal axial T1WI MR shows the right leg. The gastrocnemius forms an aponeurosis on which the soleus inserts. The plantaris tendon lies subcutaneously adjacent to the medial aspect of the gastrocnemius tendon.*

AXIAL T1 MR: RIGHT LEG

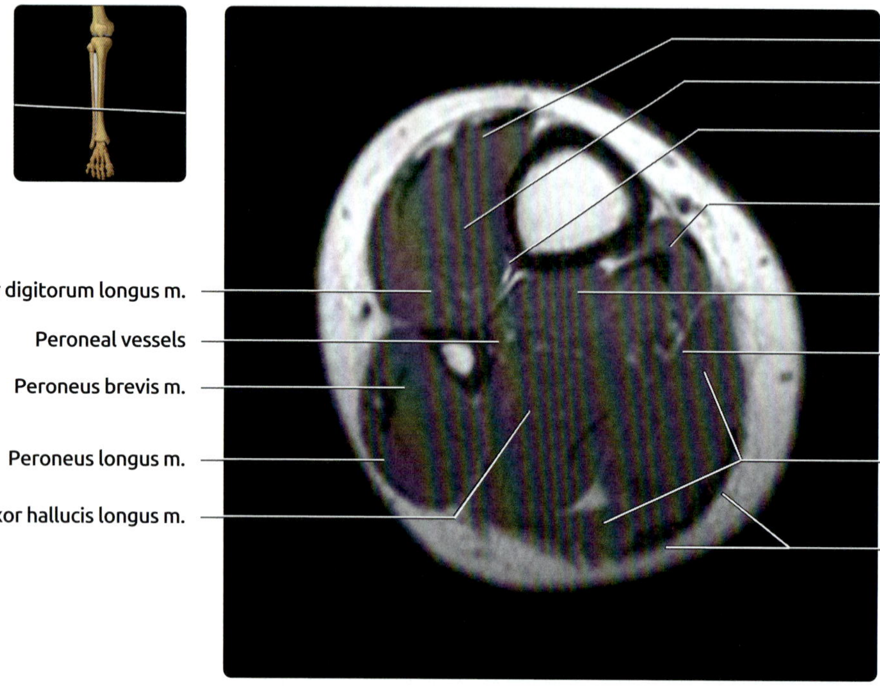

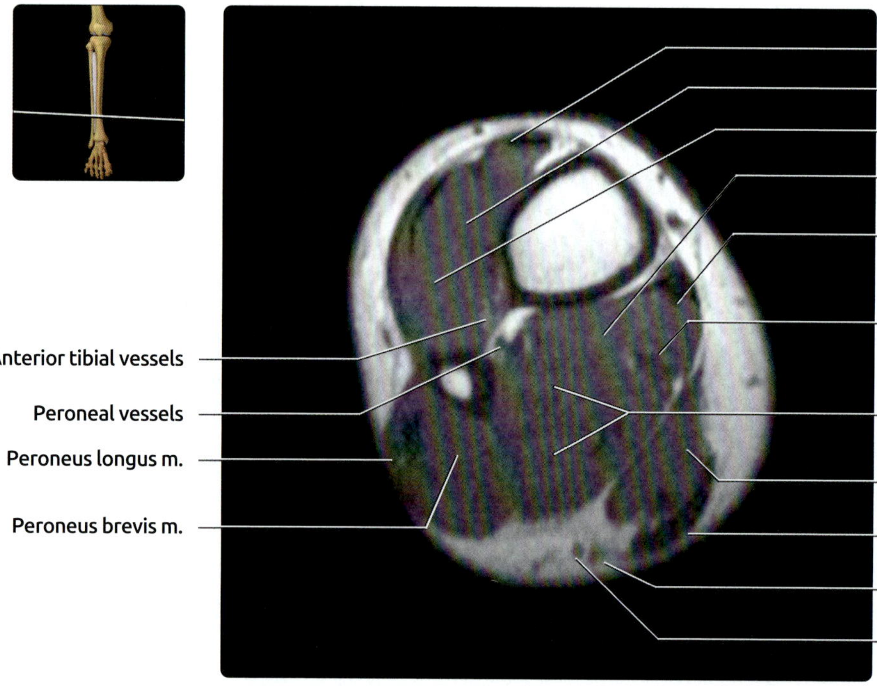

(Top) *Axial T1WI MR shows the right leg at the junction of middle and distal thirds. The deep muscles of the posterior compartment are now more prominent than the superficial.* **(Bottom)** *Slightly distal axial T1WI MR shows the right leg with the compartments more distinctly seen. The soleus is tapering and merging with the gastrocnemius tendon to form the Achilles tendon.*

AXIAL T1 MR: LEFT LEG

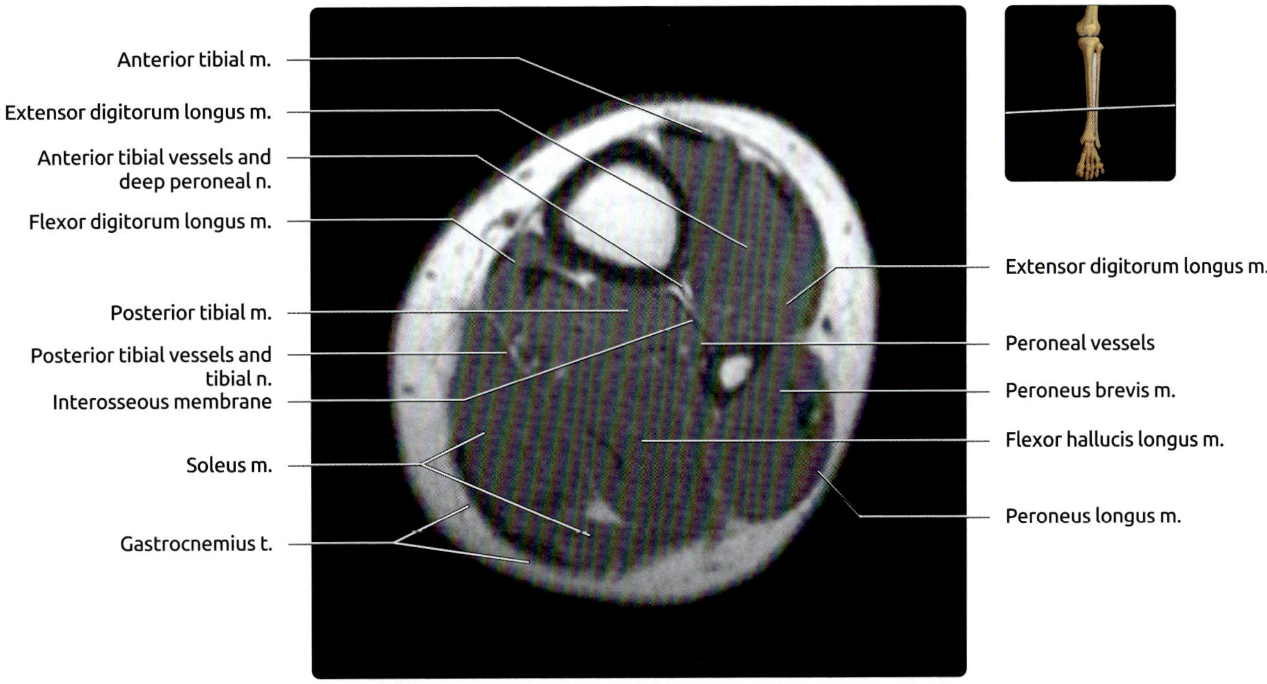

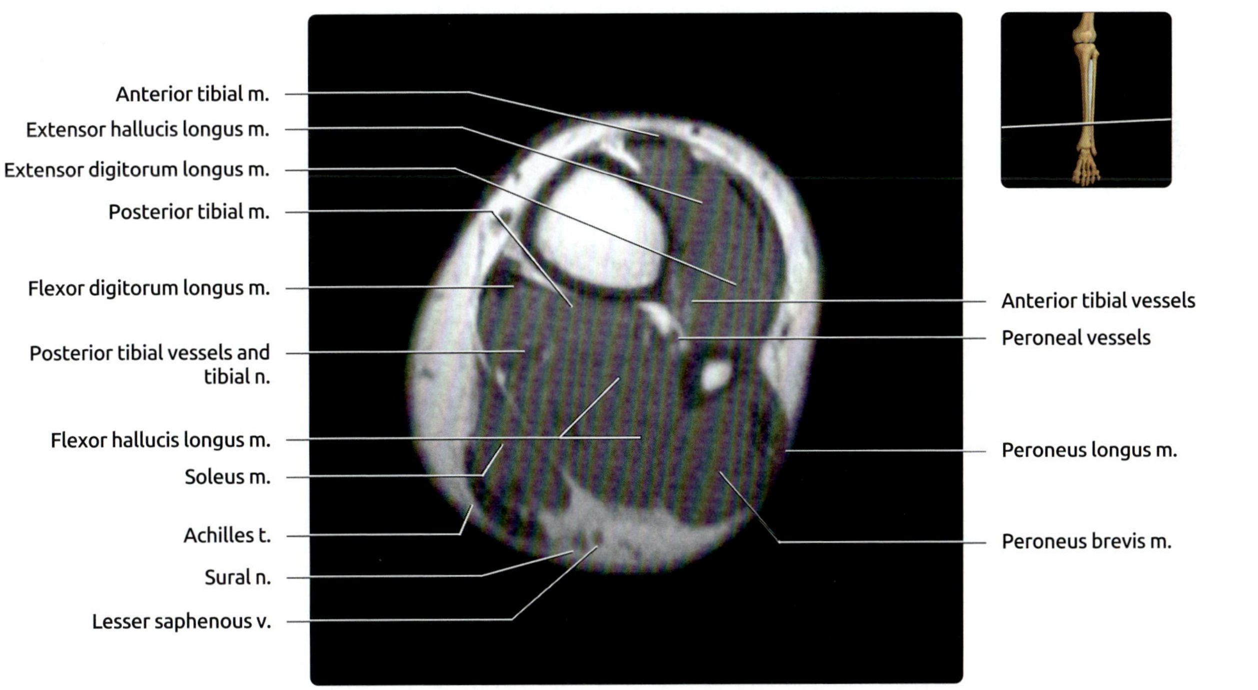

(Top) *Axial T1WI MR shows the left leg at the junction of the middle and distal thirds. The deep muscles of the posterior compartment are now more prominent than the superficial.* **(Bottom)** *Slightly distal axial T1WI MR shows the left leg with the compartments more distinctly seen. The soleus is tapering and merging with the gastrocnemius tendon to form the Achilles tendon.*

AXIAL T1 MR: RIGHT LEG

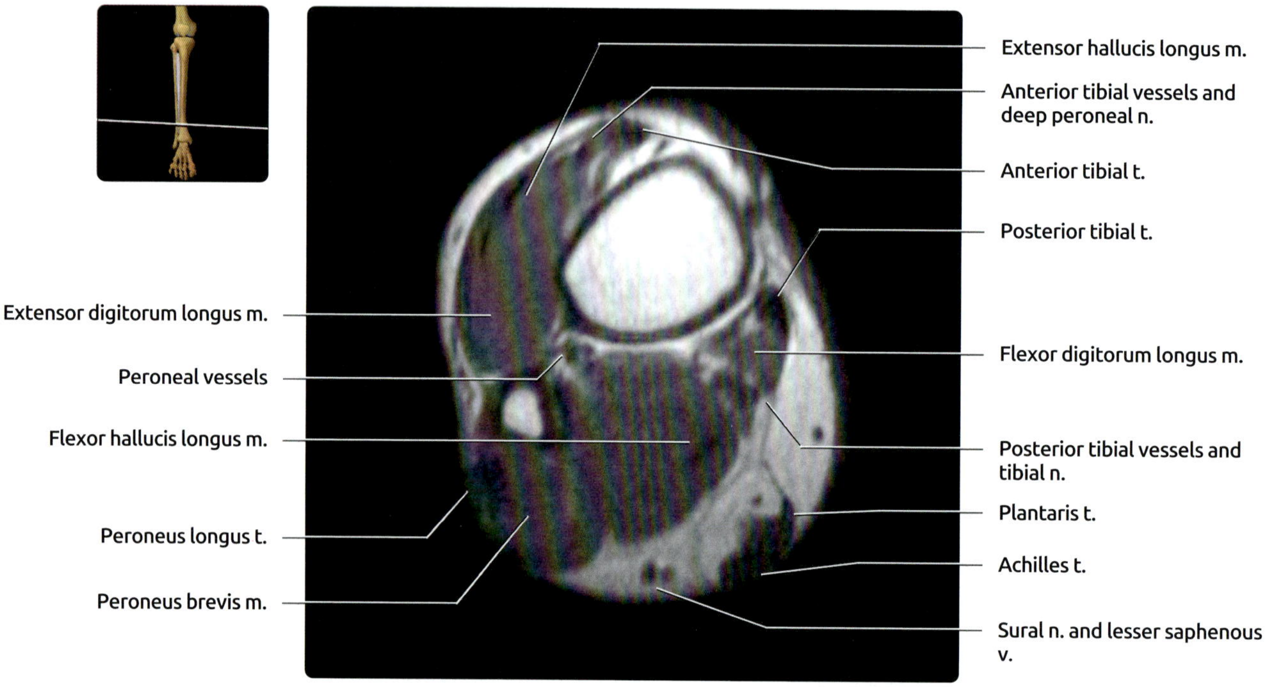

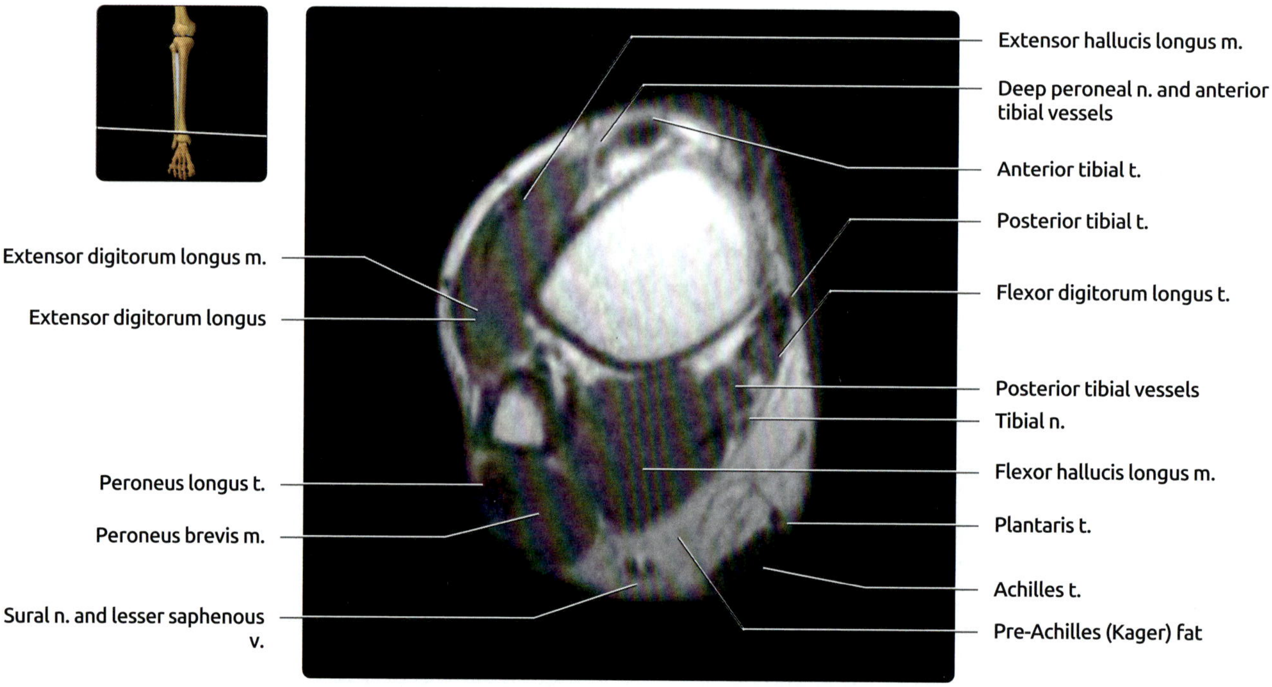

(Top) *Axial T1WI MR shows the right leg approaching the distal metaphysis. The anterior and posterior tibialis tendons are now defined, as is the Achilles tendon.* **(Bottom)** *Axial T1WI MR shows the right leg at the distal metaphysis. The major tendons of the leg are becoming more distinct. The deep flexors of the foot are separated from the Achilles tendon by the pre-Achilles fat pad, known as Kager fat pad.*

AXIAL T1 MR: LEFT LEG

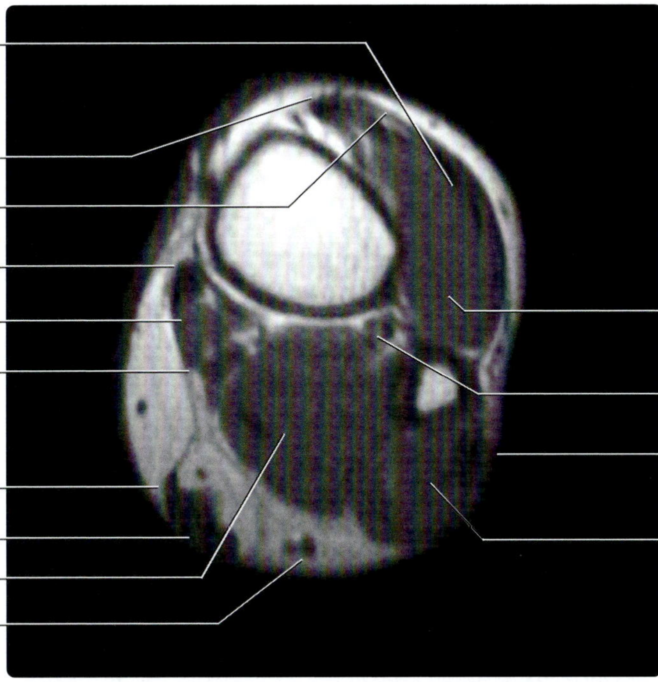

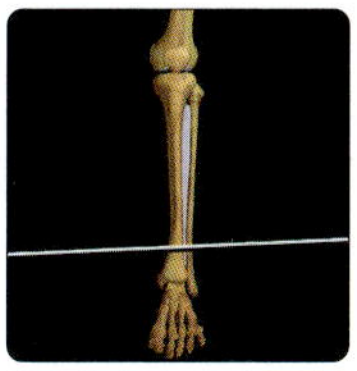

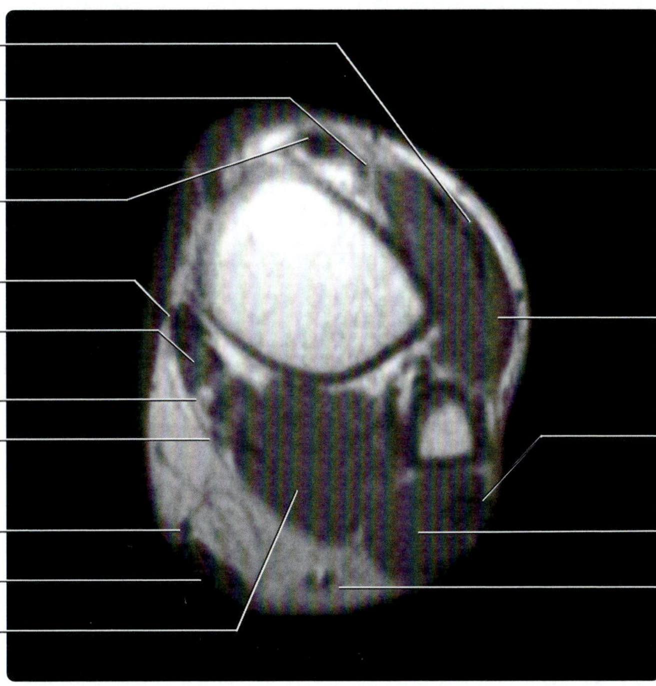

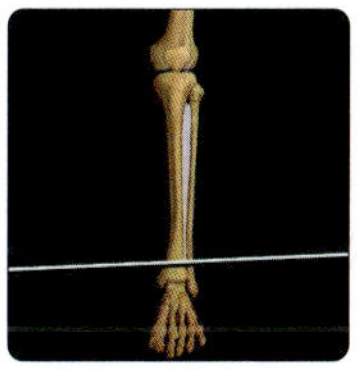

(Top) *Axial T1WI MR shows the left leg approaching the distal metaphysis. The anterior and posterior tibial tendons are now defined, as is the Achilles tendon.* **(Bottom)** *Axial T1WI MR shows the left leg at the distal metaphysis. The major tendons of the leg are becoming more distinct. The deep flexors of the foot are separated from the Achilles tendon by the pre-Achilles fat pad, known as Kager fat pad.*

AXIAL T1 MR: RIGHT LEG

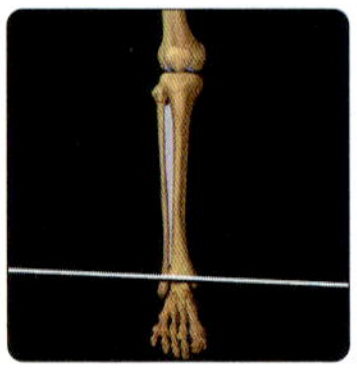

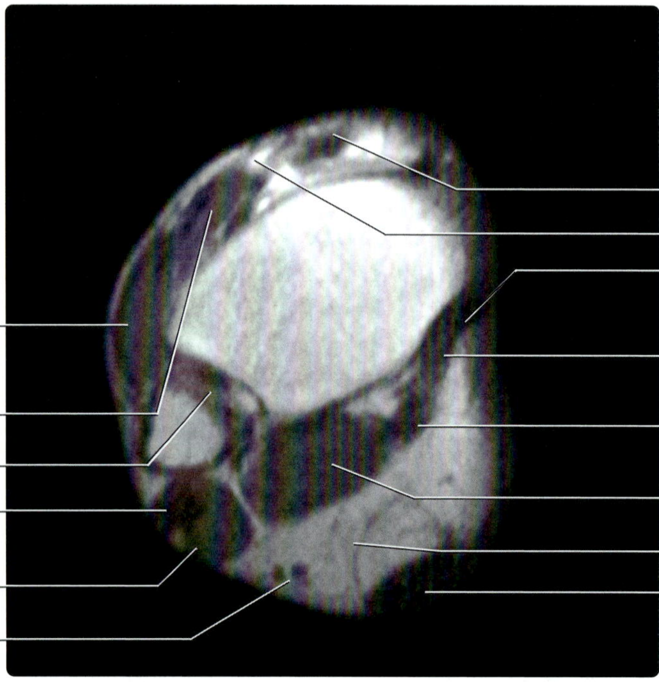

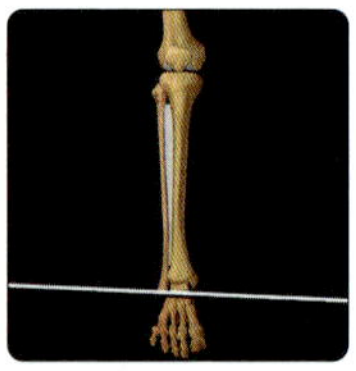

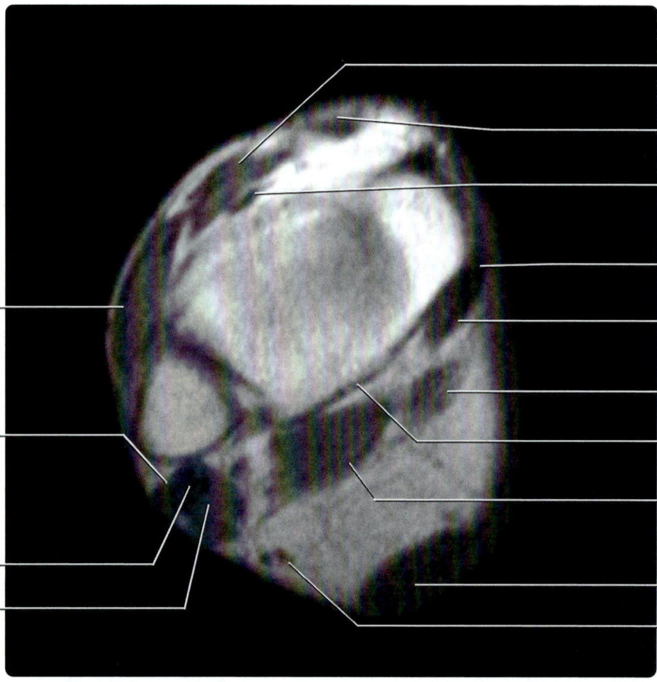

(Top) *Axial T1WI MR shows the right leg at the distal tibiofibular joint. The distal thickening of the interosseous membrane is known as the interosseous ligament. It ends about 1 cm above the tibial plafond.* **(Bottom)** *Axial T1WI MR shows the right leg at the ankle joint. The peroneus longus tendon is seen superficial to the peroneus brevis muscle and its adjacent tendon. The flexor hallucis longus is still primarily muscular, while the posterior tibial and flexor digitorum longus are tendinous.*

AXIAL T1 MR: LEFT LEG

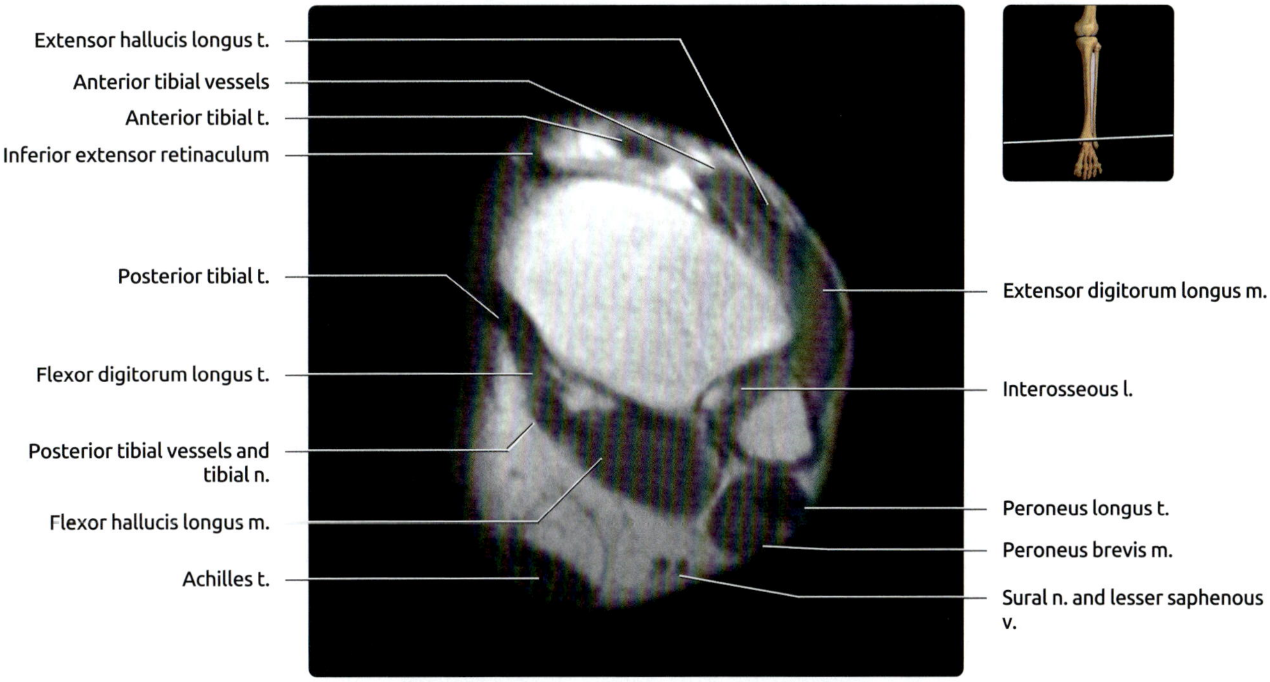

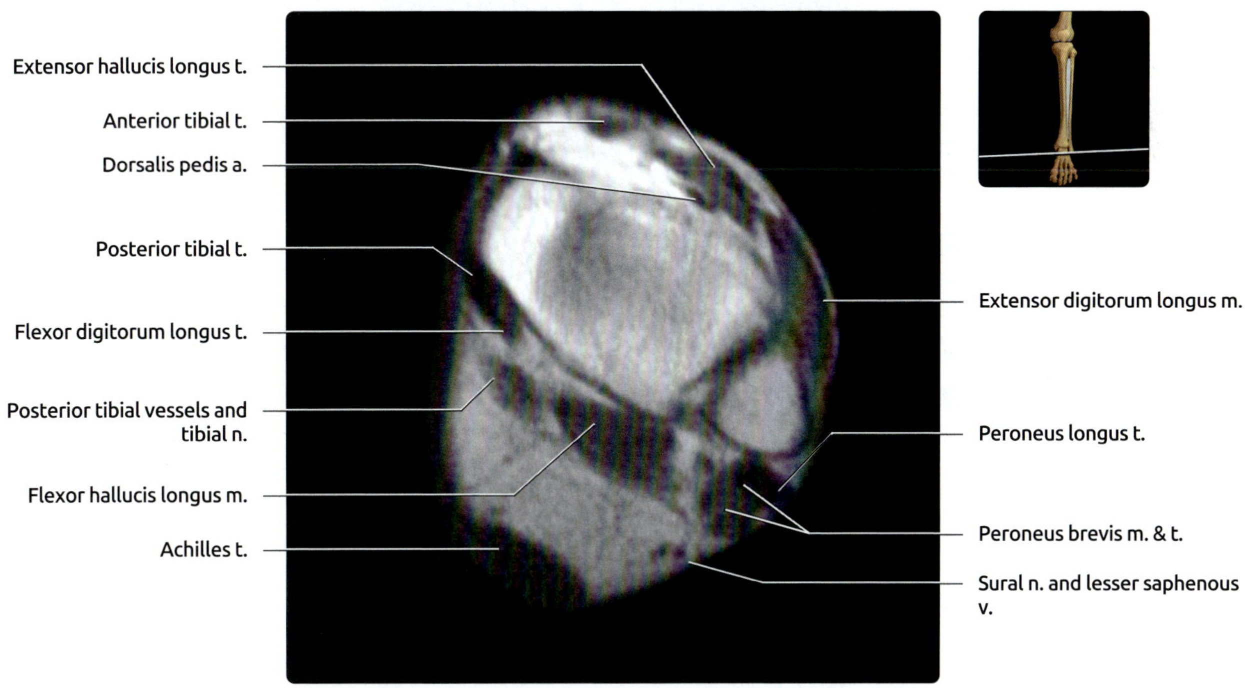

(Top) *Axial T1WI MR shows the left leg at the ankle joint. The peroneus longus tendon is seen superficial to the peroneus brevis muscle and its adjacent tendon. The flexor hallucis longus is still primarily muscular, while the posterior tibial and flexor digitorum longus are tendinous.* **(Bottom)** *Axial T1WI MR shows the right leg at the ankle joint. The peroneus longus tendon is seen superficial to the peroneus brevis muscle and its adjacent tendon. The flexor hallucis longus is still primarily muscular, while the posterior tibial and flexor digitorum longus are tendinous.*

SAGITTAL T1 MR: LEFT LEG

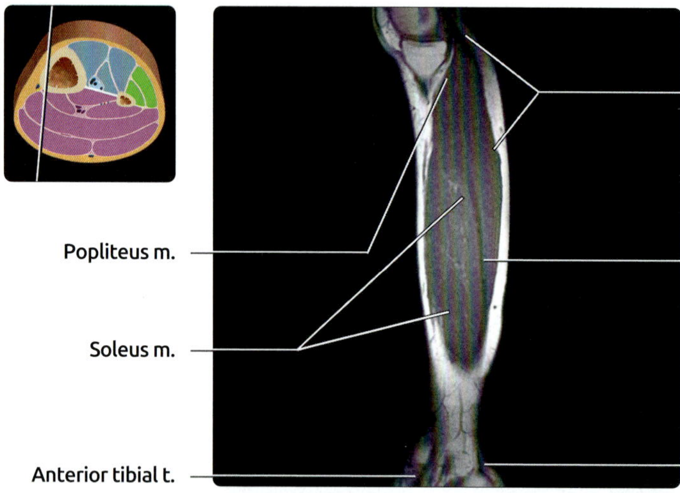

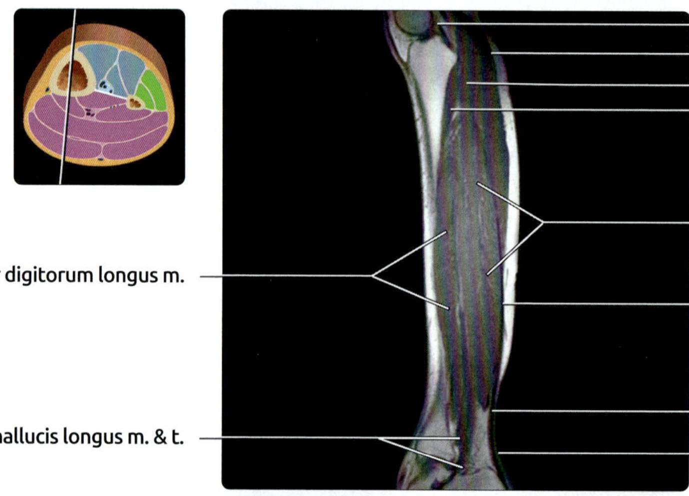

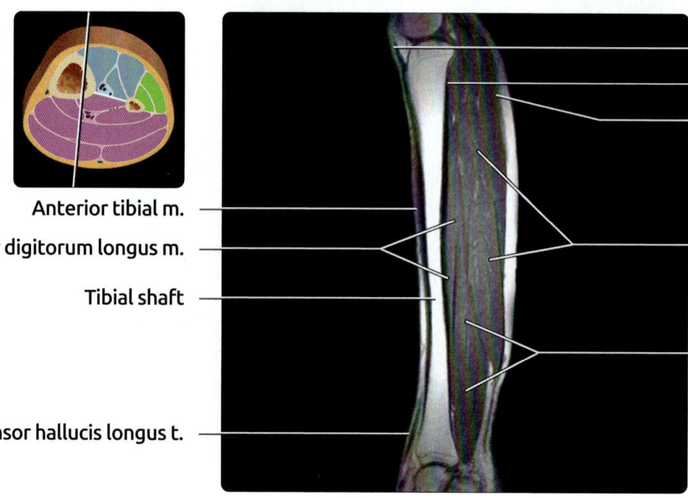

(Top) *First of 6 sagittal T1 MR images of the leg, starting medially, is shown. The bulk of the muscle here is the medial superficial posterior muscles, soleus, and gastrocnemius. The gastrocnemius has a long aponeurosis, which unites with the soleus to form the Achilles tendon.* **(Middle)** *Sagittal T1WI MR shows the medial leg. A portion of the deep posterior muscles is now seen, including the distal tendon of flexor hallucis longus. Note the distal extent of popliteus muscle and the fact that the tibial origin of the soleus is from the soleal line, along the distal site of insertion of the popliteus.* **(Bottom)** *Sagittal T1WI MR shows the midleg. The bulkiness of the flexor hallucis longus can be appreciated, along with the pre-Achilles fat pad separating it from the Achilles tendon. Note also the bare medial aspect of the shaft of the tibia, uncovered by muscle or tendon.*

SAGITTAL T1 MR: LEFT LEG

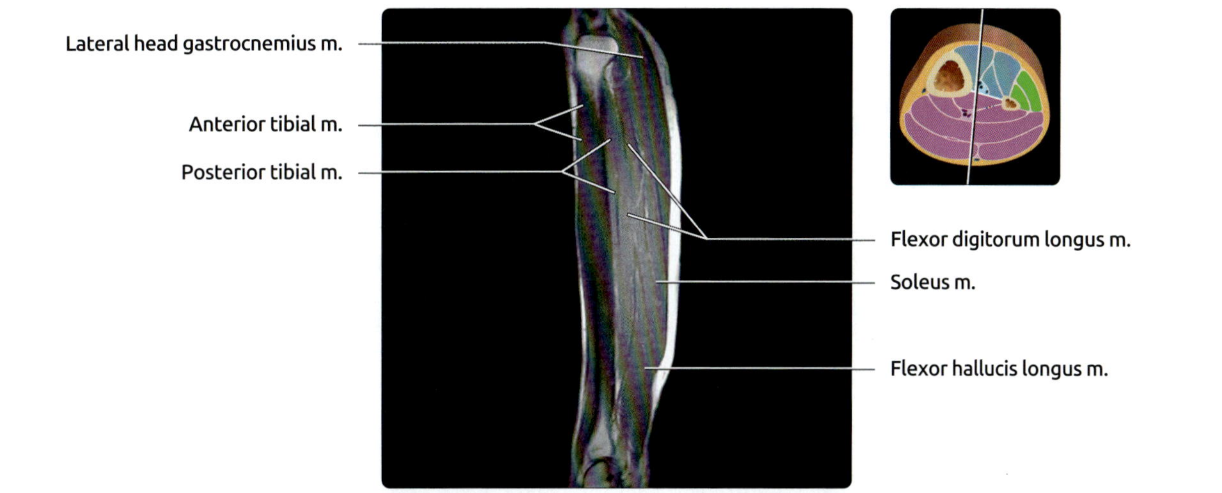

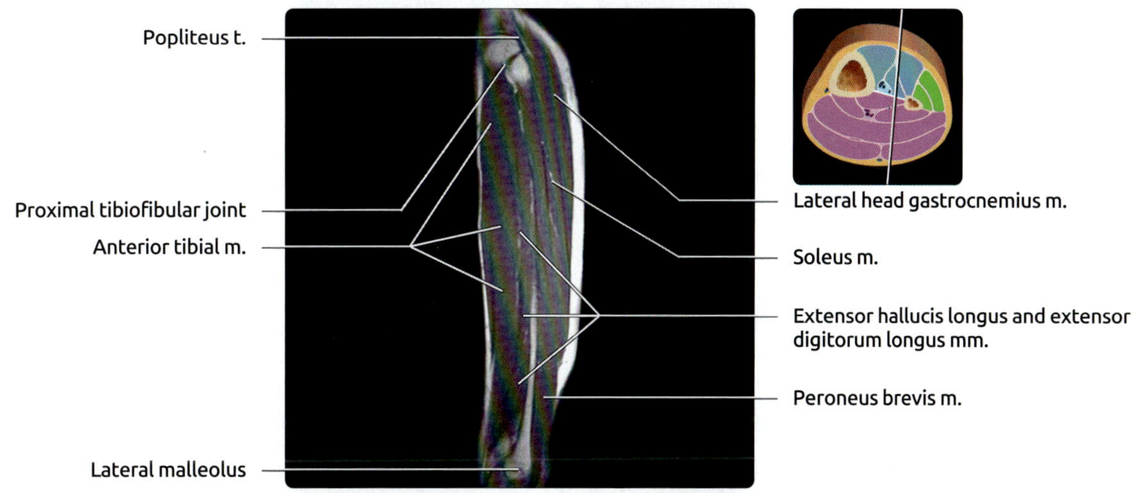

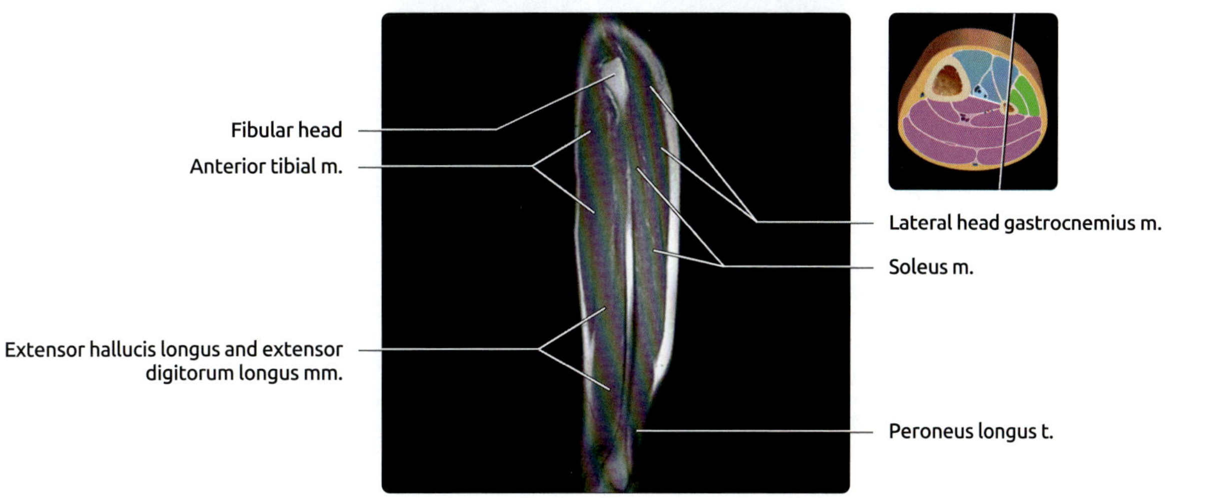

(Top) *Sagittal T1WI MR, slightly lateral in the leg, is shown. The anterior tibial (tibialis anterior) muscle is seen arising from the lateral aspect of the shaft of the tibia.* **(Middle)** *Sagittal T1WI MR is shown at the level of the fibula. The fibular origin of the soleus, as well as the peroneus and extensor digitorum, are seen.* **(Bottom)** *Sagittal T1WI MR is shown at the level of the fibula. Given the bulky muscles arising from the fibula, it is not surprising that the fibular surface is irregular. This should not be mistaken for periosteal reaction.*

CORONAL T1 MR: BOTH LEGS

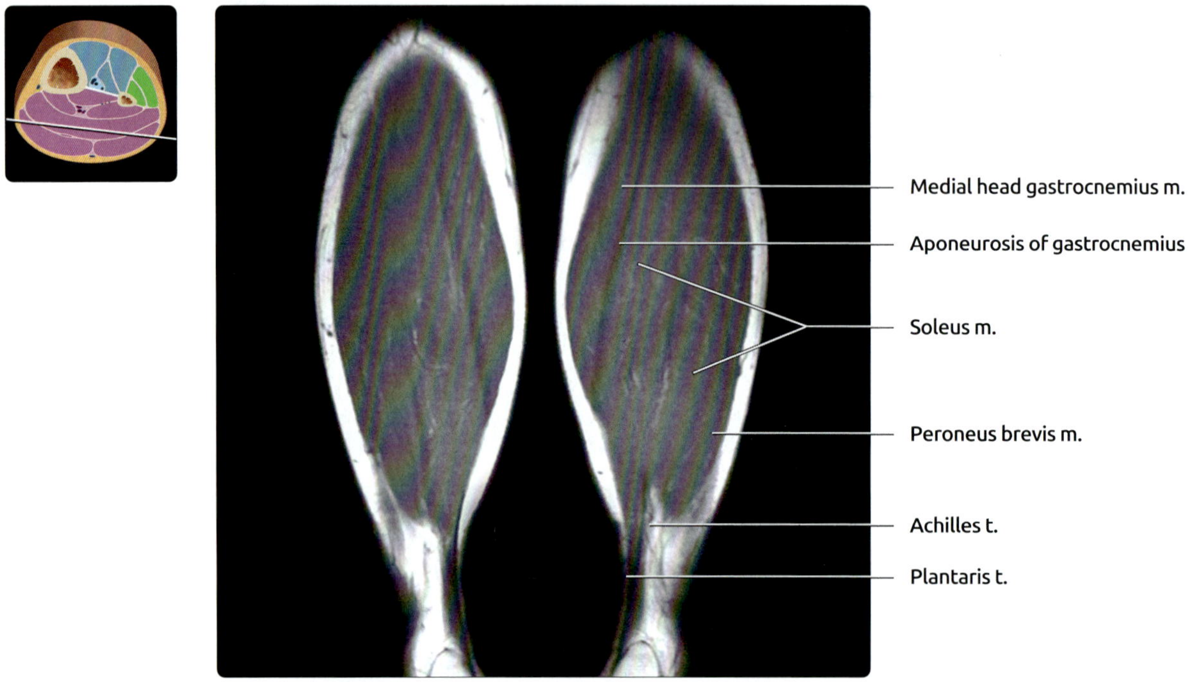

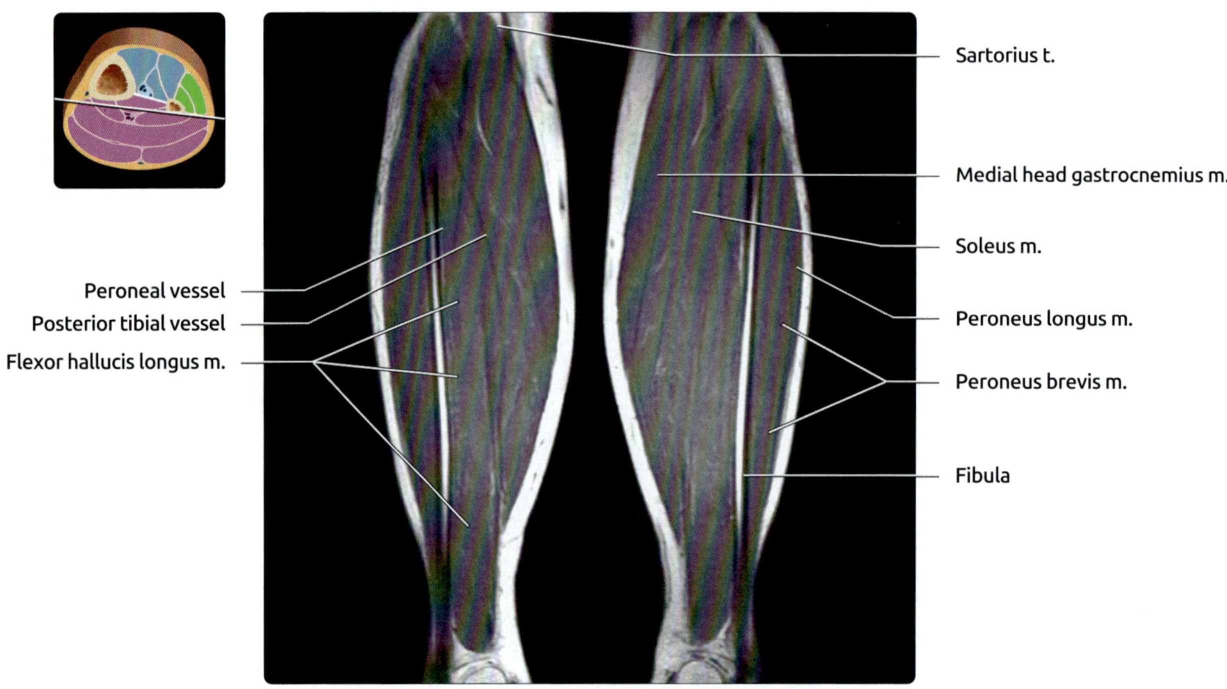

(Top) *First of 4 coronal T1 MR images of the legs is shown. This is the most posterior image, largely through the posterior superficial muscles. Note the plantaris tendon, which is seen well in the left leg, traveling and inserting medially to the Achilles tendon. The close interrelationship of the gastrocnemius and soleus is seen; the muscles are sometimes considered a single muscle, the triceps surae.* **(Bottom)** *Slightly more anterior coronal T1WI MR shows the legs, located posteriorly, through the fibula. Portions of the deep and superficial posterior compartment are seen, along with the lateral compartment.*

CORONAL T1 MR: BOTH LEGS

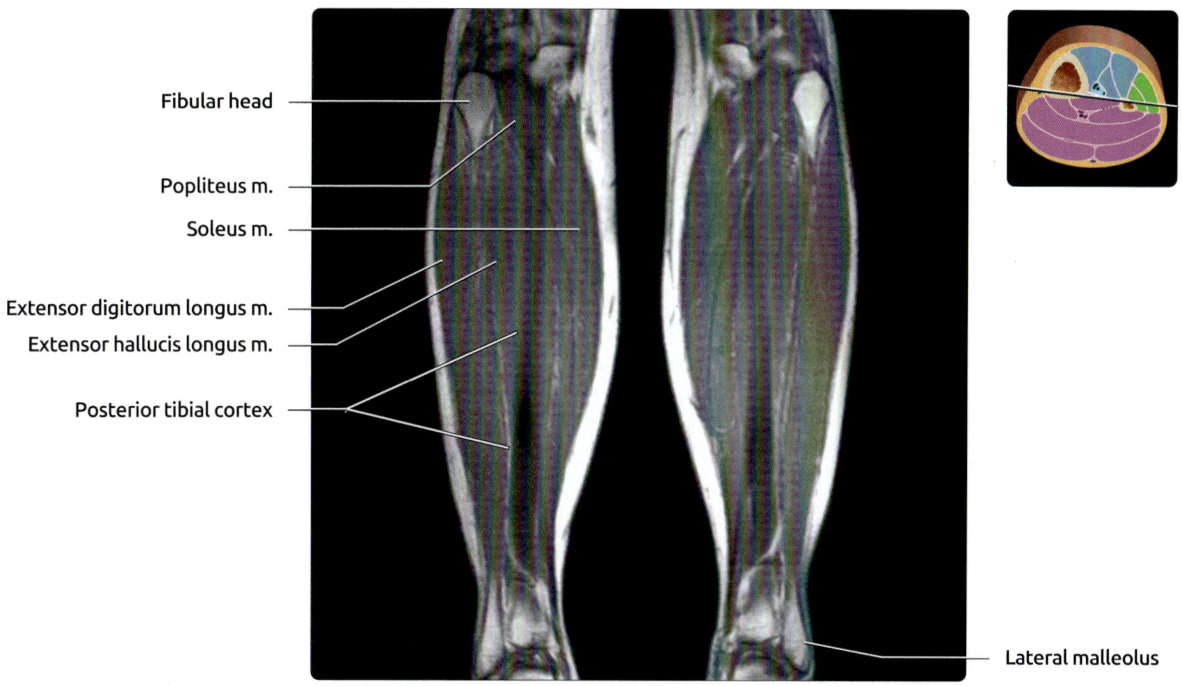

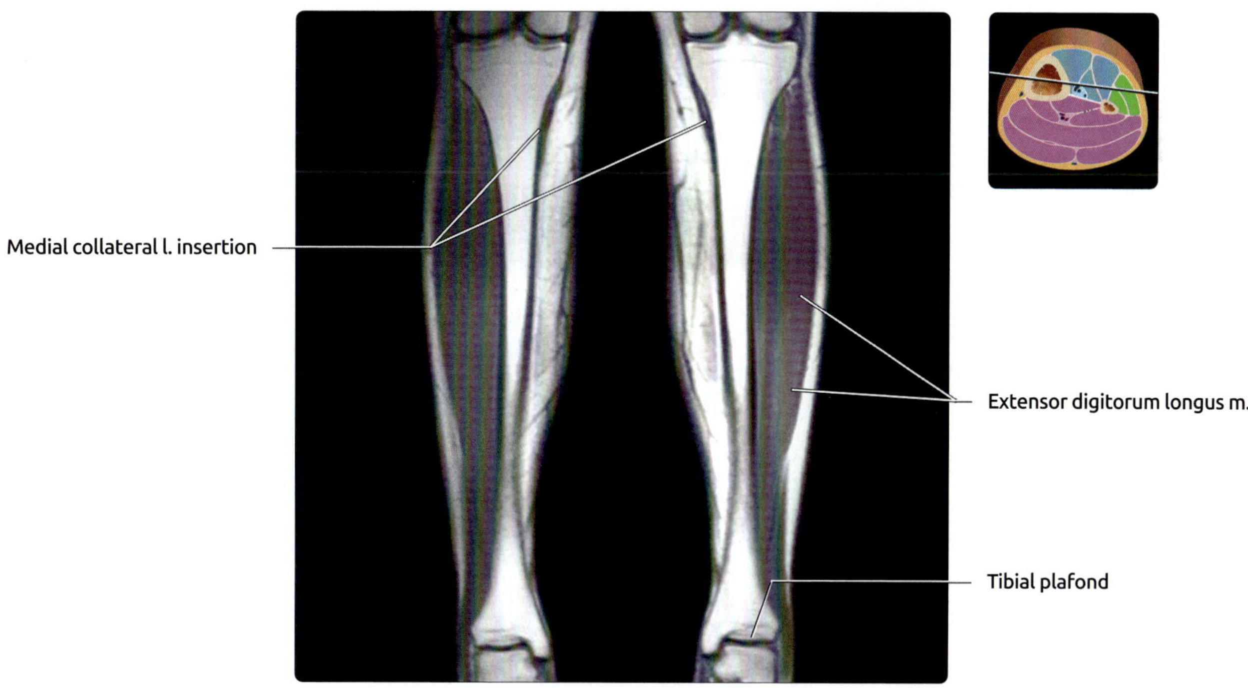

(Top) *Coronal T1WI MR shows the legs through the posterior tibial cortex. The more complex deep and superficial posterior compartments are partially seen.* **(Bottom)** *Coronal T1WI MR shows the legs, located anteriorly. Note the bare anteromedial aspect of the tibia. Because there is no overlying muscle, the blood supply is easily compromised when the tibia is fractured.*

IMAGING ANATOMY

Overview

- MR easily demonstrates large nerves, such as tibial & common peroneal nerve, but has difficulty distinguishing small nerves from vessels
- MR neurography optimal for large nerves, inadequate for smaller nerves of ankle & foot
- Nerves accompany vessels in fascial planes, highlighted by fat
- Nerves best seen on axial images; longer segments detected on coronal & sagittal images
- Normal nerves, intermediate signal on T1, mildly bright signal on fluid sensitive images
- Fascicles of larger nerves may have honeycomb appearance on axial high-resolution images

ANATOMY IMAGING ISSUES

Imaging Recommendations

- **Tibial nerve**
  - Largest, medial terminal branch of sciatic nerve
  - Arises from sciatic in posterior distal thigh
  - Descends between superficial & deep posterior leg compartments
  - In leg, supplies all posterior compartment muscles
  - Often called posterior tibial nerve in ankle
  - Curves around medial malleolus, travels in tarsal tunnel under flexor retinaculum
  - Divides in or proximal to tarsal tunnel
    - Medial calcaneal nerve: Sensory medial heel
    - Medial plantar nerve: Sensory to medial 2/3 plantar foot, motor to abductor hallucis, flexor digitorum brevis, flexor hallucis brevis, 1st lumbrical
    - Lateral plantar nerve: Sensory to lateral 1/3 of plantar foot, motor to abductor digiti minimi, quadratus plantae, adductor hallucis, flexor digiti minimi, 2nd-4th lumbricals, all interossei
  - MR anatomy of tibial nerve, branches
    - Often has honeycomb fascicular appearance on axial images
    - In knee: Well seen in abundant fat anterior to gastrocnemius muscles, posterolateral to popliteal vessels
    - In leg: Anterior to soleus, more difficult to see due to compact muscles
    - In tarsal tunnel: Lateral to vessels, closer to bone
    - In foot: Medial, lateral plantar nerves best seen on short-axis views
    - Lateral plantar nerve: Between flexor digitorum brevis & quadratus plantae
    - Medial plantar nerve follows flexor hallucis longus tendon, between abductor hallucis & flexor digitorum brevis
- **Common peroneal nerve**
  - Smaller, lateral, terminal branch of sciatic nerve
  - Arises from sciatic nerve in distal thigh
  - Descends in posterior knee between biceps femoris & lateral gastrocnemius head
  - Curves around fibular head
  - Enters anterior compartment via peroneal tunnel between fibular origins of peroneus longus
  - Provides sensory branch, lateral sural cutaneous nerve, to proximal 1/3 of lateral leg & motor branch to short head, biceps femoris
  - Trifurcates at posterior knee to
    - Articular branch: Supplies knee capsule & proximal tibiofibular joint
    - Deep peroneal nerve
    - Superficial peroneal nerve
  - MR anatomy
    - Deep & superficial peroneal divisions seen before nerve actually bifurcates
    - Common peroneal nerve easily seen in posterior knee, superficial, in abundant fat between biceps femoris & gastrocnemius muscles
    - More difficult to visualize around fibular head
- **Deep peroneal nerve**
  - Predominantly motor to extensor muscles: Tibialis anterior, extensor hallucis longus, extensor digitorum longus & brevis, peroneus tertius
  - Sensory & motor to dorsal 1st web space
  - In knee: Closer to fibular bone
  - In leg: Deep to anterolateral muscles, anterior to interosseous membrane
  - In ankle: In anterior tarsal tunnel, deep to superior & inferior extensor retinacula
  - In foot: Dorsal to talonavicular joint, 2nd cuneiform, between 1st-2nd metatarsals
  - MR anatomy
    - In knee: Anterior & closer to fibular head compared to superficial peroneal nerve
    - In leg: May be hard to see, adjacent to interosseous membrane, deep to anterior compartment muscles
    - In ankle: Deep to extensor retinacula
    - In foot: Medial branch in dorsal subcutaneous fat, lateral branch deep to extensor digitorum brevis
- **Superficial peroneal nerve**
  - In leg, migrates anteriorly between anterior & lateral compartments
  - Pierces anterior leg fascia, becomes subcutaneous 10-15 cm above ankle joint
  - MR anatomy of superficial peroneal nerve
    - May be difficult to detect in fascial plane between anterior & lateral compartments
    - Usually seen as it approaches & pierces fascia to become subcutaneous in distal leg
- **Saphenous nerve** (branch of femoral nerve)
  - Sensory to anteromedial knee, medial leg, foot
  - In knee: In medial fat plane, deep to sartorius muscle
  - In leg: Subcutaneous, lateral to greater saphenous vein
- **Sural nerve**
  - Formed by medial sural branch of tibial nerve & peroneal (sural) communicating branch of common peroneal nerve
  - Purely sensory to lateral ankle & foot, up to 5th toe base
  - Subcutaneous along posterolateral ankle
  - MR: Adjacent to lesser saphenous vein, between Achilles & peroneal tendons

GRAPHICS: TIBIAL NERVE

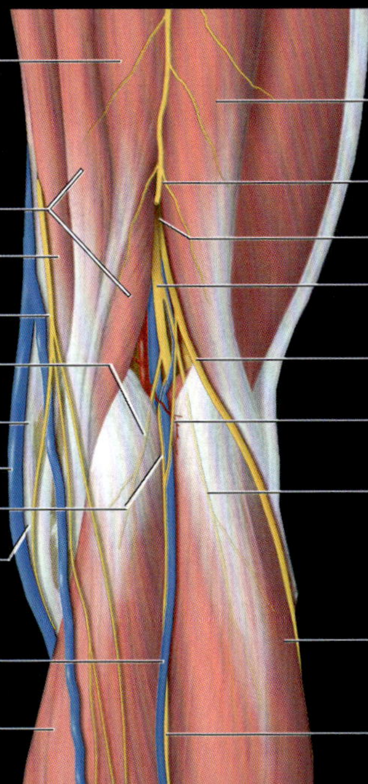

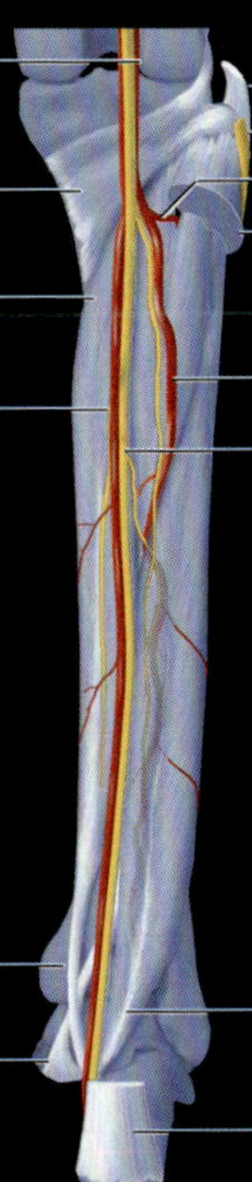

(Top) *Graphic shows the popliteal fossa. The sciatic nerve divides into tibial & common peroneal nerves in the upper popliteal fossa. The tibial nerve is initially deep to the hamstrings, but in the popliteal fossa, it becomes superficial between the semimembranosus & biceps femoris muscles. It then dives in between the medial & lateral heads of the gastrocnemius muscles to travel between the deep & superficial posterior compartments of the leg.* **(Bottom)** *The tibial nerve descends between the deep & superficial posterior leg muscles (resected here) paralleling the posterior tibial vessels. The tibial nerve controls plantar flexion, foot inversion, & toe flexion. It provides motor innervation to the muscles of the posterior superficial & deep leg compartment & plantar foot & sensation to the plantar foot. It gives articular branches to the knee joint, medial capsule, & posterior oblique ligament.*

MR: TIBIAL NERVE

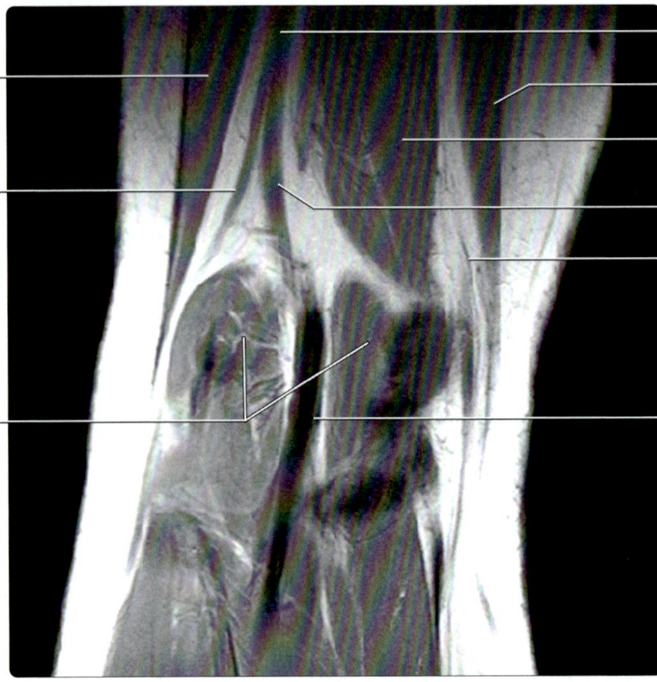

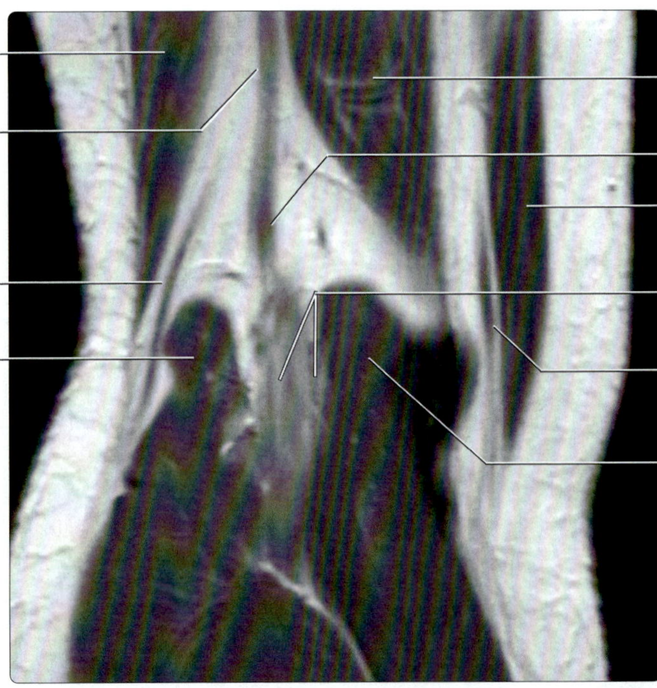

(Top) *Posterior coronal image of popliteal fossa is shown. The sciatic nerve can be seen as it terminates into the lateral common peroneal nerve & more medial & larger tibial nerve at the upper popliteal fossa. The 2 nerves are depicted as intermediate signal structures on all pulse sequences within abundant amount of fat. The division of the sciatic nerve is typically seen on coronal & axial images of the popliteal fossa. The tibial nerve continues straight downward & is difficult to visualize more distally on coronal images.* **(Bottom)** *A slightly more posterior coronal image is shown. The common peroneal nerve is visualized as it descends within fat in between the short head of the biceps femoris & lateral head of gastrocnemius muscles. The tibial nerve continues straight downward in between the medial & lateral heads of the gastrocnemius muscle.*

MR: TIBIAL NERVE

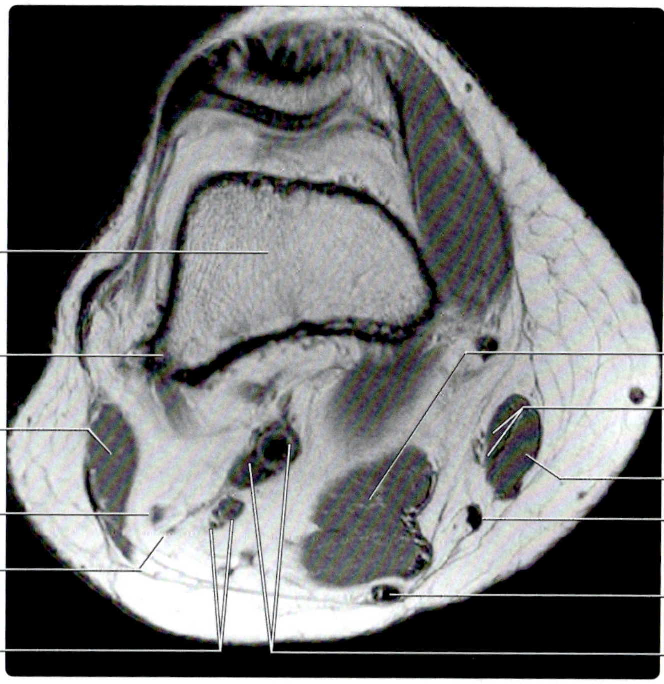

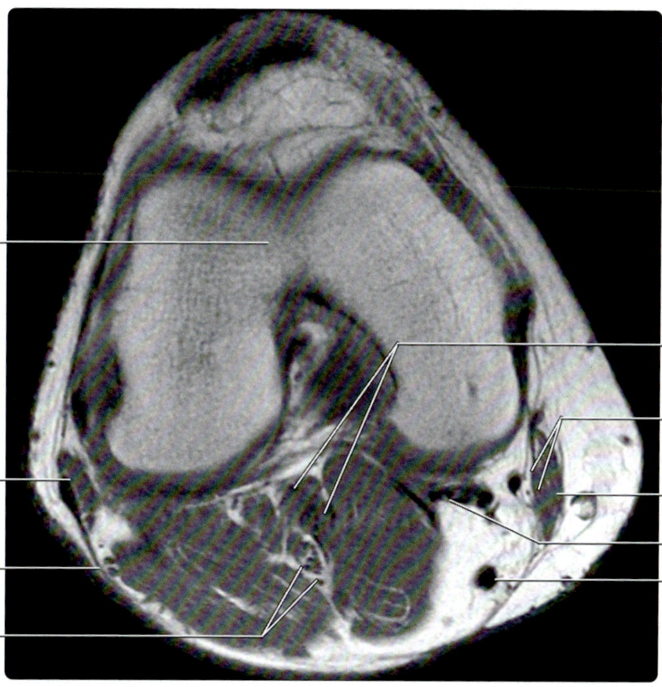

(Top) *Axial image above the knee joint is shown. The fascicles of the tibial nerve can be seen on high-resolution axial images. In the thigh & knee, the nerve is highlighted by a large amount of fat. Note that the nerve is posterolateral to the popliteal vessels & medial to the common peroneal nerve.* **(Bottom)** *Axial image more distally is shown. Multiple nerve branches of the tibial nerve are now seen. The most posterior branch is most likely the medial sural cutaneous nerve, while the ones anterior to it are probably branches to the gastrocnemius & soleus muscles. Exact labeling of these nerve branches may be difficult on routine MR studies. Note that unlike the previous image where the tibial nerve was surrounded by abundant fat, the nerve now is snugly situated between the medial & lateral heads of the gastrocnemius muscles. Note also that 2 divisions of the common peroneal nerve are clearly depicted.*

MR: TIBIAL NERVE

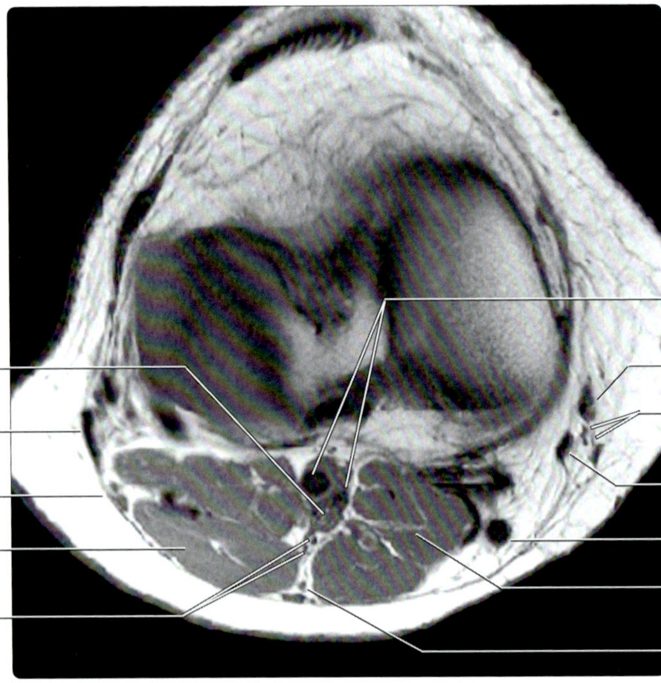

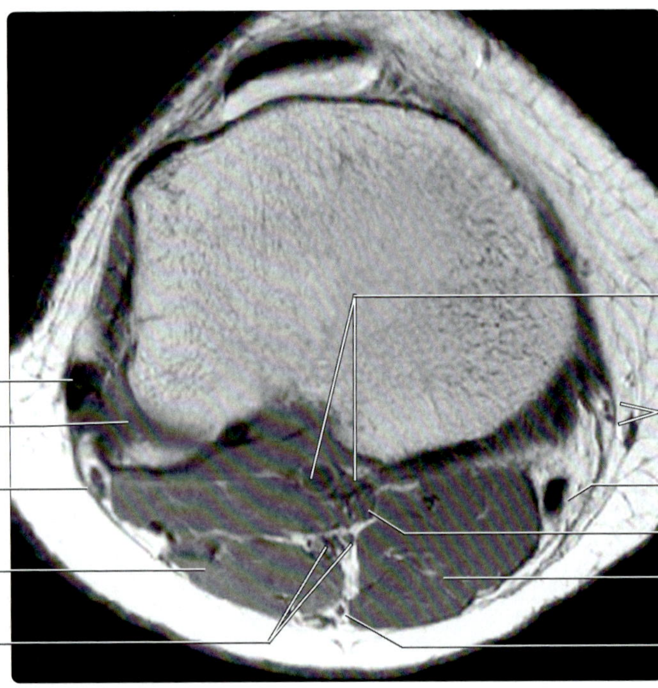

(Top) *Axial image at the knee joint is shown. The tibial nerve bisects the popliteal fossa slightly lateral to midline. Note the relative paucity of fat around the nerve & intimate relationship of the nerve with the medial & lateral heads of the gastrocnemius muscle. The relatively straight course of the nerve & its deep location protect it from direct injury. Note 2 small branches to the gastrocnemius muscle. The medial sural cutaneous nerve is approaching the posterior subcutaneous fat to form the sural nerve.* **(Bottom)** *A more distal axial image at the proximal tibial-fibular joint is shown. The tibial nerve has migrated anterior to the gastrocnemius muscle & is now found in a fat plane between the deep & superficial posterior compartments of the leg. Note the multiple branches of the nerve as they course toward the posterior leg muscles.*

MR: TIBIAL NERVE

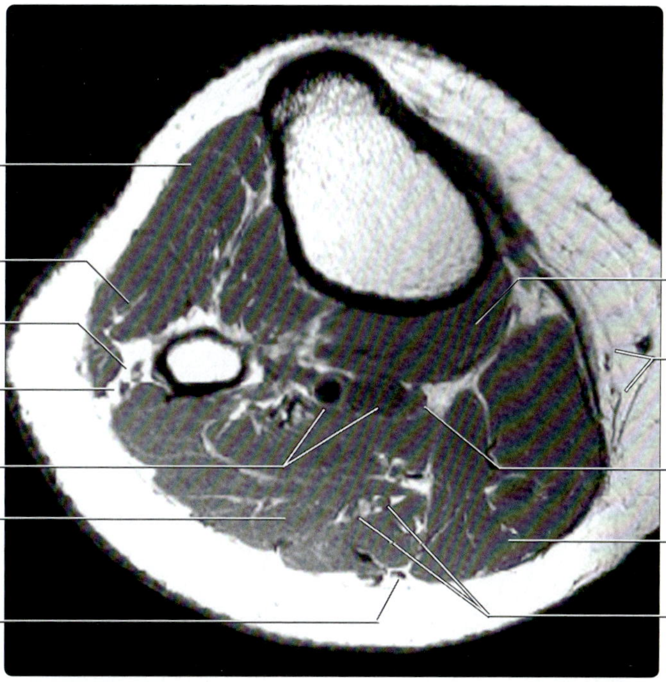

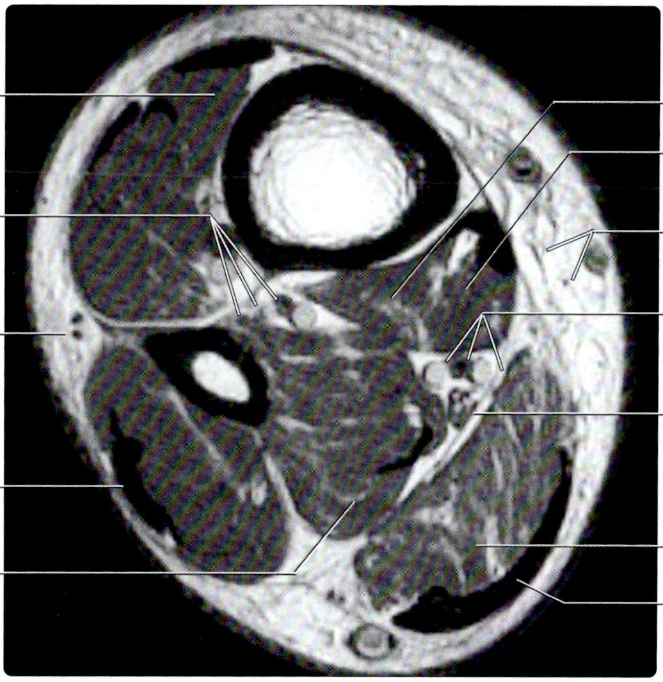

(Top) *Axial image at the proximal leg is shown. The tibial nerve is now medial to the popliteal artery & vein. Branches of the nerve, with accompanying vessels, are noted in various muscle planes of the posterior leg compartment.* **(Bottom)** *Axial image at the distal leg is shown. The tibial nerve at this level is often called the posterior tibial nerve. It descends between the superficial & deep compartments of the leg & is now more clearly visualized within a triangle of fat anterior to the soleus muscle & posterior to the flexor hallucis longus & flexor digitorum longus muscles. The nerve is still posterior to the posterior tibial artery & vein. The fascicles of the nerve are clearly seen. Note the interosseous branch of the tibial nerve adjacent to the fibula, accompanied by vessels.*

MR: TIBIAL NERVE

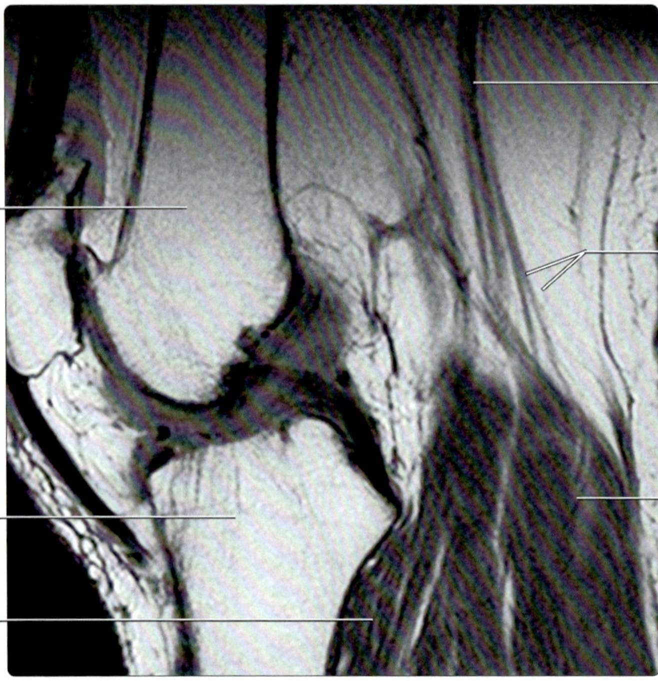

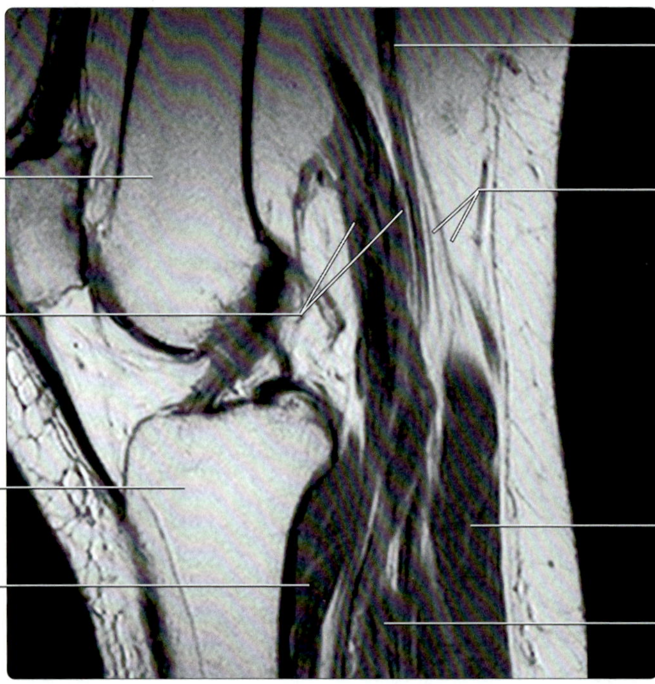

(Top) *The tibial nerve is easily depicted on sagittal images at the level of the knee. A sagittal image at the intercondylar notch area depicts the relatively straight course of the tibial nerve & a few of its posterior branches. These proximal tibial branches include the branches to the gastrocnemius & soleus muscles as well as the medial sural communicating nerve. Note the extensive amount of fat surrounding the nerve at this level.* **(Bottom)** *Note the proximity of the nerve to the popliteal vessels. Note also that the nerve becomes more difficult to visualize as it continues into the leg between the soleus & gastrocnemius muscles.*

GRAPHICS: TIBIAL NERVE, DISTAL BRANCHES

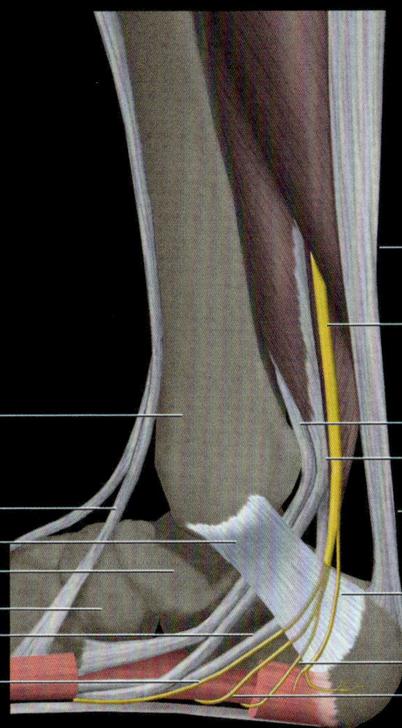

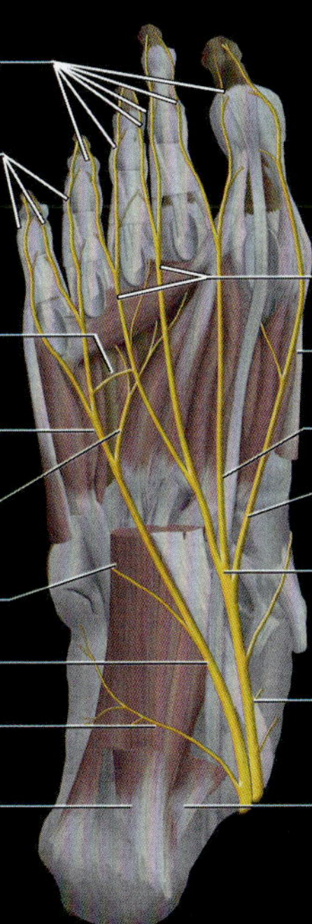

(Top) *The tarsal tunnel is traversed by the posterior tibial, flexor digitorum longus, & flexor hallucis longus tendons, posterior tibial nerve & branches, & posterior tibial vessels (not shown). The medial calcaneal nerve typically takes off from the posterior tibial nerve above the flexor retinaculum & provides sensation to the medial heel. The inferior calcaneal nerve, also called the nerve of Baxter, is the first branch of the lateral plantar nerve and innervates the abductor digiti minimi.* **(Bottom)** *Plantar foot partially dissected shows the medial plantar nerve passes between the abductor hallucis & flexor digitorum brevis. It supplies the abductor hallucis, flexor digitorum brevis, flexor hallucis brevis, & 1st lumbrical & provides sensation to medial 2/3 of foot. The lateral plantar nerve passes between the flexor digitorum brevis & quadratus plantae & supplies the quadratus plantae, abductor digiti minimi, flexor digiti minimi, adductor hallucis, 2-4 lumbricals, interossei & skin of lateral sole, 5th toe, & lateral 1/2 of 4th toe.*

MR: TIBIAL NERVE, BRANCHES TO ANKLE & FOOT

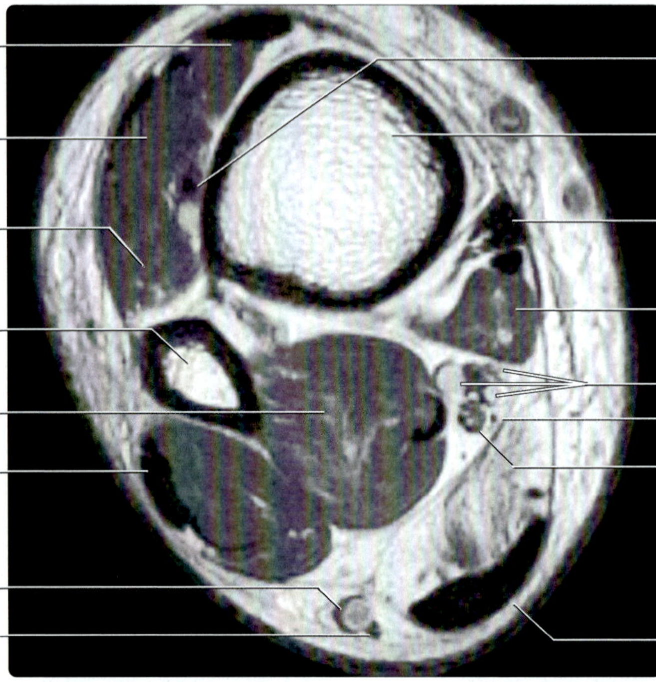

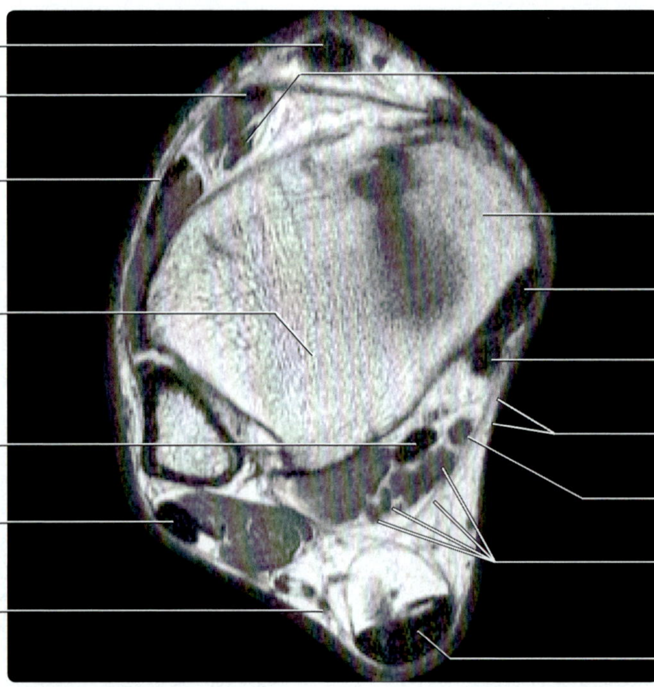

(Top) *The tibial nerve, often called the posterior tibial nerve in the ankle, is best seen on axial images in close proximity to the flexor hallucis longus tendon. In the distal leg, the nerve is posterior to vessels, but in the tarsal tunnel, it is more anterior & lateral (closer to bones). The medial calcaneal nerve can be followed on sequential axial images as a small dot branching from the posterior tibial nerve above the tarsal tunnel (as seen here), penetrating fascia & becoming subcutaneous.* **(Bottom)** *The tarsal tunnel is best seen on axial images, although segments of nerve branches are occasionally noted on sagittal images. Note that the nerves, vessels, & deep posterior compartment tendons are deep to the flexor retinaculum, while the Achilles tendon & peroneal tendons are outside the tarsal tunnel. Note also that the tibial nerve (a.k.a. posterior tibial nerve) is now anterior to the accompanying vessels.*

MR: TIBIAL NERVE, BRANCHES TO ANKLE & FOOT

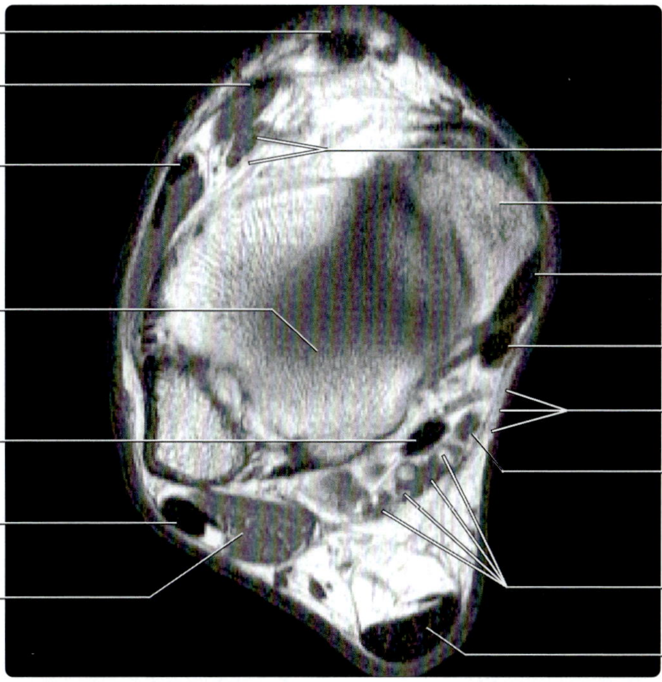

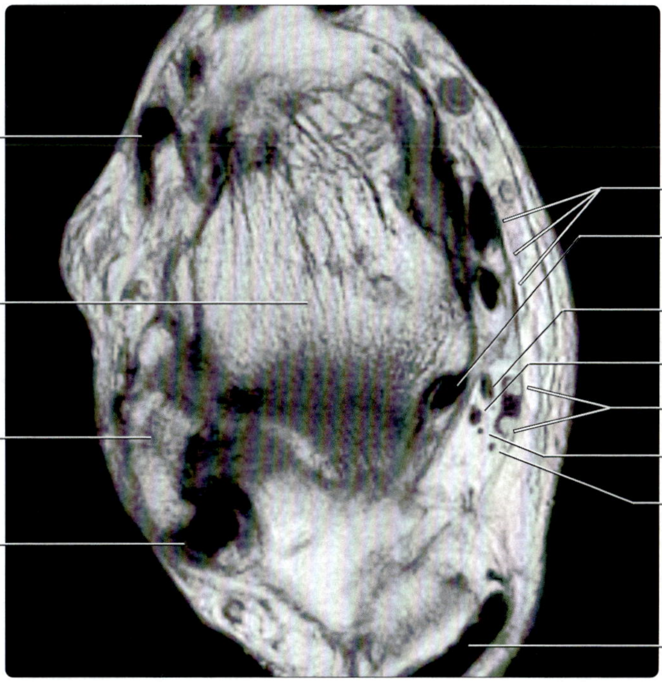

(Top) *The flexor retinaculum is a thin, low-signal structure highlighted by fat, which is best seen on axial & coronal images. The retinaculum forms the medial border of the tarsal tunnel & originates, as seen here, from the medial malleolus. Its calcaneal insertion is easier to appreciate on coronal images. The posterior tibial nerve is about to divide to the medial & lateral plantar nerves & appears bulbous on this image.* **(Bottom)** *The medial plantar & lateral plantar nerves are deep to their accompanying vessels in the tarsal tunnel. The medial plantar nerve is anterior to the lateral plantar nerve & follows the flexor hallucis longus tendon. The inferior calcaneal nerve, typically the 1st branch of the lateral plantar nerve (a.k.a. Baxter nerve) is noted here in close proximity to the lateral plantar nerve. The medial calcaneal nerve is also visualized.*

MR: TIBIAL NERVE, BRANCHES TO ANKLE & FOOT

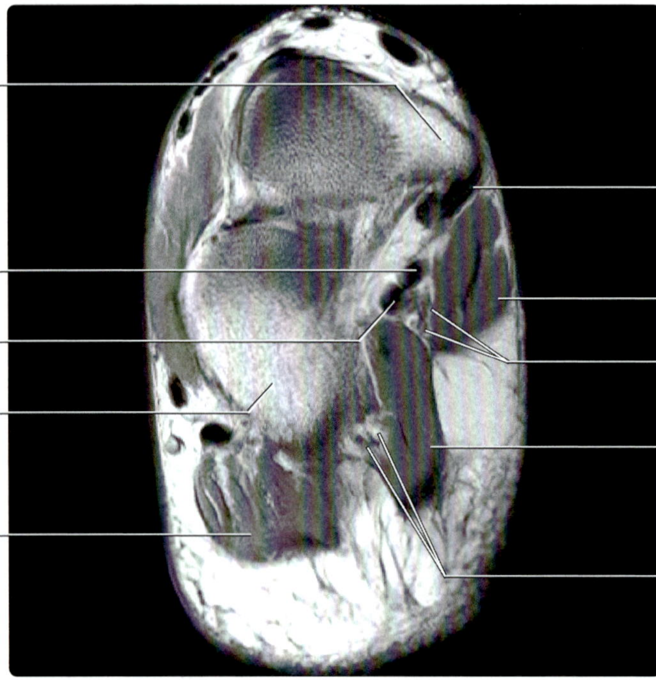

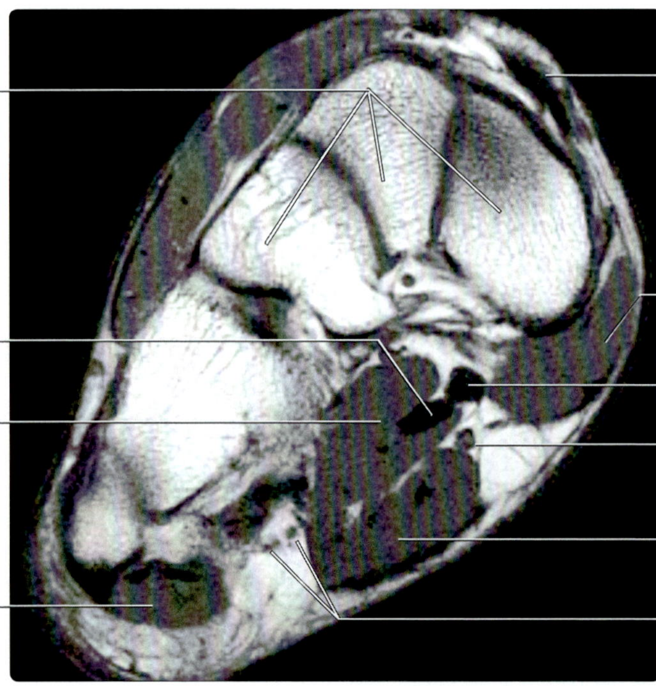

(Top) *Short-axis (oblique coronal) image at the talonavicular joint is shown. In the midfoot, the medial plantar nerve is found within a fatty triangle between the abductor hallucis & flexor digitorum brevis muscles. It is typically noted plantar to the flexor hallucis longus tendon. Note the nerve's proximity to the knot of Henry where the flexor digitorum longus & flexor hallucis longus cross each other. The lateral plantar nerve is found more posteriorly in the fat planes between the flexor digitorum brevis & quadratus plantae muscles.* **(Bottom)** *More distal short-axis image is shown. In the mid & forefoot, the plantar nerves & their branches are difficult to distinguish from adjacent vessels.*

MR: TIBIAL NERVE, BRANCHES TO ANKLE & FOOT

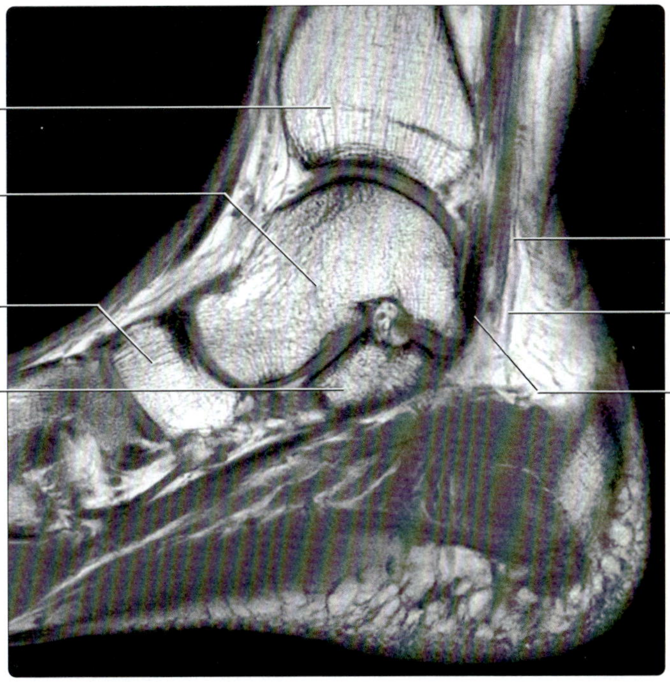

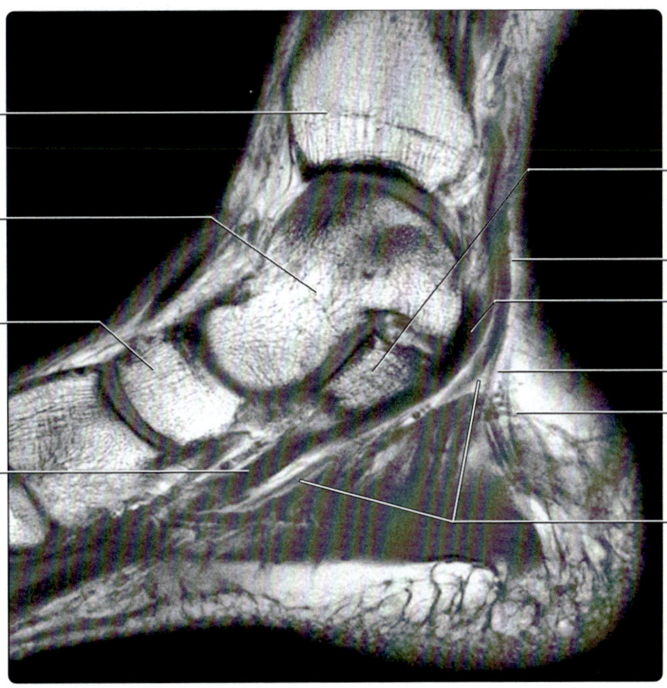

(Top) *The posterior tibial nerve & its branches are noted on far medial sagittal images of the ankle. The flexor hallucis longus tendon is found anterolateral to the nerve. The posterior tibial nerve, with its relatively straight course, can usually be distinguished from the more tortuous & more medial located vessels on sagittal images. The branching pattern of the nerves is variable. In this case, the inferior calcaneal (Baxter) nerve arises proximal to the tarsal tunnel.* **(Bottom)** *A slightly more lateral sagittal image is shown. Detection of the medial plantar nerve at the hindfoot & midfoot is made easy since it is typically posterior to the flexor hallucis longus tendon & posterior to the crossover of the flexor hallucis longus & flexor digitorum longus tendons at the knot of Henry, plantar to the navicular bone.*

MR: TIBIAL NERVE, BRANCHES TO ANKLE & FOOT

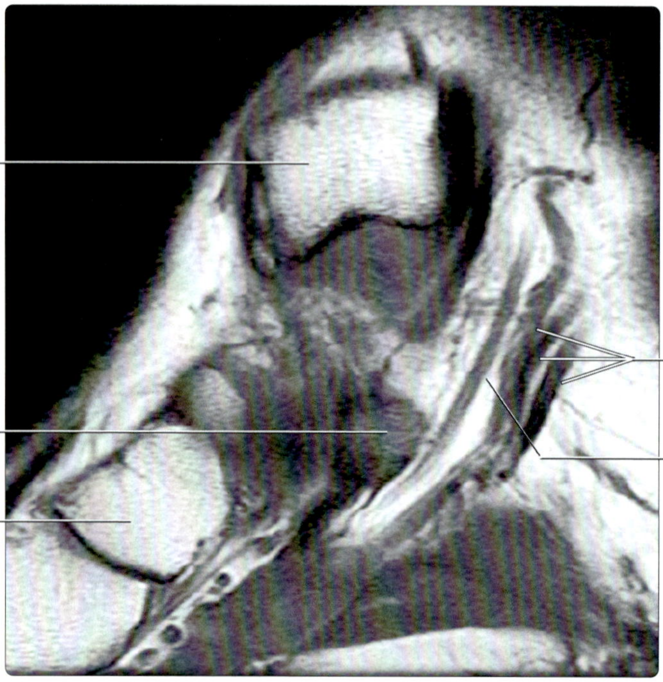

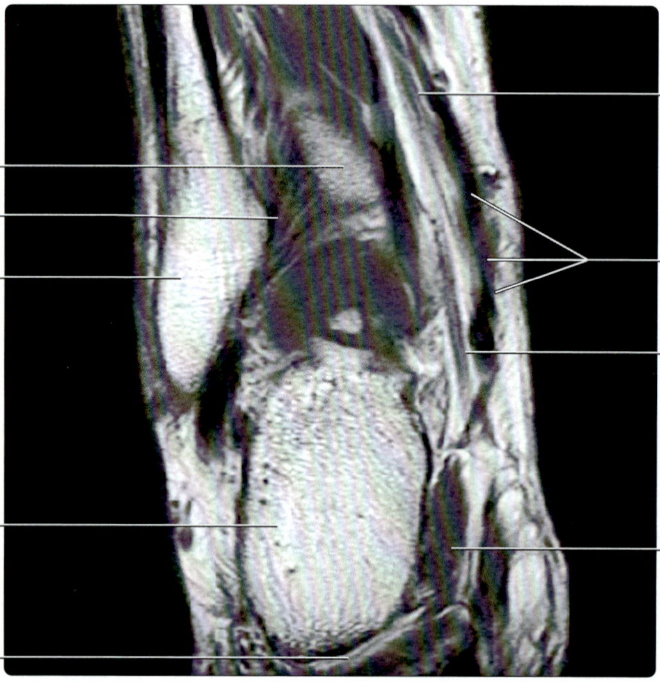

(Top) *This far medial sagittal image depicts a large portion of the medial plantar nerve as it descends down the ankle. Note that the vessels are located posterior to the nerve & are more tortuous in appearance. Prominent venous valves are typically present and are also a useful feature in distinguishing veins from nerves.* **(Bottom)** *Portions of the tibial nerve, plantar nerves, & their branches can sometimes be seen on coronal images. Note a segment of the inferior calcaneal nerve (Baxter nerve) as its proceeds across the calcaneal tubercles toward the calcaneal periosteum & abductor digiti minimi muscle.*

GRAPHICS: COMMON PERONEAL NERVE

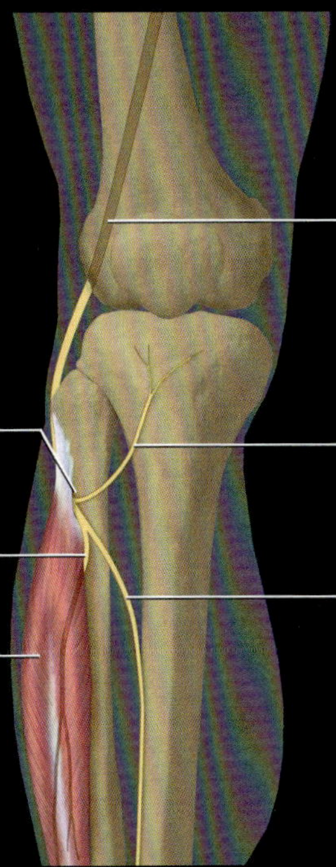

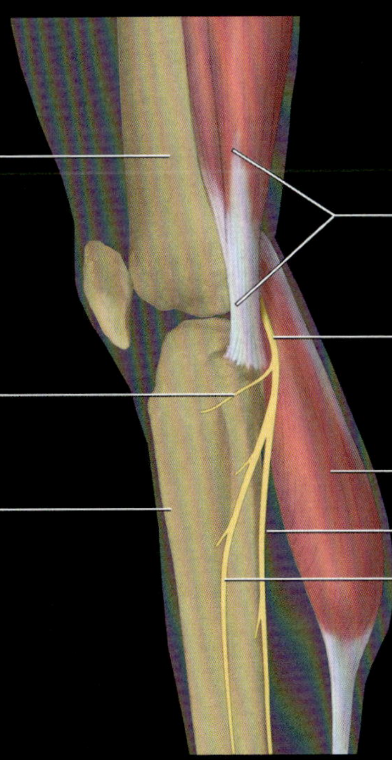

(Top) *Anterior view shows the common peroneal nerve passing into anterolateral leg compartment via a tight opening in fascia. The nerve courses around the fibular head & enters the peroneal (fibular) tunnel deep to the origin of the peroneus longus. The nerve divides proximal to or in the tunnel into deep, superficial, & recurrent (articular) peroneal branches. The deep peroneal nerve innervates the lateral leg compartment. It also gives sensory & motor innervation to the 1st web space. The superficial peroneal nerve innervates the anterior leg compartment & sensation to distal 2/3 of anterolateral leg. The recurrent articular branch supplies the anterolateral knee joint & proximal tibiofibular joint.* **(Bottom)** *Lateral view shows the deep peroneal nerve is anterior to the superficial peroneal nerve. The deep peroneal nerve descends anterior to the interosseous membrane & deep to the extensor leg muscles. The superficial peroneal nerve travels more posteriorly in fascial planes between anterior & lateral compartments of the leg.*

MR: COMMON PERONEAL NERVE

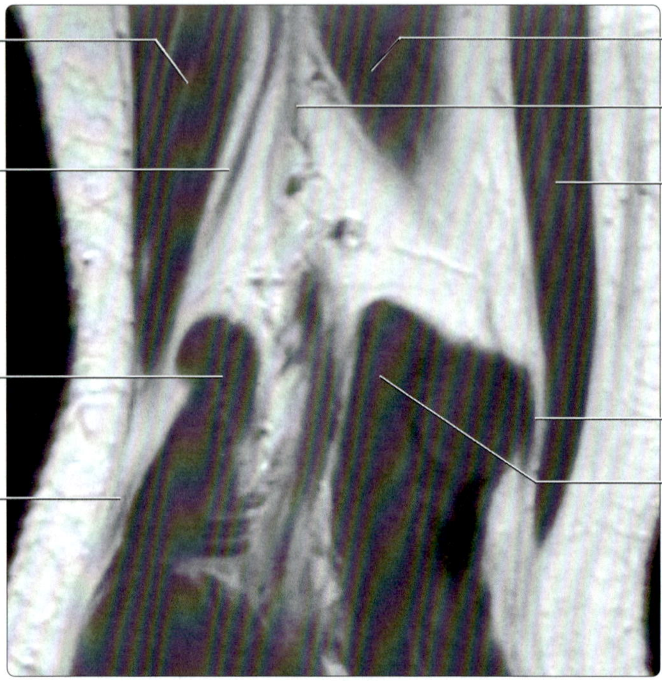

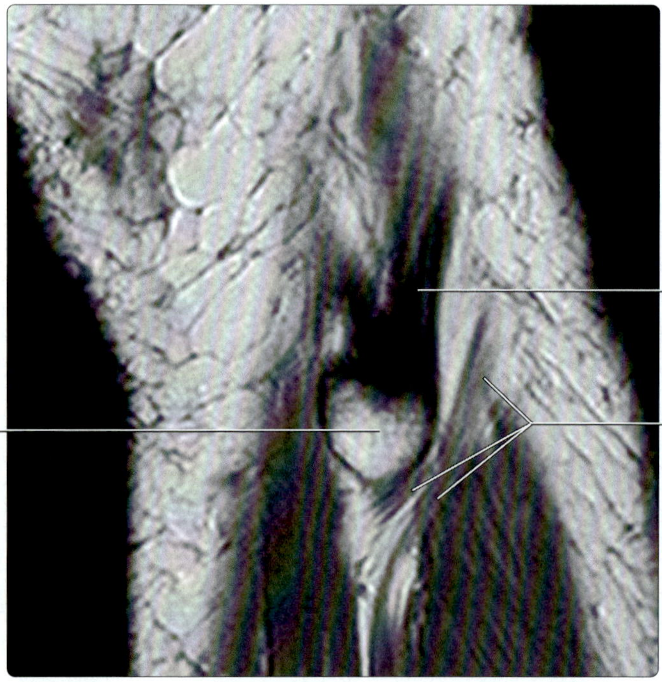

(Top) *The common peroneal nerve can be consistently visualized on coronal & axial images of the knee. Occasionally, 2 portions of the nerve may be seen on 1 coronal image as noted here: (1) Proximal portion as the nerve takes off from the sciatic nerve & (2) distal portion as the nerve curves around the fibula.* **(Bottom)** *Sagittal MR is shown. The common peroneal nerve may also be noted on far lateral sagittal images as it curves around the fibular head. Note the striation of the nerve reflecting fascicles & nerve branches. Note also the proximity of the nerve, especially the deep peroneal nerve, to the fibular head. Not surprisingly, fibular head fractures can cause laceration or entrapment of the common peroneal nerve & its branches.*

MR: COMMON PERONEAL NERVE

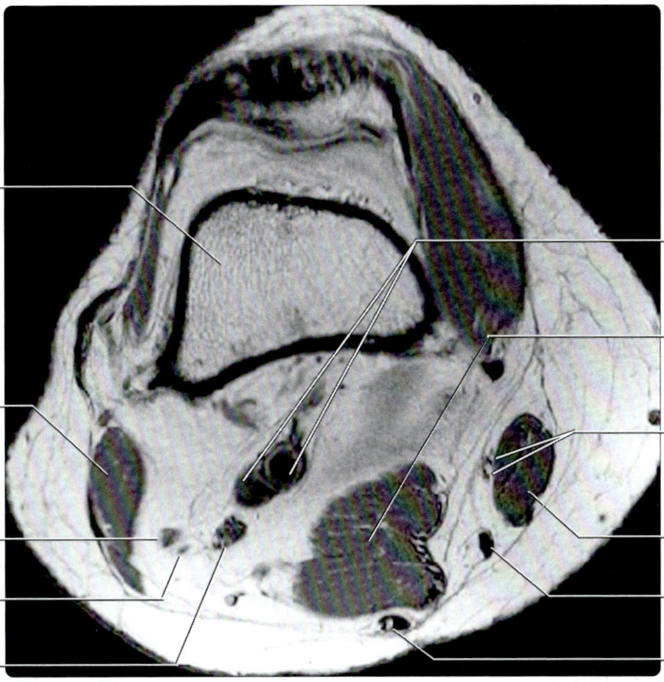

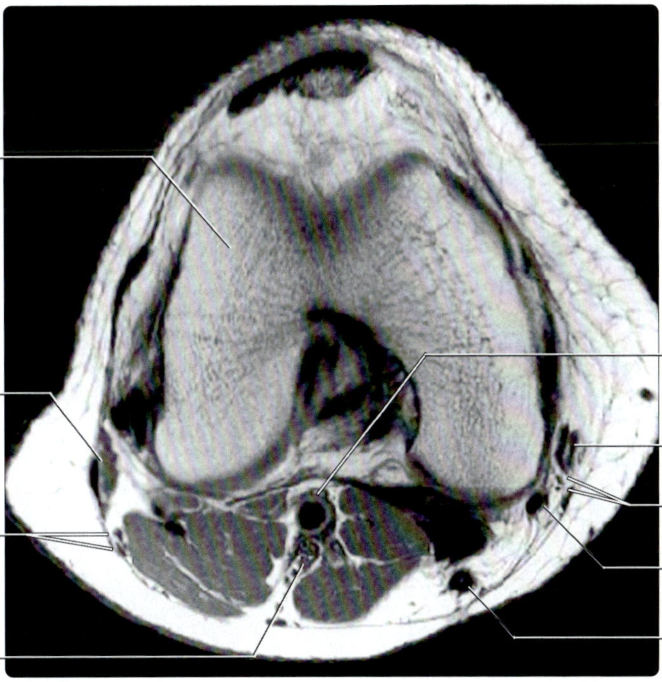

(Top) *Axial image at the upper popliteal fossa is shown. On axial images, the common peroneal nerve can be followed as it takes off from the sciatic nerve & travels toward the fibula. The nerve is consistently seen at the lateral upper popliteal fossa in abundant fat medial to the short head of the biceps femoris muscle. Note a small dot posterior to the nerve. This may be either the peroneal communicating nerve (also called the sural communicating nerve) or the lateral sural cutaneous nerve. These 2 branches often originate together via a single stem.* **(Bottom)** *Axial image just above the knee joint is shown. The common peroneal nerve is posterior to the short head of the biceps femoris & posterolateral to the lateral head of the gastrocnemius muscle. The superficial & deep branches of the common peroneal nerve are now clearly seen even though they have not yet physically separated from each other.*

MR: COMMON PERONEAL NERVE

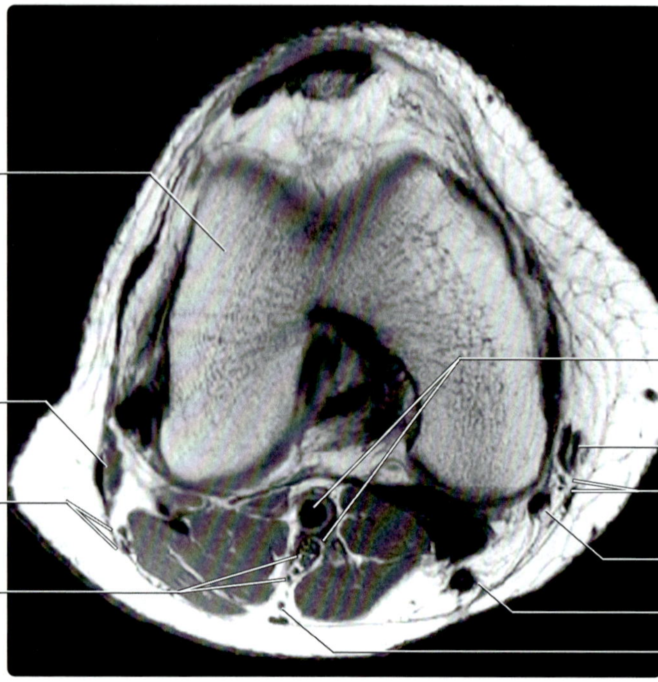

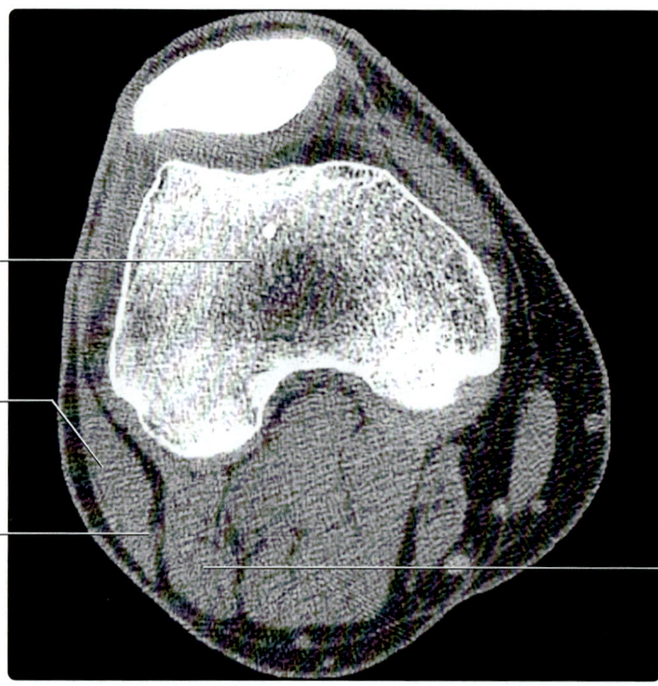

(Top) *In the knee region, the common peroneal nerve is typically posterolateral to the lateral head of the gastrocnemius as is seen in this image. In ~ 25% of individuals, as seen in next image, the common peroneal nerve traverses within a narrow passage between the short head of the biceps femoris & the lateral head of the gastrocnemius muscles.* **(Bottom)** *In this patient with anomalous 3rd head of gastrocnemius muscle, the common peroneal nerve is snugly situated between the short head of biceps femoris & the lateral head of the gastrocnemius muscles. Muscle anomalies that can predispose to entrapment of the common peroneal nerve in the knee include abnormal origins of the medial &/or lateral heads of the gastrocnemius muscle, hypertrophied short head of biceps femoris, or low lying long head of biceps femoris.*

GRAPHICS: DEEP & SUPERFICIAL PERONEAL NERVE

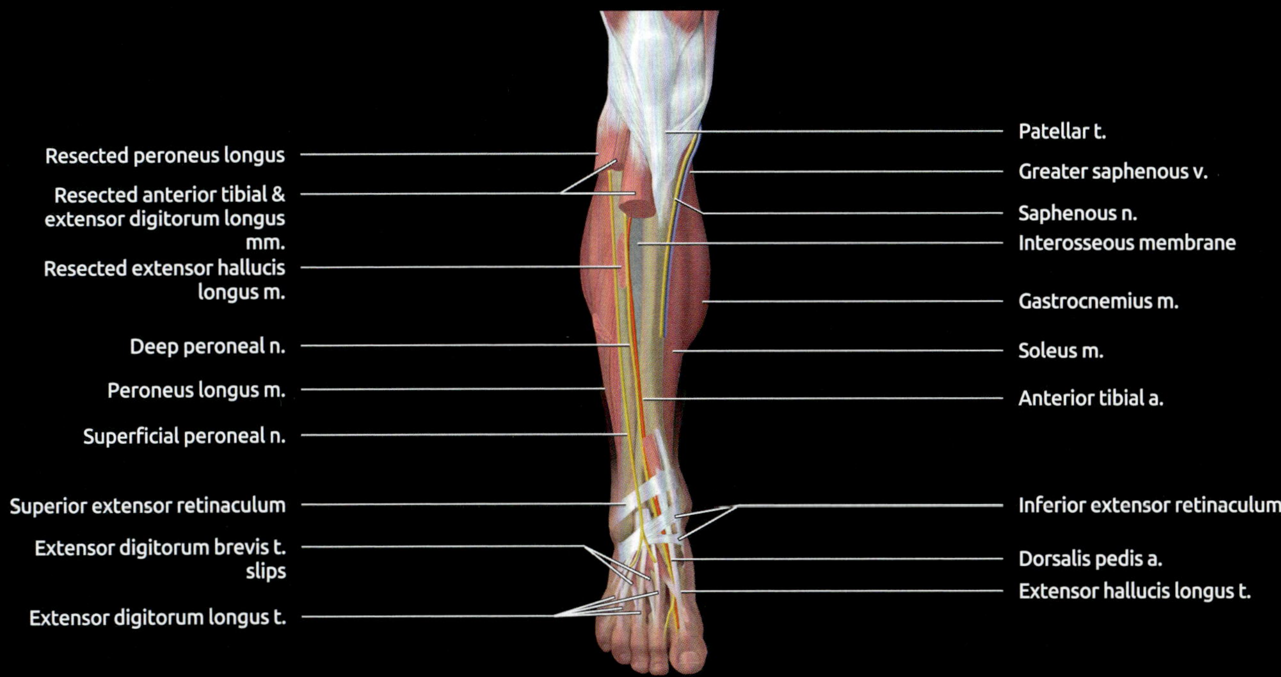

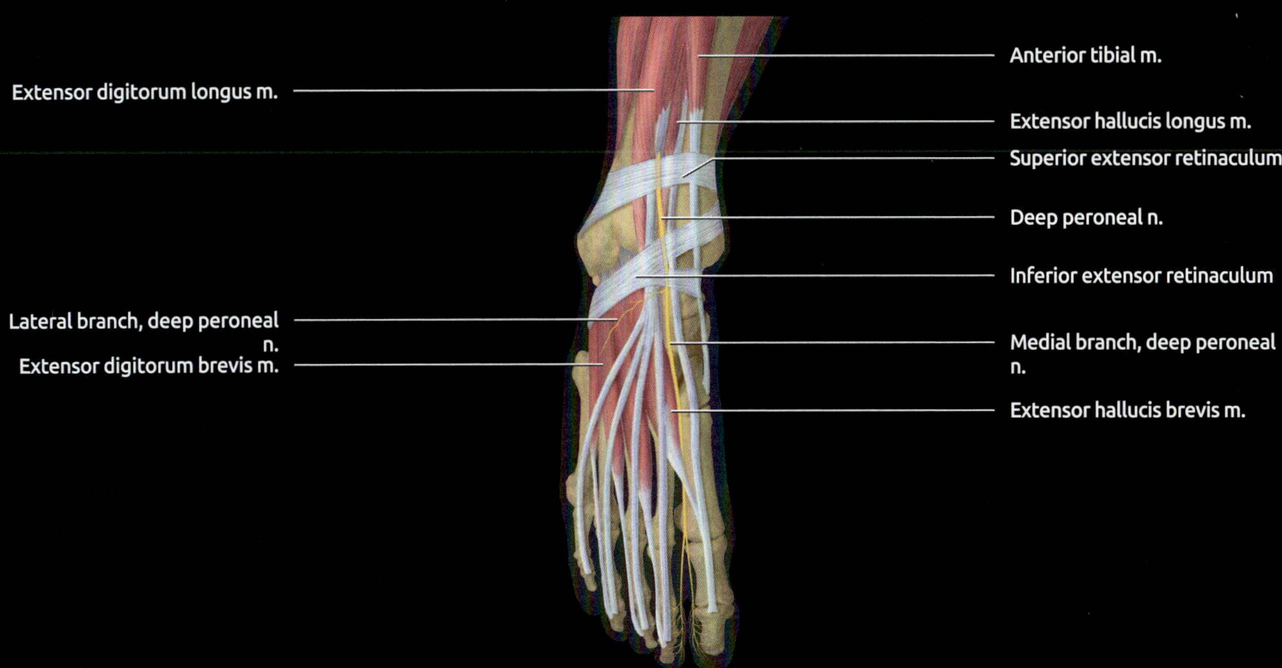

(Top) *Graphic shows the deep peroneal nerve in the leg with resected lateral & anterior compartment muscles. The deep peroneal nerve descends deep to the extensor digitorum longus muscle & anterior to the interosseous membrane in close proximity to the anterior tibial artery. In the leg, it supplies the anterior compartment muscles.* **(Bottom)** *In the ankle, the deep peroneal nerve travels deep to the extensor retinacula to enter the anterior tarsal tunnel. It terminates in 2 branches. The lateral branch innervates the extensor digitorum brevis muscle. It enlarges to become a pseudoganglion under the muscle & sends 3 tiny interosseous branches (not shown), which supply the tarsal & tarsometatarsal joints of the middle 3 toes; the 1st branch also supplies the 2nd dorsal interosseous. The medial branch continues dorsal to talonavicular joint, middle cuneiform, & in between the 1st & 2nd metatarsals to provide mostly sensory but some motor supply to the 1st web space.*

GRAPHICS: DEEP & SUPERFICIAL PERONEAL NERVE

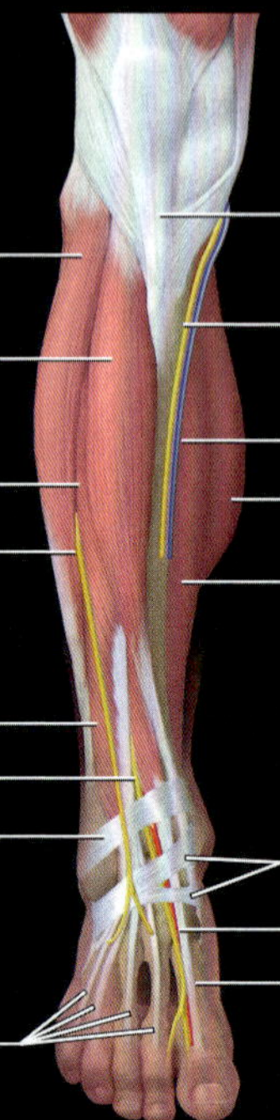

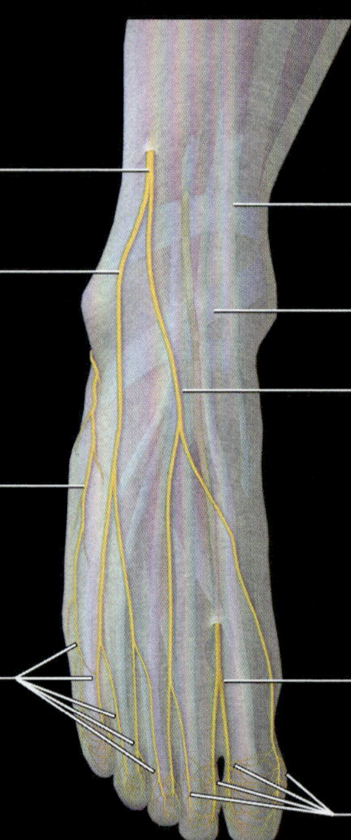

(Top) *Graphic shows the superficial peroneal nerve in the leg. It descends in the lateral leg, initially between peroneus brevis & longus muscles & then between the extensor digitorum longus & peroneus brevis muscles. In the leg, the superficial peroneal nerve supplies the lateral compartment muscles. It also provides sensory innervation to the distal 2/3 of the leg. It penetrates the anterior fascia of the leg 10-15 cm above the ankle joint to become subcutaneous.* **(Bottom)** *The superficial peroneal nerve bifurcates to the medial & intermediate dorsal cutaneous nerves. It carries sensation from the dorsal skin of all toes, except the proximal lateral foot (sural), 1st web space (deep peroneal nerve), & tips of toes (medial & lateral plantar nerves).*

MR: DEEP & SUPERFICIAL PERONEAL NERVES

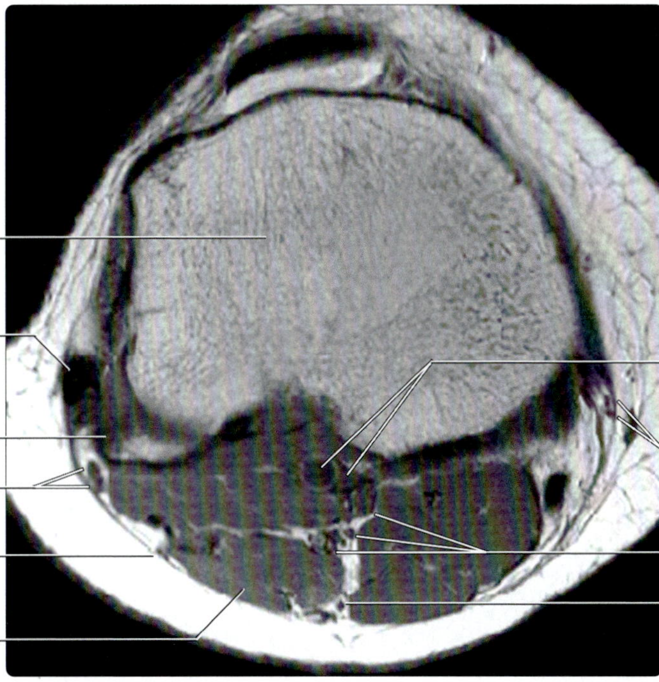

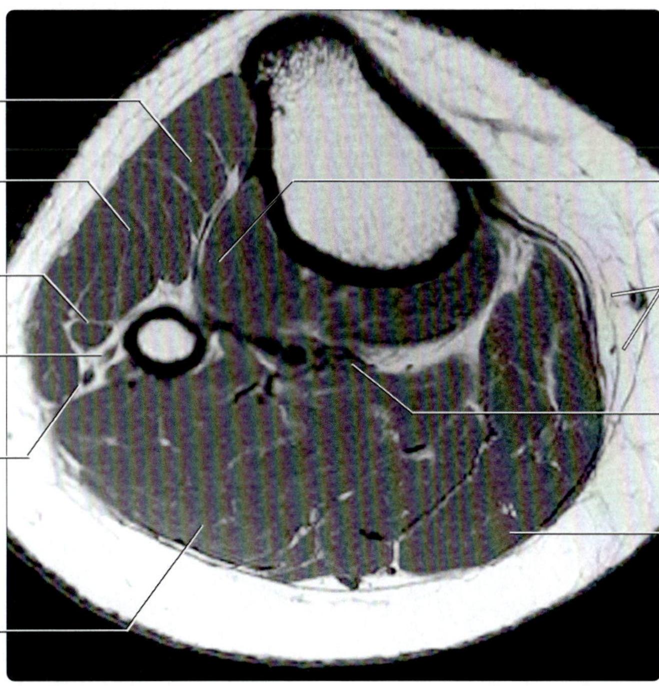

(Top) *The common peroneal nerve is approaching the fibular head. Note that the superficial & deep branches of the nerve are distinctly seen but have still not separated from each other. Note also multiple divisions of the tibial nerve. The lateral sural cutaneous nerve, a sensory branch of common peroneal nerve, is also seen.* **(Bottom)** *The common peroneal nerve has entered the peroneal or fibular tunnel under the peroneus longus muscle. The deep & superficial peroneal nerves have now separated from each other. The deep peroneal nerve is more anterior & closer to the fibular head & therefore is more susceptible to compression. Frequently, the 2 nerves are difficult to visualize in this region because of the compactness of the muscles. In this relatively slim patient, a significant amount of fat under the peroneus longus muscle allows visualization of the nerves.*

MR: DEEP & SUPERFICIAL PERONEAL NERVES

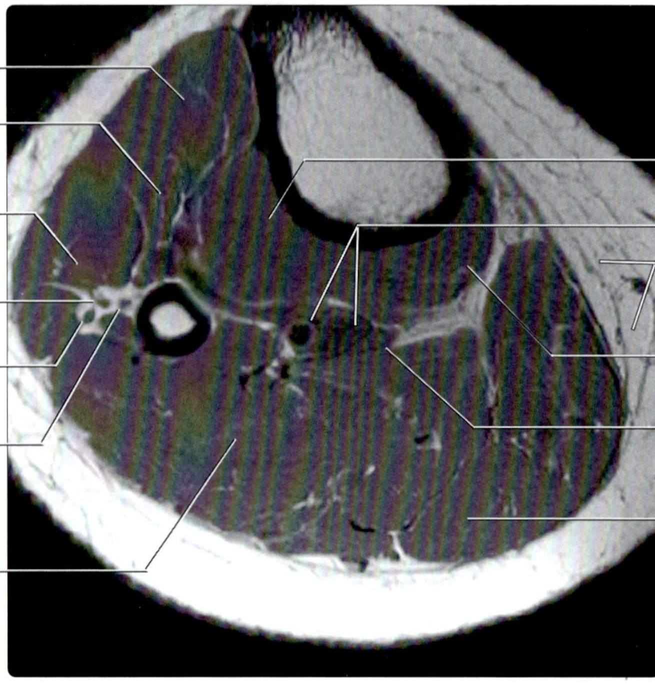

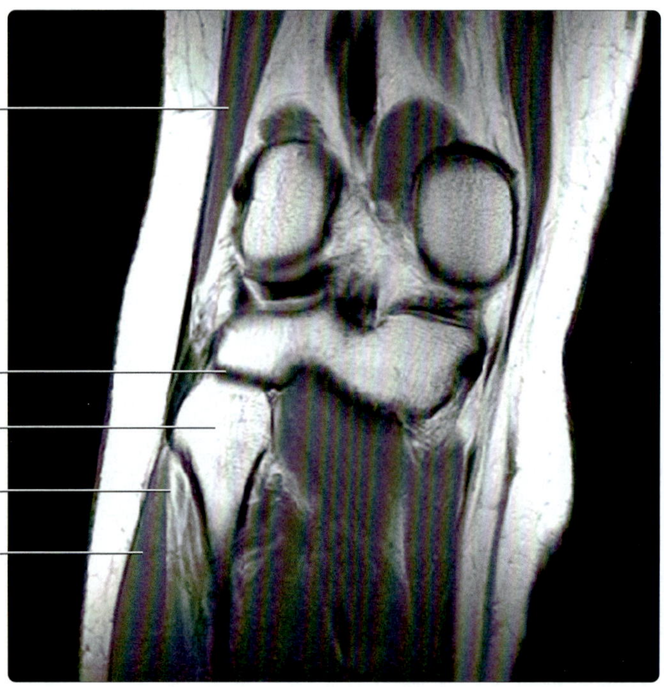

(Top) *Three separate branches of the common peroneal nerve are now visualized within the peroneal tunnel: (1) The recurrent articular nerve, most anterior & medial; (2) the deep peroneal nerve; & (3) the superficial peroneal nerve, most posterior. The nerves, highlighted by fat in this patient, are usually difficult to see in more muscular patients.* **(Bottom)** *The branches of the common peroneal nerve are noted within fat under the peroneus longus muscle.*

MR: DEEP & SUPERFICIAL PERONEAL NERVES

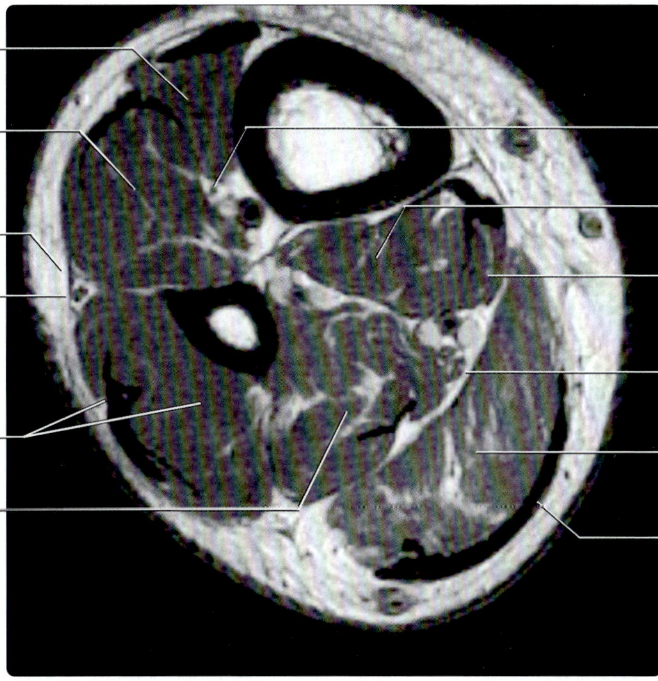

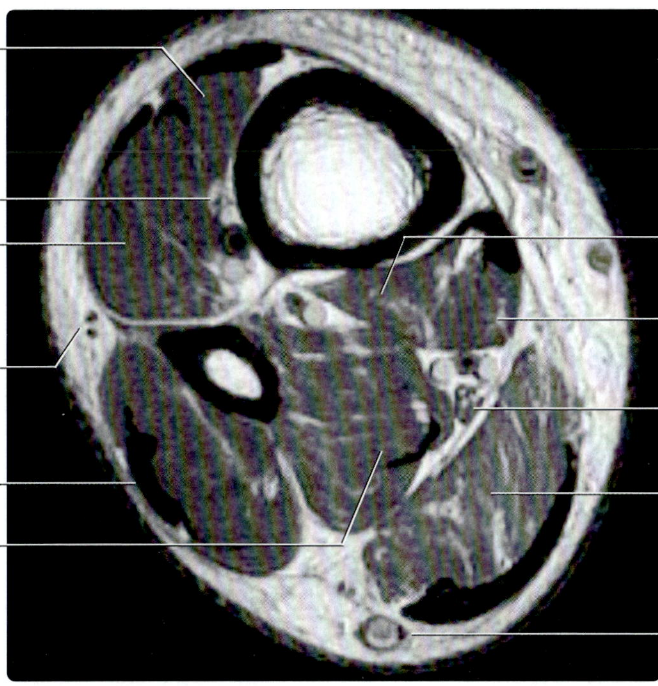

(Top) *The superficial peroneal nerve migrates from a deep to superficial location as it descends down the leg between lateral & anterior muscle compartments. As the nerve approaches the subcutaneous fat, it can be seen on axial images as a low-signal, round structure within a small, fat triangle bordered anteriorly by the extensor digitorum longus muscle, posteriorly by the peroneus brevis muscle, & laterally by linear, low-signal fascia of the leg. The deep peroneal nerve with its accompanying vessels is in a fat plane anterior to the intraosseous membrane. In muscular patients, the peroneal nerves may not be well seen in the proximal leg.* **(Bottom)** *A slightly more distal image depicts the superficial peroneal nerve & its accompanying vessels after they have penetrated the fascia within the subcutaneous fat. The deep peroneal nerve is noted deep to the anterior compartment muscles.*

MR: DEEP & SUPERFICIAL PERONEAL NERVES

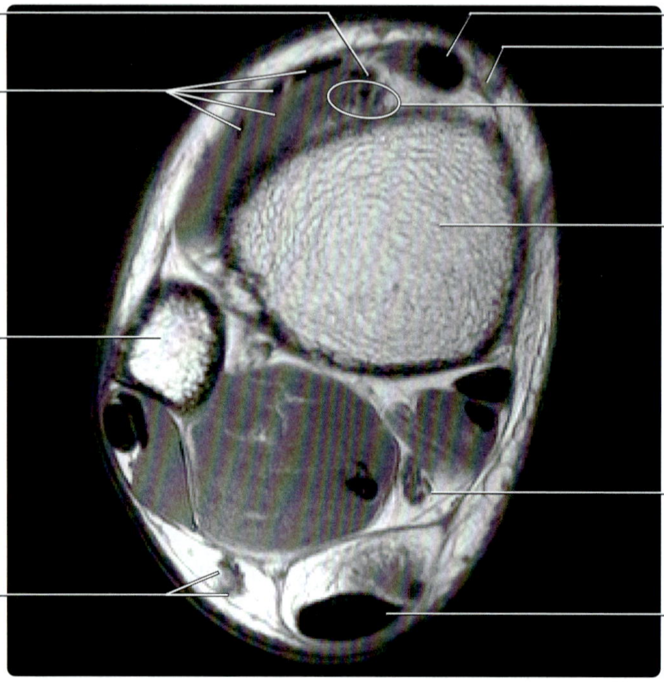

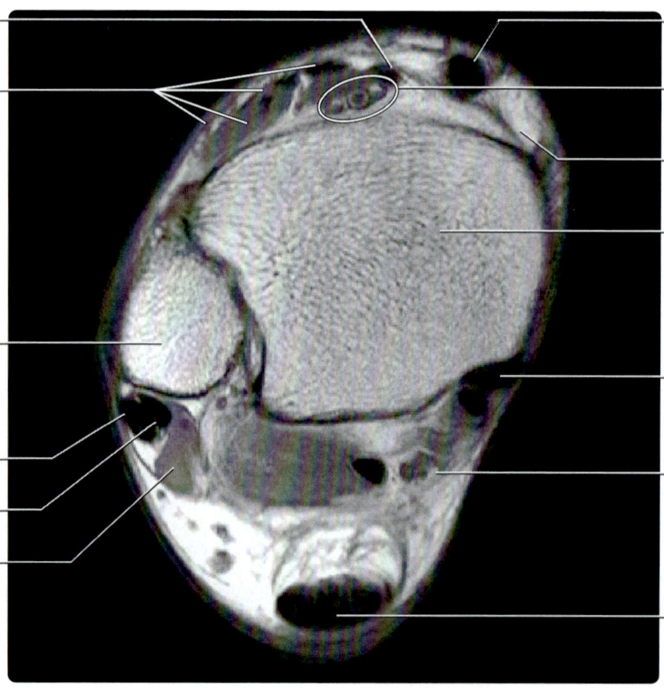

(Top) *The deep peroneal nerve dives under the superior & inferior extensor retinacula to enter the anterior tarsal tunnel. The latter is not a true tunnel but rather a flat place between medial & lateral malleoli, which is bordered superiorly by the inferior edge of the retinacula & inferiorly by the talonavicular joint. The deep peroneal nerve is best seen on axial MR images of the ankle. It is found within fat deep to the extensor retinacula. Note that the nerve in the distal leg is found deep to the extensor hallucis longus tendon. As seen in this image, it may be difficult to distinguish the nerve from the adjacent vessels.* **(Bottom)** *Just above the ankle joint, the deep peroneal nerve separates into the medial & lateral branches. Occasionally, these 2 branches may be noted on axial MR images.*

MR: DEEP & SUPERFICIAL PERONEAL NERVES

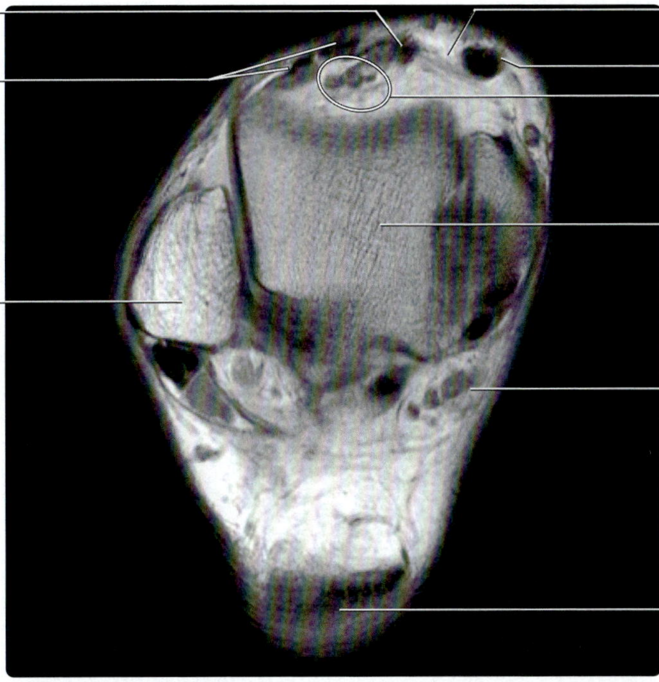

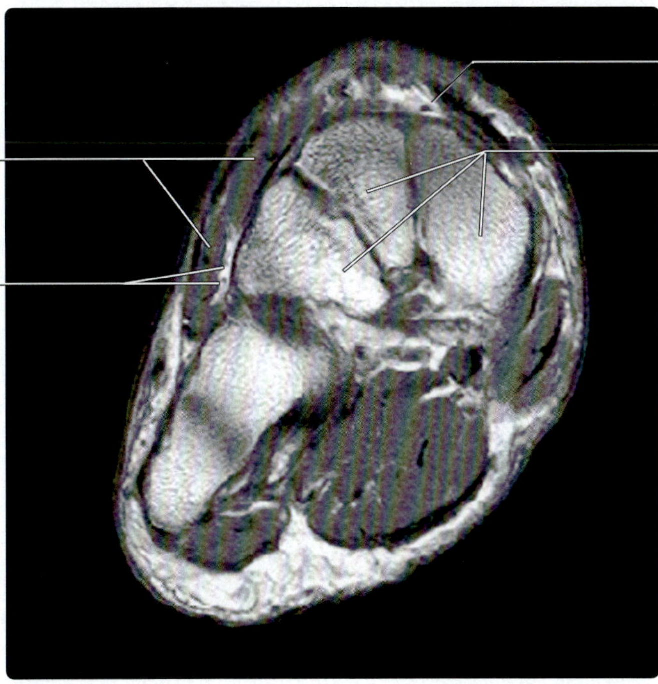

(Top) *The deep peroneal nerve & dorsalis pedis vessels are now more clearly seen since the extensor hallucis longus tendon has become more superficial. In the leg, the deep peroneal nerve is initially lateral & then anterior to the anterior tibial artery. In the ankle & foot, the nerve is lateral to the dorsalis pedis artery. Nevertheless, it may be difficult to distinguish the nerve from the vessels.* **(Bottom)** *The deep peroneal nerve can be seen in the ankle on routine axial images, but in the foot, it is better visualized on short-axis (oblique coronal) images as noted here. The medial branch of the deep peroneal nerve is usually detected in abundant fat dorsal to the 2nd cuneiform & then between the 1st & 2nd metatarsals. The lateral branch & its small interosseous branches can sometimes be seen under the extensor digitorum brevis muscle.*

GRAPHICS: CUTANEOUS INNERVATION OF LEG

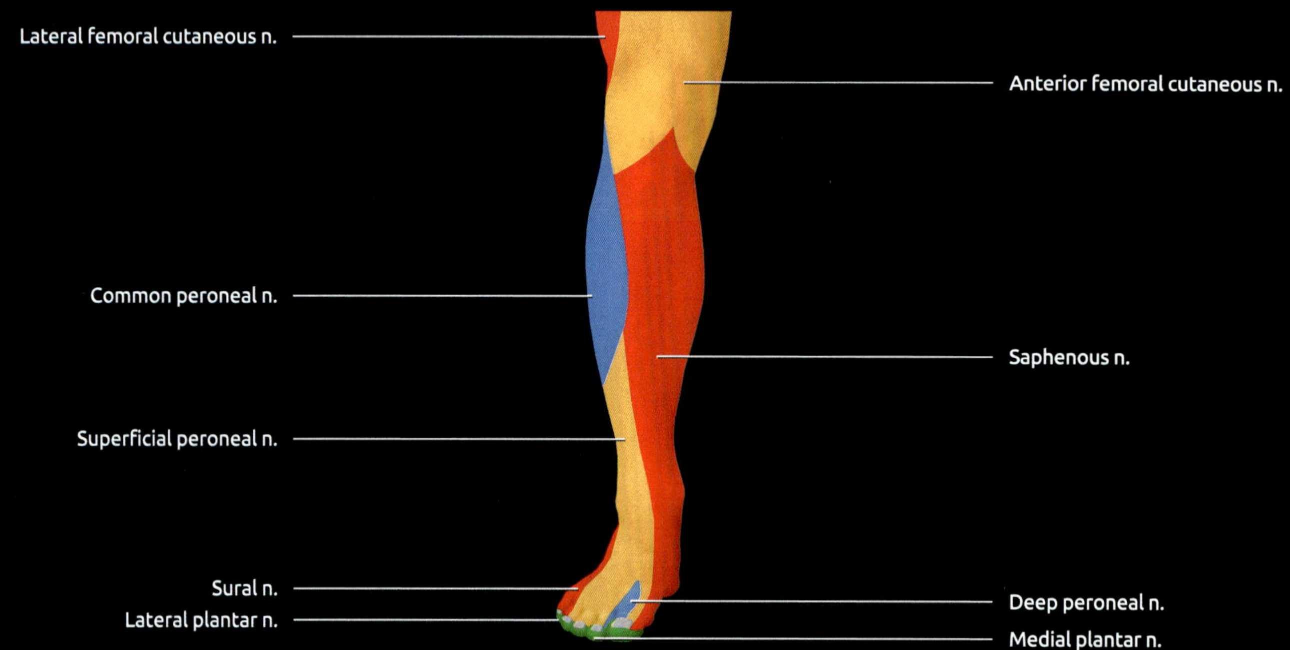

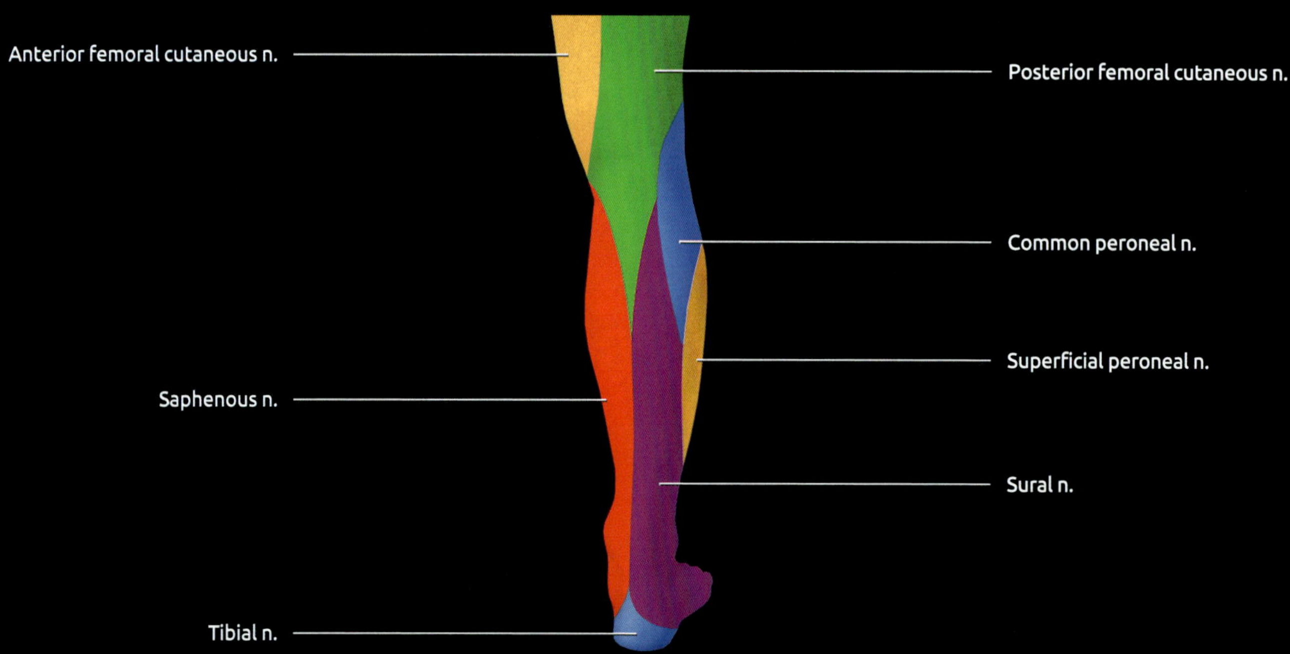

(Top) *Cutaneous innervation of the ventral (anterior) lower extremity is shown. The upper 1/3 & lower 2/3 of the lateral anterior leg are innervated by the common & superficial peroneal nerves, respectively. The anterior medial leg is supplied by the saphenous nerve (femoral nerve branch). Most dorsal foot innervation is supplied by the superficial peroneal nerve except for the 1st web space (deep peroneal nerve), medial ankle & foot (saphenous nerve), lateral ankle & foot (sural nerve), & tips of toes (medial & lateral plantar nerves). Variations & overlap in innervation are common.* **(Bottom)** *Cutaneous innervation of the dorsal (posterior) lower extremity is shown. The medial 1/2 of the posterior leg is supplied by the saphenous nerve (branch of femoral nerve), while the lateral 1/2 is supplied by the sural nerve (formed from branches of tibial & common peroneal nerve). The posterior knee is also supplied by the posterior femoral cutaneous nerve. The heel is supplied by the tibial nerve. Variations & overlap in innervation are frequent phenomena.*

GRAPHICS: CUTANEOUS INNERVATION OF LEG

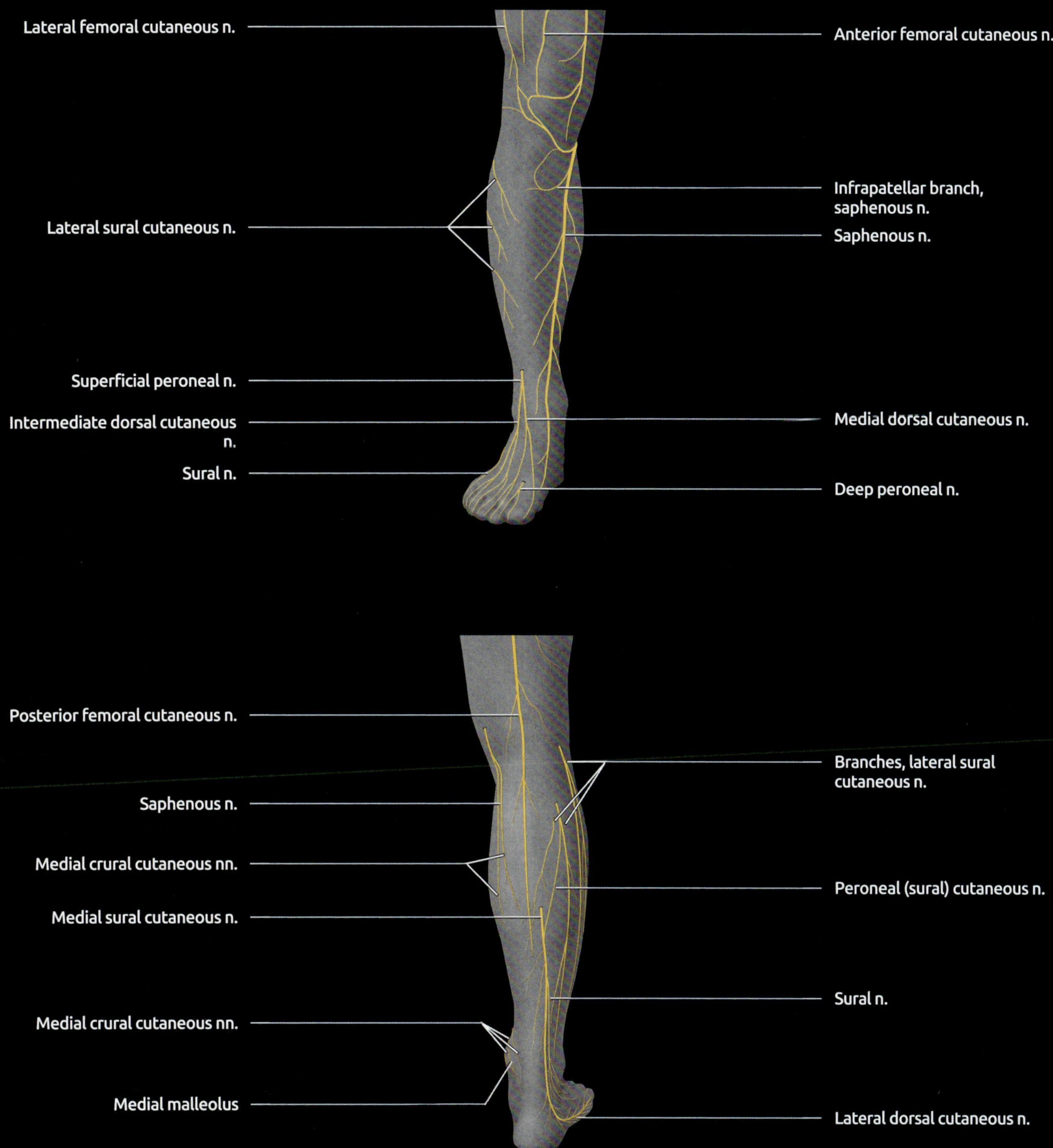

(Top) *A more detailed graphic shows cutaneous innervation of the anterior leg & foot by the saphenous nerve anteromedially, deep peroneal nerve medially, & common peroneal nerve, superficial peroneal nerve, & sural nerve laterally.* **(Bottom)** *A more detailed graphic shows cutaneous innervation of the posterior leg by the common peroneal nerve in the proximal & lateral leg (lateral sural cutaneous nerve), sural nerve in the lateral & posterior leg, & saphenous nerve in the medial leg.*

GRAPHICS: CUTANEOUS INNERVATION OF FOOT

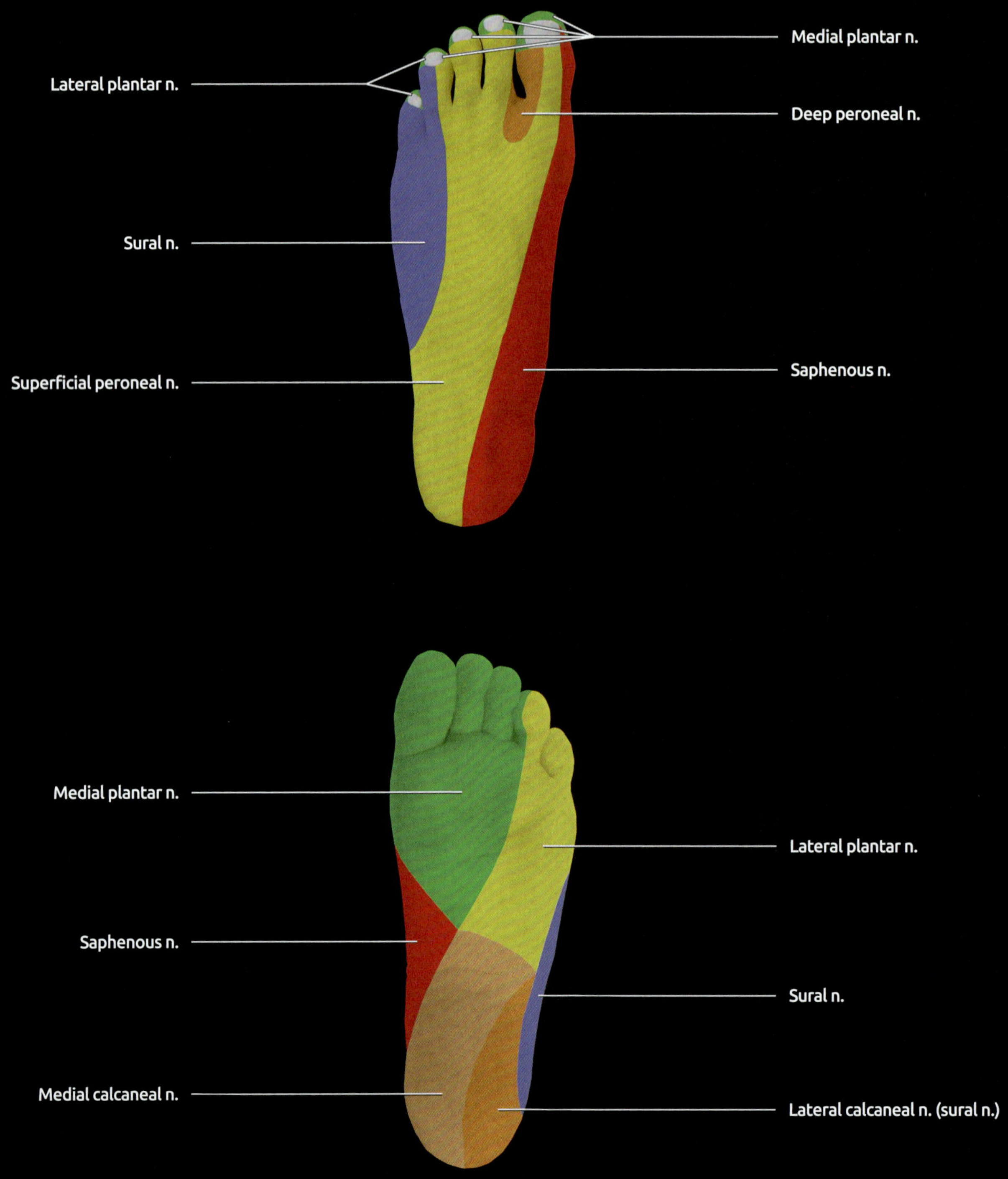

(Top) *Dorsal cutaneous innervation of the foot is shown. The dorsal cutaneous innervation is provided mainly by the superficial peroneal nerve with smaller contributions by the deep peroneal nerve to the 1st web space, sural nerve to the lateral foot up to the base of the 5th toe, & saphenous nerve to the medial foot up to the base of the 1st toe. The medial & lateral plantar nerves provide dorsal innervation to nail beds & tips of toes.* **(Bottom)** *Plantar cutaneous innervation of the foot is shown. The medial plantar nerve supplies the plantar skin of the medial 3.5 toes. The lateral plantar nerve supplies the lateral 1.5 toes. There is also plantar innervation by the sural nerve laterally & saphenous nerve medially. The skin of the heel is innervated medially by the medial calcaneal nerve (a branch of the posterior tibial nerve) & laterally by the lateral calcaneal nerve (branch of sural nerve). The lateral plantar nerve may also give rise to small branches, which pierce the plantar fascia & supply the lateral skin of the heel.*

GRAPHICS: SAPHENOUS NERVE

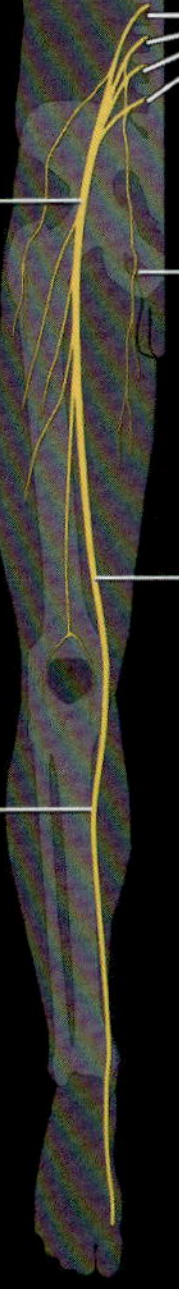

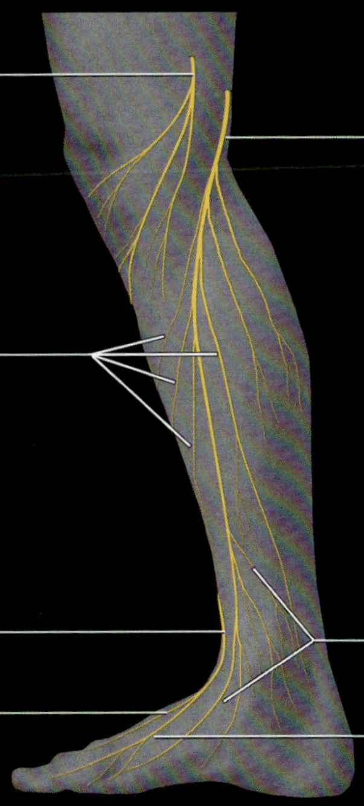

(Top) *The saphenous nerve descends along medial knee, deep to sartorius. The nerve then pierces the deep fascia of the medial knee, between the sartorius & gracilis tendons. It descends in the subcutaneous fat of the medial knee, accompanied by the greater saphenous vein, passes anterior to the medial malleolus, & terminates by the ball of the 1st toe. It supplies the skin in front of the patella (via infrapatellar branch), skin of anteromedial & posteromedial leg, & skin along the medial side of the foot as far as the head of the 1st metatarsal bone.* **(Bottom)** *The saphenous nerve (via infrapatellar branch) connects in the knee region with the medial cutaneous nerve of the thigh. The nerve supplies the medial anterior leg via many small medial crural cutaneous branches. It also sends posterior small branches supplying the posterior leg & ankle. Branches anterior to the ankle extend as far as the base of the 1st metatarsophalangeal joint.*

MR: SAPHENOUS NERVE

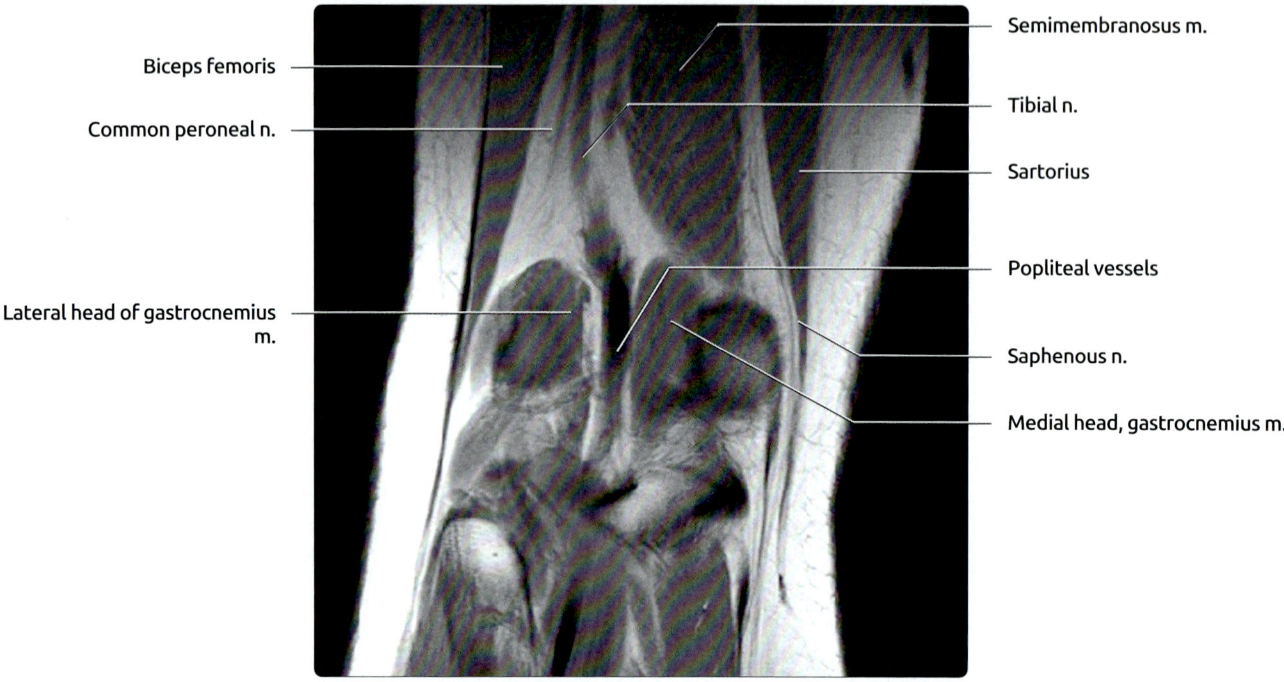

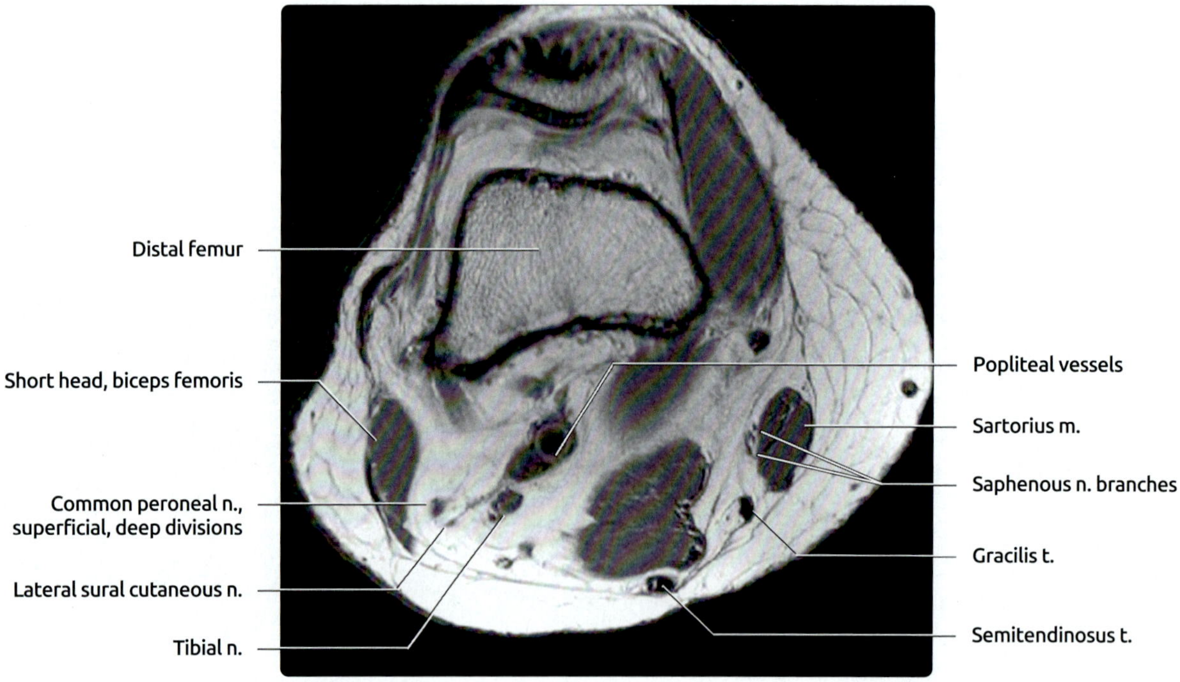

(Top) *The saphenous nerve is optimally visualized on axial images but is occasionally noted on posterior coronal images of the knee. In the thigh & knee, the nerve follows the sartorius muscle & is found within an abundant amount of fat along the lateral border of the muscle.* **(Bottom)** *Fascicles of the saphenous nerve are clearly noted on this axial image deep & lateral to the sartorius muscle.*

MR: SAPHENOUS NERVE

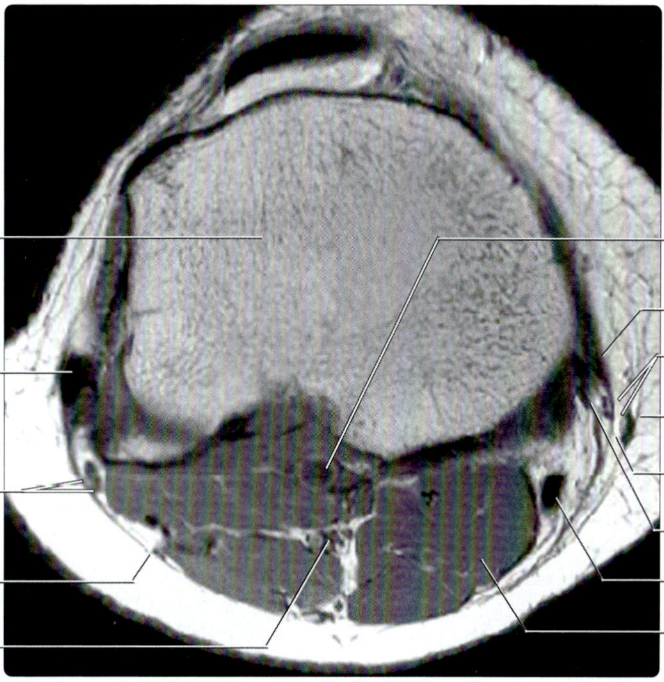

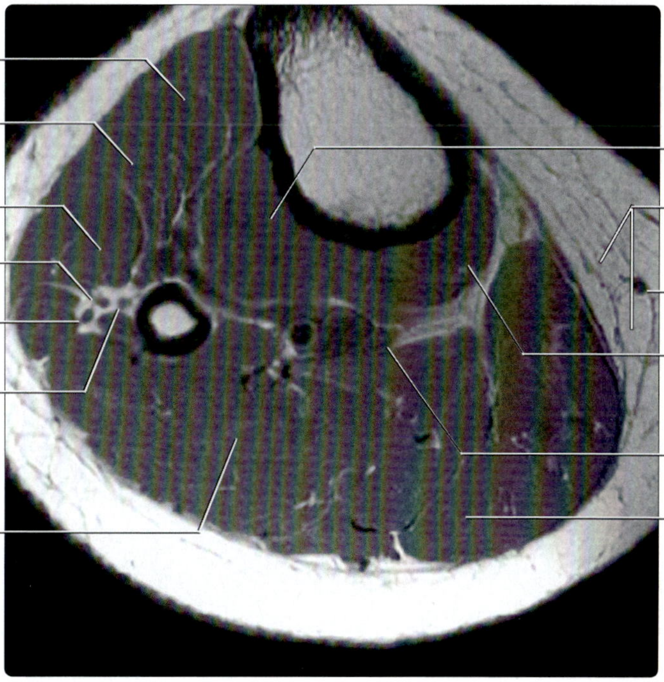

(Top) *The saphenous nerve is just about to pierce the deep medial fascia of the leg in this axial image at knee level. The nerve typically becomes subcutaneous in the medial knee area as it penetrates the fascia between the gracilis & sartorius tendons. Note that the greater saphenous vein is superficial to the deep fascia.* **(Bottom)** *Branches of the saphenous nerve are now seen in the medial subcutaneous fat of the knee. At this level, the nerve branches are minute & difficult to distinguish from adjacent vessels. The saphenous nerve descends with the greater saphenous vein, & branches continue anterior to the medial malleolus & terminate in the region of the ball of the foot. The saphenous nerve supplies the skin of the anteromedial & posteromedial leg as well as the medial aspect of the foot up to the head of the 1st metatarsal.*

MR: SAPHENOUS NERVE

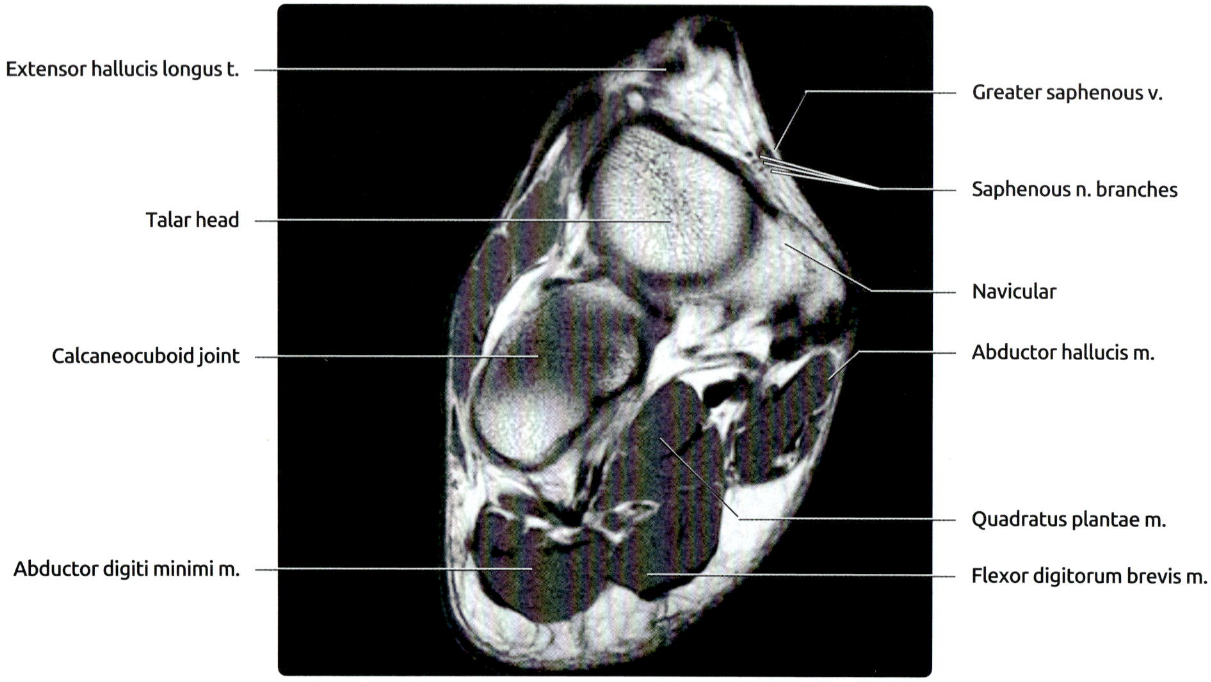

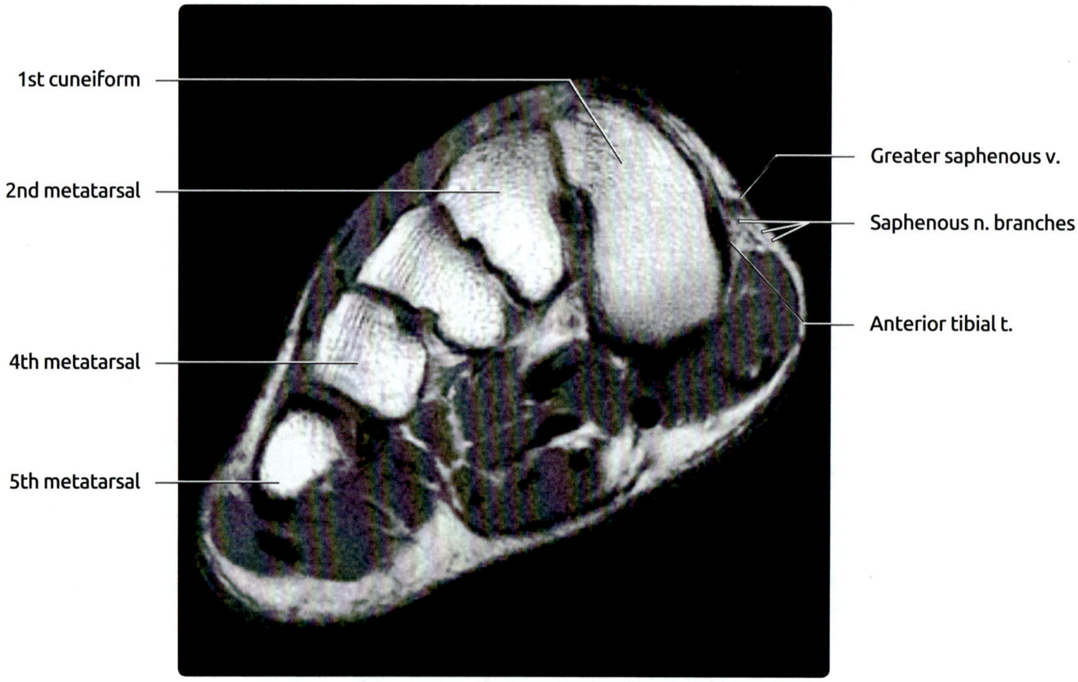

(Top) *Branches of the saphenous nerve may be seen as they travel dorsally along the medial aspect of the foot up to the base of the 1st metatarsal. The nerve branches accompany the greater saphenous vein.* **(Bottom)** *More distally, branches of the saphenous nerve are noted adjacent to the anterior tibial tendon.*

GRAPHICS: SURAL NERVE

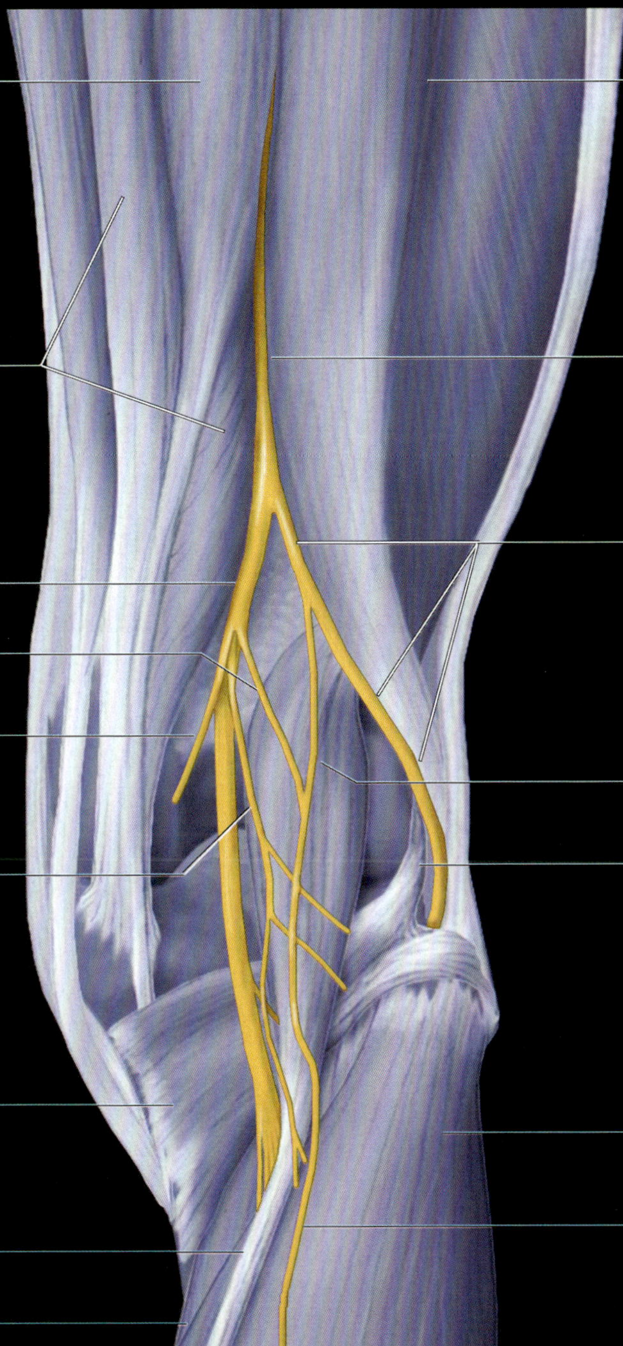

The sural nerve, a purely sensory nerve, is formed by the medial sural cutaneous branch of the tibial nerve & peroneal (sural) communicating branch of the common peroneal nerve. The latter may originate directly from the common peroneal nerve or via a common trunk with the lateral sural cutaneous nerve. The merger forming the sural nerve may occur as far down as the posterior mid leg. The sural nerve, accompanied by the lesser saphenous vein, migrates from midline to a lateral location in the distal leg & ankle & travels posterior to the lateral malleolus, between the peroneal & Achilles tendons. The nerve divides into the lateral dorsal cutaneous nerve & lateral calcaneal nerve on the dorsum of the foot & supplies the skin along the lateral border of the foot & lateral side of the little toe. Occasional the greater sensory innervation of the dorsal foot is present.

MR: SURAL NERVE

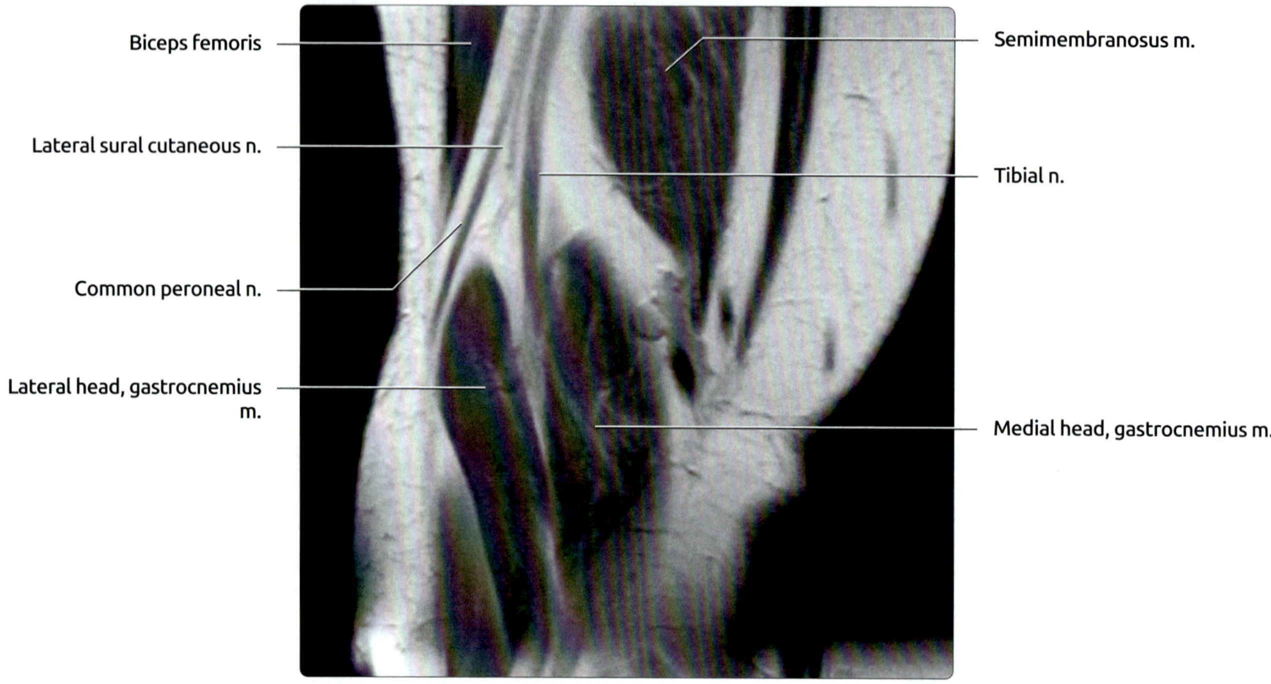

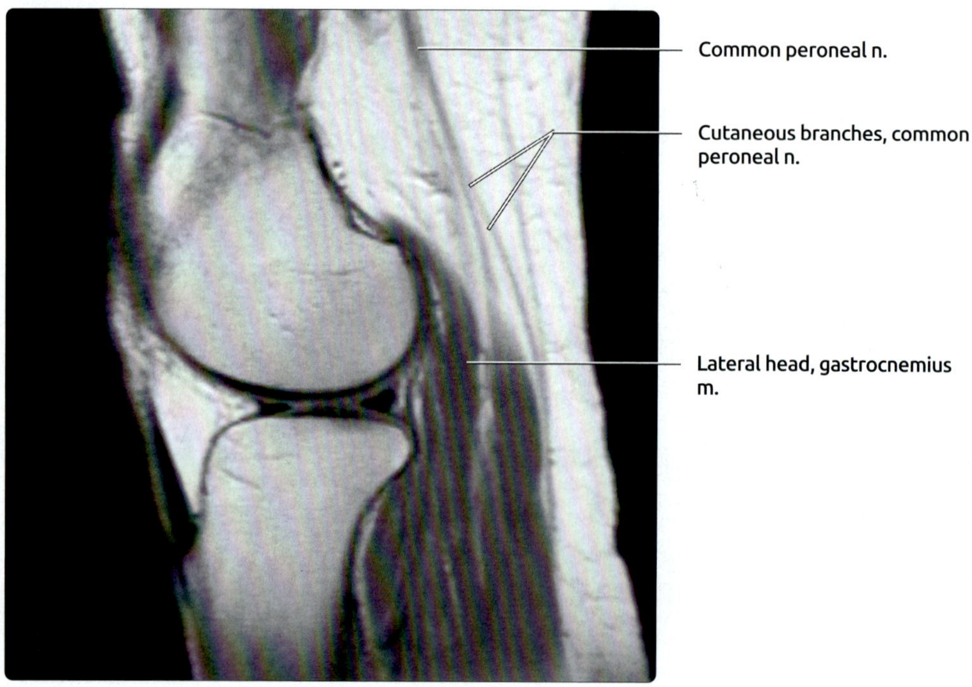

(Top) *Branches of either the tibial or common peroneal nerve forming the sural nerve are occasionally noted on axial, coronal, or sagittal MR images. In this posterior coronal MR, a branch originating from the common peroneal nerve is most likely the lateral sural cutaneous nerve.* **(Bottom)** *Note the 2 cutaneous branches of the common peroneal nerve traversing within the posterior fossa fat.*

MR: SURAL NERVE

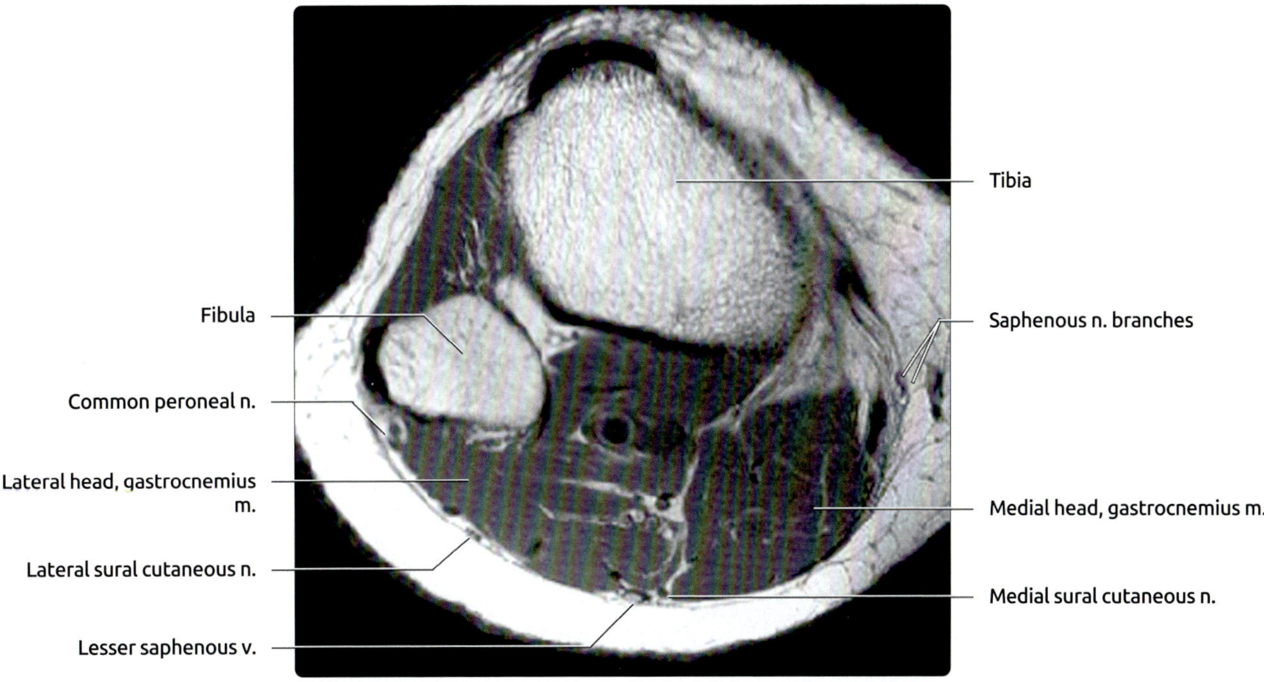

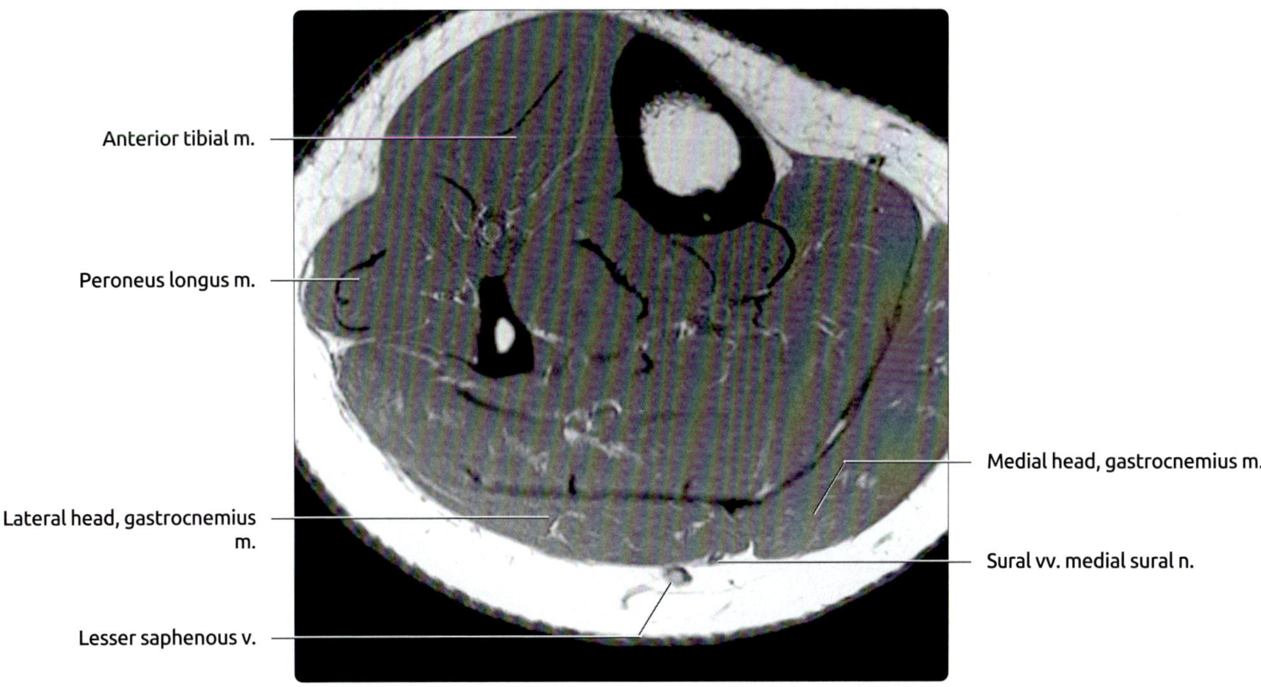

(Top) *The origin of the medial sural cutaneous nerve from the tibial nerve is occasionally seen on axial images at the knee level. More distally it is difficult to discern the medial sural cutaneous nerve from the sural nerve since the peroneal communicating branch of the common peroneal nerve is typically difficult to identify. Note proximity to the lesser saphenous vein.* **(Bottom)** *The sural nerve, easily noted on axial images of the leg, travels in abundant subcutaneous fat posterior to the medial & lateral heads of the gastrocnemius muscle.*

MR: SURAL NERVE

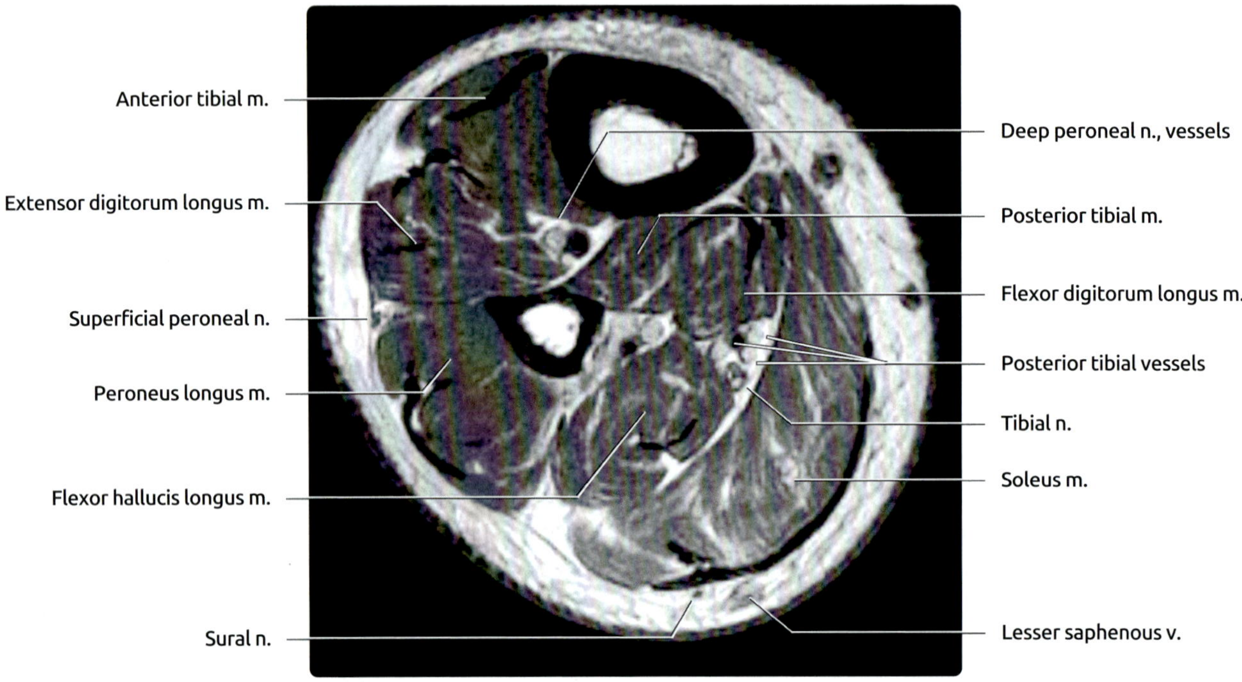

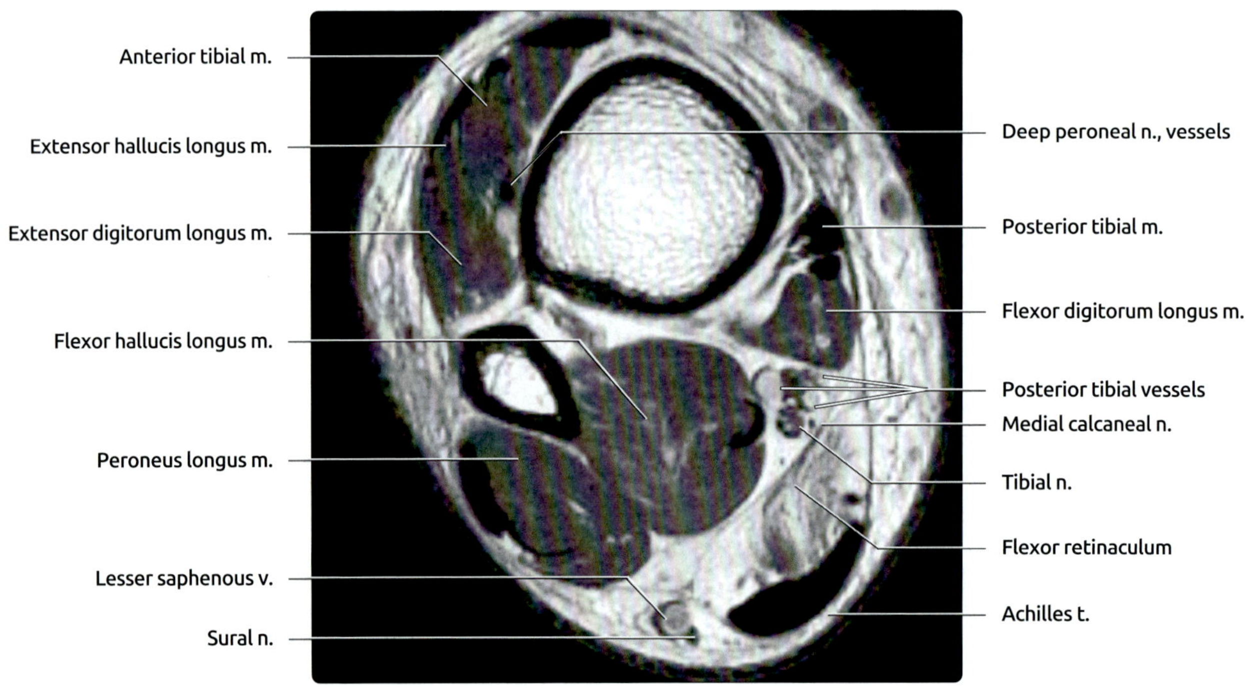

(Top) *The sural nerve is now seen posterior to the aponeurosis of the medial & lateral heads of the gastrocnemius muscle. It has migrated to a more lateral position while descending down the leg.* **(Bottom)** *In the leg, the sural nerve is posterior to the gastrocnemius aponeurosis. In the ankle, it runs between the Achilles & peroneal tendons behind & then distal to the lateral malleolus. It is accompanied by the lesser saphenous vein (usually posterior to the vein) & terminates in the lateral dorsal cutaneous & lateral calcaneal nerves. The sural nerve innervates the skin of the posterolateral distal leg, ankle, & foot up to the base of the 5th metatarsal. Significant variation in dorsal cutaneous innervation of the foot & overlap with innervation by superficial peroneal nerve exists.*

MR: SURAL NERVE

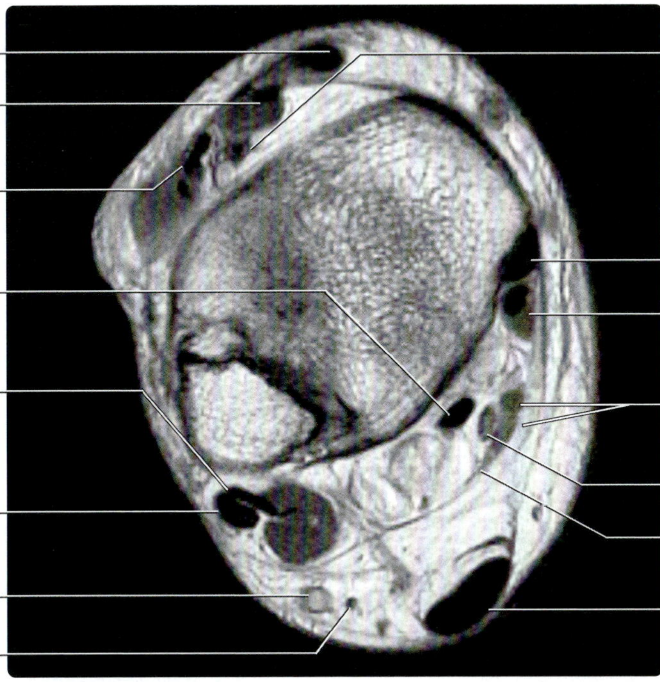

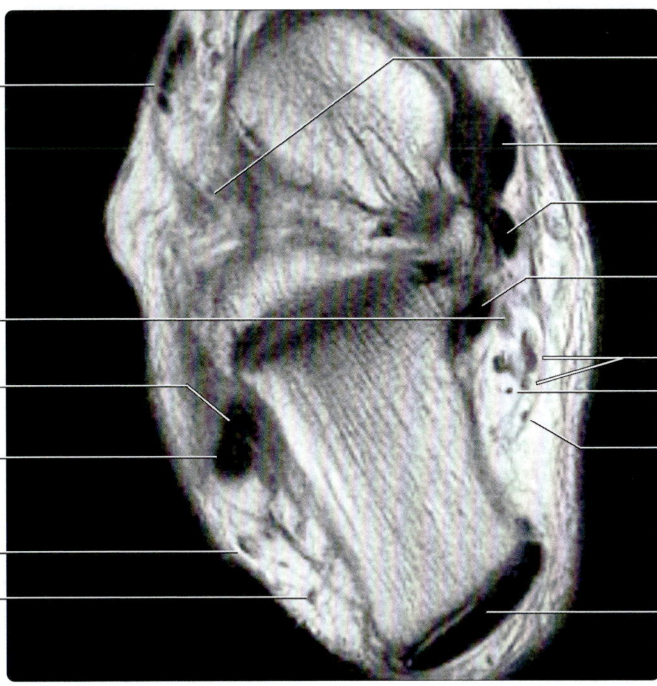

(Top) *The sural nerve, because of its small size, may sometimes be difficult to distinguish from the adjacent branches of the lesser saphenous vein. The nerve, because of its superficial location, is susceptible to direct trauma either at the ankle or the lateral leg. Fractures of the 5th metatarsal can entrap or tether the nerve.* **(Bottom)** *The sural nerve communicates with the posterior femoral cutaneous nerve in the leg & with the superficial peroneal nerve in the dorsum of the foot. The nerve is often used as a nerve graft because of its superficial location & the ease with which it can be surgically harvested.*

GROSS ANATOMY

Muscles of Leg

- **Posterior superficial compartment**
  - **Innervation**: All innervated by tibial nerve
  - **Gastrocnemius**
    - 2 heads unite to form main bulk of muscle
    - Origin: Medial and lateral heads from respective posterior femoral condyles
    - Heads separated from posterior capsule by bursa
    - Becomes tendinous in midleg, joins soleus muscle
    - Action: Plantar flexor of ankle and flexor of knee
  - **Soleus**
    - Origin: Extensive, from back of fibular head and upper 1/3 of posterior surface of shaft of fibula, from soleal line and middle 1/3 of medial border of tibia, and from tendinous arch joining these across popliteal vessels
    - Joins with tendon of gastrocnemius to form Achilles tendon
    - Action: Stabilizes ankle in standing, plantarflexes ankle
  - **Achilles tendon**
    - Conjoined tendon of gastrocnemius and soleus
    - Concave in cross section
    - Inserts on posterior margin of calcaneus
  - **Plantaris**
    - Origin: Lateral femoral condyle and oblique popliteal ligament
    - Muscle lies deep to lateral head of gastrocnemius
    - Myotendinous junction at level of origin of soleus
    - Tendon lies between medial head gastrocnemius and soleus
    - Inserts either on anteromedial Achilles or on calcaneus
    - Absent in 7-10% of general population
    - Action: Plantar flexion of ankle
- **Posterior deep compartment**
  - **Innervation**: All innervated by tibial nerve
  - **Popliteus**
    - Origin: Tendon from popliteal groove of lateral femoral condyle
    - Passes through popliteal hiatus posteriorly and medially, pierces posterior capsule of knee
    - Muscle fibers directed medially and downward to insert on posterior surface of tibia above soleal line
    - Action: Flexes knee and medially rotates tibia with respect to femur at onset of flexion (unlocking extension "screwing home" mechanism)
  - **Posterior tibial (a.k.a. tibialis posterior) muscle**
    - Origin: Interosseous membrane and adjoining parts of posterior surfaces of tibia and fibula
    - Superior end bifid; anterior tibial vessels pass forward between the 2 attachments
    - Distally, it inclines medially, under flexor digitorum longus
    - Grooves and curves around medial malleolus
    - Nerve supply: Tibial nerve
    - Action: Plantarflexes and inverts foot
  - **Flexor digitorum longus muscle**
    - Origin: Posterior surface of tibia, below popliteus, and medial to vertical ridge
    - Crosses superficial to distal part of tibialis posterior
    - Tendon grooves lower end of tibia lateral to that of tibialis posterior, passes around medial malleolus to foot
    - Action: Flexes interphalangeal and metatarsophalangeal joints of lateral 4 toes; plantarflexes and inverts foot
  - **Flexor hallucis longus muscle**
    - Origin: Posterior surface of fibula, below origin of soleus
    - Passes medially, descends down posterior to midtibia
    - Associated with os trigonum posterior to talus
    - Tendon occupies deep groove on posterior surface of talus, passes around medial malleolus, under sustentaculum tali, to great toe
    - Action: Flexes interphalangeal and metatarsophalangeal joints of great toe; plantarflexes foot
- **Lateral compartment**
  - Peroneals separated from extensors by anterior intermuscular septum and from posterior muscles by posterior septum
  - **Peroneus longus muscle**
    - Origin: Upper 2/3 lateral surface of fibula and intermuscular septa and adjacent muscular fascia
    - Becomes tendinous a few centimeters above lateral malleolus
    - Curves forward behind lateral malleolus, posterior to peroneus brevis
    - Nerve supply: Superficial peroneal
    - Action: Everts foot and secondarily plantarflexes foot
  - **Peroneus brevis muscle**
    - Origin: Lower 2/3 lateral surface of fibula and intermuscular septa and adjacent muscular fascia
    - Muscle is medial to peroneus longus at origin but overlaps peroneus longus in middle 1/3
    - Tendon curves forward behind lateral malleolus, in front of peroneus longus tendon
    - Nerve supply: Superficial peroneal
    - Action: Everts foot and secondarily plantarflexes foot
  - Synovial sheath for peroneals begins 5 cm above tip of lateral malleolus and envelops both tendons; divides into 2 sheaths at level of calcaneus
  - **Peroneus quartus muscle**
    - Accessory muscle with prevalence of 10%
    - Originates from distal leg, frequently from peroneal muscles, with variable insertion sites at foot
    - At level of malleolus, located medial or posterior to both peroneal tendons
  - **Peroneus digiti minimi muscle**
    - Accessory with prevalence of 15-36%
    - Extends from peroneus brevis muscle around medial malleolus to foot
    - Tiny tendinous slip
- **Anterior compartment**
  - **Anterior tibial (a.k.a. tibialis anterior) muscle**
    - Origin: Upper 1/2 of lateral surface of tibia and interosseous membrane
    - Tendon originates in distal 1/3; passes deep to retinaculum
    - Nerve supply: Deep peroneal and recurrent genicular
    - Action: Dorsiflexor and invertor of foot

- **Extensor digitorum longus muscle**
  - Origin: From upper 3/4 of anterior surface fibula
  - Descends behind extensor retinacula to ankle
  - Nerve supply: Deep peroneal
  - Action: Extends interphalangeal and metatarsophalangeal joints of lateral 4 toes, dorsiflexes foot
- **Peroneus tertius muscle**
  - Small, not always present
  - Origin: Continuous with extensor digitorum longus, arising from distal 1/4 of anterior surface of fibula and interosseous membrane
  - Inserts into dorsal surface at base of 5th metatarsal
  - Nerve supply: Deep peroneal
  - Action: Dorsiflexes ankle and everts foot
- **Extensor hallucis muscle**
  - Thin muscle hidden between tibialis anterior and extensor digitorum longus
  - Origin: Middle 1/2 of anterior surface of fibula and interosseous membrane
  - Tendon passes deep to retinacula to great toe
  - Nerve supply: Deep peroneal
  - Action: Extends phalanges of great toe and dorsiflexes foot

Vessels of Leg

- **Popliteal artery**
  - Continuation of superficial femoral artery after it has passed through adductor hiatus
  - Runs through fat of popliteal fossa
  - Relationships
    - Deep to artery: Femoral shaft, knee joint capsule, popliteus fascia
    - Superficial to artery: Popliteal vein, semimembranosus muscle, and gastrocnemius muscle
  - Artery lies just deep to vein in 40%, deep and medial to vein in 43%, deep and lateral to vein in 9%, and just medial or lateral to vein in 8%
  - 2 terminal branches: Anterior tibial artery and tibioperoneal trunk
- **Anterior tibial artery**
  - Smaller of the 2 terminal branches of popliteal artery
  - Origin in back of leg, at distal border of popliteus muscle
  - Passes through upper part of interosseous membrane
  - Straight course down front of leg to become dorsalis pedis artery
  - Runs on anterior surface of interosseous membrane, deep to extensor muscles
  - Muscular branches along length
  - Malleolar branches ramify over malleoli; lateral branch anastomoses with perforating branch of peroneal artery
- **Posterior tibial artery**
  - Larger of 2 terminal branches of popliteal artery
  - Main blood supply to foot
  - Passes downward and slightly medially along with tibial nerve to end in space between medial malleolus and calcaneus
  - Within calf, artery runs just deep to transverse intermuscular septum
  - Divides into lateral and medial plantar arteries in tarsal tunnel behind medial malleolus
  - Branches
    - Circumflex fibular (may arise from anterior tibial), runs laterally around neck of fibula
    - Nutrient artery to tibia
    - Muscular branches
- **Peroneal artery**
  - Largest branch of posterior tibial artery
  - Runs obliquely downward and laterally beneath soleus to fibula
  - Descends deep to flexor hallucis longus
- **Popliteal vein**
  - Paired venae comitantes of anterior and posterior tibial arteries join to form popliteal vein
  - Also receives small saphenous vein in popliteal fossa
  - Usually begins at inferior border of popliteus muscle
  - Crosses from medial to lateral side of popliteal artery as it runs in popliteal fossa, aside from always being superficial to popliteal artery
  - Ends at adductor hiatus by becoming superficial femoral vein
- **Great saphenous vein**
  - Begins at medial border of foot
  - Ascends in front of medial malleolus
  - Passes obliquely upward and backward across medial surface of distal 1/3 of tibia
  - Passes vertically upward along medial border of tibia to posterior part of medial side of knee
- **Small saphenous vein**
  - Extends behind lateral malleolus, ascends lateral to Achilles tendon
  - At midline of calf in lower popliteal region, pierces popliteal fascia, and terminates in popliteal vein

Sciatic Nerve

- Actually 2 nerves (common peroneal and tibial) bound together

Common Peroneal Nerve

- Smaller of 2 terminal divisions of sciatic nerve
- Arises from dorsal divisions of sacral plexus (L4, L5, S1, S2)
- Separates from tibial nerve midthigh, at superior angle of popliteal fossa, runs downward laterally along medial border of biceps femoris muscle and tendon
- Leaves popliteal fossa by crossing plantaris and lateral head of gastrocnemius, passes posterior and superficial to head of fibula
- Curves anteriorly over posterior aspect of head of fibula
- Winds around lateral surface of fibular neck
  - Location at fibular head/neck puts peroneal nerve at risk in several clinical situations
    - Fibular neck fracture may result in foot drop
    - Realignment during correction of chronic knee valgus deformity may stretch nerve
- Ends between lateral side of neck of fibula and peroneus longus by dividing into 3 terminal branches
  - **Recurrent articular branch**
    - To proximal tibiofibular joint
    - Occasionally acts as conduit for intraneural transmission of ganglion arising from joint
  - **Deep peroneal nerve**

- Arises on lateral side of neck of fibula, under peroneus longus
- Pierces anterior intermuscular septum and extensor digitorum longus to enter anterior compartment
- Extends down to ankle between tibialis anterior and long extensors
- Near ankle, crossed by extensor hallucis and passes to ankle midway between malleoli
- Muscular branches to anterior compartment and articular branch to ankle joint
- Deep peroneal nerve crosses over to lateral side of dorsalis pedis artery at ankle joint
- Medial and lateral terminal branches to dorsum of foot
- Medial is main terminal branch and travels distally just medial to dorsalis pedis artery

- **Superficial peroneal nerve**
  - Descends in substance of peroneus longus until it reaches peroneus brevis
  - Passes obliquely over anterior border of brevis and descends in groove between peroneus brevis and extensor digitorum longus
  - In distal 1/3 of leg, pierces deep fascia and divides into medial and lateral sensory branches to foot

Tibial Nerve

- Also called posterior tibial nerve
- Runs roughly along central axis of popliteal fossa
- Descends under fascial septum, which separates deep and superficial posterior muscle compartments
- In upper 2/3, lies on fascia of tibialis posterior and on flexor digitorum longus
- In lower 1/3, located midway between Achilles tendon and medial border of tibia
- Crosses posterior surfaces of tibia and ankle joint
- Posterior tibial vessels run with it, crossing in front of it from lateral to medial side
- At ankle, under flexor retinaculum, divides into lateral and medial plantar nerves
  - 1st branch of lateral plantar nerve is inferior calcaneal nerve (Baxter nerve)
    - Since this nerve supplies calcaneal periosteum, neuritis of this nerve can simulate plantar fasciitis
  - Medial plantar nerve can become compressed between navicular tuberosity and abductor hallucis muscle belly (jogger's foot)

Saphenous Nerve

- Longest branch of femoral nerve, arising 2 cm below inguinal ligament and descending via adductor canal
- Passes posterior to sartorius, descends posteromedial to knee where it pierces deep fascia
- In leg, accompanies great saphenous vein

Sural Nerve

- Purely sensory nerve that arises in popliteal fossa from tibial nerve
- Descends between 2 heads of gastrocnemius
- Pierces deep fascia midway between knee and ankle
- Courses superficial and posterior to peroneal tendons
- Accompanies small saphenous vein to lateral border of foot

ANATOMY IMAGING ISSUES

Imaging Recommendations

- Leg muscles
  - Relationship of different structures in posterior compartment tends to change along their courses
    - If in doubt, start from ankle level and trace structures proximally
- Leg vessels
  - Examination of lower limb vessels requires use of morphological and functional techniques
    - Morphology: Documentation of areas of stenosis or occlusion, sites of venous valves, aberrant branches, aneurysm formation, etc.
    - Functional: Combination of color and spectral Doppler examination
  - Veins require use of dynamic maneuvers
    - Valsalva: To increase abdominal pressure and accentuate reverse flow and incompetent venous valves
    - Augmentation: To increase venous return (to demonstrate venous flow and patency) by manually squeezing calf or by gently moving toes
    - Compression: To demonstrate absence of thrombus by using transducer pressure to cause complete luminal occlusion
  - Arteries require use of spectral Doppler scanning to show their phasicity; normal scan is triphasic
    - Sharp forward flow upstroke (systolic phase)
    - Small reverse flow (early diastolic phase)
    - Final smaller forward flow (late diastolic phase)
- Leg nerves
  - Use high-frequency transducers to assess nerves
  - Neural signature on ultrasound
    - Short axis: Uniformly dispersed hypoechoic dots (nerve fascicles) separated by hyperechoic epineurium
    - Long axis: Parallel hypoechoic tracts of uniform caliber
    - Overall gain control and focus settings may have to be optimized for ultrasound to demonstrate nerve well
    - Anisotropy artifact may affect scanning, especially in short axis; tilting transducer during scanning helps achieve best view
    - Distortion of this uniform appearance suggests pathology
  - Trace medium-sized nerves by following their course as they branch from their parent
  - Small (1-2 mm) nerves are difficult to identify and location may only be inferred by adjacent vessels

PANORAMIC: ANTEROLATERAL LEG

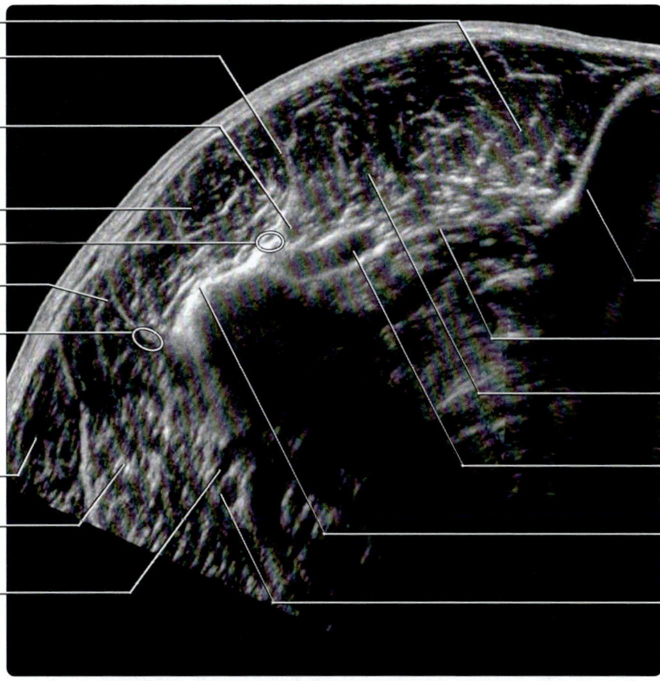

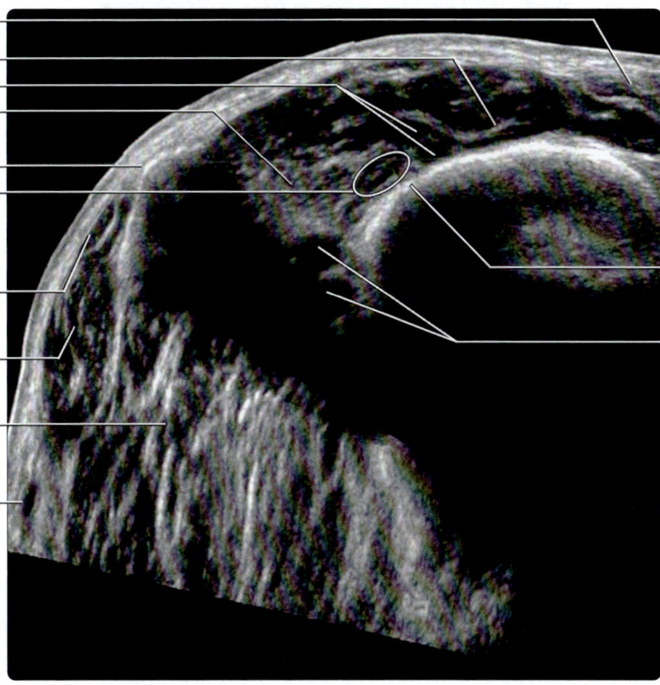

(Top) *Transverse panoramic view shows the anterior and lateral compartments of the upper leg. The crural compartments are divided by the tibia and the 2 intermuscular septa (anterior and posterior) into the anterior (extensor), lateral (peroneal), and posterior (flexor) compartments. The intermuscular septum separates the anterior from the posterior compartments.* **(Bottom)** *Transverse panoramic view shows the anterior and lateral compartments of the inferior leg. All muscles are smaller in caliber compared to those seen superiorly. An interosseous gap is still present between the tibia and fibula, but ultrasound interrogation through this gap is no longer possible, and the interosseous membrane cannot be demonstrated.*

TRANSVERSE US: ANTERIOR COMPARTMENT

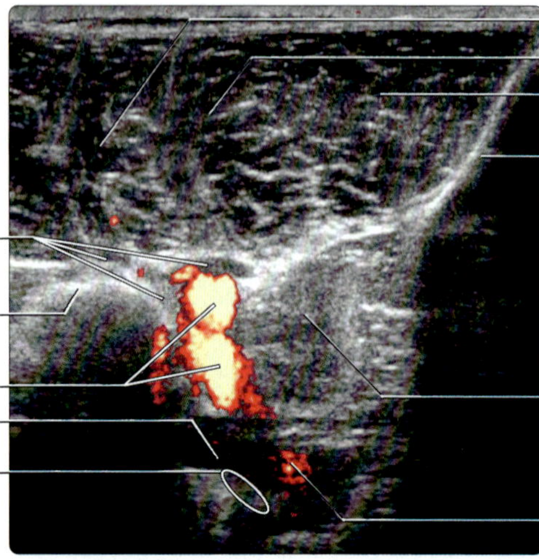

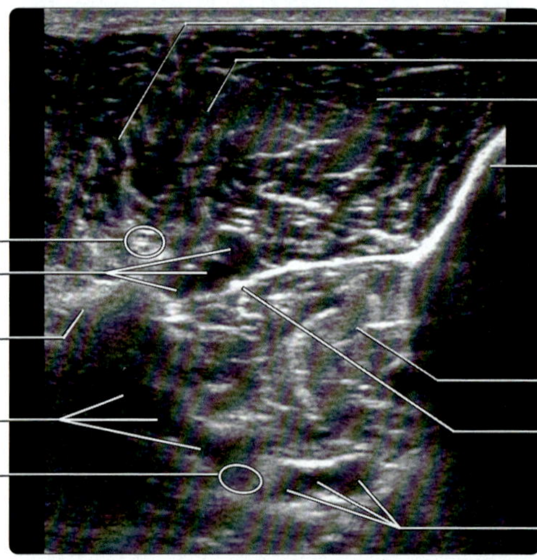

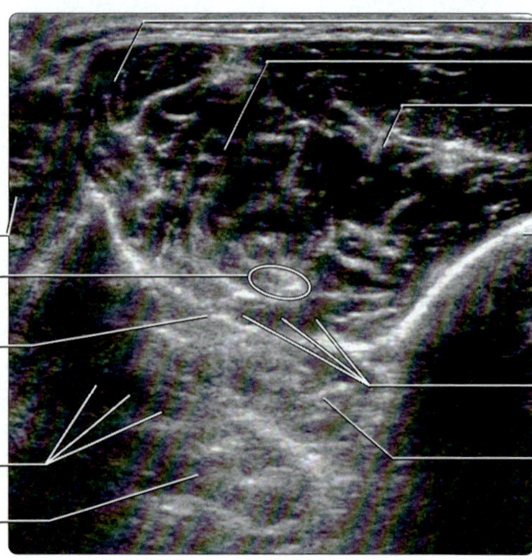

(Top) *Transverse color Doppler scan shows the anterior compartment at the upper leg level slightly below the proximal tibiofibular joint. At this level (above the superior margin of the interosseous membrane), the anterior tibial artery and vein (branches of the popliteal artery and vein) run anteriorly to supply the anterior compartment.* **(Middle)** *Transverse scan shows the anterior compartment at a slightly lower level. The tibialis anterior, extensor hallucis longus, and extensor digitorum longus muscles form the muscular component of this compartment. The deep peroneal nerve has penetrated laterally to supply this compartment. The anterior tibial vessels run on the surface of the interosseous membrane.* **(Bottom)** *Transverse scan more inferiorly shows a decrease in size of the extensor muscles and gradual migration of nerve and vessels more medially and superficially.*

SAGITTAL US: ANTERIOR COMPARTMENT

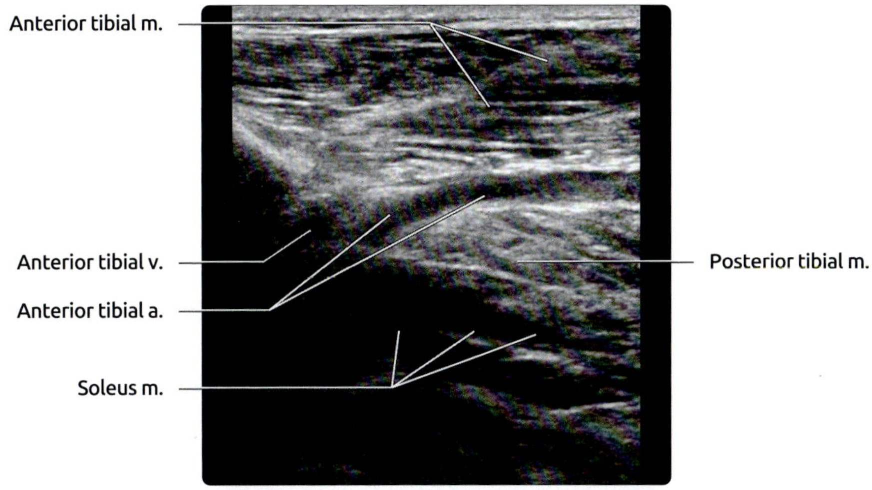

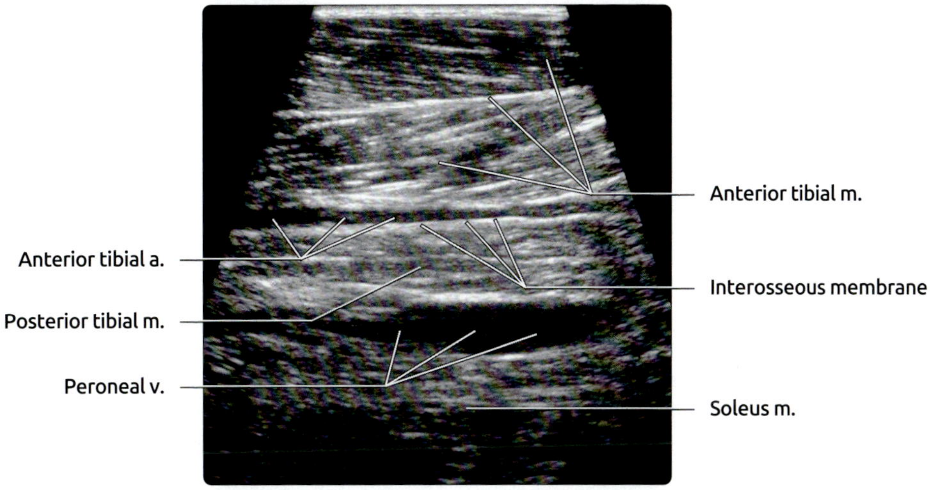

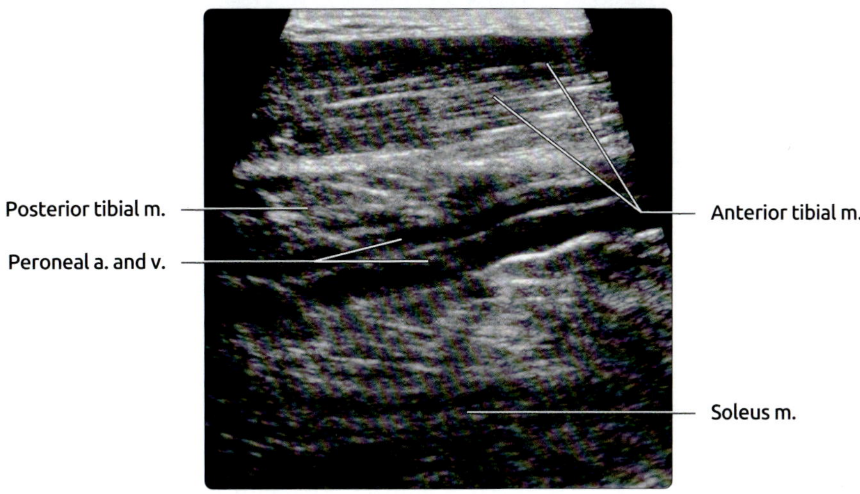

(Top) *Sagittal scan shows the anterior compartment at the upper leg level. The anterior tibial vessels pass above the superior margin of the interosseous membrane to enter the anterior compartment and supply the extensor muscles.* **(Middle)** *Sagittal scan of the anterior and posterior compartments at the midleg level shows that the interosseous gap between the tibia and fibula can be used as a window to interrogate the deep posterior structures.* **(Bottom)** *Sagittal scan shows the anterior compartment at a lower level. Within the posterior compartment, the peroneal vessels run anteriorly and just below the inferior margin of the interosseous membrane.*

TRANSVERSE US: LATERAL COMPARTMENT

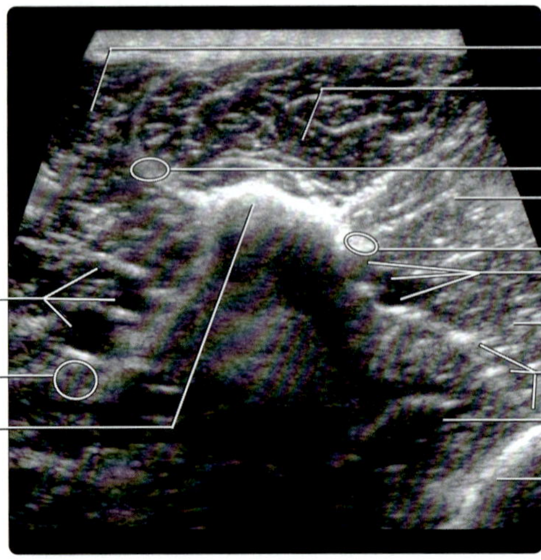

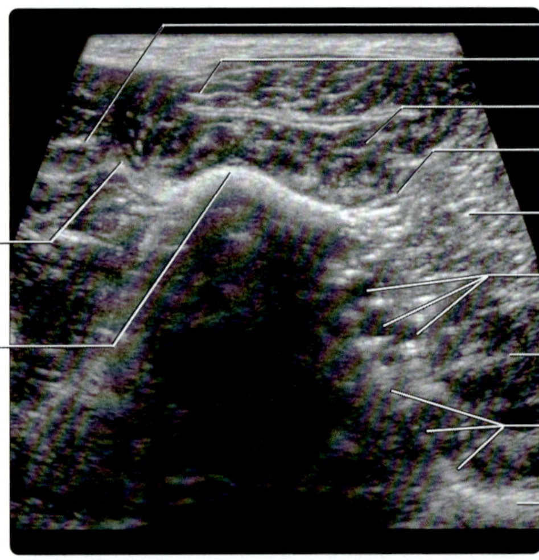

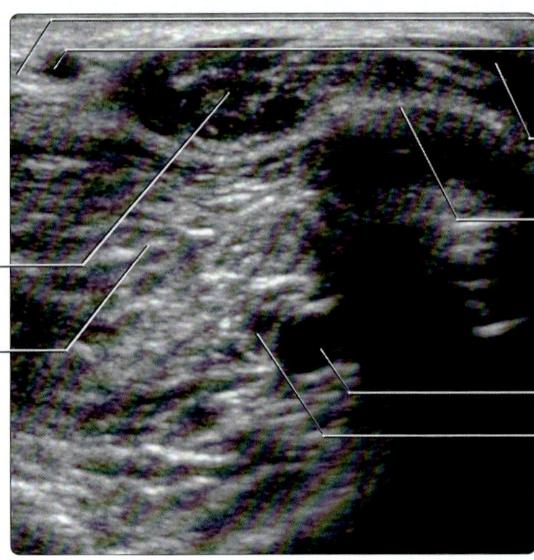

(Top) *Transverse scan shows the lateral compartment at a high level. At this level, only the peroneus longus muscle has originated and is the only muscle occupying this compartment. The superficial peroneal nerve lies on the posterior surface of the peroneus longus muscle. The deep peroneal nerve has already entered the anterior compartment after curving around the fibular neck (above this scan level).* **(Middle)** *Transverse scan at the midleg level shows that the peroneus brevis muscle has now originated and resides anterior and deep to the peroneus longus muscle. More inferiorly, the peroneus longus muscle will become smaller and turn into a tendon while the peroneus brevis will still have muscle fibers down to the level of the ankle joint.* **(Bottom)** *Transverse scan shows the level of the lateral malleolus. The peroneal tendons will run posterior to the lateral malleolus and curve around its tip to run toward the lateral foot.*

CORONAL US: LATERAL COMPARTMENT

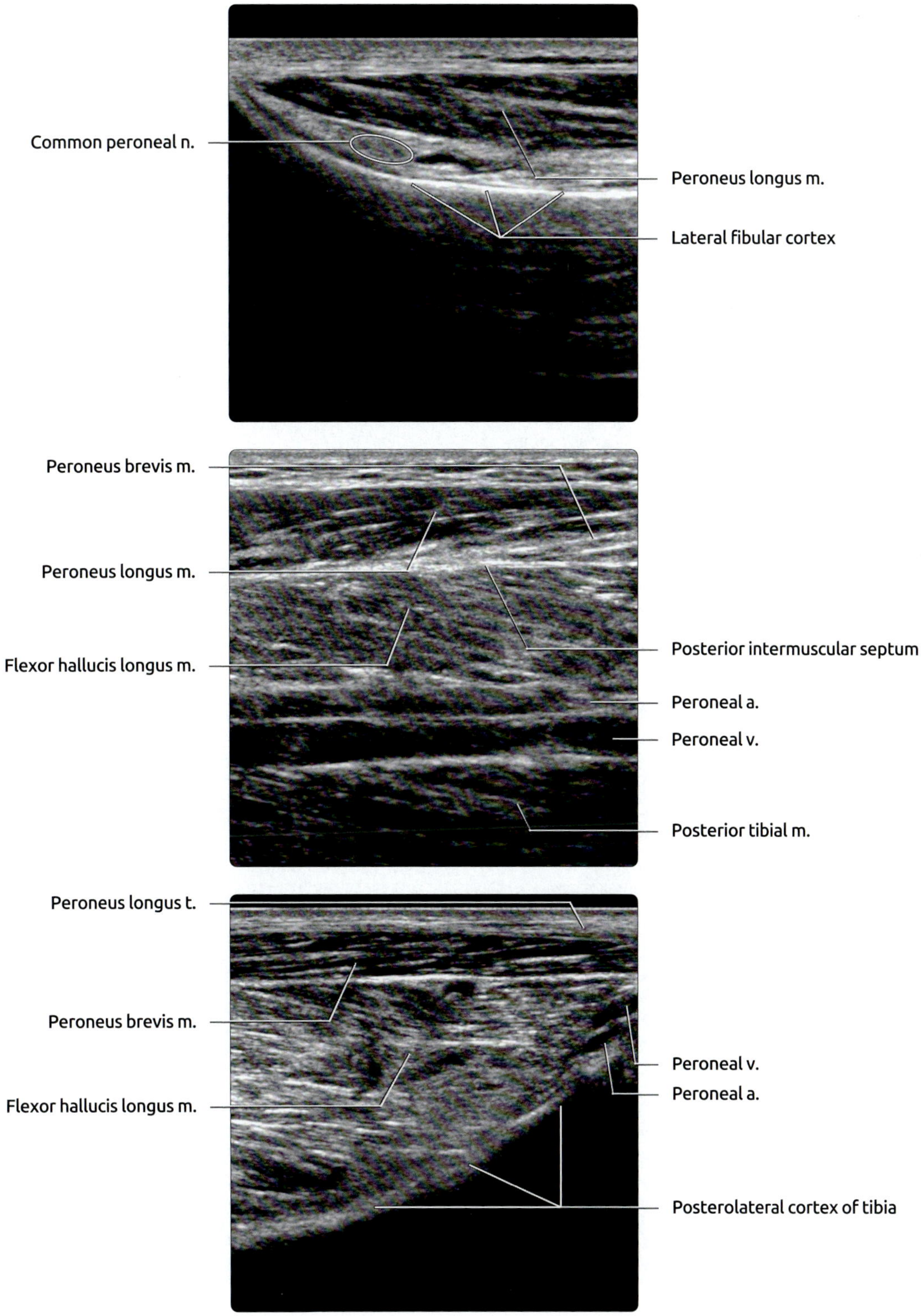

(Top) *Coronal scan shows the lateral compartment at the level of the fibular neck. The common peroneal nerve runs together with the biceps femoris tendon, then curves anteriorly around the neck of fibula to enter the lateral and then the anterior compartments.* **(Middle)** *Coronal scan of the lateral compartment at the midleg level shows the transition between the peroneus longus and peroneus brevis muscles. These are separated from the posterior compartment by the posterior intermuscular septum.* **(Bottom)** *Coronal scan further inferiorly shows that the peroneus longus muscle is now only a tendon, compared to the muscular peroneus brevis. Similarly, in the posterior compartment, the flexor hallucis longus muscle is the only muscle at this level, as the others have also become tendons.*

PANORAMIC: POSTERIOR LEG

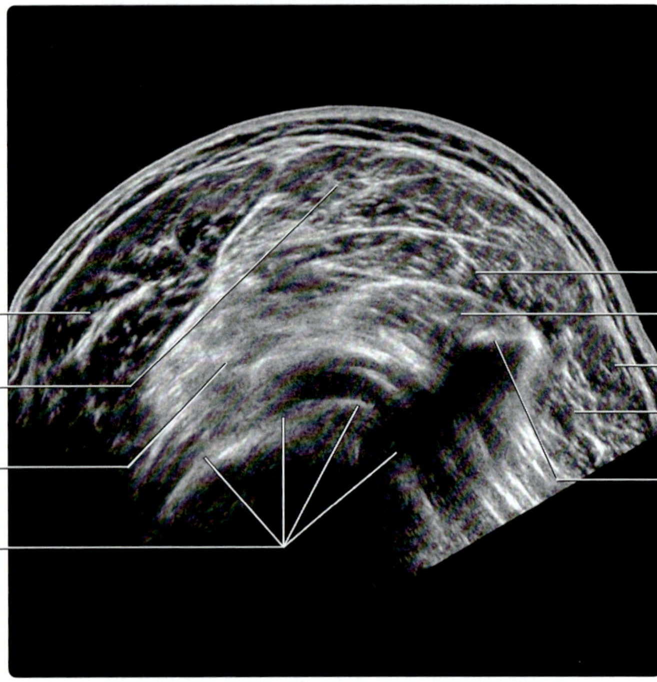

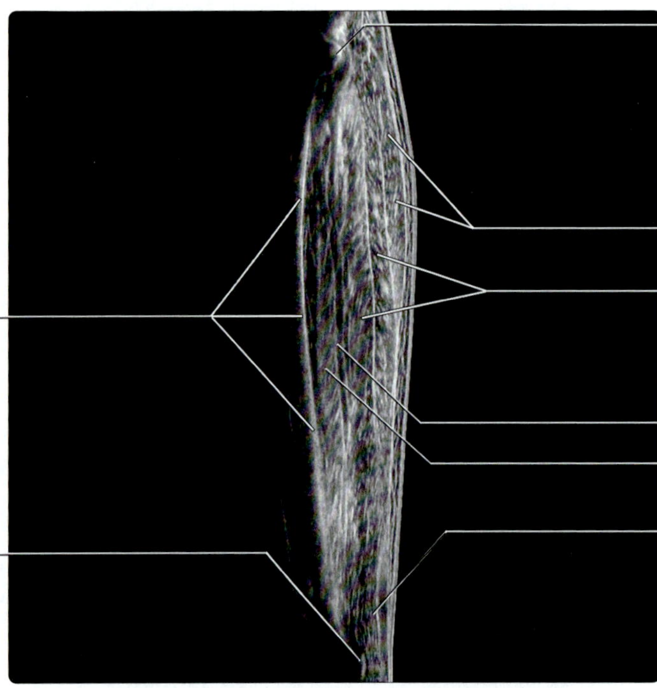

(Top) *Transverse panoramic scan shows the posterior compartment at the level of the midleg. The medial head of the gastrocnemius muscle is larger than the lateral throughout its course. From this midcalf level downward, the soleus will assume relatively more bulk as the gastrocnemius turns tendinous.* **(Bottom)** *Sagittal panoramic scan shows the posterior compartment. The gastrocnemius is muscular down to approximately the level of the midcalf. Below this level, it forms the Achilles tendon, receiving contributions from the soleus muscle. For the deep layer, the tibialis posterior muscle lies on the surface of the tibial shaft and interosseous membrane.*

TRANSVERSE US: POSTERIOR LEG

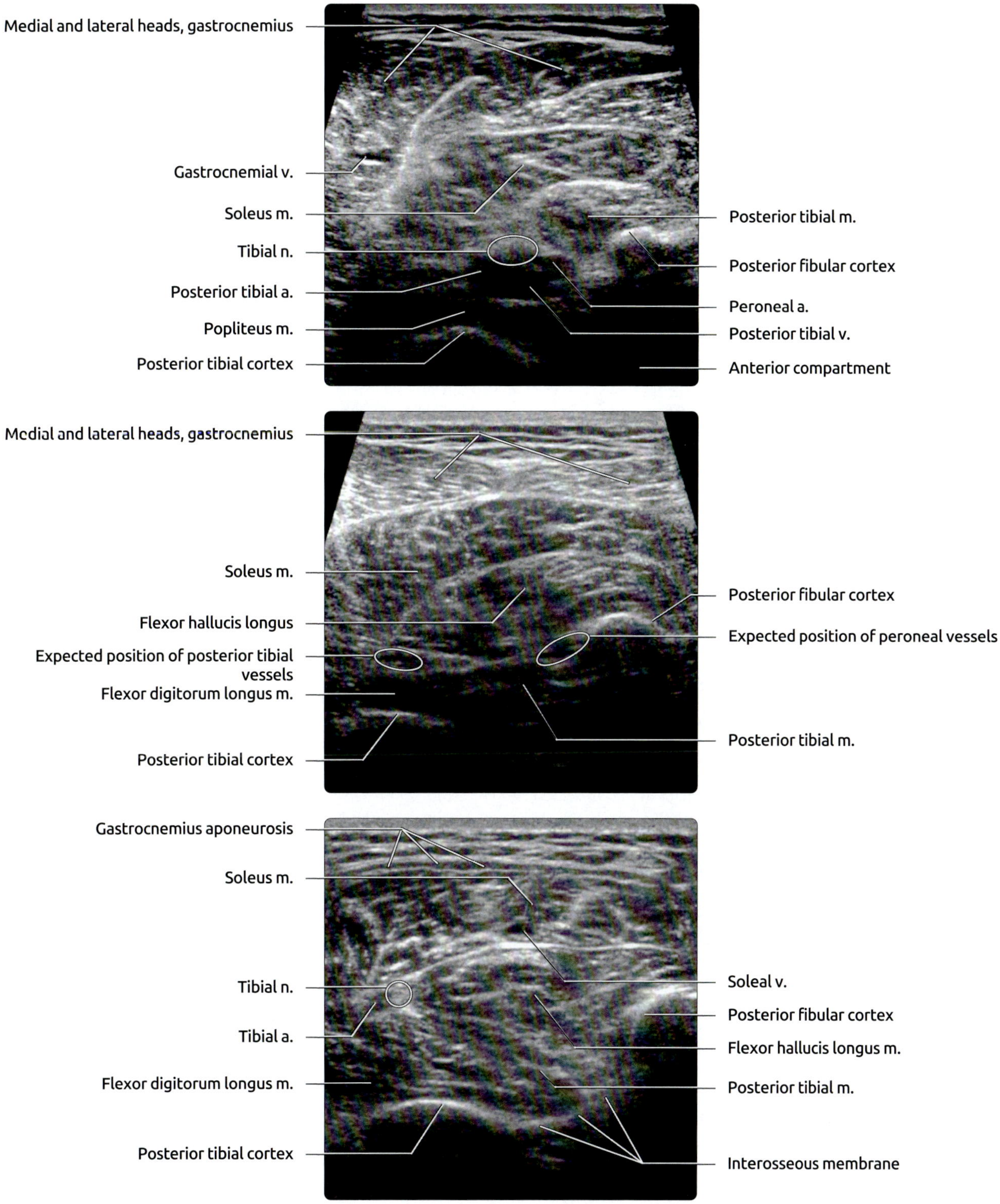

(Top) *Transverse scan is seen through the posterior compartment at the upper calf level. For this compartment, the superficial layer consists of the gastrocnemius, plantaris, and soleus muscles. The deep layer consists of the popliteus, posterior tibial, flexor digitorum longus, and flexor hallucis longus muscles.* **(Middle)** *Transverse scan shows the midcalf level. The tibial vessels have bifurcated into their peroneal and posterior tibial branches, which delineates a separation between the tibialis posterior and flexor digitorum longus from the rest of the calf muscles. Given the thickness of the gastrocnemius and soleus muscles, these deep muscles may be better seen using the anterior compartment as a window.* **(Bottom)** *Further inferiorly, the gastrocnemius has become a thin aponeurosis and together with the tendon from the soleus muscle will form the Achilles tendon.*

SECTION 3
Ankle

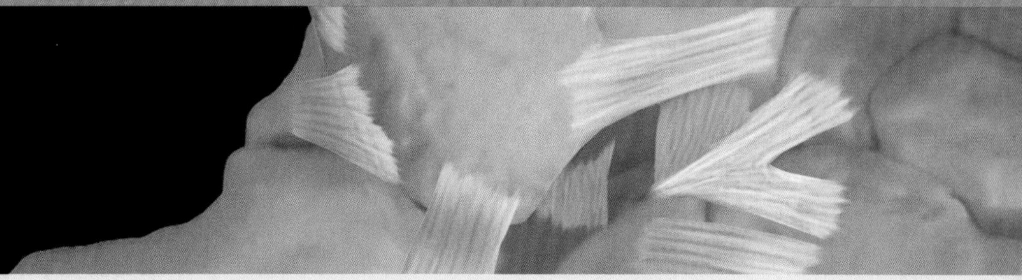

Ankle and Hindfoot Overview

TERMINOLOGY

Definitions

- Hindfoot: General term for ankle and subtalar joints, talus, and calcaneus
- Midfoot: General term for remaining tarsal bones and their articulations
  - Navicular, cuboid, cuneiforms
- Forefoot: General term for metatarsals and phalanges

GROSS ANATOMY

Osseous Structures

- **Tibia**
  - Plafond articulates with talar body
    - Slightly convex from medial to lateral, concave anterior to posterior
  - Medial malleolus articulates with medial surface of talar body
    - Forms anterior and posterior colliculi
    - Anterior colliculus extends further inferiorly than posterior colliculus
  - Posterior malleolus is broad posterior margin of tibia
- **Fibula**
  - Articulates with tibia via distal tibiofibular joint
  - Lateral malleolus articulates with lateral surface of talar body
- **Talus**
  - Articulates with tibia, fibula, calcaneus, and navicular
    - 2/3 covered by articular cartilage
    - No muscle attachments
  - Divided into body, neck, and head
  - Trochlea of body articulates with tibia
    - Term "talar dome" is misnomer
    - Slightly concave from medial to lateral, rounded convexity anterior to posterior
    - Trochlea is broader anteriorly than posteriorly
  - Posterior process projects posteriorly from body
    - Divided into medial and lateral tubercles, between which passes flexor hallucis longus tendon
    - Separate center of ossification, often remains separate ossicle in adulthood (os trigonum)
  - Lateral process projects laterally from body
    - Articulates with lateral malleolus superiorly, posterior subtalar joint inferiorly
  - Neck forms superomedial boundary of tarsal sinus
    - Major blood supply to talar body enters via neck
  - Head articulates with navicular and calcaneus
- **Calcaneus**
  - Articulates with talus (3 facets) and cuboid
  - Weightbearing, springboard for locomotion
  - Divided into posterior process, body, sustentaculum tali, anterior process

Articulations

- **Inferior tibiofibular joint**
  - Primarily fibrous joint
    - Synovial recess from ankle joint extends at least 1 cm into syndesmosis
    - May have articular cartilage at inferior portion
  - Close apposition of tibia and fibula is maintained by syndesmotic ligaments
  - Motion: Minimal superior-inferior motion and external rotation
- **Ankle (talocrural) joint**
  - Synovial joint between tibia, fibula, and talus
  - Inferior tibiofibular joint unites tibia and fibula into mortise
  - Talus is tenon within mortise of tibia + fibula
  - Motion: Hinge joint: Extension (dorsiflexion) and flexion (plantar flexion)
    - Dynamic shift of axis of rotation during dorsi and plantar flexion
  - Supported by lateral and medial collateral ligaments
- **Subtalar joint**
  - Synovial joints between talus and calcaneus
  - 3 facets: Posterior, middle, and anterior
  - Posterior facet has separate joint capsule
    - 15% communicate with ankle joint
    - 50% of weightbearing occurs through posterior subtalar joint
    - Motion: Inversion, eversion, and anteroposterior gliding
  - Middle and anterior facets communicate with each other and talonavicular joint
  - Motions: Inversion, eversion, adduction, abduction

Ligaments

- 3 sets stabilize ankle: Distal tibiofibular syndesmotic complex, lateral collateral, and deltoid ligaments
- **4 tibiofibular syndesmotic ligaments**: Maintain width of ankle mortise, stabilize against eversion
  - **Anterior and posterior inferior tibiofibular ligaments**
  - **Inferior transverse ligament**: Distal to main posterior tibiofibular ligament
  - **Interosseous ligament**: Distal thickening of syndesmotic membrane
- **3 lateral collateral ligaments**: Stabilize ankle against inversion and anterior, posterior subluxation
  - **Anterior talofibular ligament**
    - Originates 1 cm proximal to lateral malleolar tip, inserts on talar neck
    - Stabilizes talus against anterior displacement, internal rotation, and inversion
    - Weakest and 1st to tear
    - Isolated tear is common and may not result in clinical ankle instability
  - **Calcaneofibular ligament**
    - Originates from lateral malleolar tip, inserts on calcaneal trochlear eminence
    - Deep to peroneal tendons
    - Lateral restraint of subtalar joint, often tears with anterior talofibular ligament
  - **Posterior talofibular ligament**
    - Extends from lateral malleolar fossa to lateral talar tubercle
    - Strongest, rarely tears
- **Medial collateral ligament = deltoid ligament**
  - Divided into superficial and deep components
  - Superficial: From medial (superficial) margin of medial malleolus

- Fibers merge with flexor retinaculum along posteromedial margin of medial malleolus
- Multiple, variable bands, named for sites of attachment
- Anterior tibiotalar, tibiospring, and tibionavicular, deep to posterior tibial tendon
  - Tibiocalcaneal is strongest band
- Posterior tibiotalar and tibiocalcaneal
- Provide rotational stability
- Deep: Posterior and anterior tibiotalar
  - Posterior tibiotalar: Thick, striated, nearly horizontal in orientation, from posterior colliculus medial malleolus to medial fossa of talar body, prevent joint eversion
  - Anterior tibiotalar: Thin, from anterior colliculus to junction talar body and neck
- **Spring ligament (plantar calcaneonavicular ligament)**
  - Binds calcaneus to navicular, 3 components
  - Superomedial **origin**: Sustentaculum tali; **insertion**: Superomedial navicular, tibiospring band of deltoid
  - Medioplantar oblique **origin**: Calcaneal coronoid fossa; **insertion**: Plantar navicular
  - Inferoplantar longitudinal **origin**: Coronoid fossa; **insertion**: Navicular beak

Retinacula

- Focal thickening of deep fascia
- Maintain tendons in position when they change orientation
- **Superior extensor retinaculum**
  - Few cm above ankle joint
  - Attaches to anterior fibula laterally, tibia medially
  - Distally attaches to inferior extensor retinaculum
  - Prevents bowstringing of anterior compartment muscles
- **Inferior extensor retinaculum**
  - At ankle joint, Y-shaped, stem laterally, proximal, and distal bands medially
  - Stem attaches laterally to upper calcaneus
    - Loops around extensor tendons
    - Roots extend into sinus tarsi
  - Proximal medial band has deep and superficial layers, loop around extensor hallucis longus tendon and occasionally tibialis anterior tendon
  - Distal medial band superficial to extensor hallucis longus and tibialis anterior tendons
    - Attaches to plantar aponeurosis
  - Dorsalis pedis vessels, deep peroneal nerve: Deep to all layers of inferior extensor retinaculum
- **Flexor retinaculum**
  - Attaches to tubercle at posteromedial corner of medial malleolus
    - Continuous with periosteum and origin of superficial deltoid ligament
  - Proximally continuous with deep fascia of leg
  - Distally continuous with plantar aponeurosis
  - Abductor hallucis partly attached to it
  - Maintains position of extrinsic flexor tendons as they pass from leg into foot
  - Lateral border of tarsal tunnel
- **Superior peroneal retinaculum**
  - Origin: Lateral malleolus, insertions vary, most commonly to deep fascia of leg and calcaneus
  - Maintains position of peroneal tendons posterior to fibula
- **Inferior peroneal retinaculum**
  - Continuous with inferior extensor retinaculum
  - Inserts on lateral calcaneus, peroneal tubercle (trochlea)
  - Maintains position of peroneal tendons adjacent to calcaneus

Tendons

- **Anterior (extensor) compartment**: Tendons listed from medial to lateral
  - **Anterior tibial (tibialis anterior) tendon**
    - Dorsiflexes ankle, inverts foot, tightens plantar aponeurosis
    - Inserts on medial cuneiform, base of 1st metatarsal
    - Supports medial longitudinal arch during walking
  - **Extensor hallucis longus tendon**
    - Extends 1st phalanges, dorsiflexes foot and great toe
    - Inserts on dorsal base of 1st distal phalanx
  - **Extensor digitorum longus tendon**
    - Dorsiflexes ankle, extends toes, tightens plantar aponeurosis
    - Divides into 4 slips on dorsum of foot
    - Slips receive tendinous contributions from extensor digitorum brevis, lumbricals, and interosseous muscles
    - Each slip divides into 3: Central one inserts on dorsal base of middle phalanx and 2 collateral ones, which reunite and insert on bases of 2nd-5th distal phalanges
  - **Peroneus tertius tendon**
    - Typically part of extensor digitorum longus tendon
    - Inserts on dorsal base of 5th metatarsal
    - Variably present
- **Lateral compartment**
  - **Peroneus longus tendon**
    - Plantarflexes ankle, everts foot, supports longitudinal and transverse arches during walking
    - Posterolateral to peroneus brevis tendon in retrofibular groove, deep to superior peroneal retinaculum
    - Descends behind peroneal tubercle, deep to inferior peroneal retinaculum
    - Curves under cuboid sulcus, deep to long plantar ligament
    - Inserts on plantar base of 1st metatarsal, medial cuneiform
    - Os peroneum always present, ossified in ~ 20% of individuals
  - **Peroneus brevis tendon**
    - Everts foot, limits foot inversion
    - Anteromedial to peroneus longus tendon in retrofibular groove, deep to superior peroneal retinaculum
    - Descends anterior to peroneal tubercle of calcaneus, deep to inferior peroneal retinaculum
    - Inserts into base of 5th metatarsal
- **Superficial posterior compartment**
  - **Achilles tendon**
    - Main plantar flexor of ankle, foot
    - Largest and strongest tendon in body

- Conjoined tendon of medial and lateral gastrocnemius and soleus muscles
- ~ 15 cm long
- Lacks tendon sheath, enclosed by paratenon
- Inserts on posterior calcaneal tuberosity
- Retrocalcaneal bursa between distal tendon and calcaneal tuberosity

- **Plantaris tendon**
  - Vestigial, slender tendon, medial to Achilles tendon
  - Inserts on, or medial to, Achilles tendon on calcaneus
- **Deep posterior compartment** tendons are listed from medial to lateral
  - **Posterior tibial (tibialis posterior) tendon**
    - Crosses flexor digitorum longus tendon above ankle joint to become most posteromedial tendon
    - Shares tibial groove with flexor digitorum longus tendon
    - Inserts on navicular tuberosity, cuneiforms, sustentaculum tali, bases of 2nd-4th metatarsals
    - Main invertor of foot, aids in plantar flexion
    - Supports medial longitudinal arch
  - **Flexor digitorum longus tendon**
    - Lateral to tibialis posterior tendon in tibial groove
    - Crosses flexor hallucis longus tendon at master knot of Henry
    - Divides into 4 slips that give origin to lumbricals
    - Slips pass through openings in corresponding tendons of flexor digitorum brevis
    - Slips insert on bases of 2nd-5th distal phalanges
    - Flexes distal phalanges, assists in plantar flexion of ankle
  - **Flexor hallucis longus tendon**
    - Passes 3 fibroosseous tunnels: (1) Between medial and lateral talar tubercles, (2) under sustentaculum tali, (3) between 1st medial and lateral sesamoids
    - Crosses and sends slip to flexor digitorum longus at master knot of Henry
    - Inserts on base of 1st distal phalanx
    - When foot is on ground: Maintains pad of 1st toe on ground
    - When foot is off ground: Plantar flexes 1st phalanges, aids in maintaining medial longitudinal arch
    - Weak plantar flexor of ankle

Vessels

- **Anterior tibial artery** becomes **dorsalis pedis** at ankle joint
- **Posterior tibial artery** divides into medial and lateral plantar arteries in tarsal tunnel

Nerves

- **Tibial nerve**
  - Largest, medial terminal branch of sciatic nerve
  - May be called posterior tibial nerve in ankle
  - Curves around medial malleolus, travels in tarsal tunnel under flexor retinaculum
  - Divides in, or proximal to, tarsal tunnel
    - Medial calcaneal nerve: Sensory medial heel
    - Medial plantar nerve: Sensory to medial 2/3 plantar foot, motor to abductor hallucis, flexor digitorum brevis, flexor hallucis brevis, 1st lumbrical
    - Lateral plantar nerve: Sensory to lateral 1/3 of plantar foot, motor to abductor digiti minimi, quadratus plantae, adductor hallucis, flexor digiti minimi, 2nd-4th lumbricals, all interossei
  - Vulnerable to impingement in tarsal tunnel
- **Common peroneal nerve**
  - Smaller, lateral, terminal branch of sciatic nerve, divides below knee into deep and superficial peroneal nerves
- **Deep peroneal nerve**
  - Deep to extensor retinacula, in anterior tarsal tunnel
  - Predominantly motor
  - Divides just above ankle into medial (mainly sensory), lateral (mainly motor) branches
    - **Medial branch** continues dorsal to talonavicular joint, middle cuneiform, and in between 1st and 2nd metatarsals
    - **Lateral branch** ends at extensor digitorum brevis
  - In leg: Motor to anterior tibial, extensor digitorum longus, extensor hallucis longus, peroneus tertius
  - In foot: Motor to extensor digitorum brevis, sensory (and sometimes motor) to 1st web space
- **Superficial peroneal nerve**
  - Exits deep fascia 10-15 cm above ankle joint
  - Subcutaneous 6 cm above ankle, divides into subcutaneous branches
  - In leg: Motor to peroneus brevis and peroneus longus tendons, sensory to distal 2/3 lateral leg
  - In foot: Sensory to dorsal foot
- **Sural nerve**
  - Formed by medial sural branch of tibial nerve and peroneal (sural) communicating branch of common peroneal nerve
  - Purely sensory to lateral ankle and foot, up to 5th toe base
  - Subcutaneous along posterolateral ankle
- **Saphenous nerve** (branch of femoral nerve)
  - Subcutaneous, lateral to greater saphenous vein

Spaces of Ankle

- **Tarsal sinus (sinus tarsi)**
  - Lateral, funnel-shaped space between talar neck and calcaneus
  - Contains insertions of 3 bands of inferior extensor retinaculum
  - Contains cervical ligament between talar neck and calcaneus
  - Artery of tarsal sinus courses retrograde through sinus to supply talar body
- **Tarsal tunnel**
  - Roof: Flexor retinaculum
  - Floor: Medial tibia, talus, calcaneus
  - Contains tibialis posterior, flexor digitorum, and flexor hallucis tendons
  - Contains posterior tibial neurovascular bundle
    - Tibial nerve divides in tunnel into branches to calcaneus, plus medial and lateral plantar nerves
- Tarsal canal
  - Between talus and calcaneus, posteromedial extent of tarsal sinus
  - Contains interosseous ligament

GRAPHICS: TALUS

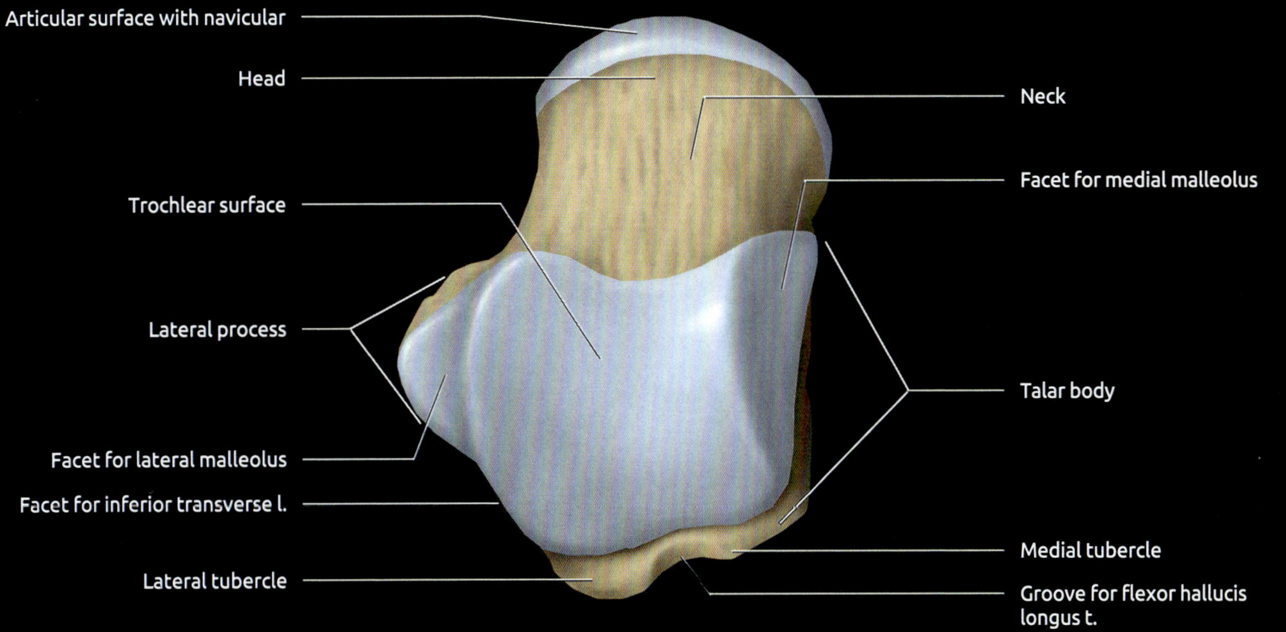

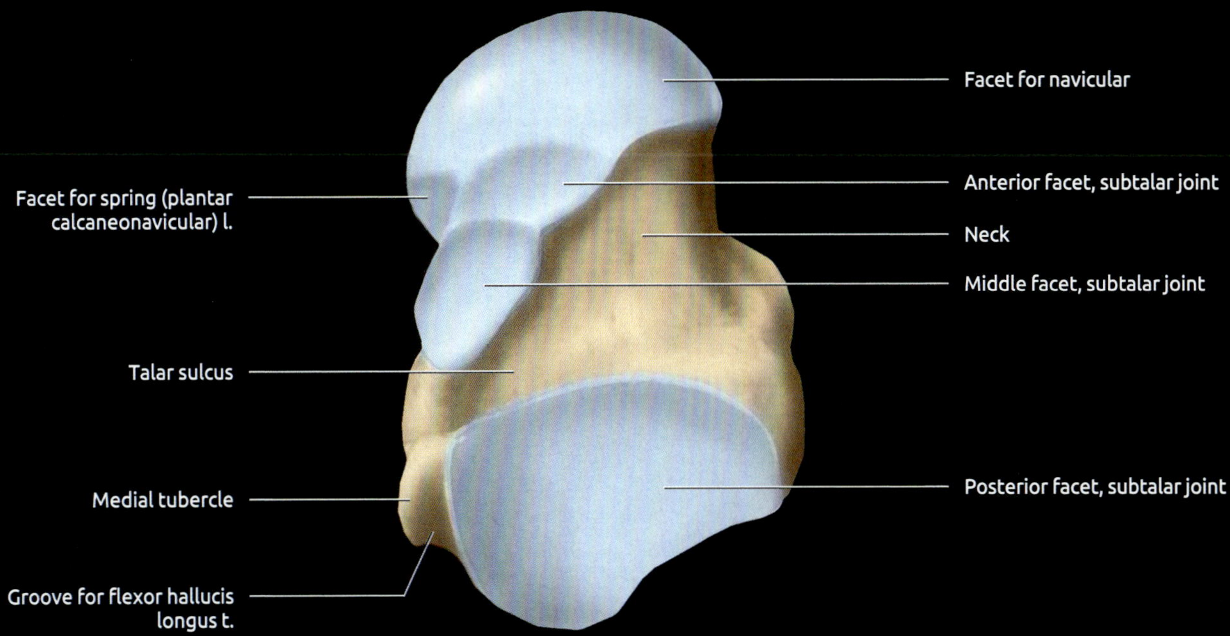

(Top) *View of the talus from above is shown. The tibia transmits body weight to the talus, which then redistributes it to the calcaneus and navicular. The talus is subdivided into body, neck, and head. The body contains the trochlea, which forms the talocrural joint with the tibia. The trochlear surface is narrower posteriorly than anteriorly. The flexor hallucis longus tendon traverses in a groove between the medial and lateral tubercles of the posterior talar process.* **(Bottom)** *Plantar view of the talus shows the articular facets for the subtalar joint and the talonavicular joint. The cervical and interosseous ligaments insert into the plantar talar neck. The talar sulcus and calcaneal sulcus together form the tarsal canal and sinus tarsi space.*

GRAPHICS: TALUS

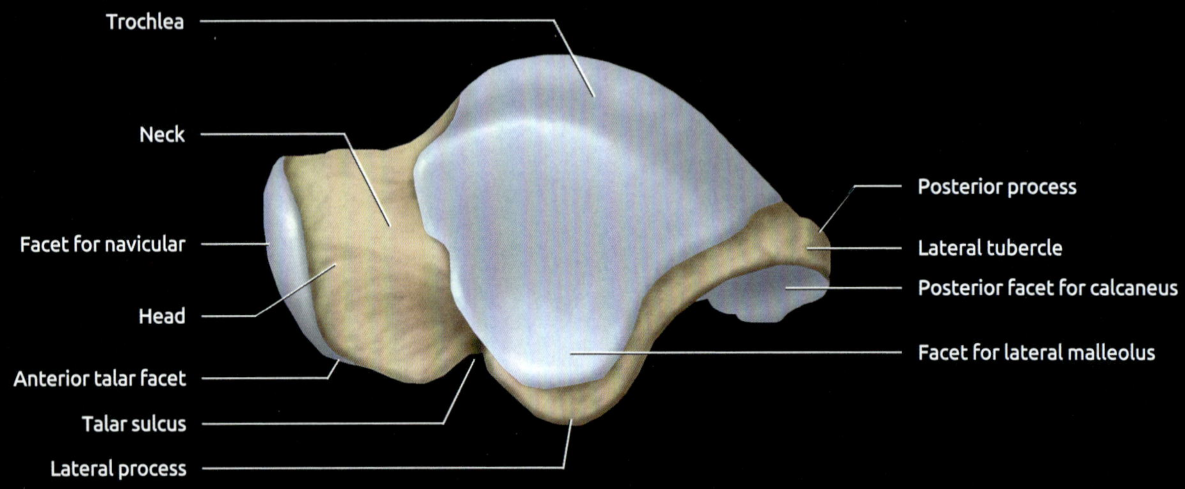

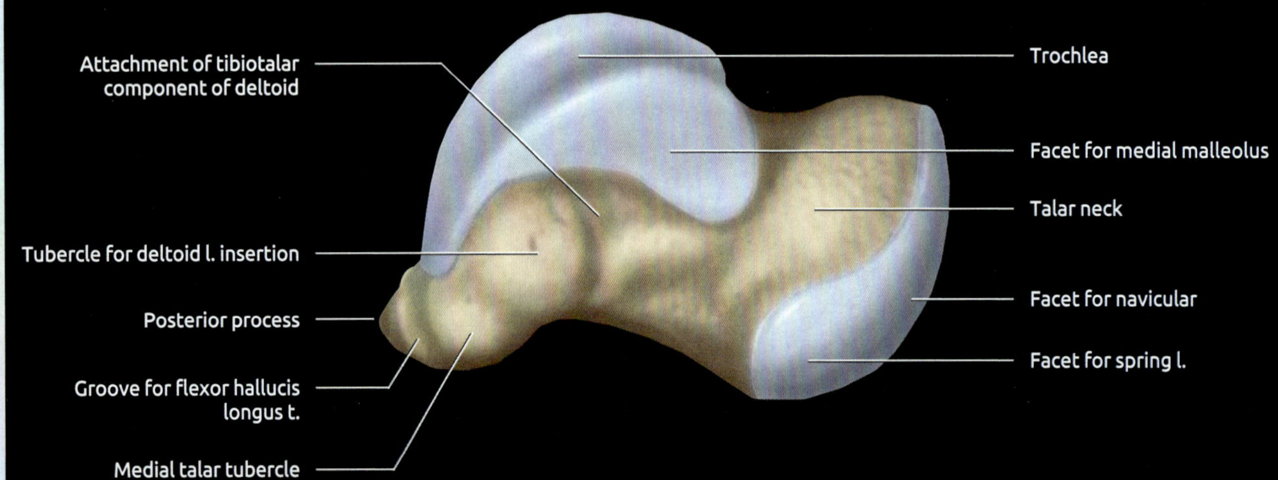

(Top) *A lateral view of the talus is shown. The talar facet for the lateral malleolus is quite large and covers most of the lateral process of the talus. The lateral facet is obliquely oriented. It is also larger and extends more posteriorly than the medial facet. When elongated, the lateral tubercle is termed a Stieda process. An os trigonum is an unfused lateral talar tubercle, which forms a synchondrosis with the posterior process of talus. The talus has no muscles or tendons attaching to it and 2/3 of its surface is covered with cartilage (blue).* **(Bottom)** *Medial view of the talus shows the short facet for the medial malleolus. The deltoid ligament inserts onto the fovea of the talus below the facet. The trochlea has a central indentation that increases and stabilizes the articular contact with the tibia.*

GRAPHICS: CALCANEUS

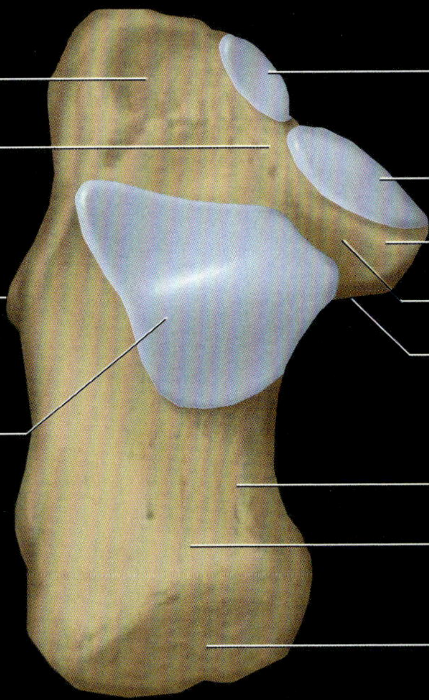

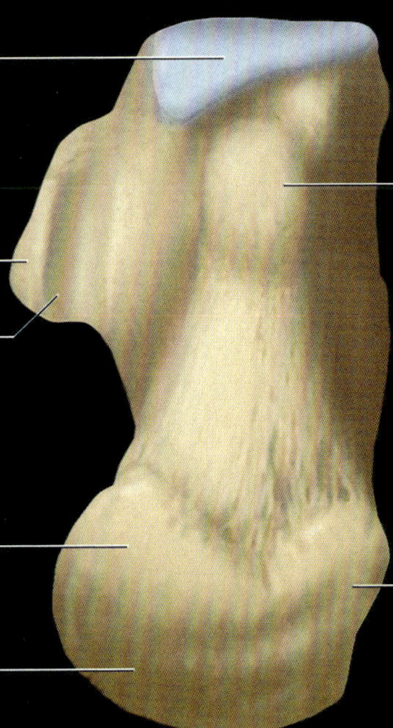

(Top) *View of the calcaneus from above is shown. The calcaneus is subdivided into anterior process, body, and tuberosity. The calcaneus articulates with the talus via 3 facets: Anterior, middle, and posterior. The anterior and middle facets are often confluent. The anterior process of the calcaneus is the site of origin of the bifurcate ligament, which inserts on the navicular and cuboid.* **(Bottom)** *Plantar view of the calcaneus is shown. The plantar calcaneus has a rough surface, especially proximally. It gives origins to the lateral, medial, and anterior tubercle (processes). These serve as attachments for the superficial layer of foot muscles and plantar ligaments. The medial tubercle is broader than the lateral tubercle. The anterior tubercle marks the distal attachment of the long plantar ligament. The flexor hallucis longus traverses in a groove along the plantar surface of the sustentaculum tali.*

GRAPHICS: CALCANEUS

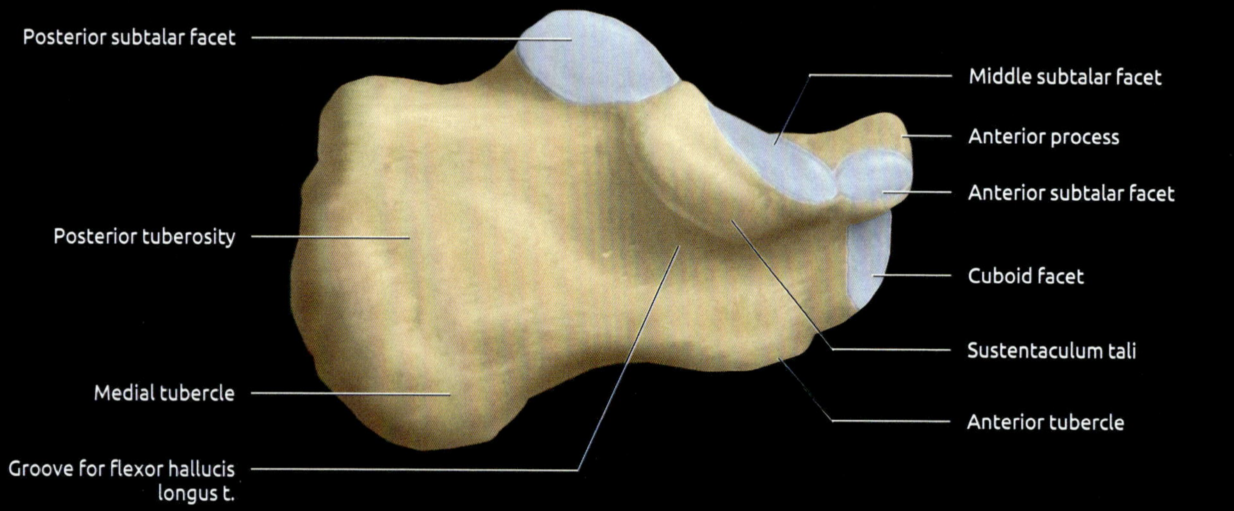

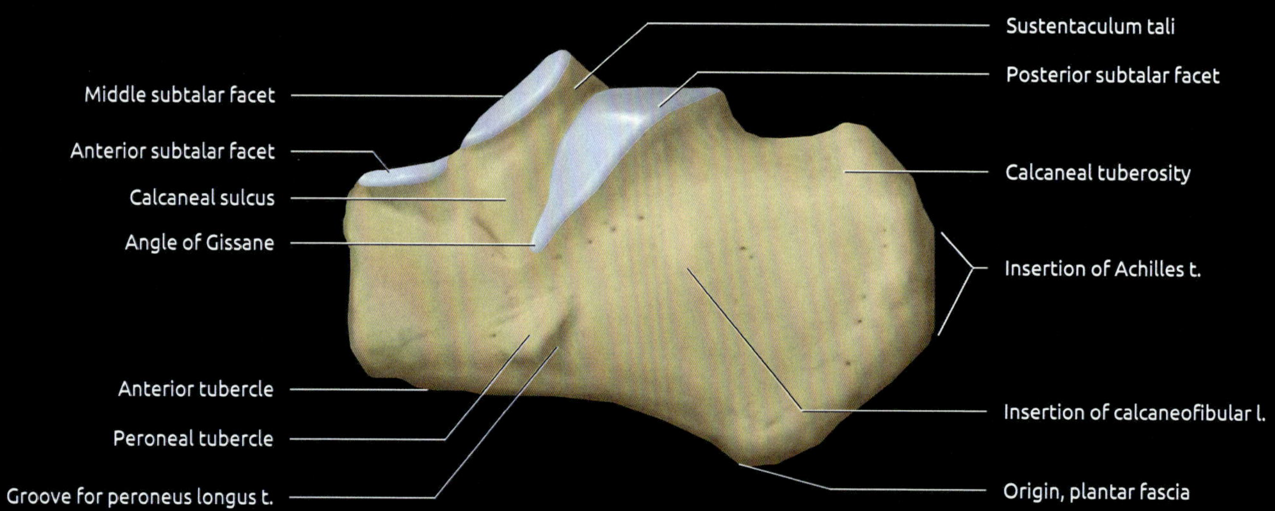

(Top) *Medial view of calcaneus is shown. The calcaneus has a medial, shelf-like process termed sustentaculum tali, which projects medially and superiorly from the upper border of the distal calcaneus. The sustentaculum tali provides medial support to the talus and has a plantar groove for the flexor hallucis longus and, less frequently, for the flexor digitorum longus tendons.* **(Bottom)** *A lateral view of the calcaneus is shown. The Achilles and plantaris tendons insert into the calcaneus at the posterior calcaneal tuberosity. The peroneal tendons descend along the lateral aspect of the calcaneus, separated from one another by the peroneal tubercle (present in 40% of people) and inferior peroneal retinaculum.*

GRAPHICS: MUSCLE ATTACHMENTS TO HINDFOOT

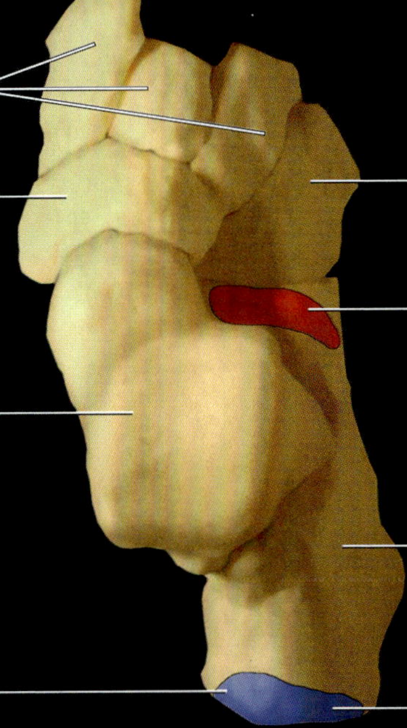

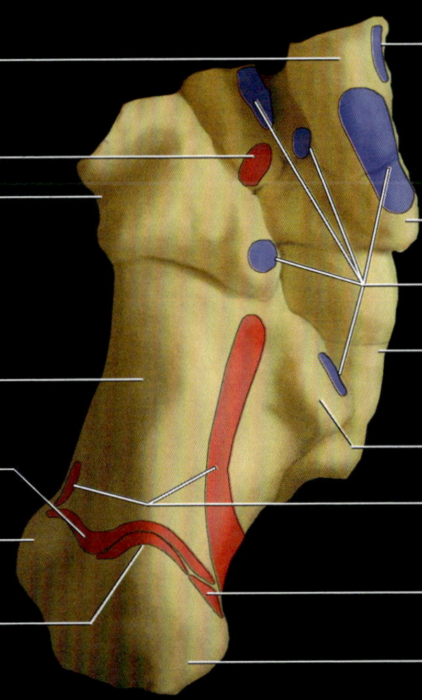

(Top) *Dorsal muscle attachments are shown. The posterior tuberosity of the calcaneus has a broad ridge, inferior to its superior posterior margin, for Achilles and plantaris tendon attachments. A retrocalcaneal bursa is interposed between the Achilles tendon and calcaneus above insertion. The extensor digitorum brevis originates from the dorsolateral aspect of the anterior process of calcaneus, just distal to the calcaneal articulation with the talus. Note that the talus has no dorsal muscular attachments.* **(Bottom)** *Plantar muscle attachments are shown. Four muscles originate from the calcaneus: Abductor hallucis from the medial tubercle, flexor digitorum brevis from the medial tubercle, and abductor digiti minimi from the medial and lateral tubercles. The quadratus plantae originates more distally via 2 heads from the medial and lateral plantar calcaneal surfaces. Note the multiple insertions of the posterior tibial (tibialis posterior) tendon. Its primary insertion is on the navicular.*

GRAPHICS: HINDFOOT LIGAMENTS

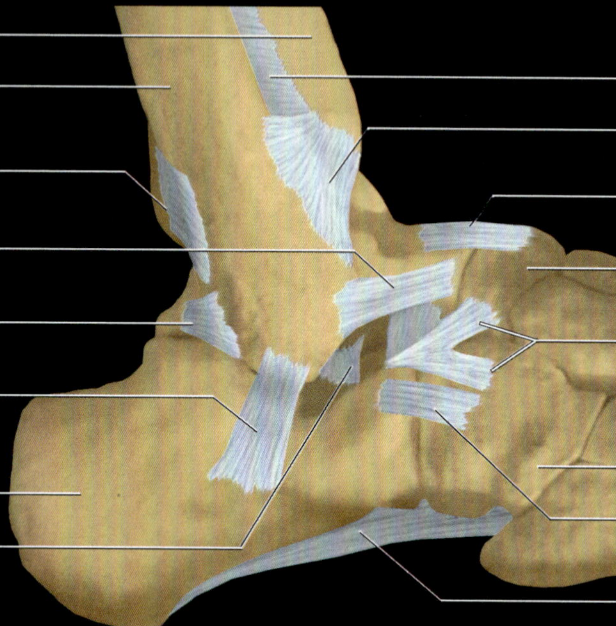

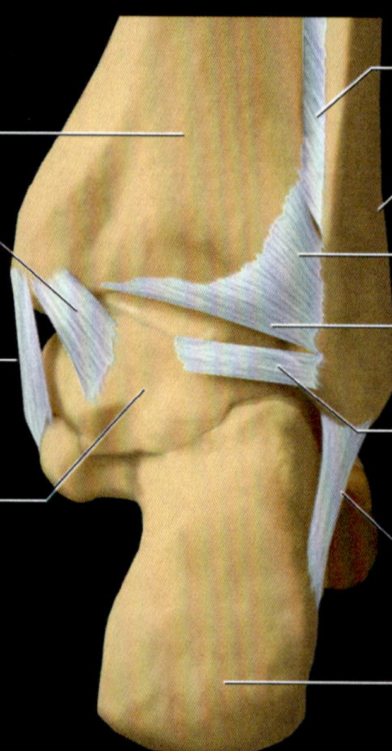

(Top) *Lateral view of the ankle is shown. Two groups of lateral ligaments support the ankle: (1) The syndesmotic ligaments, including the anterior tibiofibular, posterior tibiofibular, and syndesmotic ligaments and (2) the lateral collateral ligaments, including the anterior talofibular, posterior talofibular, and calcaneofibular ligaments. Other ligaments that bind the lateral hindfoot include the talocalcaneal ligaments, talocalcaneal interosseous ligament, and cervical ligament in the sinus tarsi. Note the bifurcate ligament, which extends from the calcaneus to the navicular and cuboid.* **(Bottom)** *Posterior view of the ankle is shown. The tibiofibular ligaments are obliquely oriented and their fibular origin is above the fibular fossa. The inferior transverse ligament, which is the inferior aspect of the posterior tibiofibular ligament, extends distal to the tibial posterior surface.*

GRAPHICS: HINDFOOT LIGAMENTS

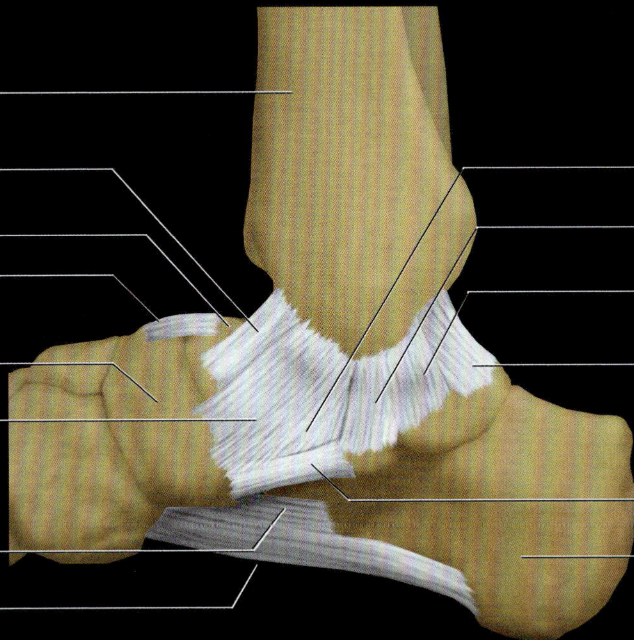

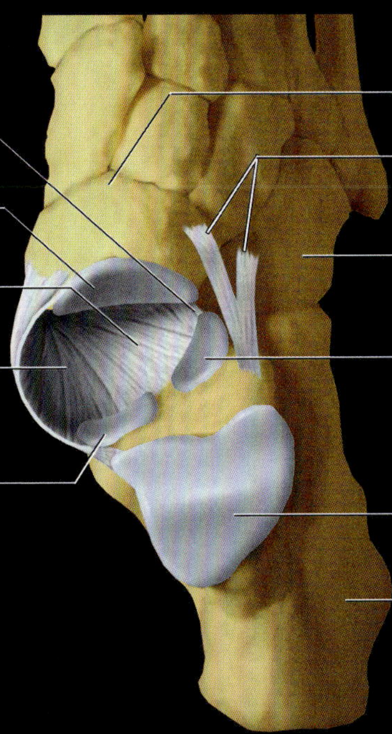

(Top) *Medial view of the ankle is shown. The deltoid ligament is the major supporter of the ankle. It has many variable components, but a commonly accepted division includes the deep anterior and posterior tibiotalar and superficial anterior and posterior tibiotalar, tibiocalcaneal, tibiospring and tibionavicular bands. Note that the superficial deltoid is band-like, and distinction between its various components relies on the sites of origins and insertions.* **(Bottom)** *Spring ligament is shown from above with the talus removed. The ligament forms a sling supporting the talar head and is composed of the superomedial, medioplantar oblique, and inferoplantar longitudinal bands. It originates from the sustentaculum tali, tibiospring, and coronoid fossa and inserts onto the plantar navicular. The bifurcate ligament originates on the anterosuperior corner of the calcaneus and inserts onto the navicular and cuboid.*

GRAPHICS: RETINACULA

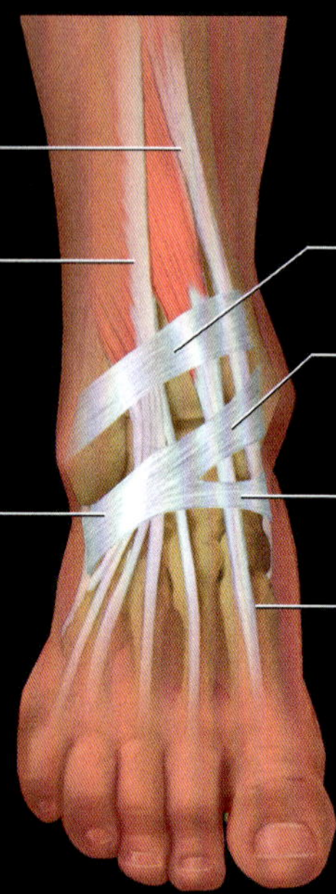

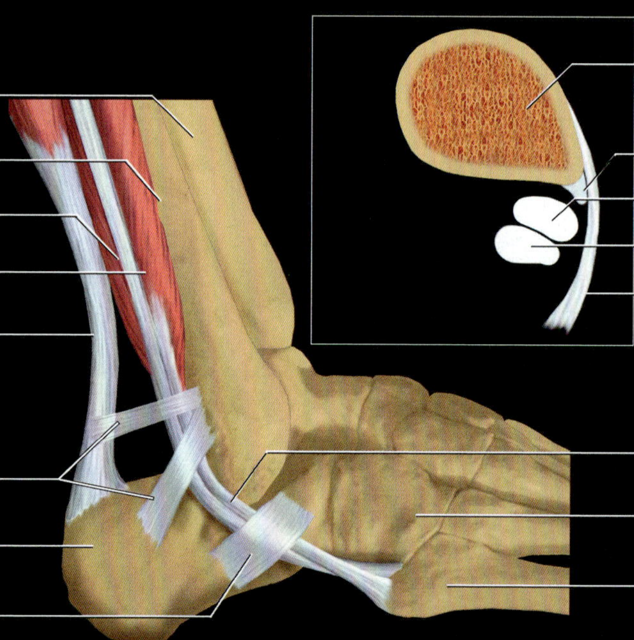

(Top) *Extensor retinacula is shown. The superior and inferior extensor retinacula loop over and bind the anterior compartment tendons. The superior extensor retinaculum is above the ankle joint. The inferior extensor retinaculum is Y-shaped and is composed of lateral stem and 2 medial limbs. The stem originates at the calcaneus, and the medial limbs attach to the medial malleolus and plantar aponeurosis.* **(Bottom)** *Peroneal retinacula is shown. The superior peroneal retinaculum holds the peroneal tendons in the retrofibular groove. The retinaculum has variable insertions but typically inserts on the deep fascia of leg and on the calcaneus. The inferior peroneal retinaculum holds the peroneal tendons against the calcaneus.*

GRAPHICS: ANKLE TENDONS

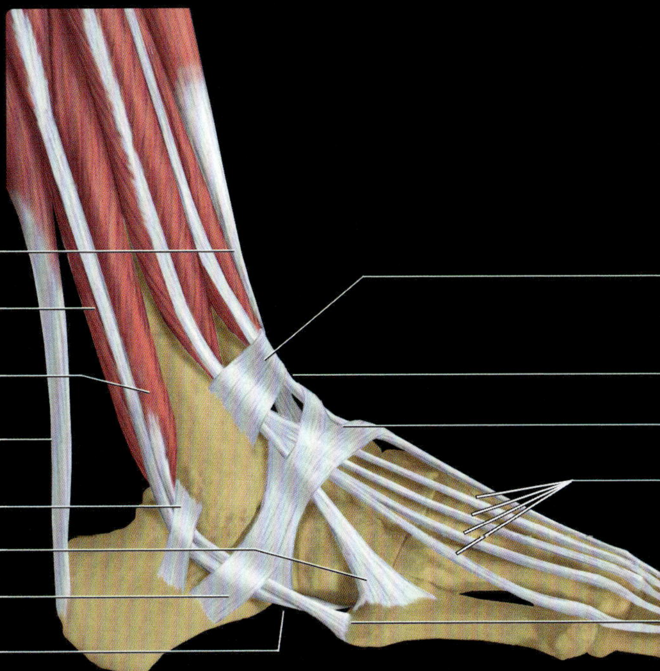

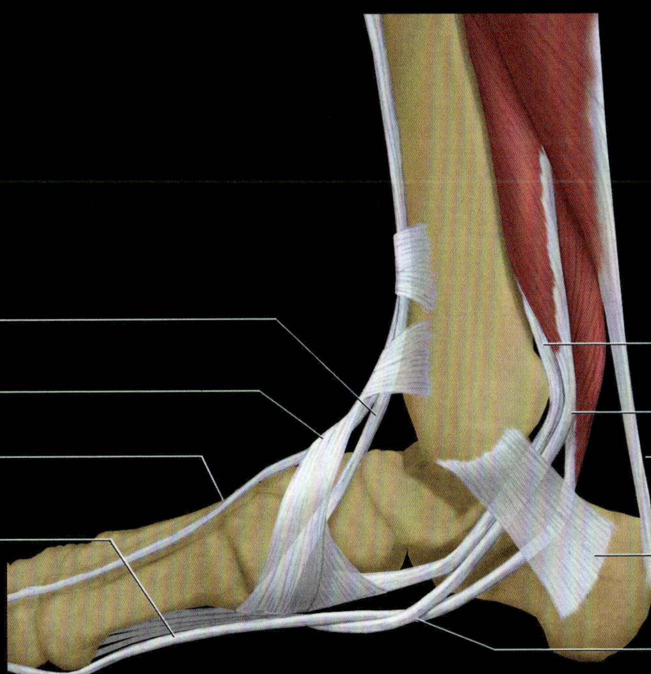

(Top) *Lateral view shows how the peroneus brevis and peroneus longus tendons descend posterior to the fibula, maintained within the retromalleolar groove by the superior peroneal retinaculum, and continue along the lateral wall of calcaneus, held in place by the inferior peroneal retinaculum. Fibers of the inferior peroneal retinaculum insert and separate the 2 tendons. The peroneus longus tendon curves around the cuboid to enter the sole of the foot. Both the peroneus brevis and peroneus tertius tendons insert on the 5th metatarsal base.* **(Bottom)** *Medial view shows the posterior tibial, flexor digitorum longus, and flexor hallucis longus tendons traversing under the flexor retinaculum within the tarsal tunnel. The flexor digitorum longus and flexor hallucis longus tendons cross each other under the navicular. The extensor tendons descend deep to the extensor retinacula.*

GRAPHICS: ANKLE NERVES

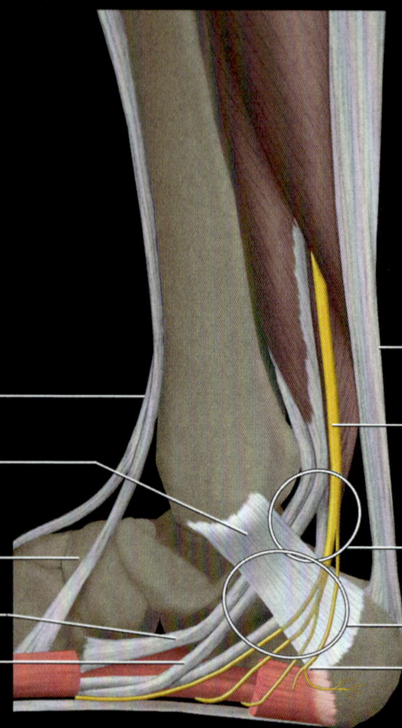

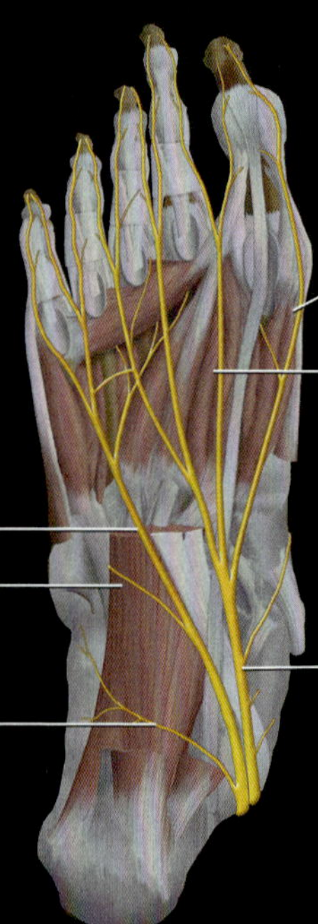

(Top) *The tarsal tunnel is traversed by the posterior tibial, flexor digitorum longus, and flexor hallucis longus tendons, tibial nerve and branches, and posterior tibial vessels (not shown). The roof of the tunnel is the flexor retinaculum, and the floor is the subjacent bones.* **(Bottom)** *The medial plantar nerve passes between the abductor hallucis and flexor digitorum brevis (removed) and supplies the abductor hallucis, flexor digitorum brevis, flexor hallucis brevis, and 1st lumbrical and provides sensation to medial 2/3 of foot. The lateral plantar nerve passes between the flexor digitorum brevis and quadratus plantae and divides into the superficial branch (divides into 2 common digital nerves) and deep branch (runs deep to flexor tendons). The latter sends a communicating branch to the 3rd digital nerve. The lateral plantar nerve supplies the quadratus plantae, abductor digiti minimi, flexor digiti minimi, adductor hallucis, 2-4 lumbricals, interossei and skin of lateral sole, 5th toe, and lateral 1/2 of 4th toe.*

GRAPHICS: ANKLE NERVES

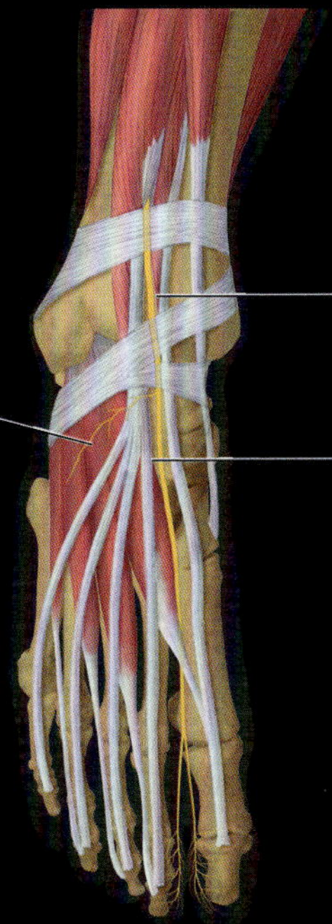

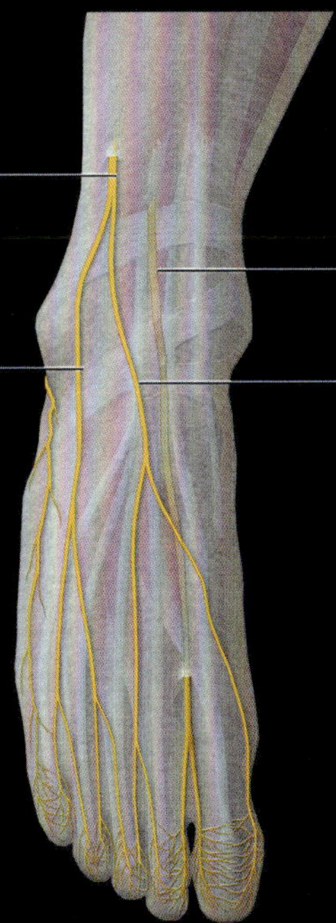

(Top) *The deep peroneal nerve travels deep to the extensor retinacula and terminates in 2 branches. The lateral branch innervates the extensor digitorum brevis muscle. It sends 3 tiny interosseous branches (not shown), which supply the tarsal and tarsometatarsal joints of the middle 3 toes; the 1st branch also supplies the 2nd dorsal interosseous. The medial branch continues dorsal to talonavicular joint, middle cuneiform, and in between the 1st and 2nd metatarsals to provide mostly sensory but some motor supply to the 1st web space.* **(Bottom)** *In the distal leg, the superficial peroneal nerve bifurcates to the medial and intermediate dorsal cutaneous nerves. The medial dorsal cutaneous nerve, via 2 dorsal digital nerves, supplies the 1st-3rd toes and communicates with the saphenous and deep peroneal nerve. The intermediate dorsal cutaneous nerve, also via digital branches, supplies 3rd-5th toes and skin of the lateral ankle and communicates with the sural nerve (not shown).*

GRAPHICS: CUTANEOUS INNERVATION

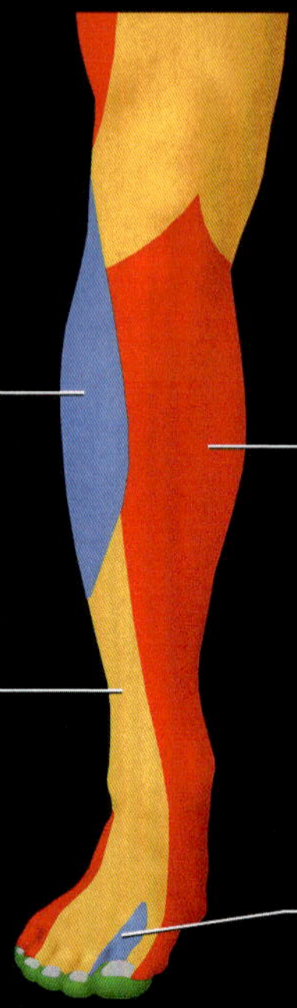

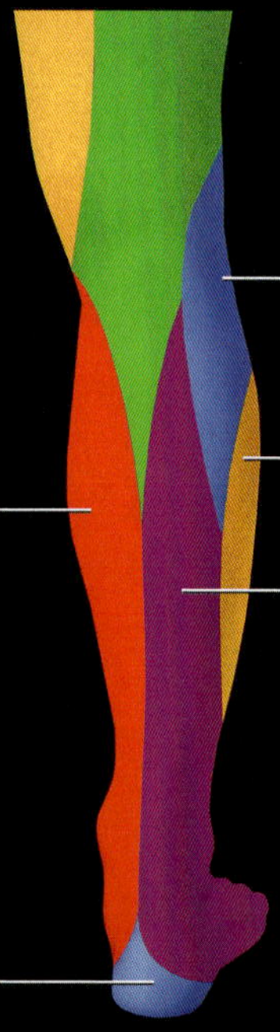

(Top) *Cutaneous innervation of the ventral (anterior) leg is shown. The upper 1/3 and lower 2/3 of the lateral anterior leg are innervated by the common and superficial peroneal nerves, respectively. The anterior medial leg is supplied by the saphenous nerve (femoral nerve branch). Most dorsal foot innervation is supplied by the superficial peroneal nerve except for the 1st web space (deep peroneal nerve), medial ankle and foot (saphenous nerve), lateral ankle and foot (sural nerve), and tips of toes (medial and lateral plantar nerves). Variations and overlap in innervation are common.* **(Bottom)** *Cutaneous innervation of the dorsal (posterior) leg is shown. The medial 1/2 of the posterior leg is supplied by the saphenous nerve (branch of femoral nerve), while the lateral 1/2 is supplied by the sural nerve (formed by a merger of branches of the tibial and common peroneal nerve). The heel is supplied by the tibial nerve. Variations and overlap in innervation are frequent phenomena.*

GRAPHICS: CUTANEOUS INNERVATION

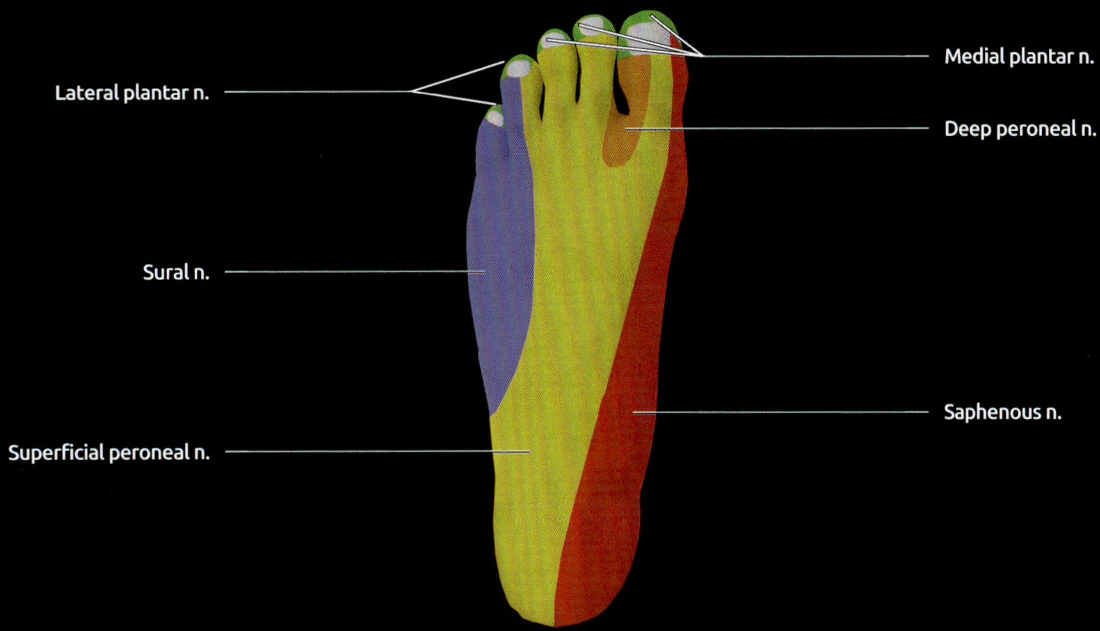

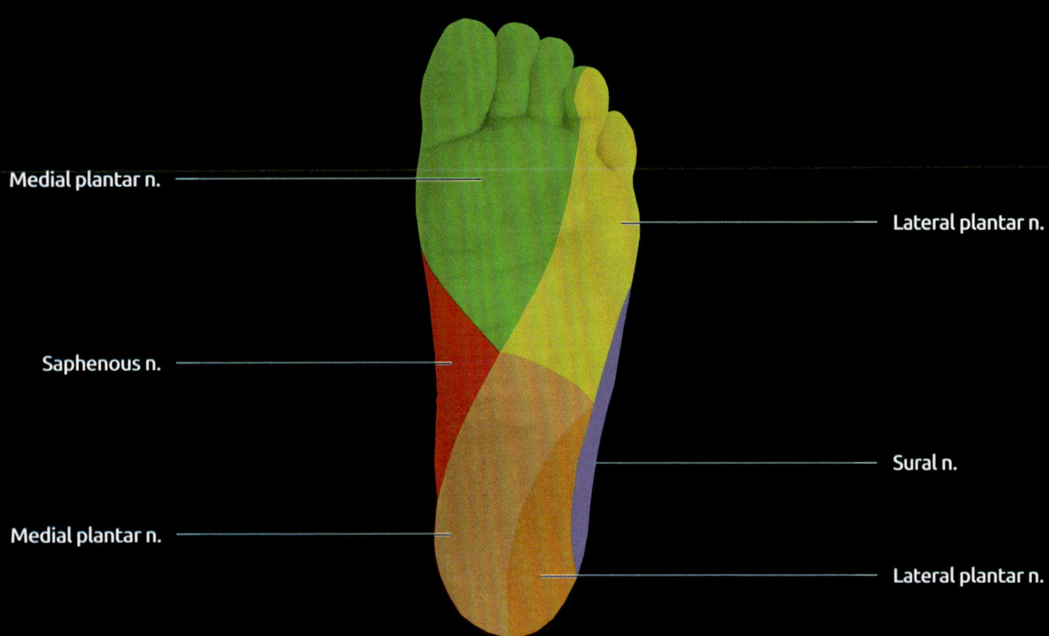

(Top) *The dorsal cutaneous innervation is provided mainly by the superficial peroneal nerve, with contributions by the deep peroneal nerve, sural nerve, and saphenous nerve. The medial and lateral plantar nerves provide dorsal innervation to the nail beds and tips of toes.* **(Bottom)** *The medial plantar nerve supplies the plantar skin of the medial 3.5 toes. The lateral plantar nerve supplies the lateral 1.5 toes. There is typically communication between the medial and lateral plantar nerves at the level of the 3rd and 4th common digital nerves. There is also plantar innervation by the sural nerve laterally and saphenous nerve medially. The skin of the heel is innervated medially by the medial calcaneal nerve (a branch of the posterior tibial nerve) and laterally by the lateral calcaneal nerve (branch of sural nerve). The lateral plantar nerve may also give rise to small branches, which pierce the plantar fascia and supply the lateral skin of the heel.*

IMAGING ANATOMY

Overview

- Images should be obtained with patient standing when possible
- Anteroposterior (AP) view of ankle
  - Obtained in same plane as AP of knee
  - Since ankle is externally rotated relative to knee, this view does not show mortise joint of ankle in profile
  - Imaging finding of correct positioning: Fovea of talus seen in profile
  - Anterior colliculus projects inferior to posterior colliculus
    - Inferior cortex of posterior colliculus seen through anterior colliculus should not be mistaken for fracture
- Mortise view of ankle
  - Ankle internally rotated 15-20°; malleoli should be same distance from film
  - Foot is dorsiflexed
    - Brings larger, anterior portion of talar trochlea into view
  - Imaging finding of correct positioning: Mortise seen in profile
  - Medial, superior, and lateral joint spaces should be equal
- Lateral view of ankle
  - Oriented to axis of hindfoot
  - Imaging findings of correct positioning
    - Medial malleolus not anterior to tibial plafond
    - Fibula at posterior 1/3 of tibial plafond
    - 2 sides of talar trochlea superimposed
- Inversion stress view
  - Talar trochlea may tilt into 5° of varus normally
  - Bilateral symmetry useful
- Eversion or external rotation stress view
  - Loss of congruity of medial ankle gutter is abnormal
- Gravity stress view
  - Patient lies in lateral decubitus position, affected side down
  - Pillow under knee, leg beyond end of table
  - Imaging cassette placed posterior to ankle
  - Image obtained from anterior to posterior (cross-table AP)
  - Reportedly equal in accuracy to manual stress view
- Lateral stress view
  - Lateral view with anterior stress applied
  - Evaluates for anterior subluxation of talus (anterior drawer sign)
- Broden view
  - Evaluation of posterior subtalar joint
  - Ankle in 45° internal rotation
- Os calcis (tangential calcaneal) views
  - May be obtained supine or standing
  - Standing: Patient stands on cassette, leg bent forward, beam angled 45° anteriorly to plantar surface of foot
  - Supine: Cassette posterior to ankle, patient dorsiflexes foot, beam angled 45° cephalad from plantar surface of foot
- Hindfoot alignment view
  - Patient standing, foot straight forward, toes at imaging cassette
  - Imaging cassette 20° from vertical, top margin away from patient's toes
  - X-ray tube parallel to imaging cassette
  - Lead strip at back of heel, perpendicular to axis of foot
  - Normal: Axis of tibia falls within 8 mm of most inferior point on calcaneus

ANATOMY IMAGING ISSUES

Imaging Pitfalls

- Poorly positioned mortise view may mimic syndesmotic injury
  - Useful guideline: If medial body of talus overlaps medial malleolus of tibia, exam is overly rotated and cannot accurately measure overlap of tibia and fibula
- Stress views are often false-negative for instability unless performed under anesthesia

Arthrography

- Anterior approach to ankle
- Patient may be in supine or lateral decubitus position
  - Lateral decubitus position aids in visualization of anterior lip of tibia
  - Useful if lacking C-arm to allow cross-table lateral imaging
- Needle between anterior tibial tendon and extensor hallucis longus tendons
- Start needle trajectory slightly distal to ankle join line, angle cephalad
  - Allows needle to extend under dorsal lip of tibia
- Contrast should flow away from needle, fill anterior and posterior joint spaces
- Air can be used as contrast agent for therapeutic injections
- MR arthrogram: Gadolinium contrast diluted 1:200 with lidocaine, bupivacaine, iodinated contrast, and normal saline
- 15% of patients have communication with posterior subtalar joint
- Flexor hallucis longus normally communicates with ankle joint, may or may not fill with contrast
- Abnormal extension of contrast used as sign of ligament tear
  - Contrast around peroneal tendons indicates calcaneofibular ligament tear
  - Contrast along lateral talar neck indicates anterior talofibular ligament tear
  - Contrast along posterior tibial tendon sheath indicates superficial deltoid ligament detachment and detachment of medial periosteum

SELECTED REFERENCES

1. Golanó P et al: Ankle anatomy for the arthroscopist. Part II: role of the ankle ligaments in soft tissue impingement. Foot Ankle Clin. 11(2):275-96, v-vi, 2006
2. Oh CS et al: Anatomic variations and MRI of the intermalleolar ligament. AJR Am J Roentgenol. 186(4):943-7, 2006
3. Bartonícek J: Anatomy of the tibiofibular syndesmosis and its clinical relevance. Surg Radiol Anat. 25(5-6):379-86, 2003
4. Lee SH et al: Ligaments of the ankle: normal anatomy with MR arthrography. J Comput Assist Tomogr. 22(5):807-13, 1998
5. Burks RT et al: Anatomy of the lateral ankle ligaments. Am J Sports Med. 22(1):72-7, 1994

RADIOGRAPHS: ANKLE

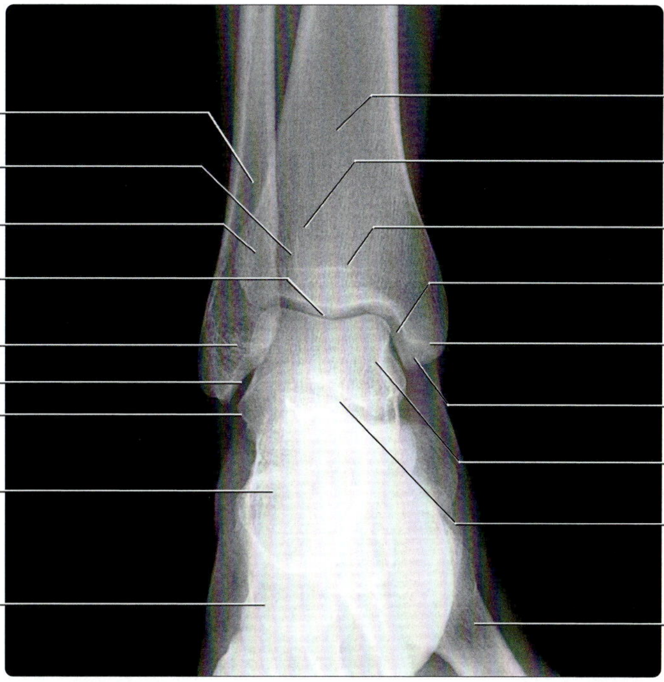

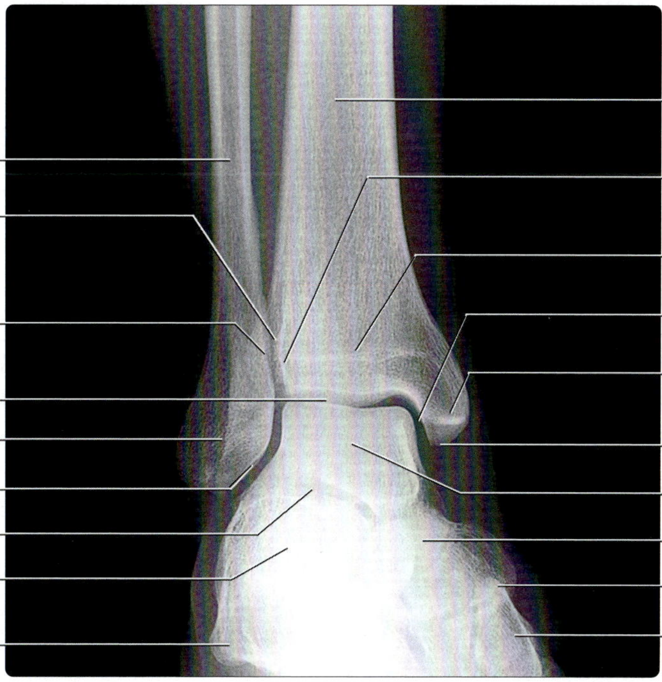

(Top) *Routine non-weight-bearing AP view of the ankle is obtained with the patient supine, the heel on the cassette and the toes pointed upward. The x-ray beam is directed at the center of the ankle joint. The talus overlaps the distal fibula obscuring the lateral ankle mortise. Note that the anterior margin of the fibular groove extends further laterally compared to the posterior margin. Similarly, the anterior colliculus of the medial malleolus extends more distally than the posterior colliculus.* **(Bottom)** *Non-weight-bearing ankle mortise view (oblique) is obtained with the patient supine and the foot internally rotated until the medial and lateral malleoli are equidistant from the cassette. The lateral ankle mortise is now visualized. The talus should be equidistant from the tibial plafond on both the AP and ankle mortise views.*

RADIOGRAPHS: ANKLE

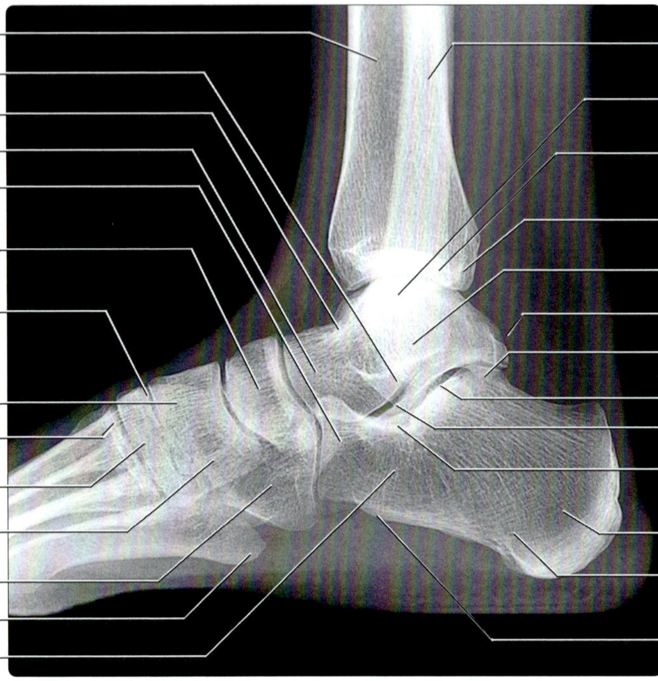

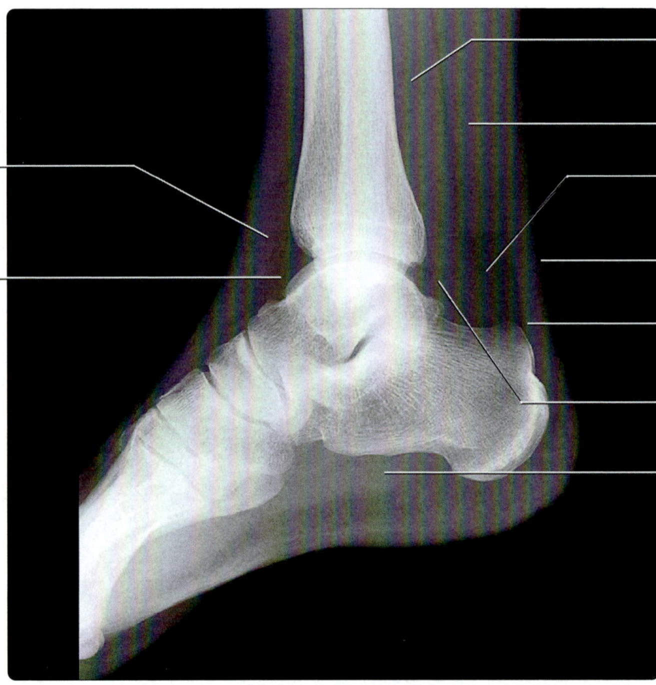

(Top) *Non-weight-bearing lateral view of the ankle depicts both the calcaneus and talus in profile. The posterior, medial, and lateral malleoli are superimposed over one another and over the talus, potentially obscuring fractures at those locations. The lateral view should include the base of the 5th metatarsal. The middle subtalar facet should be seen in tangent on any view which also shows the posterior subtalar facet in tangent.* **(Bottom)** *The soft tissues of the ankle are emphasized on this lateral view. The Achilles tendon should be uniform in diameter and sharply demarcated. It is separated from the deep flexors by the pre-Achilles fat pad. A small retrocalcaneal fat pad, location of retrocalcaneal bursa, is found between the tendon & calcaneus. Anterior displacement of the small fat pad anterior to the anterior joint line is consistent with joint effusion. Flexor hallucis longus muscle posterior to the ankle should not be mistaken for a joint effusion.*

RADIOGRAPHS: ANKLE

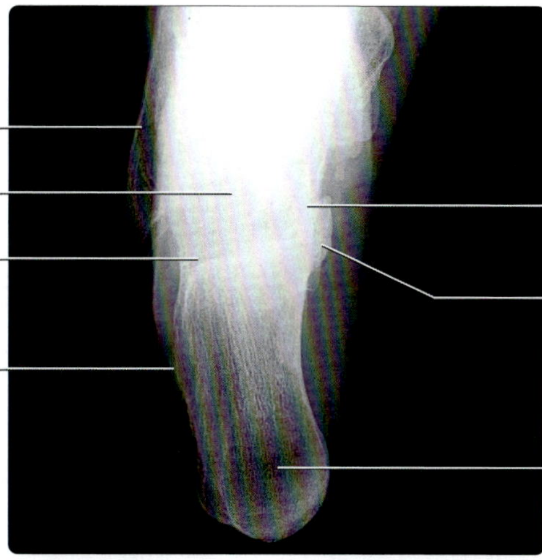

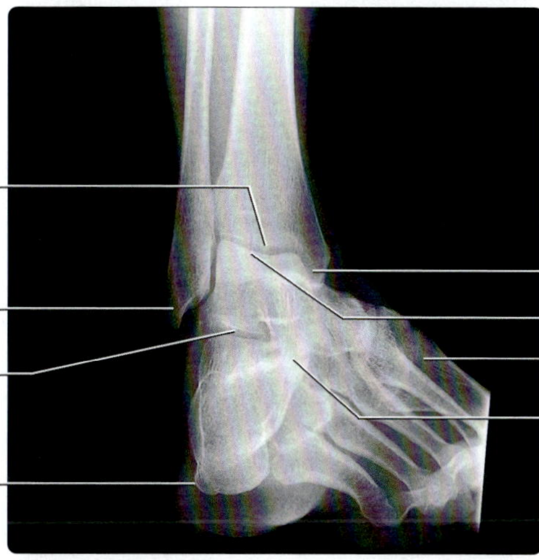

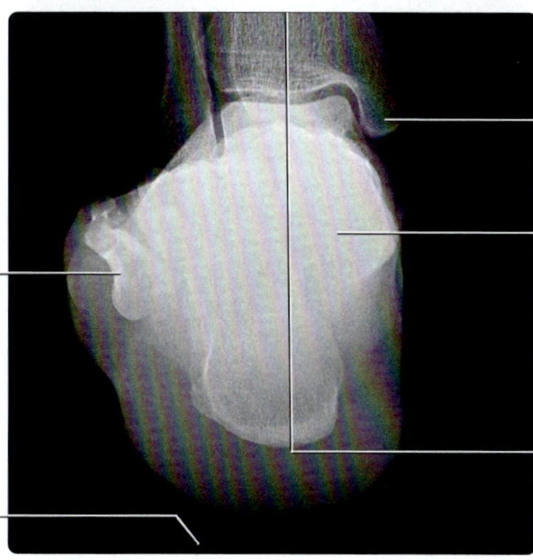

(Top) *The calcaneus (Harris) view is obtained with the patient supine or standing and the foot in maximum dorsiflexion. The view depicts the middle and posterior subtalar joints.* **(Middle)** *Broden views are obtained with the patient supine, foot in 45° of internal rotation and 10°, 20°, 30°, and 40° of tube angulation. The views afford visualization of the posterior subtalar joint but have become somewhat obsolete as computed tomography is used more frequently for problem solving in the ankle.* **(Bottom)** *Hindfoot alignment view assesses the relative position of the most inferior portion of the posterior calcaneal process relative to the axis of the tibia, measured as shown above. The most inferior portion of the calcaneal posterior process should lie within 8 mm from the tibial axis.*

ARTHROGRAPHIC ANATOMY: ANKLE

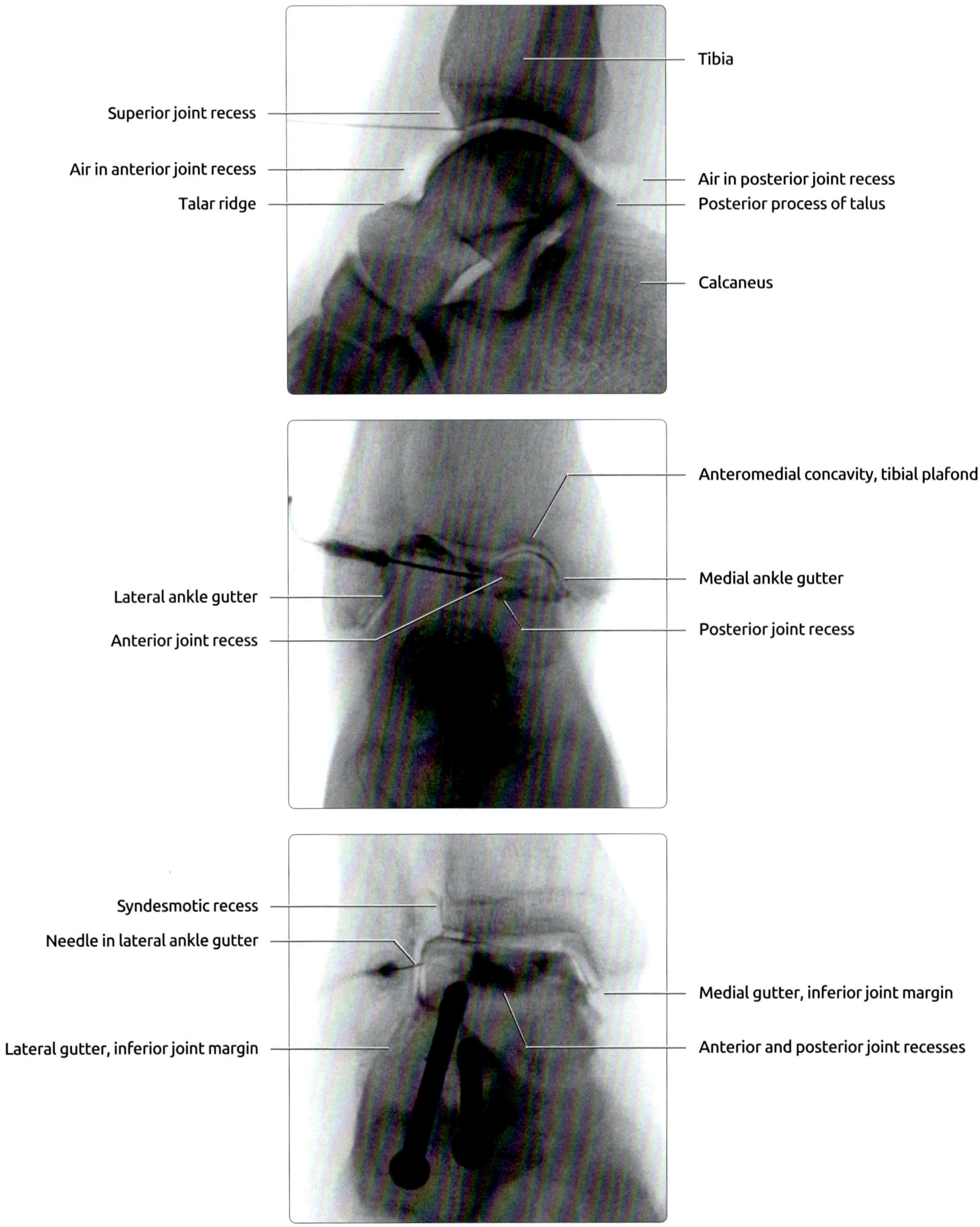

(Top) *Lateral ankle air arthrogram shows normal contour of the ankle joint with the anterior recess extending to talar ridge and the posterior recess extending posterior to the posterior process of talus. Anteriorly, a superior recess extends slightly above the joint line. Air is useful for therapeutic arthrograms as it avoids the joint irritation and allergic reaction, which can be seen with use of iodinated contrast.* **(Middle)** *AP ankle arthrogram shows the normal extent of filling of medial and lateral joint gutters. The medial gutter does not fill completely due to the presence of the deep deltoid ligament.* **(Bottom)** *Mortise view arthrogram shows a normal ankle joint in a patient who had prior subtalar fusion. Approach in this case was via the lateral ankle gutter.*

AXIAL MR ARTHROGRAM: ANKLE

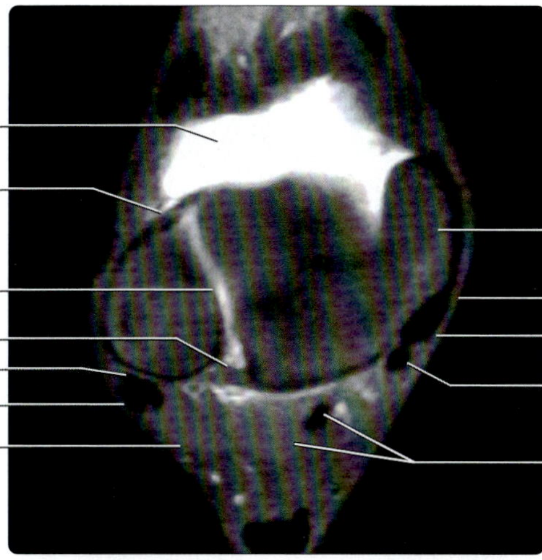

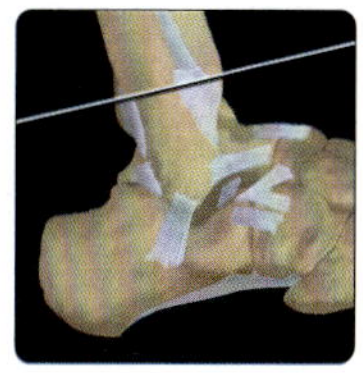

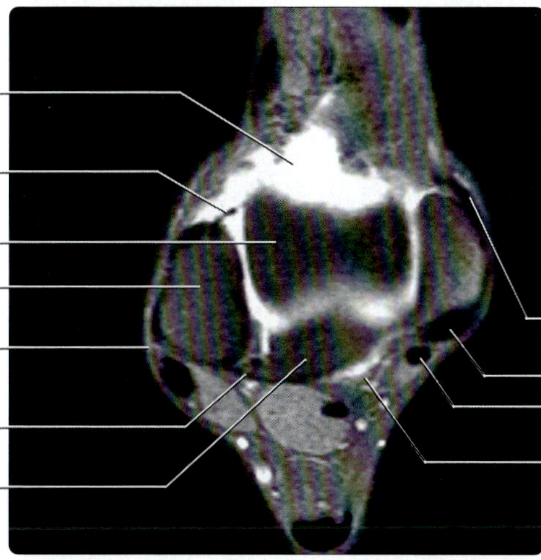

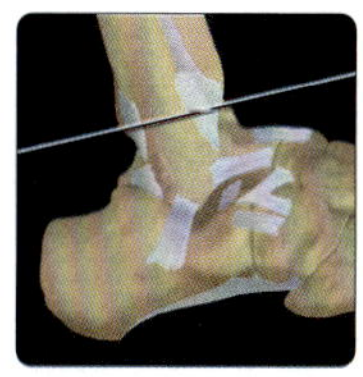

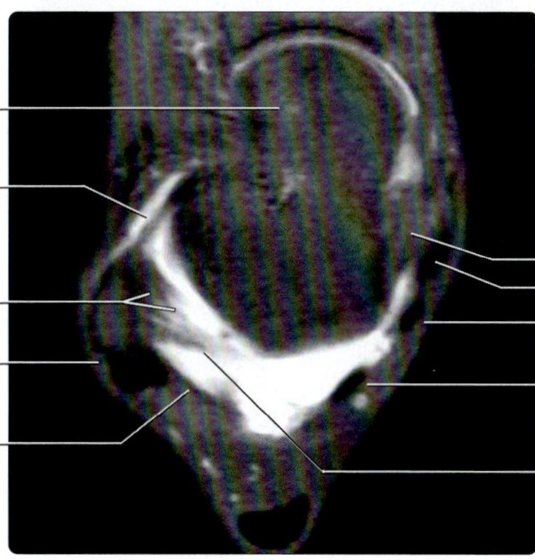

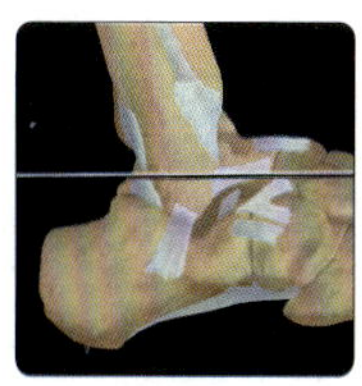

(Top) *Selected axial T1WI FS MR arthrograms from different patients through the ankle joint are arranged from superior to inferior. At the level of the tibial plafond, axial image shows the anterior and posterior ligaments. Fluid extends between the tibia and fibula ~ 1 cm cephalad to the plafond in normal syndesmotic recess. Note the rounded anterior joint recess, which extends ~ 5-10 mm above the plafond.* **(Middle)** *At the level of the talar dome, the accessory tibiotalar ligament (Bassett ligament) is seen arising from the fibula. It courses superiorly and medially and inserts on the anterolateral corner of the tibial plafond.* **(Bottom)** *At the superior margin of the talar neck, the anterior talofibular ligament is seen attaching to the anterolateral corner of the talar body. The posterior talofibular ligament is much broader and thicker than the anterior talofibular ligament. It has a fan-shaped appearance with striations similar to those seen in the anterior cruciate ligament.*

AXIAL MR ARTHROGRAM: ANKLE

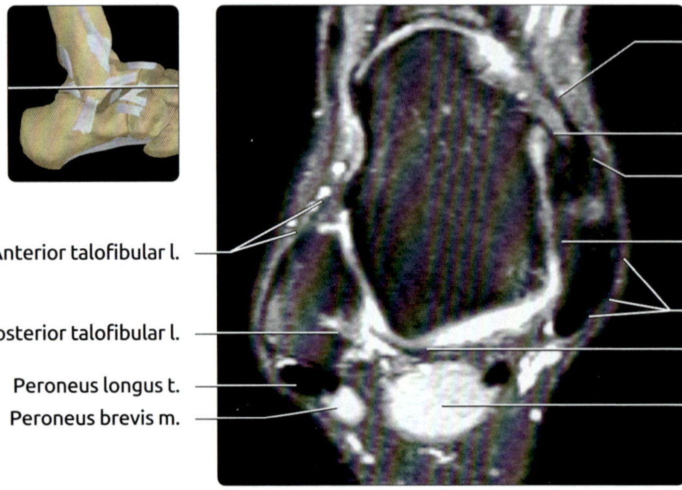

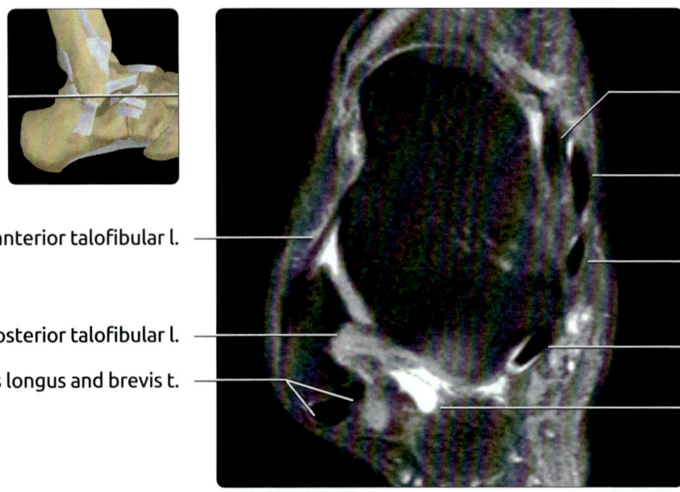

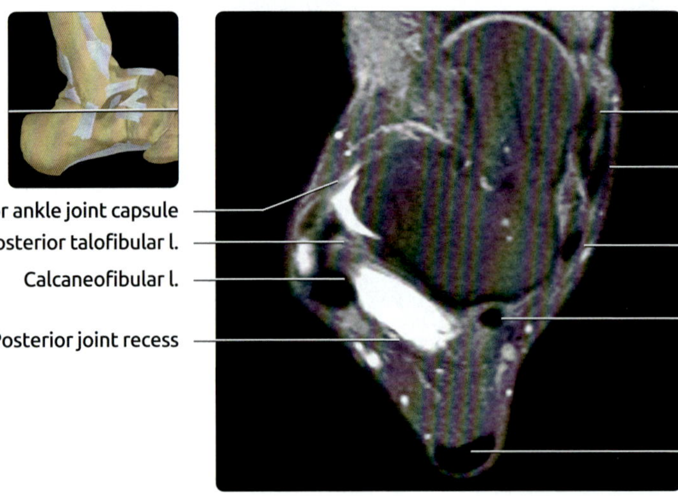

(Top) *Deltoid ligament bands are named for attachments. Deep anterior tibiotalar ligament attaches to the small bony prominence at the midtalar neck. The tibionavicular ligament attaches to the medial eminence of the navicular. Note that the anterior talofibular ligament in this patient is thin and redundant, consistent with prior injury.* **(Middle)** *The accessory anterior talofibular ligament is inferior to the main portion of the ligament and appears continuous with it on MR. Anterior deltoid fibers course deep to the posterior tibial tendon.* **(Bottom)** *At the level of the fibular tip, the calcaneofibular ligament is seen extending posteriorly and inferiorly deep to the peroneal tendons. In this patient, the posterior joint recess was continuous with the subtalar joint. This image shows the anterior lateral joint capsule inferior to the anterior talofibular ligament.*

SAGITTAL MR ARTHROGRAM: ANKLE

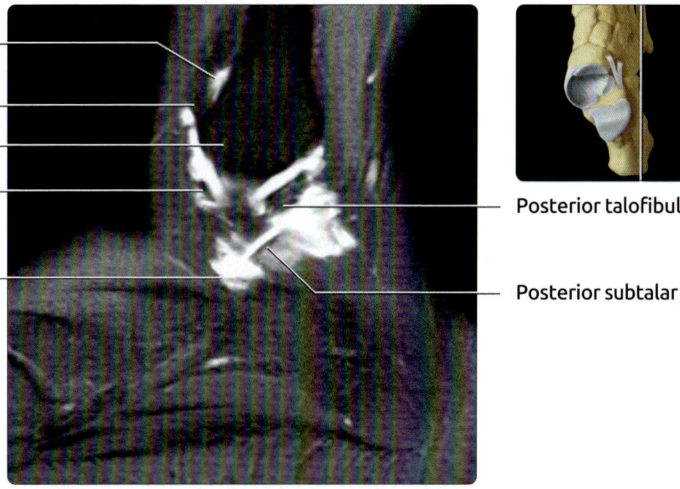

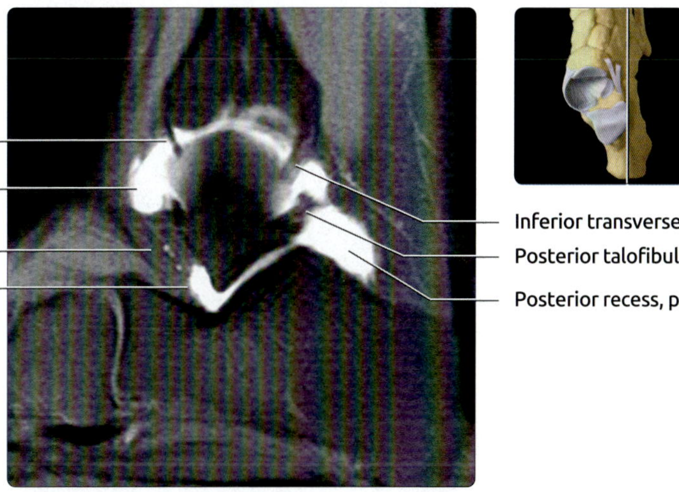

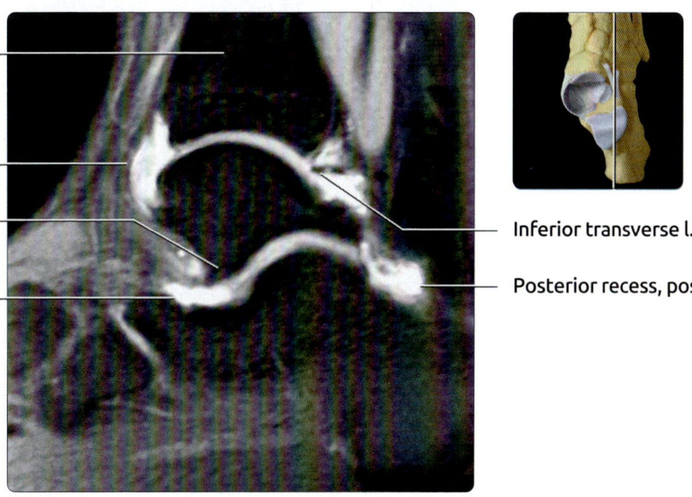

(Top) *Selected sagittal T1WI FS MR arthrograms from different patients were taken through the ankle joint from lateral to medial. On the far lateral image, collateral ligaments are outlined by distended joint recesses. Subtalar joint filling is a normal variant.* **(Middle)** *The oblique course of the Bassett ligament, the accessory anterior tibiofibular ligament inferior to main anterior tibiofibular ligament, is well seen on this image. Note also the oblique course of the inferior transverse ligament.* **(Bottom)** *Inferior transverse ligament forms meniscoid structure; in cross section, it may mimic a loose body.*

SAGITTAL MR ARTHROGRAM: ANKLE

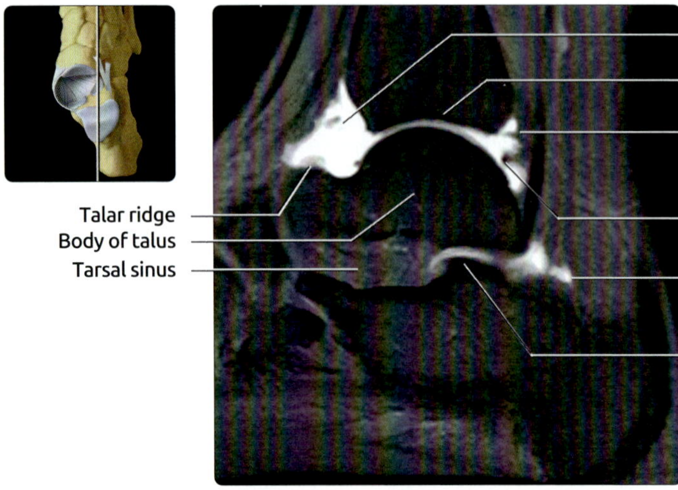

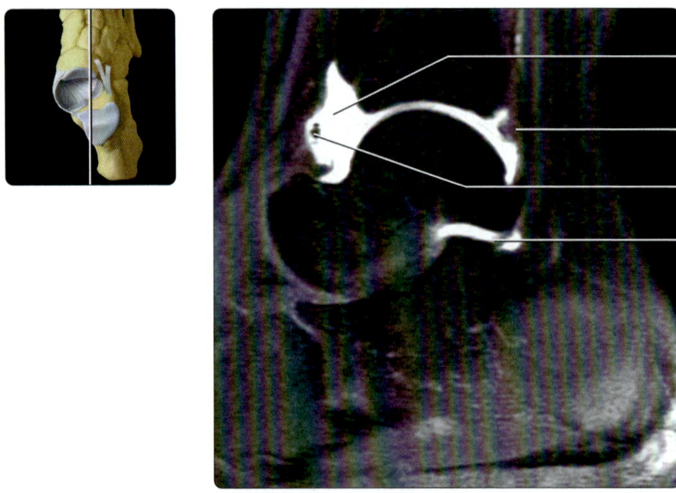

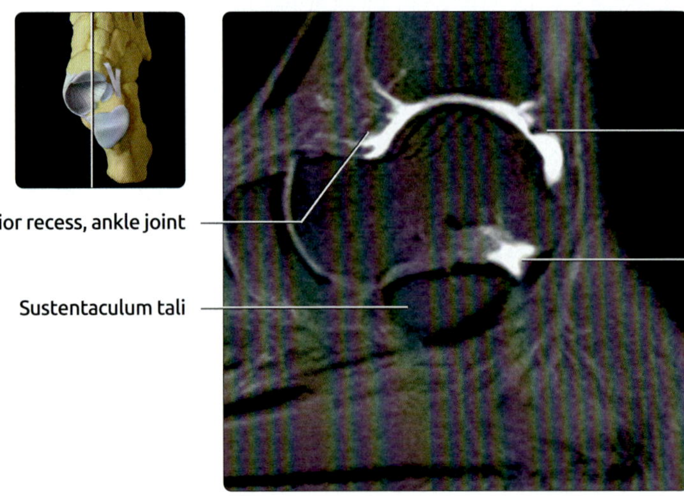

(Top) *The anterior joint recess is large, allowing for a wide range of motion.* **(Middle)** *The anterior tibial attachment of the joint capsule in this patient is slightly high compared to average; some variability should be expected. Distally, the joint capsule attaches to the talar ridge at the junction of the talar neck and head. Air bubble is iatrogenic, introduced at time of arthrography.* **(Bottom)** *At the medial aspect of the ankle joint, the inferior transverse ligament is approaching the tibia. The posterior inferior tibiofibular ligament has already inserted and is no longer visible.*

CORONAL MR ARTHROGRAM: ANKLE

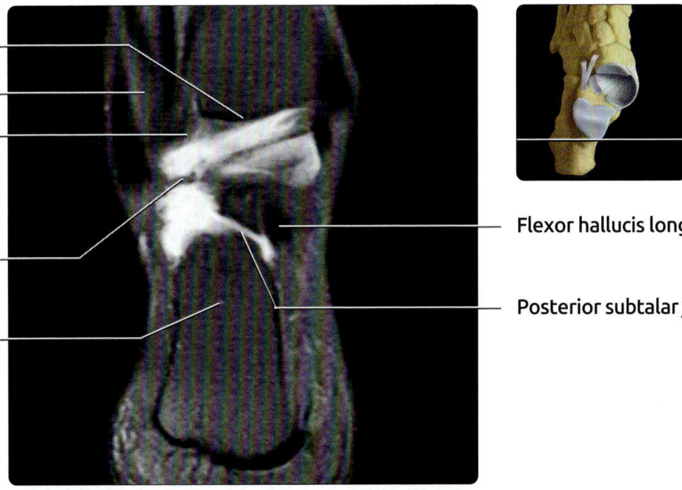

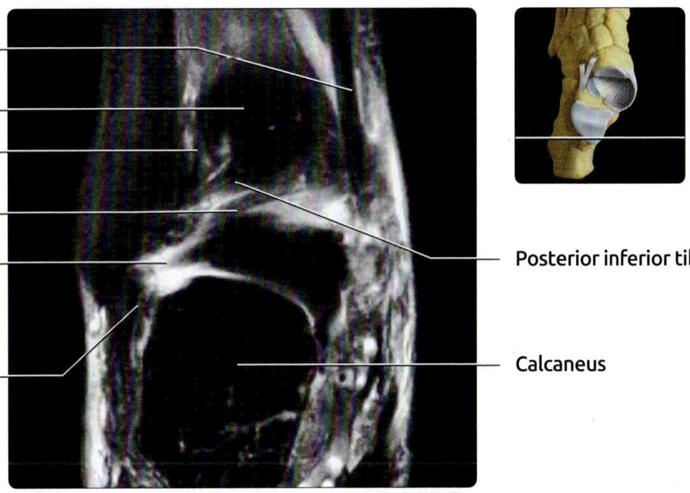

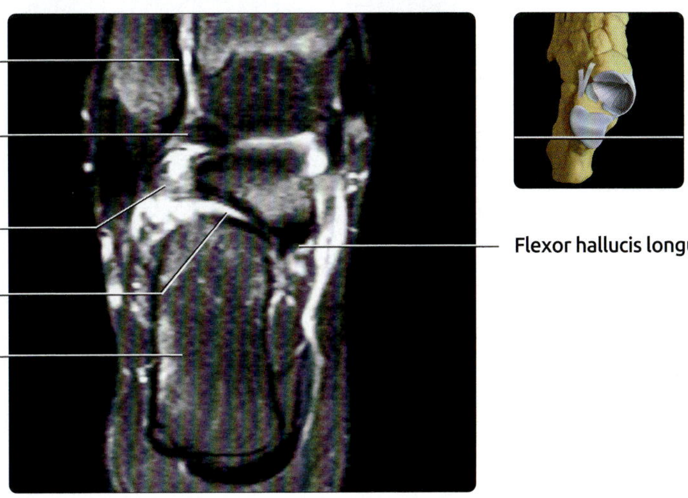

(Top) *Selected coronal T1WI FS MR arthrograms from different patients show the ankle joint from posterior to anterior. The posterior inferior tibiofibular ligament extends from the posterior malleolus and lateral aspect of the tibia to the fibula, at the level of the plafond. The inferior transverse (intermalleolar) ligament is more inferior and extends from the medial margin of the posterior tibia to the fibula, forming a labrum-like structure across the joint.* **(Middle)** *Slightly more anteriorly, portions of the posterior tibiofibular ligament are visible, and the posterior talofibular ligament comes into view inferior to tibiofibular ligaments.* **(Bottom)** *This young, skeletally immature soccer player has an unusually large syndesmotic recess, which may reflect old trauma, but was asymptomatic at time of examination. Although anatomy books usually state the recess is < 1 cm in superoinferior dimension, greater extension proximally is a common incidental finding.*

CORONAL MR ARTHROGRAM: ANKLE

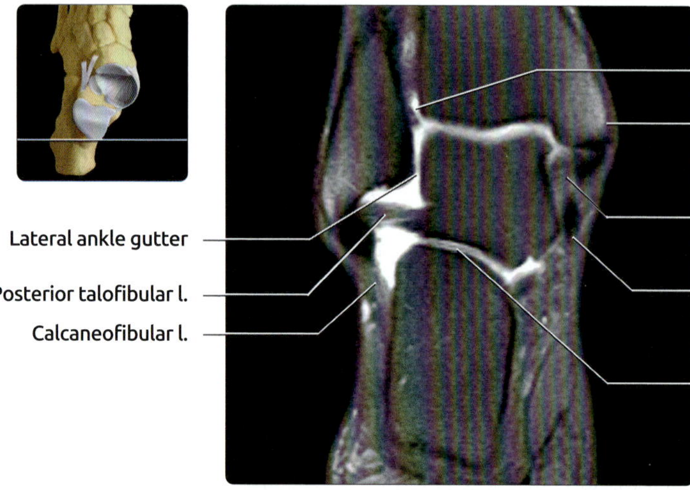

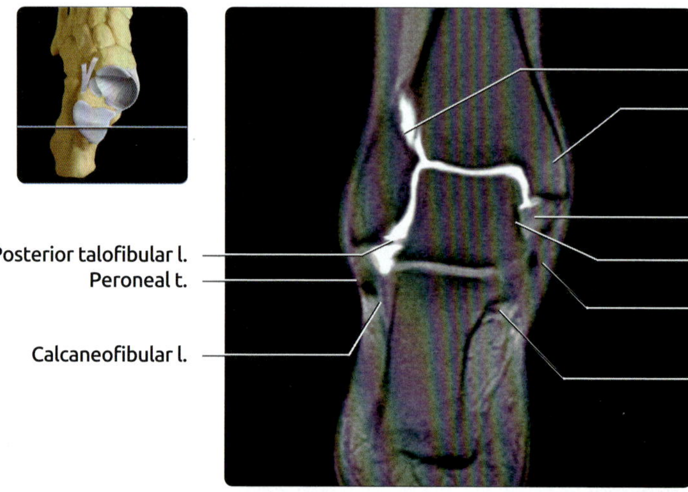

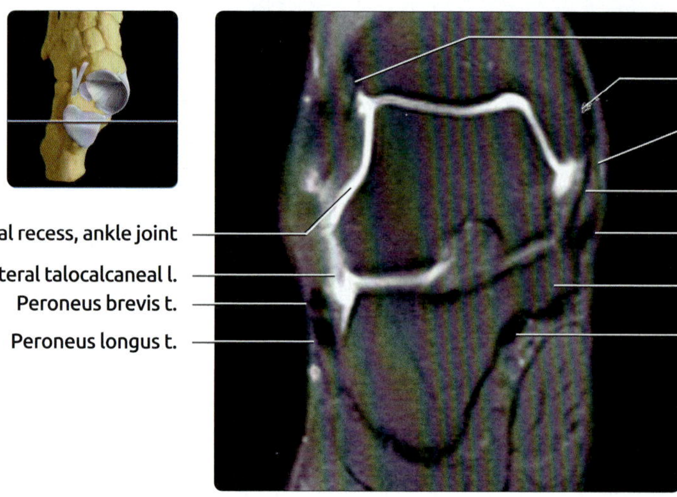

(Top) *Posterior deep fibers of the deltoid ligament arise primarily from the posterior surface of the anterior colliculus of the medial malleolus and also from the posterior colliculus. The fibers travel slightly inferiorly to insert on the concavity at the medial aspect of the body of the talus. Contrast deep to calcaneofibular ligament has extended from the subtalar joint. The lateral ankle gutter is often called the lateral "clear space."* **(Middle)** *Note normal contrast filling of the medial and lateral ankle gutters. This outlines the full extent of hyaline cartilage investing articular surfaces. The entire lateral surface of the talar body is covered by cartilage. The cartilage on the medial surface ends at the fovea for the insertion of the deep deltoid ligament.* **(Bottom)** *Anterior bands of superficial deltoid ligament diverge at the level of the anterior colliculus of the medial malleolus. The syndesmotic ligaments are variably designated. Some authors would call the ligament labelled as anterior inferior tibiofibular ligament simply the "anterior tibiofibular ligament."*

CORONAL MR ARTHROGRAM: ANKLE

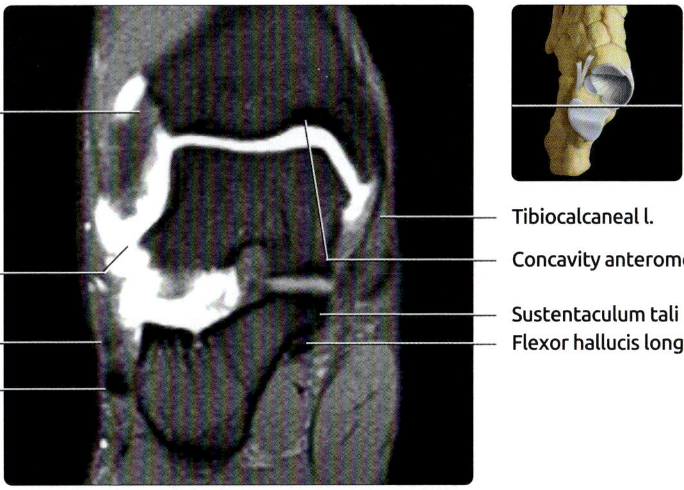

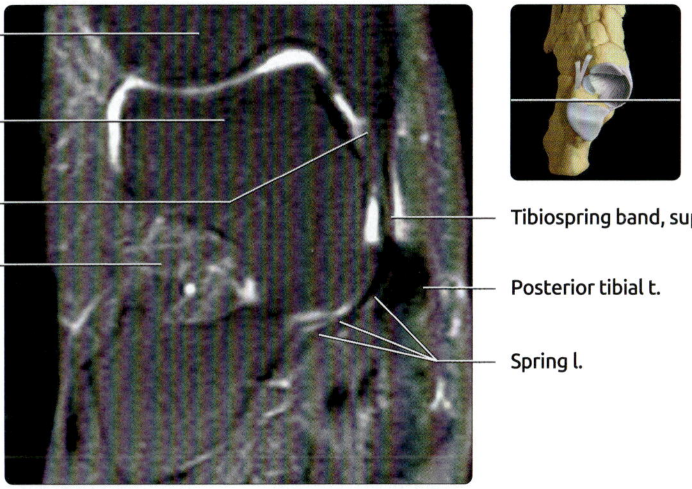

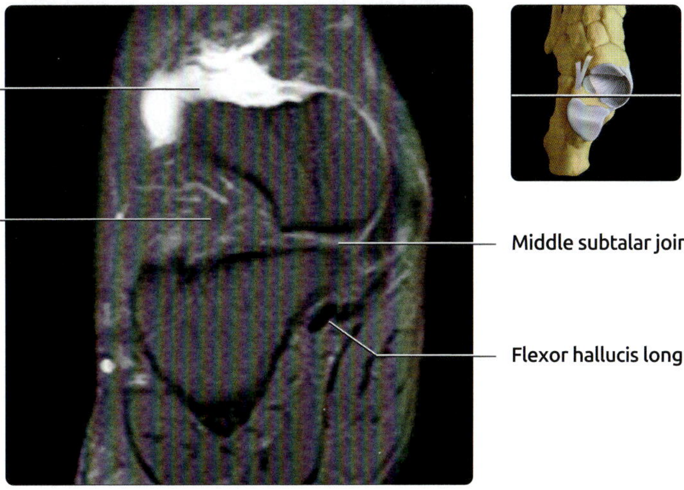

(Top) *The entire oblique course of the anterior tibiofibular ligament is unusually well seen in this patient. The anterolateral joint recess is larger than normal, reflecting an old anterior talofibular ligament injury. The anteromedial portion of the tibial plafond forms a bowl-shaped concavity, which is covered with cartilage.* **(Middle)** *The anterior deep tibiotalar ligament inserts on the proximal talar neck, while the tibiospring ligament superficial to it is continuous with the spring ligament.* **(Bottom)** *The anterior recess of the talar joint ends at the talar neck. The anterior superficial deltoid fibers continue anteriorly to insert on the spring ligament, talar neck, and median eminence of the navicular.*

IMAGING ANATOMY

Anatomy Relationships

- Anatomy of joint capsules
  - Ankle joint capsule communicates with flexor hallucis longus tendon sheath
  - Posterior subtalar joint has separate joint capsule
    - 10-15% of cases show continuity with ankle joint capsule
  - Middle, anterior subtalar joint share joint capsule with talonavicular joint
    - Sometimes called talocalcaneonavicular joint
- Deep and superficial deltoid components have different functions
  - Deep deltoid ligament protects against eversion
  - Superficial deltoid ligament protects against twisting injury

Patient Positioning

- Axial imaging may be performed in straight axial position (continuation of plane of leg)
  - Foot is usually plantar flexed when patient is lying comfortably in MR scanner
  - Straight axial imaging results in oblique images through hindfoot
- May angle axial images along axis of talus
  - Same orientation as for axial MR of foot
  - Distal tibia and fibula will be seen at slightly oblique angle
- Choose angle of slices based on area of concern
  - Straight axial: To evaluate distal tibia or Achilles tendon
  - Angled axial: To evaluate remainder of hindfoot
- Coronal imaging has similar issues
  - Usually best to angle perpendicular to axis of talus

Structures Optimally Seen in Axial Plane

- Anterior talofibular ligament (ATFL) reliably evaluated only in this plane
  - Fibular attachment: 1 cm above fibular tip
  - Talar attachment: Most superior image (or next image), which includes talar neck
- Calcaneofibular ligament
  - Majority of ligament well seen
  - Fibular attachment to inferior border of fibular tip is not visible in axial plane
- Extrinsic tendons of ankle and foot
  - Achilles tendon should have concave margin anteriorly
  - Posterior tibial tendon should be 2x size of flexor digitorum longus
- Ankle retinacula
  - Flexor retinaculum
    - Thin sheet of fibrous tissue
    - Attaches medially to pointed prominence at posteromedial margin of tibia
    - Merges laterally with fascia overlying flexor hallucis longus muscle
    - Extends inferiorly to form roof of tarsal tunnel (this portion better seen on coronal images)
  - Peroneal retinaculum
    - Thin sheet of fibrous tissue
    - Attaches laterally to posterolateral border of fibula
    - Attaches medially to lateral margin of calcaneus and Achilles aponeurosis
- Syndesmotic ligaments
  - Obliquely oriented
  - Must evaluate on multiple slices
- Posterior margin of fibula
  - Should be concave
  - Convex posterior margin is associated with peroneal tendon dysfunction
    - Due to increased stress on peroneal retinaculum
- Posterior talofibular ligament
  - Thick, striated appearance
  - Often appears lax in axial plane

Structures Optimally Seen in Sagittal Plane

- Talar dome
  - Small osteochondral lesions may be masked by partial volume artifact on axial, coronal images
- Achilles tendon and pre-Achilles space
- Subtalar joint
- Chopart joint
- Plantar fascia

Structures Optimally Seen in Coronal Plane

- Tarsal sinus ligaments
  - Cervical ligament and extensor retinaculum bands may be confused on sagittal images
  - Cervical ligament anterior to extensor retinaculum
- Hindfoot portions of flexor and peroneal tendons
- Deltoid ligament

ANATOMY IMAGING ISSUES

Imaging Recommendations

- Always include T1 sequence in axial plane in every ankle MR
  - Improves visualization of accessory muscles
  - Helpful in confirming ligament integrity

Imaging Pitfalls

- Anterior inferior tibiofibular ligament
  - Axial images slice obliquely through ligament + accessory Bassett ligament
    - May mimic ligament discontinuity
    - Correlate with coronal images
- ATFL
  - Joint capsule inferior to ligament often thickens after ATFL tear
  - Do not mistake thickened inferior capsule for intact ATFL
- Accessory muscles
  - Easily overlooked on MR because normal muscle signal intensity
  - Can be symptomatic
  - Clinically can be mistaken for mass
- Posterior tibial tendon dislocation
  - Tendon displaced medially, anteriorly
  - Often overlooked because tendon is normal in signal intensity
- Tarsal sinus
  - Difficult to distinguish cervical ligament from bands of extensor retinaculum in tarsal sinus
  - Cervical ligament is anterior to extensor retinaculum

GRAPHICS: MUSCLES AND TENDONS OF ANKLE

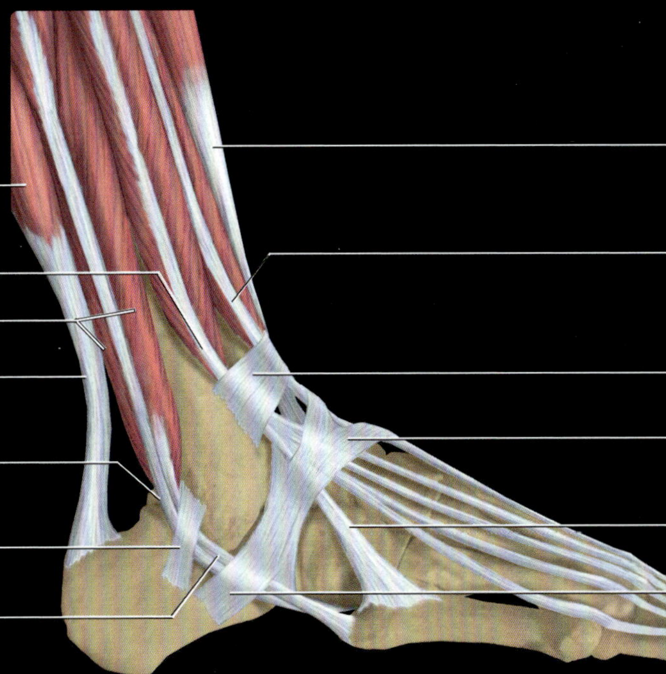

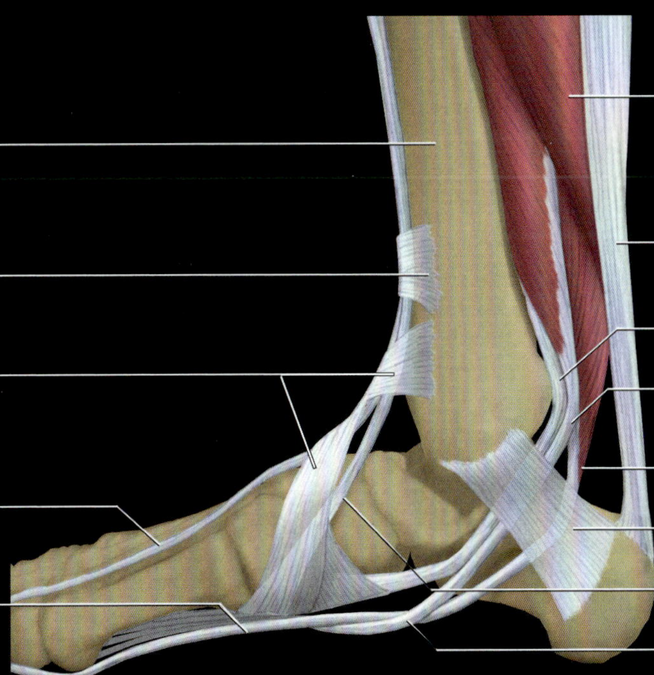

(Top) *Lateral view shows the tendons of the ankle. The peroneus brevis and peroneus longus tendons occupy the lateral compartment. They descend posterior to the fibula, held by the superior peroneal retinaculum, and continue along the lateral wall of calcaneus, held by the inferior peroneal retinaculum. Fibers of the inferior peroneal retinaculum insert either into the peroneal tubercle or calcaneal wall and separate the 2 tendons. The peroneus longus tendon curves around the cuboid to enter the sole of the foot. Both the peroneus brevis and peroneus tertius insert on the 5th metatarsal base.* **(Bottom)** *Flexor retinaculum is shown. The retinaculum extends from the medial malleolus to the plantar aponeurosis. It binds the posterior compartment tendons and forms the lateral border of tarsal tunnel. More superior fibers of the retinaculum (not shown) are transversely oriented and extend from the posterior margin of the medial malleolus to merge with the deep flexor fascia.*

AXIAL T1 MR: RIGHT ANKLE

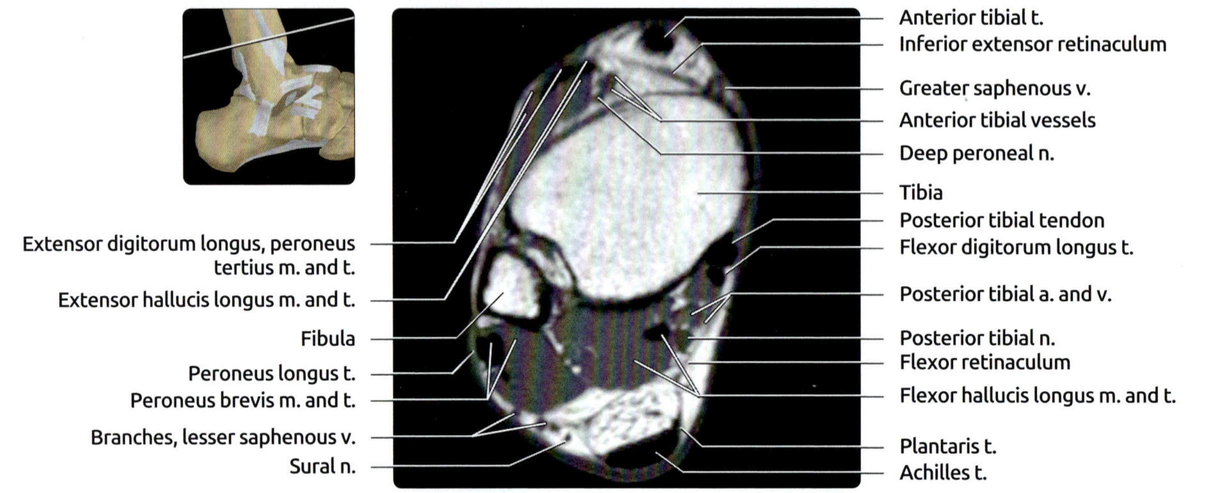

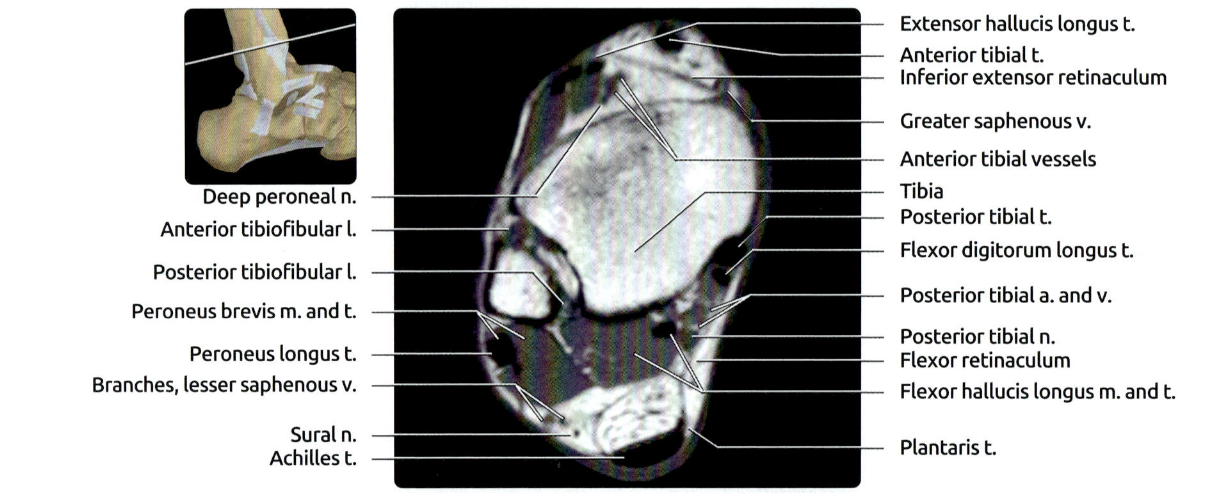

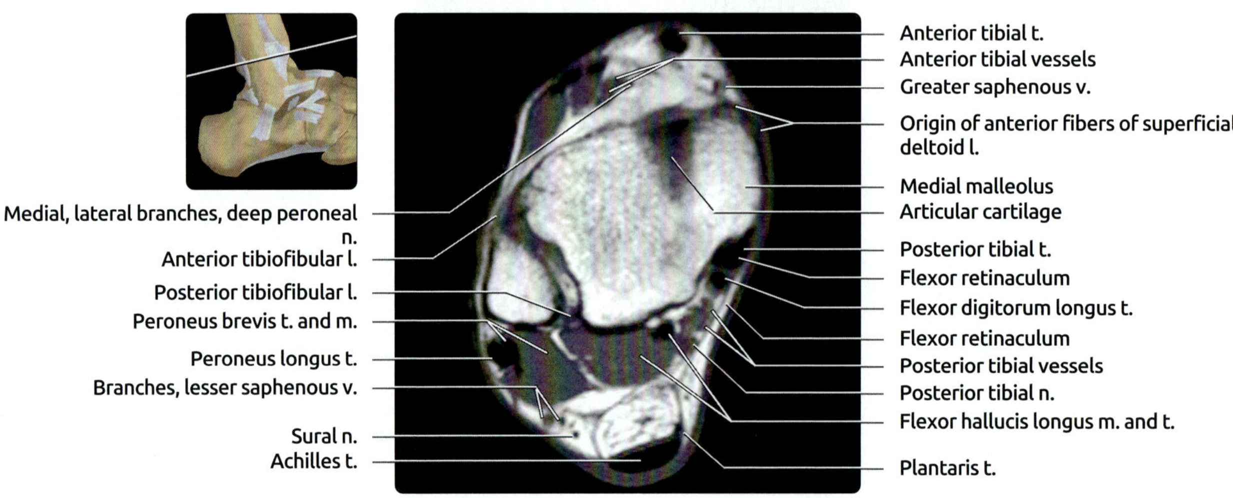

(Top) *First in a series of 18 axial T1 MR images of the right ankle is shown. The cut is just above the tibial plafond and is perpendicular to the long axis of the tibia.* **(Middle)** *The anterior and posterior tibiofibular ligaments extend from the distal tibia to the fibula and, along with the interosseus ligament, support the distal tibiofibular joint. The anterior surface of the Achilles tendon is flat. The tendon is partially surrounded by a paratenon. The plantaris tendon is found just medial to the Achilles tendon.* **(Bottom)** *Posterior tibial and flexor digitorum longus tendons lie in a groove posterior to the medial malleolus. They are held in place by the overlying flexor retinaculum. The posterior tibial tendon is 2x the diameter of the flexor digitorum longus tendon.*

AXIAL T1 MR: LEFT ANKLE

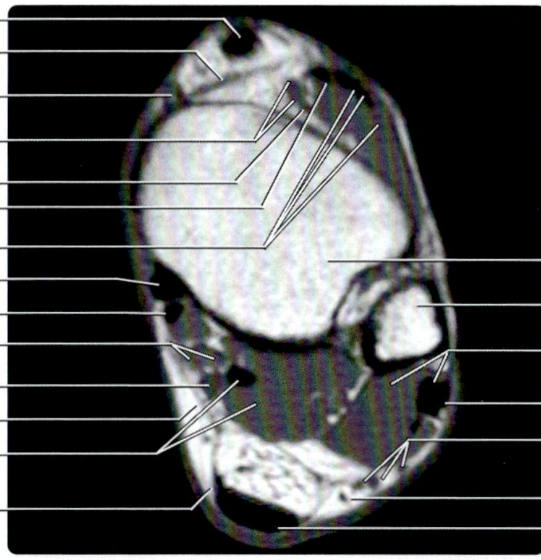

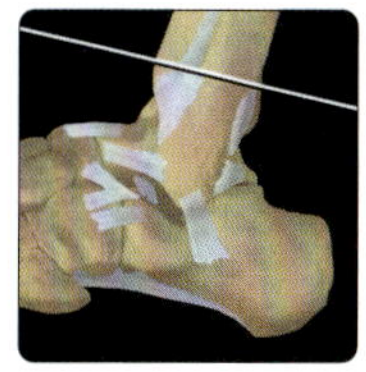

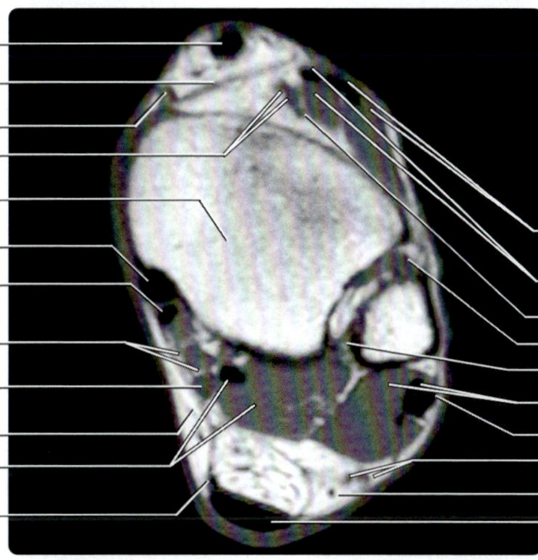

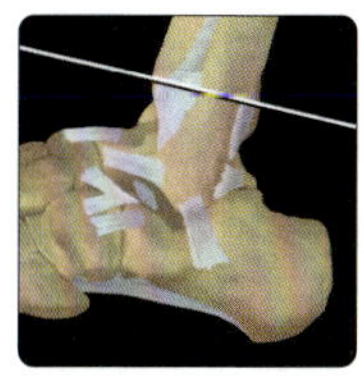

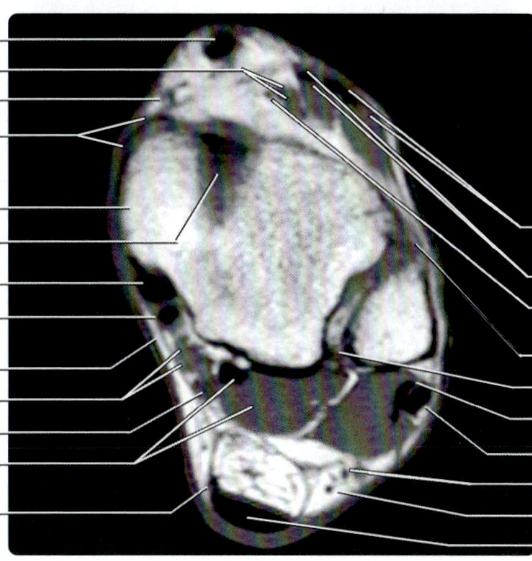

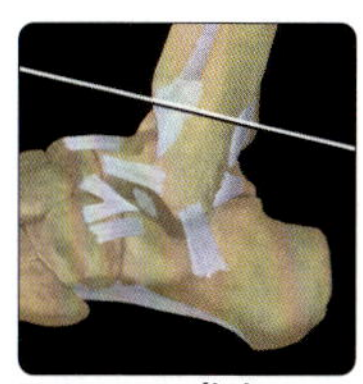

(Top) *First in a series of 18 axial T1 MR images of the left ankle is shown. The cut is just above the tibial plafond and is perpendicular to the long axis of the tibia.* **(Middle)** *The anterior and posterior tibiofibular ligaments extend from the distal tibia to the fibula and, along with the interosseous ligament, support the distal fibrous tibiofibular joint. The anterior surface of the Achilles tendon is flat. The tendon is partially surrounded by a paratenon. The plantaris tendon is found just medial to the Achilles tendon.* **(Bottom)** *Posterior tibial and flexor digitorum longus tendons lie in a groove posterior to the medial malleolus. They are held in place by the overlying flexor retinaculum. The posterior tibial tendon is 2x the diameter of the flexor digitorum longus tendon.*

AXIAL T1 MR: RIGHT ANKLE

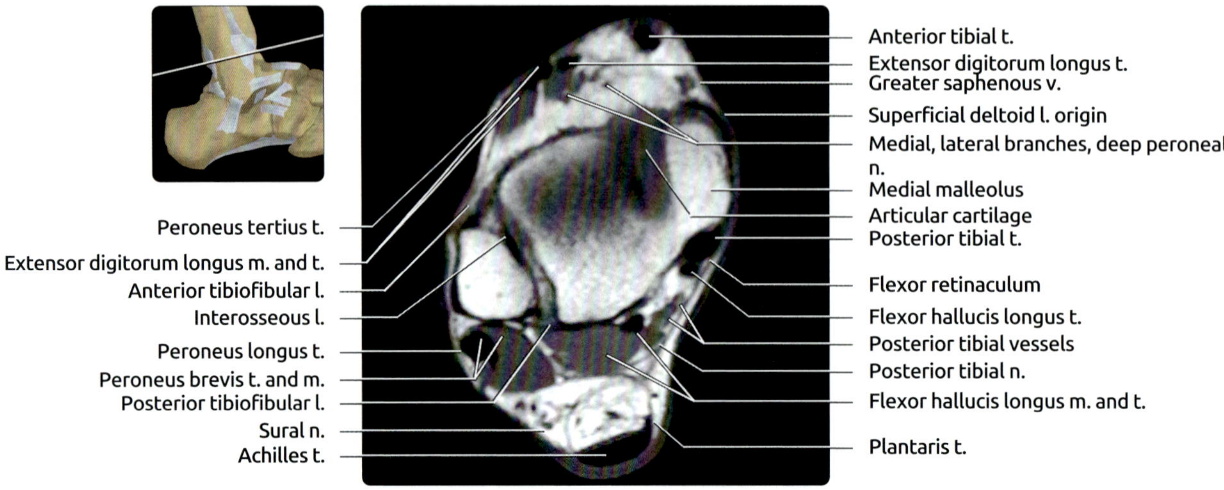

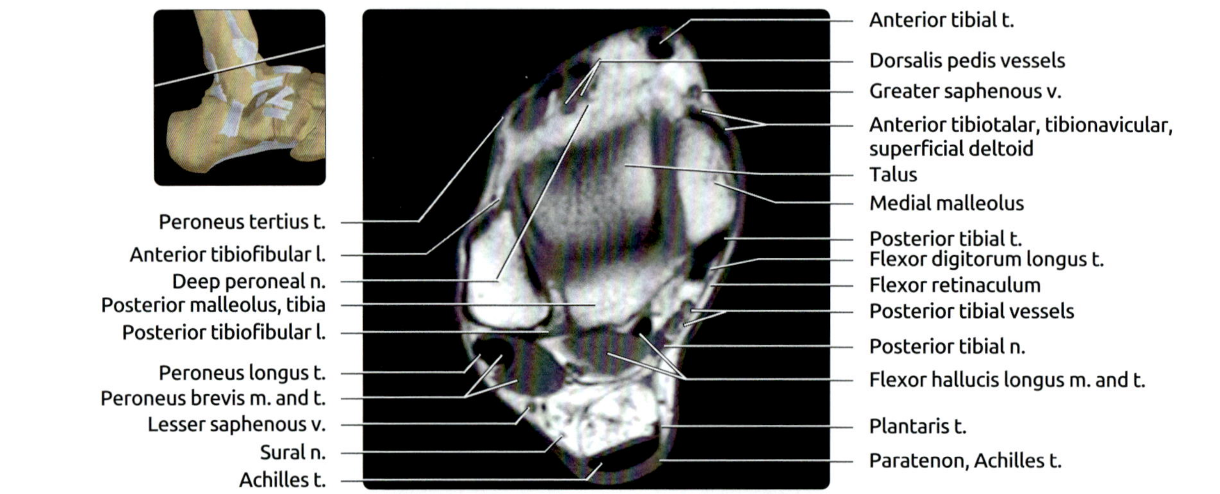

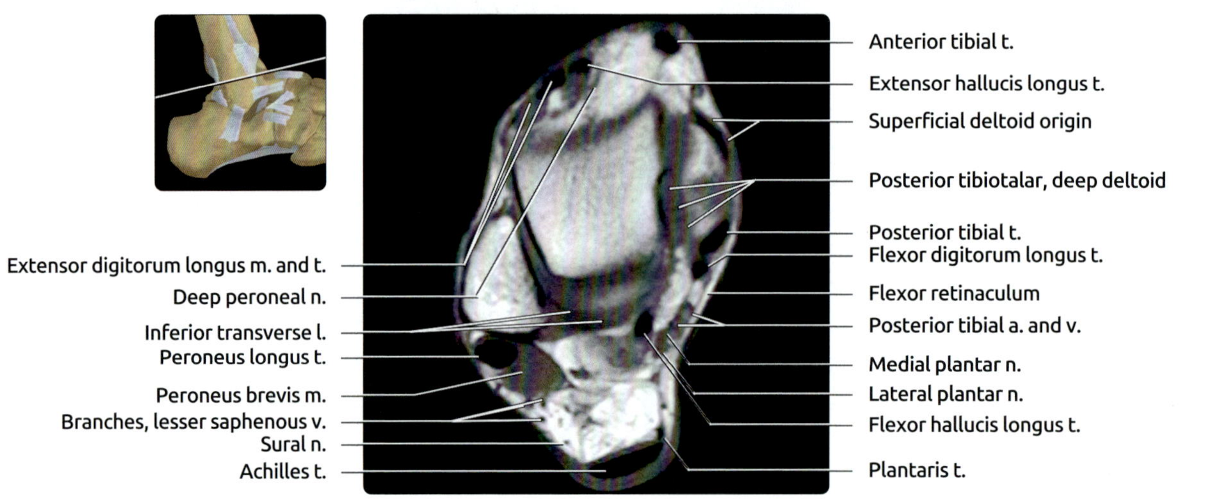

(Top) *The interosseous ligament is visualized in between the tibia and fibula. This ligament, a thickening of the interosseous membrane, is variable and may be perforated or absent.* **(Middle)** *The relative position of soft tissue structures posterior to the medial malleolus can be remembered by the mnemonic Tom, Dick, and a very nervous Harry. These signify the posterior tibial tendon, the flexor digitorum tendon, artery, vein, nerve, and flexor hallucis longus tendon.* **(Bottom)** *The deep posterior tibiotalar component of the deltoid ligament originates from the posterior colliculus and is typically striated. The inferior transverse ligament, the very inferior aspect of the posterior tibiofibular ligament, extends distal to the tibial posterior surface.*

AXIAL T1 MR: LEFT ANKLE

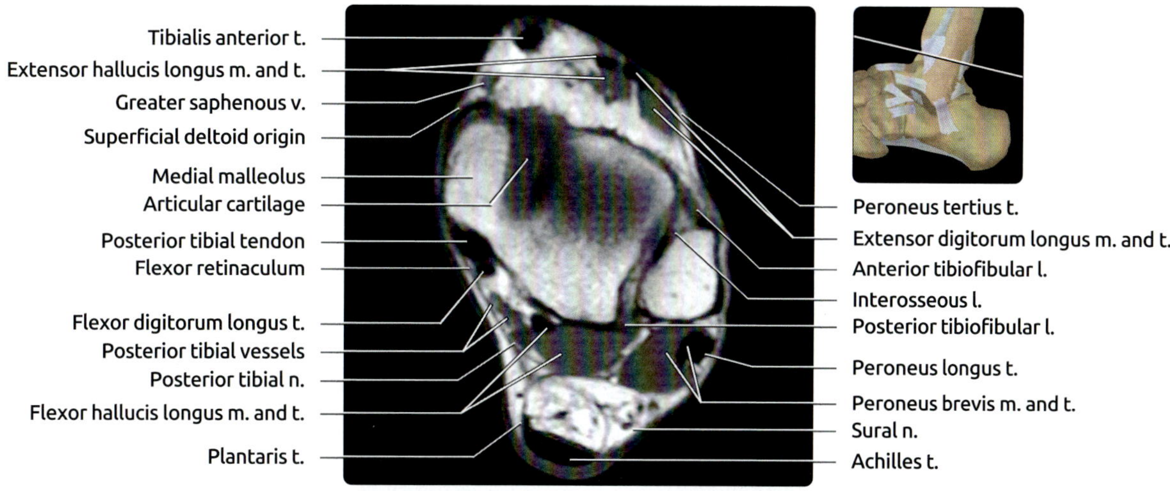

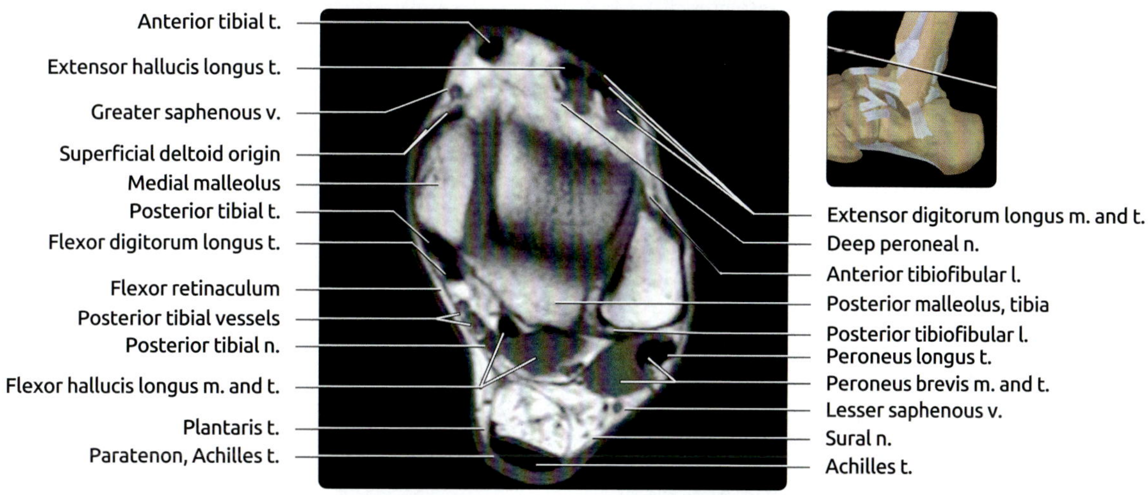

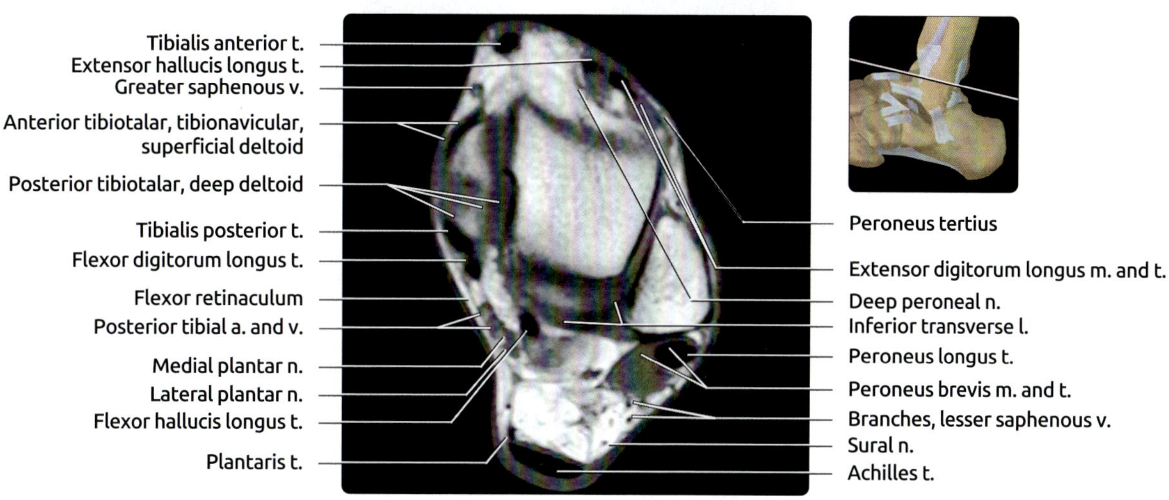

(Top) *The interosseous ligament is visualized in between the tibia and fibula. This ligament, a thickening of the interosseous membrane, is variable and may be perforated or absent.* **(Middle)** *The relative position of soft tissue structures posterior to the medial malleolus can be remembered by the mnemonic Tom, Dick, and a very nervous Harry. These signify the posterior tibial tendon, the flexor digitorum tendon, artery, vein, nerve, and flexor hallucis longus tendon.* **(Bottom)** *The deep posterior tibiotalar component of the deltoid ligament originates from the posterior colliculus and is typically striated. The inferior transverse ligament, the very inferior aspect of the posterior tibiofibular ligament, extends distal to the tibial posterior surface.*

AXIAL T1 MR: RIGHT HINDFOOT AXIS

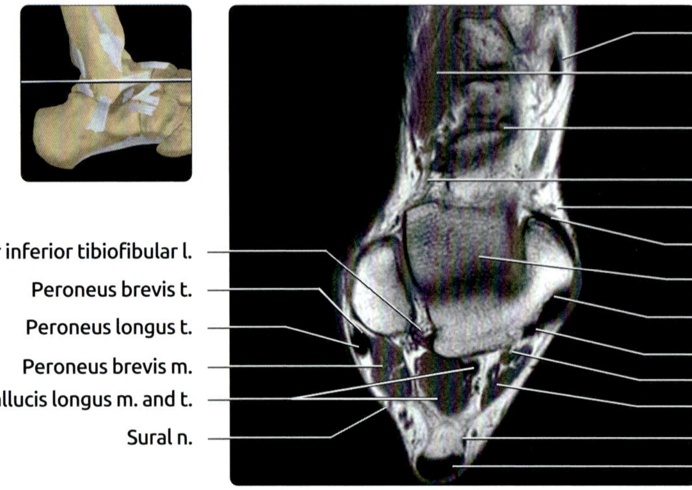

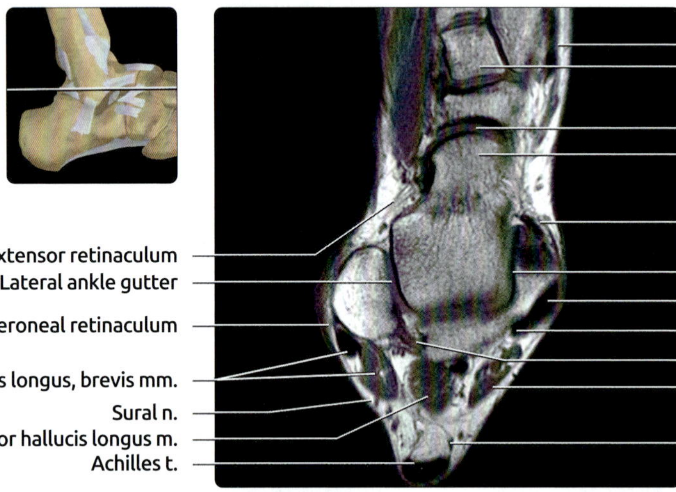

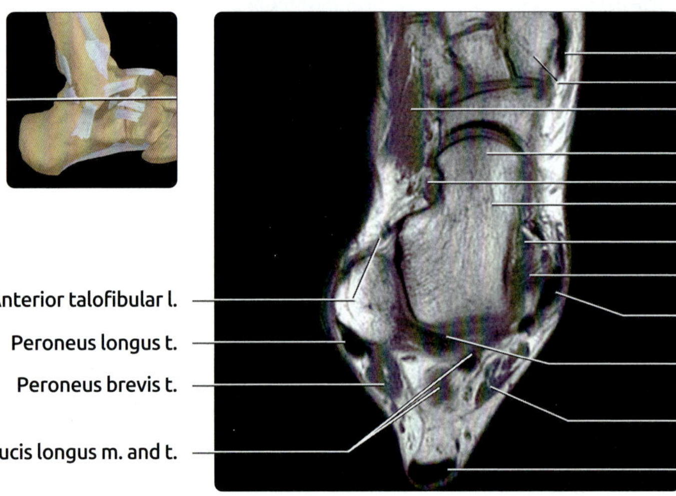

(Top) *The axial images from this point inferiorly are angled along the axis of the talus to optimize visualization of hindfoot structures. Note this patient has an accessory flexor muscle.* **(Middle)** *The ankle joint includes vertically oriented portions between the talar body and the malleoli. These may be called the ankle gutters or the ankle clear spaces.* **(Bottom)** *The deep deltoid ligament has 2 bands. The larger band occupies part of the medial ankle gutter, extending from the deep surface of the anterior colliculus of the medial malleolus to the fovea of the talus. This band is usually referred to as the deep deltoid ligament, disregarding the anterior band. The small anterior band is variably present; it extends from the medial malleolus to the talar neck. Anterior talofibular ligament inserts on a squared prominence at the lateral junction of the talar body and neck.*

AXIAL T1 MR: LEFT HINDFOOT AXIS

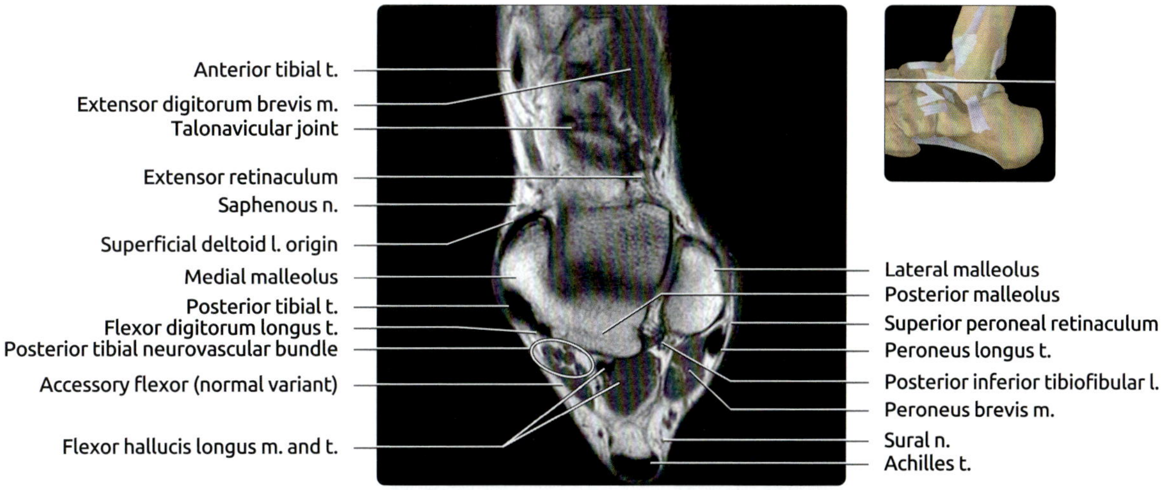

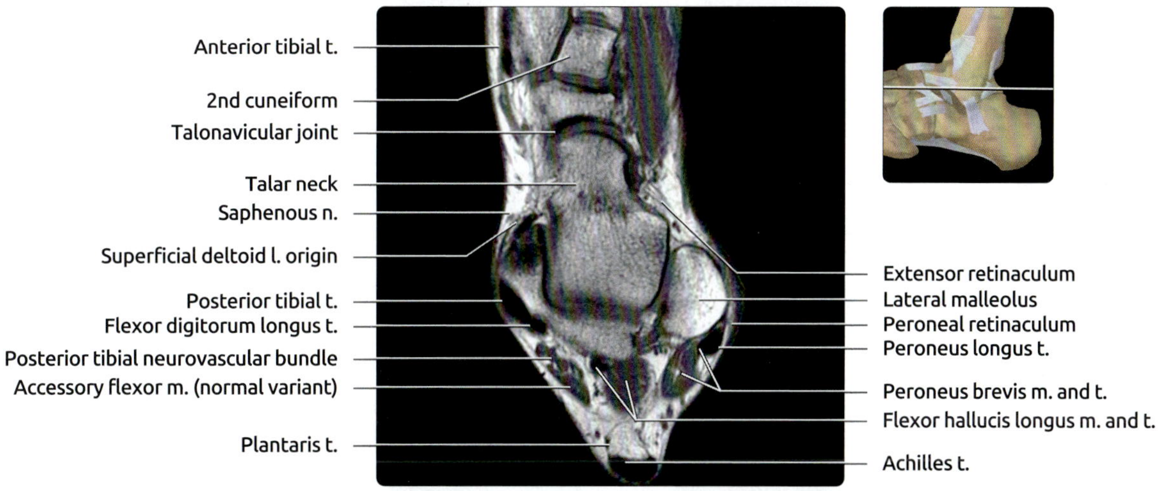

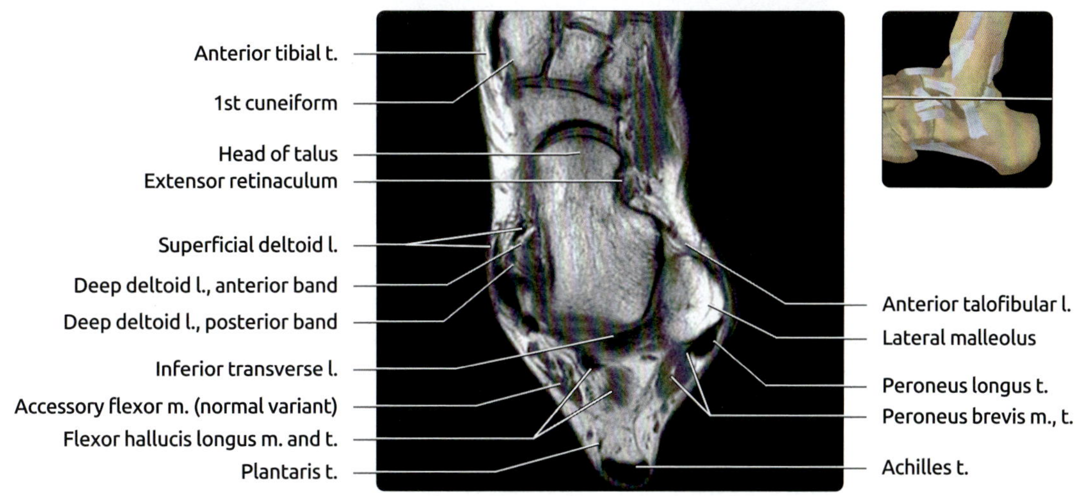

(Top) *The axial images from this point inferiorly are angled along the axis of the talus to optimize visualization of hindfoot structures. Note this patient has an accessory flexor muscle.* **(Middle)** *The ankle joint includes vertically oriented portions between the talar body and the malleoli. These may be called the ankle gutters or the ankle clear spaces.* **(Bottom)** *The deep deltoid ligament has 2 bands. The larger band occupies part of the medial ankle gutter, extending from the deep surface of the anterior colliculus of the medial malleolus to the fovea of the talus. This band is usually referred to as the deep deltoid ligament, disregarding the anterior band. The small anterior band is variably present; it extends from the medial malleolus to the talar neck. Anterior talofibular ligament inserts on a squared prominence at the lateral junction of the talar body and neck.*

AXIAL T1 MR: RIGHT HINDFOOT AXIS

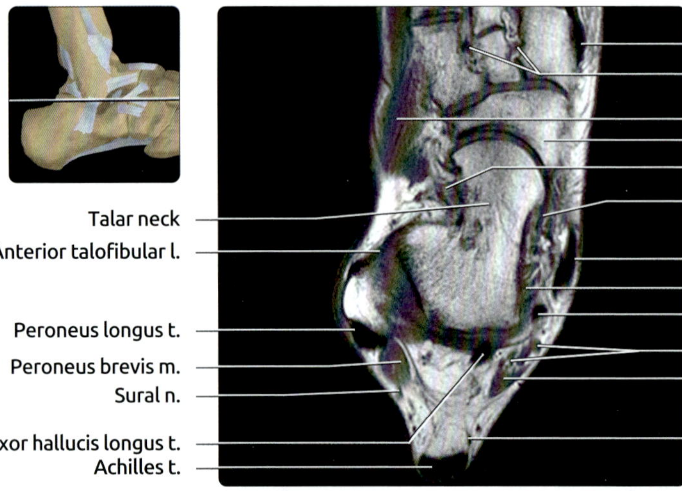

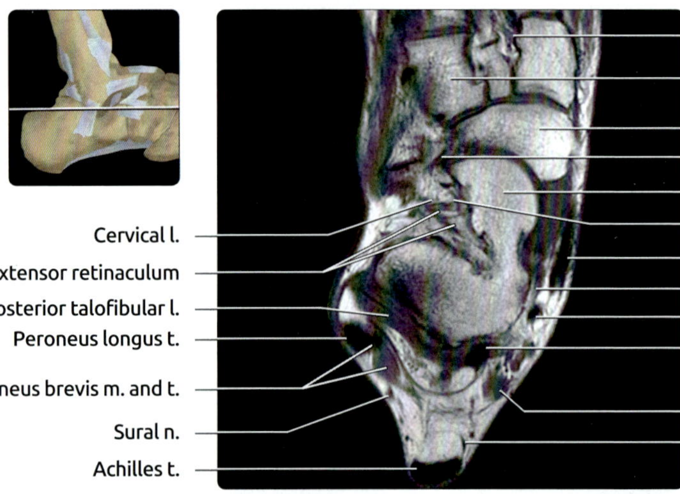

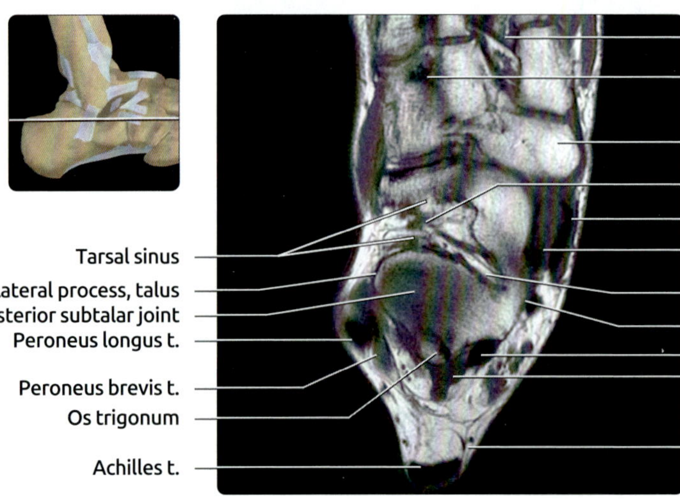

(Top) *Because of the oblique course of the deep deltoid ligament, fibers are seen inserting on the talus inferior to the medial malleolus.* **(Middle)** *The extensor retinaculum has 3 bands: Lateral, middle, and medial. They traverse the tarsal sinus and insert on the dorsal surface of the calcaneus, posterior to the cervical ligament.* **(Bottom)** *The funnel shape of the tarsal sinus is well seen on this image. The tarsal sinus lies between the talus and calcaneus, lateral to the sustentaculum tali. It is primarily filled with fat through which pass ligaments and the artery of the tarsal sinus. Posteromedially, it flows into a narrow space, the tarsal canal, which contains the tibiocalcaneal interosseous ligament.*

AXIAL T1 MR: LEFT HINDFOOT AXIS

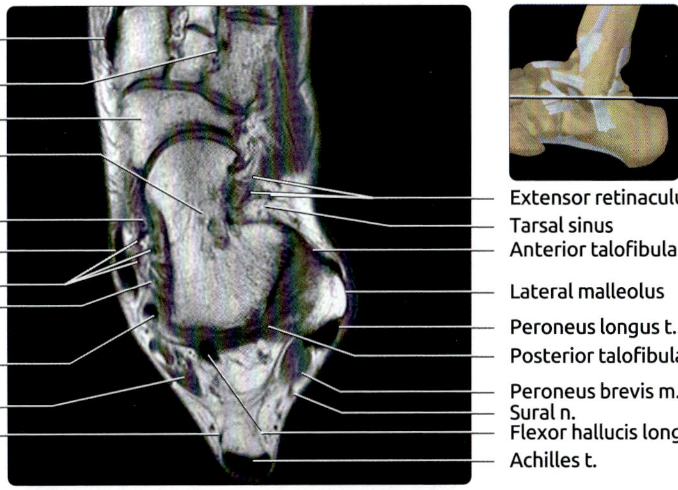

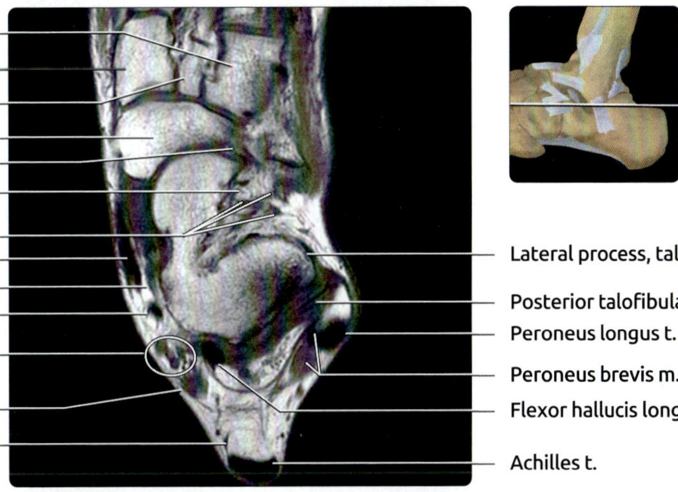

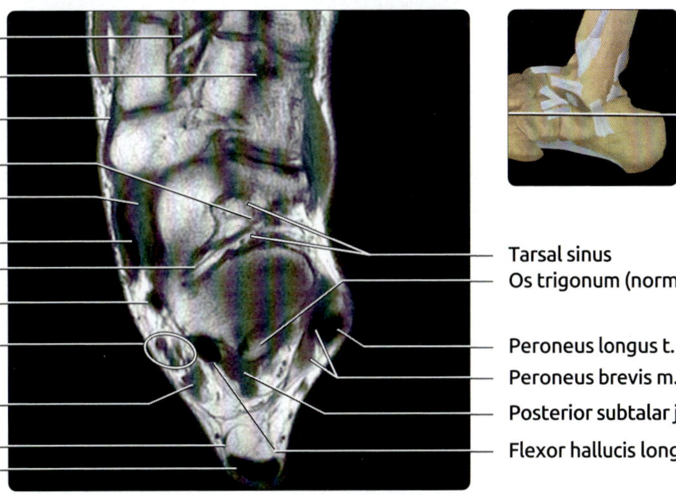

(Top) *Because of the oblique course of the deep deltoid ligament, fibers are seen inserting on the talus inferior to the medial malleolus.* **(Middle)** *The extensor retinaculum has 3 bands: Lateral, middle, and medial. They traverse the tarsal sinus and insert on the dorsal surface of the calcaneus, posterior to the cervical ligament.* **(Bottom)** *The funnel shape of the tarsal sinus is well seen on this image. The tarsal sinus lies between the talus and calcaneus, lateral to the sustentaculum tali. It is primarily filled with fat through which pass ligaments and the artery of the tarsal sinus. Posteromedially, it flows into a narrow space, the tarsal canal, which contains the tibiocalcaneal interosseous ligament.*

AXIAL T1 MR: RIGHT HINDFOOT AXIS

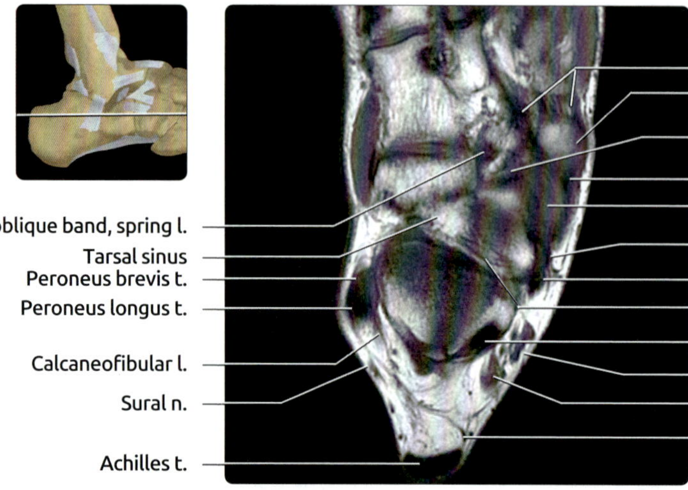

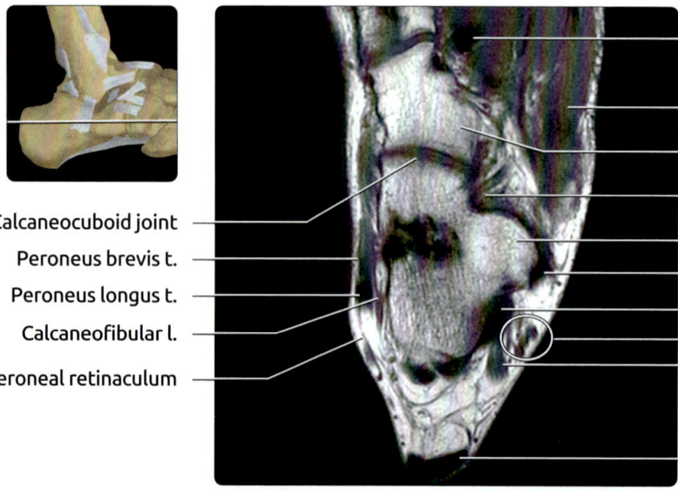

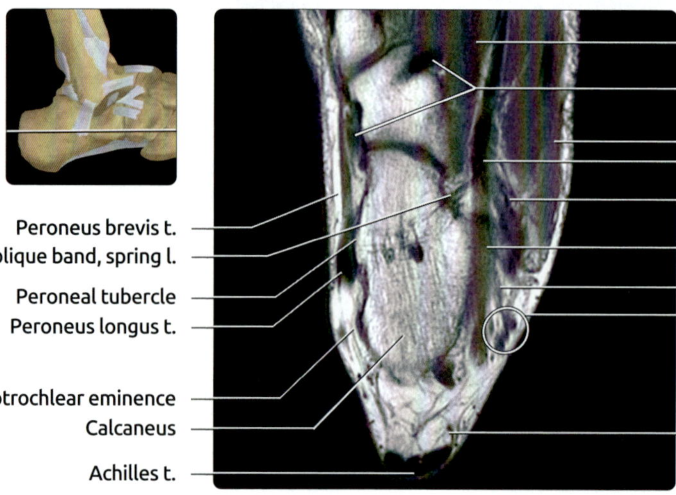

(Top) *Medioplantar oblique band of spring ligament arises from the coronoid fossa, a portion of the calcaneus just anterior to the sustentaculum tali.* **(Middle)** *On this image, the patient's normal variant accessory flexor muscle is seen inserting on the flexor hallucis longus tendon, and so it can be designated as an accessory flexor hallucis longus. Accessory flexor muscles are fairly common, and they can be named according to the muscle they most closely follow or according to their site of insertion. The important points are to recognize them as normal muscles rather than masses and to realize they may result in ankle impingement or even exertional compartment syndromes.* **(Bottom)** *The tibial nerve divides in the tarsal tunnel giving rise to calcaneal branches as well as medial and lateral plantar branches. The points at which the branches divide are variable. The lateral plantar nerve moves laterally and inferiorly as it extends to the lateral side of the foot. Baxter nerve is its 1st branch, innervating the abductor digiti minimi.*

AXIAL T1 MR: LEFT HINDFOOT AXIS

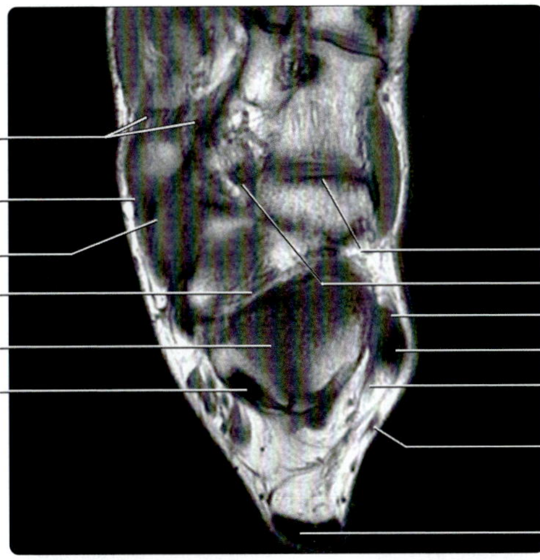

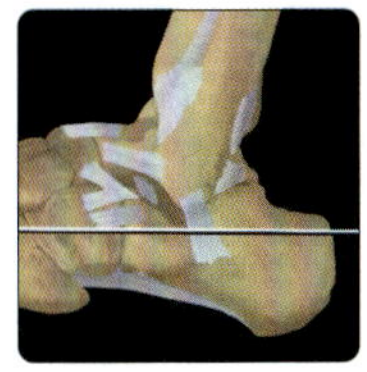

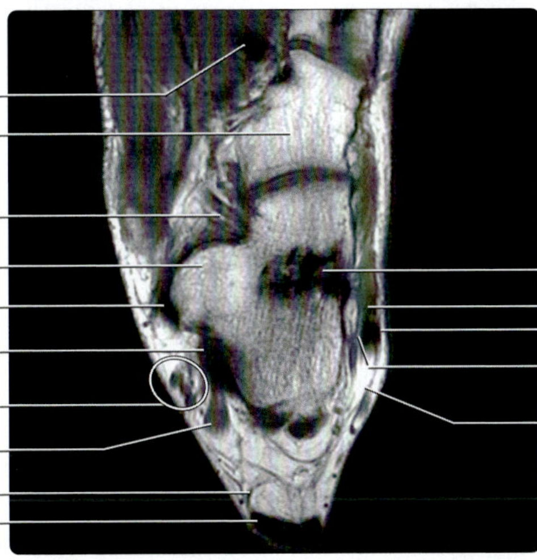

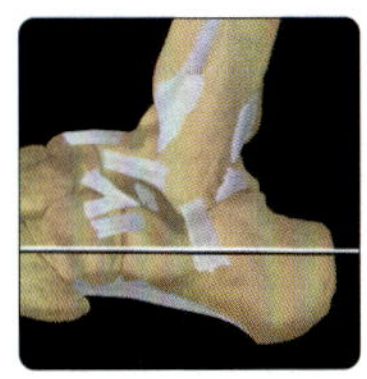

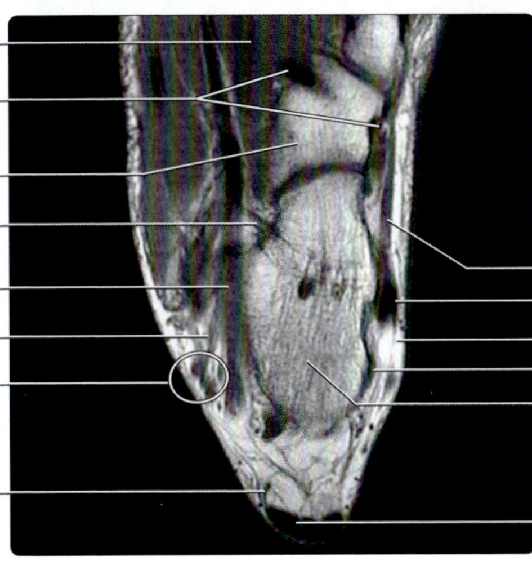

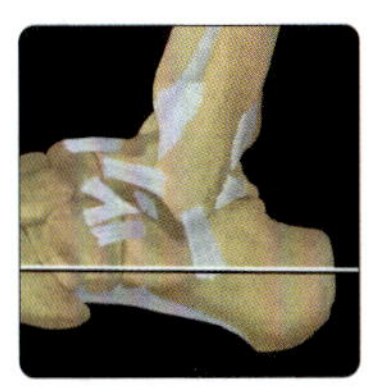

(Top) *Medioplantar oblique band of spring ligament arises from the coronoid fossa, a portion of the calcaneus just anterior to the sustentaculum tali.* **(Middle)** *On this image, the patient's normal variant accessory flexor muscle is seen inserting on the flexor hallucis longus tendon, and so it can be designated as an accessory flexor hallucis longus. Accessory flexor muscles are fairly common, and they can be named according to the muscle they most closely follow or according to their site of insertion. The important points are to recognize them as normal muscles rather than masses and to realize they may result in ankle impingement or even exertional compartment syndromes.* **(Bottom)** *The tibial nerve divides in the tarsal tunnel giving rise to calcaneal branches as well as medial and lateral plantar branches. The points at which the branches divide are variable. The lateral plantar nerve moves laterally and inferiorly as it extends to the lateral side of the foot. Baxter nerve is its 1st branch, innervating the abductor digiti minimi.*

AXIAL T1 MR: RIGHT HINDFOOT AXIS

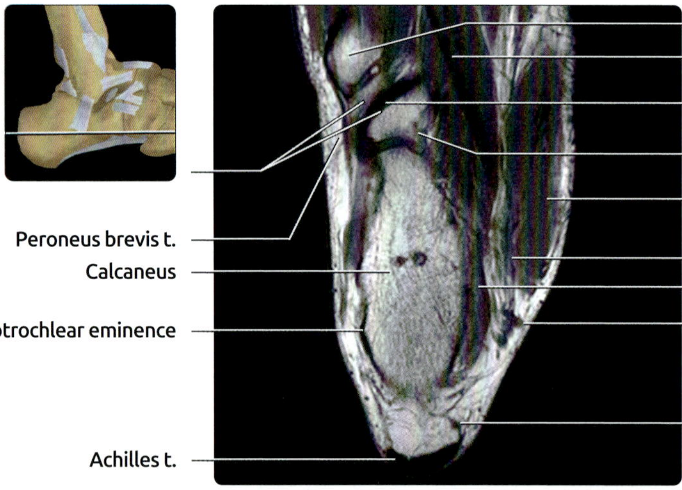

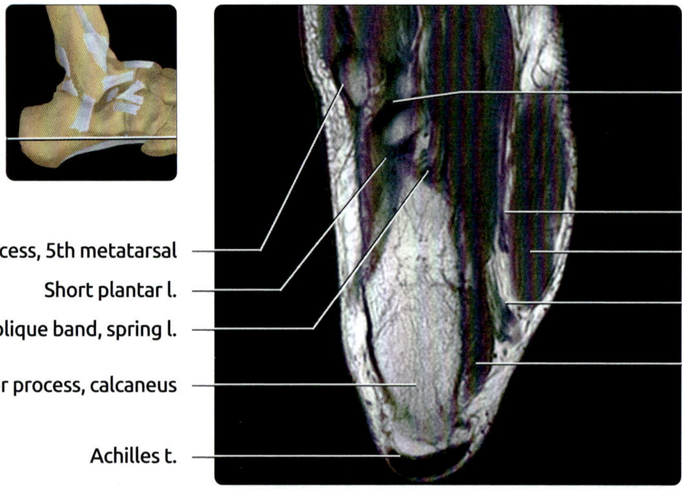

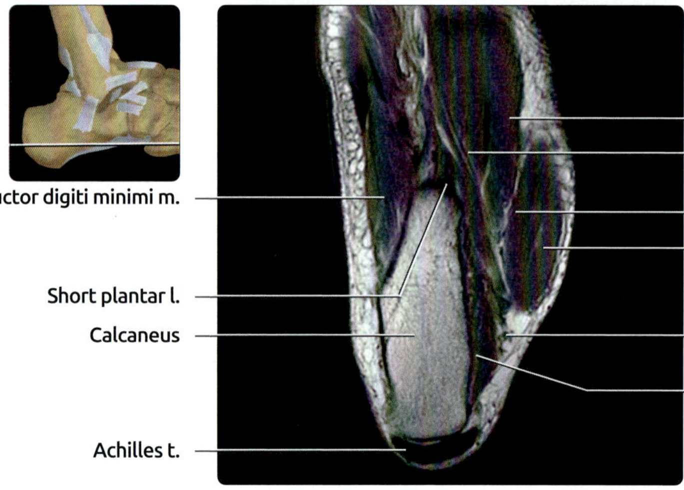

(Top) *Peroneus longus tendon is seen coursing through the cuboid sulcus. The sites of branching of the tibial nerve and its branches are fairly variable. Quadratus plantae muscle inserts on the flexor digitorum longus tendon, and lumbrical muscles originate on the tendon.* **(Middle)** *The short plantar ligament, a.k.a. the plantar calcaneocuboid ligament, ends at the proximal margin of the cuboid. The long plantar ligament, superficial to it, forms the floor of the cuboid tunnel in which the peroneus longus tendon lies. It is best seen on sagittal images. The roof of the tunnel is the cuboid sulcus.* **(Bottom)** *The lateral plantar nerve lies between the quadratus plantae and flexor digitorum brevis muscles. It divides into deep and superficial branches. The medial plantar nerve lies between the abductor hallucis and flexor digitorum brevis muscles.*

AXIAL T1 MR: LEFT HINDFOOT AXIS

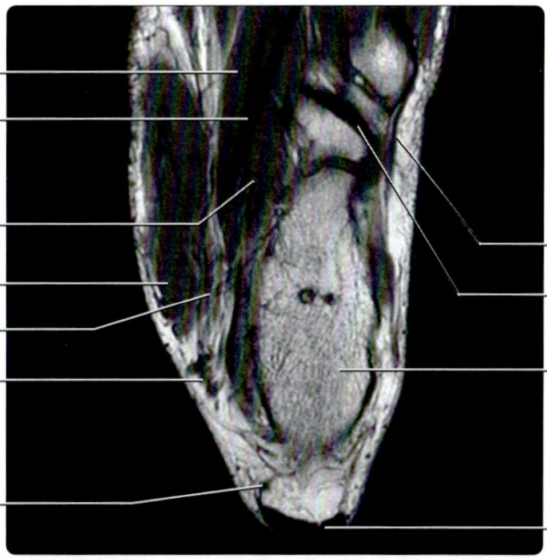

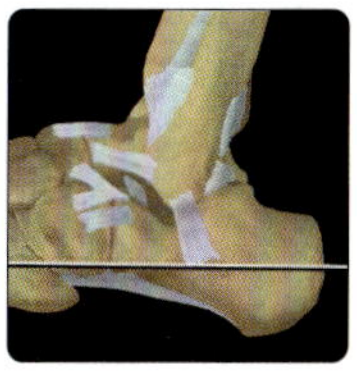

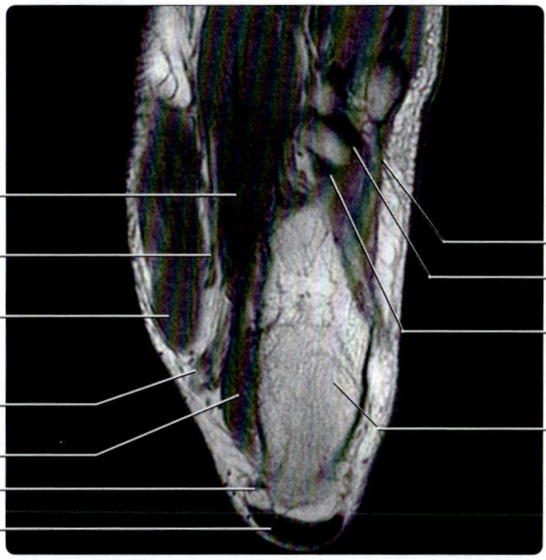

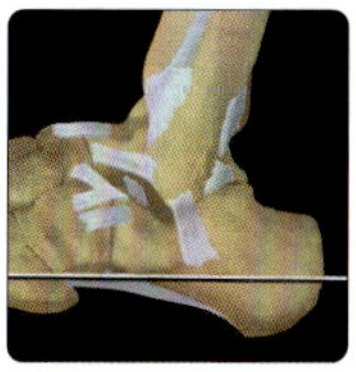

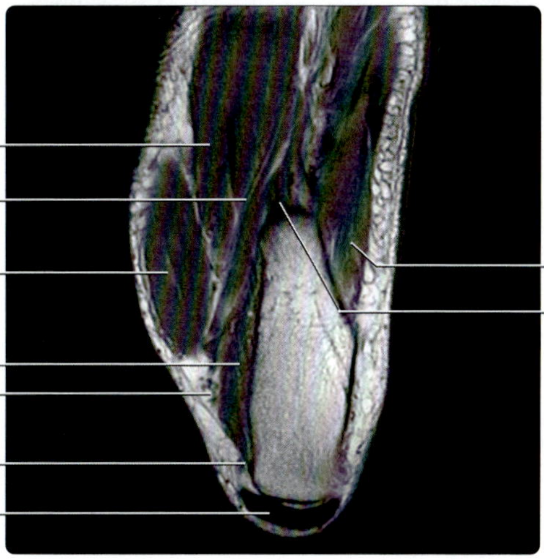

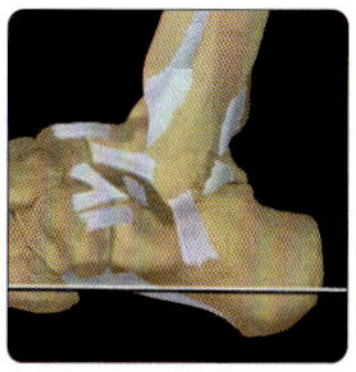

(Top) *Peroneus longus tendon is seen coursing through the cuboid sulcus. The sites of branching of the tibial nerve and its branches are fairly variable. Quadratus plantae muscle inserts on the flexor digitorum longus tendon, and lumbrical muscles originate on the tendon.* **(Middle)** *The short plantar ligament, a.k.a. the plantar calcaneocuboid ligament, ends at the proximal margin of the cuboid. The long plantar ligament, superficial to it, forms the floor of the cuboid tunnel in which the peroneus longus tendon lies. It is best seen on sagittal images. The roof of the tunnel is the cuboid sulcus.* **(Bottom)** *The lateral plantar nerve lies between the quadratus plantae and flexor digitorum brevis muscles. It divides into deep and superficial branches. The medial plantar nerve lies between the abductor hallucis and flexor digitorum brevis muscles.*

CORONAL T1 MR: RIGHT ANKLE

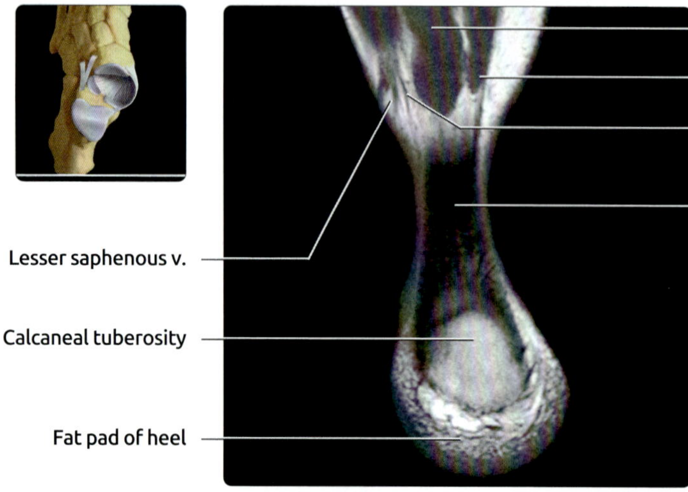

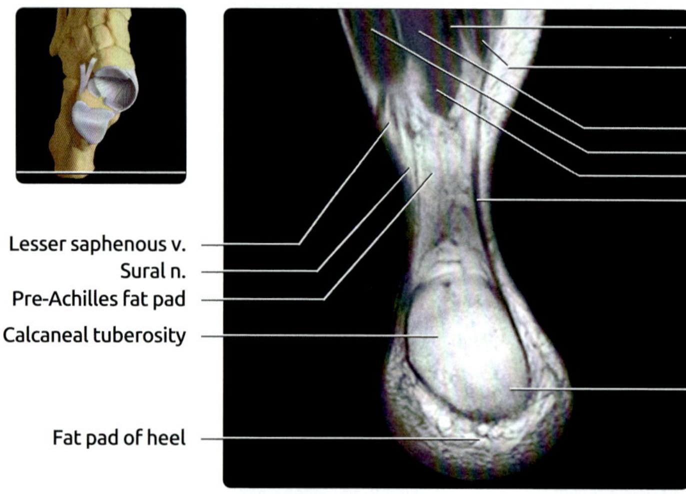

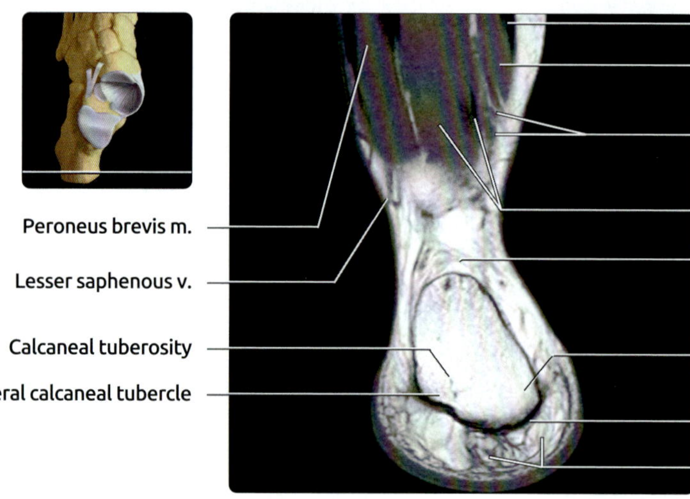

(Top) *The ankle can be imaged in a straight coronal plane or angled with the axis of the foot. For the most posterior structures, the straight coronal is optimal, as shown here. More anterior images in this series will be angled perpendicular to the talus, as shown on accompanying scout images. This improves visualization of the subtalar joint and other hindfoot structures.* **(Middle)** *The Achilles tendon is the largest tendon in the body. It inserts into the posterior margin of the calcaneal tuberosity slightly below its superior apex. The plantaris tendon runs along the medial margin of the Achilles tendon and inserts separately along the medial border of the calcaneus.* **(Bottom)** *The flexor hallucis longus muscle is broad and remains muscular more distally than the other muscles of the posterior compartment of the leg; it may be seen down to the ankle joint. The peroneus brevis muscle also descends down to the ankle joint, whereas the peroneus longus muscle is no longer visualized at that level.*

CORONAL T1 MR: LEFT ANKLE

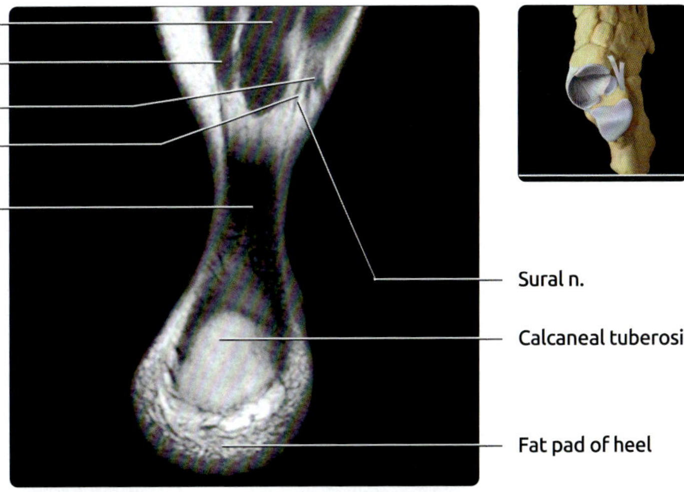

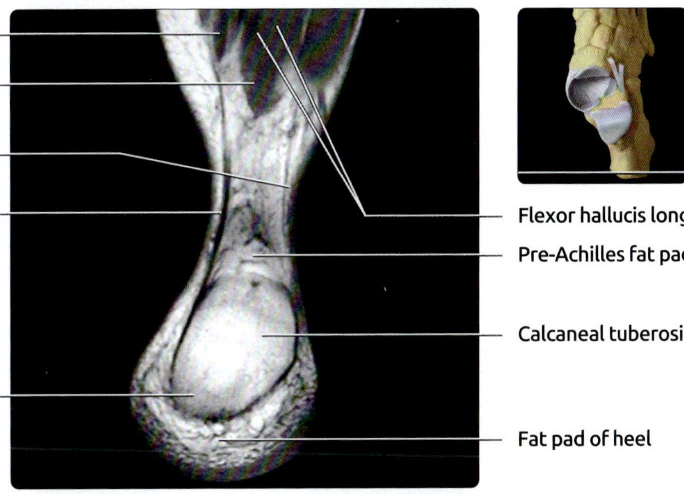

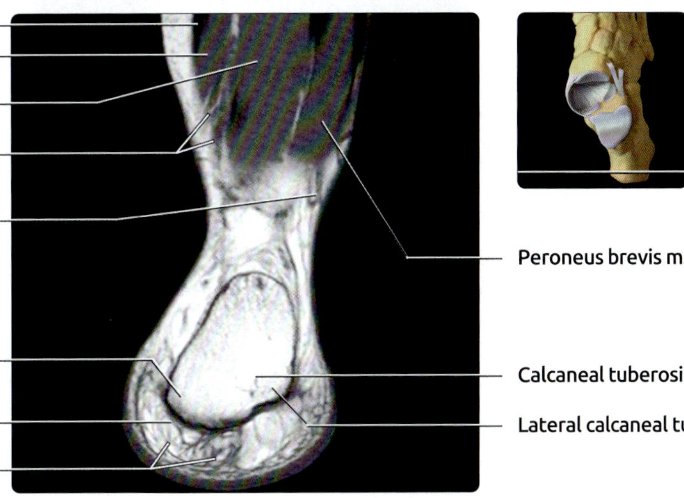

(Top) *The ankle can be imaged in a straight coronal plane or angled with the axis of the foot. For the most posterior structures, the straight coronal is optimal, as shown here. More anterior images in this series will be angled perpendicular to the talus, as shown on accompanying scout images. This improves visualization of the subtalar joint and other hindfoot structures.* **(Middle)** *The Achilles tendon is the largest tendon in the body. It inserts into the posterior margin of the calcaneal tuberosity slightly below its superior apex. The plantaris tendon runs along the medial margin of the Achilles tendon and inserts separately along the medial border of the calcaneus.* **(Bottom)** *The flexor hallucis longus muscle is broad and remains muscular more distally than the other muscles of the posterior compartment of the leg; it may be seen down to the ankle joint. The peroneus brevis muscle also descends down to the ankle joint, whereas the peroneus longus muscle is no longer visualized at that level.*

CORONAL T1 MR: RIGHT ANKLE

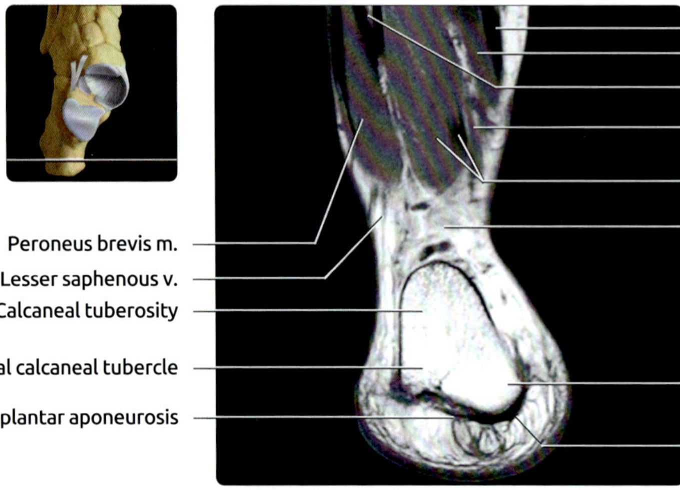

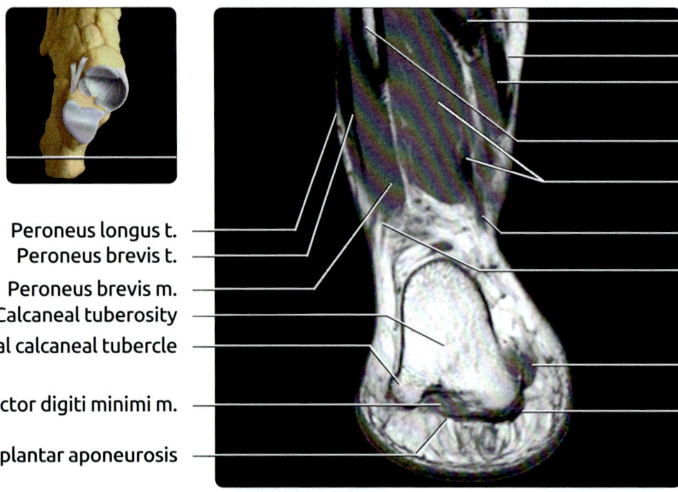

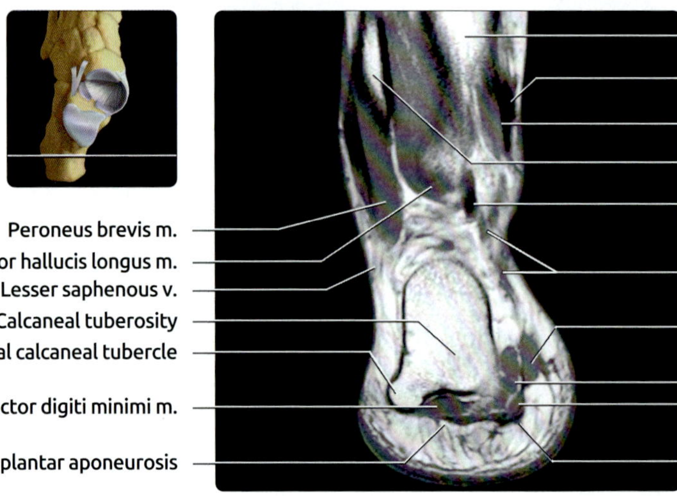

(Top) *In the ankle, the posterior tibial nerve and its accompanying vessels descend within a fat plane between the flexor digitorum longus and flexor hallucis longus. The nerve is lateral to the artery and veins.* **(Middle)** *The medial and lateral tubercles of the calcaneus give origin to the 1st layer of intrinsic muscles of the foot and to the plantar aponeurosis. The abductor digiti minimi muscle originates from the lateral tubercle and the flexor digitorum brevis; abductor hallucis and abductor digiti minimi muscles originate from the medial tubercle.* **(Bottom)** *The plantar fascia (aponeurosis) is now coming into view. It has 3 proximal parts: A strong, broad, and thick central band covering the flexor digitorum brevis muscle, a lateral band covering the abductor digiti minimi, and a thin band covering the abductor hallucis muscle and continuous with the flexor retinaculum.*

CORONAL T1 MR: LEFT ANKLE

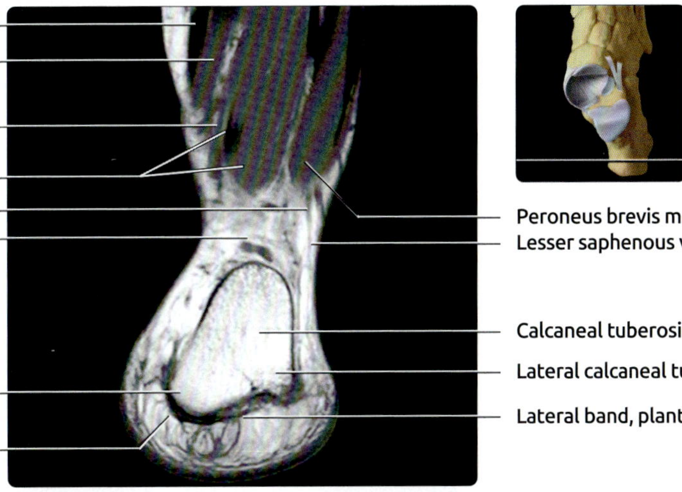

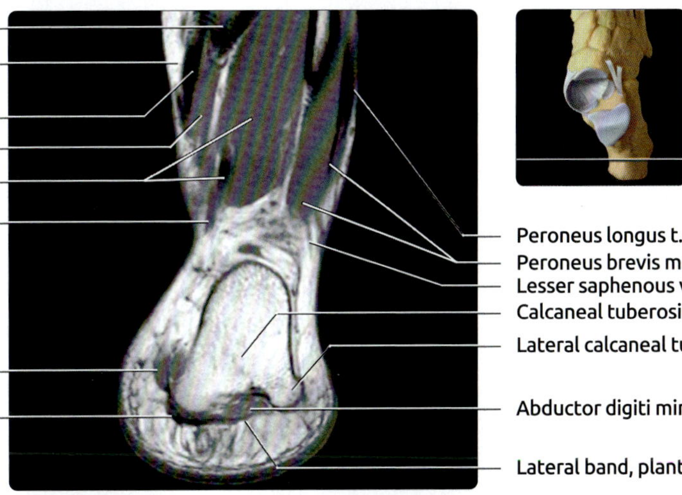

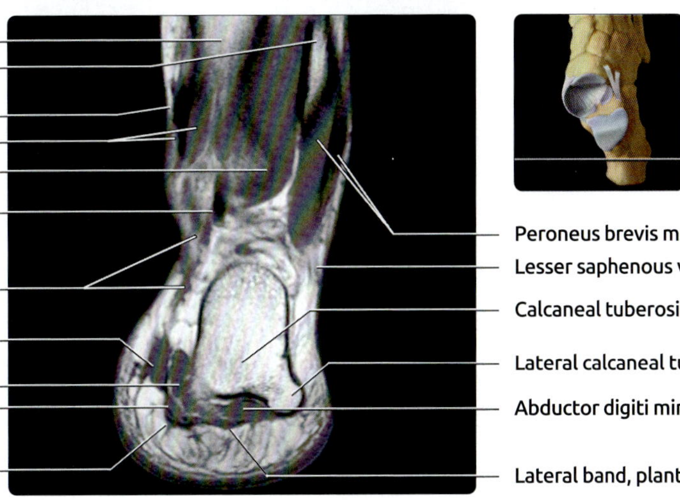

(Top) *In the ankle, the posterior tibial nerve and its accompanying vessels descend within a fat plane between the flexor digitorum longus and flexor hallucis longus muscles. The nerve is lateral to the artery and veins.* **(Middle)** *The medial and lateral tubercles of the calcaneus give origin to the 1st layer of intrinsic muscles of the foot and to the plantar aponeurosis. The abductor digiti minimi muscle originates from the lateral tubercle and the flexor digitorum brevis; abductor hallucis and abductor digiti minimi muscles originate from the medial tubercle.* **(Bottom)** *The plantar fascia (aponeurosis) is now coming into view. It has 3 bands: A strong, broad, and thick central band covering the flexor digitorum brevis muscle, a lateral band covering the abductor digiti minimi, and a thin band covering the abductor hallucis muscle and continuous with the flexor retinaculum.*

CORONAL T1 MR: RIGHT ANKLE

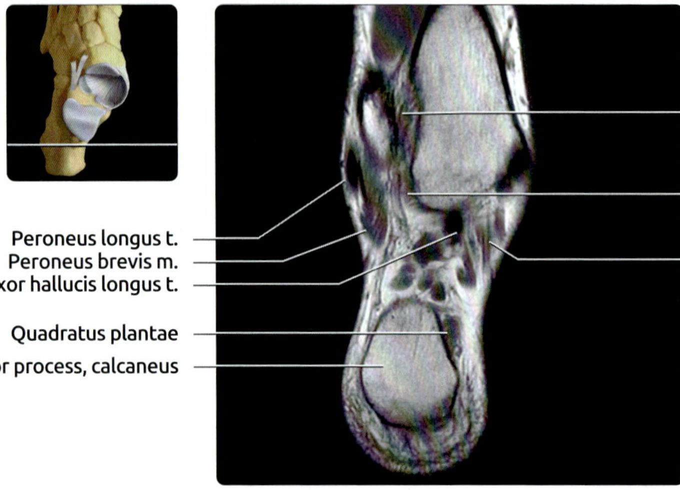

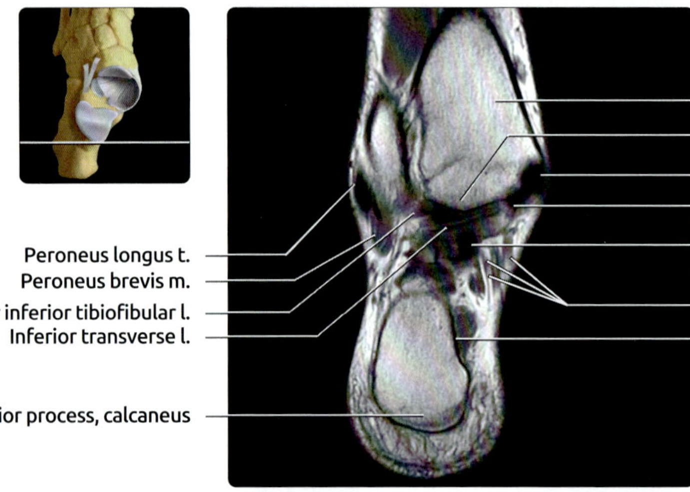

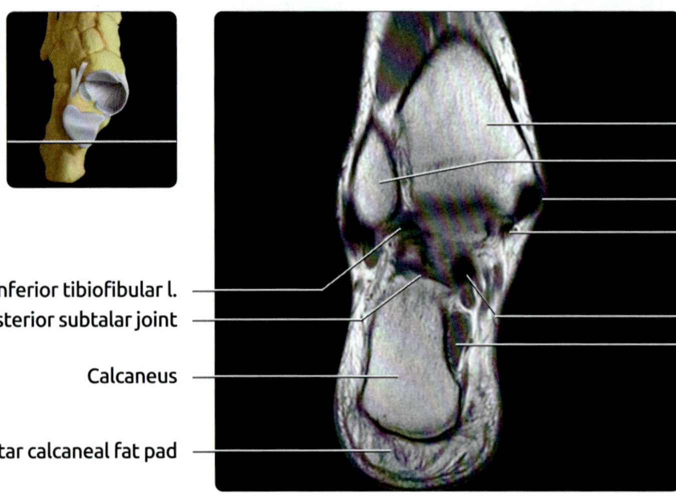

(Top) *The coronal images are angled perpendicular to the talus, which improves visualization of hindfoot structures. For that reason, the calcaneus is seen at a more posterior portion than on the previous images.* **(Middle)** *The posterior inferior tibiofibular ligament originates from the posterior malleolus and inserts into the fibula above the malleolar fossa. The inferior transverse ligament extends distal to the tibial posterior surface and inserts quite far medially, close to the medial malleolus.* **(Bottom)** *The posterior subtalar joint is broad and curved. Inversion, eversion, and gliding motion occur at this joint.*

CORONAL T1 MR: LEFT ANKLE

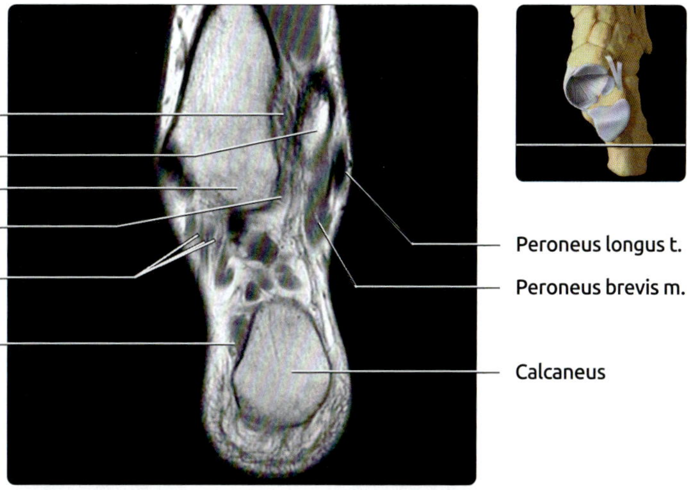

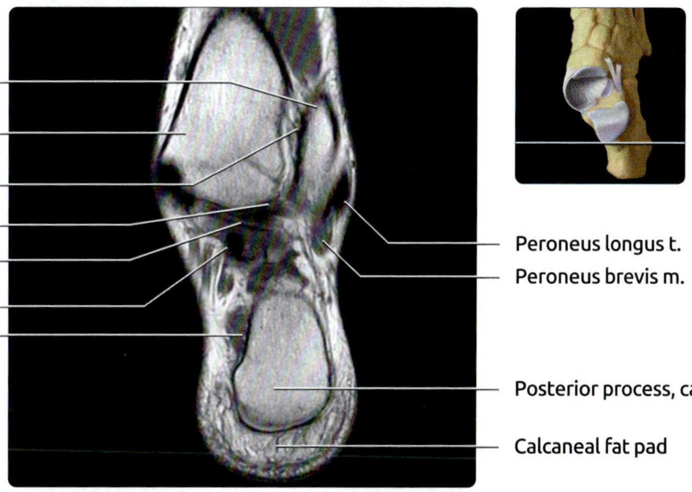

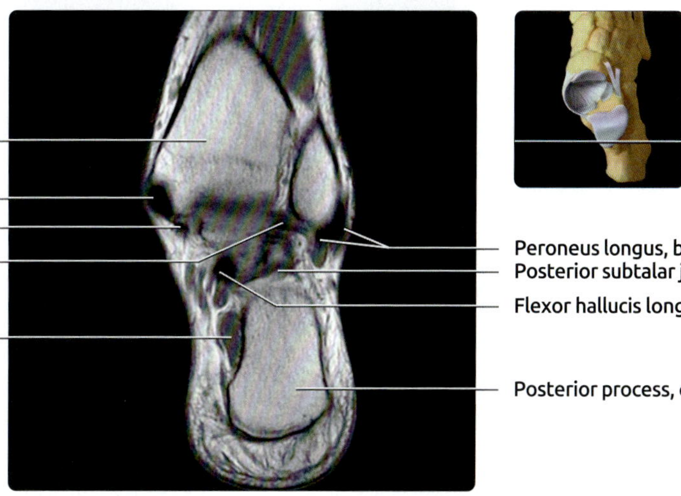

(Top) *The coronal images are angled perpendicular to the talus, which improves visualization of hindfoot structures. For that reason, the calcaneus is seen at a more posterior portion than on the previous images.* **(Middle)** *The posterior inferior tibiofibular ligament originates from the posterior malleolus and inserts into the fibula above the malleolar fossa. The inferior transverse ligament extends distal to the tibial posterior surface and inserts quite far medially close to the medial malleolus.* **(Bottom)** *The posterior subtalar joint is broad and curved. Inversion, eversion, and gliding motion occur at this joint.*

CORONAL T1 MR: RIGHT ANKLE

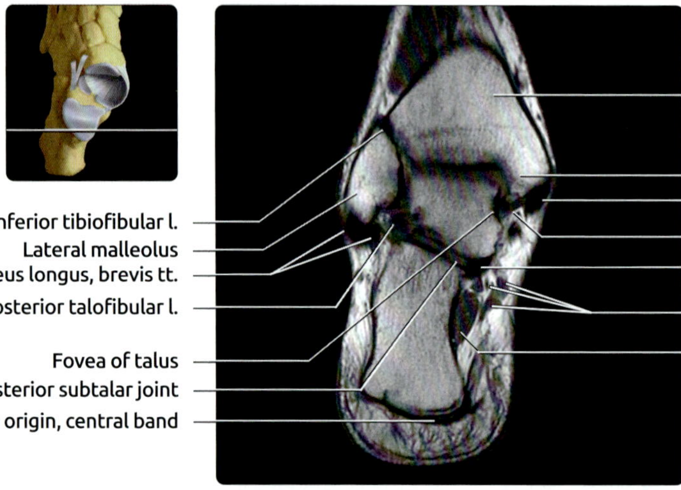

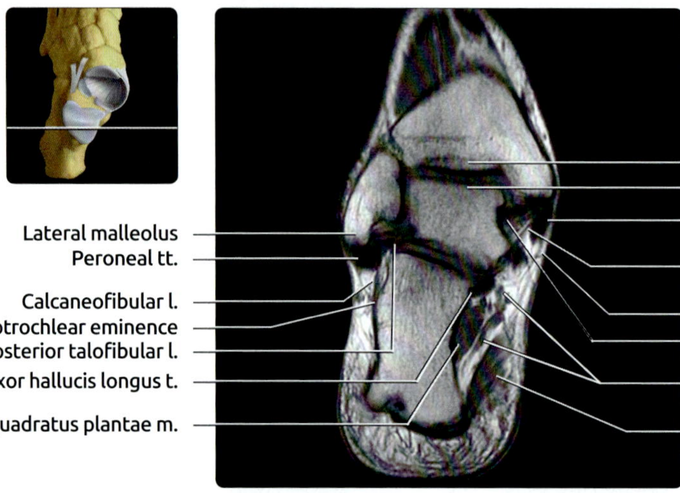

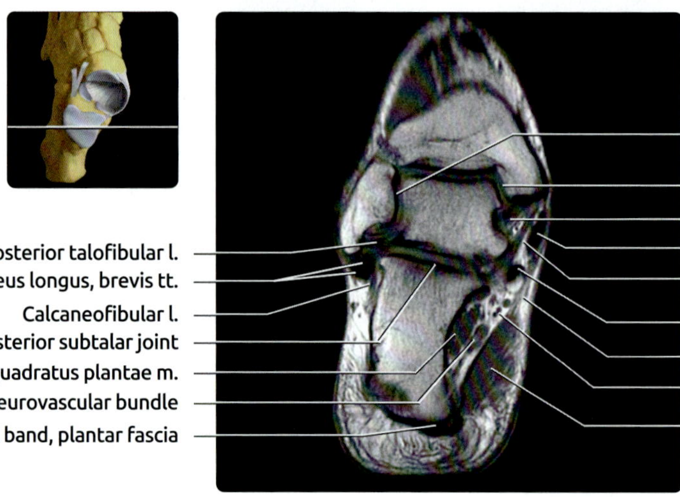

(Top) *The deep deltoid ligament is now coming into view. It has 2 bands. The posterior band is the constant and strong portion and is often referred to simply as deep deltoid ligament. It arises from the posterior border of the anterior colliculus, as well as a small portion of the posterior colliculus of the medial malleolus, and inserts on the fovea at the medial margin of the talar body.* **(Middle)** *The calcaneofibular ligament is consistently seen on coronal images of the hindfoot deep to the peroneal tendons. It arises from the tip of the lateral malleolus and courses posteriorly, inferiorly, and medially to insert on the retrotrochlear eminence of the calcaneus.* **(Bottom)** *The contents of the tarsal tunnel, deep extrinsic flexor tendons and posterior tibial neurovascular bundle with its branches, are held beneath the flexor retinaculum. The medial osseous structures provide the floor of the tunnel.*

CORONAL T1 MR: LEFT ANKLE

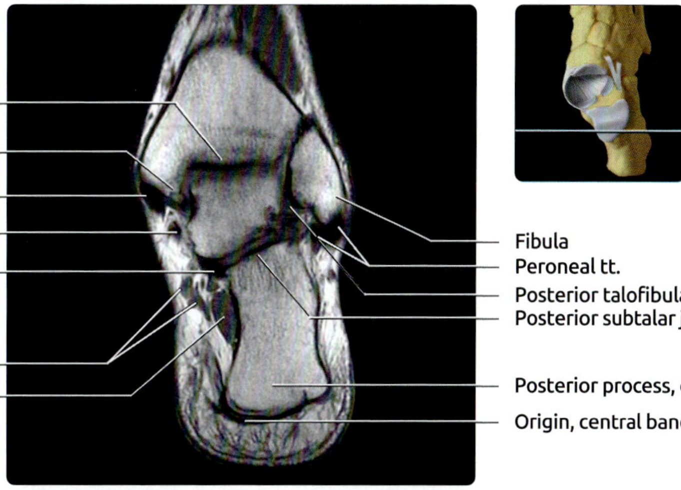

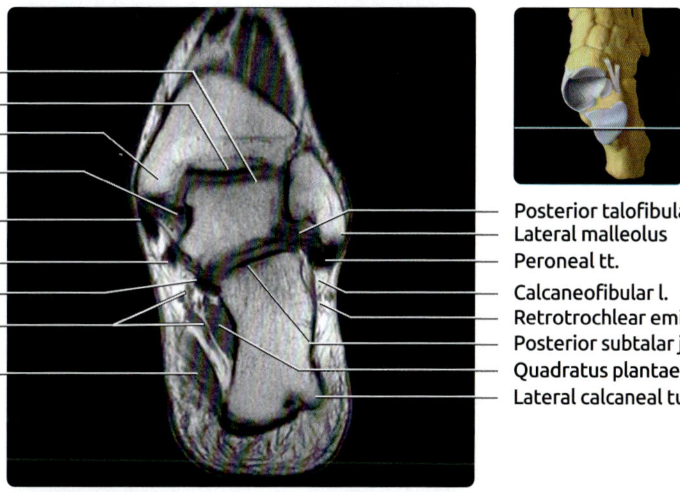

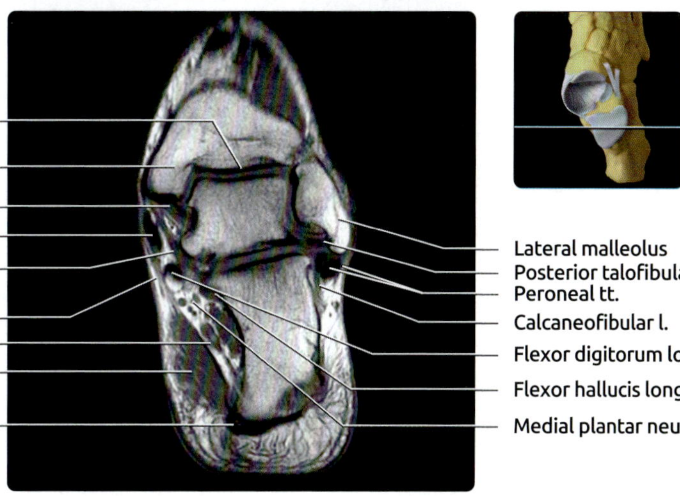

(Top) *The deep deltoid ligament is now coming into view. It has 2 bands. The posterior band is the constant and strong portion and is often referred to simply as deep deltoid ligament. It arises from the posterior border of the anterior colliculus, as well as a small portion of the posterior colliculus of the medial malleolus, and inserts on the fovea at the medial margin of the talar body.* **(Middle)** *The calcaneofibular ligament is consistently seen on coronal images of the hindfoot deep to the peroneal tendons. It arises from the tip of the lateral malleolus and courses posteriorly, inferiorly, and medially to insert on the retrotrochlear eminence of the calcaneus.* **(Bottom)** *The contents of the tarsal tunnel, deep extrinsic flexor tendons and posterior tibial neurovascular bundle with its branches, are held beneath the flexor retinaculum. The medial osseous structures provide the floor of the tunnel.*

CORONAL T1 MR: RIGHT ANKLE

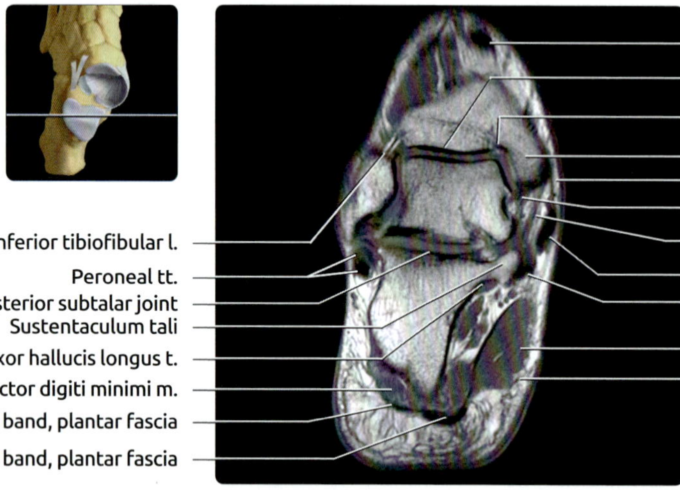

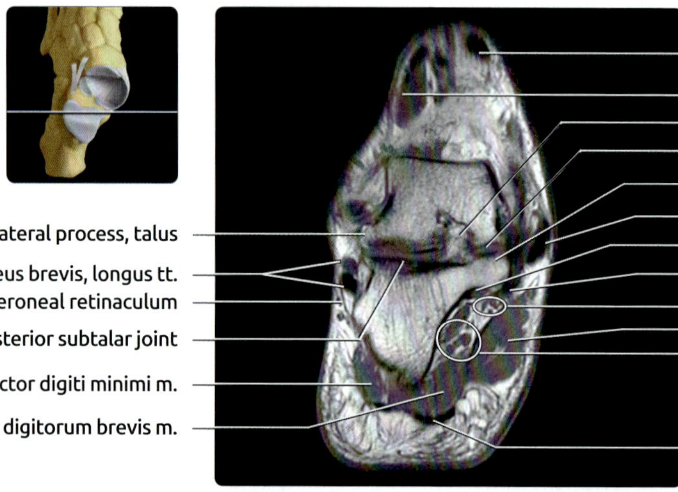

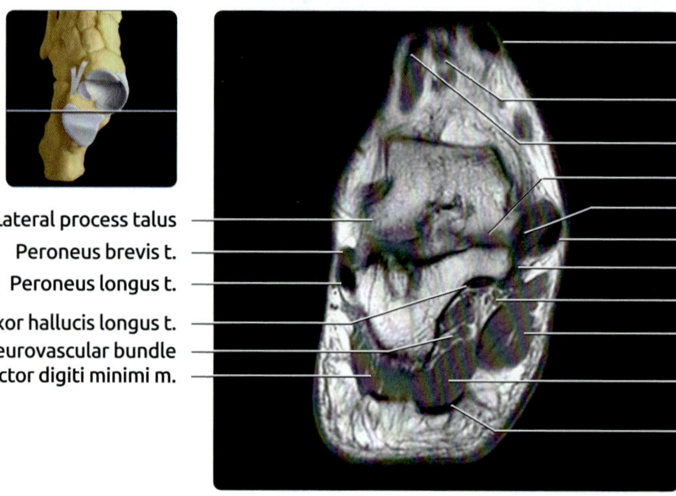

(Top) *The notch of Harty is a small elevation in the tibial medial surface, often associated with low-signal sclerosis above it, that should not be mistaken for tibial osteochondral lesion. The sustentaculum tali is a medial protuberance of the calcaneus; its most posterior portion, seen here, is nonarticular. More anteriorly it forms the inferior margin of the middle subtalar joint.* **(Middle)** *The majority of the sustentaculum tali articulates with a medial projection of the talus. The flexor hallucis longus tendon is seen coursing beneath the sustentaculum tali. Both it and the peroneus brevis show slightly increased signal intensity due to magic angle artifact.* **(Bottom)** *The tibialis anterior tendon is the largest extensor tendon. It can be followed on sequential coronal images and inserts on the 1st cuneiform and base of the 1st metatarsal. The posterior tibial nerve has split into the medial and lateral plantar nerves. The medial plantar nerve travels superior to the lateral plantar nerve and close to the flexor hallucis longus tendon.*

CORONAL T1 MR; LEFT ANKLE

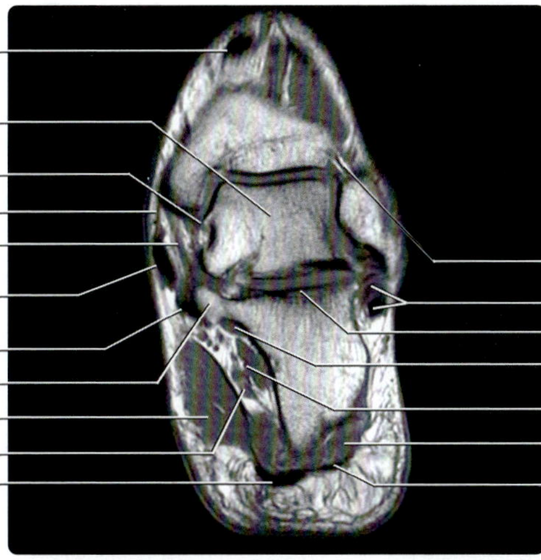

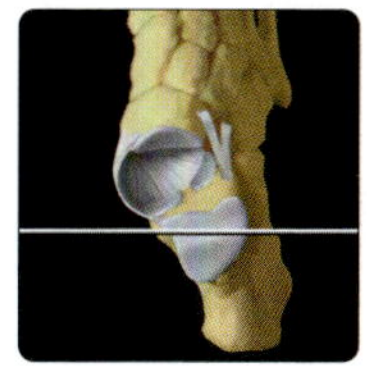

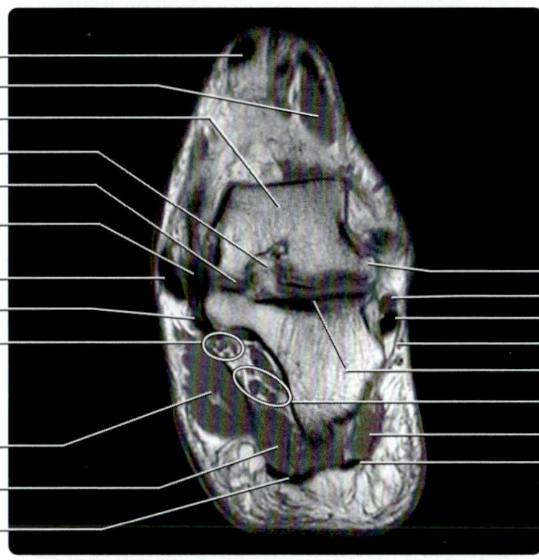

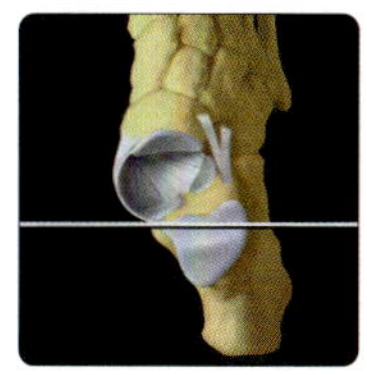

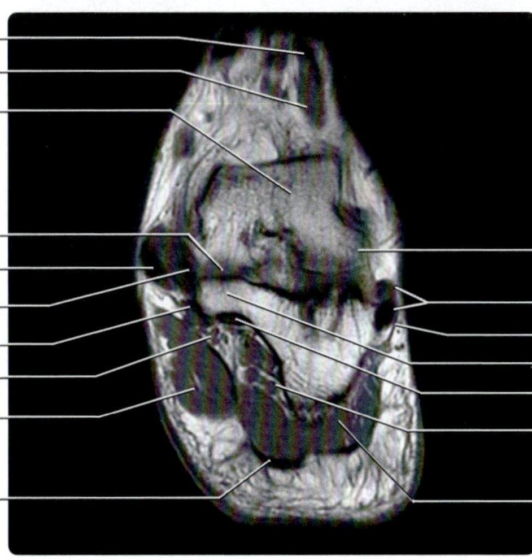

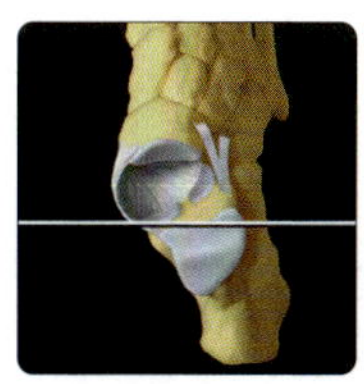

(Top) *The notch of Harty is a small elevation in the tibial medial surface, often associated with low-signal sclerosis above it, that should not be mistaken for tibial osteochondral lesion. The sustentaculum tali is a medial protuberance of the calcaneus; its most posterior portion, seen here, is nonarticular. More anteriorly it forms the inferior margin of the middle subtalar joint.* **(Middle)** *The majority of the sustentaculum tali articulates with a medial projection of the talus. The flexor hallucis longus tendon is seen coursing beneath the sustentaculum tali. Both it and the peroneus brevis show slightly increased signal intensity due to magic angle artifact.* **(Bottom)** *The tibialis anterior tendon is the largest extensor tendon. It can be followed on sequential coronal images and inserts on the 1st cuneiform and base of the 1st metatarsal. The posterior tibial nerve has split into the medial and lateral plantar nerves. The medial plantar nerve travels superior to the lateral plantar nerve and close to the flexor hallucis longus tendon.*

CORONAL T1 MR: RIGHT ANKLE

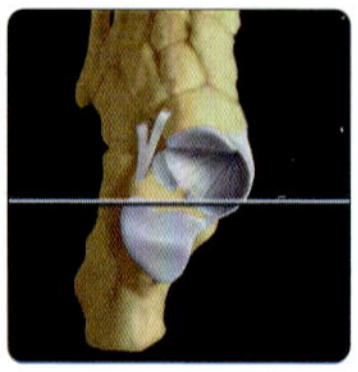

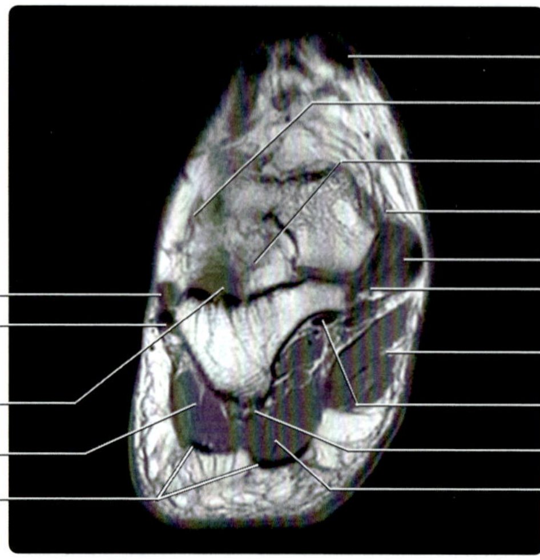

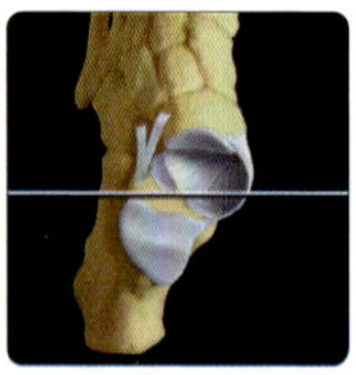

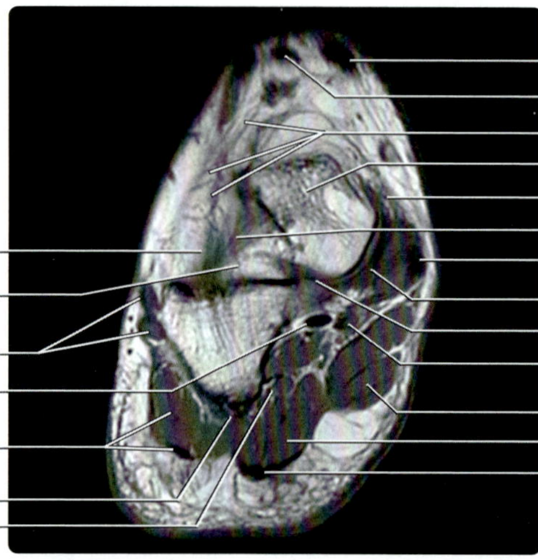

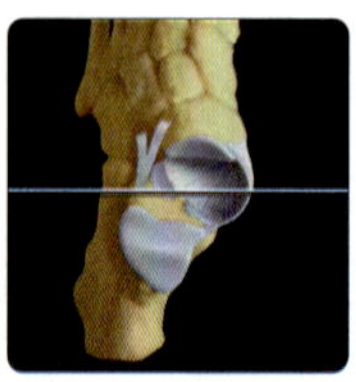

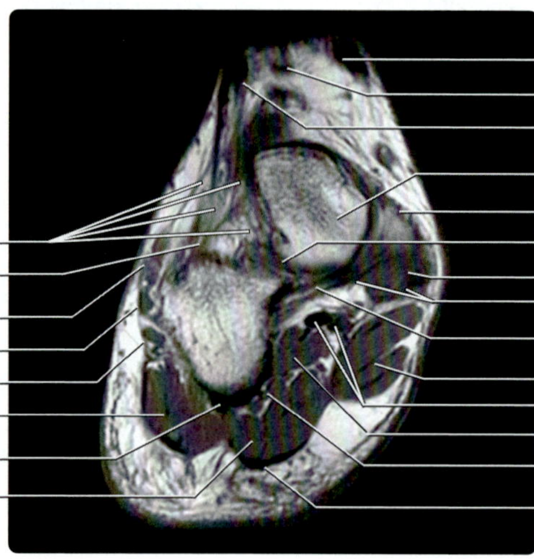

(Top) *The sinus tarsi is a lateral, funnel-shaped space between the talus and calcaneus, which is continuous with the tarsal canal located posteromedial to it. A joint recess from the posterior subtalar joint extends into the posteroinferior portion of the tarsal sinus.* **(Middle)** *Three bands of extensor retinaculum extend into tarsal sinus crossing the cervical ligament. The subcutaneous fat between the abductor hallucis and flexor digitorum brevis muscle is typically not traversed by the septa and therefore can be mistaken for a lipoma.* **(Bottom)** *The flexor digitorum longus and flexor hallucis longus tendons approximate and then cross each other under the navicular at the knot of Henry. The cervical ligament crosses the insertions of the extensor retinaculum in the tarsal sinus. Medioplantar oblique band of spring ligament originates from calcaneus immediately anterior to sustentaculum tali. Medioplantar oblique and superomedial bands arise from the sustentaculum.*

CORONAL T1 MR: LEFT ANKLE

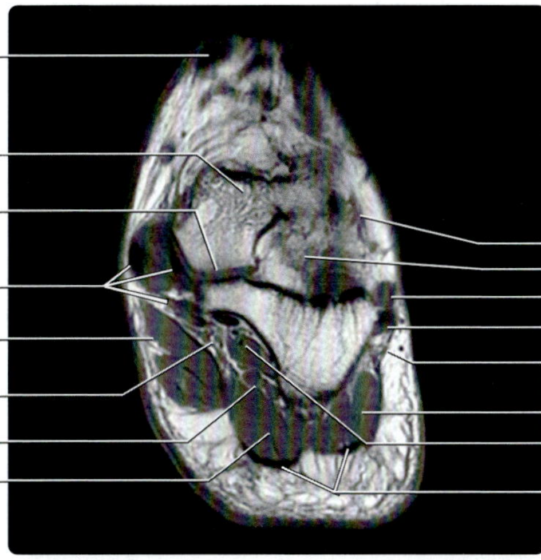

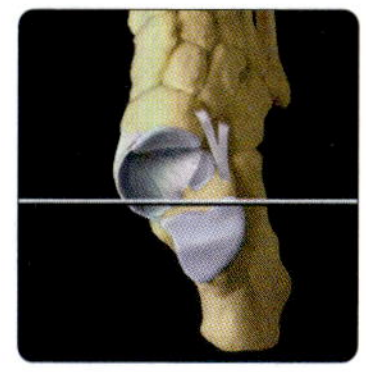

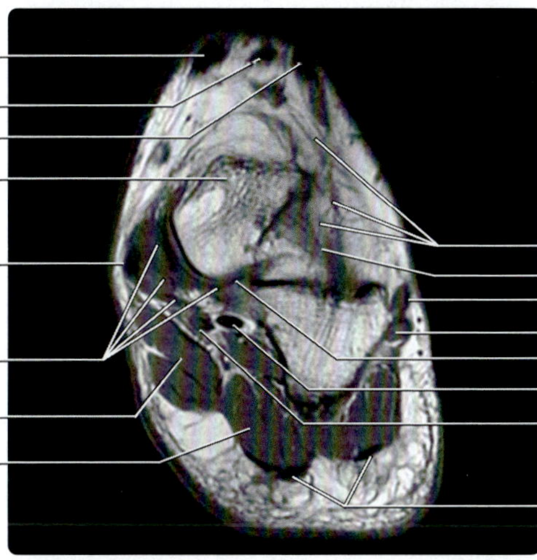

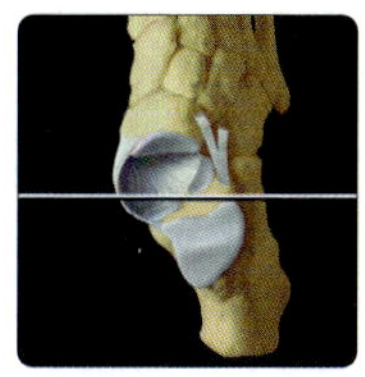

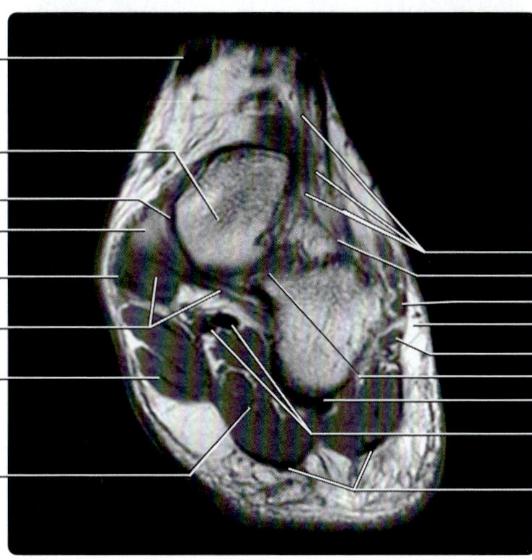

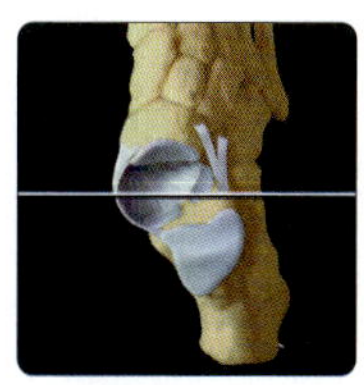

(Top) *The sinus tarsi is a lateral, funnel-shaped space between the talus and calcaneus, which is continuous with the tarsal canal located posteromedial to it. A joint recess from the posterior subtalar joint extends into the posteroinferior portion of the tarsal sinus.* **(Middle)** *Three bands of extensor retinaculum extend into tarsal sinus crossing the cervical ligament. The subcutaneous fat between the abductor hallucis and flexor digitorum brevis muscle is typically not traversed by the septa and therefore can be mistaken for a lipoma.* **(Bottom)** *The flexor digitorum longus and flexor hallucis longus tendons approximate and then cross each other under the navicular at the knot of Henry. The cervical ligament crosses the insertions of the extensor retinaculum in the tarsal sinus. Medioplantar oblique band of spring ligament originates from calcaneus immediately anterior to sustentaculum tali. Medioplantar oblique and superomedial bands arise from the sustentaculum.*

CORONAL T1 MR: RIGHT ANKLE

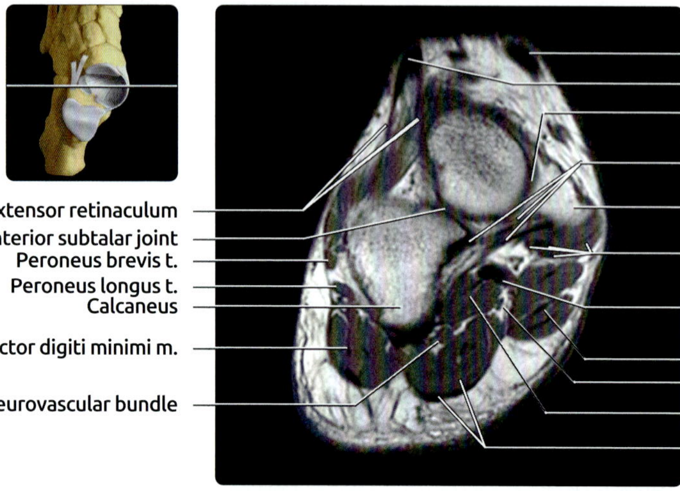

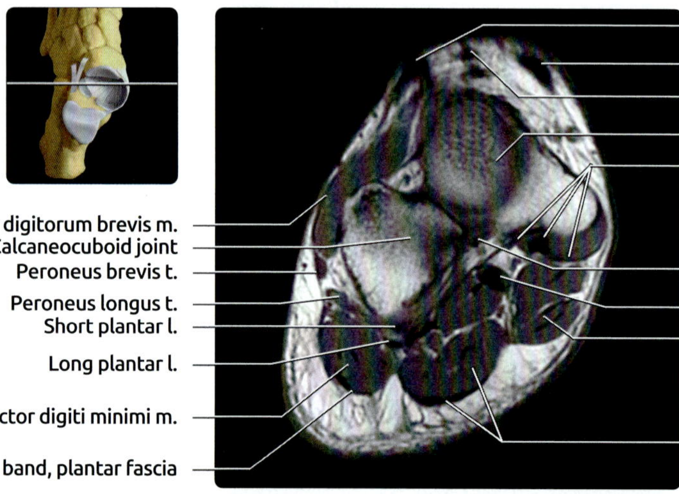

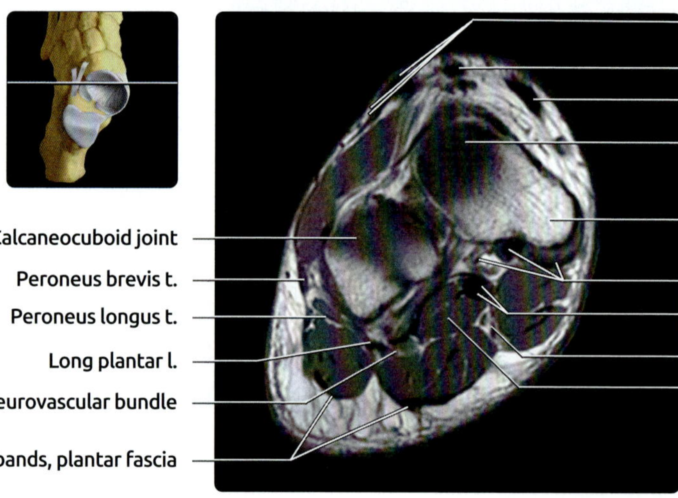

(Top) *The anatomy of the spring ligament is complex. Fortunately for practical reading of MR, tears are usually attritional, chronic, and involve all components.* **(Middle)** *Portions of the calcaneocuboid and talonavicular joints are seen en face. Peroneal tendons are diverging. Peroneus brevis tendon will become a thin ribbon as it inserts on the 5th metatarsal base. Peroneus longus is coursing medially and inferiorly toward the cuboid tunnel.* **(Bottom)** *Flexor hallucis and digitorum longus tendons have crossed. Quadratus plantae will insert on flexor digitorum longus. Anterior tibial tendon is starting to wrap around the medial side of the foot to its insertions on the 1st cuneiform and 1st metatarsal.*

CORONAL T1 MR: LEFT ANKLE

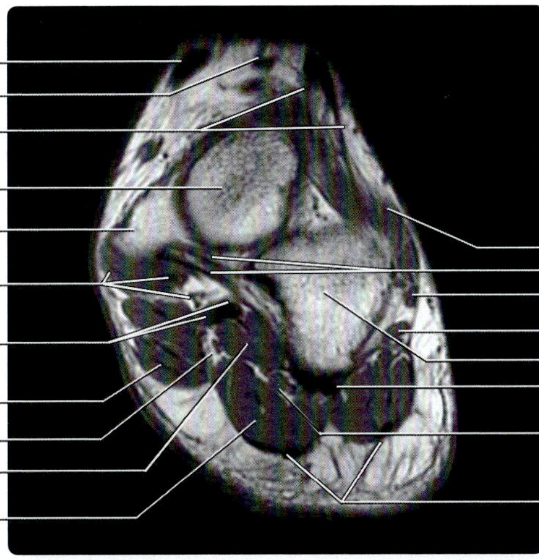

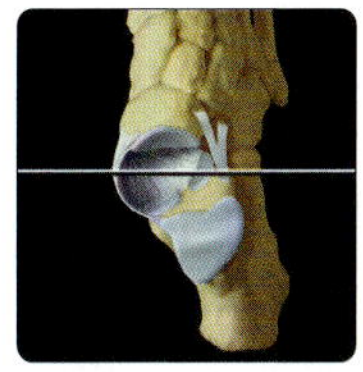

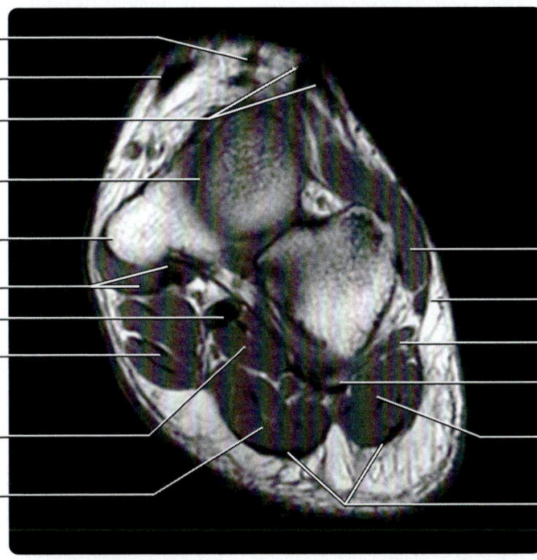

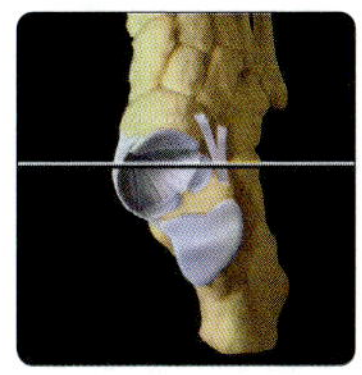

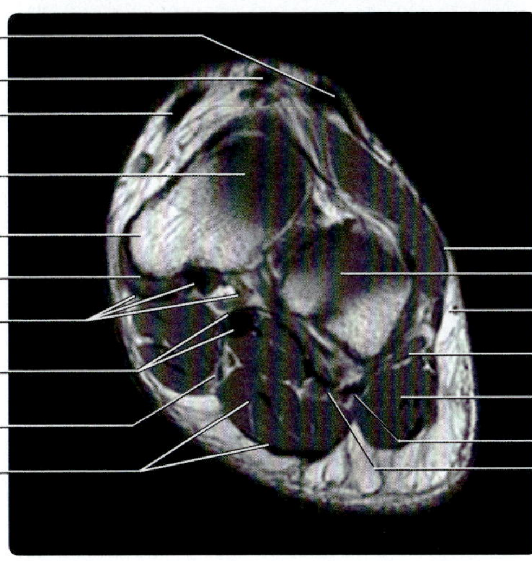

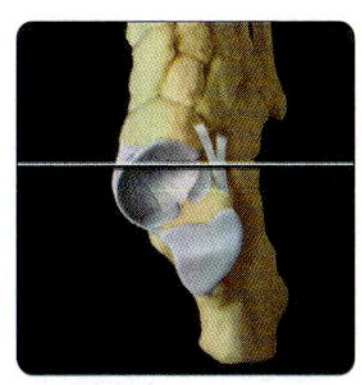

(Top) *The anatomy of the spring ligament is complex. Fortunately for practical reading of MR, tears are usually attritional, chronic, and involve all components.* **(Middle)** *Portions of the calcaneocuboid and talonavicular joints are seen en face. Peroneal tendons are diverging. Peroneus brevis tendon will become a thin ribbon as it inserts on the 5th metatarsal base. Peroneus longus is coursing medially and inferiorly toward the cuboid tunnel.* **(Bottom)** *Flexor hallucis and digitorum longus tendons have crossed. Quadratus plantae will insert on the flexor digitorum longus. Anterior tibial tendon is starting to wrap around the medial side of the foot to its insertions on the 1st cuneiform and 1st metatarsal.*

SAGITTAL T1 MR: ANKLE

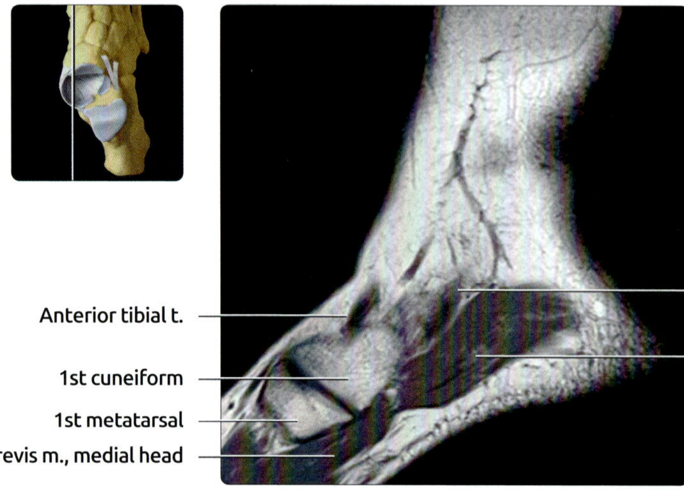

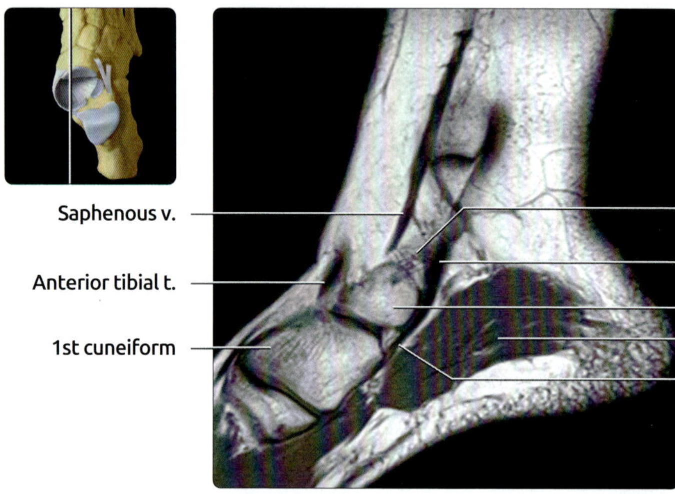

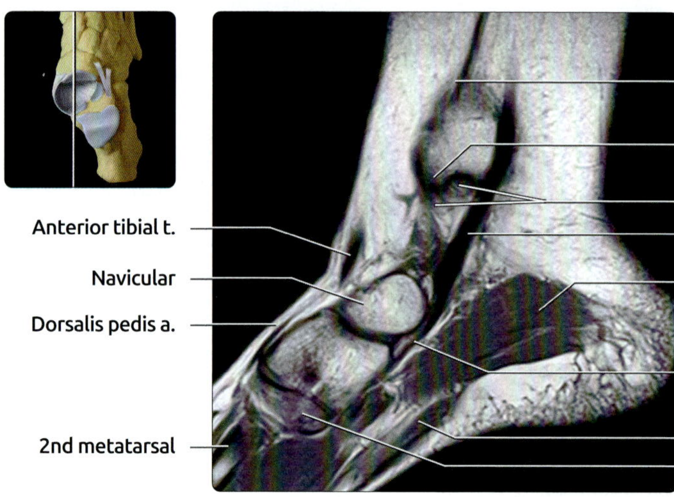

(Top) *Serial sagittal T1 MR images show the ankle from medial to lateral. On this furthest medial image, the anterior tibial tendon is seen wrapping around the medial margin of the 1st cuneiform. It will insert on the plantar-medial margin of the 1st cuneiform and metatarsal.* **(Middle)** *There is a sturdy slip of posterior tibial tendon extending from the navicular to the 1st cuneiform. Superomedial band of spring ligament is partly visible.* **(Bottom)** *A few fibers of the anterior portions of the superficial deltoid ligament are visible arising from the medial surface of the medial malleolus. The bands are named for their attachments: Anterior and posterior tibiotalar, tibiocalcaneal, tibiospring, and tibionavicular.*

SAGITTAL T1 MR: ANKLE

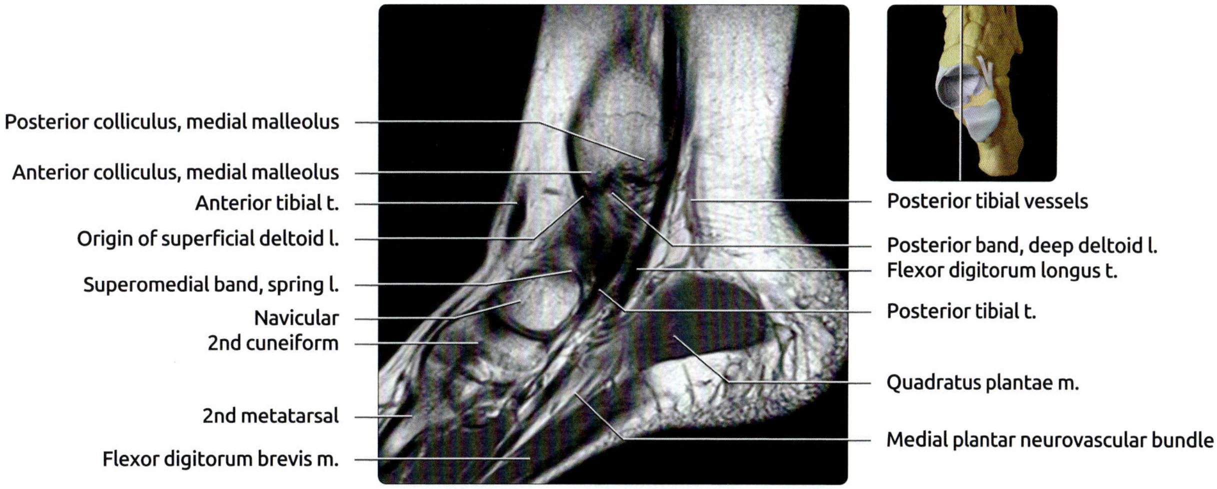

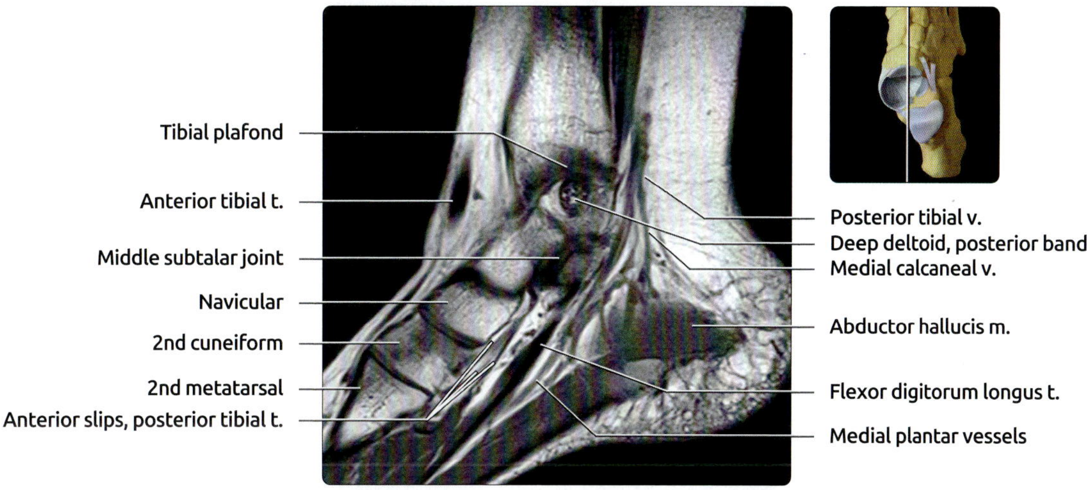

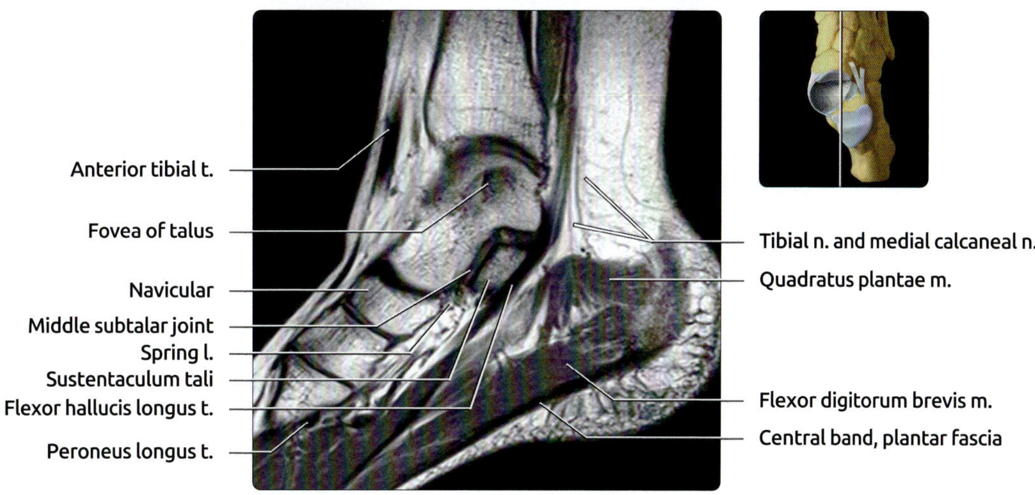

(Top) *Posterior tibial artery and vein lie medial to tibial nerve. All of the superficial deltoid ligament bands arise from the anterior and superficial surface of the medial malleolus.* **(Middle)** *The bulbous valves on veins help to distinguish them from arteries and nerves. The distinction is more readily apparent on fluid-sensitive sequences as the vessels are usually higher signal intensity than the nerves.* **(Bottom)** *The fovea of the talus, inferior to the cartilaginous portion of the joint, is the site of insertion of the posterior band of the deep deltoid ligament.*

SAGITTAL T1 MR: ANKLE

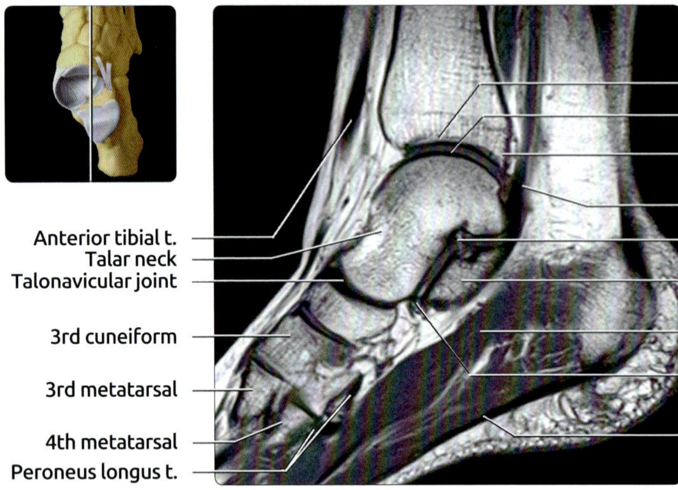

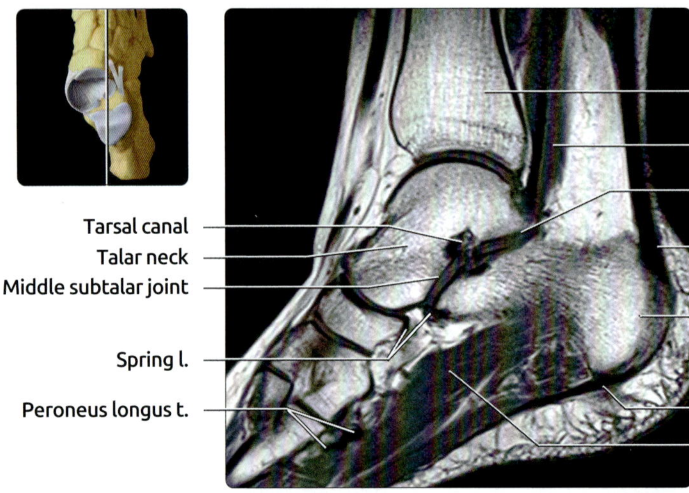

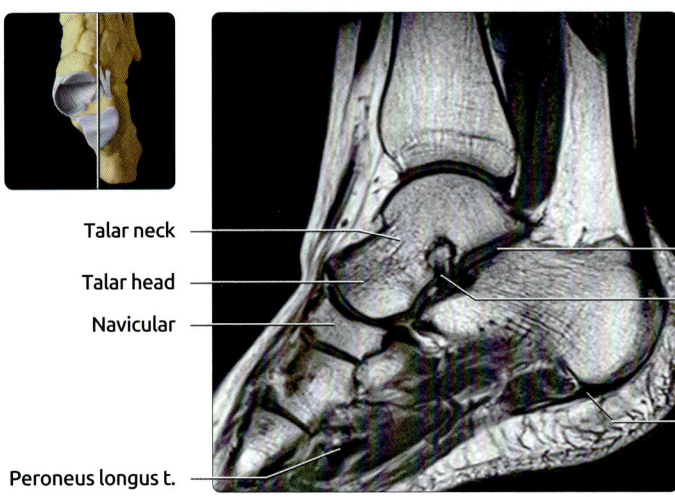

(Top) *The talar trochlea, miscalled the talar dome, articulates with the tibial plafond. The plafond extends further inferiorly in its posterior portion, a broad expansion of the tibia called the posterior malleolus.* **(Middle)** *The posterior subtalar joint is shorter in anteroposterior dimension medially than it is laterally. The middle subtalar joint lies anterior to it and also extends further medially.* **(Bottom)** *The interosseous talocalcaneal ligament lies in the tarsal canal, the narrow posteromedial extension of the tarsal sinus.*

SAGITTAL T1 MR: ANKLE

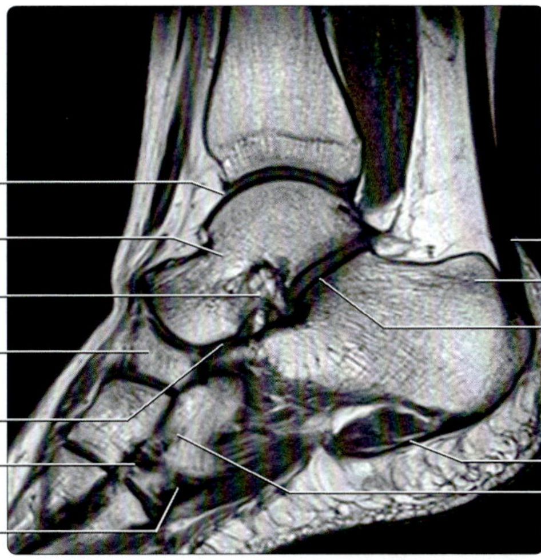

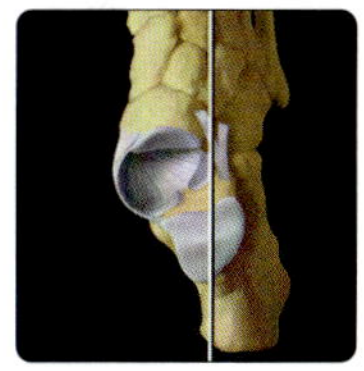

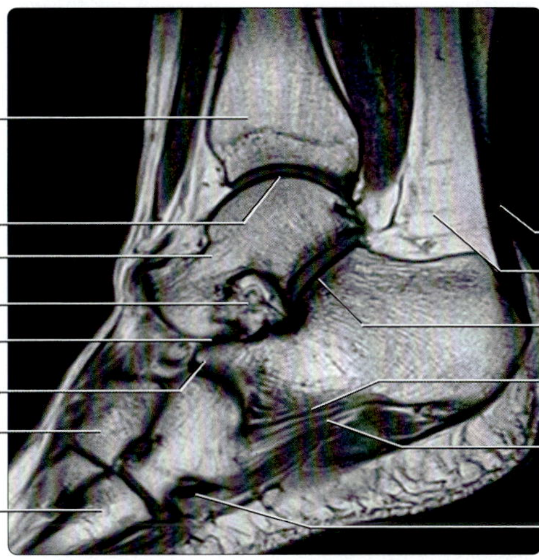

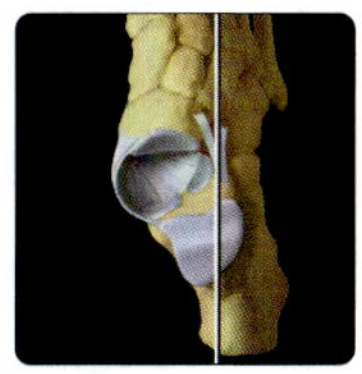

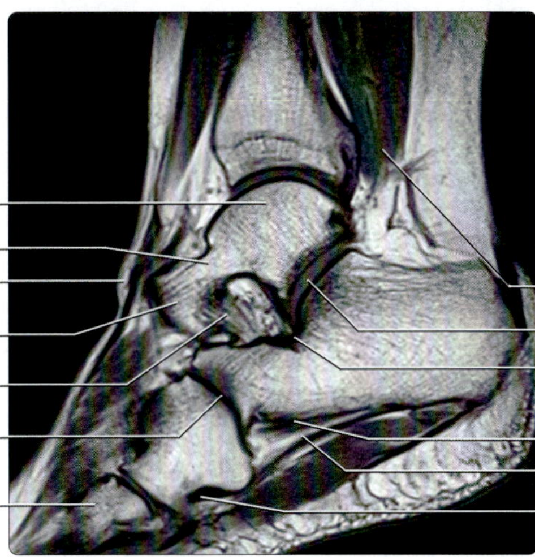

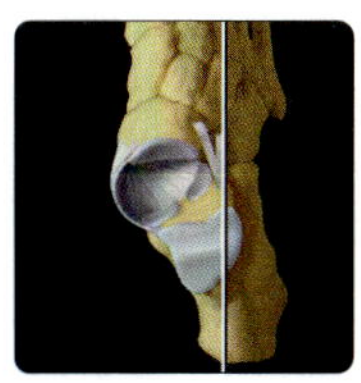

(Top) *The funnel-shaped tarsal sinus begins to be visible at this level. It will widen farther laterally.* **(Middle)** *The short and long plantar ligaments are coming into view.* **(Bottom)** *Note that when the foot is not weight bearing, the calcaneocuboid joint normally appears subluxated. The joint has a sinusoidal contour. The calcaneus moves inferiorly relative to the cuboid when a person stands.*

SAGITTAL T1 MR: ANKLE

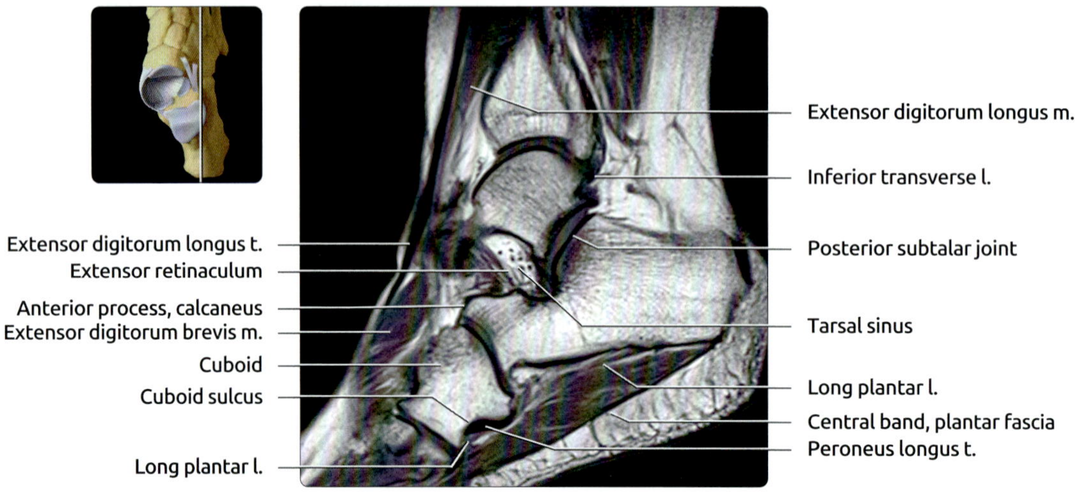

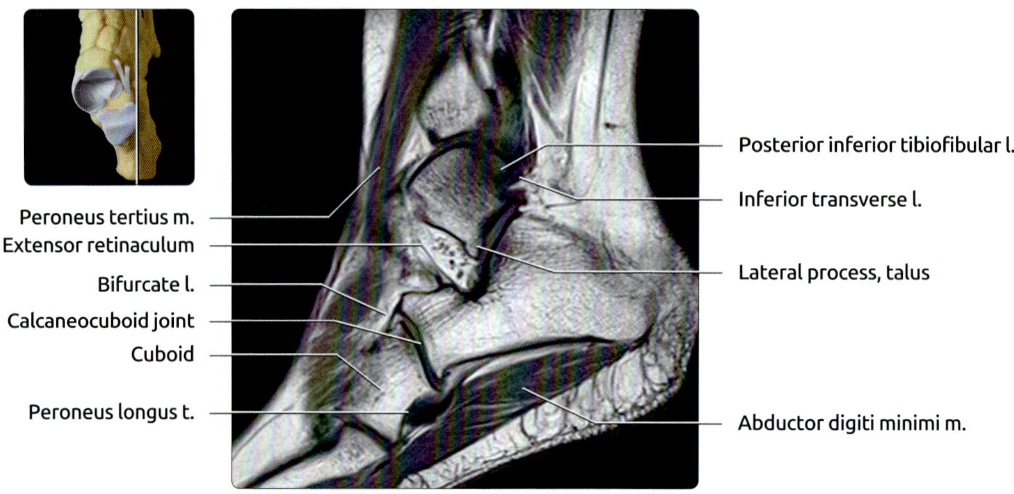

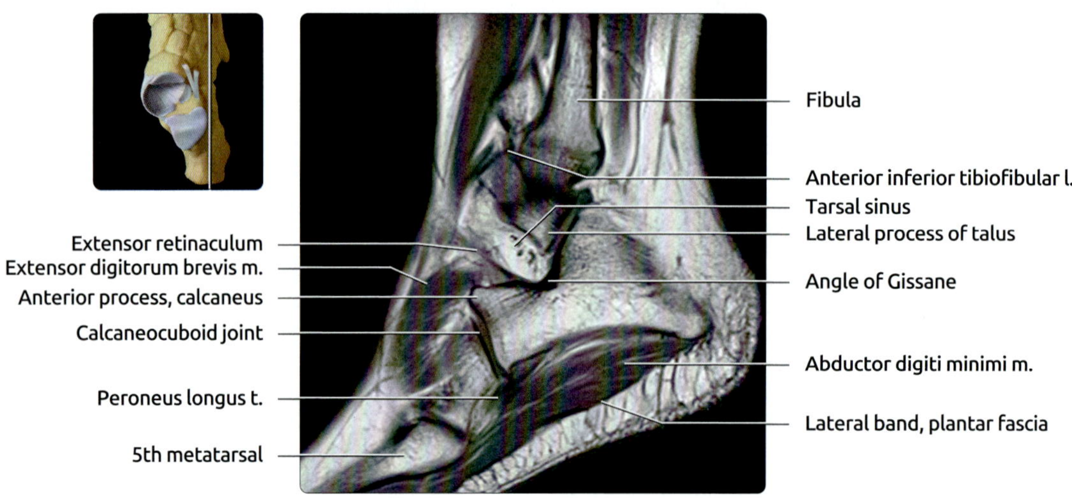

(Top) *The long plantar ligament converts the cuboid sulcus into a tunnel through which passes the peroneus longus tendon.* **(Middle)** *The inferior transverse ligament can mimic a loose body. It extends from the posteromedial tibia to the tip of the fibula. The calcaneocuboid limb of the bifurcate ligament is also well seen on this image.* **(Bottom)** *Extensor retinaculum is seen coursing over the dorsum of the hindfoot. It sends 3 limbs into the tarsal sinus.*

SAGITTAL T1 MR: ANKLE

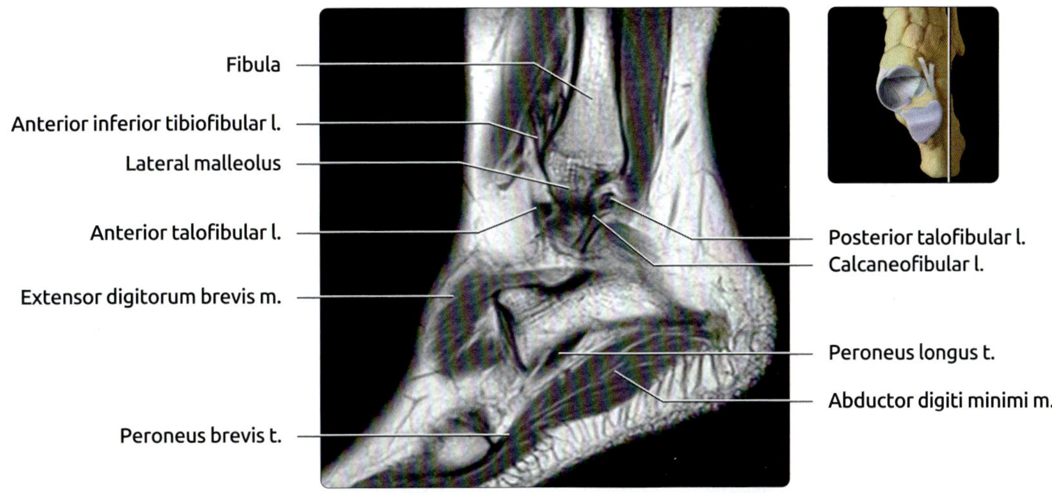

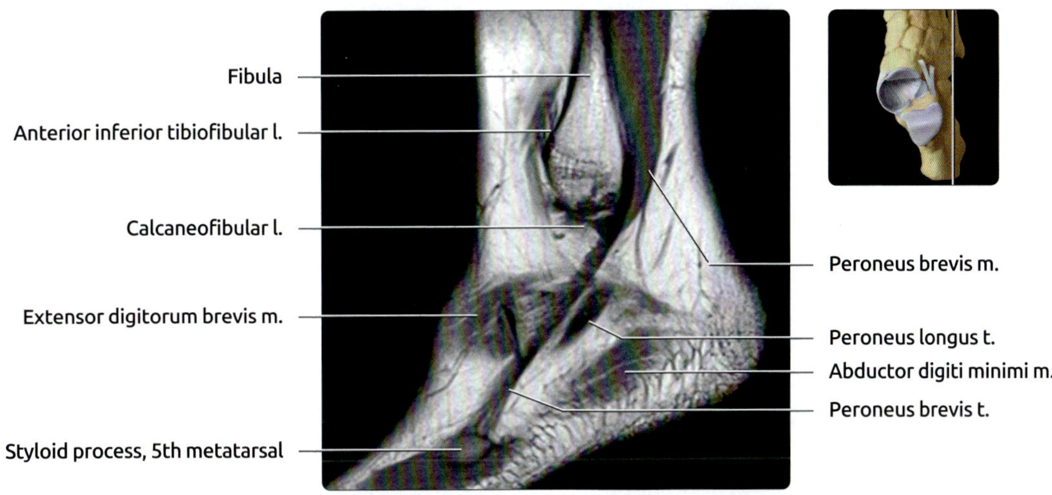

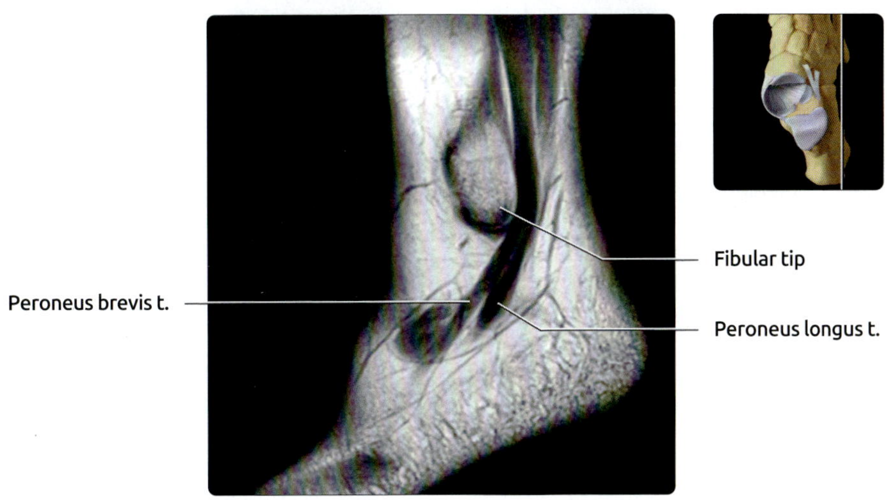

(Top) *The striated appearance of the anterior inferior tibiofibular ligament is well shown. The most inferior fascicle, the Bassett ligament, is reportedly a normal variant but is almost always visible on MR.* **(Middle)** *The peroneus brevis tendon is anterior to the longus in the foot. It is seen attaching to the styloid process of the 5th metatarsal.* **(Bottom)** *The farthest lateral image in this sequence shows the divergence of the peroneus brevis and longus tendons.*

GROSS ANATOMY

Organizing Anatomy

- Muscles originate at knee or leg, become tendinous around ankle, tendons insert in foot
- 3 compartments: Anterior, lateral, and posterior
- Anterior compartment from medial to lateral contains anterior tibial, extensor hallucis longus, extensor digitorum longus, and peroneus tertius (variably present) tendons
- Posterior compartment has deep and superficial compartments
  - Superficial: Achilles and plantaris tendons
  - Deep from medial to lateral contains posterior tibial, flexor digitorum longus, & flexor hallucis longus tendons
- Lateral compartment contains peroneus longus and brevis tendons

Transition From Leg to Foot

- Tendons (except Achilles) all dramatically change course from leg to foot
- Positions are maintained by retinacula, fibrous bands, which hold tendons close to underlying bones and joints
  - Extensor retinaculum
    - Bursa usually present deep to inferior extensor retinaculum
  - Flexor retinaculum
  - Peroneal retinaculum

Tendon Sheaths

- All tendons of ankle except Achilles have sheaths
- Achilles surrounded by loose tissue called paratenon
- Flexor hallucis longus tendon sheath communicates with ankle joint

Anterior Compartment: Innervation by Deep Peroneal Nerve

- Anterior tibial
  - Largest tendon of anterior compartment
  - Origin: Upper 2/3 lateral tibia, interosseous membrane, intermuscular septum
  - Insertion: Medial margin of 1st cuneiform and 1st metatarsal
  - Action: Dorsiflexion, inversion
  - Variant: Tendon may be bifid; may have small accessory muscle (of Gruber)
  - Variant: May insert on navicular or more distally on 1st digit
- Extensor hallucis longus
  - Origin: Proximal fibula and interosseous membrane
  - Insertion: Distal phalanx, 1st toe (sometimes to proximal phalanx)
  - Action: Dorsiflexion of 1st toe and foot
- Extensor digitorum longus
  - Origin: Lateral tibial condyle, upper 3/4 fibula, upper interosseous membrane
  - Insertion: 2nd-5th toes, join extensor digitorum brevis
  - Action: Dorsiflexion of toes
- Peroneus tertius
  - Origin: Distal fibula and interosseous membrane
  - Insertion: Dorsal margin of 5th metatarsal base
  - Variably present

Lateral Compartment: Innervation by Peroneal Nerve

- Peroneus longus
  - Origin: Proximal fibula
  - Insertion: 1st cuneiform and 1st metatarsal base
  - Action: Plantar flexion and eversion
  - Travels from lateral to medial plantar surface of foot through cuboid sulcus
- Peroneus brevis
  - Origin: Lower 2/3 fibula, deep to peroneus longus
  - Insertion: 5th metatarsal styloid process (also called tuberosity)
  - Action: Plantar flexion and eversion
  - Muscle normally terminates at tip of fibula, but muscle belly may be low-lying
- Peroneus quartus (variably present)
  - Origin: Distal, lateral fibula
  - Insertion: Variable, usually on peroneus brevis or calcaneus

Superficial Posterior Compartment: Innervation by Tibial Nerve

- Achilles tendon
  - Conjoined tendon of gastrocnemius and soleus muscles
  - Insertion: Posterior tuberosity of calcaneus
  - Action: Plantar flexion of foot
  - Anterior margin is concave; AP diameter < 6 mm on axial images
  - Soleus muscle may be low-lying and extend nearly to calcaneus
- Plantaris
  - Origin: Posterior margin of lateral femoral condyle
  - Insertion: Posterior process calcaneus, medial to Achilles
  - Action: Plantar flexion of foot

Deep Posterior Compartment: Innervation by Tibial Nerve

- Posterior tibial
  - Origin: Posterior tibia, fibula, and interosseous membrane
  - Insertion: Median eminence of navicular
    - Small slips extend anteriorly to 1st-3rd cuneiforms, cuboid, 2nd-4th metatarsals (± 5th metatarsal)
  - Action: Inversion, plantar flexion of foot
- Flexor digitorum longus
  - Origin: Posterior tibia and intermuscular septum with posterior tibial muscle
  - Note: Crosses lateral to posterior tibial muscle above ankle
  - Insertion: 2nd-5th toes
  - Quadratus plantae inserts onto it, flexor digitorum brevis slips arise from it
- Flexor hallucis longus
  - Origin: Posterior fibula and interosseous membrane
  - Insertion: Distal phalanx of 1st toe
  - Action: Plantar flexion of 1st toe
  - Note: Communicates with ankle joint; fluid in tendon sheath is normal
  - Note: Intersects with flexor digitorum longus tendon at master knot of Henry, in midfoot

GRAPHICS: LATERAL ANKLE TENDONS AND SHEATHS

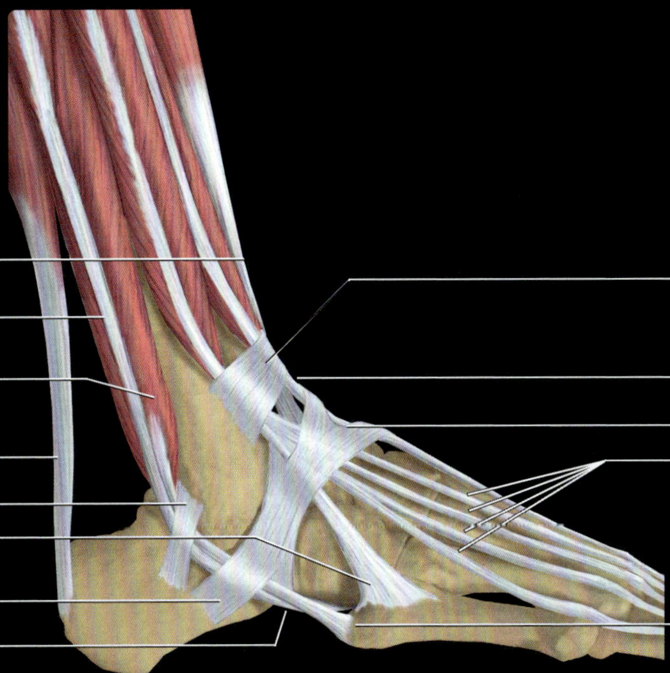

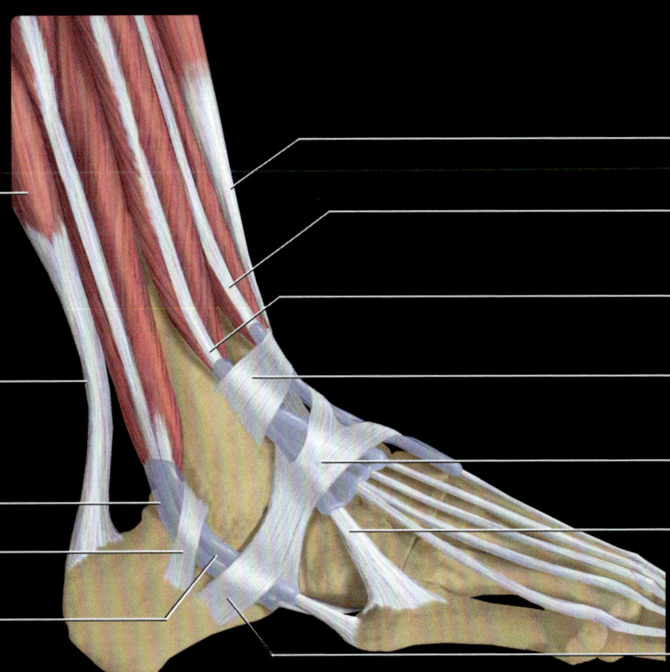

(Top) *Lateral view shows how the peroneus brevis and peroneus longus tendons descend posterior to the fibula, maintained within the retromalleolar groove by the superior peroneal retinaculum and continue along the lateral wall of calcaneus, held in place by the inferior peroneal retinaculum. Fibers of the inferior peroneal retinaculum insert and separate the 2 tendons. The peroneus longus tendon curves around the cuboid to enter the sole of the foot. Both the peroneus brevis and peroneus tertius tendons insert on the 5th metatarsal base.* **(Bottom)** *Lateral view shows the tendon sheaths, which provide tendons with vascularity, smooth gliding, and greater freedom of movement. The Achilles tendon is the only ankle tendon without a tendon sheath; it is surrounded by paratenon. The peroneal tendons share a common sheath above the inferior peroneal retinaculum. More distally each tendon is enveloped by its own sheath. The peroneus longus tendon has a 2nd sheath under the sole of the foot.*

GRAPHICS: TENDONS OF ANKLE

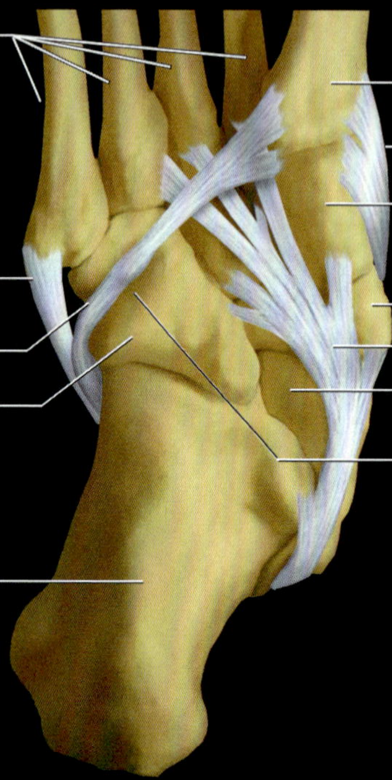

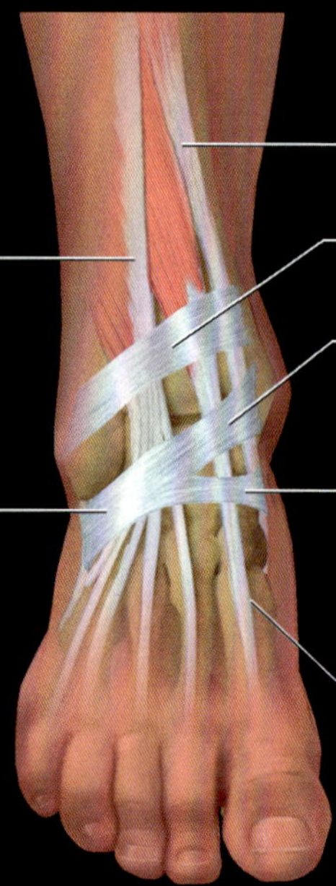

(Top) *Graphic shows the insertions of long tendons on the plantar foot. The posterior tibial tendon inserts on all the tarsal bones (excluding talus) and on 2nd-4th metatarsal bases. The posterior and anterior tibial tendons and peroneus longus tendon insertions together form a sling supporting the medial longitudinal arch.* **(Bottom)** *Anterior view shows the extrinsic tendons held by the superior and inferior extensor retinacula and extending to their insertions.*

GRAPHICS: TENDONS AND SHEATHS

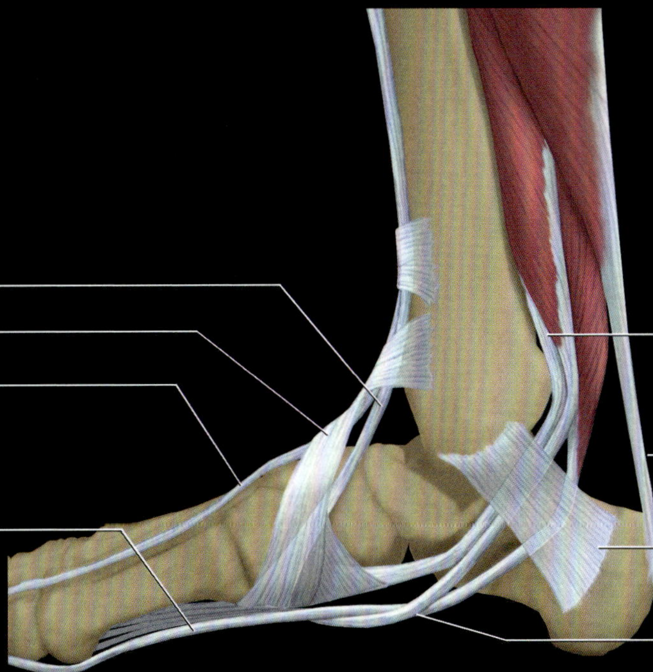

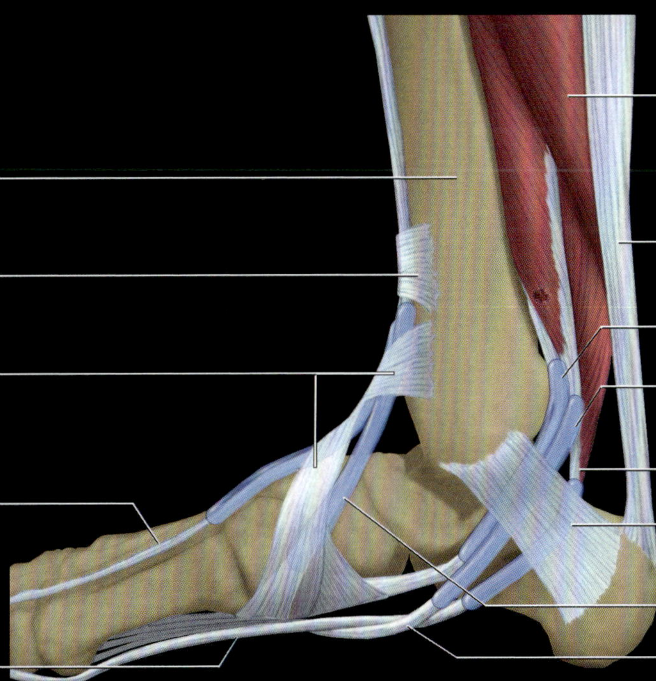

(Top) *Medial view shows the posterior tibial, flexor digitorum longus, and flexor hallucis longus tendons traversing under the flexor retinaculum within the tarsal tunnel. The flexor digitorum longus and flexor hallucis longus tendons cross each other under the navicular. The extensor tendons descend deep to the extensor retinacula.* **(Bottom)** *The sheath of posterior tibial tendon ends approximately 1-2 cm proximal to its navicular insertion. Minimal tendon sheath fluid is normal except in the flexor hallucis longus sheath where a large amount of fluid is common due to normal communication with the ankle joint.*

AXIAL MR: ACHILLES TENDON

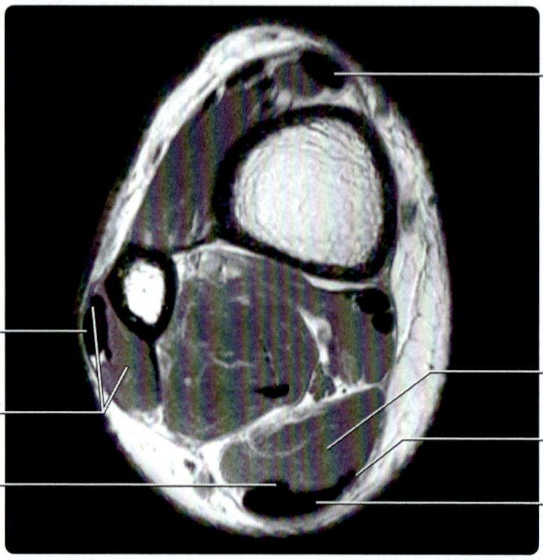

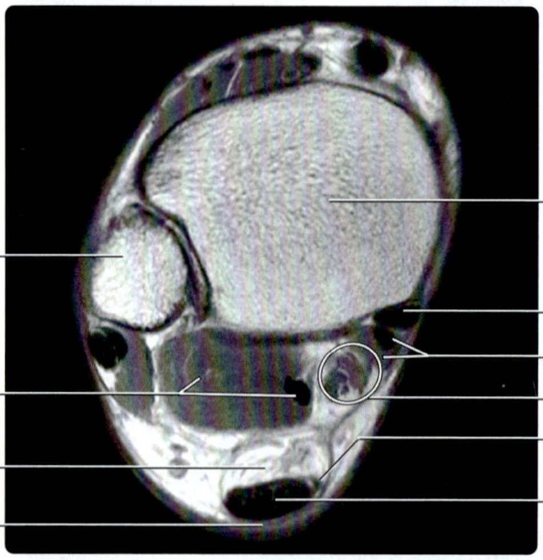

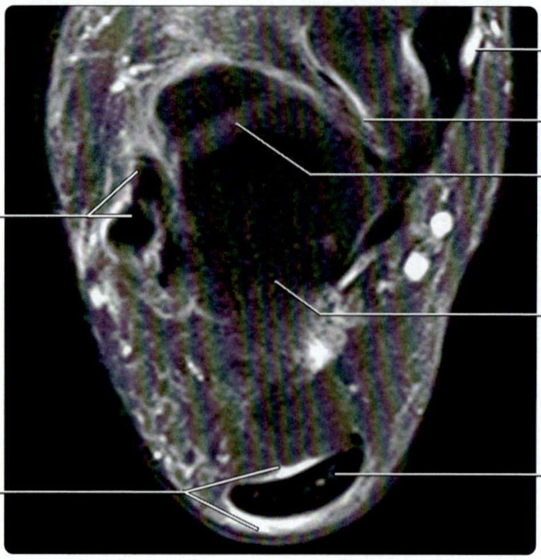

(Top) *As the soleus tendon joins the gastrocnemius aponeurosis, it forms a lateral bump on the anterior surface of the Achilles tendon, as seen on this axial image. The Achilles tendon spirals as it descends down the calf so that the gastrocnemius contribution is mainly on the lateral and posterior surface of the tendon.* **(Middle)** *The anterior surface of the Achilles tendon is now flat to slightly concave. Note the subtle normal heterogeneity of the tendon. The large pre-Achilles (Kager) fat pad separates the Achilles tendon from the deep posterior compartment tendons. This fat pad is typically traversed by fine, low-signal vessels and septa. Note the plantaris tendon descending along the medial aspect of the Achilles tendon.* **(Bottom)** *Axial PD FS MR shows the paratenon, the tissue surrounding the Achilles tendon in lieu of a tendon sheath. Note that the tendon has a normal, concave anterior contour and thickness (< 6 mm). There is also a small amount of fluid in the posterior tibial tendon sheath, an incidental finding.*

AXIAL MR: ACHILLES TENDON

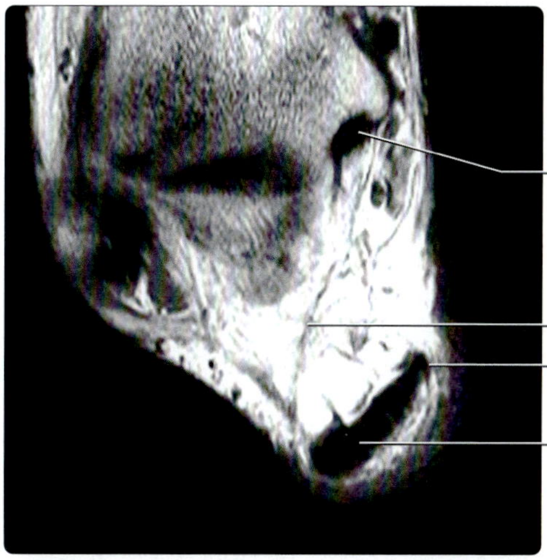

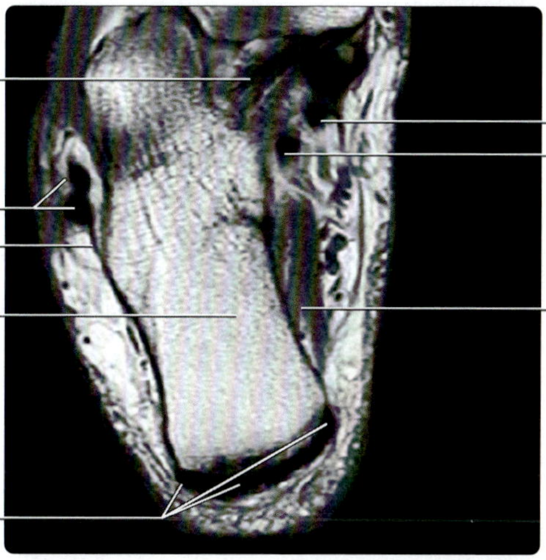

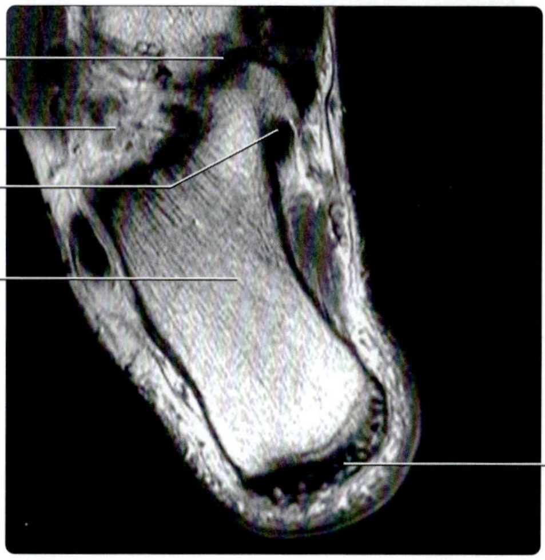

(Top) *The Achilles tendon inserts into a large rough area on the posterior calcaneus, a few millimeters below the apex of the calcaneal tuberosity. The tendon develops a flat contour approximately 4 cm above its insertion as seen in this image. Note the normal heterogeneity of the tendon. The tendon may be cartilaginous at its very distal aspect.* **(Middle)** *Note the broad insertion of the Achilles tendon to the calcaneus.* **(Bottom)** *Note the interdigitation of the bone and tendon at the insertion of the Achilles tendon to the calcaneus.*

SAGITTAL MR: ACHILLES TENDON

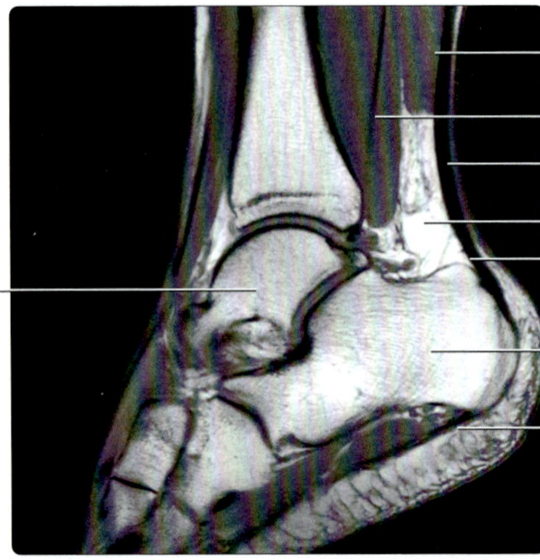

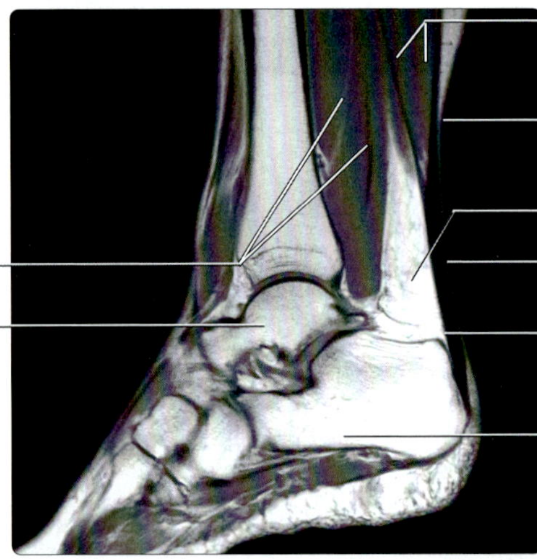

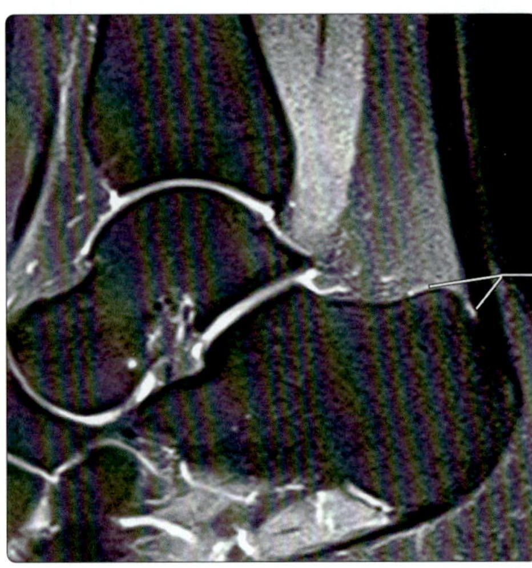

(Top) *The Achilles tendon measures approximately 15 cm in length. The soleus muscle may be low-lying, however, extending nearly to the tendon insertion on the calcaneus (not seen in this case).* **(Middle)** *Note the merger of the soleus tendon with the gastrocnemius tendon/aponeurosis. Tears of the Achilles tendon typically occur 2-6 cm above the insertion of the Achilles tendon, an area that is well seen on routine sagittal ankle images. Tears of the Achilles musculotendinous junction, however, may require imaging more proximally.* **(Bottom)** *The pre-Achilles bursa is also known as the retrocalcaneal bursa. It is normal to see a small amount of fluid in the bursa, as shown here. The retro-Achilles bursa is an adventitious bursa due to impingement of the heel, usually related to shoes.*

AXIAL MR: POSTERIOR TIBIAL TENDON

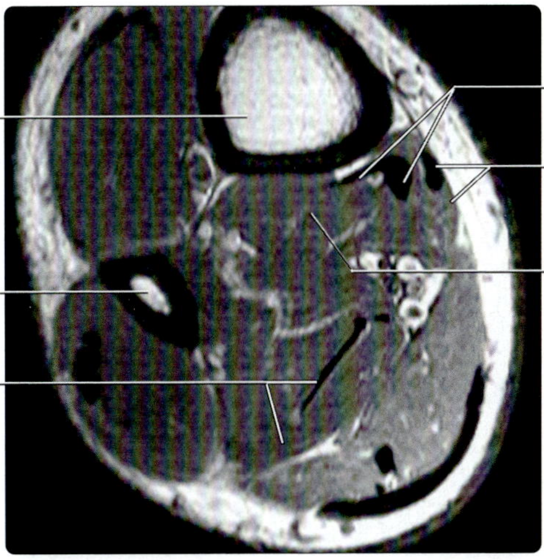

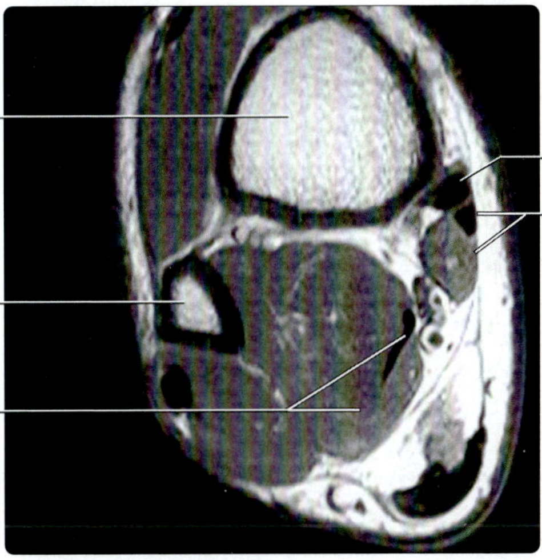

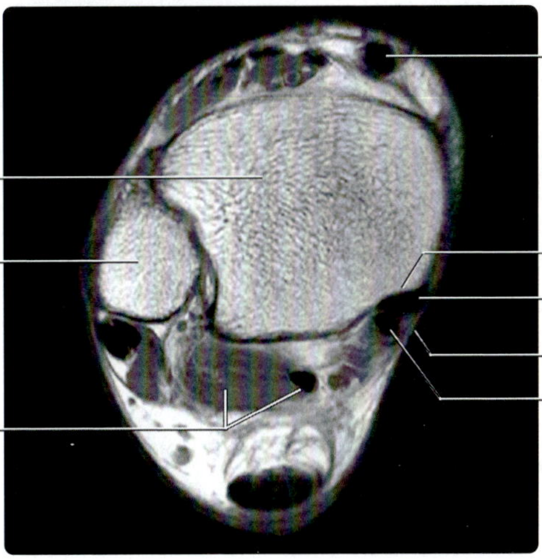

(Top) *In the distal leg, the posterior tibial muscle lies between the flexor hallucis longus and flexor digitorum longus muscles. Often, the muscle has 2 tendinous slips (as seen here), which typically fuse into 1 slip by the time the tendon reaches the ankle joint. Occasionally, the 2 tendon slips are still seen at the ankle joint and should not be mistaken for a torn tendon.* **(Middle)** *A few centimeters above the ankle joint, the posterior tibial tendon crosses deep to the flexor digitorum longus tendon to become the most medial tendon of the deep posterior compartment.* **(Bottom)** *Just above the ankle joint, the posterior tibial and flexor digitorum longus tendon lie deep to the flexor retinaculum, within a common retrotibial groove, posterior to the tibia and medial malleolus. Each tendon, however, is enclosed within its own separate tendon sheath. The flexor retinaculum holds the tendons in place within the retrotibial groove. The posterior tibial tendon is 2x the size of the flexor digitorum longus tendon.*

CORONAL MR: POSTERIOR TIBIAL TENDON

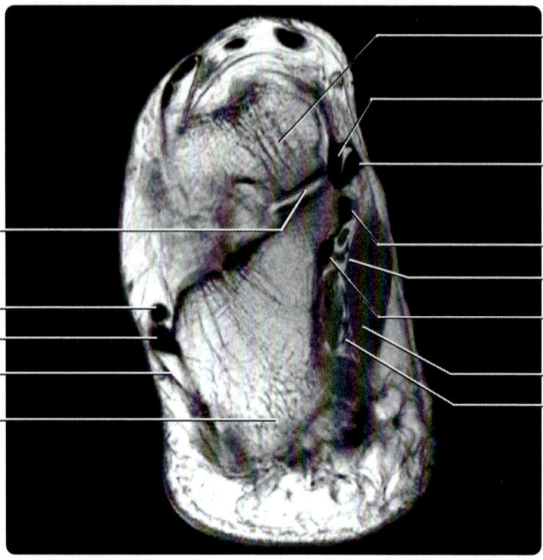

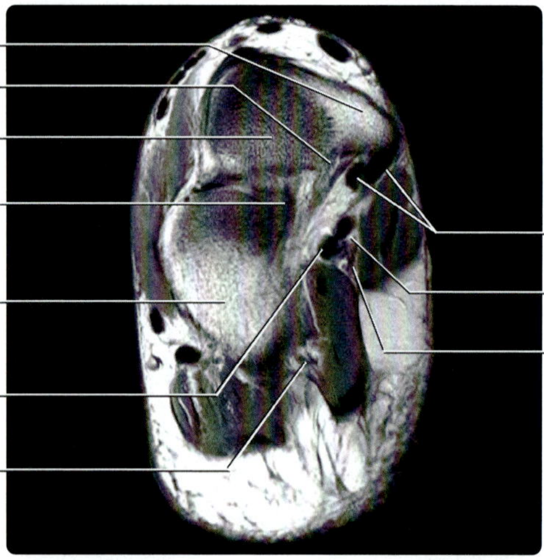

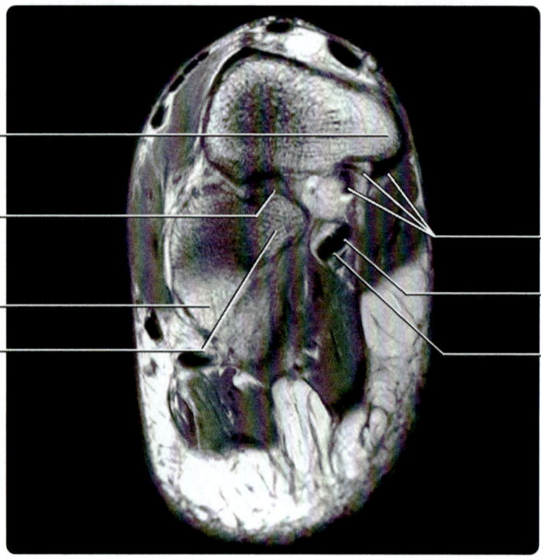

(Top) *Coronal MR through the hindfoot shows that as the posterior tibial tendon courses anteriorly, medial to the talar head, it lies superficial to the deltoid ligament.* **(Middle)** *In the foot, the posterior tibial tendon divides into 2 major components, as seen in this image: (1) Larger, more medial division inserts directly into the navicular tuberosity and (2) lateral, smaller division inserts to all other tarsal bones (excluding talus) and 2nd-4th metatarsal bases. The posterior tibial tendon may appear heterogeneous at its navicular insertion due to the magic angle phenomenon or partial volume averaging of tendon slips.* **(Bottom)** *Coronal T1WI MR is anterior to the main portion of the posterior tibial tendon onto the navicular. Several small slips are seen extending anteriorly.*

MR: POSTERIOR TIBIAL TENDON DISTAL SLIPS

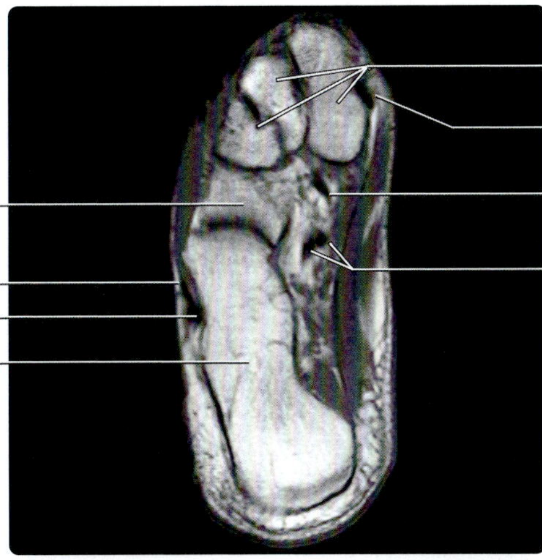

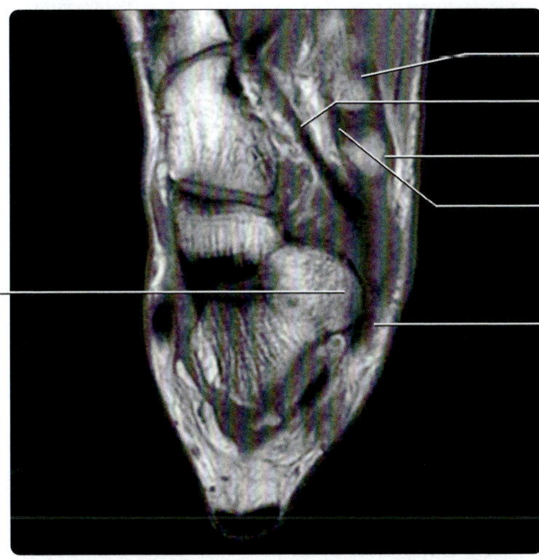

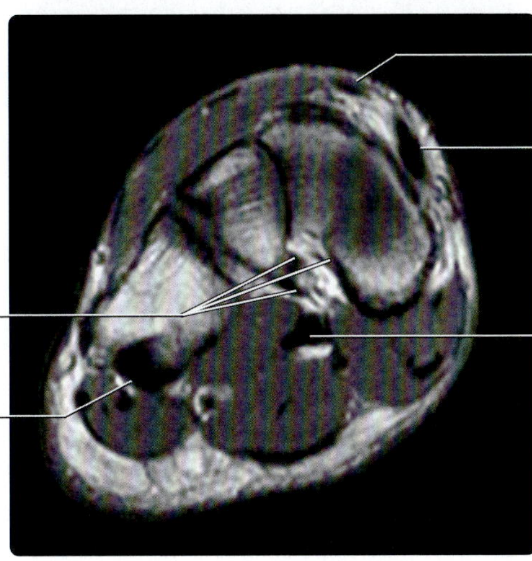

(Top) *Oblique axial T1WI MR shows one of the distal tibialis posterior tendon slips approaching the bases of the 2nd cuneiform.* **(Middle)** *Axial T1WI MR shows that the lateral anterior slip of the posterior tibial tendon diverges from the main tendon insertion slightly before its insertion on the plantar margin of the median eminence of the navicular. A medial slip extends directly anterior from the plantar margin of the navicular, inserting on the 1st cuneiform. The role of these slips in maintaining the arch of the foot is evident on this image.* **(Bottom)** *Coronal T1WI MR in the same patient shows 3 slips of tibial tendon attaching to 1st and 3rd cuneiforms. Anterior slips are variable in size.*

MR: DISTAL POSTERIOR TIBIAL TENDON

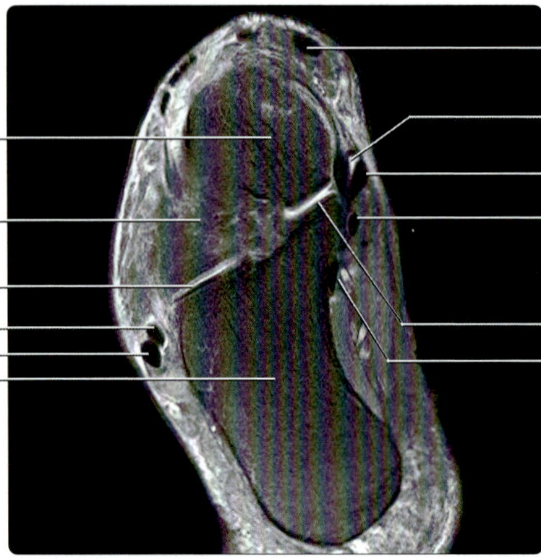

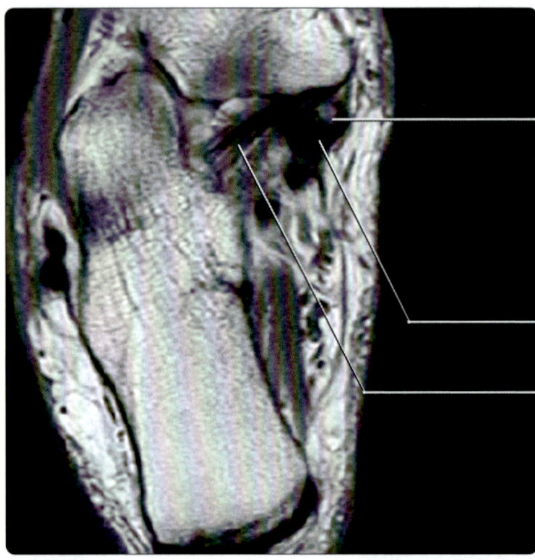

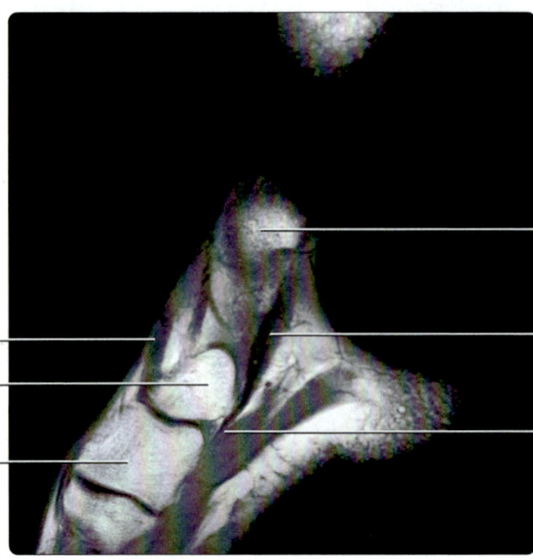

(Top) *Oblique axial PD FS shows a minimal amount of fluid within the posterior tibial tendon sheath. This is normal and should not be misinterpreted as tenosynovitis.* **(Middle)** *Heterogeneity at the insertion of the posterior tibial tendon may be related to the presence of type 1 accessory navicular. Three types of ossifications can occur at the navicular tuberosity (median eminence). Type 1 is a small sesamoid bone embedded in the posterior tibial tendon. Type 2 is a large triangular ossification representing a nonfused accessory ossification of the navicular. A synchondrosis is present between the ossification and the navicular. Most of the fibers of the posterior tibial tendon insert into the accessory ossification center rather than to the navicular; this weakens the tendon's actions and causes stress on the synchondrosis. Type 3 is a fused accessory ossification producing a cornuate navicular.* **(Bottom)** *Sagittal T1WI MR shows the posterior tibial tendon inserting on the inferior surface of the median eminence of the navicular.*

AXIAL MR: FLEXOR HALLUCIS LONGUS TENDON

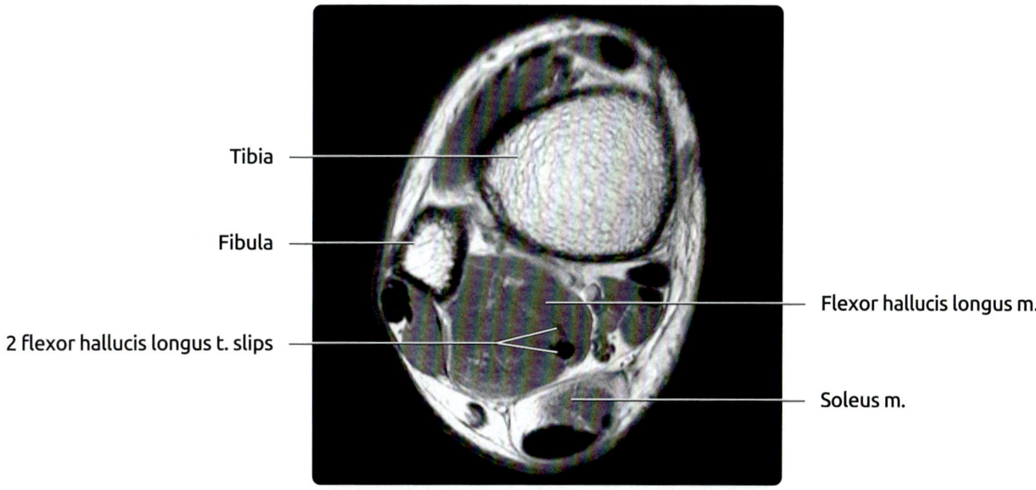

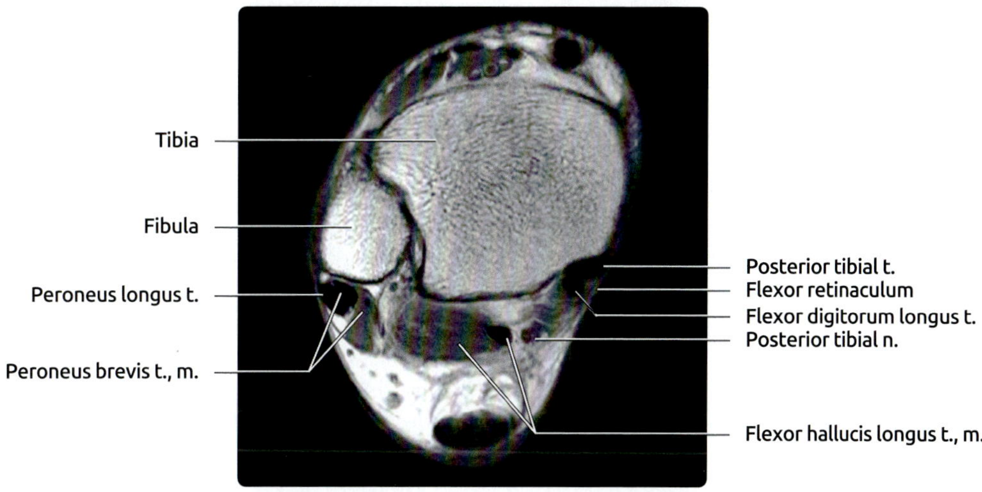

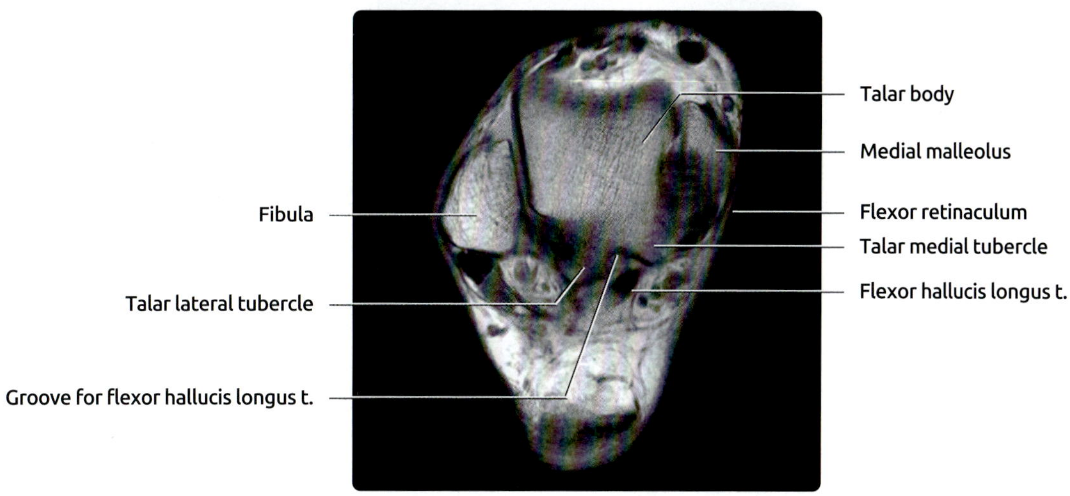

(Top) *The flexor hallucis longus tendon descends down the distal leg within the posterior aspect of its muscle. Not infrequently, the tendon is formed by 2 major tendon slips, which usually merge into a single tendon above the ankle joint but sometimes remain separate quite far distally. The secondary irregularity and heterogeneity of the tendon should not be misinterpreted for disease.* **(Middle)** *The flexor hallucis longus tendon and muscle are seen just above the tibial plafond. The posterior tibial and flexor digitorum are purely tendinous at this level.* **(Bottom)** *The flexor hallucis longus tendon traverses 2 major tunnels in the ankle and hindfoot. The 1st tunnel is between the medial and lateral tubercles of the talus. A fibrous band converts the groove into a tunnel. The 2nd tunnel is under the sustentaculum tali of the calcaneus.*

MR: FLEXOR HALLUCIS LONGUS TENDON

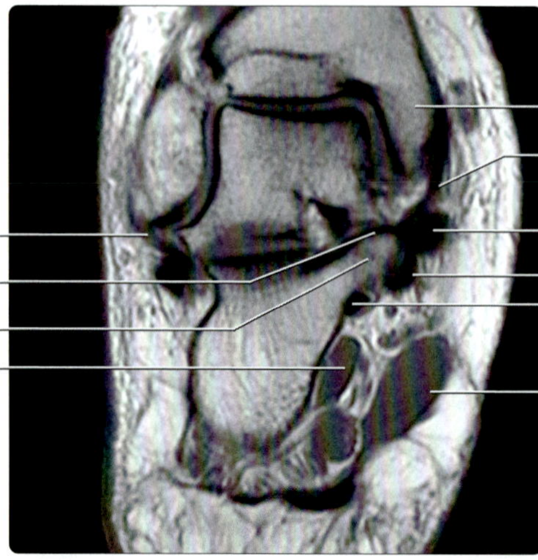

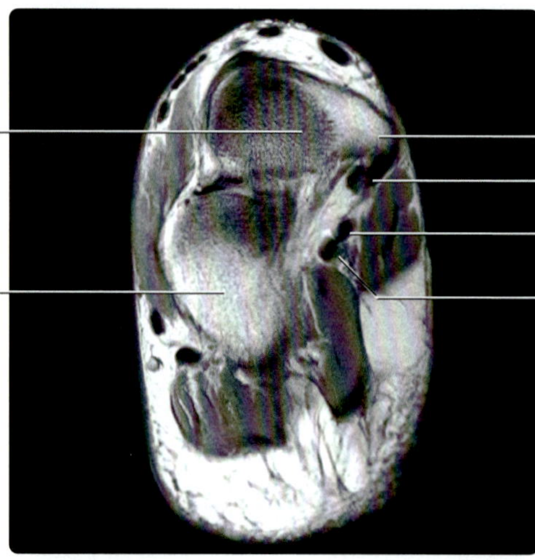

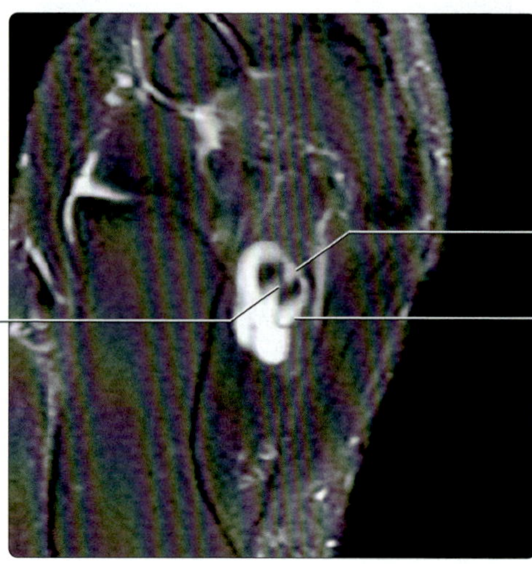

(Top) *Coronal T1WI MR at the level of the sustentaculum tali shows the flexor hallucis longus tendon inferior to the sustentaculum, the flexor digitorum longus at the medial margin of the sustentaculum, and the posterior tibial tendon (the most superior of the tendons).* **(Middle)** *Plantar to the navicular tuberosity (median eminence), the flexor hallucis longus tendon 1st approaches and then crosses the flexor digitorum longus tendon at the master knot of Henry.* **(Bottom)** *Fluid within the flexor hallucis longus tendon sheath may extend quite far distally into the knot of Henry. This is typically an incidental finding and of no clinical significance. Isolated fluid in this area, however, without fluid proximal to it, may indicate tenosynovitis. The medial plantar nerve follows the flexor hallucis longus tendon and may be impinged upon by the fluid.*

CORONAL MR: FLEXOR HALLUCIS LONGUS TENDON

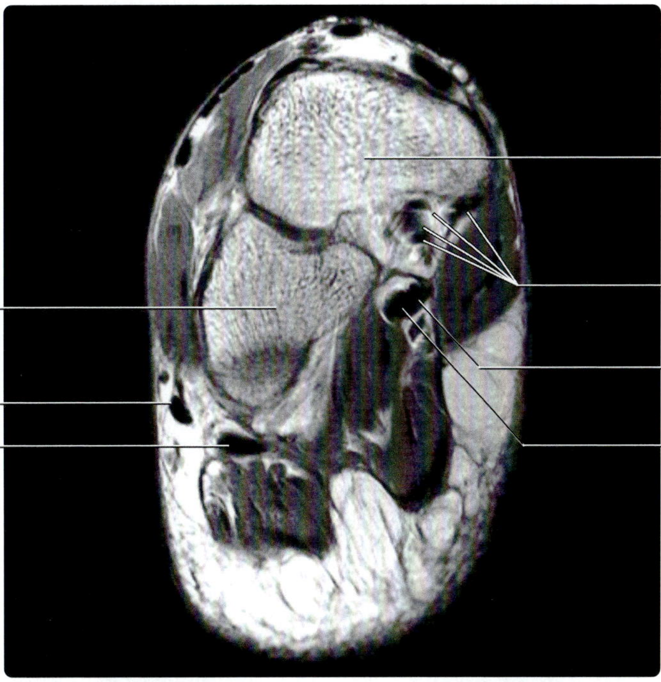

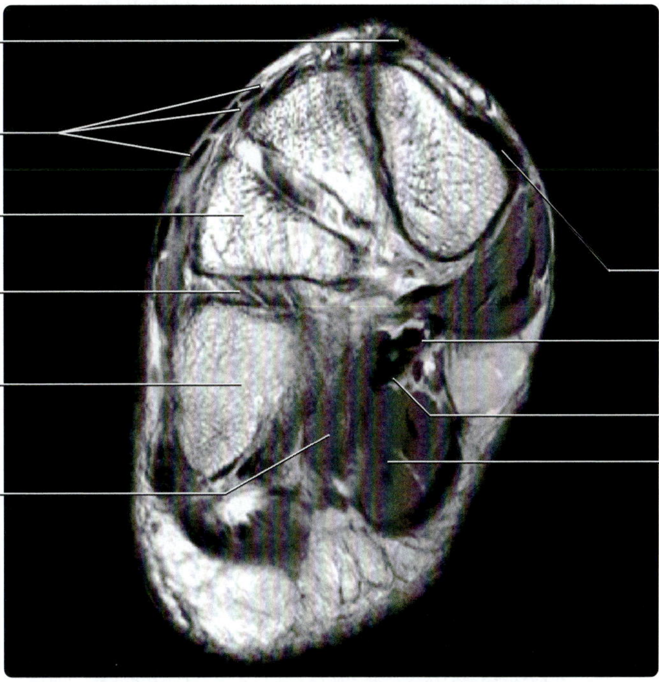

(Top) *As the flexor hallucis longus tendon crosses the flexor digitorum longus tendon (under the navicular tuberosity, at the knot of Henry), it sends a fibrous slip to the latter tendon. This slip prevents the flexor hallucis longus tendon from significant proximal retraction if it tears distal to the knot of Henry.* **(Bottom)** *Distal to the knot of Henry, the flexor hallucis longus tendon is located superiorly and medially to the flexor digitorum longus tendon.*

MR: FLEXOR HALLUCIS LONGUS TENDON

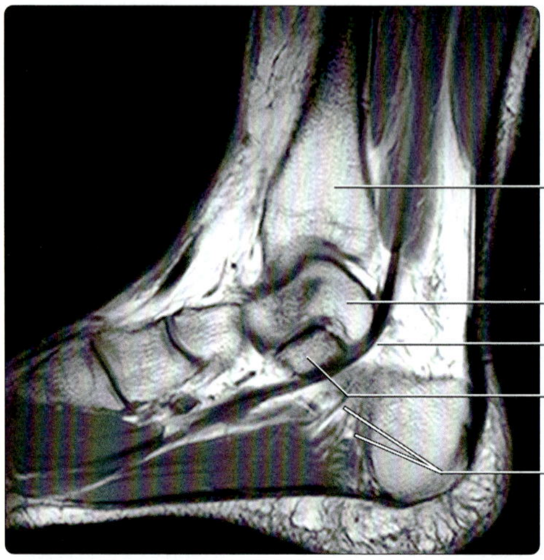

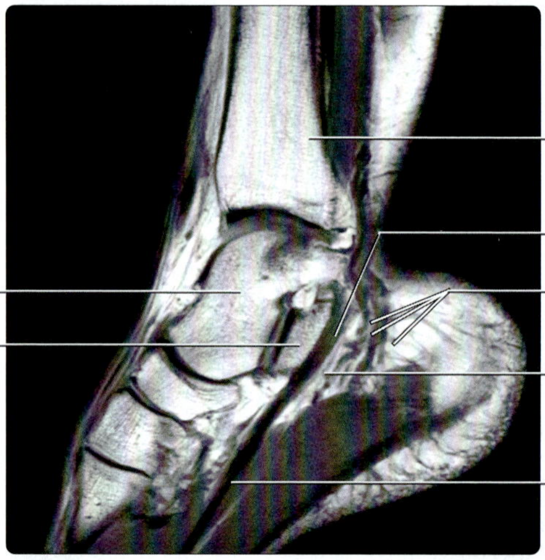

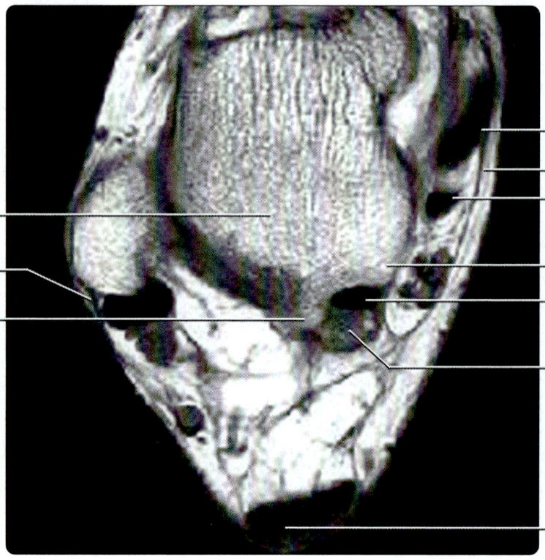

(Top) *The flexor hallucis longus tendon is well seen on sagittal images of the ankle as it descends under the sustentaculum tali.* **(Middle)** *Note that the distal flexor digitorum longus tendon is typically seen on the same sagittal image in which the flexor hallucis longus tendon is noted to descend under the sustentaculum tali. This is due to the crossing over of the tendons in the knot of Henry under the navicular tuberosity. Note also the medial plantar nerve's proximity to the flexor hallucis longus tendon.* **(Bottom)** *Typically, the muscle of the flexor hallucis longus extends to the ankle joint and is not seen at the level of the talar groove. In a low-lying flexor hallucis longus muscle, as in this patient, muscle tissue extends into the groove and may produce impingement symptoms.*

AXIAL MR: PERONEAL TENDONS

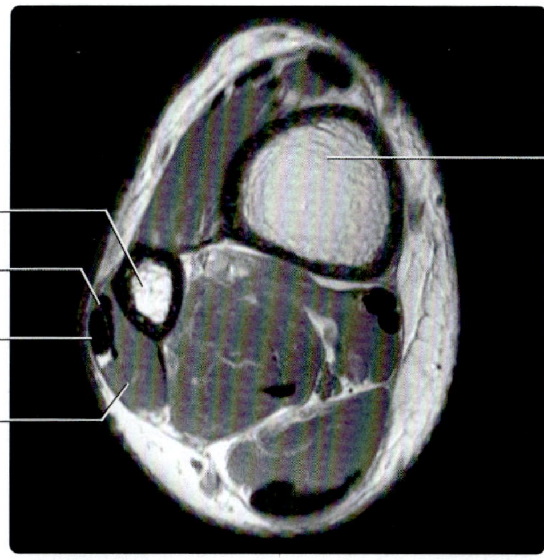

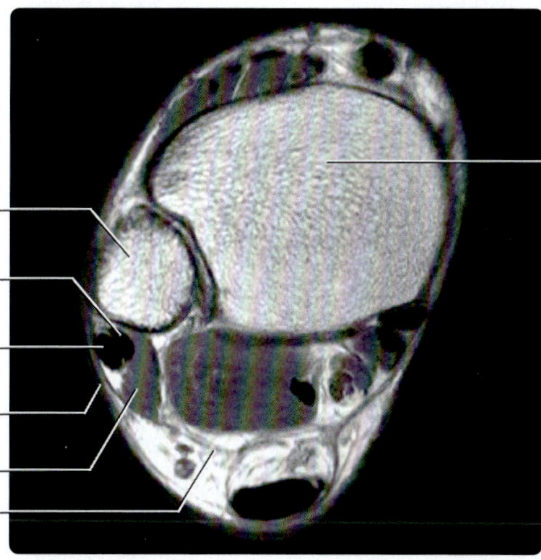

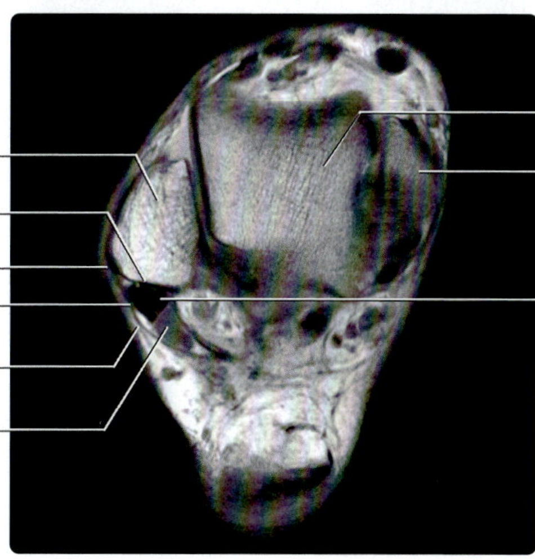

(Top) *The peroneal tendons descend together in the lateral compartment of the leg. In the distal leg, the peroneus longus muscle has become entirely tendinous, while both the muscle and tendon of the peroneus brevis are visualized. Note that in the distal leg, the peroneal tendons are lateral rather than posterior to the fibula; this should not be misinterpreted as subluxation of the tendons.* **(Middle)** *More distally, peroneal tendons lie directly posterior to the distal fibula. The peroneus brevis tendon is typically crescentic in shape and is located anteromedial to the peroneus longus tendon. The superior peroneal retinaculum extends from the distal fibula to the calcaneus and deep leg fascia and maintains the peroneal tendons within the retromalleolar groove.* **(Bottom)** *The superior peroneal retinaculum is a reinforcement of the leg aponeurosis. It is seen as a low-signal band originating from the lateral distal fibula, at the retromalleolar groove, approximately 1 cm above the fibular tip. It can be followed to its insertion to the deep fascia of the leg.*

AXIAL MR: PERONEAL TENDONS

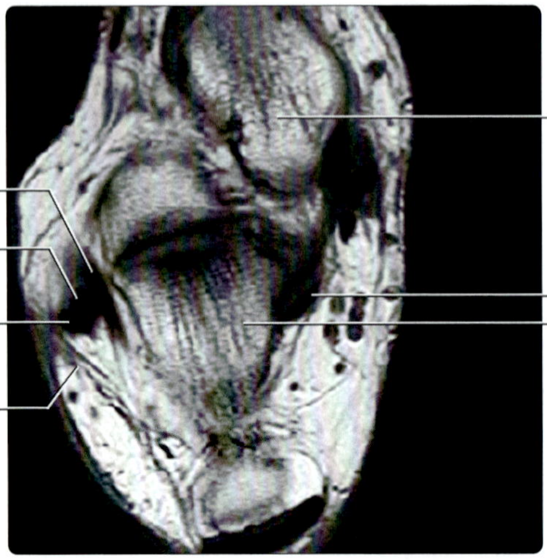

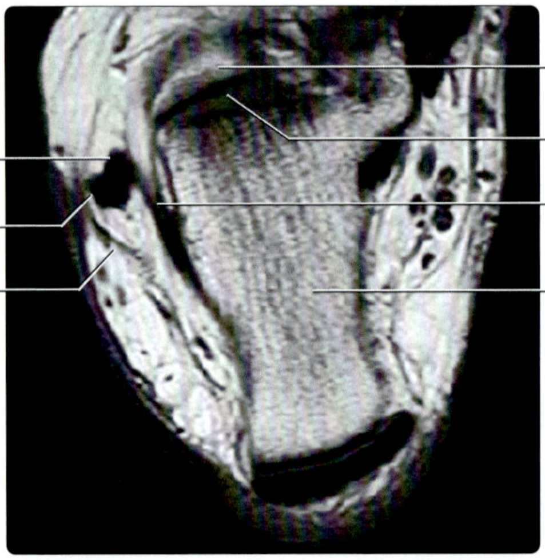

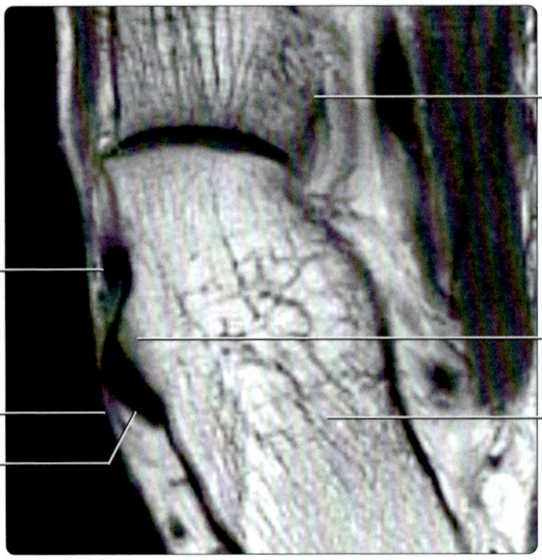

(Top) *The calcaneofibular ligament is obliquely oriented from the tip of the fibula posteriorly and inferiorly. It inserts on the calcaneus deep to the peroneal tendons.* **(Middle)** *The peroneal retinaculum is superficial to the peroneal tendons, while the calcaneofibular ligament lies deep to the tendons.* **(Bottom)** *The peroneal tubercle, a normal variant, is a calcaneal wall protuberance that separates the peroneal tendons. Hypertrophy of the tubercle predisposes to peroneus longus tendon tear.*

MR: PERONEAL TENDONS

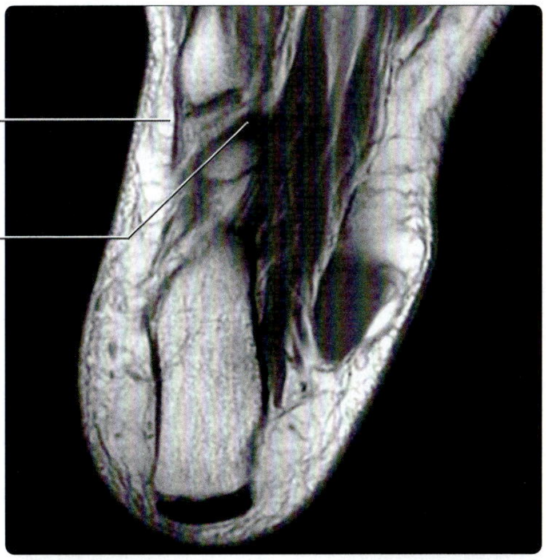

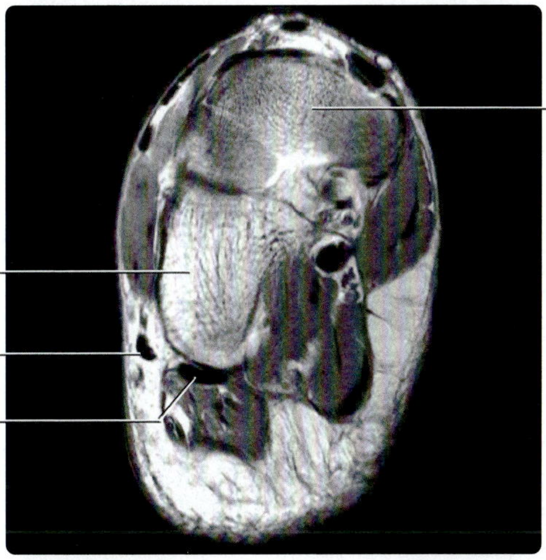

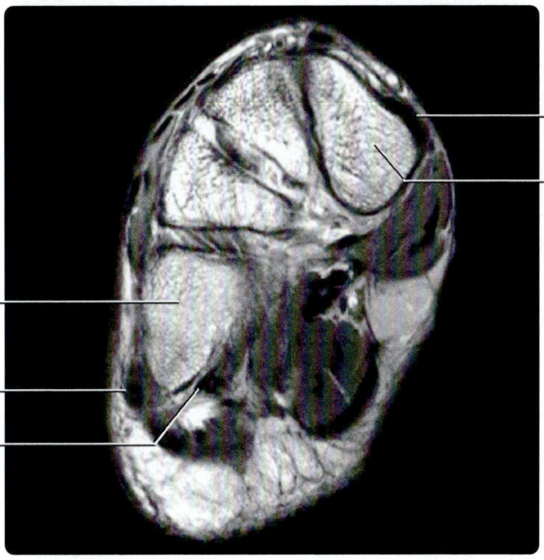

(Top) *Peroneus brevis tendon becomes a thin ribbon as it approaches its insertion on the styloid process of the 5th metatarsal. Peroneus longus tendon is seen coursing anteromedially in the cuboid sulcus toward its attachment on the medial plantar surface of the foot.* **(Middle)** *Coronal MR shows the peroneus brevis tendon continuing toward its insertion on the 5th metatarsal base. The peroneus longus tendon enters the cuboid tunnel, plantar to the cuboid, and continues along the sole of the foot toward its insertion on 1st cuneiform and 1st metatarsal base.* **(Bottom)** *The distal course of the peroneus longus tendon along the plantar surface of the foot is best seen on short-axis midfoot images but may also be seen on distal axial images of the ankle. The tendon is often suboptimally seen on T1WI due to the magic angle effect. Note the insertion of the anterior tibial tendon on the 1st cuneiform.*

CORONAL MR: PERONEAL TENDONS

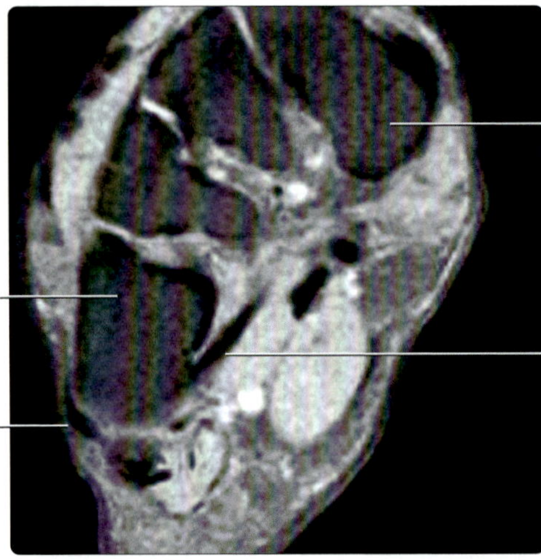

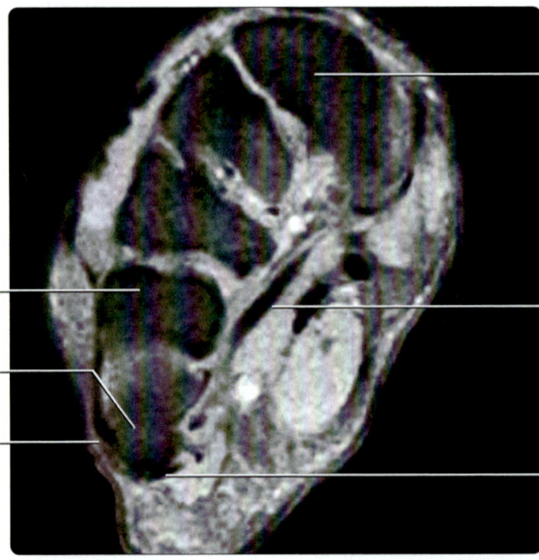

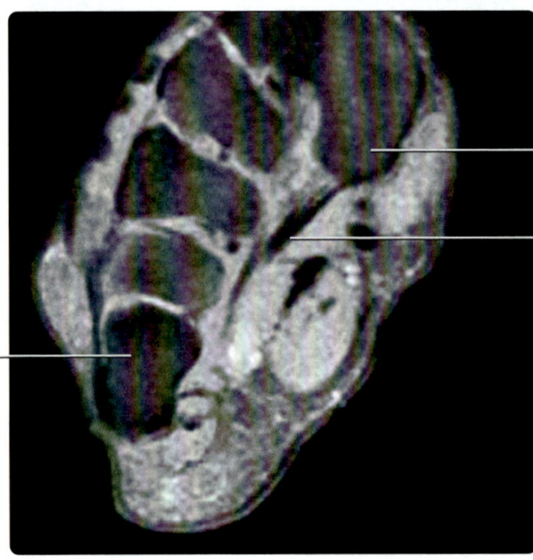

(Top) *The course of the peroneus longus tendon along the plantar surface of the foot is frequently better seen on axial T2WI FS MR due to the relative lack of the magic angle effect.* **(Middle)** *On a more distal axial image, the peroneus longus tendon continues deep to the 3rd compartment muscles. Note the insertion of the peroneus brevis tendon on the base of the 5th metatarsal. The peroneus brevis and plantar fascia insert onto the plantar base of the 5th metatarsal, while the peroneus tertius tendon inserts on the dorsal base of the 5th metatarsal.* **(Bottom)** *Note the normal striation of the very distal peroneus longus tendon as it divides into slips to several insertion sites.*

SAGITTAL MR: PERONEAL TENDONS

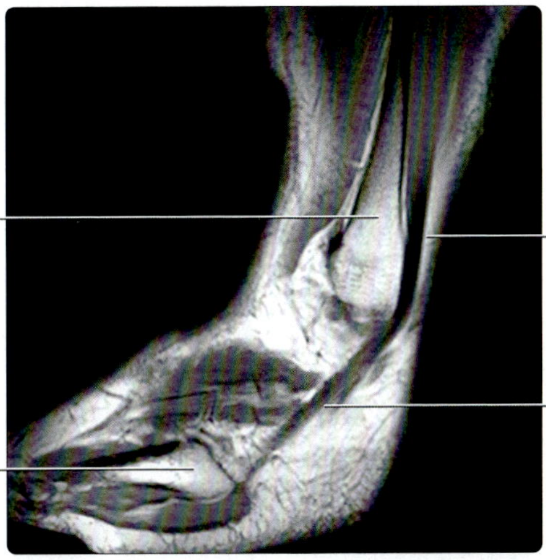

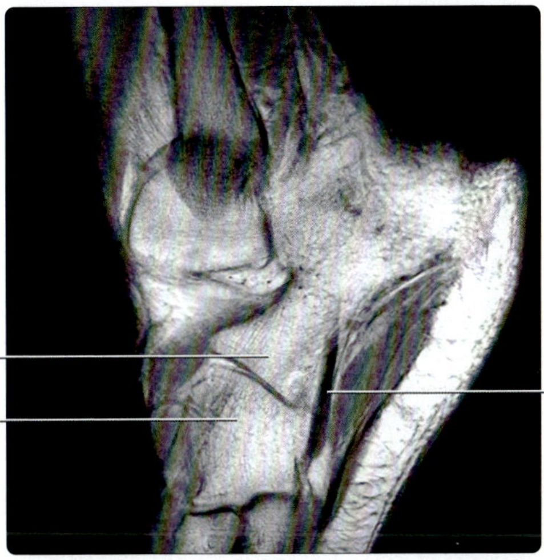

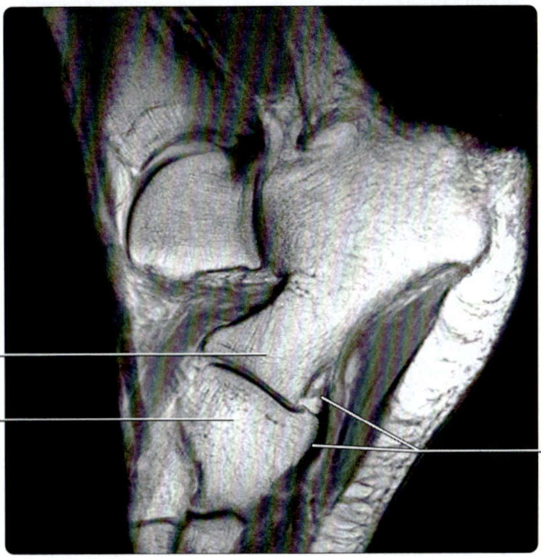

(Top) *The peroneal tendons are optimally assessed on axial images but may be followed on sagittal images as they proceed toward their insertion sites. The peroneus brevis tendon is predisposed to friction and tearing as it descends within the fibular retromalleolar groove.* **(Middle)** *The peroneus longus tendon traverses within 2 fibroosseous tunnels. It 1st shares the retromalleolar groove with the peroneus brevis tendon. It then descends along the lateral wall of the calcaneus where it can undergo friction posterior to the peroneal tubercle. Its final tunnel is plantar to the cuboid within the cuboid tunnel. In this image, the peroneus longus tendon descends along the lateral wall of the calcaneus approaching its cuboid tunnel.* **(Bottom)** *In this image, the peroneus longus is seen starting to curve under the plantar surface of the cuboid to enter the cuboid tunnel.*

SAGITTAL MR: PERONEAL TENDONS

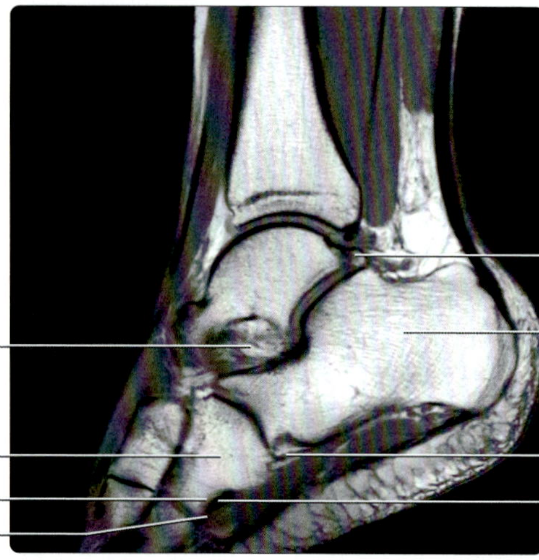

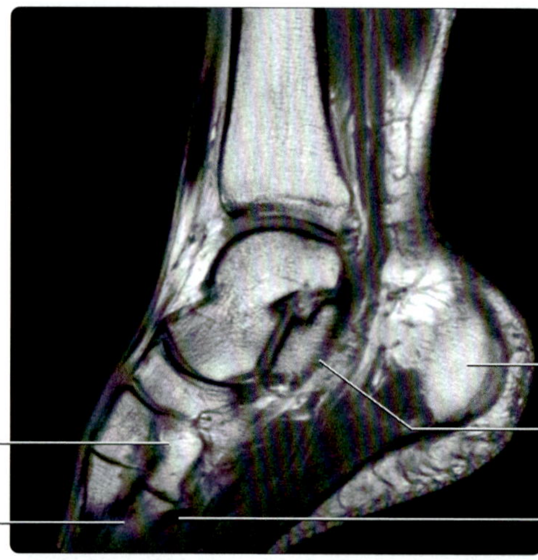

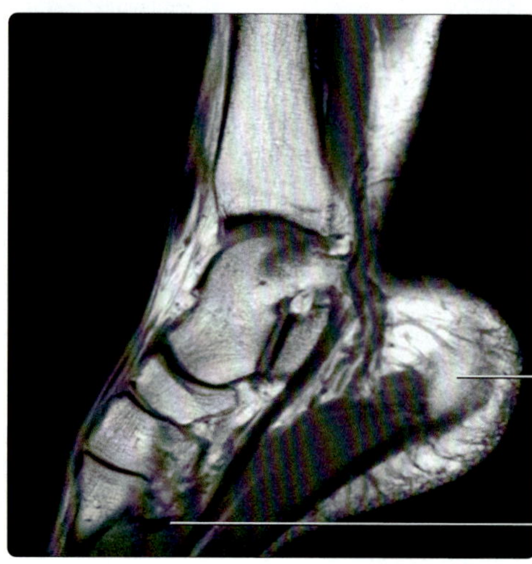

(Top) *The peroneus longus tendon has now entered the tunnel under the cuboid. The tendon is held in place by a strong fibrous band derived from the long plantar ligament. Sequential sagittal images allow visualization of the peroneus longus tendon as it obliquely crosses the sole of the foot. The tendon is typically seen in cross section as a small, linear, low-signal structure deep to the plantar muscles.* **(Middle)** *The peroneus longus tendon is seen obliquely traversing the plantar surface of the sole toward its insertion.* **(Bottom)** *The peroneus longus tendon is now under the 2nd metatarsal base. The insertion to the metatarsal is not always well seen on T1WI due to striation and magic angle effect.*

MR: PERONEAL TENDONS

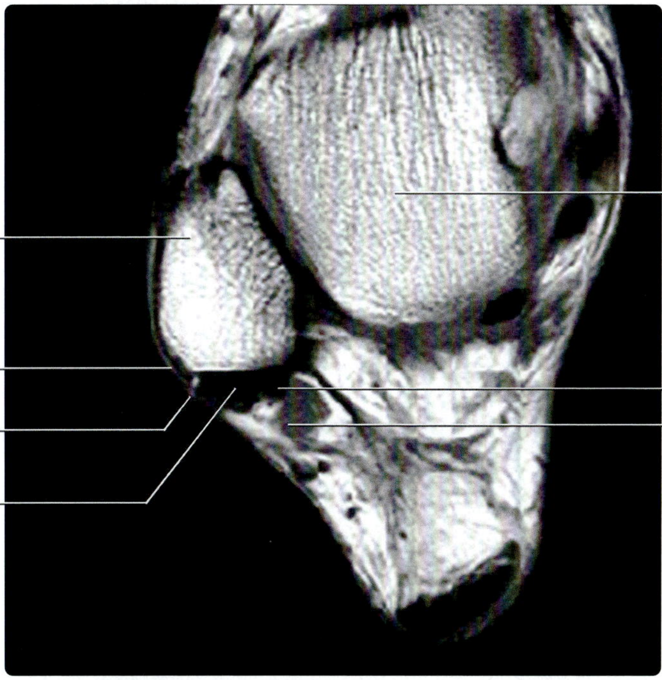

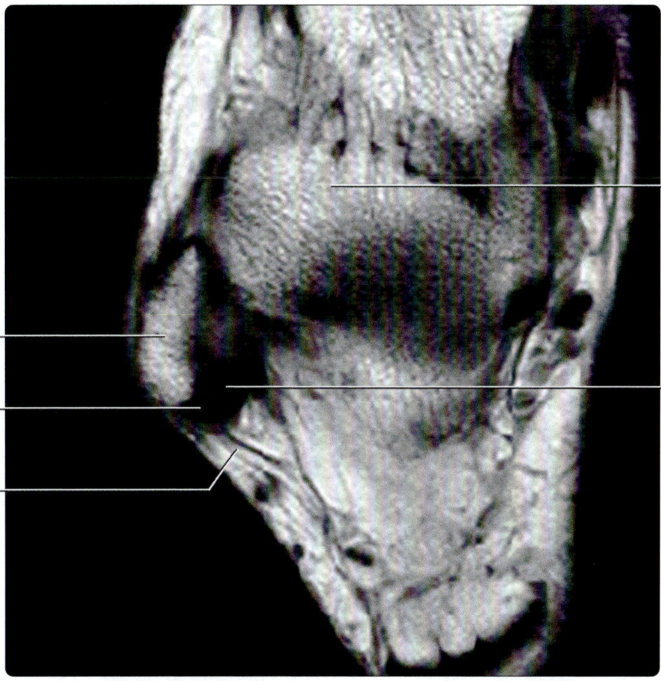

(Top) *Usually, the peroneus brevis tendon is anteromedial to the peroneus longus tendon within the retromalleolar groove. Occasionally, however, the peroneus brevis tendon is located medial to the peroneus longus tendon. In those instances, as the tendons descend distally, the peroneus brevis tendon may appear medially subluxed relative to the distal fibular tip. This is a normal finding that should not be misinterpreted for disease.* **(Bottom)** *Note the pseudosubluxation of the peroneus brevis tendon relative to the distal fibular tip. This is a normal finding.*

AXIAL MR: ANTERIOR TIBIAL TENDON

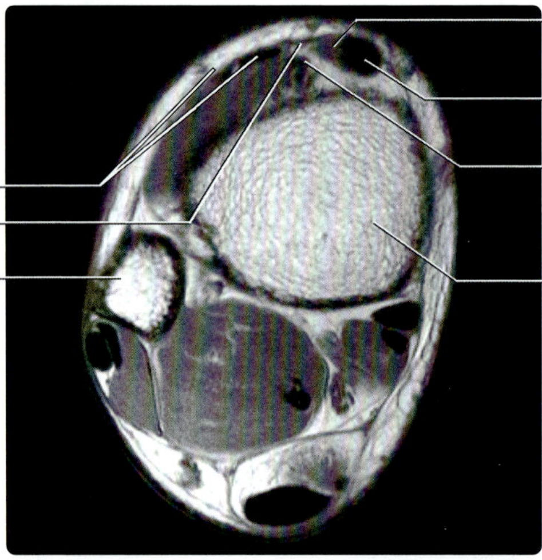

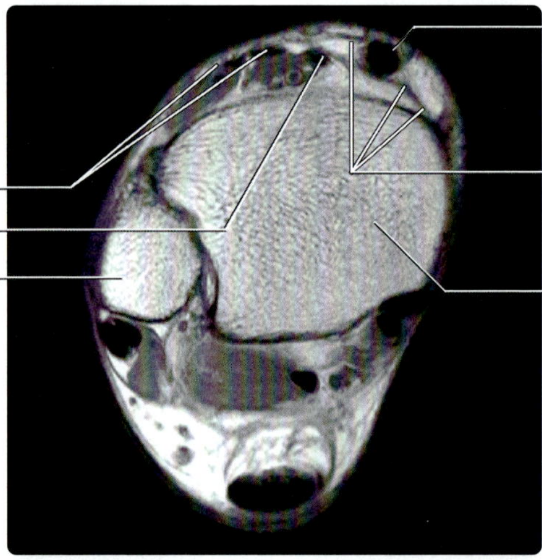

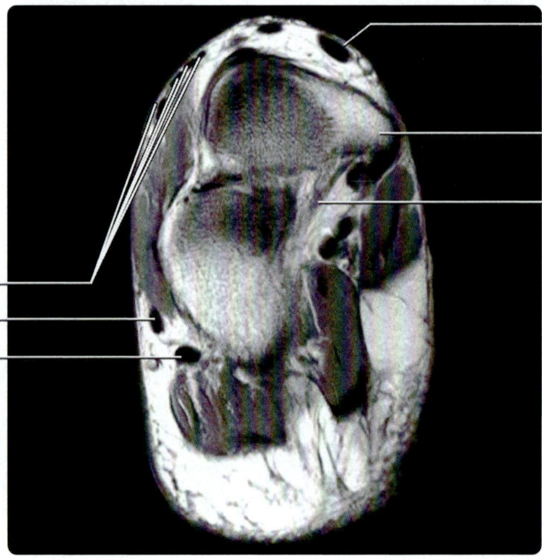

(Top) *The anterior tibial muscle becomes completely tendinous at the level of the ankle. At the ankle, the tendon is enveloped by the superior and inferior extensor retinacula. It descends obliquely and medially to insert on the medial and inferior surfaces of the 1st cuneiform and base of the 1st metatarsal.* **(Middle)** *Note the limbs of the inferior extensor retinaculum superficial and deep to the anterior tibial tendon. This tendon is rarely injured, except by direct laceration. Attritional tears are rarely seen and primarily seen in elderly women.* **(Bottom)** *The tibialis anterior tendon is quite superficial and can be easily palpated under the skin in the medial ankle. It is the most commonly injured tendon of the extensor compartment tendons. It usually undergoes chronic degeneration, often related to impingement by the enveloping retinacula or, more commonly, by osteophytes originating from the talonavicular or navicular-cuneiform joints. Bony irregularities of the medial surface of the 1st cuneiform can also predispose the tendon to tears.*

MR: ANTERIOR TIBIAL TENDON

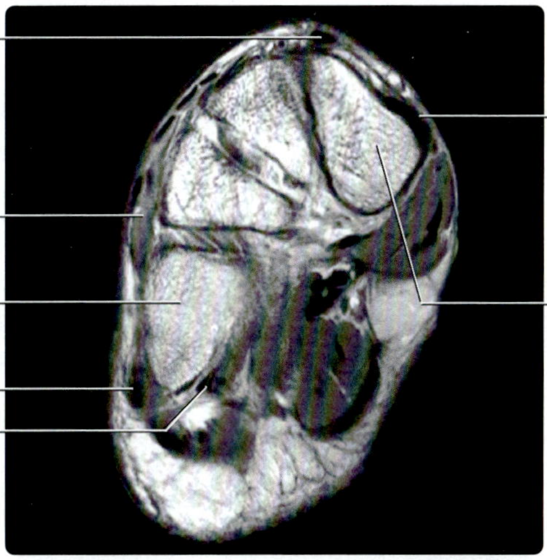

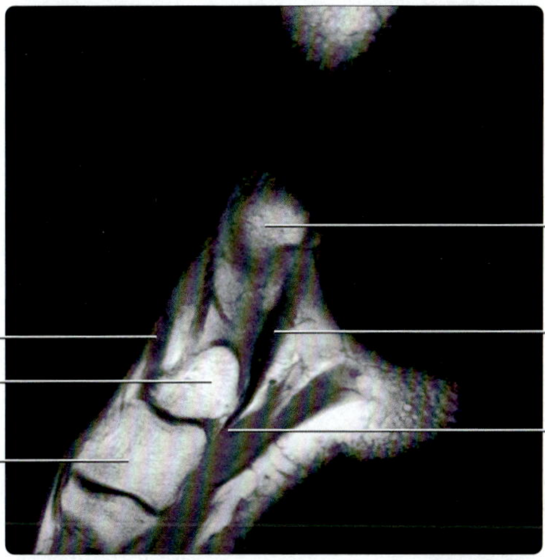

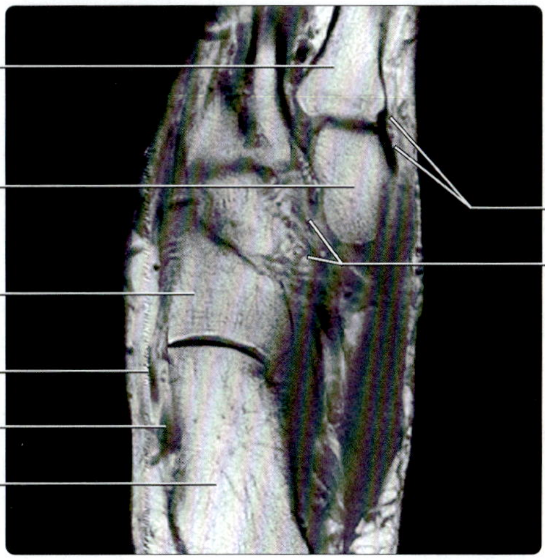

(Top) *Note the insertion of the anterior tibial tendon to the medial surface of the 1st cuneiform. The insertion to the 1st metatarsal is usually less prominent on MR ankle images and may be better depicted on oblique axial midfoot images.* **(Middle)** *The anterior tibial tendon is seen wrapping around the navicular toward its insertion on the 1st cuneiform and 1st metatarsal. Careful evaluation of this area sometimes reveals tendinosis of the tibialis anterior, which can be overlooked on routine axial images of the ankle. The tibialis anterior, tibialis posterior, and peroneus longus tendons form a sling around the medial axis of the midfoot supporting the medial longitudinal arch.* **(Bottom)** *Note the insertion of the anterior tibial tendon to both the 1st cuneiform and 1st metatarsal on this axial ankle view.*

GROSS ANATOMY

Syndesmotic Tibiofibular Ligaments

- Stabilize against eversion
- **Anterior inferior tibiofibular**: Oblique course from anterior lateral corner tibia inferiorly and laterally to fibula
    - Bassett ligament: Separate fascicle, usually present inferior to main band
- **Posterior inferior tibiofibular**
    - Main band oriented horizontally from posterior malleolus to posterior margin of fibula
    - Inferior transverse (or intermalleolar) band: Oblique course from medial, posterior tibia to fibular tip
- **Interosseous ligament**: Thickening of interosseous membrane, which extends length of tibial and fibular shafts
    - Extends to ~ 1 cm above tibial plafond (variable)
    - Synovial recess of ankle joint present inferior to ligament

Lateral Collateral Ligaments

- **3 separate ligaments**
- Stabilize against inversion, internal rotation, anterior subluxation
- Anterior talofibular: Oblique course from 1 cm above fibular tip to superior margin of talar neck
    - Reliably seen on axial images only
    - Inserts on talus on 1st or 2nd superior axial images, which includes talar neck
- Calcaneofibular: Oblique course from fibular tip posteriorly and inferiorly to lateral margin of calcaneus
    - Deep to peroneal tendons; well seen on axial and coronal images
- Posterior talofibular: Horizontal course from lateral talar body to medial margin of fibula
    - Striated appearance should not be mistaken for tear
    - Well seen on coronal and axial images

Deltoid Ligament

- Well seen on axial and coronal images
- **Deep deltoid ligament**
    - Stabilizes against eversion
    - Main (posterior) band
        - Most structural important portion of deltoid
        - Originates primarily from posterior border of anterior colliculus of medial malleolus
        - Courses inferiorly, medially, and anteriorly
        - Inserts on medial fovea of talar body
        - Has striated appearance
    - Anterior band is small, variably present, and of doubtful clinical importance
        - Originates at anterior margin of medial malleolus
        - Inserts on medial talus at junction of body and neck
- **Superficial deltoid ligament**
    - Stabilizes against rotation
    - Multiple bands, named for their attachments
    - Anterior superficial components originate from anterior corner medial malleolus as continuous band; continuous with periosteum and flexor retinaculum
    - Tibiocalcaneal: Inserts at sustentaculum tali; strongest band
    - Tibiospring: Merges with spring ligament
    - Tibionavicular: Inserts on medial border of navicular, deep to posterior tibial tendon
    - Posterior tibiotalar band: Variably present; originates more posteriorly on medial malleolus, inserts posterior talar body

Tarsal Canal and Tarsal Sinus Ligaments

- **Cervical ligament**: Stabilizes subtalar joint
    - Oblique course in tarsal sinus from inferolateral talar neck to superolateral calcaneus
    - Best seen on coronal images
    - On sagittal and axial images, it may be confused with bands of extensor retinaculum
- **Talocalcaneal interosseous ligament**: Stabilizes subtalar joint
    - Short, vertical ligament in tarsal canal
- **Roots, inferior extensor retinaculum**: 3 bands attach in tarsal sinus
    - Medial: Medial calcaneal insertion in posterior tarsal sinus, anterior to talocalcaneal interosseous ligament
    - Intermediate: Middorsal calcaneal insertion adjacent to cervical ligament
    - Lateral: Lateral margin calcaneal insertion lateral to extensor digitorum brevis muscle origin
    - Best seen on coronal images

Spring Ligament

- 3 bands
- From calcaneus to navicular, supports talar head and medial longitudinal arch
- **Superomedial**: Strongest, hammock-shaped, best seen on axial images
    - Origin: Sustentaculum tali and tibiospring band of deltoid
    - Insertion: Superomedial navicular
    - Deep to posterior tibial tendon
- **Medioplantar oblique**
    - Best seen on axial images
    - Origin: Coronoid fossa of calcaneus
    - Insertion: Plantar, medial navicular
    - Striated appearance, oblique course
- **Inferoplantar longitudinal**
    - Best seen on axial and sagittal images
    - Origin: Coronoid fossa; insertion: Navicular beak
    - Short, straight course

Bifurcate Ligament

- Best seen on sagittal images
- Origin: Dorsal margin of calcaneal anterior process; insertion via 2 limbs to navicular and cuboid

Short and Long Plantar Ligaments

- Best seen on sagittal and axial images
- Support longitudinal arch

Short Plantar Ligament (Plantar Calcaneocuboid)

- Origin: Calcaneal anterior tubercle; insertion: Cuboid

Long Plantar Ligament: Superficial to Short Plantar Ligament

- Origin: At and anterior to medial, lateral, anterior tubercles; insertion: Cuboid, bases 2nd-5th metatarsals

GRAPHICS: HINDFOOT LIGAMENTS

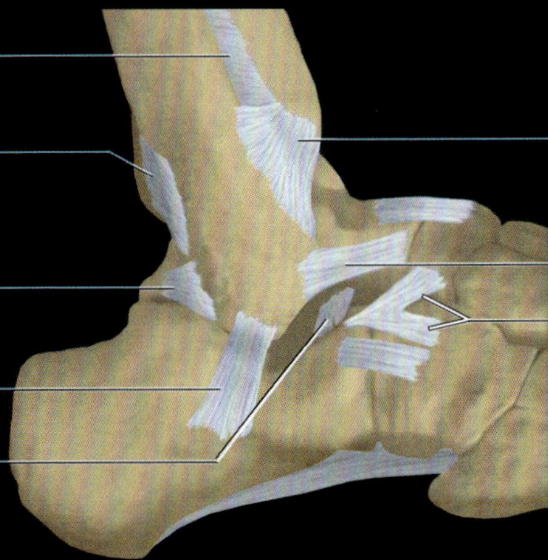

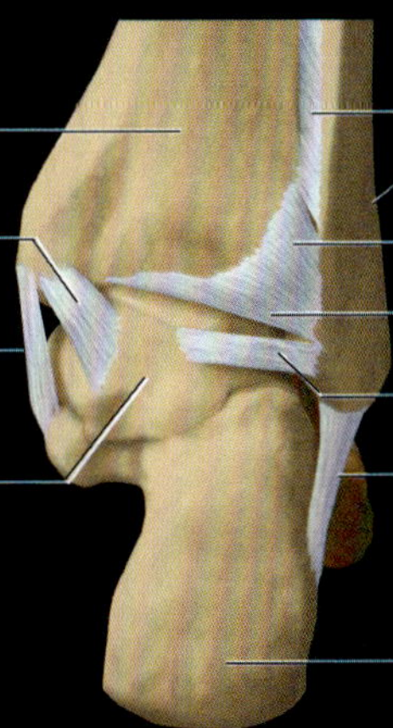

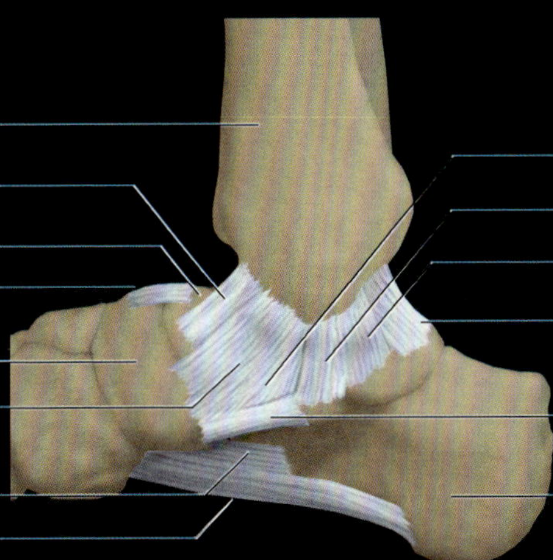

(Top) *Lateral view of the ankle is shown. Syndesmotic ligaments, including the anterior inferior tibiofibular, posterior inferior tibiofibular, and interosseous ligaments stabilize against eversion injury. Lateral collateral ligaments, including the anterior talofibular, posterior talofibular, and calcaneofibular ligaments stabilize against inversion and anteroposterior translation. The subtalar joint is stabilized by the cervical ligament and interosseous ligament (not shown). The bifurcate ligament stabilizes against inversion. Plantar ligaments stabilize the longitudinal arch.* **(Middle)** *Posterior graphic of the ankle is shown. The tibiofibular ligaments are obliquely oriented, and their fibular origin is above the fibular malleolar fossa. The inferior transverse ligament (the inferior portion of the posterior tibiofibular ligament) extends distal to the tibial posterior surface.* **(Bottom)** *Medial graphic of the ankle is shown. The superficial deltoid originates from the superficial margin of the medial malleolus. The bands are named for their insertions.*

AXIAL T1 MR: TIBIOFIBULAR SYNDESMOTIC LIGAMENTS

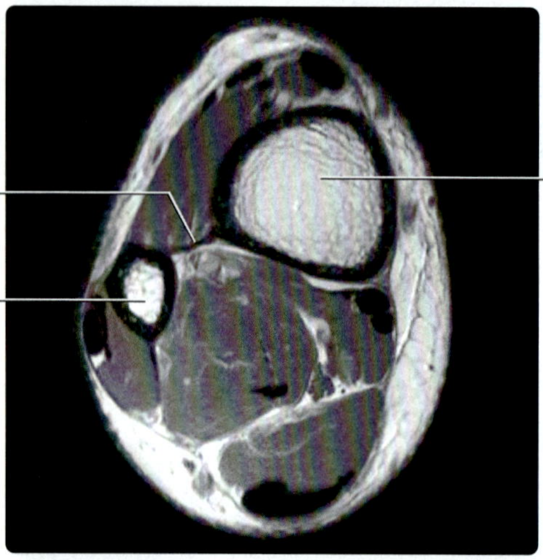

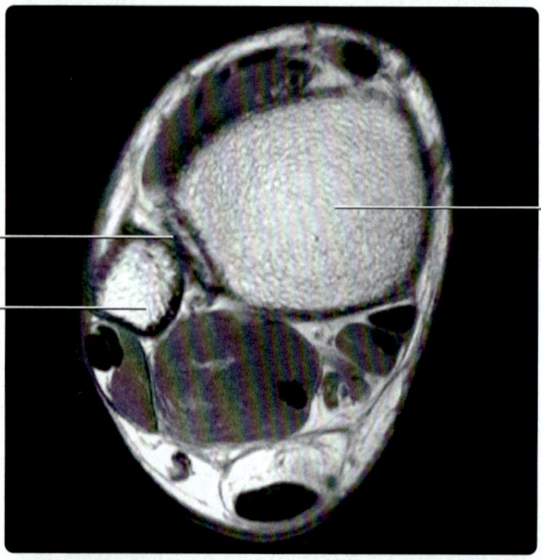

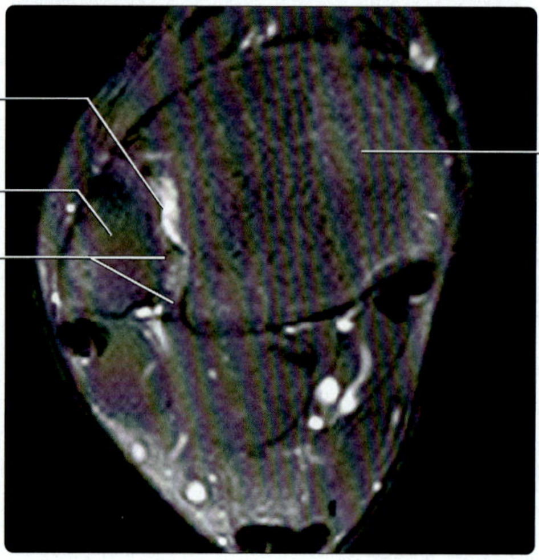

(Top) *The tibiofibular interosseous membrane is shown. The membrane is typically visualized as a well-defined, low-signal structure, binding the tibia and fibula. Its distal thickening is the interosseous ligament. Just above the ankle joint, the membrane becomes less defined and may even be discontinuous.* **(Middle)** *The tibiofibular interosseous ligament is shown. The ligament is a distal thickening of the tibiofibular membrane. Occasionally, it may be visualized as a distinct structure, as in this image, but often it may be poorly defined, discontinuous, and even absent.* **(Bottom)** *A fluid-filled recess measuring between 0.5-1.0 cm extends from the ankle joint into the tibiofibular fibrous joint. The tibiofibular ligament is frequently present at the superior margin of the recess. In this particular case, it extends posterior to the recess.*

AXIAL T1 MR: TIBIOFIBULAR SYNDESMOTIC LIGAMENTS

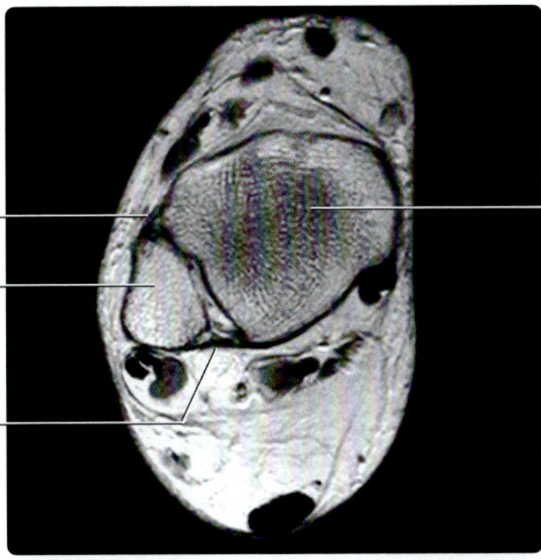

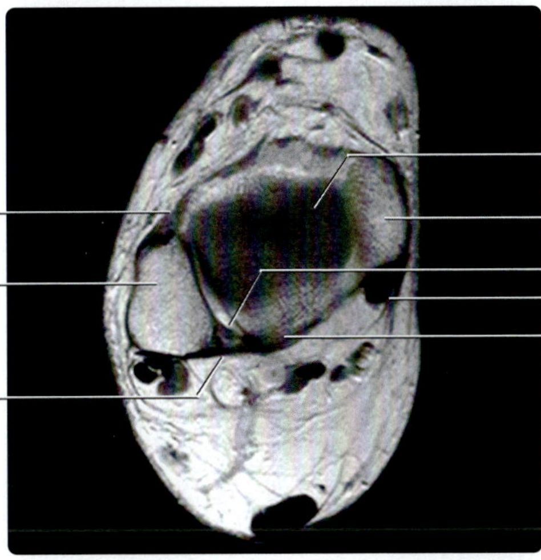

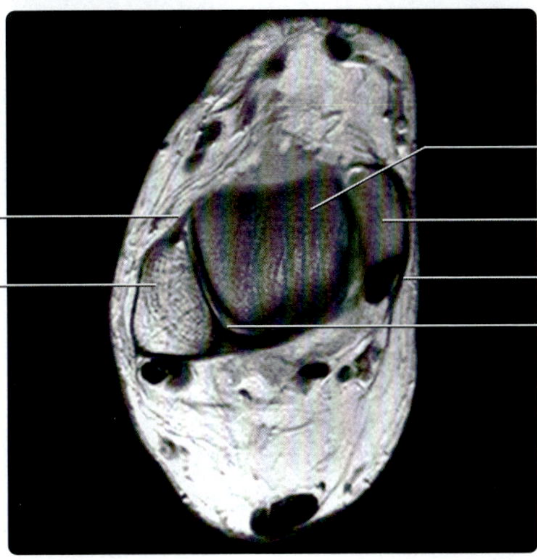

(Top) *The anterior and posterior inferior tibiofibular ligaments above the ankle joint are shown. The ligaments are optimally seen on axial images. The anterior inferior tibiofibular ligament may appear discontinuous due to fat between the ligament and the accessory Bassett ligament.* **(Middle)** *Anterior and posterior tibiofibular ligaments at the ankle joint are shown. The ligaments are visualized at, or slightly below, the ankle joint. Note that at this level, the fibula is round, without the more distal medial indentation of the malleolar fossa.* **(Bottom)** *The anterior and posterior tibiofibular ligaments at the talar dome (talus is square at this level) are shown. The very inferior aspect of the anterior tibiofibular ligament has been coined the Bassett ligament. The inferior transverse ligament is continuous with the posterior inferior tibiofibular ligament but extends distal to the posterior tibial articular surface.*

CORONAL T1 MR: TIBIOFIBULAR SYNDESMOTIC LIGAMENTS

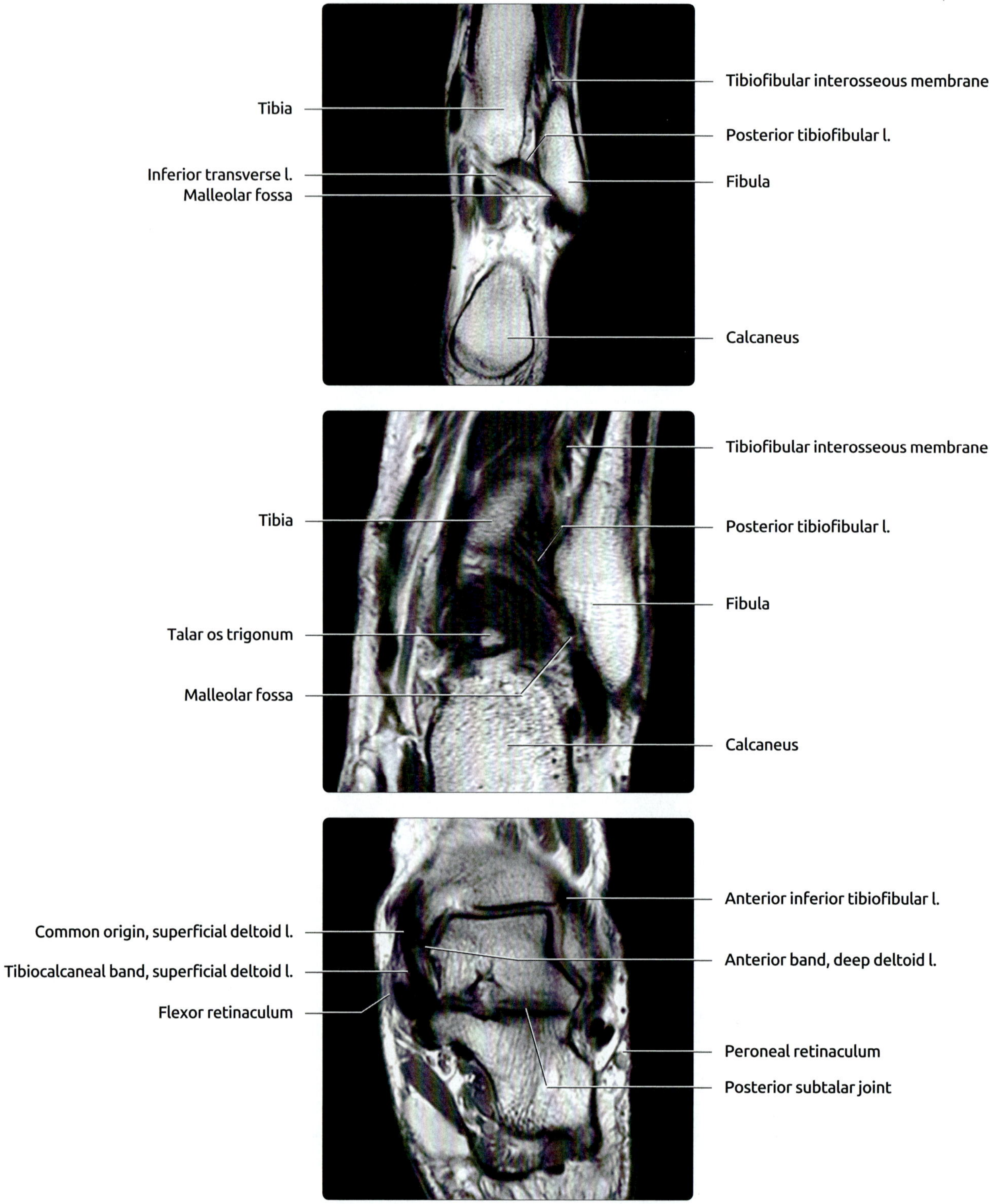

(Top) *Coronal T1WI MR of the left ankle shows the posterior inferior tibiofibular ligament. The downward oblique course of the ligament is best appreciated on coronal images. The ligament descends from its superior position on the tibia toward its more inferior fibular insertion. Note that the ligament inserts on the fibula above the malleolar fossa.* **(Middle)** *Coronal T1WI MR of the left ankle shows the posterior inferior tibiofibular ligament. The striation of the ligament is due to fat interposed between its fascicles and should not be misinterpreted as a tear on axial images.* **(Bottom)** *The anterior inferior tibiofibular ligament has an oblique from the anterior margin of the tibia, inferiorly and laterally to the fibula. The Bassett ligament forms a separate fascicle inferior to the main portion of the ligament.*

CORONAL T2 FS MR: TIBIOFIBULAR SYNDESMOTIC LIGAMENTS

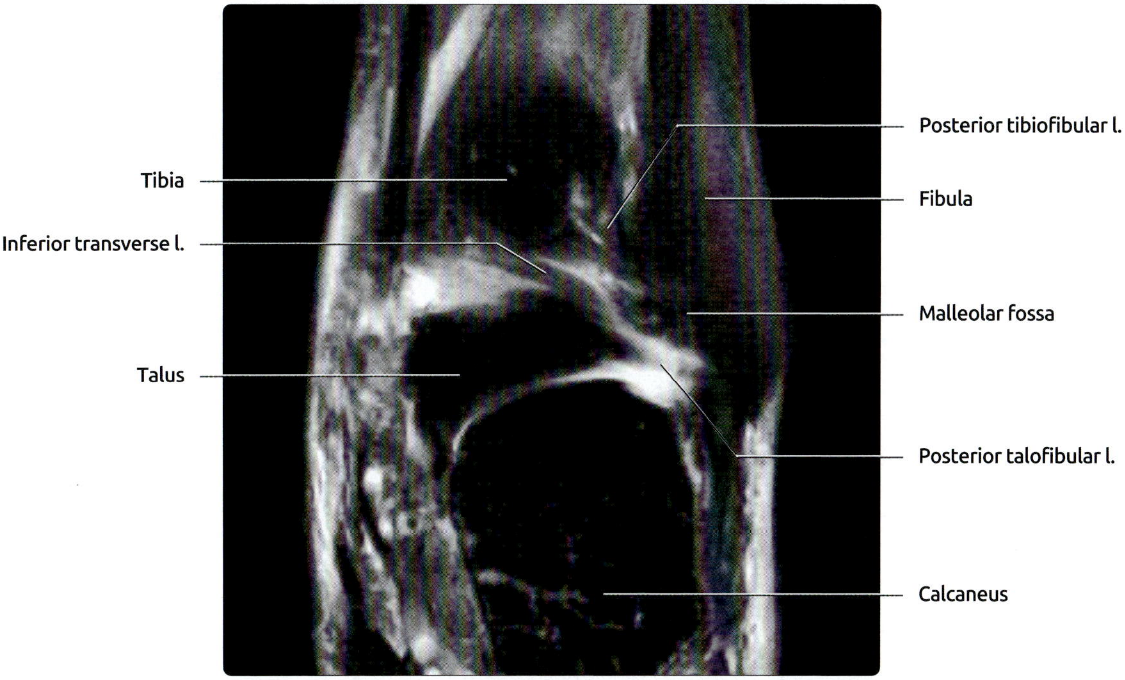

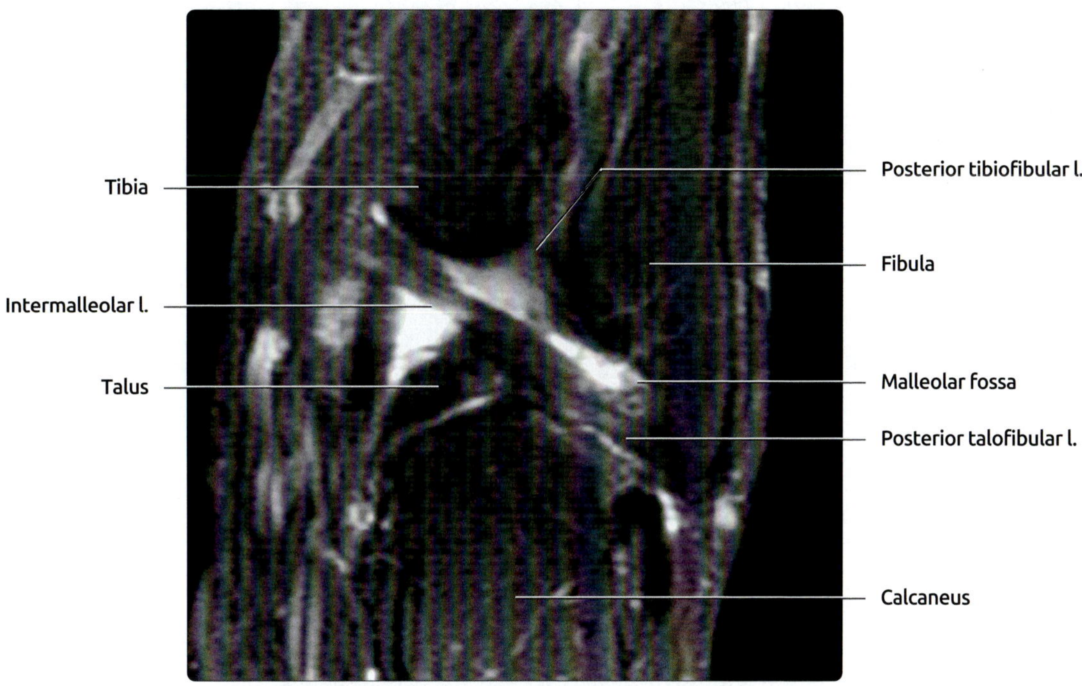

(Top) *The posterior inferior tibiofibular ligament is seen on this coronal fluid-weighted, fat-suppressed image. Note that the inferior transverse ligament extends distal to the posterior tibia, forming a posterior labrum and deepening the posterior ankle joint. Its tibial insertion is quite far medial, almost to the level of the medial malleolus. The tibiofibular ligaments insert onto the fibula above the malleolar fossa, while the talofibular ligaments insert below it.* **(Bottom)** *The intermalleolar ligament is seen on this coronal fluid-weighted, fat-suppressed image. The intermalleolar ligament, also called the tibial slip, is a normal variant that extends from the posterior talofibular ligament almost to the tibial medial malleolus. This ligament is found between the inferior transverse and posterior talofibular ligaments. It may be difficult to distinguish it from the inferior transverse ligament.*

SAGITTAL MR: TIBIOFIBULAR SYNDESMOTIC LIGAMENTS

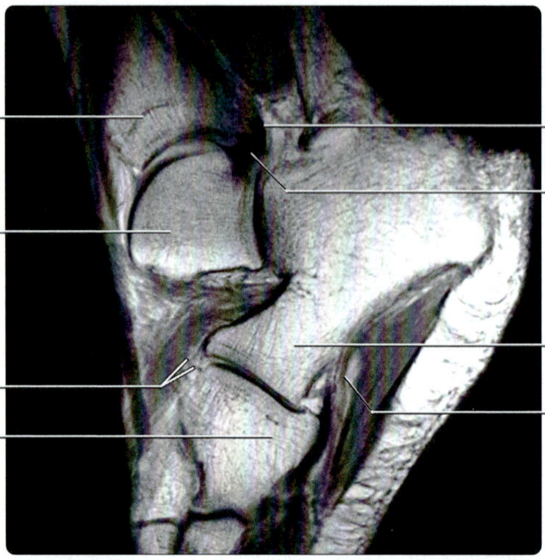

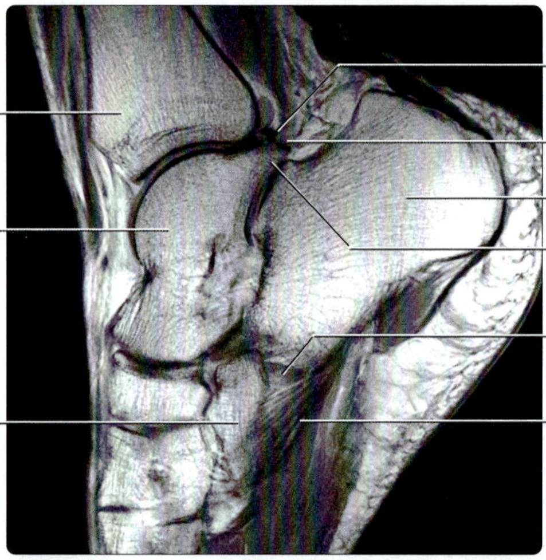

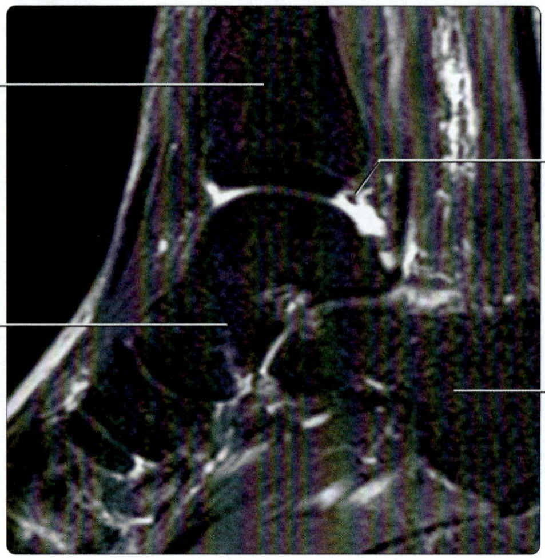

(Top) *Sagittal T1WI MR shows the inferior extent of the tibiofibular ligament distal to the tibial posterior surface. The sagittal images are suboptimal for visualizing the tibiofibular and talofibular ligaments.* **(Middle)** *On sagittal images, the tibiofibular and talofibular ligaments are typically seen in cross section as small, low signal intensity, oval structures posterior to the talus and should not be misinterpreted as intraarticular bodies. Following the ligaments on sequential images will obviate this problem. Note that the posterior talofibular ligament is barely visualized as it originates from the lateral tubercle of the talus.* **(Bottom)** *Sagittal STIR MR depicts the inferior transverse ligament surrounded by fluid, simulating an intraarticular body.*

SAGITTAL & AXIAL MR: TIBIOFIBULAR SYNDESMOTIC LIGAMENTS

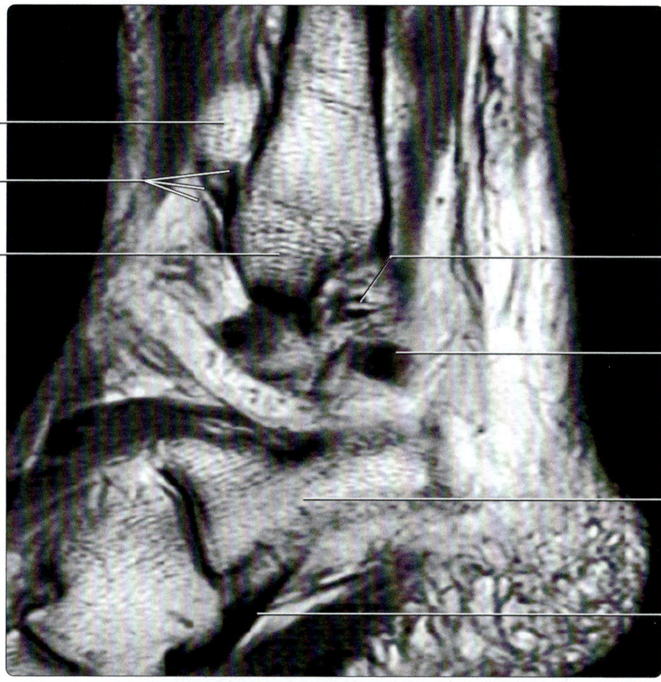

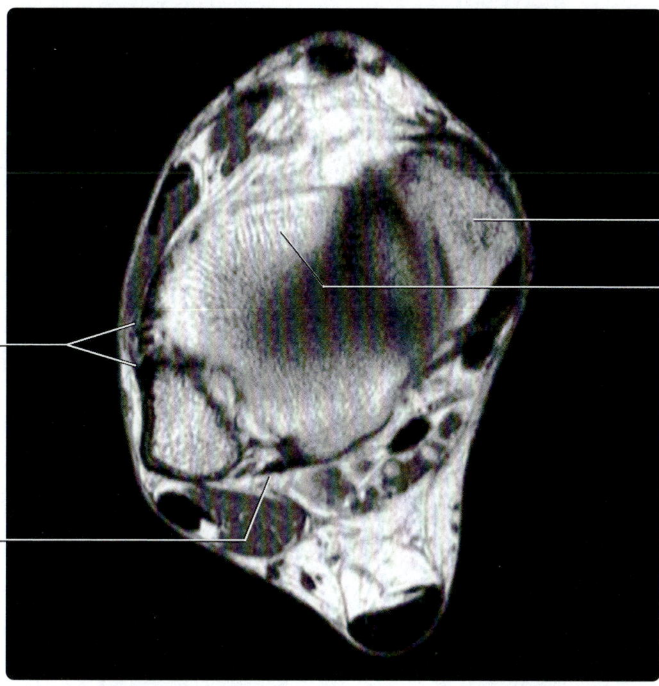

(Top) *A far lateral sagittal T1WI MR allows a glimpse of the anterior tibiofibular ligament traversing between the tibia and fibula. Note the striation of the ligament. The calcaneofibular ligament is also visualized.* **(Bottom)** *Normal striation of the anterior inferior tibiofibular ligament is seen on this axial T1WI MR. Because of the oblique descent of the anterior tibiofibular ligament and the fat interposed between its fascicles, it may appear discontinuous. When the fibers are followed on adjacent images, their continuity is evident.*

AXIAL T2 FS MR: DELTOID AND SYNDESMOTIC LIGAMENTS

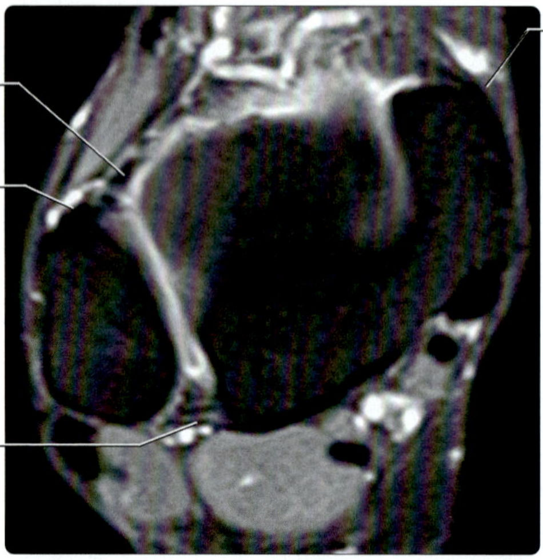

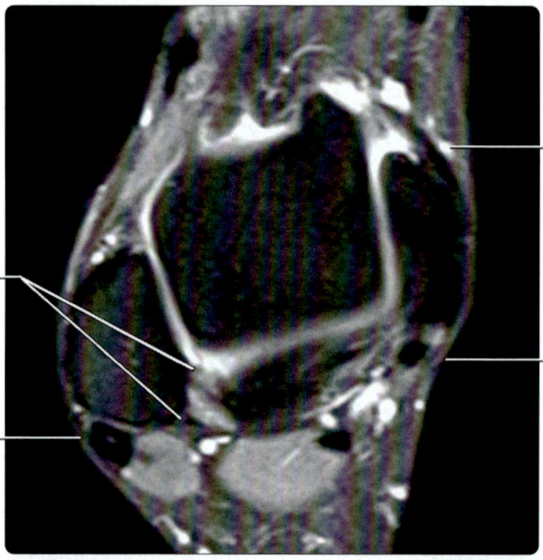

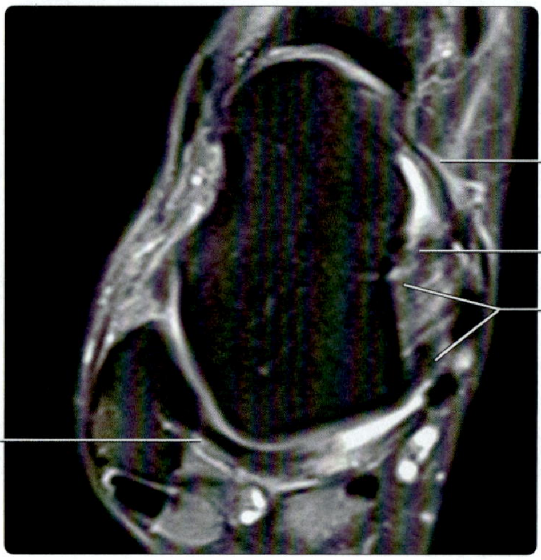

(Top) *Axial T2WI FS MR shows the common origin of the anterior bands of the superficial ligament from the medial malleolus. Laterally, the image includes portions of the anterior inferior tibiofibular ligament and the Basset ligament. The juxtaposition of the 2 ligamentous bands can be mistaken for a ligament tear.* **(Middle)** *Axial T2WI FS MR shows fibers of the superficial deltoid ligament. The ligament bands are not distinguishable at this point. The posterior inferior tibiofibular ligament is thick and striated.* **(Bottom)** *Axial T2WI FS MR demonstrates the broad extent of the deep deltoid ligament from anterior to posterior. A striated appearance, with taut individual fibers, is normal. The ligament is slightly oblique in orientation, from anteromedial to posterolateral. The tibionavicular band of the superficial deltoid is outlined here by joint effusion.*

CORONAL T2 FS MR: DELTOID LIGAMENT

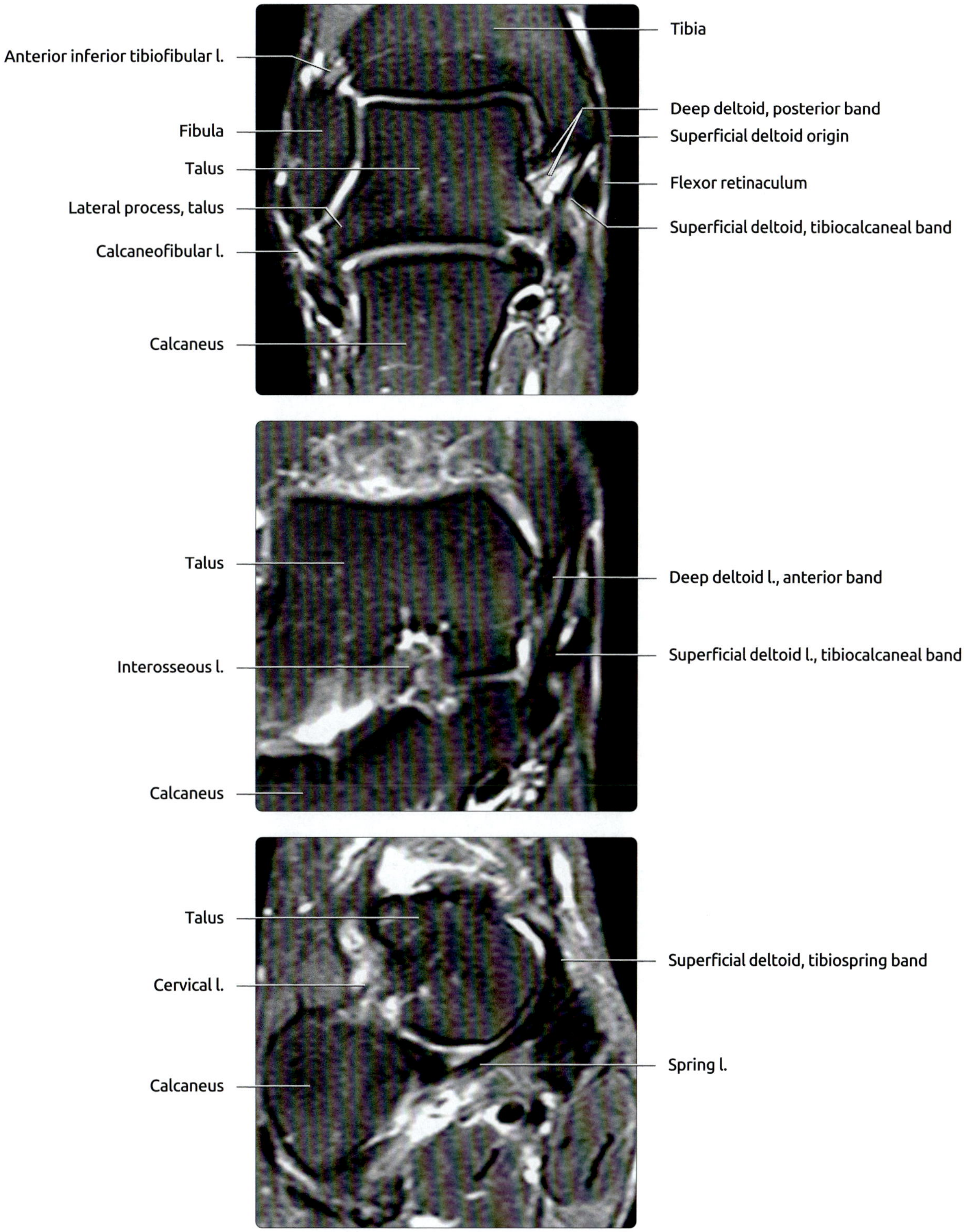

(Top) *Coronal T2WI FS MR shows the fan-shaped deep deltoid extending from the medial malleolus to the medial fovea of the talar body. The normal ligament has a striated appearance and does not completely fill the fovea. The posterior band is the primary band of the deep deltoid ligament. The anterior inferior tibiofibular ligament has a short, oblique course.* **(Middle)** *Coronal T2WI FS MR shows the anterior band of the deep deltoid ligament. This small band is of doubtful significance and variably present. The tibiocalcaneal band of the superficial deltoid is the strongest component of the superficial deltoid.* **(Bottom)** *Coronal T2WI FS MR at the level of the talar head shows the tibiospring band of the superficial deltoid ligament continuous with the spring ligament.*

CORONAL T1 MR: DEEP DELTOID LIGAMENT

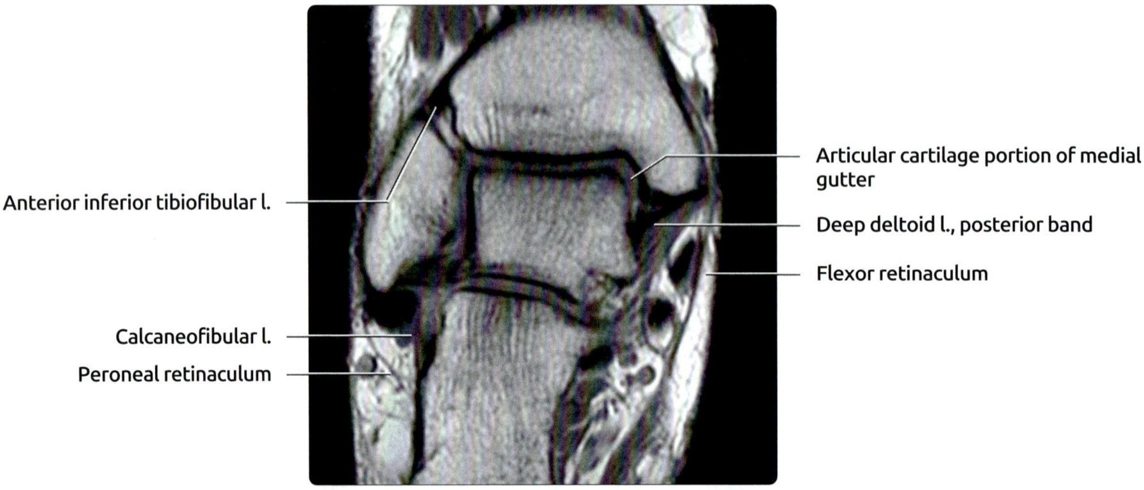

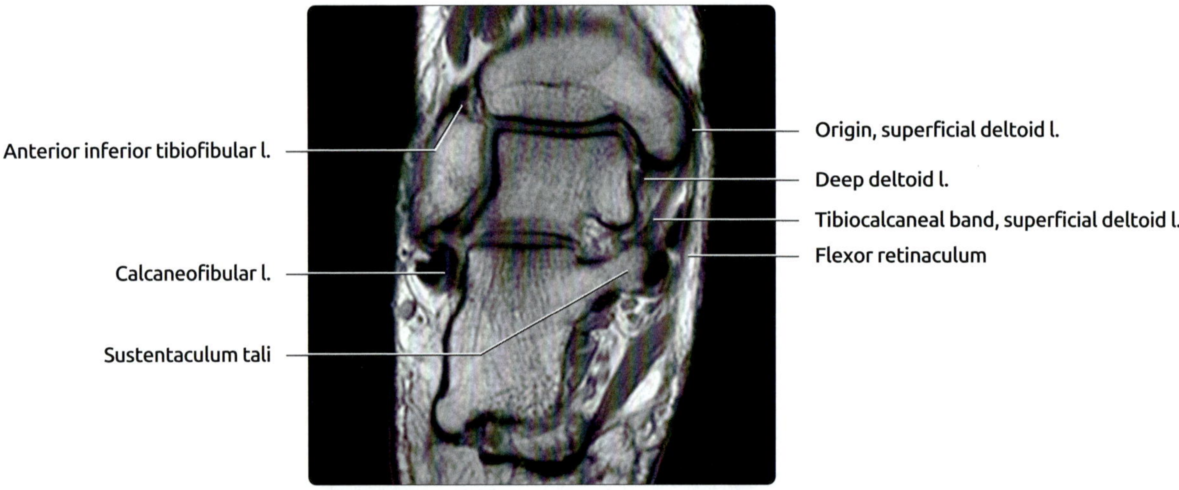

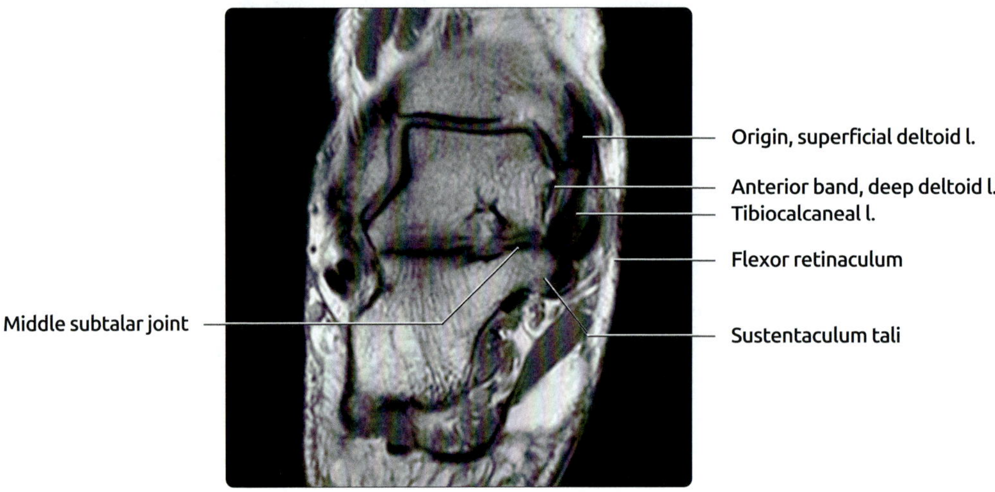

(Top) *The posterior band of the deep deltoid ligament is often simply designated as the deep deltoid, disregarding the small, variably present anterior band. It has a striated appearance and an oblique course from the posterior margin of the anterior colliculus of the medial malleolus and the posterior colliculus to the fovea at the medial talus.* **(Middle)** *The anterior bands of the superficial deltoid have a common origin from the superficial, medial, and anterior margins of the medial malleolus. The tibiocalcaneal band is the strongest band. It inserts on the sustentaculum tali of the calcaneus.* **(Bottom)** *The tibiocalcaneal band of the superficial deltoid is always present in uninjured patients. In this normal volunteer, it is slightly thicker than is usually seen.*

CORONAL T2 MR: LATERAL COLLATERAL LIGAMENTS

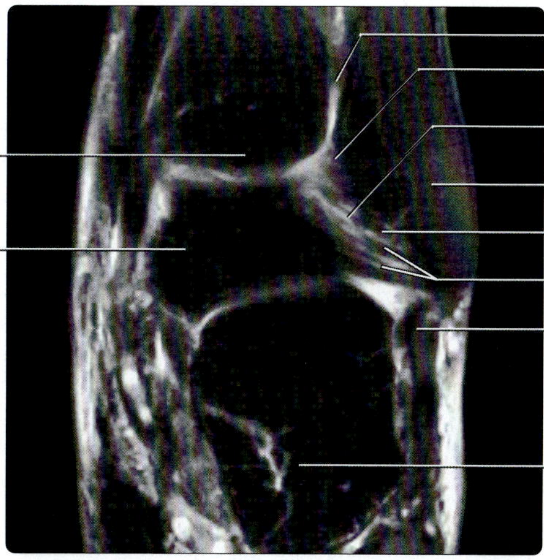

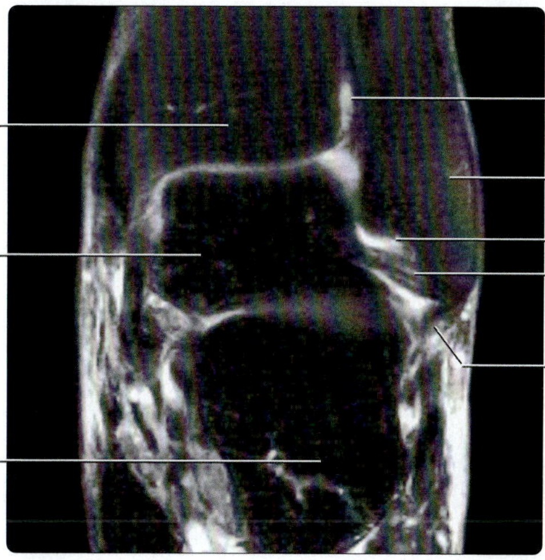

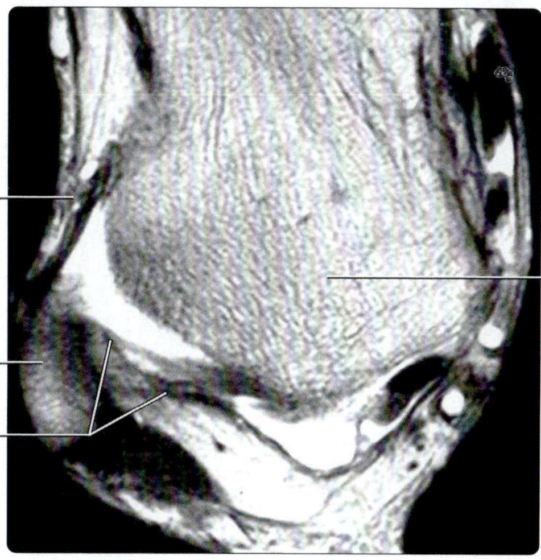

(Top) *Coronal T2WI FS MR shows the lateral collateral ligaments. The lateral collateral ligaments consist of anterior and posterior talofibular, as well as calcaneofibular ligaments. Although they are in close proximity to the syndesmotic ligaments, their function, protecting against inversion, internal rotation, and anterior subluxation are very different.* **(Middle)** *A slightly more anterior coronal T2WI FS MR is shown. The posterior talofibular ligament is visualized as a distinct structure from the posterior tibiofibular ligament.* **(Bottom)** *Lateral collateral ligaments are shown on this axial T2WI MR. The ligaments are optimally seen on axial images. Since these ligaments are thickening of the capsule, they are highlighted by fluid. Note the fan-shaped and striated fibular insertion of the posterior talofibular ligament, which should not to be mistaken for a tear.*

CORONAL T1 MR: LATERAL COLLATERAL LIGAMENTS

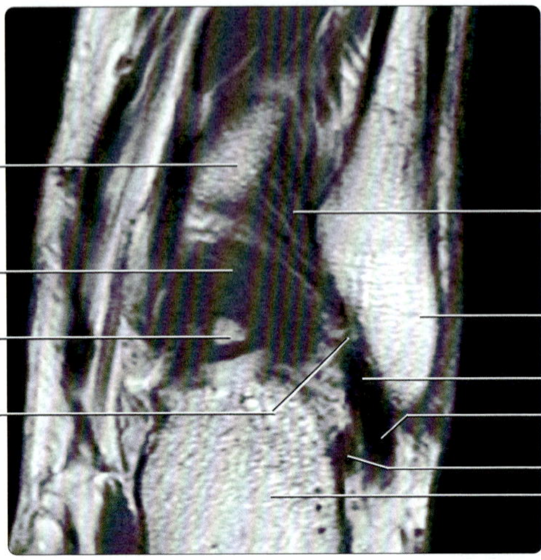

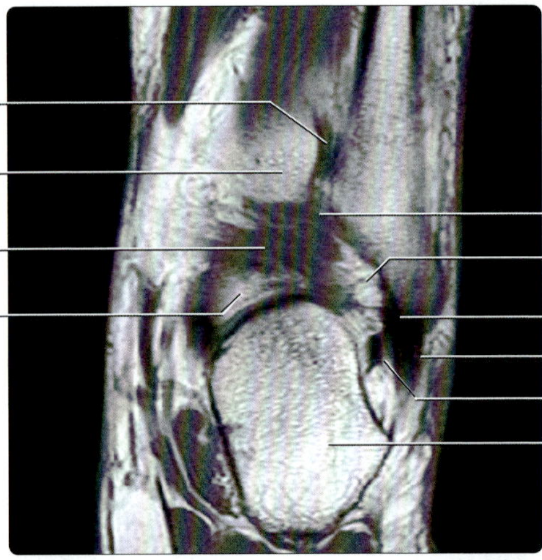

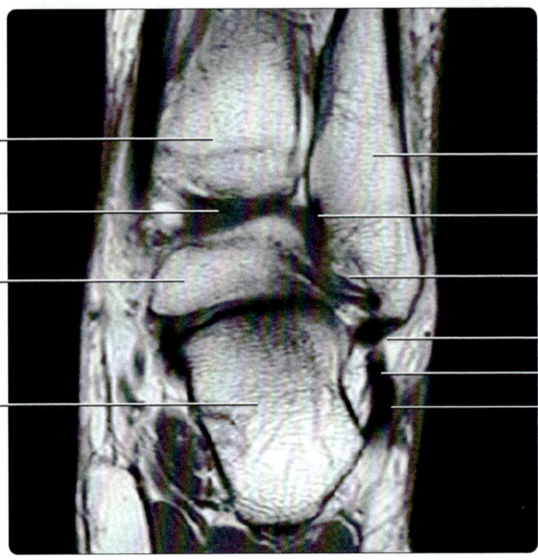

(Top) *Coronal posterior T1WI MR shows the calcaneal insertion of the calcaneofibular ligament. The ligament can be followed on sequential coronal images from its fibular origin to its calcaneal insertion.* **(Middle)** *The calcaneofibular ligament is seen on a more anterior coronal T1WI MR. Note proximity of the ligament to peroneal tendons, which can be used to locate the ligament. A tear of the ligament may produce reactive fluid within the common peroneal tendon sheath; this should not to be mistaken for peroneal tenosynovitis.* **(Bottom)** *In a more anterior image, the origin of the calcaneofibular ligament from the tip of the fibula is visualized.*

AXIAL & SAGITTAL MR: LATERAL COLLATERAL LIGAMENTS

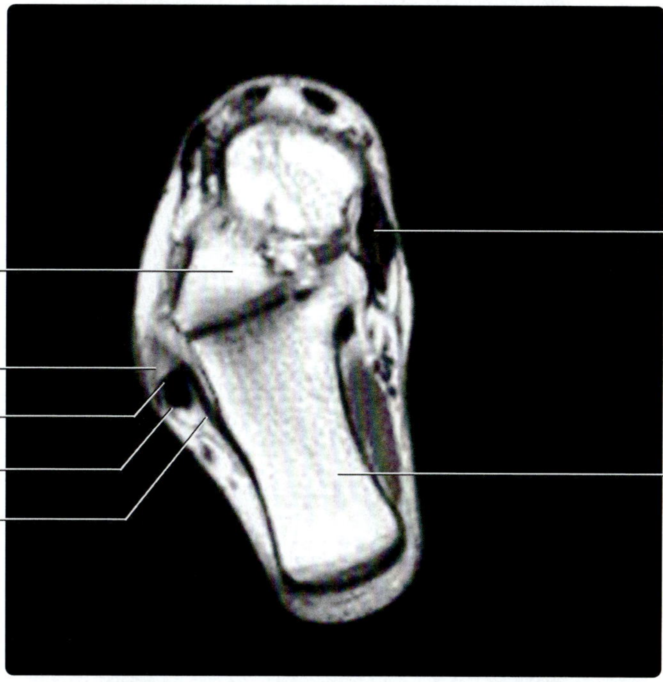

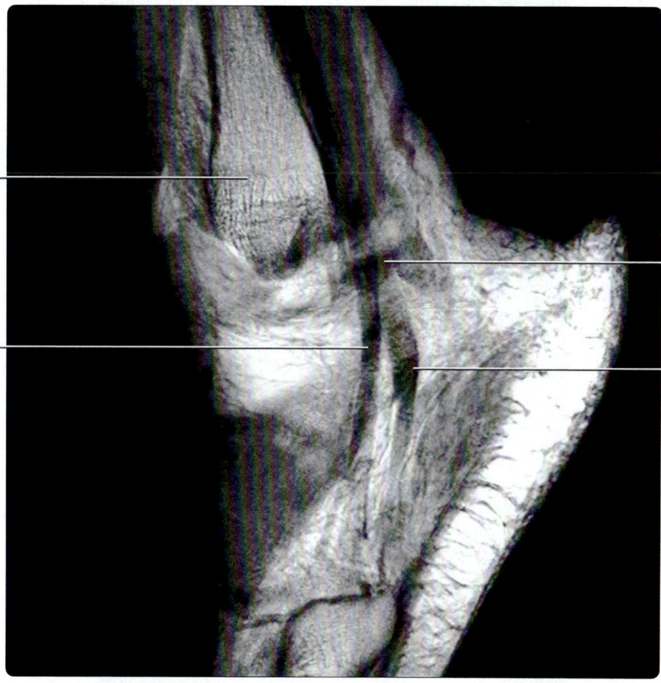

(Top) *The calcaneofibular ligament is seen on this axial oblique T1WI MR. The calcaneofibular ligament changes orientation with ankle movements. In mild plantar flexion, the ligament becomes close to horizontal in orientation and may be visualized on axial images as it hugs the calcaneus deep to the peroneal tendons. Its location deep to the peroneal tendons is a clue in locating this ligament.* **(Bottom)** *On this far lateral sagittal MR, the calcaneofibular ligament may be visualized, due to partial volume averaging, as a low-signal shadow superimposed on the peroneal tendons. Note that in this patient, scanned in plantarflexion, the calcaneofibular ligament is relatively horizontal. In general, mild plantar flexion of the ankle aids in detecting the calcaneofibular ligament on axial images.*

SAGITTAL T1 MR: LATERAL COLLATERAL LIGAMENTS

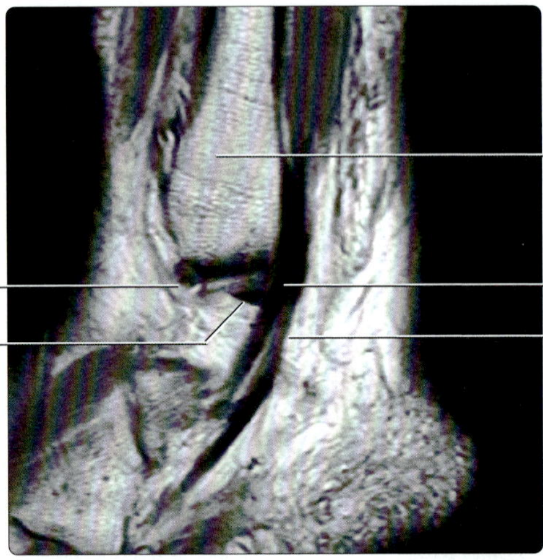

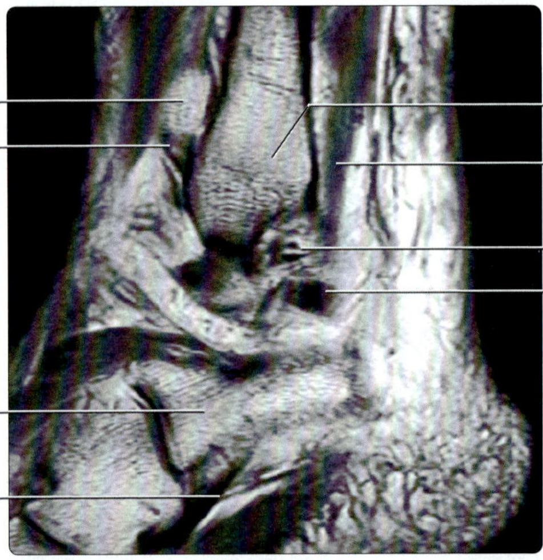

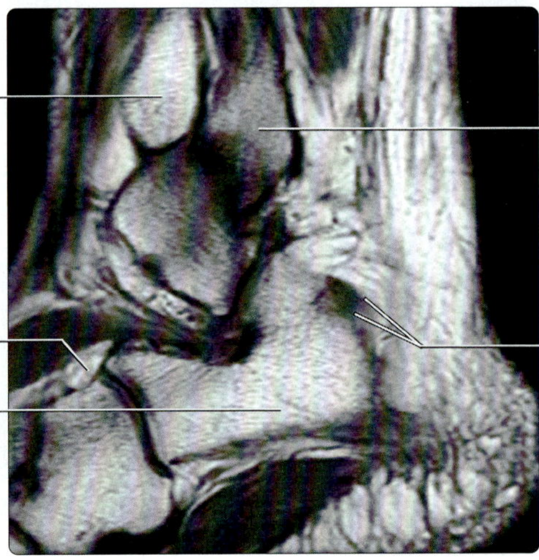

(Top) *Sequential sagittal T1 MR images show the calcaneofibular ligament, lateral to medial. Occasionally, the ligament may be visualized on sequential sagittal images from its fibular origin to its posterior calcaneal insertion.* **(Middle)** *The calcaneofibular ligament is now visualized as it is traversing the region deep (medial) to the peroneal tendons (peroneals are not well seen in this image). Note also the striated posterior talofibular ligament behind (posterior to) the fibula.* **(Bottom)** *Sagittal T1WI MR shows the calcaneofibular ligament. The calcaneofibular ligament is now seen in cross section as it inserts onto the calcaneus.*

AXIAL T1 MR: DELTOID LIGAMENT

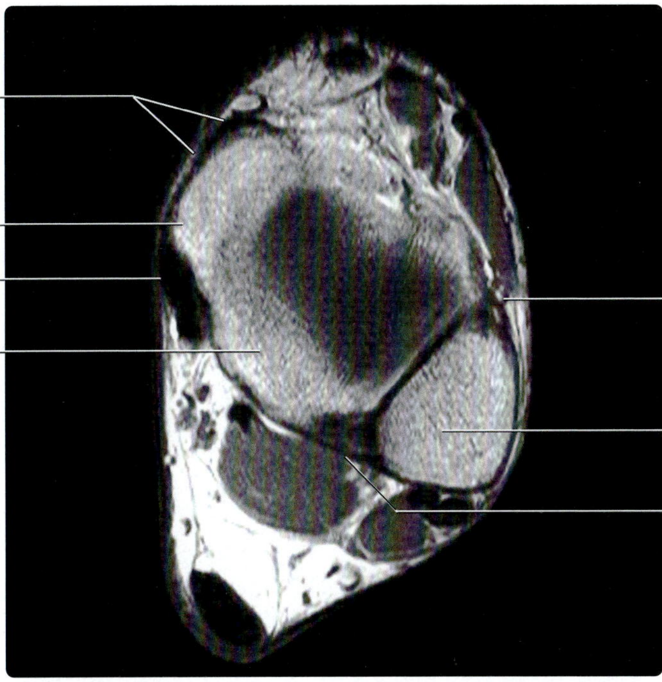

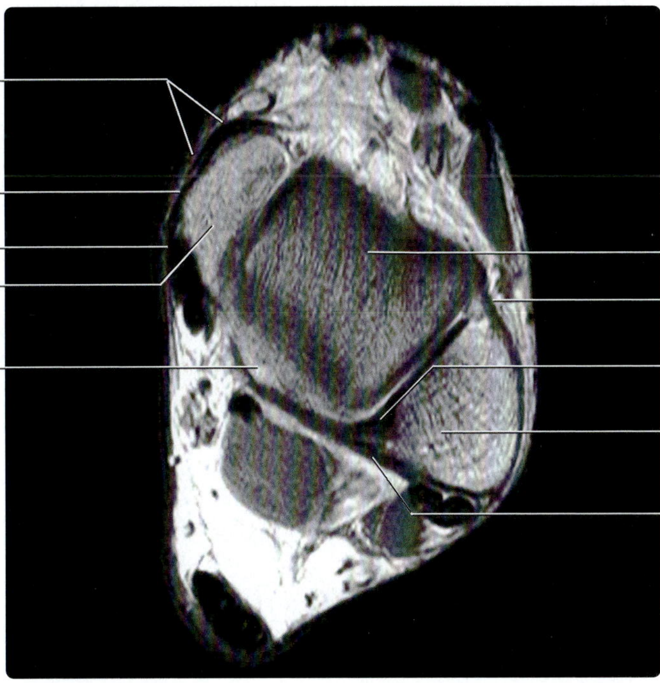

(Top) *The origin of the superficial deltoid ligament is seen on this axial T1WI MR. The superficial deltoid ligament is continuous with the periosteum of the medial malleolus, which is continuous with the flexor retinaculum origin.* **(Bottom)** *Axial T1WI MR, located slightly more distally, depicts the origin of the superficial deltoid. Its continuity with the periosteum of the medial malleolus, and the flexor retinaculum, is evident. This entire fascial layer may be avulsed from anterior to posterior due to twisting injury.*

AXIAL T2 MR: DELTOID LIGAMENT

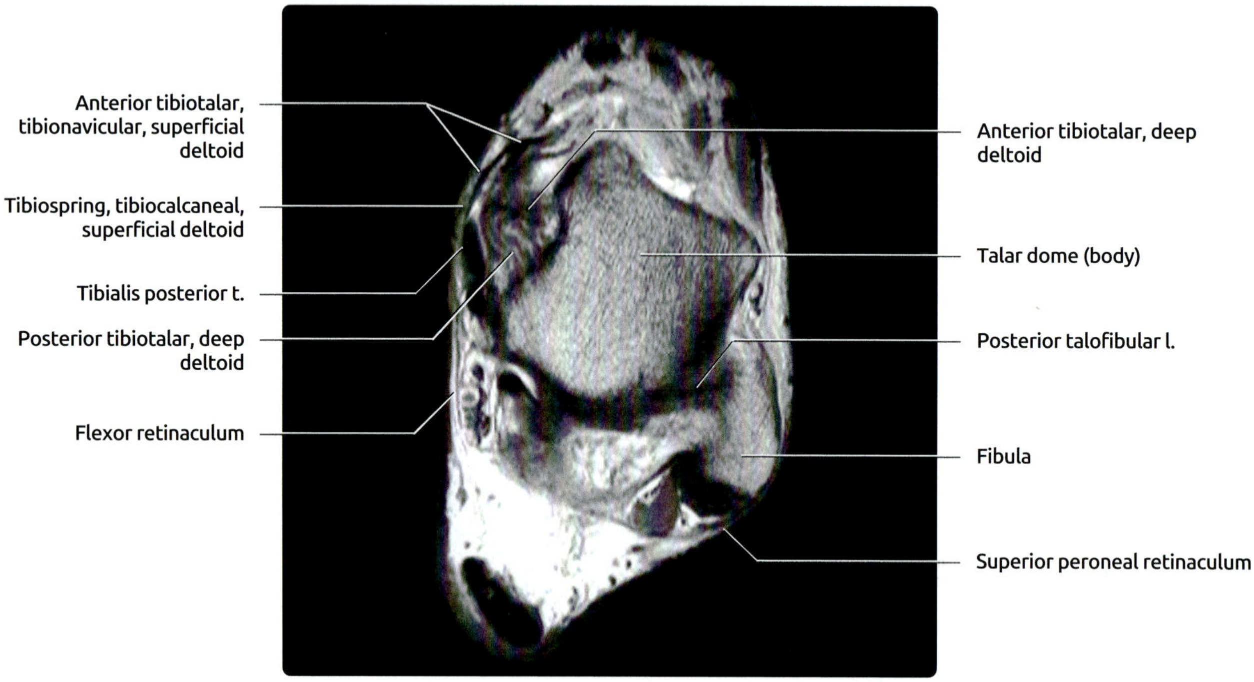

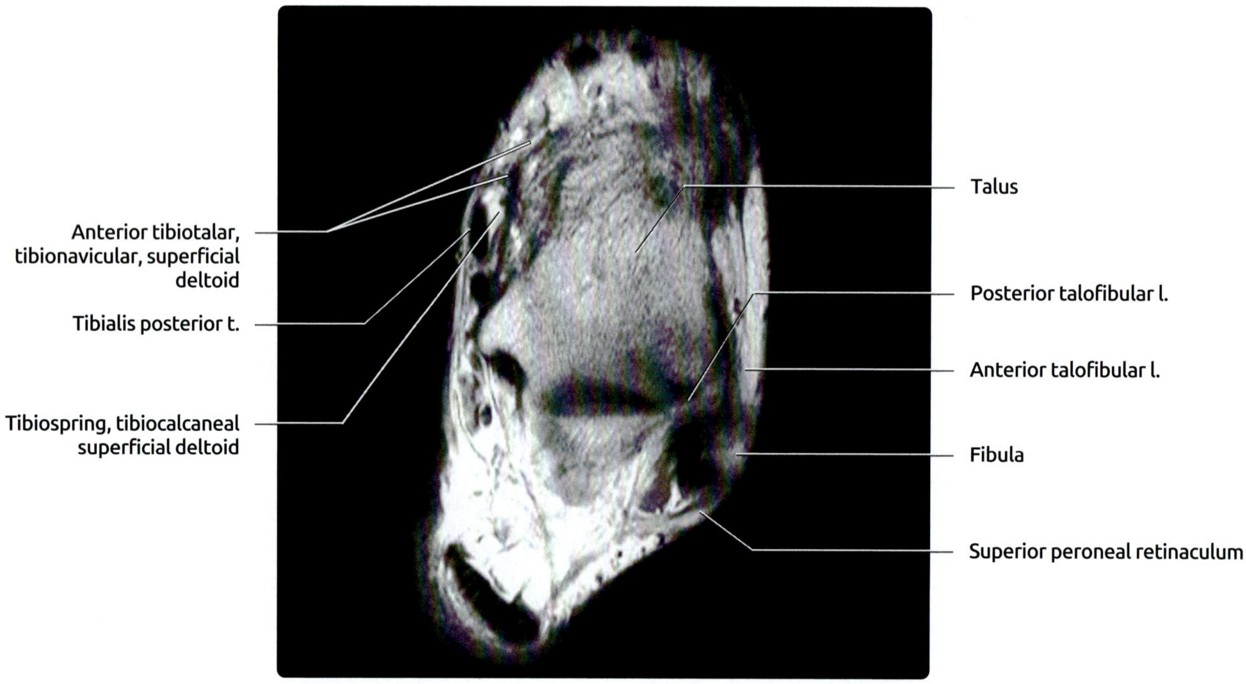

(Top) *Axial T2WI MR, at the level of talar dome, depicts the superficial deltoid bands diverging toward their insertions. The striated appearance of the deep deltoid ligament is well seen.* **(Bottom)** *Axial T2WI MR, located slightly more distally, depicts the tibiocalcaneal and tibiospring ligaments of the deltoid. The tibiospring ligament is slightly anterior to the tibiocalcaneal band and merges with the spring ligament.*

GRAPHICS: TARSAL CANAL & SINUS TARSI LIGAMENTS

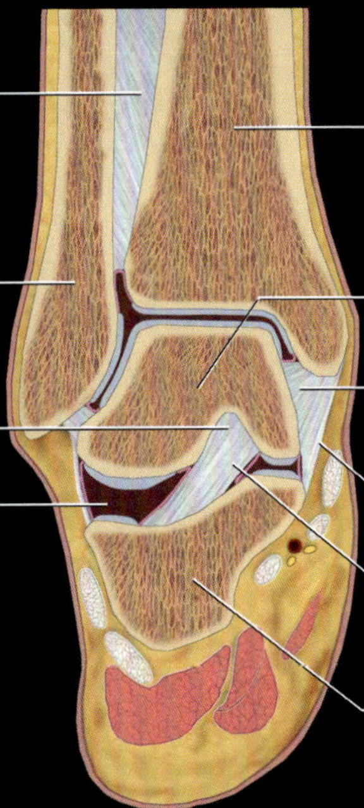

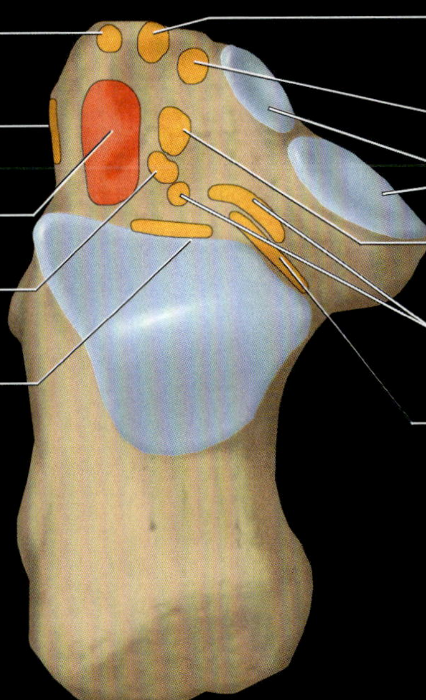

(Top) *Tarsal canal ligaments are shown. The tarsal canal is a space between the posterior subtalar joint and sustentaculum tali, traversed by the talocalcaneal interosseous ligament. The sinus tarsi is a more lateral space between the talus and calcaneus, which is continuous with the tarsal canal. The sinus tarsi is traversed by the roots of the inferior extensor retinaculum and by the cervical ligament.* **(Bottom)** *Calcaneal insertions of sinus tarsi ligaments are shown. The talocalcaneal interosseous ligament is most medial and posterior, while the cervical ligament is most anterior. The intermediate root of the inferior extensor retinaculum is immediately posterior to the cervical ligament, while the lateral root is lateral to the origin of the extensor digitorum brevis muscle. The medial root has 2 calcaneal and 1 talar insertions.*

CORONAL & SAGITTAL MR: TARSAL CANAL & TARSAL SINUS LIGAMENTS

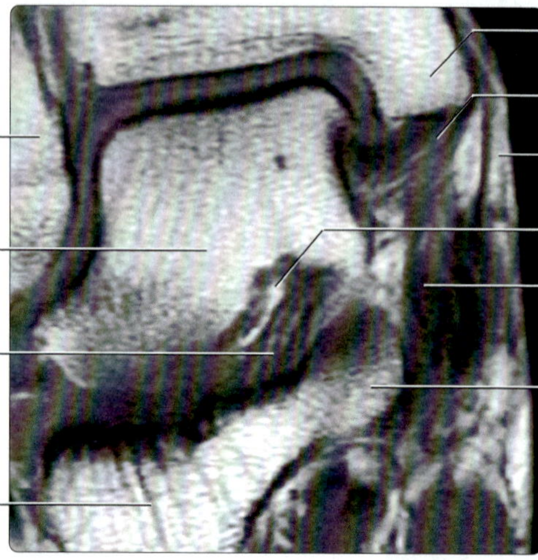

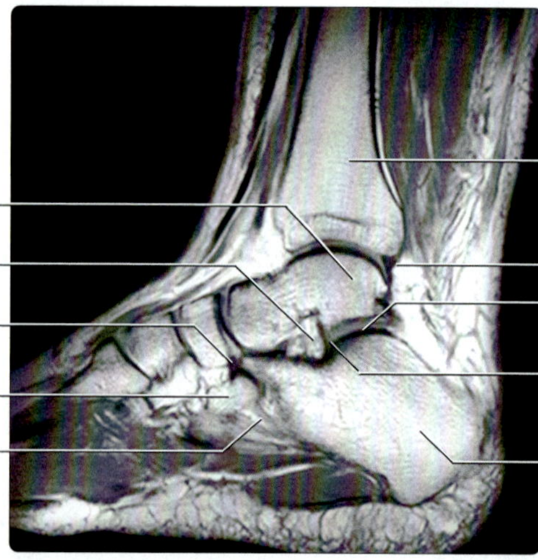

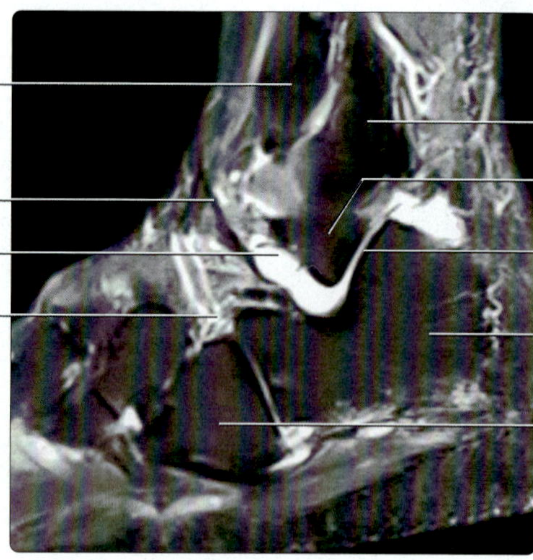

(Top) *Coronal MR shows the talocalcaneal interosseous ligament. The ligament's calcaneal insertion is just anterior to the posterior subtalar joint. The ligament then traverses the tarsal canal and ascends obliquely and medially to insert on the talar sulcus. The talocalcaneal interosseous ligament is best identified on coronal and sagittal images as the most posterior and medial of sinus tarsi ligaments.* **(Middle)** *Sagittal T1WI MR depicts the interosseous ligament as a band extending from the talus to the calcaneus, found anterior to the posterior subtalar joint. This ligament is typically found on the most medial sagittal images of the sinus tarsi.* **(Bottom)** *Tarsal sinus fluid often implies acute or chronic disease. However, a fluid-filled recess may extend from the posterior subtalar joint into the sinus tarsi. This should not be misinterpreted as pathology of the sinus tarsi.*

CORONAL & SAGITTAL MR: TARSAL CANAL & TARSAL SINUS LIGAMENTS

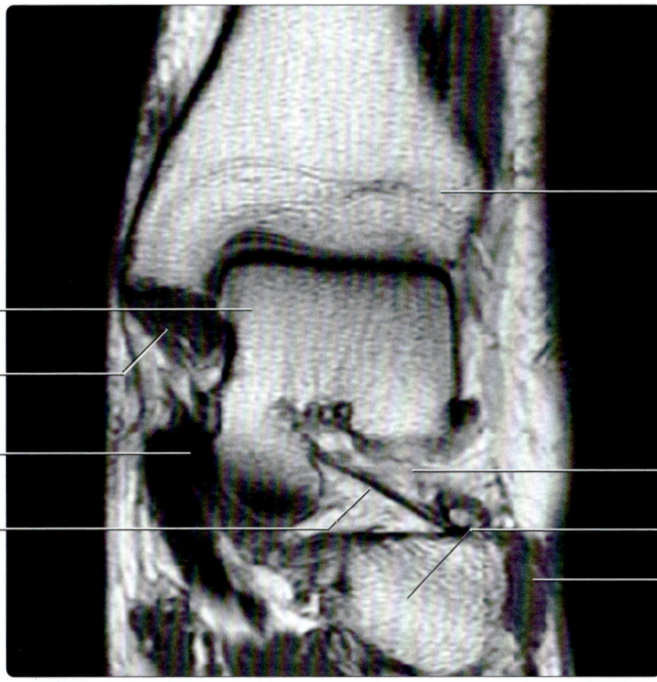

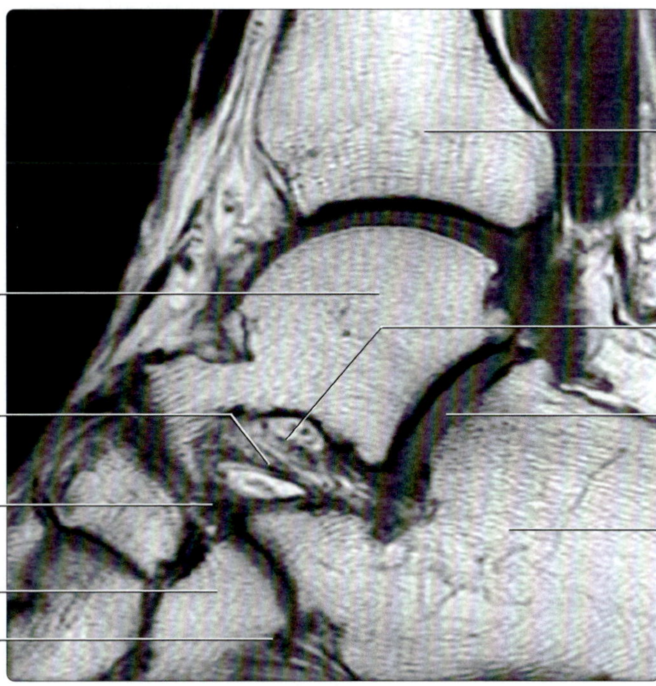

(Top) *Coronal T1WI MR shows the cervical ligament. The cervical ligament is the strongest ligament connecting the talus to the calcaneus. It is also the most anterior ligament of the sinus tarsi. Its calcaneal origin is medial to the origin of the extensor digitorum brevis muscle. The ligament ascends upward anteriorly and medially to insert on the inferior aspect of the talar neck. The ligament becomes more horizontal in valgus and more vertical in varus position of the calcaneus.* **(Bottom)** *Sagittal T1WI MR shows the cervical ligament. The ligaments anterior course from the calcaneus to the talus is better appreciated on sagittal images. Note the intermediate root of the inferior extensor retinaculum located immediately posterior to the cervical ligament.*

SAGITTAL MR: TARSAL CANAL & TARSAL SINUS LIGAMENTS

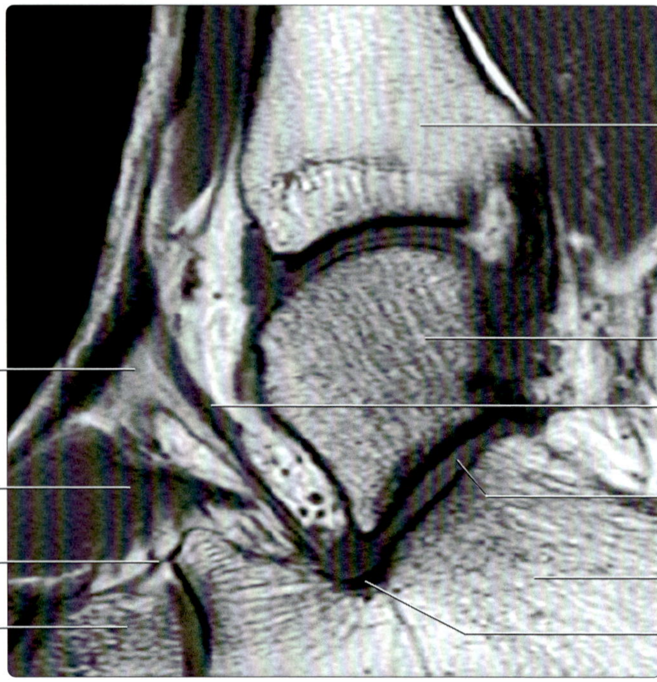

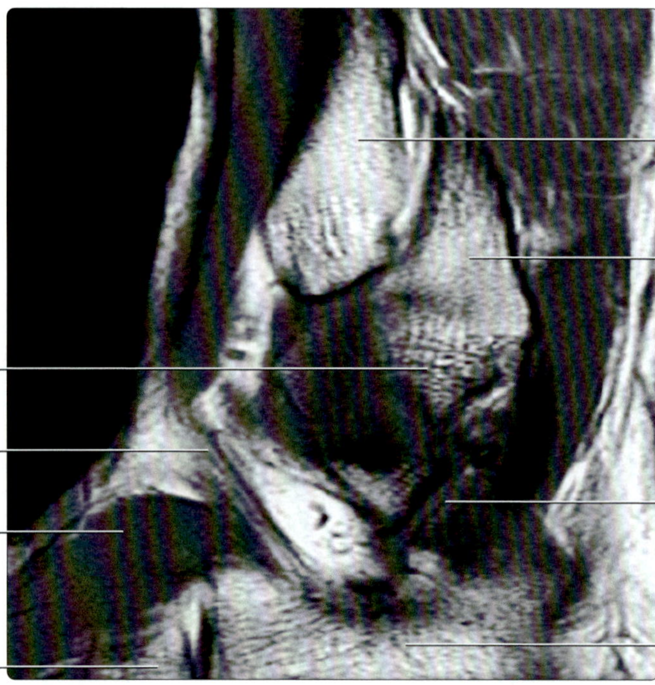

(Top) *Sagittal MR shows roots of the extensor retinaculum. The intermediate root inserts into the calcaneus slightly posterior to the cervical ligament. The medial root has medial and lateral calcaneal insertions and 1 talar insertion. The intermediate root and lateral component of the medial root may insert very close to each other on the calcaneus, but the latter is found closer to the posterior subtalar joint.* **(Bottom)** *Sagittal T1WI MR shows the lateral root of the inferior extensor retinaculum. The root inserts into the calcaneus lateral to the origin of the extensor digitorum brevis muscle. It is continuous with the inferior peroneal retinaculum and deep fascia. The ligament is found on very far lateral sagittal images of the sinus tarsi.*

GRAPHIC & CORONAL MR: SPRING LIGAMENT

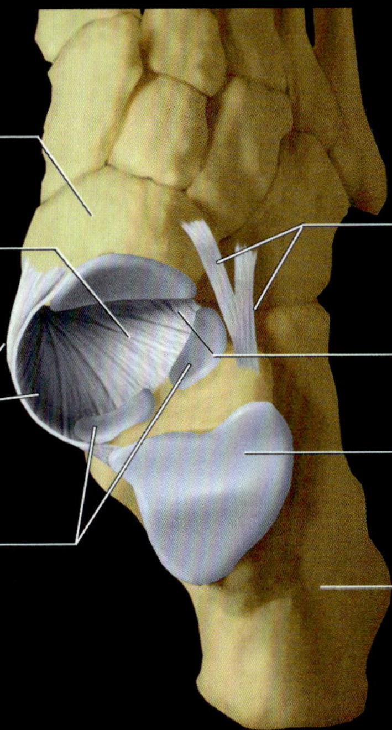

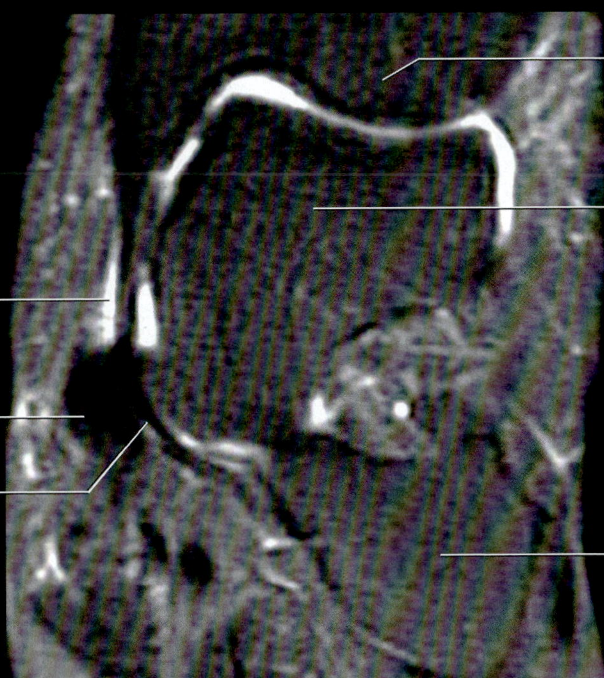

(Top) *The spring ligament is a hammock-shaped structure, which supports the talar head and medial longitudinal arch. Coronal oblique and sagittal images provide optimal visualization of the components of the spring ligament; however, routine ankle images are also useful. The superomedial component originates from the sustentaculum tali and inserts into superomedial navicular and the tibiospring ligament. It is best seen on coronal and axial images and occasionally on a far medial sagittal image. The medioplantar oblique is best seen on axial images, while the inferoplantar longitudinal is seen on both axial and sagittal images.* **(Bottom)** *Coronal T2WI FS MR shows the superomedial spring ligament. The ligament hugs the talar head and is contiguous with the tibiospring component of the deltoid ligament. Note the proximity of the tibialis posterior tendon to the ligament.*

AXIAL T1 MR: SPRING LIGAMENT

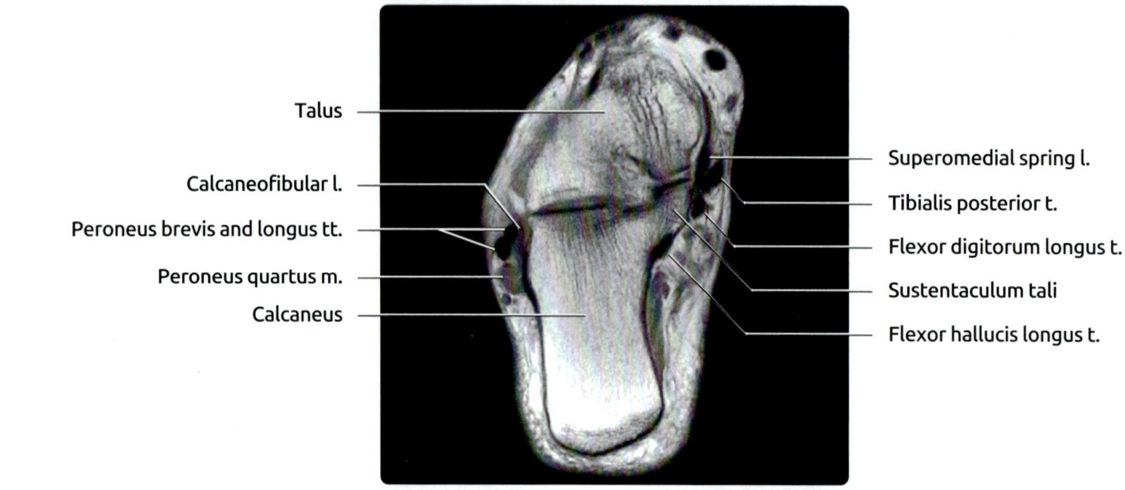

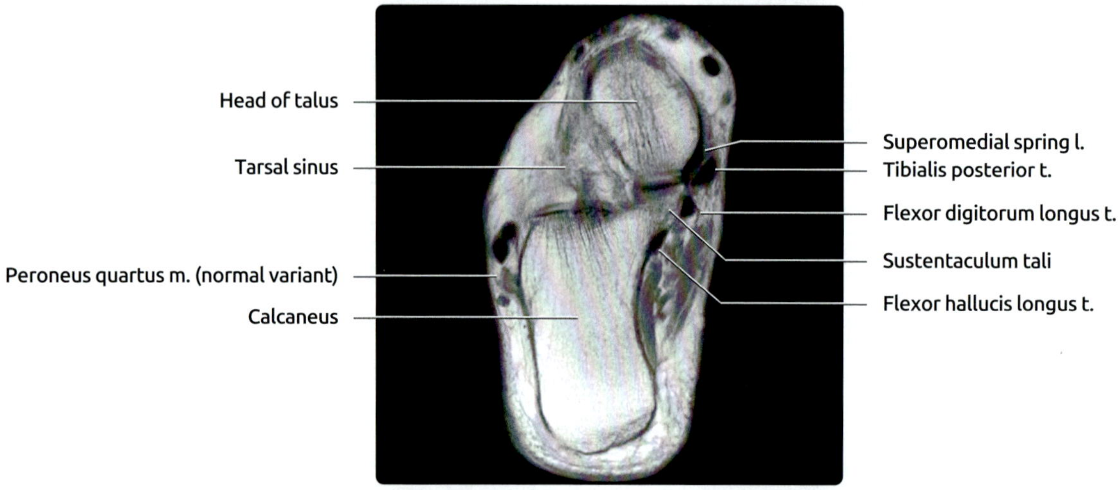

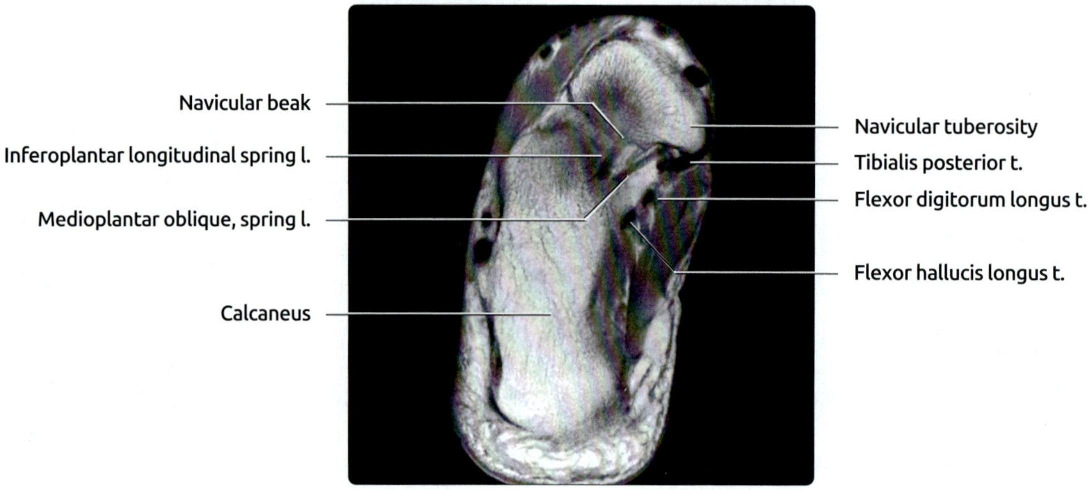

(Top) *Axial T1WI MR shows the superomedial spring ligament. The superomedial spring is seen on axial images as it originates from the sustentaculum tali and curves around the talar head toward its navicular insertion (latter not seen). Notice the proximity of the tibialis posterior tendon.* **(Middle)** *A more distal axial T1WI MR shows the superomedial spring ligament.* **(Bottom)** *A more distal axial T1WI MR is shown. The medioplantar oblique and inferoplantar longitudinal components of the spring ligament originate from the calcaneus at the coronoid fossa (between the sustentaculum tali and anterior calcaneal process). The medioplantar oblique is consistently seen as it inserts into the plantar navicular, just lateral to the navicular tuberosity and tibialis posterior tendon. The inferoplantar longitudinal inserts on the beak of the navicular.*

AXIAL T1 MR: SPRING LIGAMENT

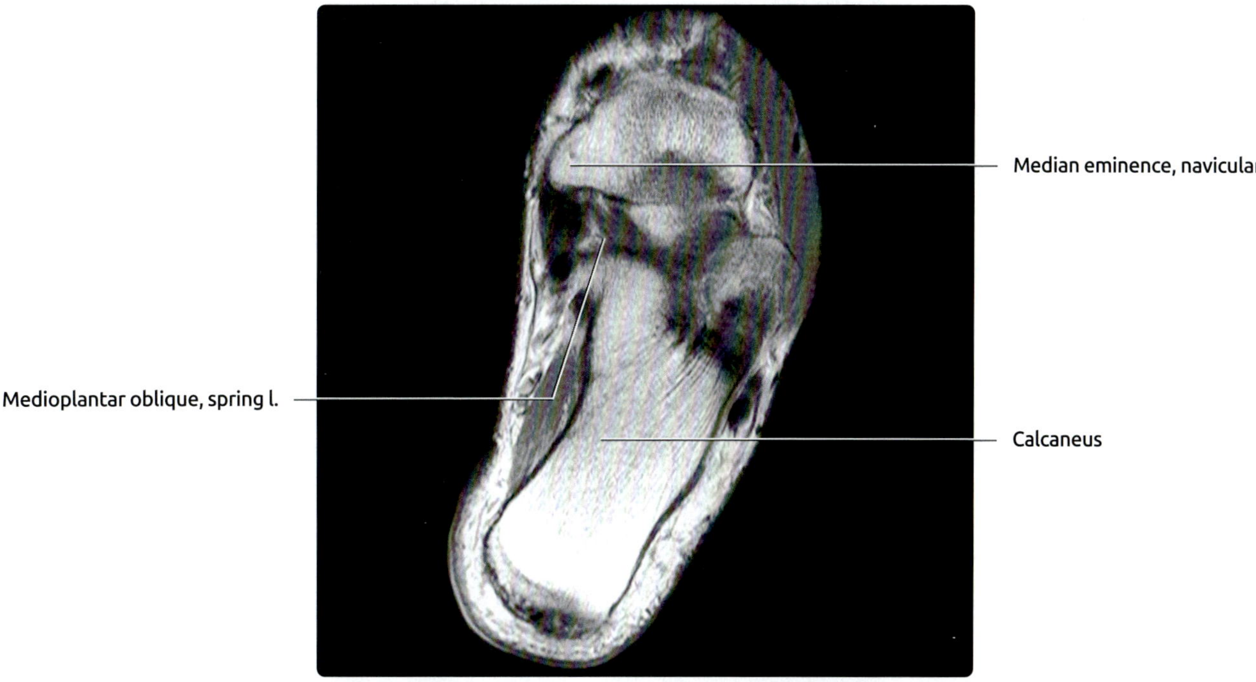

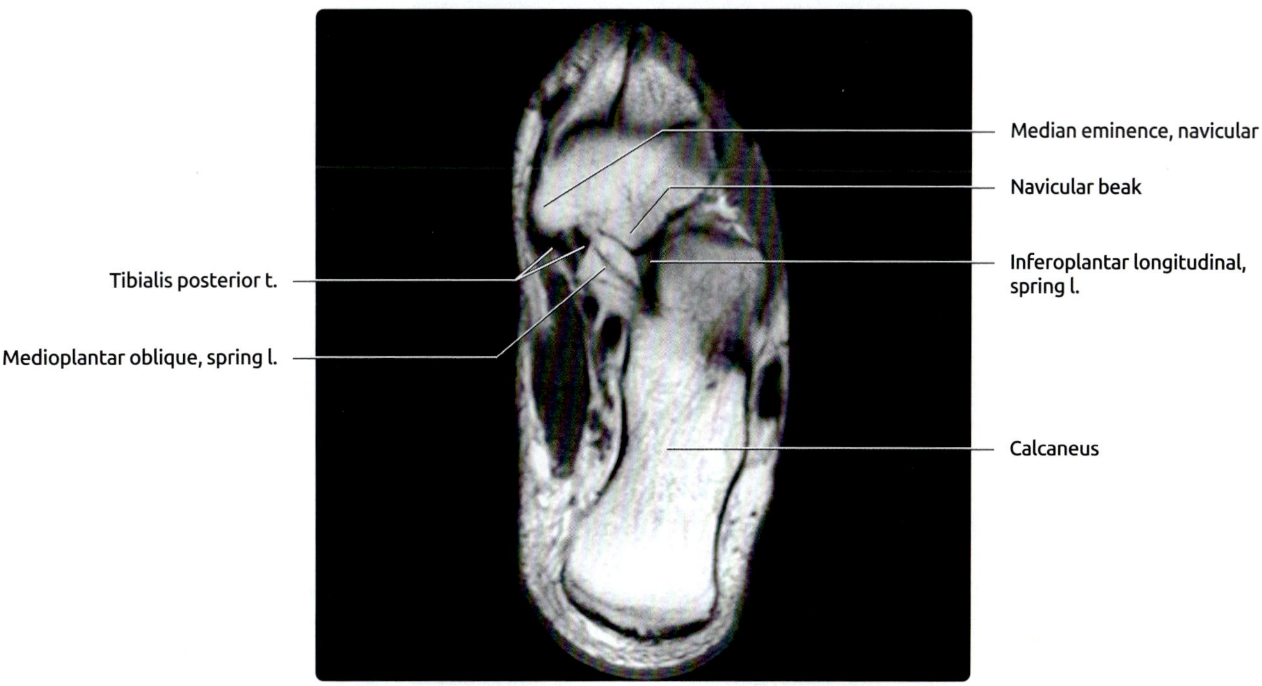

(Top) *Axial T1WI MR shows the medioplantar oblique component of the spring ligament. The ligament is frequently striated and is often relatively thick.* **(Bottom)** *A more distal axial T1WI MR is shown. Note the navicular beak at the insertion of the inferoplantar component of the spring ligament. Because of the straight course of the inferoplantar longitudinal component of the spring ligament, it is often seen on axial and sagittal images.*

SAGITTAL T1 MR: SPRING LIGAMENT

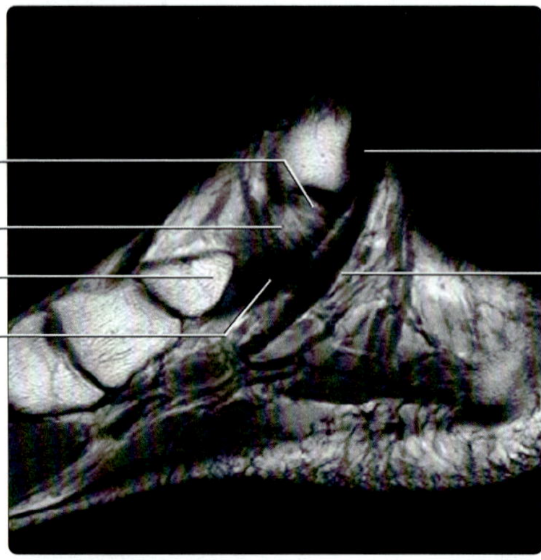

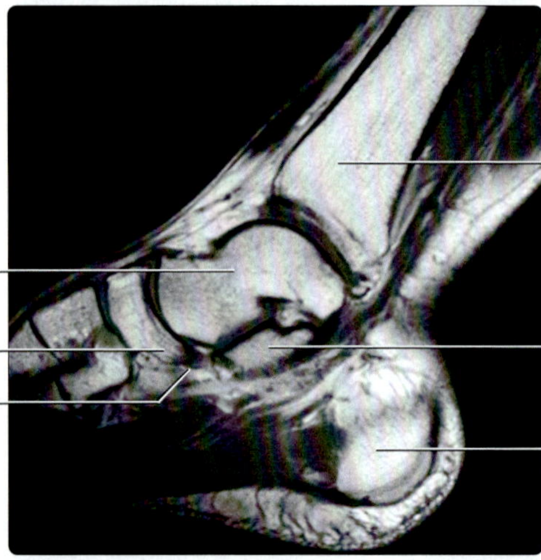

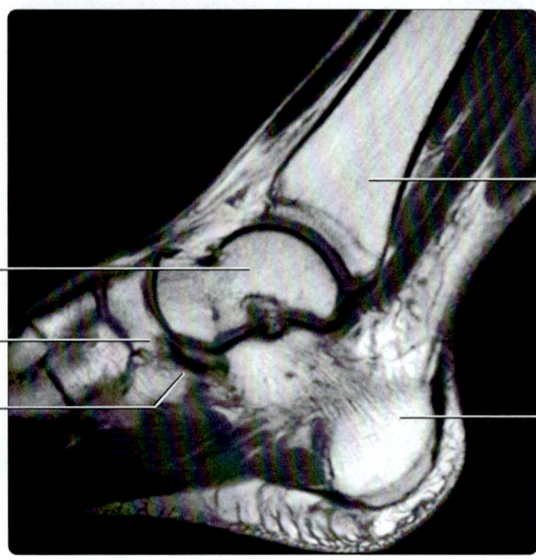

(Top) *The superomedial component of the spring ligament is sometimes seen on a far medial image as a low-signal band medial to the talar head and lateral to the tibialis posterior tendon.* **(Middle)** *The inferoplantar longitudinal band of the spring ligament is shown. Because of its oblique course, the medioplantar oblique component of the spring ligament is difficult to identify on routine sagittal images and may been seen on cross section as an oval, low-signal structure. However, the inferoplantar longitudinal component, because of its straight and short course, is frequently seen on sagittal images. Visualization of the beak of the navicular aids in identifying the ligament.* **(Bottom)** *Inferoplantar longitudinal ligament is shown. The ligament is a low-signal band extending from the navicular beak to the coronoid fossa of the calcaneus.*

SAGITTAL & AXIAL MR: BIFURCATE LIGAMENT

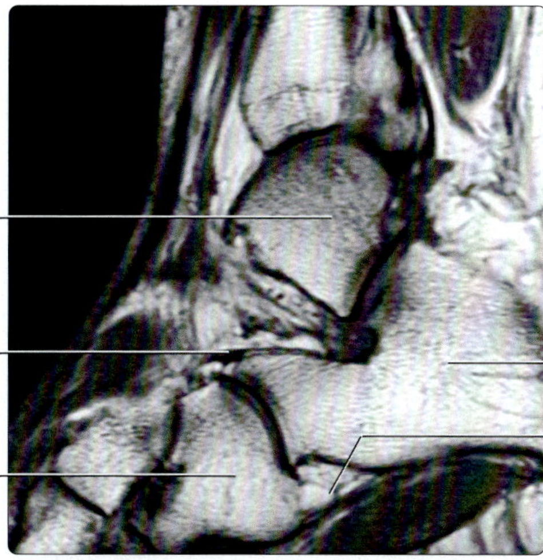

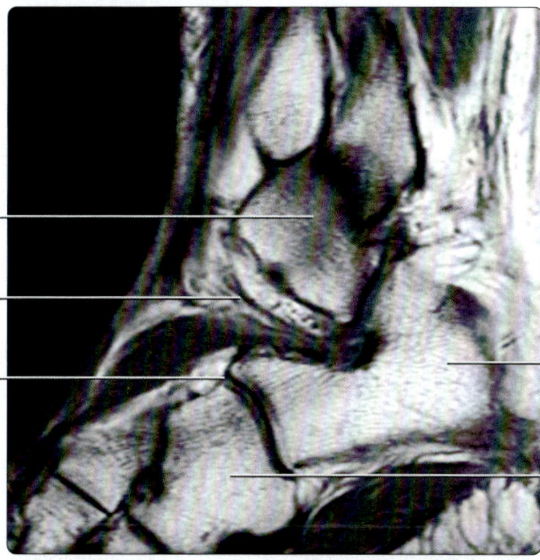

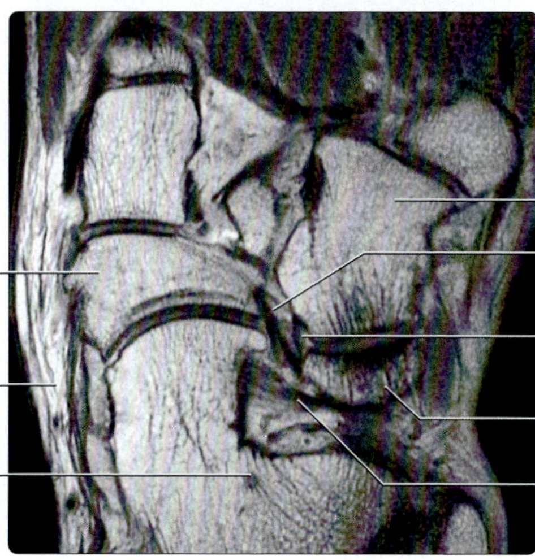

(Top) *The lateral calcaneonavicular ligament of the bifurcate ligament is best seen on a sagittal image just lateral to the origin of the inferoplantar longitudinal component of the spring ligament. It is seen as a fine, curved, low-signal structure originating from the anterior process of the calcaneus.* **(Middle)** *The medial calcaneocuboid component of the bifurcate ligament originates lateral to the lateral calcaneonavicular component. It is often quite a delicate, low signal intensity structure, which may be absent in some individuals.* **(Bottom)** *The bifurcate ligament is occasionally seen on axial oblique images of the hindfoot.*

AXIAL T1 MR: LONG & SHORT PLANTAR LIGAMENTS

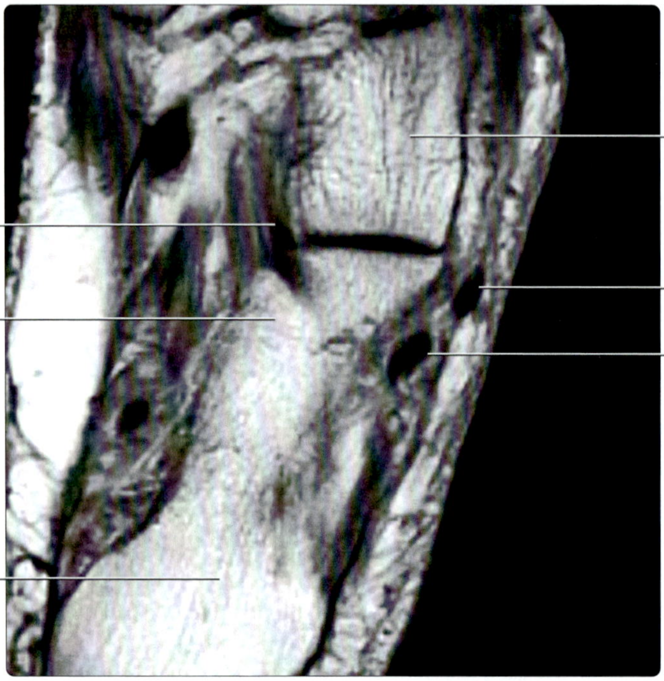

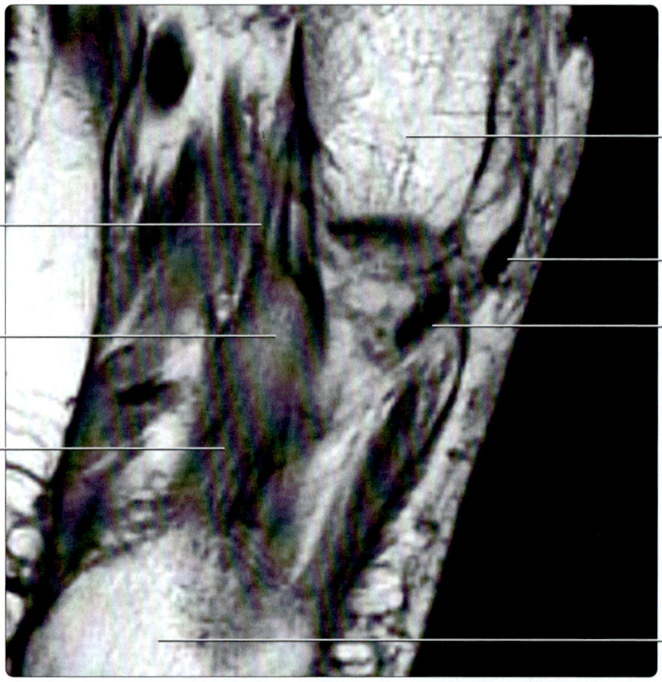

(Top) *The plantar calcaneocuboid ligament is subdivided into short, deep, and long superficial plantar ligaments. The short plantar ligament, also called the short plantar calcaneocuboid ligament, is more medial than the long plantar ligament. It originates from the anterior tubercle of the calcaneus and inserts on the entire posterior plantar surface of and on the beak of the cuboid.* **(Bottom)** *A more distal (plantar) axial image in the same patient is shown. The long plantar ligament originates from the anterior tubercle and more posteriorly from the anterior aspect and intertubercular segment of the posterior calcaneal tuberosities. Its deeper fibers, representing the bulk of the ligament, insert on the cuboid crest, and its superficial fibers form a thinner layer, which forms the roof of the cuboid tunnel of the peroneus longus tendon and inserts on the 2nd-5th metatarsal bases.*

SAGITTAL T1 MR: LONG & SHORT PLANTAR LIGAMENTS

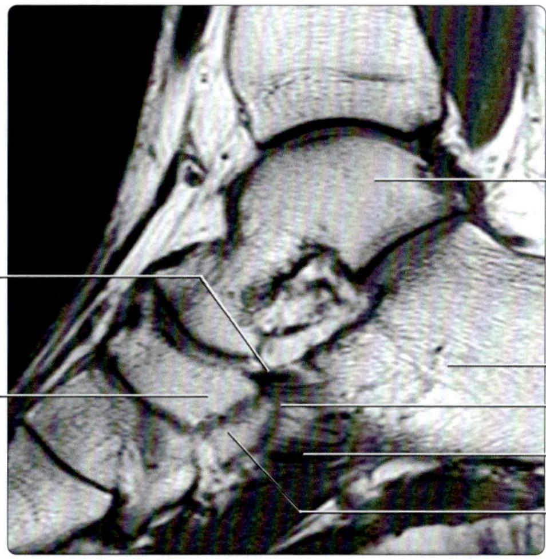

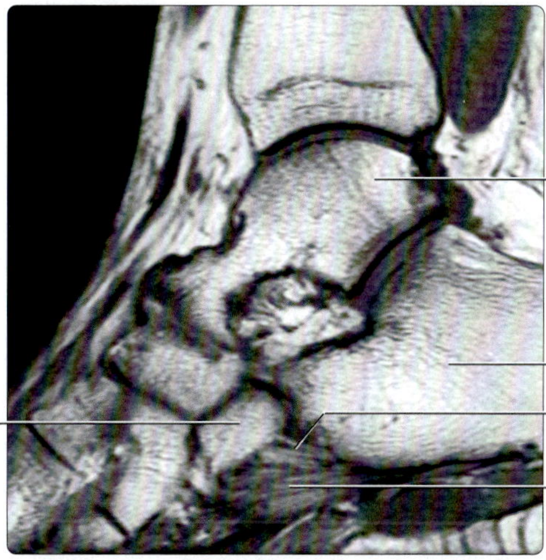

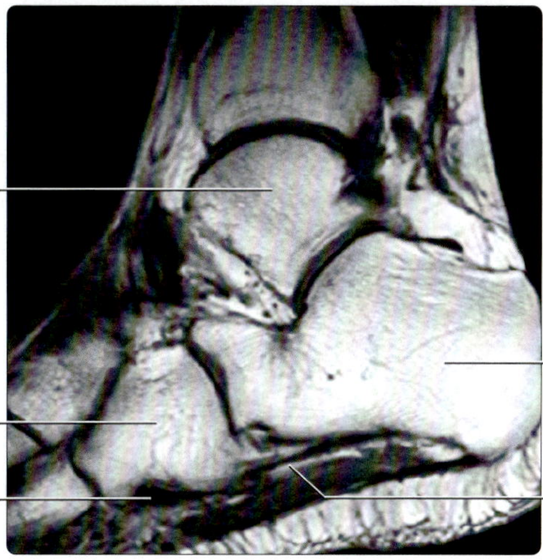

(Top) *Note the proximity of the plantar component of the spring ligament to the short plantar ligament on this image. The inferoplantar longitudinal ligament inserts into the beak of the navicular. The short plantar ligament is found more plantarly and is deeper than the long plantar ligament. It inserts on the cuboid.* **(Middle)** *A more lateral sagittal image in the same patient is shown. Note the marked striation of both the short and long plantar ligaments.* **(Bottom)** *A more lateral sagittal image in a different patient is shown. The superficial fibers of the long plantar ligament continue distal to the cuboid to insert onto the bases of the 2nd-5th metatarsals, and thus form the roof of the peroneus longus tunnel under the cuboid.*

GROSS ANATOMY

Ligaments

- 3 sets bind ankle: Distal tibiofibular syndesmotic complex, lateral collateral ligaments, and deltoid ligaments
- **Tibiofibular syndesmotic ligaments**
  - Anterior, posterior, and interosseous
  - At level of tibial plafond
    - Inferior transverse band of posterior ligament extends more inferiorly to tip of fibula
  - Obliquely oriented from superomedial to inferolateral
  - Prevent eversion, lateral translation of talus
- **Lateral collateral ligaments**
  - Anterior and posterior talofibular, calcaneofibular
  - Anterior talofibular
    - From 1 cm above tip of tibula to shoulder of talar body, at junction of body and neck
  - Calcaneofibular
    - Deep to peroneal tendons
    - From tip of fibula posteriorly and inferiorly to calcaneus
  - Posterior talofibular: From deep surface of fibula to lateral margin of talar body
  - Prevent inversion, internal rotation of ankle
- **Deltoid ligament (medial collateral ligament)**
  - Deep and superficial components
  - Deep: Medial surface of medial malleolus to fovea of talus
  - Superficial: Multiple bands named for attachments
    - Common origin from superficial surface of medial malleolus
    - Talocalcaneal band: Strongest, inserts on sustentaculum tali
    - Tibiospring: Merges with spring ligament
    - Tibiotalar: Small anterior and posterior bands
    - Tibionavicular: Merges with spring ligament
  - Prevent eversion, lateral translation, rotation of ankle
- **Spring ligament**
  - Only superomedial band is well seen on US
  - From sustentaculum tali to navicular
  - Plantar bands are deep, difficult to identify sonographically

Retinacula

- **Superior extensor retinaculum**
  - Slightly above ankle joint line
  - Attaches to anterior fibula laterally, tibia medially
  - Binds down anterior compartment muscles
- **Inferior extensor retinaculum**
  - At ankle joint, Y-shaped, stem laterally, proximal and distal bands medially
  - Stem attaches laterally to upper calcaneus
  - Dorsalis pedis vessels, deep peroneal nerve: Deep to all layers of inferior extensor retinaculum
- **Flexor retinaculum**
  - Attaches to posteromedial corner of medial malleolus, deep fascia of flexor compartment, calcaneus
  - Maintains position of deep flexor tendons
  - Forms roof of tarsal tunnel
- **Superior peroneal retinaculum**
  - Attaches to posterolateral corner of fibula, calcaneus, crural fascia
  - Maintains position of peroneal tendons behind fibula
- **Inferior peroneal retinaculum**
  - Continuous with inferior extensor retinaculum
  - Inserts on lateral calcaneus, peroneal tubercle (trochlea)
  - Binds peroneus brevis, peroneus longus tendons to calcaneus

Tendons

- **Anterior (extensor) compartment**
  - From medial to lateral: Anterior tibial, extensor hallucis longus, extensor digitorum longus, and (variably present) peroneus tertius
- **Lateral compartment: Peroneus longus and brevis tendons**
  - Peroneus longus is superficial to brevis in leg, inferior to it in foot
  - They cross beneath lateral malleolus
  - Both act to evert foot
  - Tendons share tendon sheath proximal to peroneal tubercle of calcaneus
  - Peroneus brevis becomes ribbon-like toward its insertion on 5th metatarsal styloid process
  - Peroneus brevis muscle normally extends to tip of fibula
    - If muscle seen more distally, consider peroneus quartus muscle vs. low-lying peroneus brevis muscle
- **Superficial posterior compartment**
  - **Achilles tendon**
    - Conjoint tendon of medial and lateral gastrocnemius and soleus muscles
    - Lacks tendon sheath, partially enclosed by paratenon
    - Inserts into posterior calcaneal tuberosity
    - Retrocalcaneal bursa between distal tendon and calcaneal tuberosity
    - Main plantarflexor of ankle, foot
    - Anterior contour is concave (kidney bean shape)
    - Normal size < 6 mm AP dimension
- **Plantaris tendon**
  - Vestigial, slender tendon, medial to Achilles tendon
  - Inserts on Achilles tendon or calcaneus
- **Deep posterior (flexor) compartment**
  - From medial to lateral: Posterior tibial, flexor digitorum longus, flexor hallucis longus
  - Posterior tibial is 2x size of flexor digitorum brevis
  - Flexor hallucis longus still has muscular portion at level of ankle

Tarsal Tunnel

- Fibroosseous tunnel in medial ankle
- Roof: Flexor retinaculum
- Floor: Medial malleolus, talus, calcaneus
- Contains: Deep flexor tendons, tibial nerve and its branches, posterior tibial artery & vein and their branches
- Tibial nerve is vulnerable to compression due to mass-occupying lesion or scar in tarsal tunnel

GRAPHICS: ANKLE

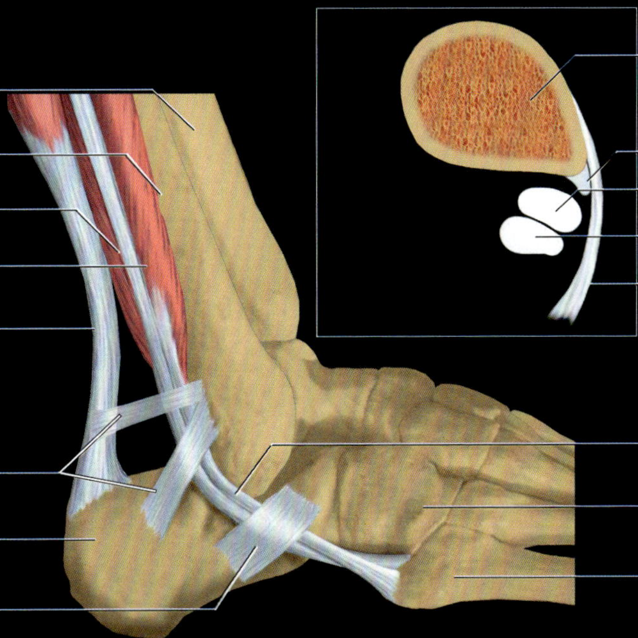

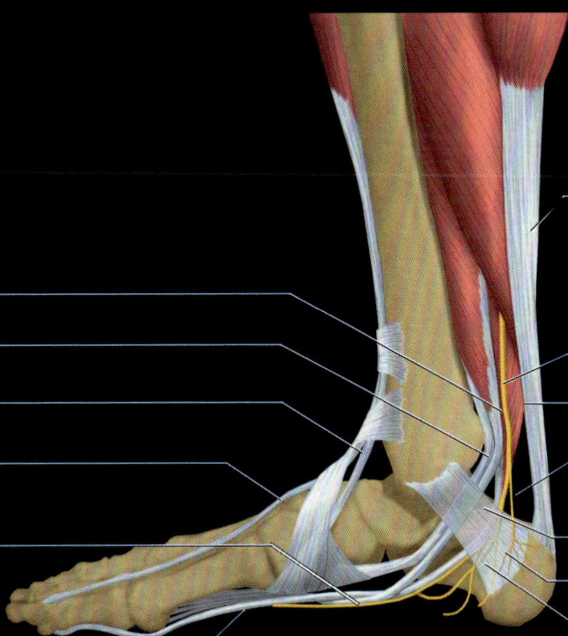

(Top) *Peroneal retinacula are shown. The superior peroneal retinaculum holds the peroneal tendons in the retrofibular groove. The superior retinaculum maintains the position of the peroneal tendons posterior to the fibula. The inferior peroneal retinaculum holds the peroneal tendons against the calcaneus.* **(Bottom)** *Tarsal tunnel is seen accommodating the posterior tibial neurovascular bundle. The medial calcaneal nerve supplies skin of the medial heel. The medial plantar nerve supplies the flexor hallucis brevis, abductor hallucis, flexor digitorum brevis, and 1st lumbrical. It carries sensation from medial 2/3 of the plantar foot. The lateral plantar nerve supplies all other plantar muscles, including 2nd-4th lumbricals and all interossei, plus sensation from lateral 1/3 of mid and forefoot.*

LONGITUDINAL US: ANTERIOR ANKLE

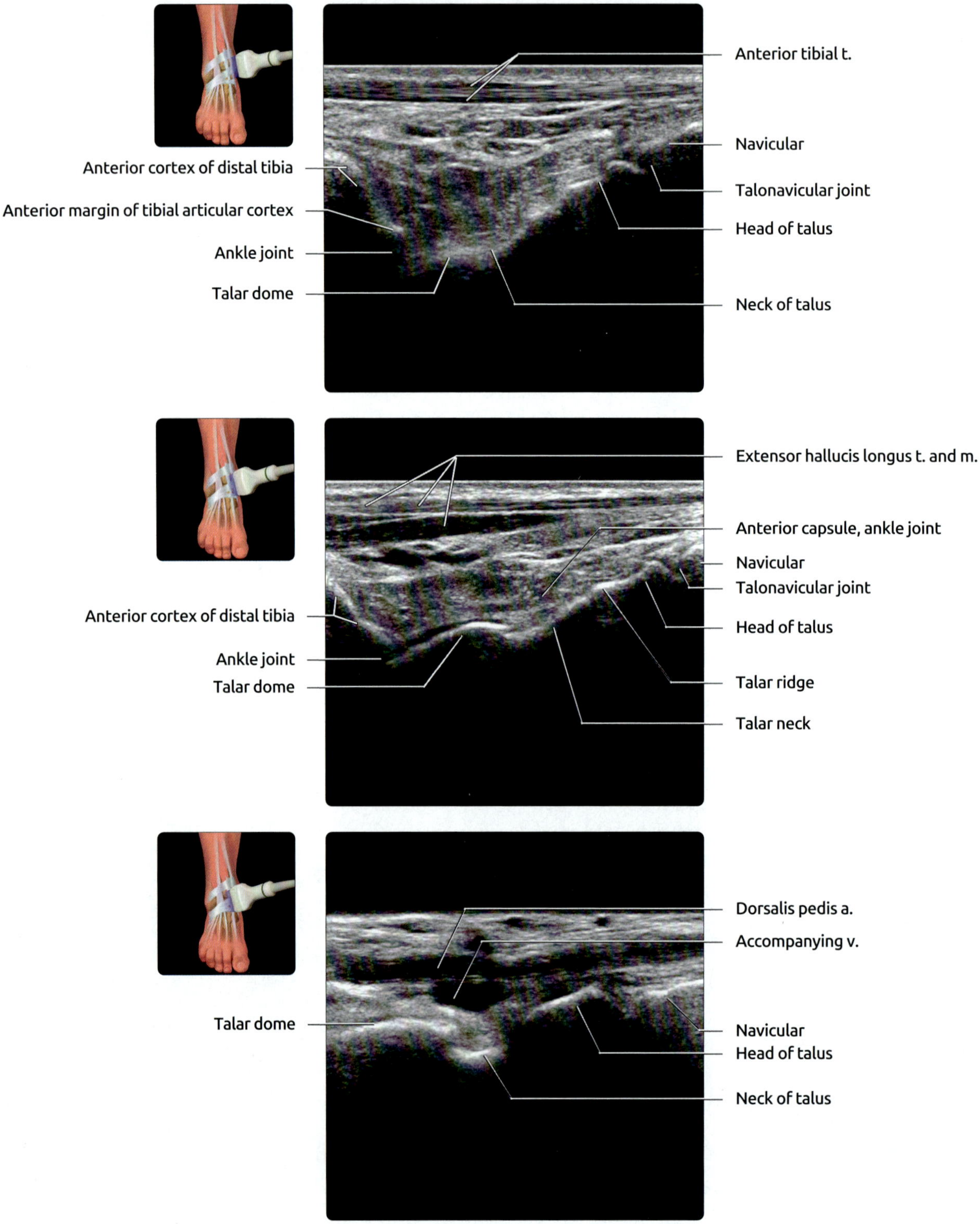

(Top) *Longitudinal scan of the anterior aspect of the ankle shows the course of the anterior tibial tendon. A thin hypoechoic synovial layer can be seen enveloping the tendon. Note that the distal tibial cortex curves posteriorly from the metaphysis to the articular surface.* **(Middle)** *Slightly more laterally, this sagittal scan shows the extensor hallucis longus tendon and muscle. The talar ridge is the site of insertion of the anterior joint capsule.* **(Bottom)** *Further laterally, the dorsalis pedis artery and the accompanying vein(s) come into view. At this point, the subcutaneous tissue is thinnest, a result of the transverse arch of the midfoot with the apex roughly coinciding with the site of this artery. This creates a shallow bony backing for palpating the artery.*

TRANSVERSE US: ANTERIOR ANKLE

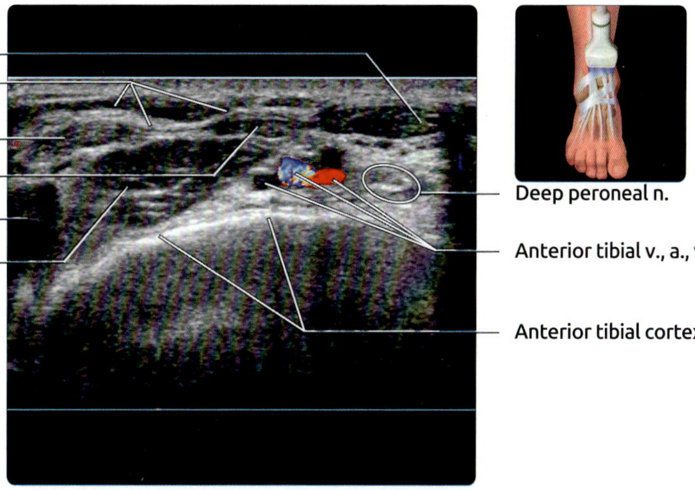

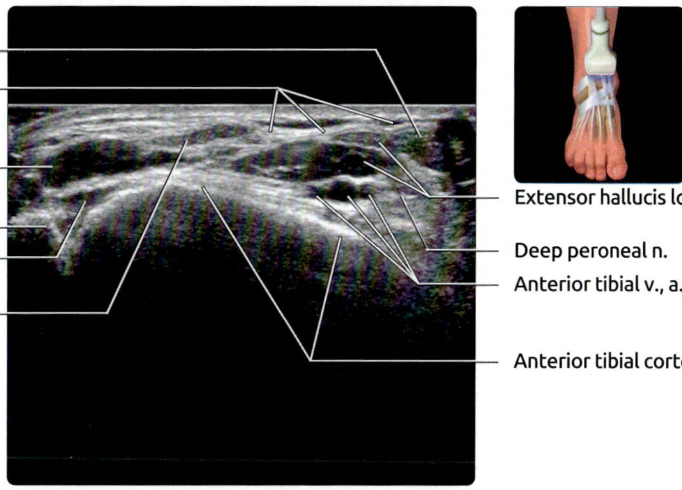

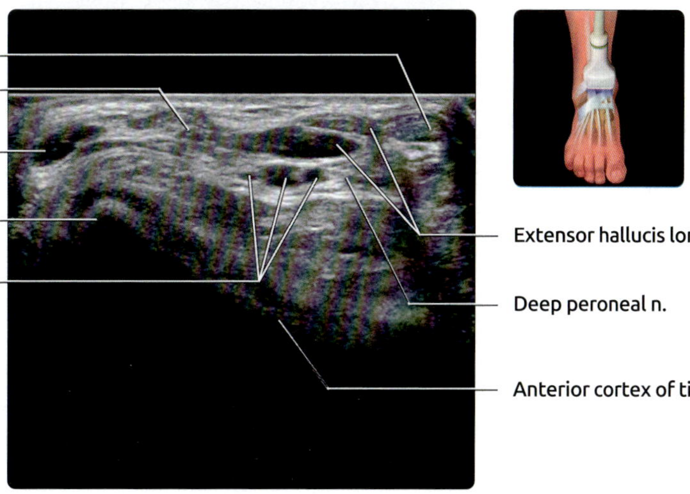

(Top) *Anterior transverse color Doppler scan above level of the ankle joint is shown. The basic relationship of the main structures of the anterior ankle hold true here and down through the ankle joint. From medial to lateral, the structures are: Anterior tibial, extensor hallucis longus, nerve and vessels, and extensor digitorum longus (mnemonic: Tom, Harry, and Dick).* **(Middle)** *Transverse scan of the ankle joint at the level of the anterior tibiofibular ligament is shown. The anterior tibiofibular ligament, like most ankle ligaments, runs an oblique course and, therefore, may appear irregular or interrupted on a straight axial scan. This can be corrected by scanning obliquely along the long axis of the ligament.* **(Bottom)** *Transverse scan more inferiorly shows the deep peroneal nerve medial to the dorsalis pedis vessels and deep to the extensor hallucis longus tendon.*

LONGITUDINAL US: POSTERIOR ANKLE

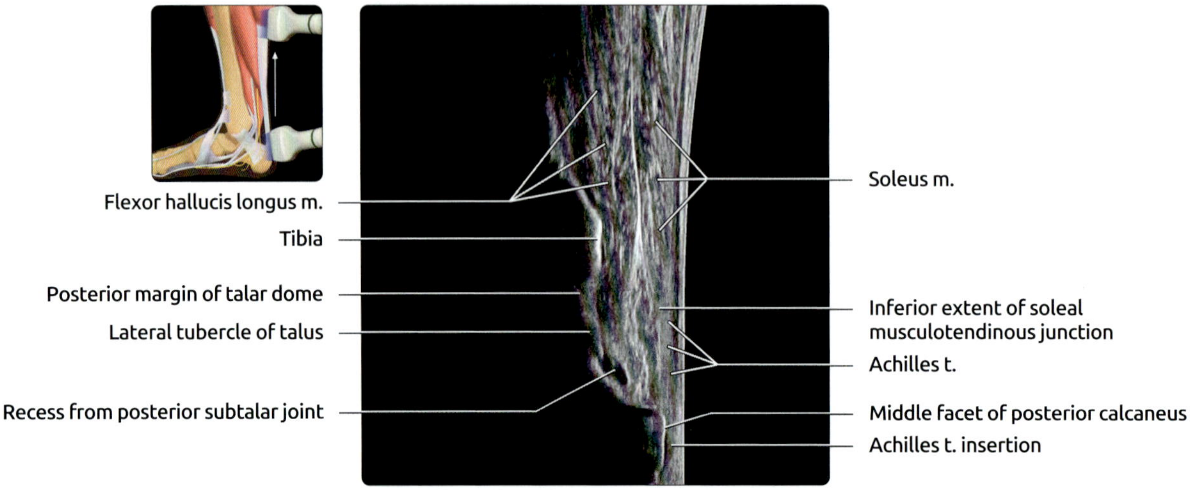

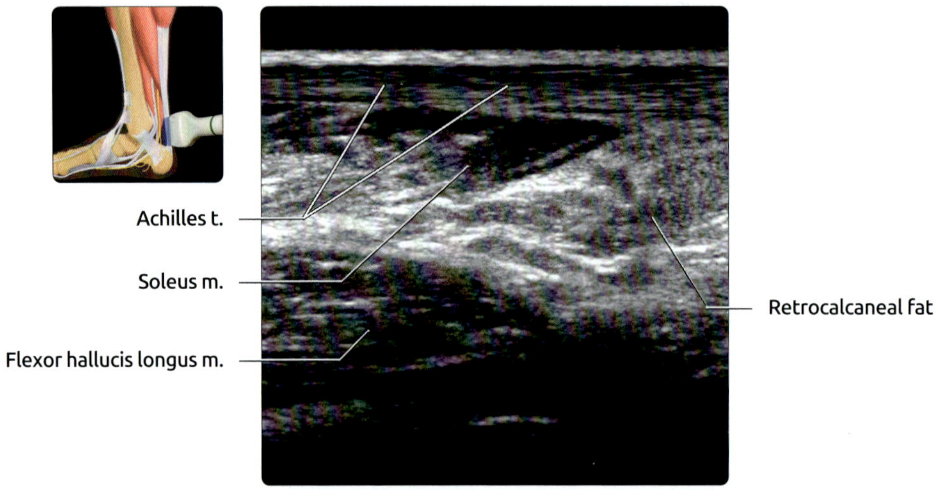

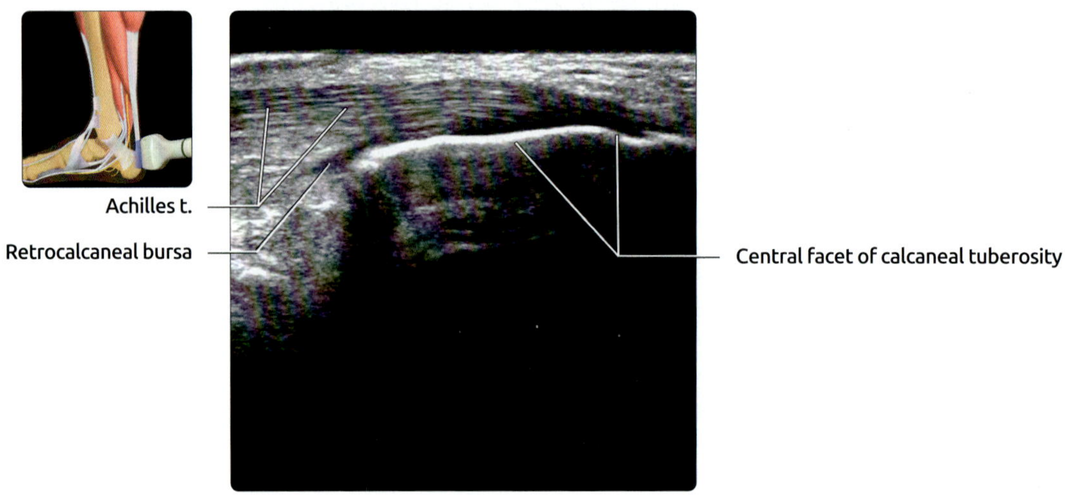

(Top) *Sagittal panoramic view shows the posterior ankle. The dominant structure in the posterior ankle is the Achilles tendon, the largest tendon in the body. The ankle should be in dorsiflexion to tighten this tendon during examination so that the organization of its fibers and continuity can be assessed. Deep to the Achilles tendon is the flexor hallucis longus muscle.* **(Middle)** *Sagittal scan of the lower posterior leg shows the musculotendinous junction between the soleus muscle and the Achilles tendon. These structures join at an angle with a crisp border.* **(Bottom)** *Sagittal scan more distally shows the insertion of the Achilles tendon onto the middle facet of the posterior calcaneal surface. The retrocalcaneal bursa separates the Achilles tendon from the superior facet of the posterior calcaneal surface. This bursa usually contains a tiny amount of fluid detectable on ultrasound.*

TRANSVERSE US: ACHILLES TENDON

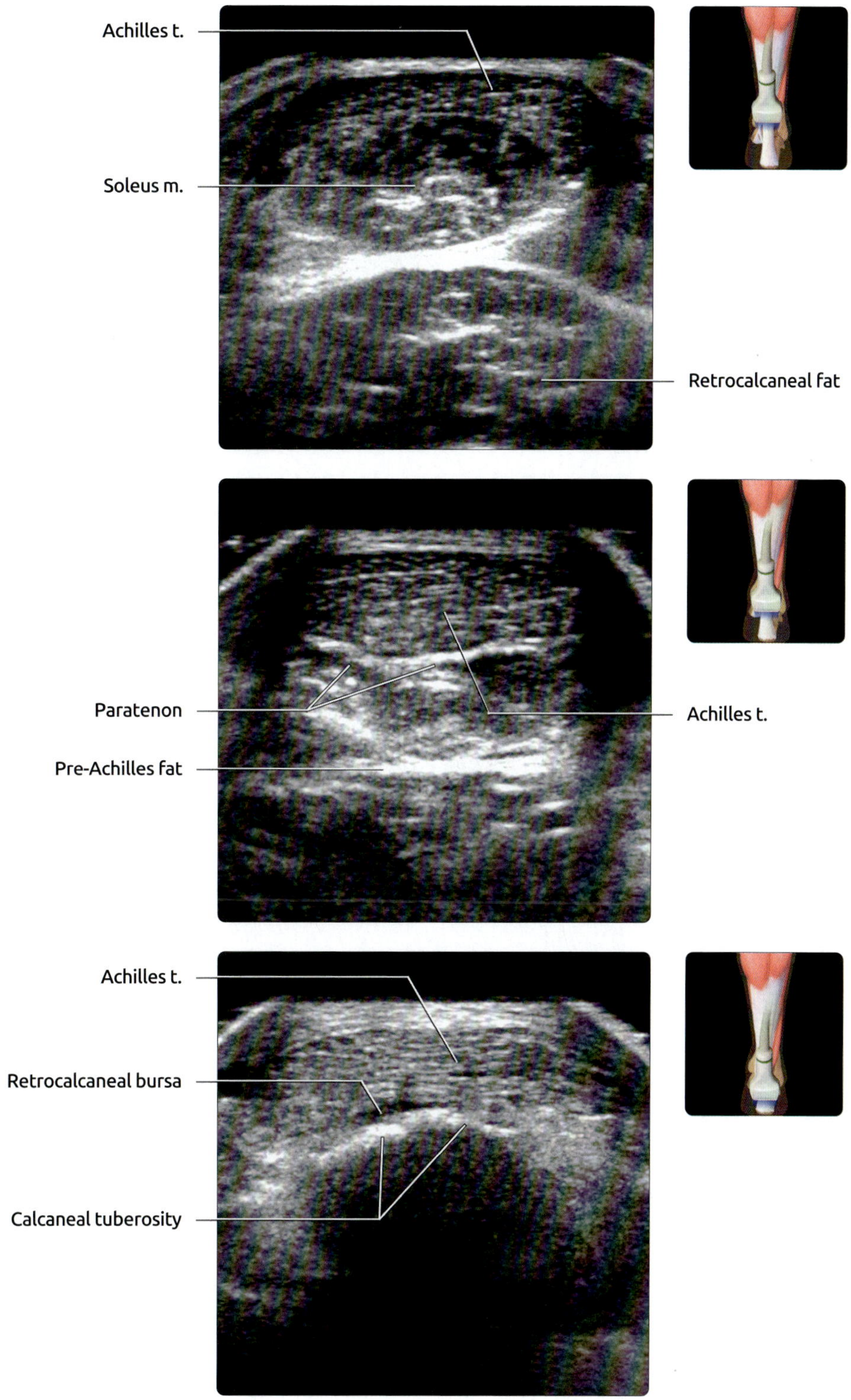

(Top) *Series of transverse scans through the Achilles tendon is shown. At a superior level, the soleus muscle can be seen deep to the Achilles tendon. The Achilles tendon begins superiorly as a continuation of the gastrocnemius aponeurosis, which then joins with the soleus tendon to form the Achilles tendon.* **(Middle)** *Transverse scan shows the Achilles tendon at its midportion. The tendon now assumes an oval shape. The fibrils within the tendon produce a coarsely dotted appearance. Focal hypoechogenicity or change in shape of this tendon should suggest tear/rupture or tendinosis. The tendon does not have a sheath, and is surrounded by loose tissue called a paratenon. Pre-Achilles fat, also called Kager's fat, separates the tendon from the deep flexors of the foot.* **(Bottom)** *At a lower level before its insertion onto the calcaneal tuberosity, the Achilles tendon becomes flattened. A small amount of fluid is frequently seen in the retrocalcaneal bursa deep to the tendon.*

US: POSTEROMEDIAL ANKLE

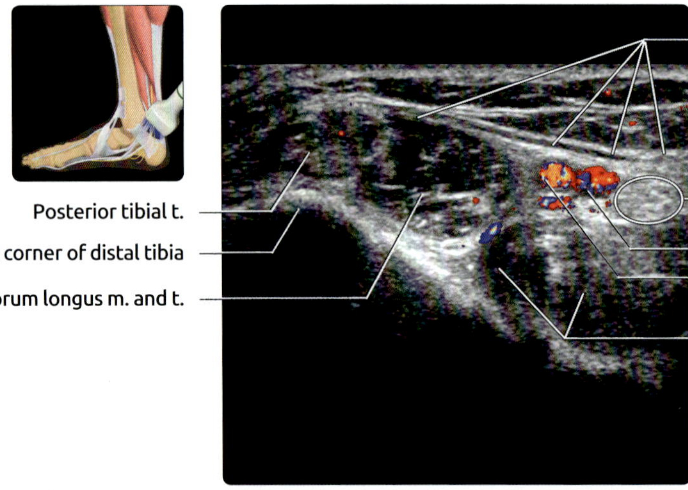

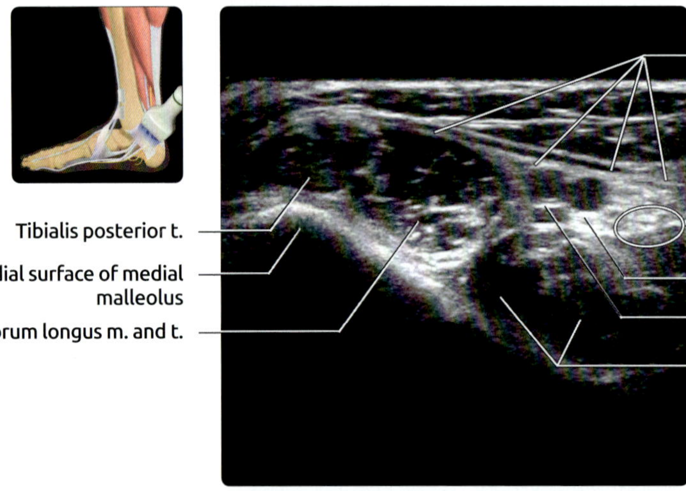

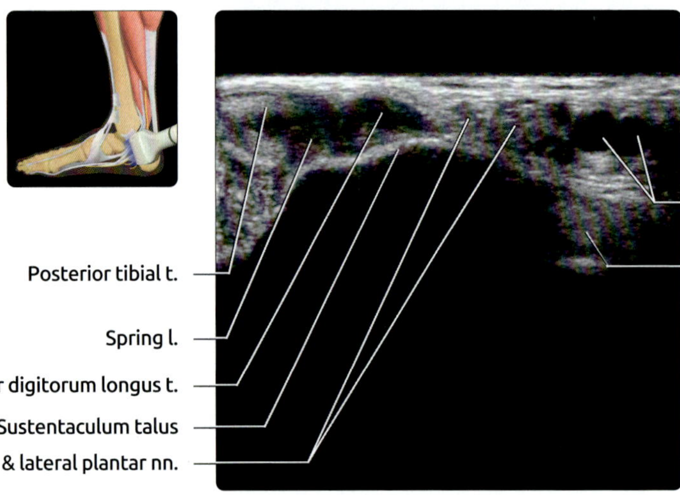

(Top) *Transverse color Doppler scan shows the posterior aspect of the distal tibia just above the medial malleolus. This area is held down by the flexor retinaculum and termed the tarsal tunnel. Within this tunnel are the tibialis posterior, flexor digitorum longus, posterior tibial artery, vein, nerve, and flexor hallucis longus (mnemonic: Tom, Dick, and a very nervous Harry).* **(Middle)** *Corresponding grayscale transverse scan just above the medial malleolus is shown. Image is less grainy without simultaneous color Doppler interrogation, and the nerve fibers (hypoechoic dots) give the typical neural signature.* **(Bottom)** *More inferiorly, this oblique coronal scan through the sustentaculum tali of the calcaneus shows that the mnemonic of Tom, Dick, and Harry still holds (tibialis posterior superior to flexor digitorum longus and flexor hallucis longus). The flexor hallucis longus tendon now runs in a groove inferior to the sustentaculum tali.*

CORONAL US: MEDIAL ANKLE

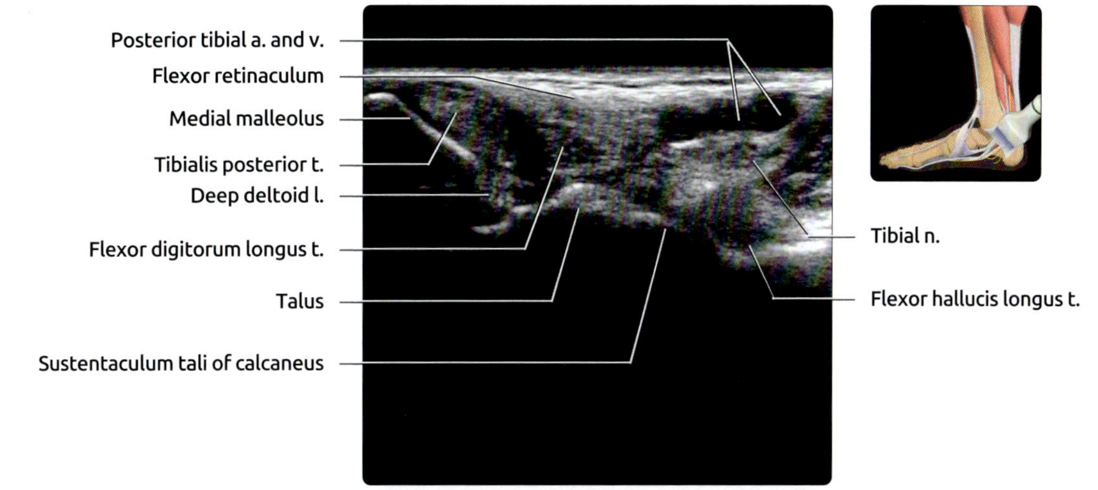

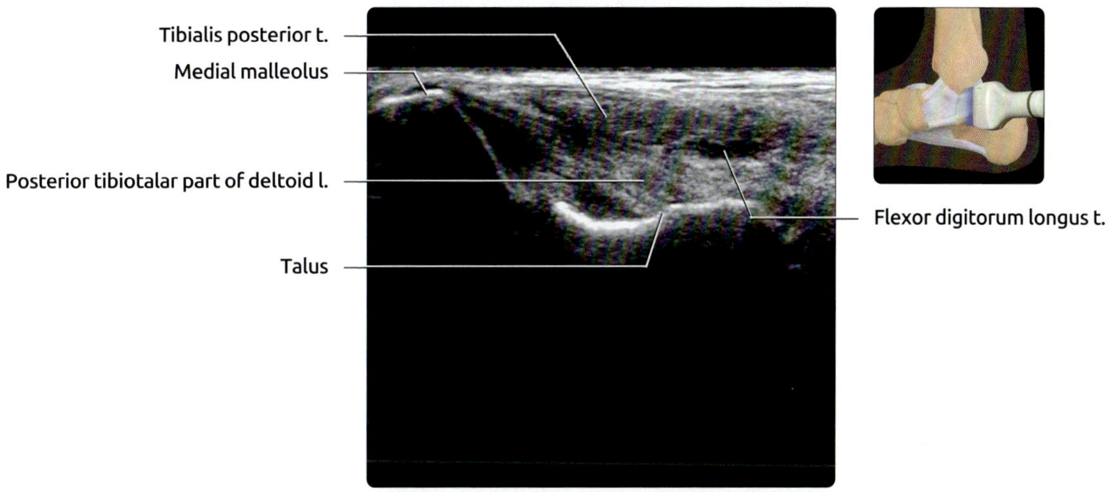

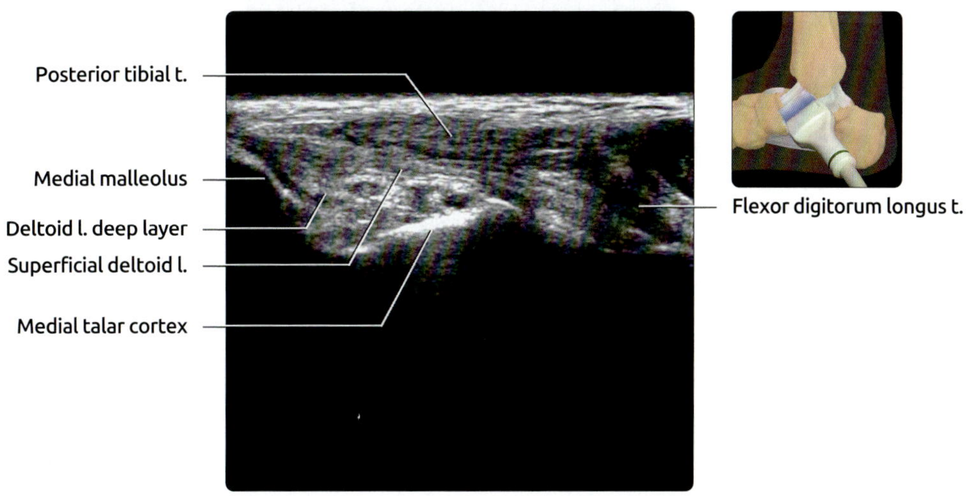

(Top) *Coronal scan through the posterior portion of the tarsal tunnel is shown. All structures within the tunnel curve around the medial malleolus to run forward to the midfoot. The posterior tibial tendon runs on the surface of the deltoid ligament, flexor digitorum longus on the talus, and flexor hallucis longus on the calcaneus under the sustentaculum tali.* **(Middle)** *Coronal scan slightly anterior to the prior image is seen through the posterior (posterior tibiotalar) portion of deltoid ligament, which runs from the medial malleolus to the talus. The tibialis posterior and flexor digitorum longus tendons run superficial to this ligament.* **(Bottom)** *Coronal scan is seen anterior to the prior image. The superficial layer (tibiospring) runs from the malleolus to the spring ligament, the deep component to the talus. Posterior tibial tendon is seen obliquely on this image as it courses both anteriorly and inferiorly toward its insertion on the inferomedial margin of the navicular.*

TRANSVERSE US: MEDIAL ANKLE

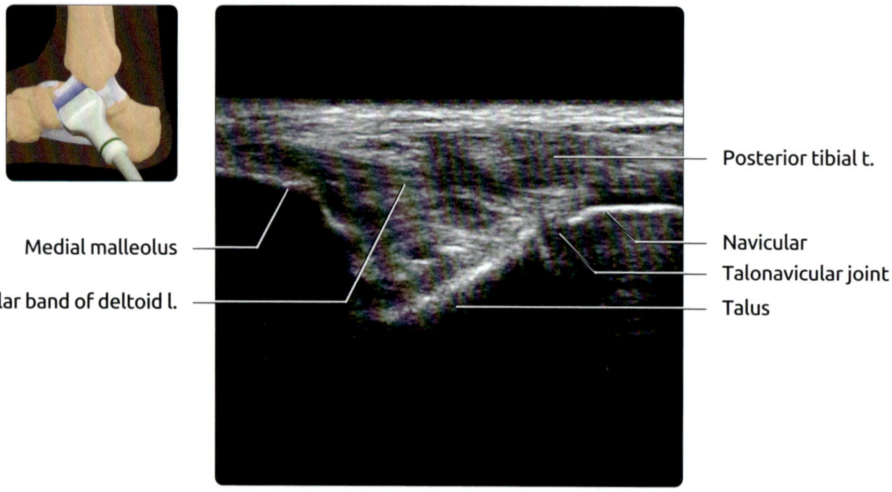

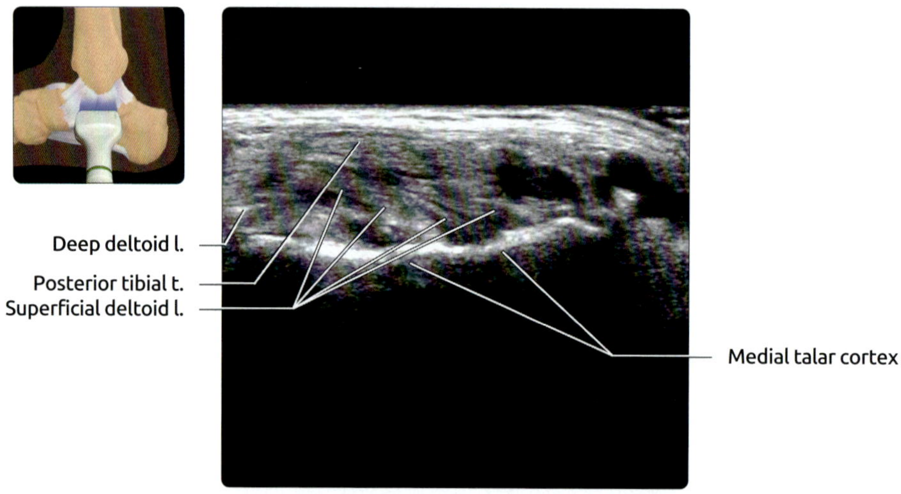

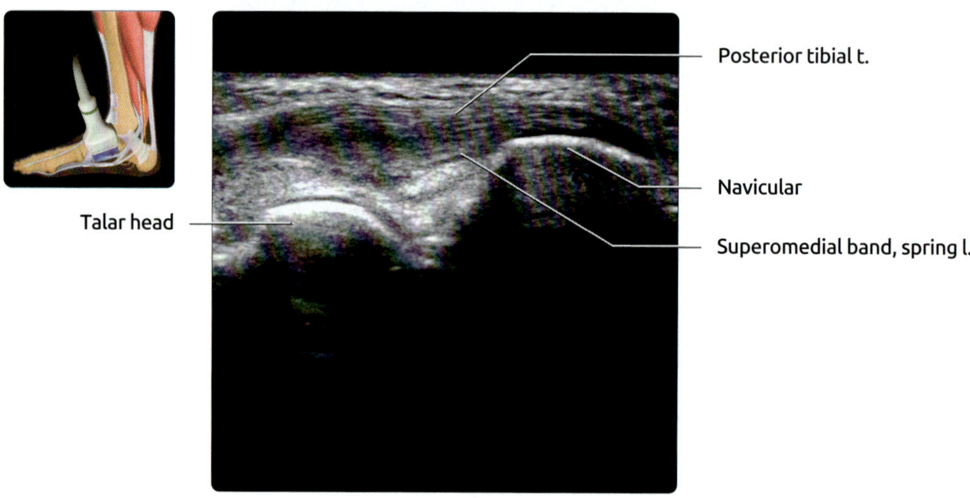

(Top) *Transverse scan is seen through the anterior portion of deltoid ligament; a superficial layer (talonavicular) runs from the malleolus to the navicular.* **(Middle)** *Transverse scan through medial wall of the talus shows deep and superficial components of the deltoid ligament. The bands of the superficial deltoid ligament are named for their bony attachments and are best distinguished by following them on a dynamic ultrasound. The posterior tibial tendon runs superficial to this ligament.* **(Bottom)** *Transverse scan shows the long axis of the tibialis posterior tendon inserting onto the median eminence of the navicular. Deep to the tendon is the superomedial band of the spring ligament, which merges slightly more dorsally with the tibionavicular band of the deltoid ligament.*

TRANSVERSE US: LATERAL ANKLE

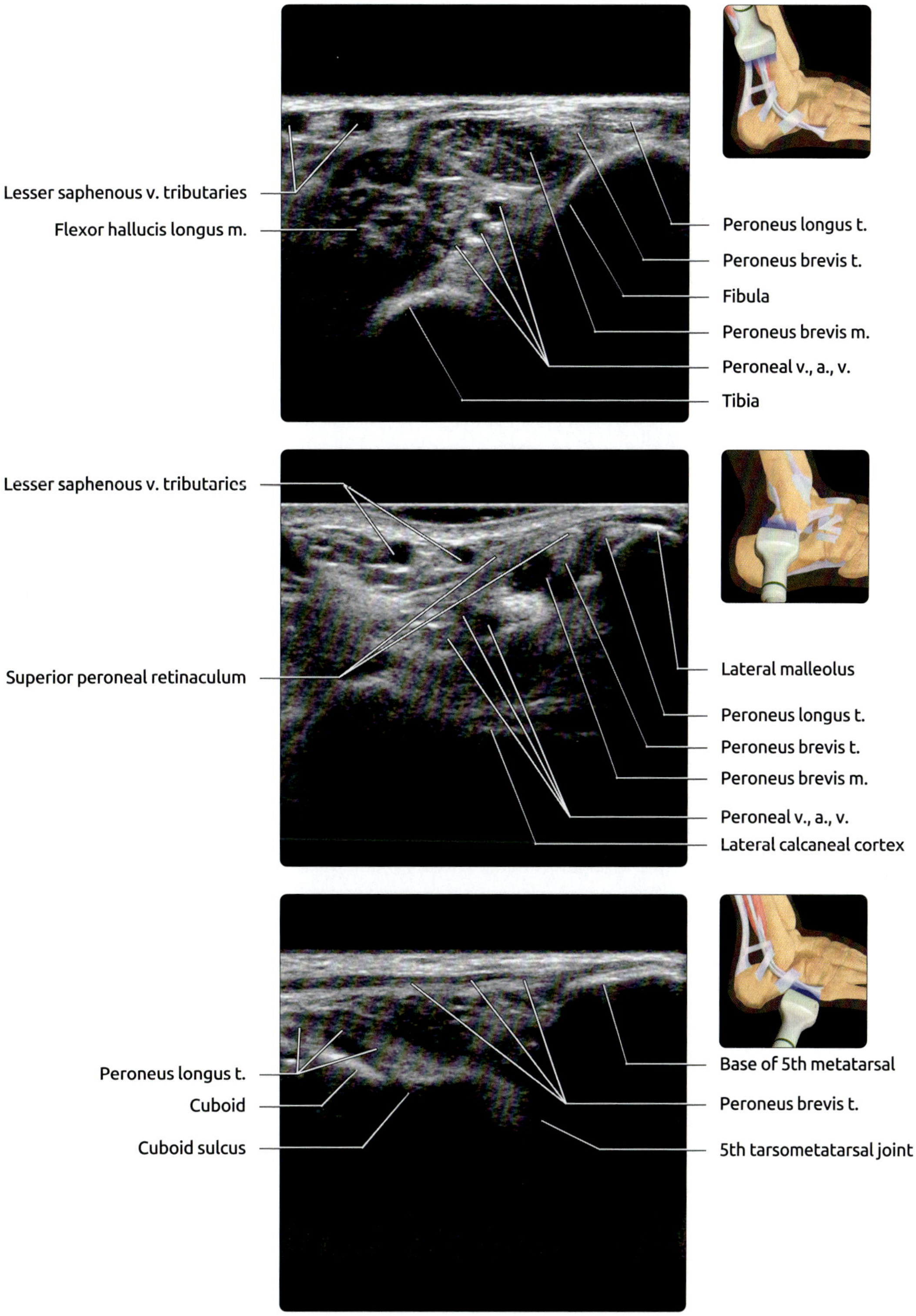

(Top) *Transverse scan of the posterior aspect of the distal fibula shows the distal peroneal muscles. The peroneus longus tendon runs superficial to the peroneus brevis. The peroneus brevis still maintains a muscular portion, which lies posterior to the tendon and continues to just above the tip of the lateral malleolus.* **(Middle)** *Transverse scan is shown at the level just above the tip of the lateral malleolus. The peroneal tendons are now held down by the superior peroneal retinaculum, which prevents tendon subluxation (bowstringing). There is still a residual component of the peroneus brevis muscle.* **(Bottom)** *Transverse scan of the lateral aspect of the foot shows insertion of the peroneus brevis tendon onto the base of the 5th metatarsal bone. Also shown here is the peroneus longus tendon turning under the cuboid sulcus, after which it extends to its attachments on the 1st and 2nd metatarsal bases and medial cuneiform.*

US: PERONEAL TENDONS

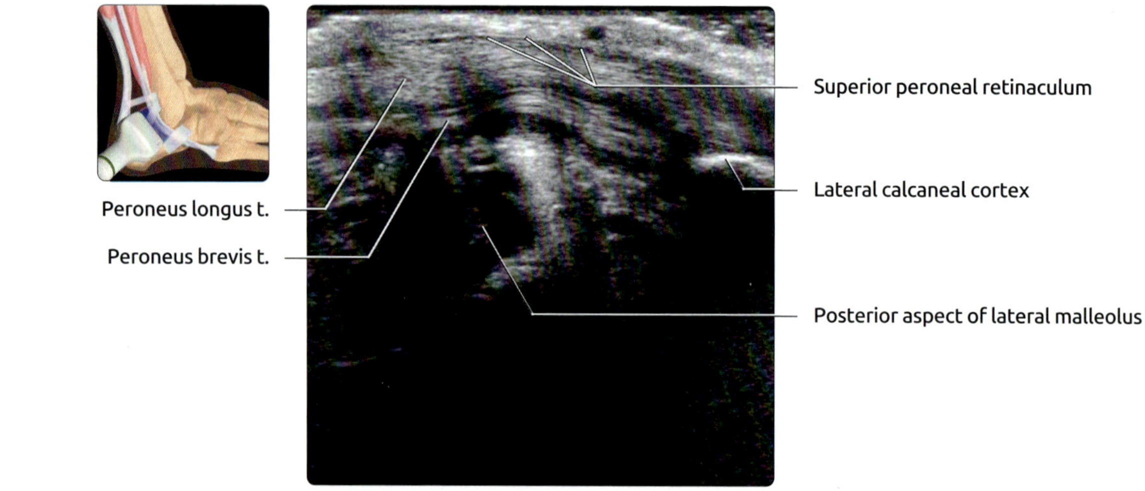

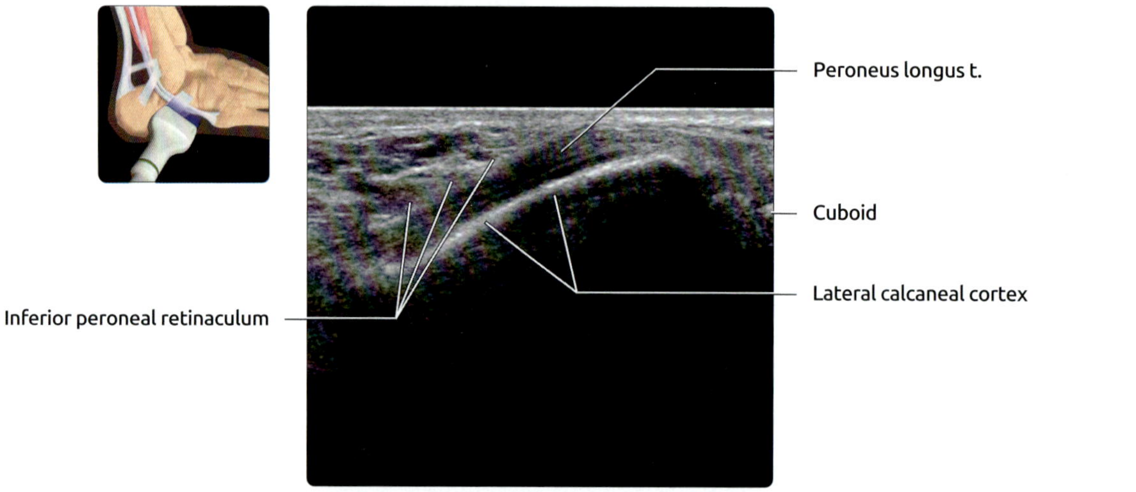

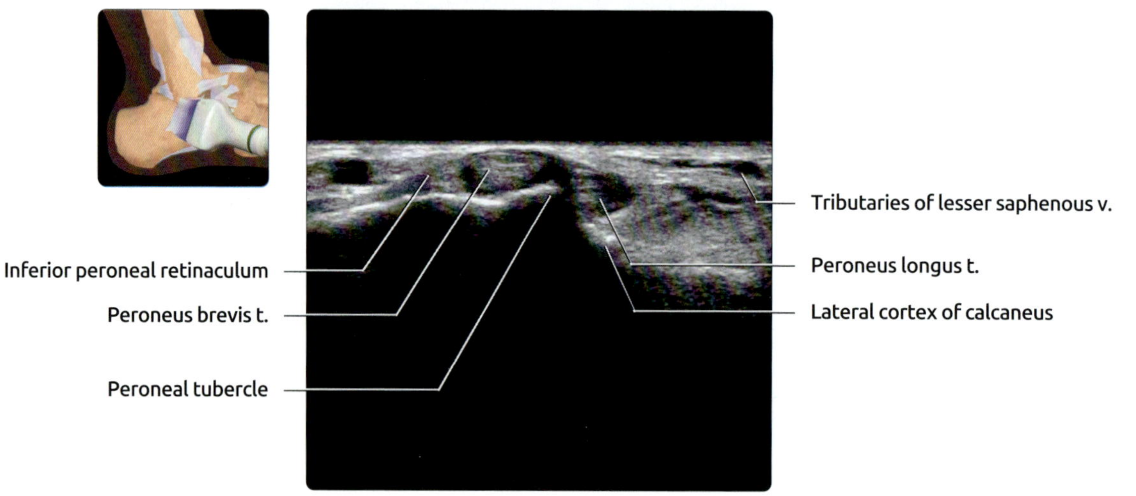

(Top) *Oblique coronal scan of the posterior aspect of the lateral malleolus shows the longitudinal course of the peroneal tendons. Both tendons run inferior onto the lateral surface of the calcaneus, passing over the calcaneal fibular ligament on the way.* **(Middle)** *Oblique transverse scan shows the lateral aspect of the calcaneus along the course of the peroneus longus tendon. The peroneus longus lies inferior to the peroneus brevis in the foot.* **(Bottom)** *Coronal scan of the lateral surface of the calcaneus shows the peroneal tendons held down by the inferior peroneal retinaculum but partially separated by peroneal tubercle, a protuberance on the lateral calcaneal cortex. A large peroneal tubercle can result in impingement on the peroneal tendons.*

US: LATERAL COLLATERAL LIGAMENT

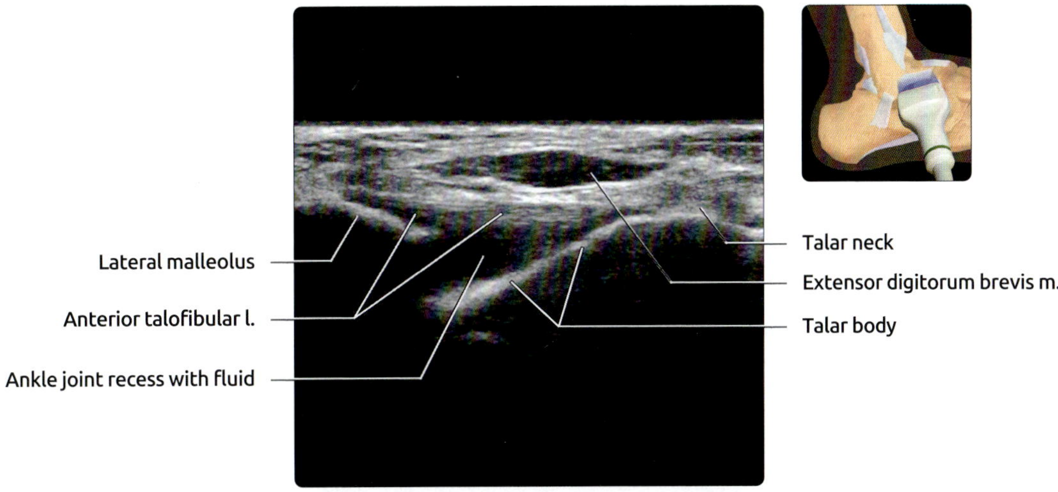

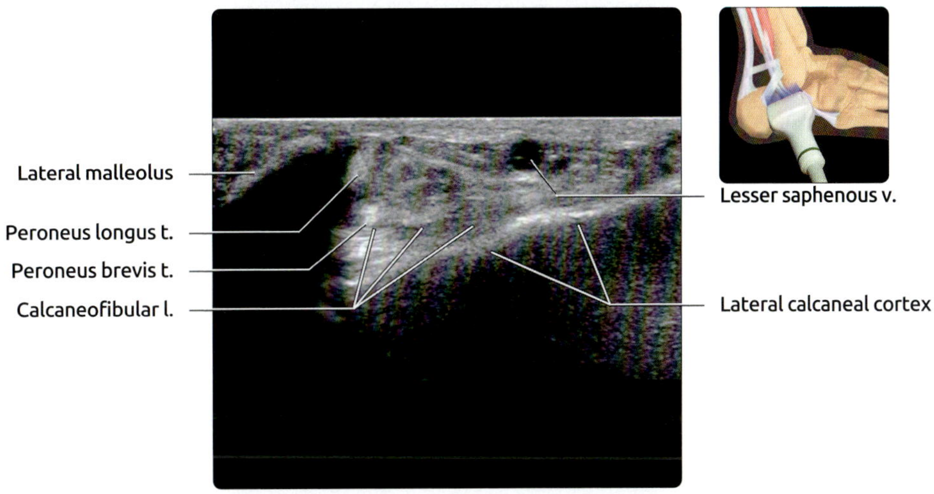

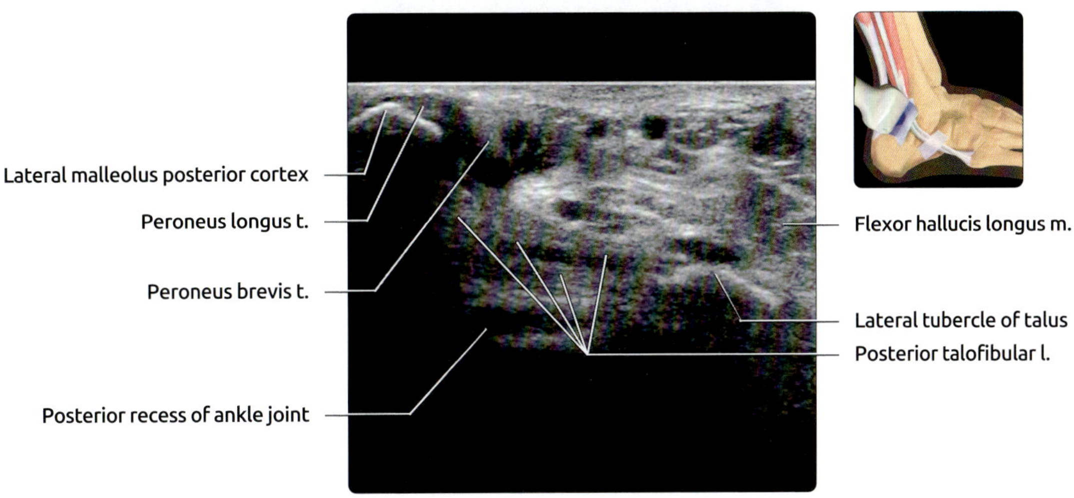

(Top) *Oblique transverse scan shows the lateral ankle along the course of the anterior talofibular ligament. An anterolateral ankle joint recess exists deep to this ligament, making it a good area to look for small effusions. The lateral fibers of the extensor digitorum brevis muscle run on the surface of this ligament.* **(Middle)** *Oblique coronal scan along the long axis of the calcaneofibular ligament is shown. The ligament forms the floor of the peroneal tendon sheath, and fluid can be seen extending from the joint around the peroneal tendons when the ligament is torn.* **(Bottom)** *Transverse scan of the posterior aspect of the lateral malleolus shows the posterior talofibular ligament. Deep to this ligament is the posterior recess of the ankle joint.*

SECTION 4

Foot

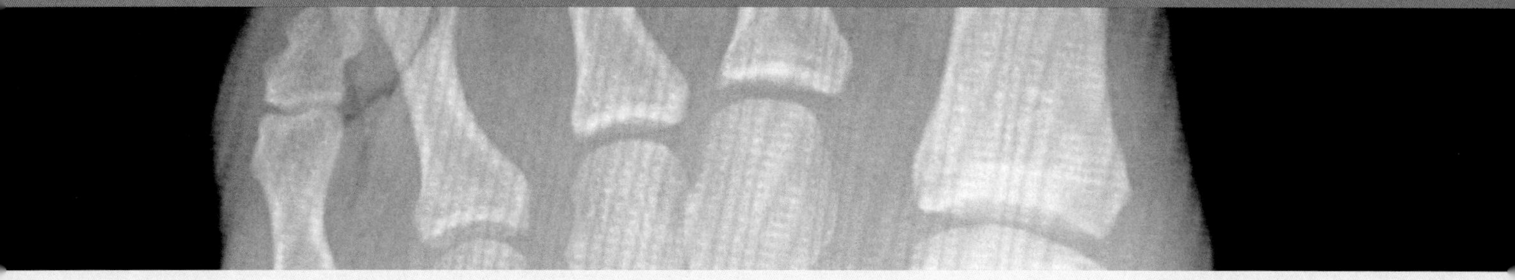

TERMINOLOGY

Definitions

- **3 major divisions from proximal to distal**
  - **Hindfoot**: Calcaneus and talus
  - **Midfoot**: Navicular, cuneiforms, and cuboid
  - **Forefoot**: Metatarsals and phalanges
- **2 columns**
  - **Medial column**: Talus, navicular, cuneiforms 1-3, digits 1-3
  - **Lateral column**: Calcaneus, cuboid, digits 4 and 5

IMAGING ANATOMY

Arches of Foot

- Foot is arched from posterior to anterior and from medial to lateral
- **Transverse arch of foot**
  - Triangular cuneiform bones and metatarsal bases form arch
  - Major supporting structures of transverse arch
    - Spring ligament, Lisfranc ligament, intermetatarsal and intertarsal ligaments
- **Longitudinal arch of foot**
  - From posterior process calcaneus to metatarsal heads, apex in midfoot
  - Medial side is higher than lateral
  - Metatarsals slant downward from apex of arch to metatarsophalangeal (MTP) joint
    - This is called inclination angle
    - Inclination angle decreases from 20° at 1st to 5° at 5th metatarsal
  - Major supporting structures of longitudinal arch: Plantar fascia, long and short plantar ligaments, spring ligament, posterior tibial tendon, peroneus longus tendon

Distribution of Weight-Bearing

- 50% of weight borne on subtalar joint and calcaneus
- Remainder transmitted to MTP joints, greatest weight on 1st toe

Bony Anatomy

- **Cuboid bone**
  - Roughly cuboidal shape
  - 1 ossification center: Ossifies between 9th fetal month and 6 months age
  - Articulates with calcaneus, navicular, 3rd cuneiform, 4th and 5th metatarsals, rarely head of talus
    - Dorsal ligaments (calcaneocuboid, cubonavicular, cuneocuboid, cubometatarsal) strengthen each of these articulations
    - Short and long plantar ligaments attach to plantar surface
  - Sulcus at lateral margin, under which passes peroneus longus tendon
- **Navicular bone**
  - Curved shape, concave proximally and convex distally
  - 1 ossification center: Ossifies in 3rd year of life
  - Articulates with talus, cuboid, cuneiforms
    - Single facet proximally for articulation with head of talus
    - 3 facets distally for cuneiform articulations
    - 1 facet laterally for articulation with cuboid
    - Connected to anterior process of calcaneus by bifurcate ligament
    - Connected to sustentaculum tali by spring ligament
  - Large median eminence (tuberosity) for attachment of posterior tibial tendon is located plantar to main body of navicular
- **Cuneiform bones**
  - Wedge-shaped, with base of wedge at dorsal surface of 2nd and 3rd cuneiforms, dorsomedial surface 1st cuneiform
  - 1st cuneiform (medial cuneiform)
    - Articulates with navicular, 2nd cuneiform, 1st metatarsal
    - 1 or 2 ossification centers: Ossify in 2nd year of life
  - 2nd cuneiform (middle or intermediate cuneiform)
    - Articulates with navicular, 1st and 3rd cuneiforms, 2nd metatarsal
    - 1 ossification center: Ossifies in 3rd year of life
  - 3rd cuneiform (lateral cuneiform)
    - Articulates with navicular, 2nd cuneiform, cuboid, 3rd metatarsal
- **Metatarsal bones**
  - 2 ossification centers: Shaft ossifies in 9th prenatal week, epiphysis in 3rd-4th years of life
    - 1st metatarsal has epiphysis at proximal end, others at distal end
  - 2nd-5th metatarsals have articulations at bases with adjacent metatarsals
  - 1st metatarsal
    - Articulates with 1st cuneiform, 1st proximal phalanx, sesamoids of metatarsal head
    - Variable articulation with 2nd metatarsal base
  - 2nd-3rd metatarsals
    - Articulate with respective cuneiforms and proximal phalanges
    - 2nd metatarsal base recessed relative to 1st and usually 3rd
  - 4th-5th metatarsals
    - Articulate with cuboid and respective proximal phalanges
    - Styloid process of 5th metatarsal extends lateral to cuboid
- **Phalanges**
  - 1st toe is biphalangeal, other toes are triphalangeal
  - 5th toe sometimes has failure of segmentation of middle and distal phalanges
  - 2 ossification centers: Shaft ossifies in 9th-15th prenatal weeks, epiphysis during 2nd-8th years

Musculature

- **Plantar muscles**: 4 layers
  - 1st layer: Abductor hallucis, flexor digitorum brevis, abductor digiti minimi, peroneus brevis
  - 2nd layer: Quadratus plantae (flexor accessorius), flexor digitorum and hallucis longus, lumbricals
  - 3rd layer: Flexor hallucis brevis, adductor hallucis, flexor digiti minimi brevis, tibialis posterior
  - 4th layer: Plantar interossei (3), dorsal interossei (4)
  - Peroneus longus courses across all layers, from superficial plantar laterally to deep plantar medially

- **Dorsal muscles**: 2 muscle layers
  - Superficial layer: Tibialis anterior, extensor hallucis longus, extensor digitorum longus, peroneus tertius
  - Deep layer: Extensor hallucis brevis, extensor digitorum brevis
  - In forefoot, long and short extensors run side by side in single layer

Compartments

- **4 plantar compartments** divided by fascial layers
- **Medial plantar compartment**
  - Contains abductor hallucis, flexor hallucis longus, and flexor hallucis brevis
- **Central plantar compartment**
  - Superficial subcompartment: Contains flexor digitorum brevis, distal portion of flexor digitorum longus
  - Intermediary subcompartment: Contains proximal plantar portion of flexor digitorum longus, quadratus plantae, lumbricals
  - Deep subcompartment: Limited to forefoot, contains adductor hallucis
- **Lateral plantar compartment**
  - Contains abductor and flexor digiti minimi
- **Interosseous compartment**
  - Contains plantar and dorsal interosseous muscle
- **Dorsal compartment**
  - Superficial layer: Extrinsic extensor tendon
  - Deep layer: Intrinsic extensor muscle

Major Ligaments

- Plantar fascia (aponeurosis): 3 portions extend from tuberosity of calcaneus to transverse metatarsal ligaments of toes
  - Medial band: Thin structure superficial to abductor hallucis muscle
  - Central band: Thick, strong structure superficial to flexor digitorum brevis
    - Divides into separate bands to each toe; these are linked by transverse bands
    - Distally sends septa superficially into subcutaneous fat and deep to MTP joints
  - Lateral band: Thin structure superficial to abductor digiti minimi
  - Medial and lateral bands sometimes terminate at level of mid metatarsals
- Long plantar ligament: Originates calcaneal tuberosity, inserts cuboid and bases 2nd-4th metatarsals
  - Forms tunnel roof for peroneus longus tendon
- Short plantar (plantar calcaneocuboid) ligament: Deep to long ligament, inserts more proximally on cuboid
- Plantar calcaneocuboid (spring) ligament: Originates sustentaculum tali, inserts plantar aspect navicular
- Bifurcate ligament: Originates anterior process of calcaneus dorsally, inserts navicular and cuboid
- Lisfranc ligament: Originates 1st cuneiform, inserts base 2nd metatarsal
- Intermetatarsal ligaments: Dorsal and plantar ligaments between 2nd-5th metatarsal bases
- Transverse metatarsal ligaments: Superficial and deep ligaments between metatarsal heads

Nerves

- **Tibial nerve** divides into medial calcaneal, medial, and lateral plantar branches at level of tarsal tunnel
  - **Medial calcaneal nerve**: Sensory to skin of heel, medial hindfoot
  - **Medial plantar nerve**
    - Between 1st and 2nd muscle layers, accompanies medial plantar artery
    - Motor branches: Abductor hallucis, flexor digitorum and hallucis brevis, 1st lumbrical
    - Plantar digital nerves to 1st-3rd toes, medial aspect 4th toe
  - **Lateral plantar nerve**: Has deep and superficial divisions
    - Motor branches: Flexor digiti minimi brevis, lumbricals, interossei, adductor hallucis
    - Superficial lateral plantar nerve: Between 1st and 2nd muscle layers
    - Plantar digital nerves to 5th toe, lateral aspect 4th toe
    - Deep lateral plantar nerve: Between 3rd and 4th muscle layers; accompanies lateral plantar artery
- **Deep peroneal nerve**: Dorsum of foot, between tibialis anterior and extensor hallucis longus
  - Motor branch: Extensor digitorum brevis
- **Superficial peroneal nerve**: Divides into medial and lateral branches at dorsum of foot
  - Sensory branches to dorsal foot
- **Sural nerve**: Lateral, superficial branch of tibial nerve
  - Extends along lateral margin of foot
  - Sensory branches to lateral foot

Arteries

- Posterior tibial artery divides into medial and lateral plantar arteries at level of tarsal tunnel
  - Plantar arteries accompany medial and deep lateral plantar nerves
- Peroneal artery accompanies superficial peroneal nerve down anterolateral aspect ankle
  - May join or replace posterior tibial artery
- Anterior tibial artery continues into foot as dorsalis pedis artery, deep to extensor retinaculum
  - Divides into multiple branches in midfoot, forming arcade

Bursae

- Extensor digitorum brevis: Between muscle and 2nd cuneiform and metatarsal bases
- Extensor hallucis longus: Between tendon and 1st cuneiform and metatarsal bases
- Abductor digiti minimi: Between muscle and tuberosity of 5th metatarsal
- MTP joints: Bursa located dorsally, between metatarsal heads, and medial to 1st metatarsal head

Foot Motion

- **Supination**: Elevation of medial arch of foot; inversion + adduction
- **Pronation**: Depression of medial arch of foot; eversion + abduction

GRAPHICS: NERVES & ARTERIES OF FOOT

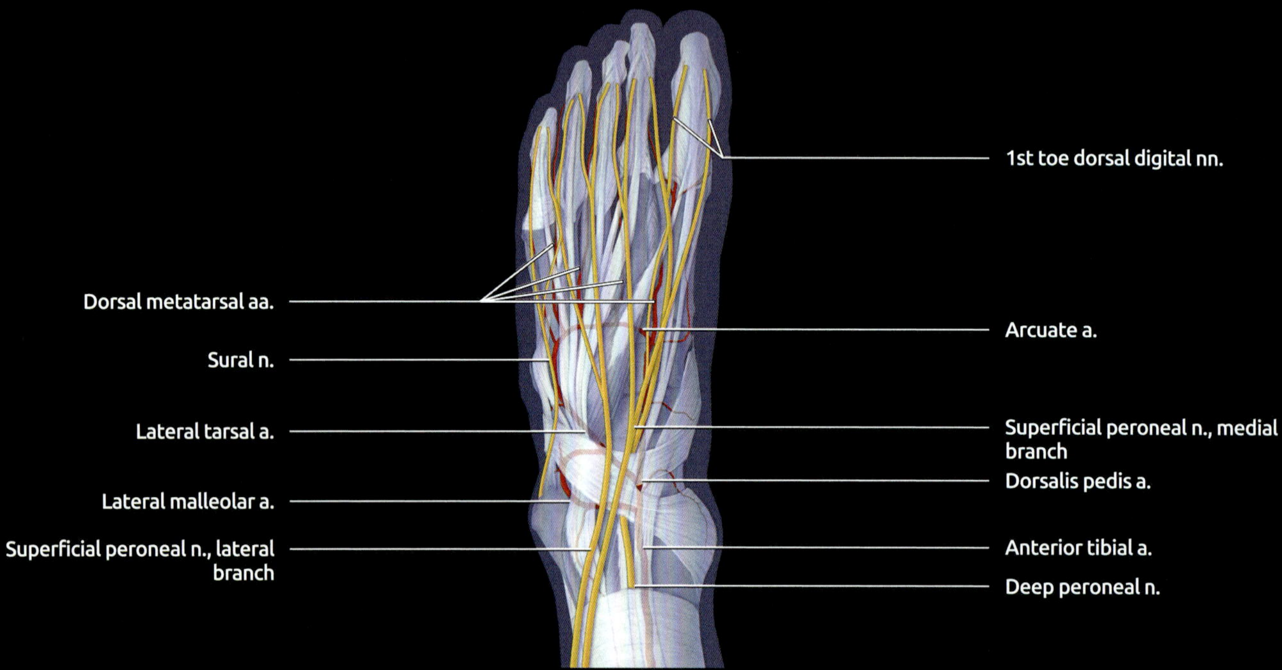

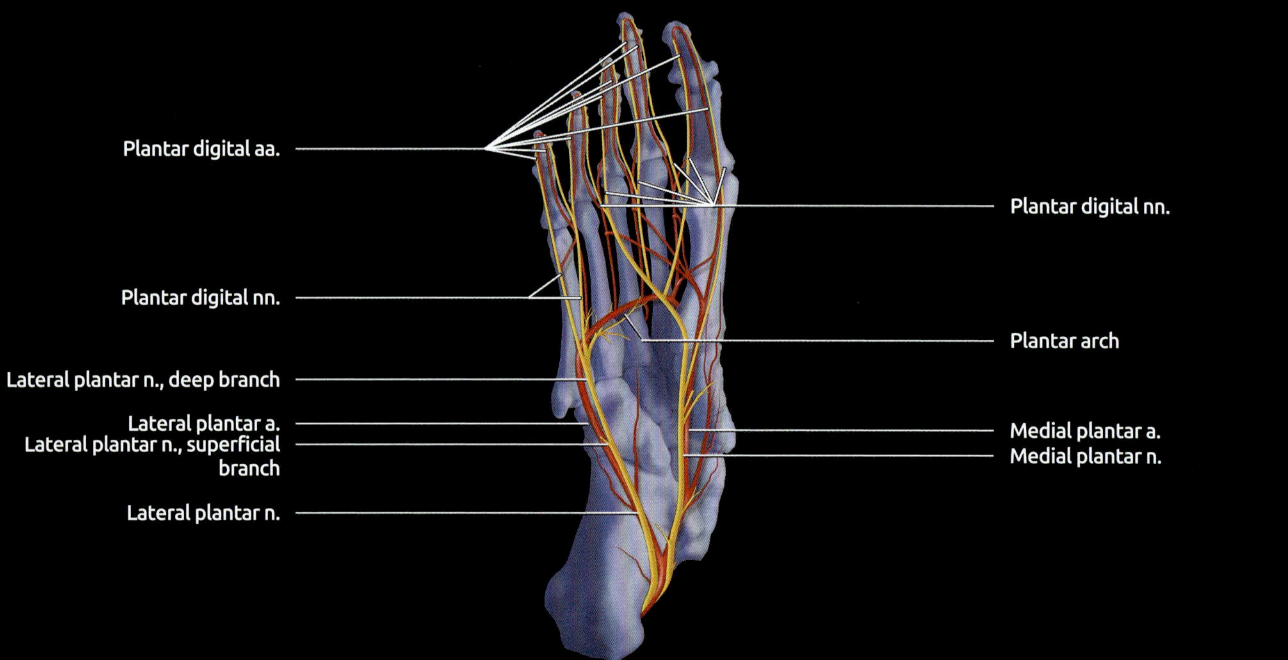

(Top) *Graphic shows arteries and nerves at the dorsal aspect of the foot. The deep peroneal nerve accompanies the anterior tibial artery. The superficial peroneal nerve divides into medial and lateral branches in the distal 1/3 of the leg. The anterior tibial artery is called the dorsalis pedis in foot. It terminates in the arcuate artery, which communicates with the plantar arterial arch and in digital vessels.* **(Bottom)** *Graphic shows arteries and nerves at the plantar aspect of the foot. The posterior tibial nerve and artery divide into medial and lateral plantar branches. These divide further into digital branches to medial and lateral aspects of each toe. The plantar arch sends vessels dorsally, as well as to plantar aspect of toes.*

GRAPHICS: LIGAMENTS OF FOOT

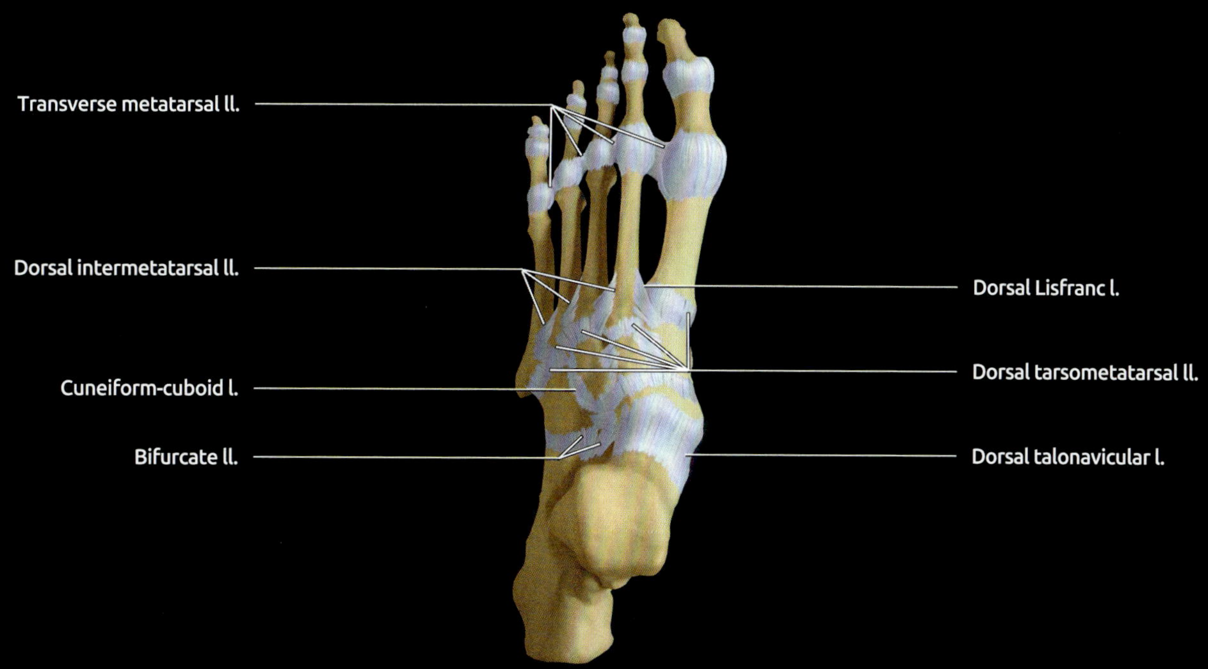

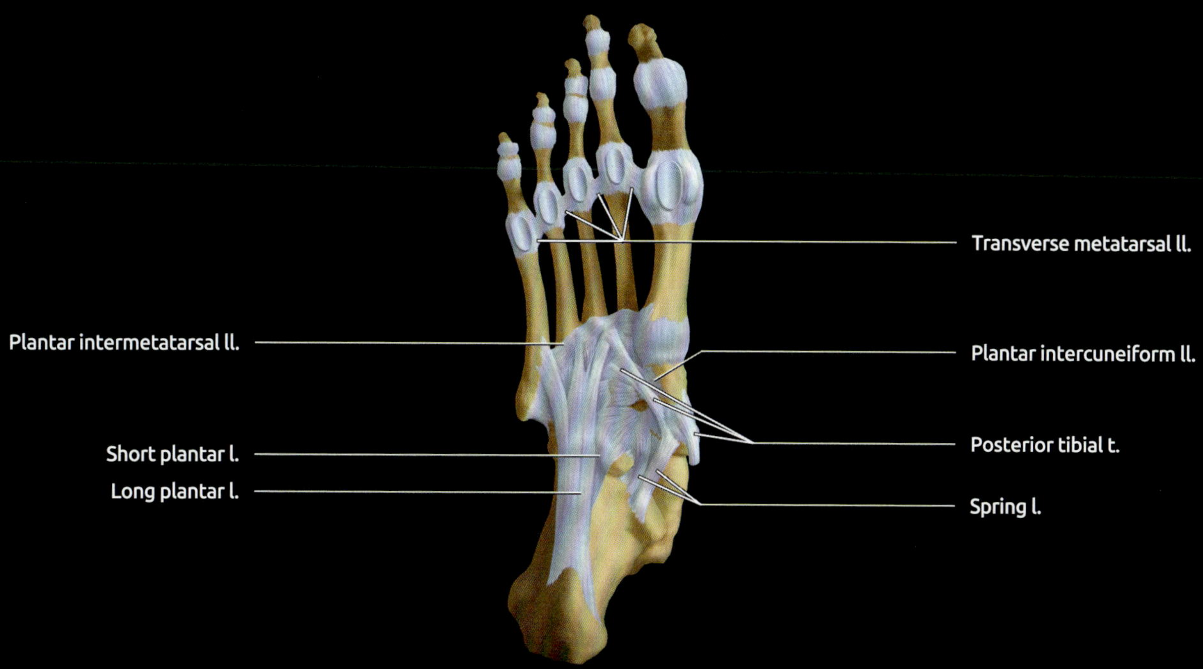

(Top) *Graphic of dorsal ligaments shows dense ligaments between the tarsal bones and between the tarsals and metatarsals. Ligaments are generally named for the bones they bridge. Exceptions are the bifurcate ligament, which extends from the anterior process calcaneus to the cuboid and navicular, and the dorsal Lisfranc ligament, which extends from the 1st cuneiform to 2nd metatarsal.* **(Bottom)** *Graphic of plantar ligaments shows ligaments deep to the plantar fascia, as well as the navicular, cuneiform, and metatarsal insertions of the posterior tibial tendon. The spring ligament, also known as the plantar calcaneonavicular ligament, originates on the sustentaculum tali and anterior calcaneus and inserts on the navicular. Deep intertarsal ligaments are also shown and are named for bones they bridge.*

GRAPHICS: COLUMNS & LONGITUDINAL ARCH

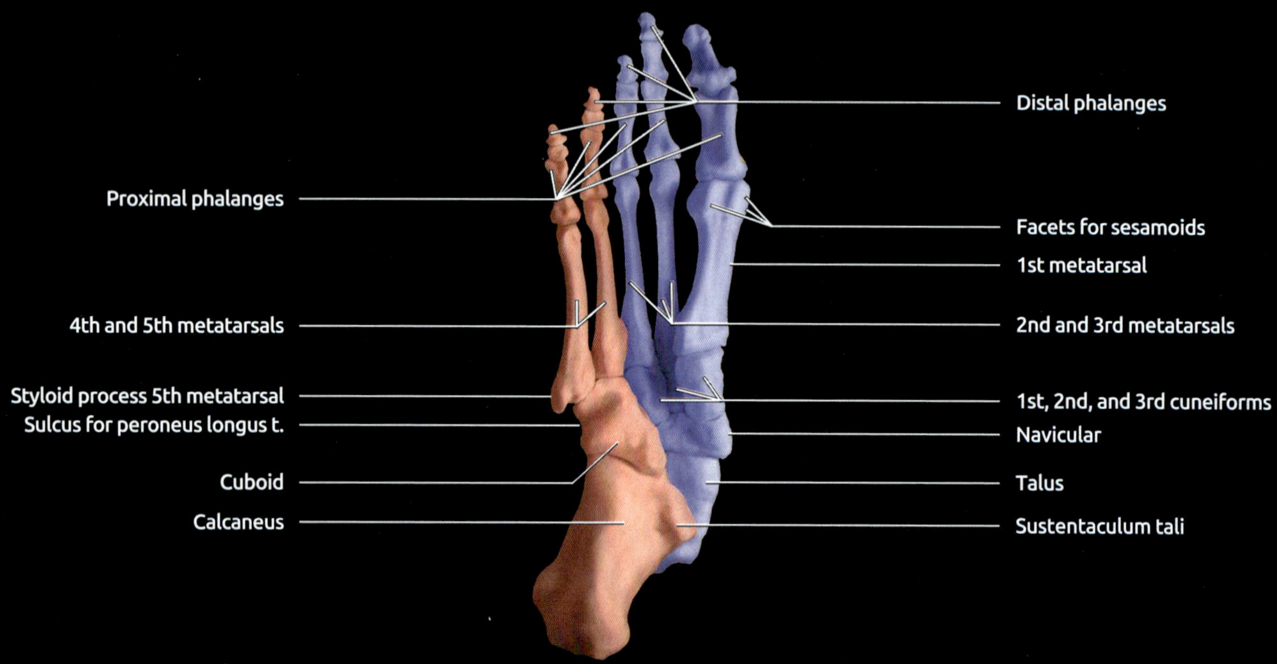

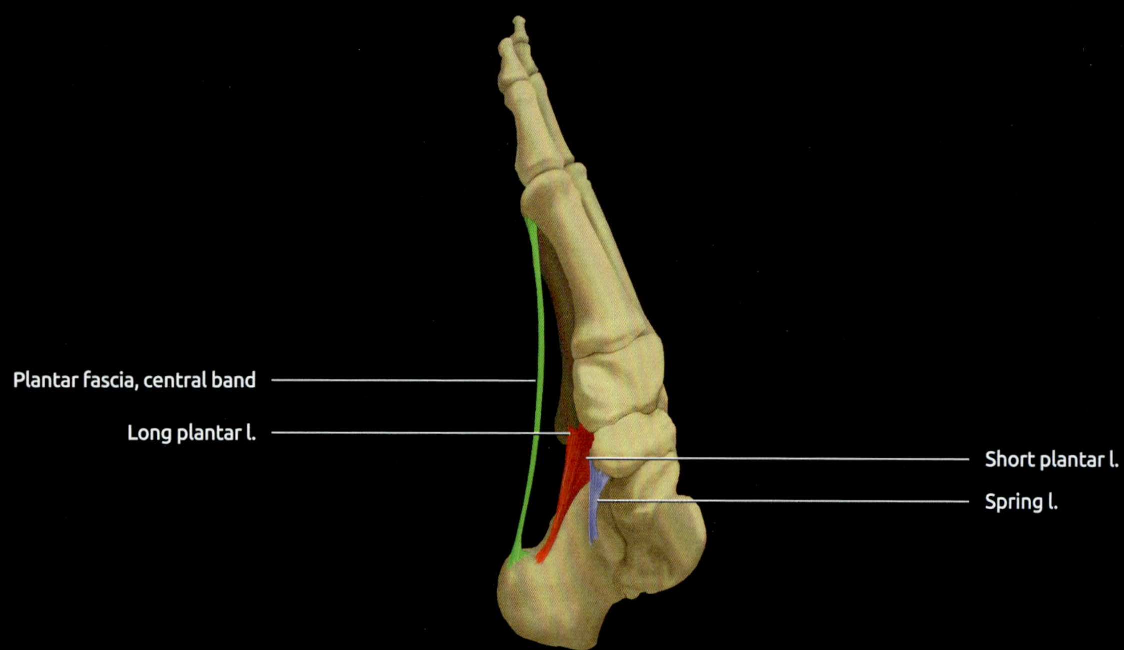

(Top) *Plantar view of foot shows the lateral column in pink and the medial column in blue. This plantar diagram is also useful for showing the appearance of the transverse arch created by wedge-shaped cuneiform bones. Plantar margins of cuneiforms are closely apposed, and the 2nd cuneiform is recessed.* **(Bottom)** *Graphic shows the longitudinal arch of the foot from the medial side together with a schematic representation of the major plantar ligaments helping maintain the longitudinal arch. The plantar fascia is the most important structure for maintaining the arch. It acts like a tie beam between the ends of the arch: Calcaneal tuberosity and metatarsal heads. Long and short plantar ligaments originate on the calcaneus with the short plantar ligament deep to the long plantar ligament. Both insert on the cuboid. The long plantar ligament also sends fibers to metatarsal bases. The spring ligament extends from the sustentaculum tali and adjacent anteromedial calcaneus to the plantar surface of navicular.*

GRAPHICS: TRANSVERSE ARCH

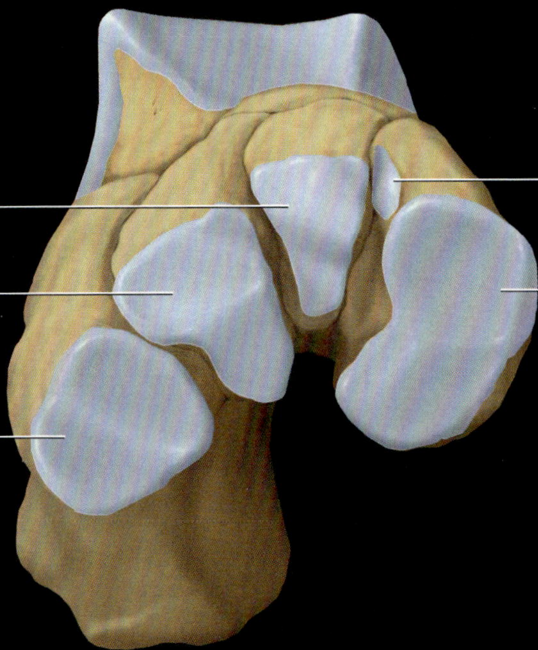

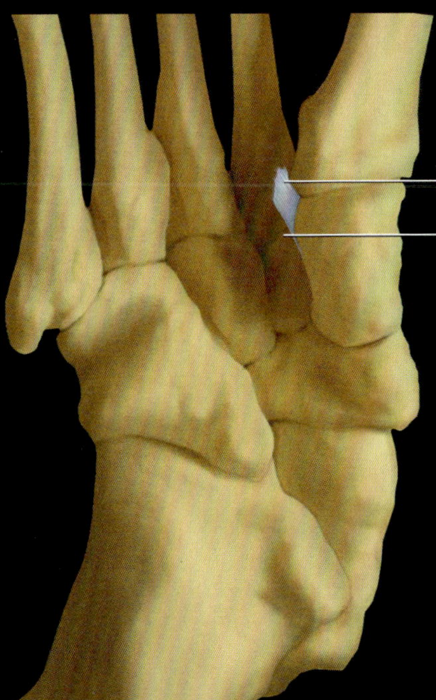

(Top) *Graphic shows the transverse arch formed by the cuneiforms and cuboid. The 1st cuneiform is largest, and the 2nd is smallest. The arch is continued anterior to this image by configuration of the proximal portions of the metatarsals. Interosseous and intercuneiform ligaments maintain the shape of the arch together with the peroneus longus tendon. Note the multifaceted articular surfaces at the tarsometatarsal joint.* **(Bottom)** *Graphic shows the transverse arch from the plantar side of the foot. The arch is formed by bones, but stability is dependent on ligaments. Lisfranc ligaments are critically important in maintaining the arch. There are 3 distinct Lisfranc ligaments extending from the 1st cuneiform to the base of 2nd metatarsal: Dorsal, interosseous, and plantar. The interosseous ligament is the strongest of them and is structurally most important.*

GRAPHICS: MUSCULATURE OF FOOT

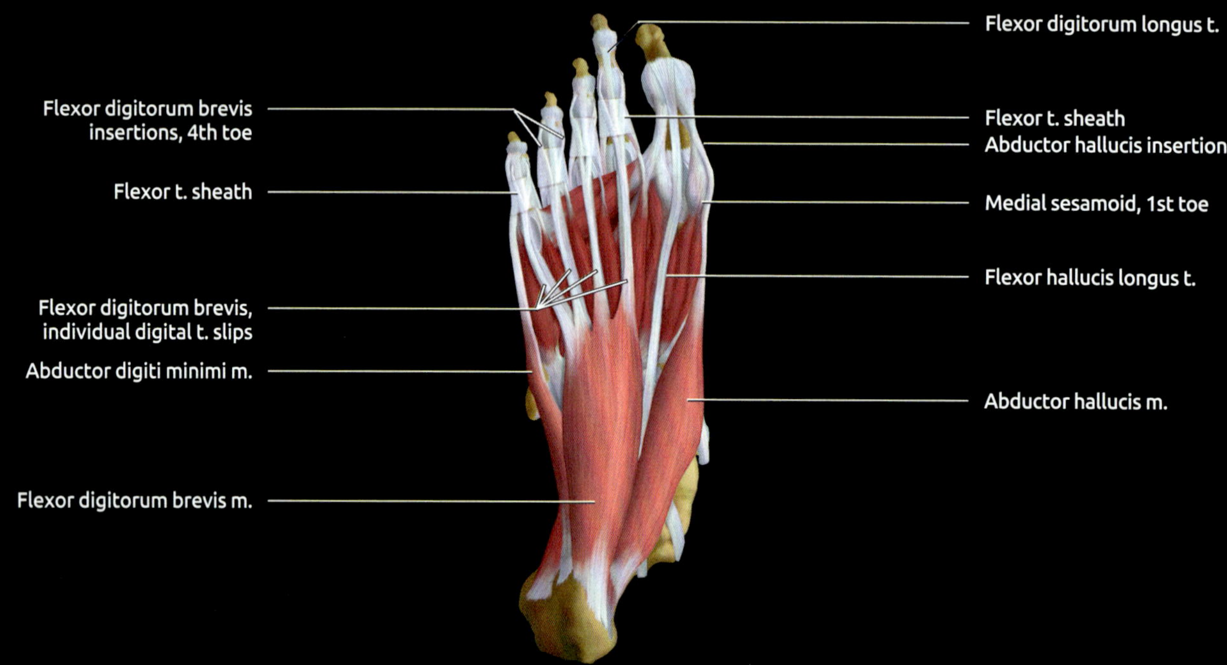

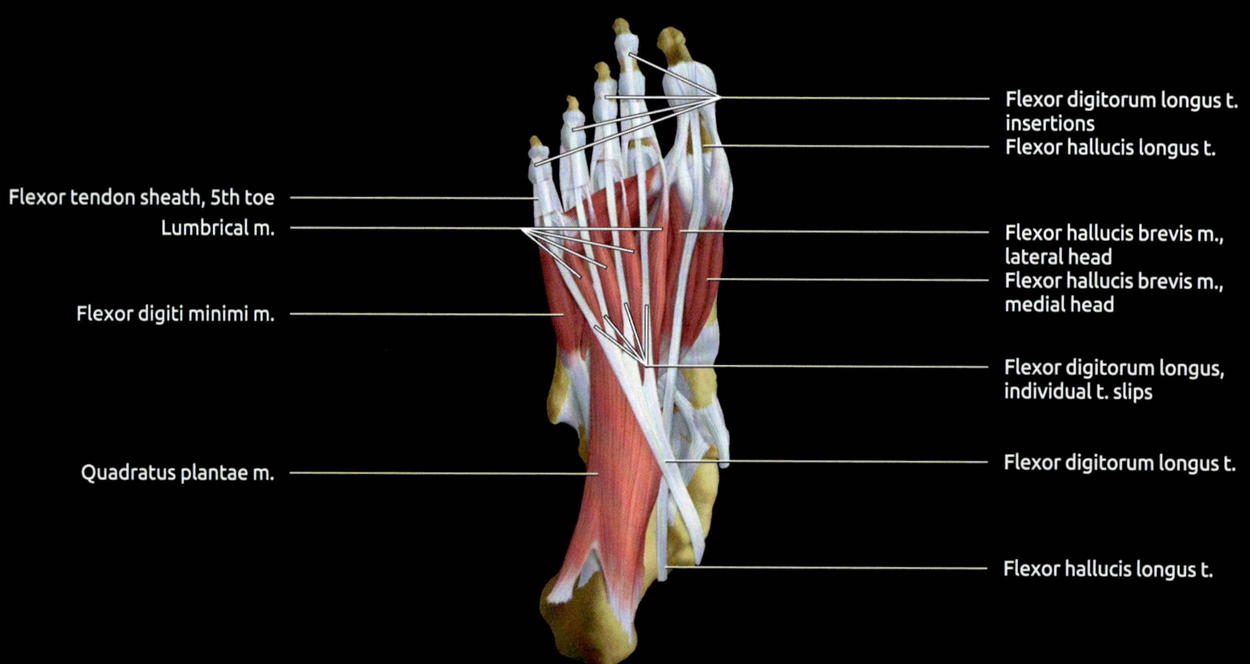

(Top) *Graphic shows the superficial layer of plantar foot muscles: Abductor digiti minimi, flexor digitorum brevis, and abductor hallucis. The deep muscles are partially visible deep to the superficial layer. Flexor digitorum brevis tendons split in each digit (4th digit labeled) attaching at the lateral aspects of the middle phalangeal bases. Flexor tendon sheaths hold the flexor mechanism in close proximity to the phalanges.* **(Bottom)** *Graphic shows the 2nd layer of the plantar muscles. The interesting arrangement of interactions between the flexors is well seen: Quadratus plantae inserting on the flexor digitorum longus tendon and lumbricals arising from individual flexor digitorum longus tendon slips. In the toes, the flexor tendons are contained with fibrous tendon sheaths.*

GRAPHICS: MUSCULATURE OF FOOT

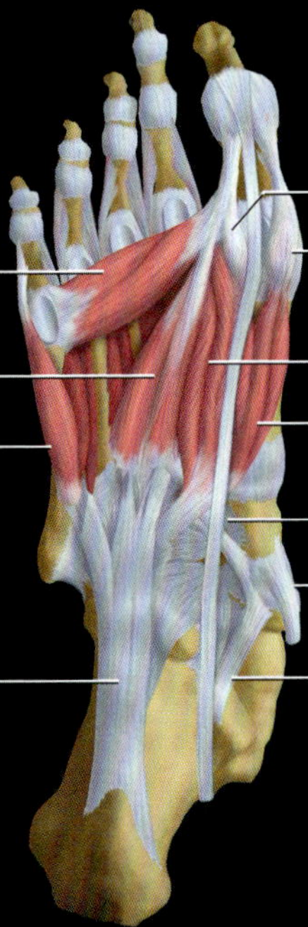

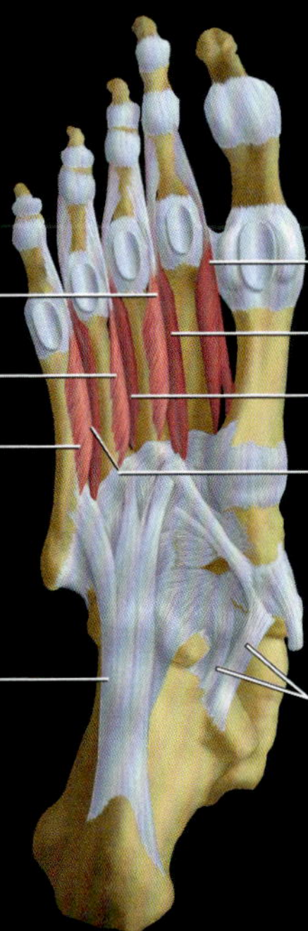

(Top) *Graphic shows the 3rd layer of plantar muscles. This layer contains the flexor hallucis brevis and flexor digiti minimi, as well as the adductor hallucis muscle. The oblique head of the adductor hallucis is thick and broad, whereas the transverse head is thin and occasionally congenitally absent.* **(Bottom)** *Graphic shows the 4th layer of plantar muscles, the interosseous muscles. There are 4 dorsal interossei. They have bipennate origins from 2 adjacent metatarsals. The 1st dorsal interosseous inserts on the medial side of the 2nd proximal phalanx. Remaining dorsal interossei insert on the lateral side of the corresponding proximal phalanx. There are 3 plantar interossei. The 1st plantar interosseous muscle originates from medial side of 3rd metatarsal and inserts on medial side of 3rd proximal phalanx. The 2nd and 3rd plantar interossei originate on medial sides of 4th and 5th metatarsals, respectively, and insert on medial side of corresponding proximal phalanx.*

TERMINOLOGY

Definitions

- Chopart joint: Talonavicular & calcaneocuboid joint
- Lisfranc joint: Tarsometatarsal joint

IMAGING ANATOMY

Internal Contents

- **Subtalar joint (talocalcaneal joint)**: 3 facets, 2 joint capsules
  - **Posterior subtalar facet**
    - 50% of weight-bearing across this joint
    - Wider laterally than medially
    - Oriented diagonally from posterosuperior to anteroinferior
    - Articular surfaces also form shallow cephalad arc
    - Joint capsule communicates with ankle joint 15% of time
    - Joint capsule does not communicate with middle, anterior subtalar joints
    - Anterior joint recess extends into tarsal sinus
  - Middle and anterior facet joints communicate with talonavicular joint
    - Functionally part of talocalcaneonavicular joint
  - **Middle subtalar facet**
    - Between sustentaculum tali of calcaneus and medial projection from talus
    - Horizontally oriented
    - Medial to tarsal sinus
    - Anterior and medial to posterior subtalar joint
  - **Anterior subtalar facet**
    - Small, continuous with middle subtalar facet, but oriented more obliquely
- **Talonavicular joint**
  - Convex talar head articulates with concave proximal navicular
- **Talocalcaneonavicular joint**
  - Single joint cavity for talonavicular, middle, and anterior subtalar facets
- **Calcaneocuboid joint**
  - Separate joint cavity
  - Acts together with talonavicular joint as Chopart joint
  - Anterior process of calcaneus at superior margin of joint does not articulate with navicular
    - Joined to navicular and cuboid by bifurcate ligament
- **Naviculocuneiform joint**
  - 3 navicular facets, 1 for each cuneiform, but 1 joint capsule
  - Navicular is convex anteriorly, cuneiforms form concave surface
- **Intercuneiform joints**
  - Variable communications with each other, naviculocuneiform joint, tarsometatarsal joint
  - Obliquely oriented, reflecting triangular shape of cuneiform bones
- **Tarsometatarsal joint**: 3 separate joint capsules
  - 1st tarsometatarsal joint
  - 2nd-3rd tarsometatarsal joints
  - 4th-5th tarsometatarsal joints
  - May communicate with intercuneiform joints
- **Metatarsophalangeal joints**
  - Tight capsule medially, superiorly, and laterally
    - Well-defined medial and lateral collateral ligaments
    - From head of metatarsal to base of proximal phalanx
  - Large plantar recess
    - From metatarsal neck to base proximal phalanx
    - Allows dorsiflexion
  - Plantar plate
    - Thickening in plantar side of joint capsule
    - Attaches proximally to metatarsal neck, distally to base proximal phalanx
- **1st metatarsophalangeal joint**
  - Differs from other metatarsophalangeal joints in its sesamophalangeal apparatus
    - Sesamophalangeal apparatus: Sesamoids + tendons attaching to sesamoids + plantar plate
    - Medial (also called tibial) and lateral (fibular) sesamoids
    - Medial sesamoid: In medial head of flexor hallucis brevis & abductor hallucis
    - Lateral sesamoid: In lateral head of flexor hallucis brevis & adductor hallucis
    - Tendons attach to medial and lateral margins, respectively, of 1st proximal phalanx
    - Plantar plate merges with tendons

ANATOMY IMAGING ISSUES

Imaging Recommendations

- Foot alignment can only be evaluated accurately on weight-bearing radiographs
  - Calcaneocuboid, talonavicular joints often appear subluxated on nonweight-bearing lateral, but normal on weight-bearing lateral
  - If pes planus is seen on nonweight-bearing view this is true-positive finding
  - If pes cavus is seen on nonweight-bearing view this may be false-positive finding
- Care must be taken to have patients stand naturally
- Patients may pronate foot instead of holding natural stance unless both feet are side-by-side
- Standard series consists of AP, lateral, and oblique views of foot
- Helpful to have steps and elevated platform for patients to stand while films obtained
  - Allows x-ray beam to be centered on foot
- Sesamoid view
  - Patient prone, toes dorsiflexed against plate, x-ray beam from posterior to anterior **or**
  - Patient supine, toes dorsiflexed by band holding them in position **or**
  - Patient standing, toes dorsiflexed against plate, x-ray beam angled toward sesamoids from posterior to anterior
- Toe films
  - Helpful to cone down on region of concern
  - Use pencil or other device to move overlapping toes out of view on lateral radiograph

AP & OBLIQUE FOOT RADIOGRAPHS

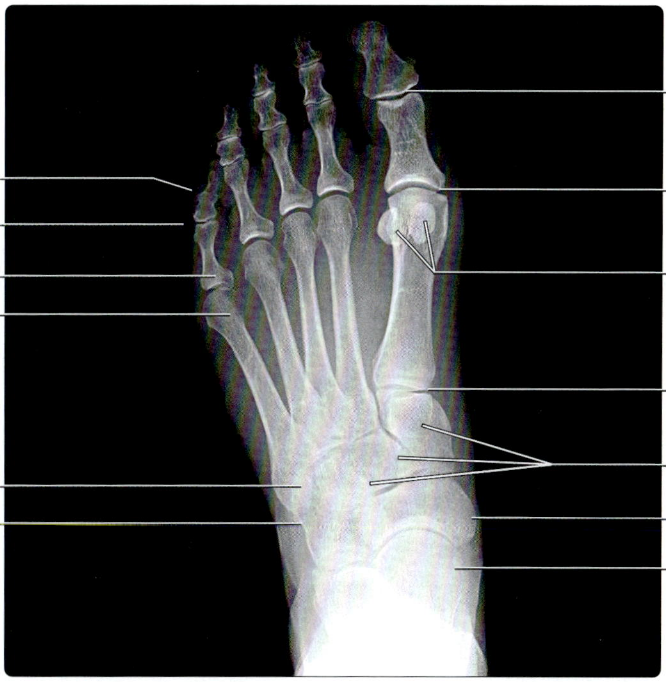

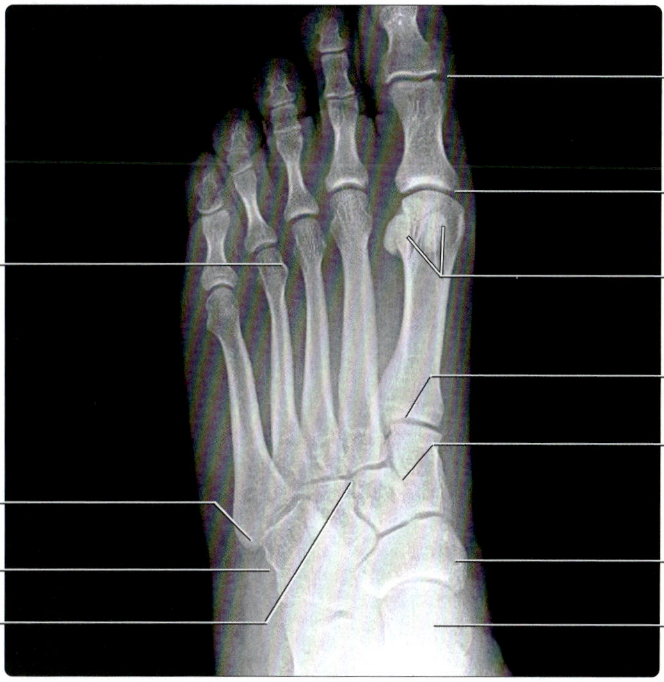

(Top) *Anteroposterior weight-bearing radiograph of the foot shows a normal amount of overlap of the bones of the midfoot. Articulations between cuboid and navicular, between cuneiforms, and between cuboid and lateral cuneiform are not seen in profile. Tarsometatarsal (TMT) joints are sometimes in profile, but joints may not be visible due to obliquity of joint; this should not be mistaken for joint fusion.* **(Bottom)** *On oblique view, intercuneiform joints, TMT joints, and styloid process (also called tuberosity) at the base of the 5th metatarsal are usually better seen than on anteroposterior view. A normal notch at the medial margin of the metatarsal heads is often thrown into profile on this view and should not be mistaken for erosion.*

LATERAL FOOT: WEIGHT BEARING AND NONWEIGHT BEARING

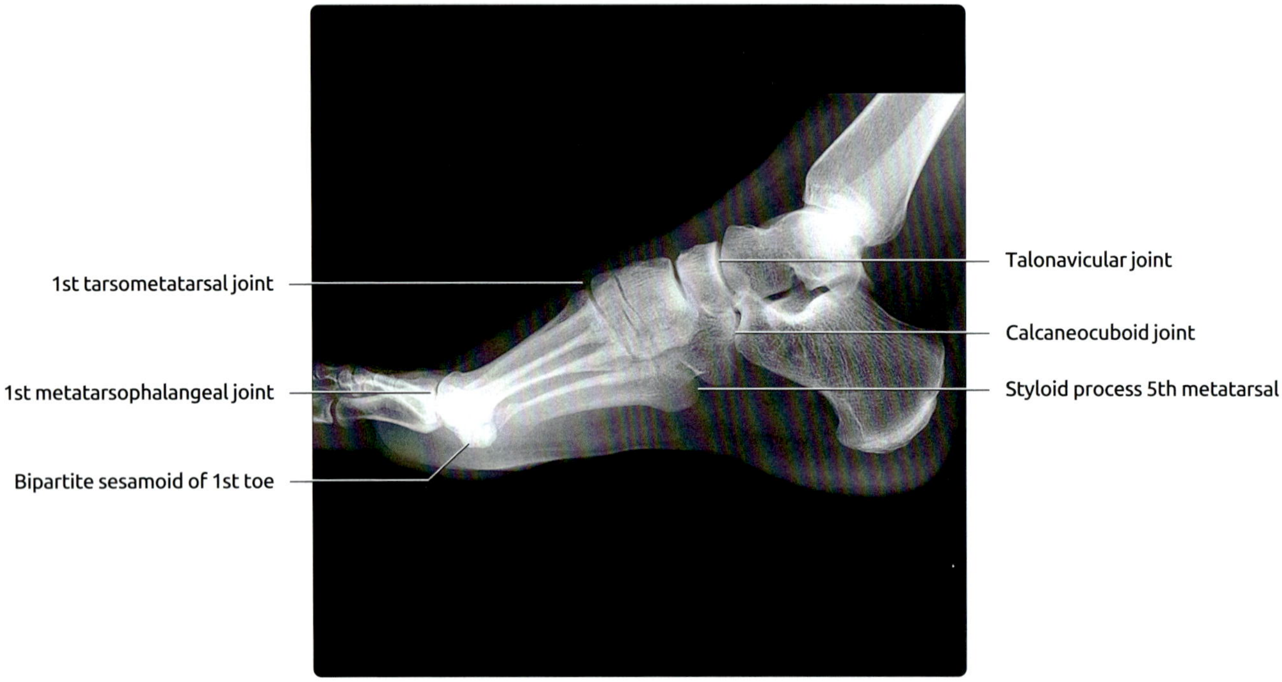

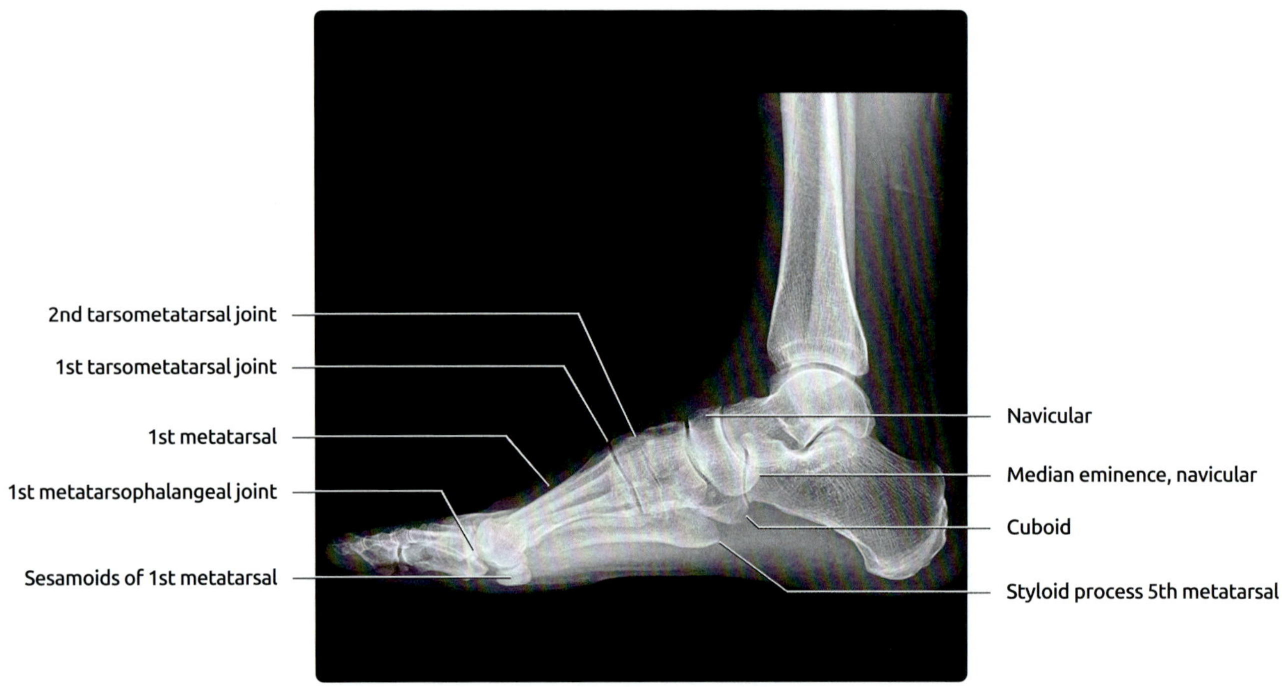

(Top) *On this nonweight-bearing lateral radiograph, the longitudinal arch of the foot usually appears higher than on a weight-bearing view. The calcaneocuboid and talonavicular joints appear subluxated inferiorly on this view but that is a normal finding, which resolves on weight-bearing radiographs.* **(Bottom)** *Lateral weight-bearing radiograph shows the longitudinal arch of the foot, from the posterior process of calcaneus to the 1st MTP joint. Note the relatively plantar position of the median eminence (tuberosity) of the navicular. The line drawn along the center of the talar axis will continue along the axis of the 1st metatarsal in a normally aligned foot. The 1st and 2nd metatarsal bases are both at the dorsal aspect of the foot; they can be distinguished by the more proximal position of the 2nd metatarsal.*

POSTERIOR SUBTALAR JOINT ARTHROGRAPHY

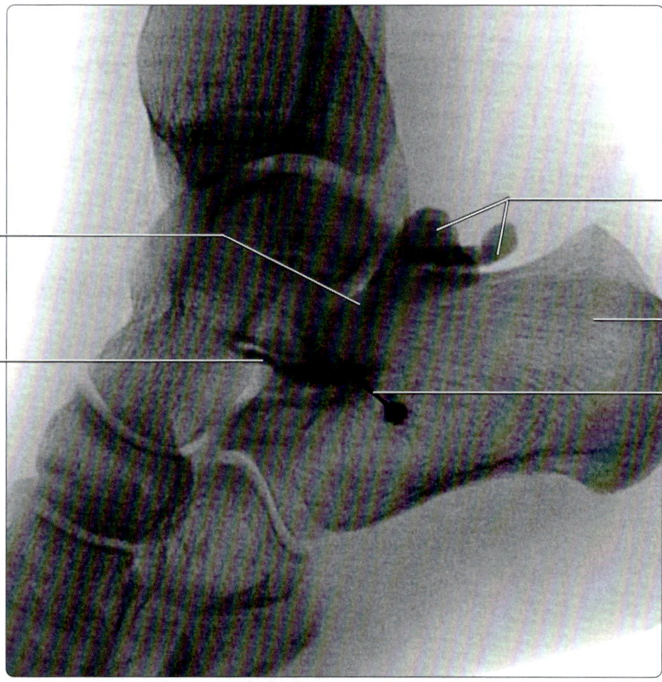

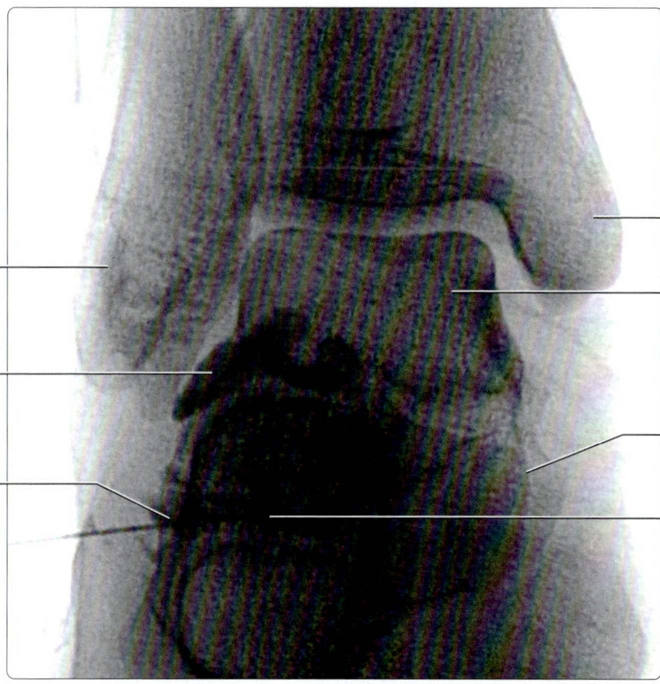

(Top) *Lateral spot radiograph from a posterior subtalar arthrogram shows the anterior and posterior joint recesses, which are variable in size. The anterior recess normally extends into the posterior portion of the sinus tarsi, as in this case.* **(Bottom)** *Anteroposterior spot radiograph from the same posterior subtalar joint arthrogram shows the joint recesses superimposed on the talus. The joint is difficult to see on this view, which is useful primarily for confirming needle position. Note that the lateral margin of the joint is well below the level of the fibular tip.*

POSTERIOR SUBTALAR JOINT MR ARTHROGRAPHY

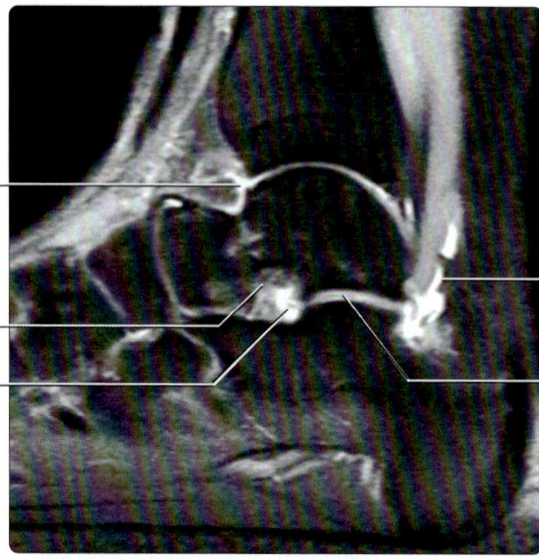

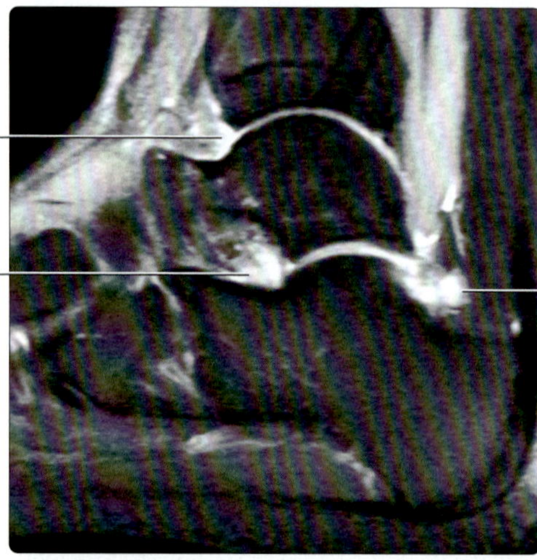

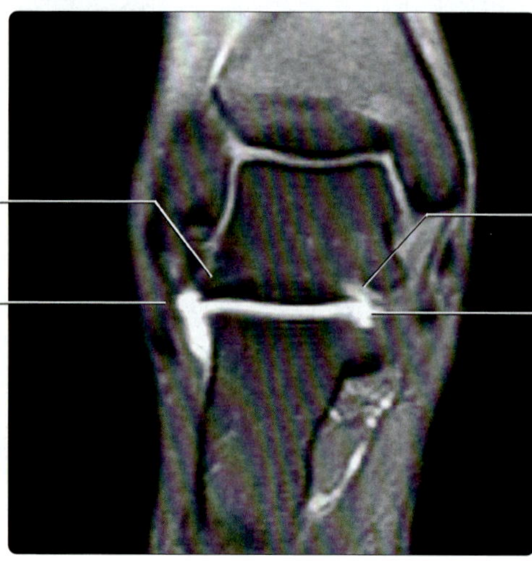

(Top) *Sagittal T1WI PD FS MR at the medial margin of the posterior subtalar joint shows the relatively small size of the joint compared to its size laterally. Contrast in the flexor hallucis longus tendon sheath and tibiotalar joint are normal variants present in 15% of the population.* **(Middle)** *Sagittal PD FS MR shows fluid filling the normal anterior and posterior recesses of the posterior subtalar joint.* **(Bottom)** *Coronal T1WI FS MR through the posterior subtalar joint shows the normal recess into the tarsal canal. Laterally, contrast often extends to the undersurface of the calcaneofibular ligament. In other patients, a well-defined talocalcaneal ligament contains contrast closer to the joint.*

TALOCALCANEONAVICULAR JOINT ARTHROGRAPHY

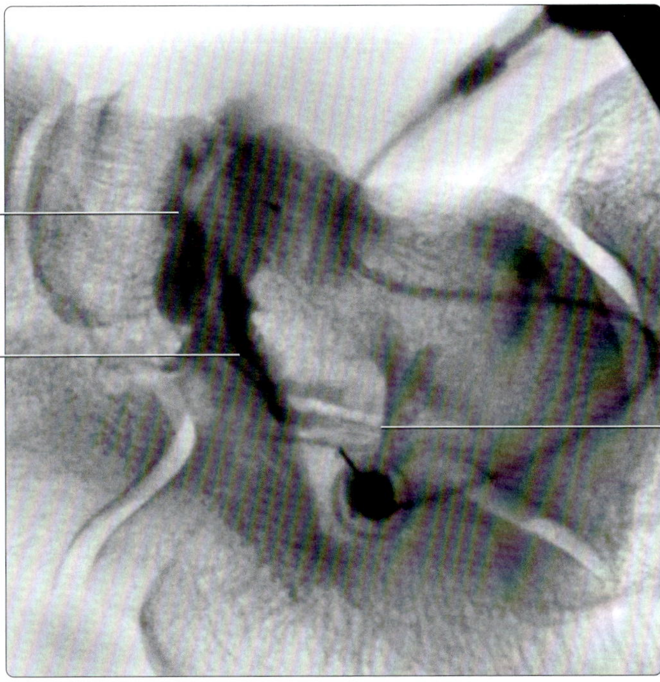

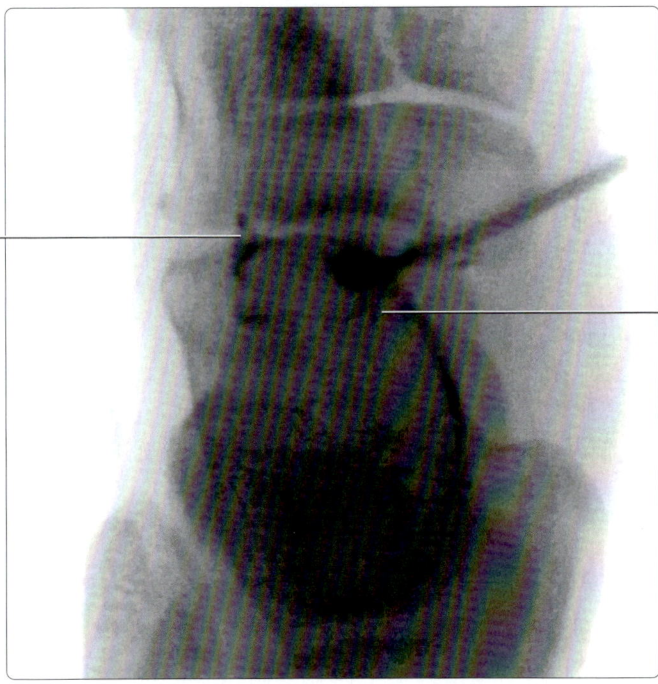

(Top) *Lateral spot radiograph obtained after middle subtalar joint injection is shown. The talonavicular joint, anterior subtalar facet, and middle subtalar facet form a common joint cavity.* **(Bottom)** *Anteroposterior spot radiograph in a different patient from a talonavicular joint injection shows contrast in joint recesses. The rounded talar head articulates with the disc-shaped navicular.*

CALCANEOCUBOID JOINT ARTHROGRAPHY

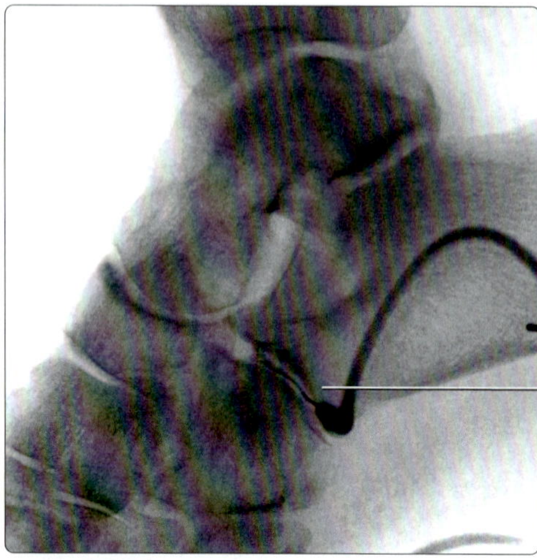

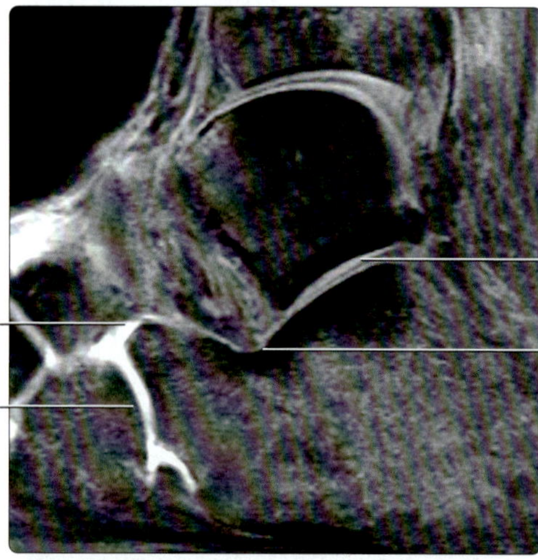

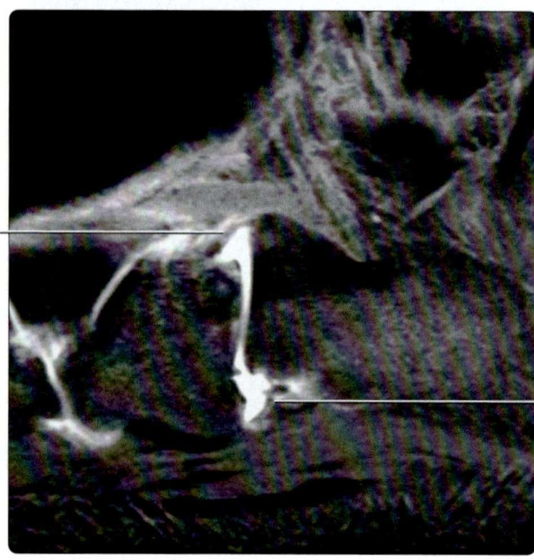

(Top) *Lateral spot radiograph from calcaneocuboid injection is shown. The calcaneocuboid joint has an S-shaped contour. On nonweight-bearing films, the cuboid usually appears to be subluxated slightly inferior to the calcaneus.* **(Middle)** *Sagittal MR arthrography of the calcaneocuboid joint shows contrast outlining joint surfaces and joint recesses. The anterior process of the calcaneus forms a triangular tip and does not articulate with the navicular.* **(Bottom)** *Sagittal MR arthrography lateral to the previous image shows the bifurcate ligament extending from the anterior process of the calcaneus to the cuboid and navicular. Apparent joint incongruity is a normal finding on nonweight-bearing images.*

NAVICULOCUNEIFORM JOINT ARTHROGRAPHY

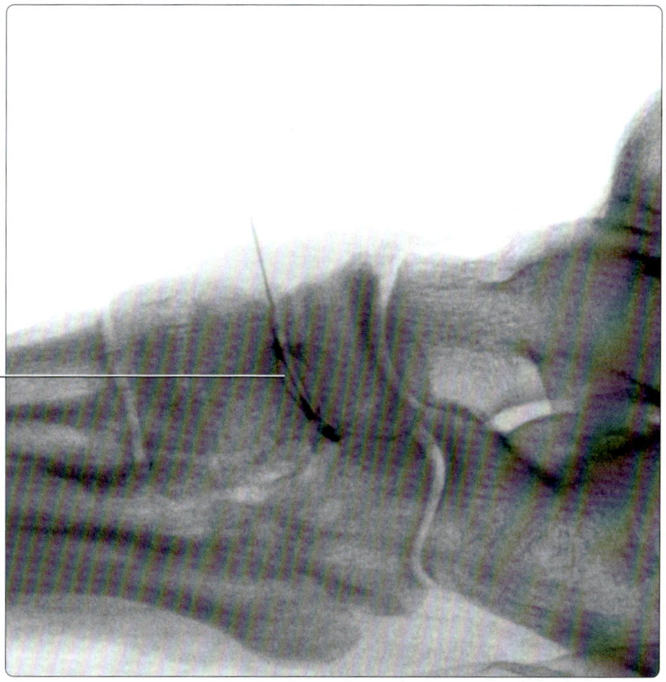

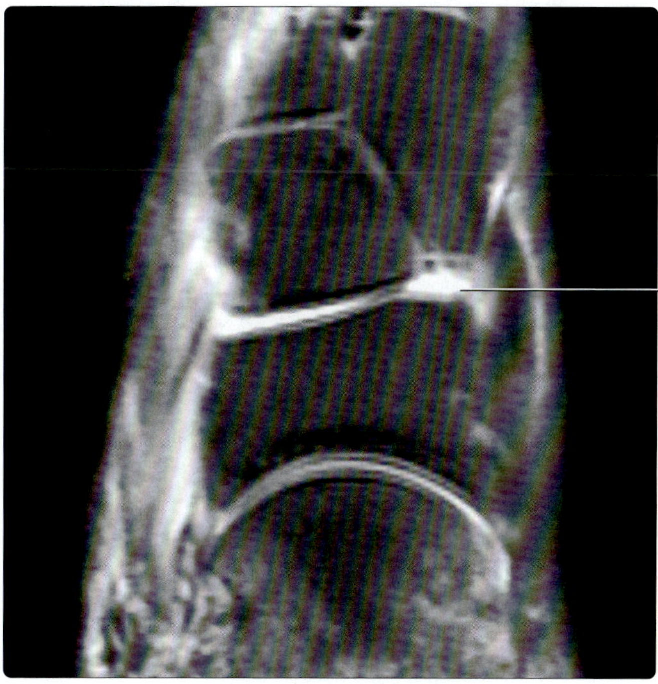

(Top) *Lateral spot radiograph of naviculocuneiform arthrogram shows that the naviculocuneiform joint has a contour similar to that of the talonavicular joint. It often communicates with intercuneiform joints.* **(Bottom)** *Axial naviculocuneiform MR arthrography shows that the naviculocuneiform joint has 3 contiguous facets for articulation with each of the cuneiforms.*

INTERCUNEIFORM & TARSOMETATARSAL JOINTS

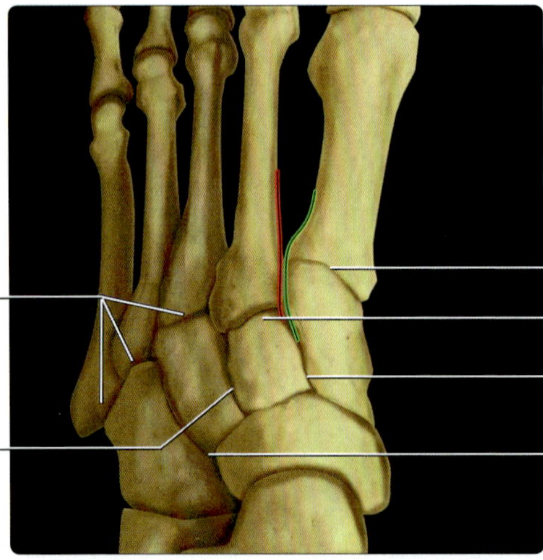

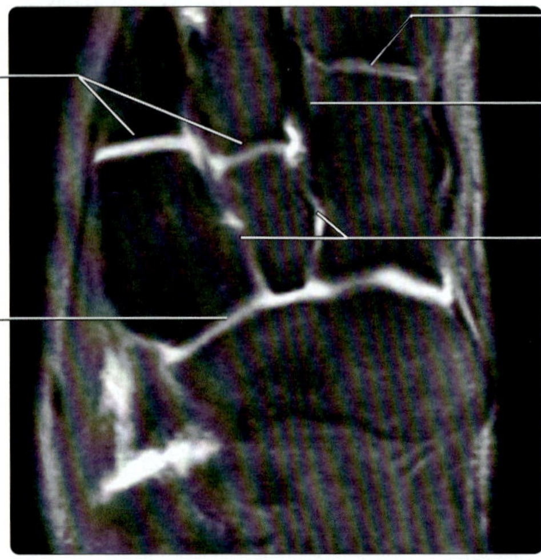

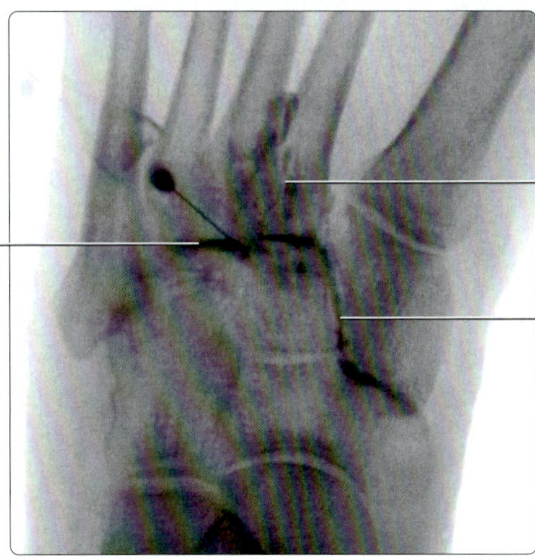

(Top) *Graphic shows that the TMT joint forms a shallow arc from medial to lateral. It is stabilized by the recessed position of the 2nd TMT and by the Lisfranc ligament between the 1st cuneiform and 2nd metatarsal base. The 1st cuneiform is centered on the 1st metatarsal; the medial margin of the 2nd cuneiform is aligned with the medial margin of the 2nd metatarsal; the 5th metatarsal extends beyond the cuboid.* **(Middle)** *Axial MR arthrography with contrast filling intercuneiform, naviculocuneiform, and 2nd and 3rd TMT joints shows variable communications between the intercuneiform joints, TMT joints, and naviculocuneiform joints.* **(Bottom)** *The 2nd and 3rd TMT joints form a single joint cavity, also communicating with the 2nd intermetatarsal joint. The communication seen here, with the 1st intercuneiform joint, is uncommon.*

1ST METATARSOPHALANGEAL JOINT ARTHROGRAPHY

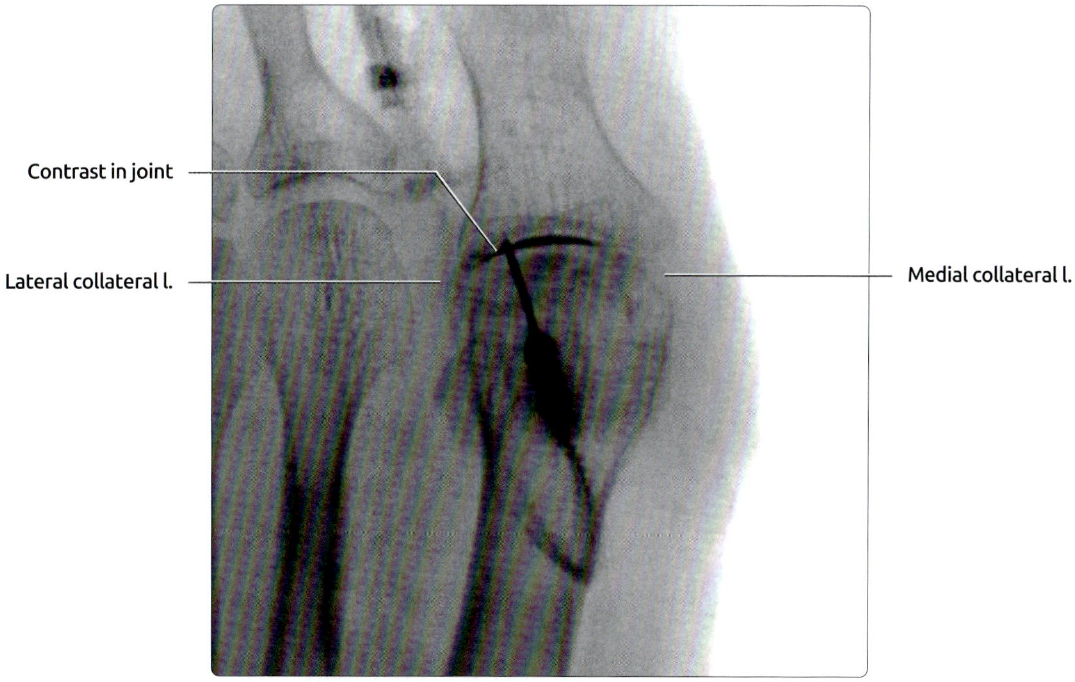

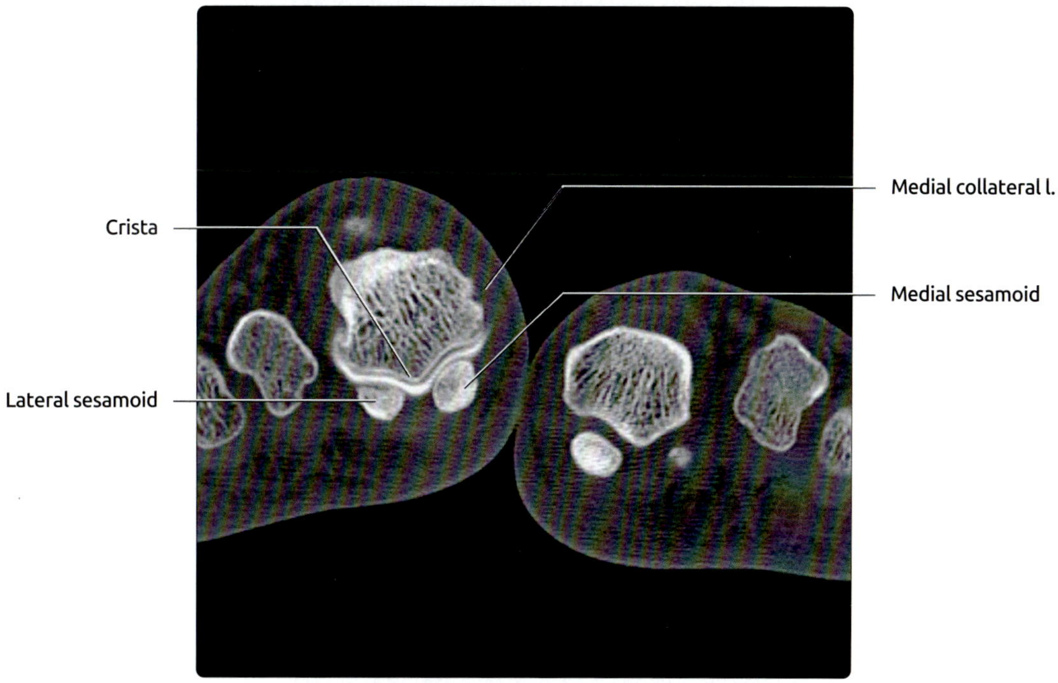

(Top) *Anteroposterior spot radiograph from the 1st MTP arthrography shows contrast filling the joint space, limited medially and laterally by collateral ligaments.* **(Bottom)** *Coronal CT arthrogram shows the normal synovial articulation between the sesamoids and 1st metatarsal head.*

1ST METATARSOPHALANGEAL MR ARTHROGRAPHY

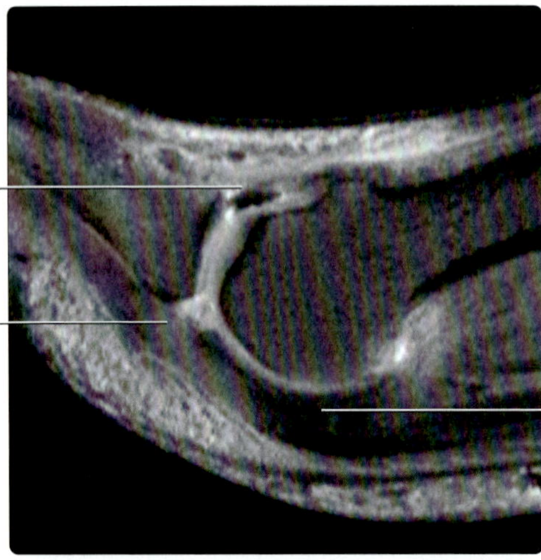

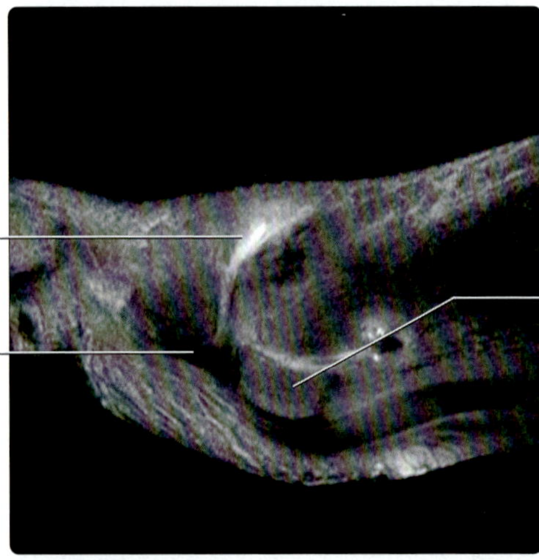

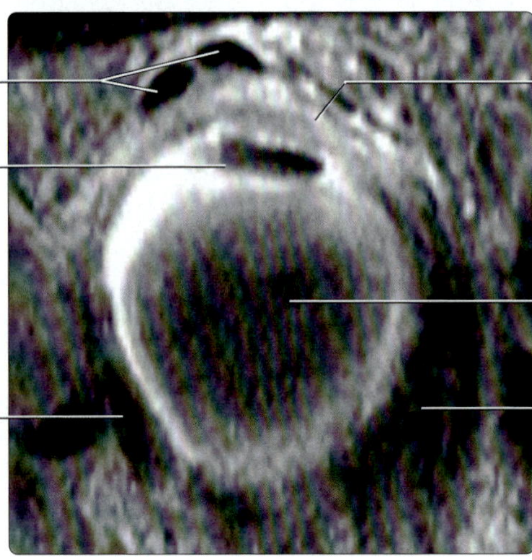

(Top) *Sagittal T1WI FS MR arthrography through the 1st metatarsophalangeal joint shows relationships of the joint capsule and the medial sesamoid. The sesamophalangeal apparatus includes the plantar plate, sesamoids, and tendons in which sesamoids sit. It attaches to the base of the proximal phalanx.* **(Middle)** *Sagittal T1WI FS MR arthrography through the lateral margin of 1st metatarsophalangeal joint shows relationships of the joint capsule and the lateral sesamoid. Sesamophalangeal apparatus is shown attaching to lateral, plantar margin of 1st proximal phalangeal base.* **(Bottom)** *Coronal T1WI FS MR arthrography shows the sesamophalangeal apparatus at the periphery of the plantar aspect of the joint, close to the distal attachments.*

2ND METATARSOPHALANGEAL JOINT

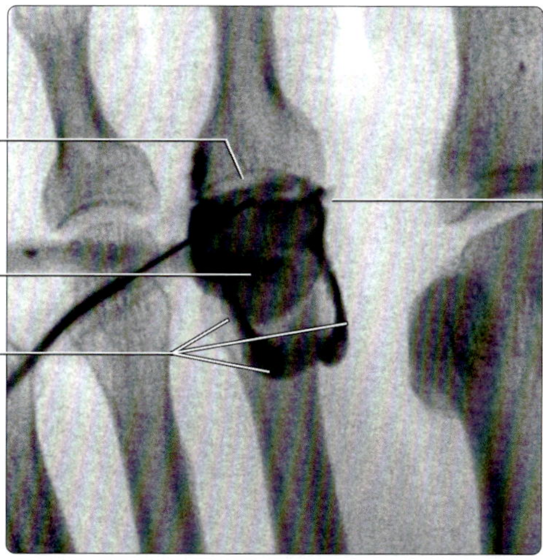

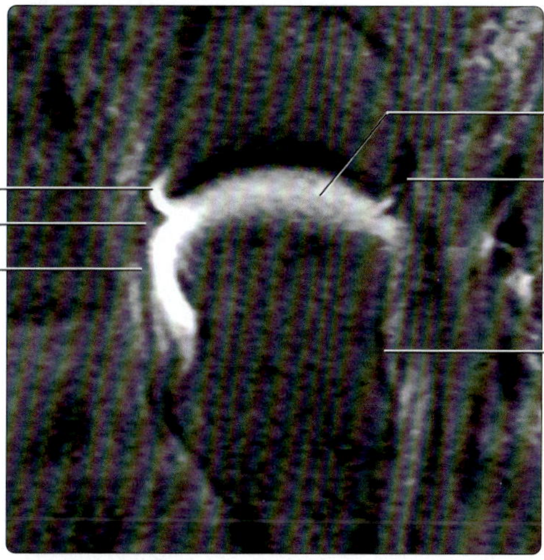

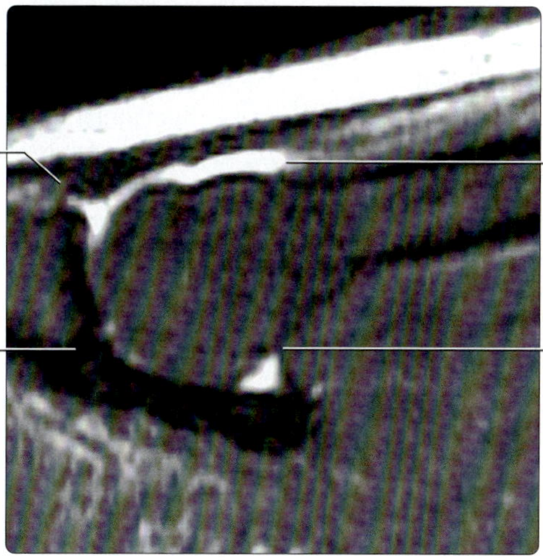

(Top) *Anteroposterior spot radiograph from the 2nd metatarsophalangeal arthrography shows normal filling of the capacious plantar recesses. The joint capsule is tightly adherent at the medial and lateral collateral ligaments.* **(Middle)** *Axial T1WI MR arthrography shows the collateral ligaments and articular cartilage outlined by contrast. Small, meniscoid structures are visible.* **(Bottom)** *Sagittal T1WI MR arthrogram through the 2nd metatarsophalangeal joint shows attachment of the plantar plate to the metatarsal neck. The plantar and dorsal joint recesses are normally fairly redundant, unlike the tight attachments at the base of the proximal phalanges.*

TERMINOLOGY

Definitions

- Axial (horizontal) plane of foot
  - Long axis of foot
  - Slightly oblique compared to axial plane in leg
  - Hindfoot: Images angled along long axis of talus
  - Midfoot and forefoot: Images angled along long axis of 2nd metatarsal
- Coronal plane of foot
  - Short axis of foot
  - Hindfoot: Images angled perpendicular to neck of talus
  - Midfoot and forefoot: Images angled perpendicular to long axis of 2nd metatarsal

IMAGING ANATOMY

Structures Best Seen in Axial Plane

- Lisfranc ligament (3 separate bands, from 2nd cuneiform to 1st metatarsal base)
  - Dorsal band: Most superior slice through 2nd cuneiform and 1st metatarsal
  - Interosseous band: Thick band centrally located, must have taut appearance
  - Plantar band: Thinnest band, at plantar margin of 2nd cuneiform
- Spring ligament (plantar bands)
  - From calcaneus to navicular
  - Medioplantar oblique: Originates on coronoid fossa of calcaneus, anterior to sustentaculum tali, inserts on navicular lateral to posterior tibial tendon
  - Inferoplantar longitudinal: Short, straight course from coronoid fossa of calcaneus to navicular beak

Structures Best Seen in Coronal Plane

- Tarsal tunnel
  - Fibroosseous tunnel in medial hindfoot
    - Roof: Flexor retinaculum
    - Floor: Medial margins of talus and calcaneus
  - Contains: Posterior tibial neurovascular bundle and branches, posterior tibial tendon, flexor hallucis longus and flexor digitorum longus tendons
  - Importance: Mass, venous varicosity, cyst, or anomalous muscle may cause impingement on tibial nerve or its branches
    - Results in tarsal tunnel syndrome: Pain, numbness, muscle weakness, and atrophy
- Tarsal sinus
  - Funnel-shaped space between talar neck and dorsal margin of calcaneus
  - Contains: Cervical ligament, limbs of extensor retinaculum, artery of tarsal sinus
  - Importance: Injury may lead to fibrosis, pain at lateral hindfoot, subjective instability
- Tarsal canal
  - Posteromedial extension of tarsal sinus
  - Contains: Interosseous ligament
  - Significance: Ligament tear can be associated with subtalar instability
- Spring ligament, superomedial band
  - Strongest portion of spring ligament
  - Originates on sustentaculum tali, tibiospring band of superficial deltoid ligament
  - Inserts on medial navicular
- Intrinsic muscles
  - Interrelationships of muscle layers usually best seen on coronal images
- Compartments of foot
  - 4 plantar compartments divided by fascial layers
  - Medial, middle (superficial & deep), lateral
  - Significance: Infection usually limited to 1 compartment unless patient has had prior surgery

Structures Best Seen in Sagittal Plane

- Tarsometatarsal joints
  - Due to obliquity of joints, partial volume averaging may cause interpretative difficulties in other planes
  - Significance: Joint disorders, instability
- Plantar plate of metatarsophalangeal joints
  - Plantar thickening of joint capsule
  - Extends from metatarsal neck to base of proximal phalanx
  - 1st metatarsophalangeal plantar plate incorporates its sesamoids
  - Significance: Injury to plantar plate can result in dorsal subluxation or dislocation at joint
- Phalanges
  - Due to their normally flexed position, difficult to localize abnormalities on axial, coronal images
  - Significance: Osteomyelitis often involves terminal phalanges, best seen on sagittal images

MR Protocol

- Use dedicated foot coil or knee coil
- Usually patient supine, some authors prefer patient prone, foot plantar flexed
  - Prone position results in some distortion of normal anatomy
- Usually angle along 2nd metatarsal axis for sagittal images
  - Modify for other regions of interest
- Coronal should be perpendicular to metatarsals
- Axial should be along plane of 2nd metatarsal
- High-density pad around forefoot often improves image quality
- T1-weighted imaging usually obtained in sagittal, axial planes
- Fluid-sensitive imaging in coronal, sagittal planes
- For osteomyelitis, obtain T1-weighted images in all 3 planes

ANATOMY IMAGING ISSUES

Imaging Pitfalls

- Talonavicular joint recess between plantar bands of spring ligament can be confused with ligament rupture
- Bursae between metatarsal heads may be mistaken for neuromas
- Divergence of metatarsals may create confusion on sagittal images as to exact digit being imaged
- Flexion of toes may mimic abnormality due to partial volume averaging

GRAPHICS: DORSAL AND PLANTAR FOOT LIGAMENTS

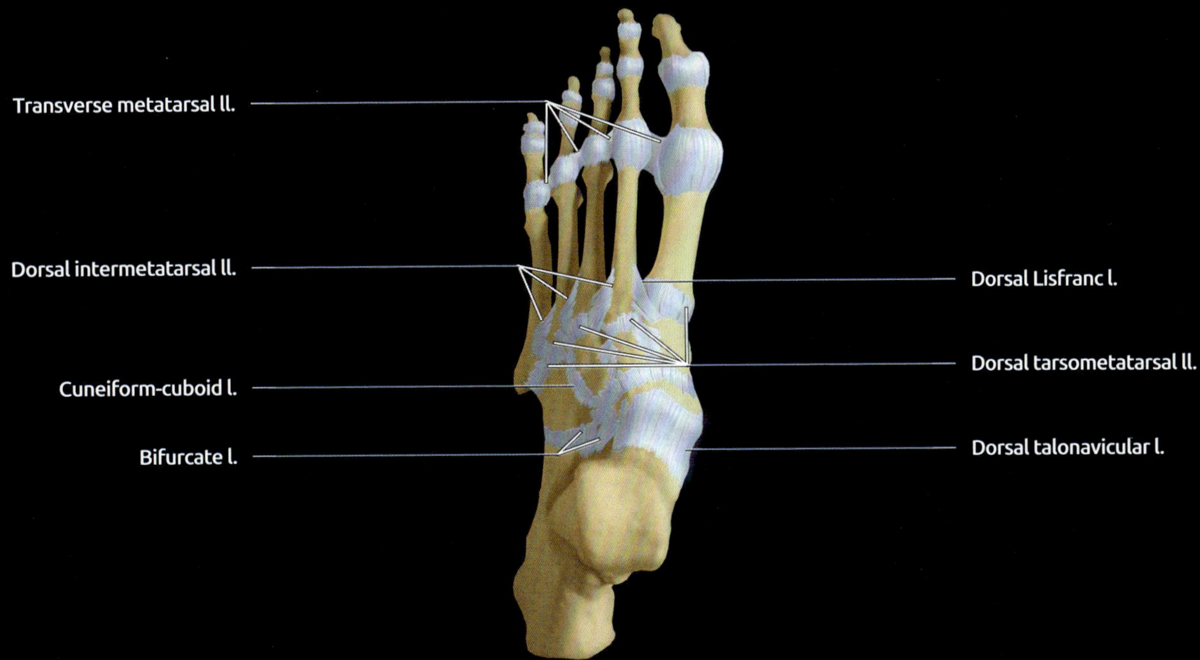

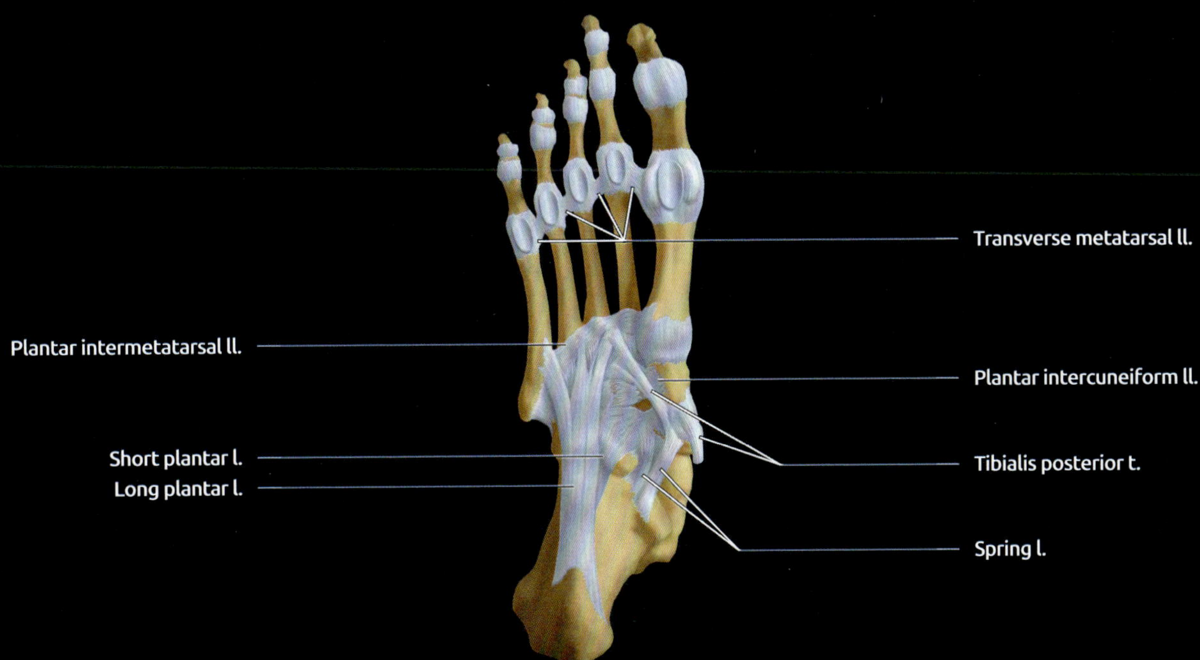

(Top) *Graphic of dorsal ligaments shows dense ligaments between tarsal bones and between tarsals and metatarsals. Ligaments are generally named for the bones they bridge. Exceptions are the bifurcate ligament, which extends from the anterior process calcaneus to the cuboid and navicular, and the dorsal Lisfranc ligament, from the 1st cuneiform to 2nd metatarsal.* **(Bottom)** *Graphic of plantar ligaments shows ligaments deep to the plantar fascia as well as proximal and distal attachments of the tibialis posterior tendon. The spring ligament, a.k.a. the plantar calcaneonavicular ligament, originates on the sustentaculum tali and anterior calcaneus and inserts on the navicular. Deep intertarsal ligaments are also shown and are named for bones they bridge.*

AXIAL LONG-AXIS T1 MR: RIGHT FOOT

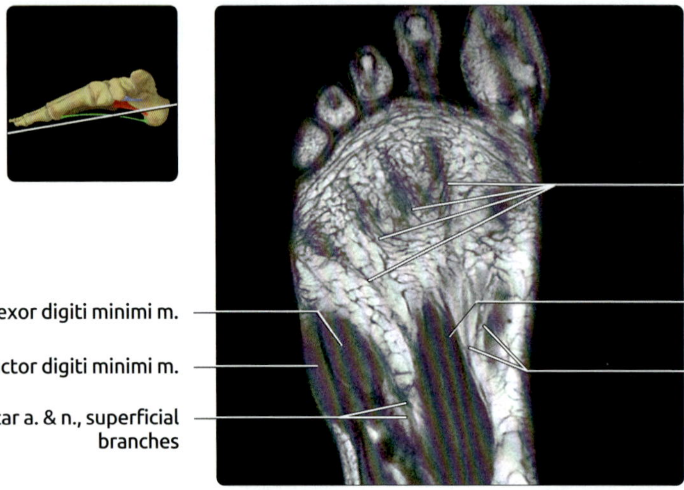

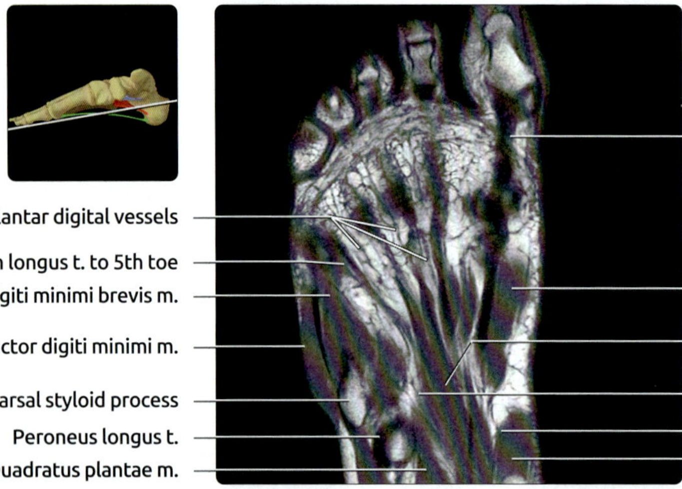

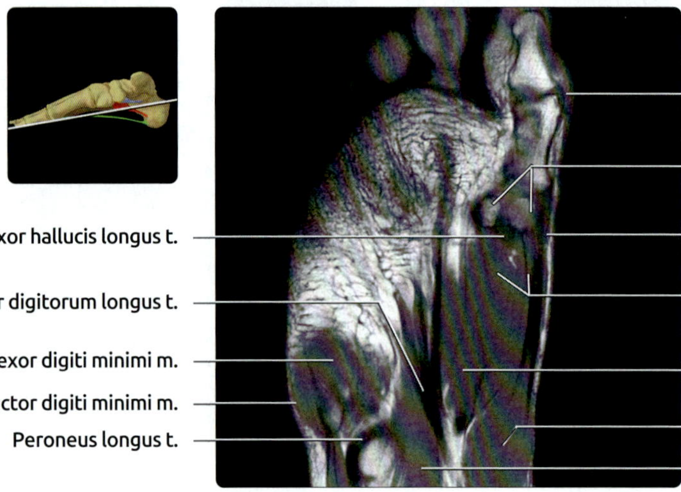

(Top) *First in a series of axial long-axis T1 MR images shows the right foot from plantar to dorsal. Plantar fascia, superficial to the flexor digitorum brevis muscle, is seen dividing into digital bands in the forefoot.* **(Middle)** *The medial plantar nerve courses lateral to the medial plantar artery, between the abductor hallucis and flexor digitorum brevis. The lateral plantar nerve courses between the flexor digitorum brevis muscle and quadratus plantae muscle and continues laterally, dividing into deep and superficial branches at the level of the 5th metatarsal base, between the flexor digitorum brevis and abductor digiti minimi.* **(Bottom)** *Medial and lateral heads of flexor digitorum brevis muscle are seen attaching to sesamoids of the 1st toe. Their distal insertion onto the base of the 1st proximal phalanx is not seen on this image.*

AXIAL LONG-AXIS T1 MR: LEFT FOOT

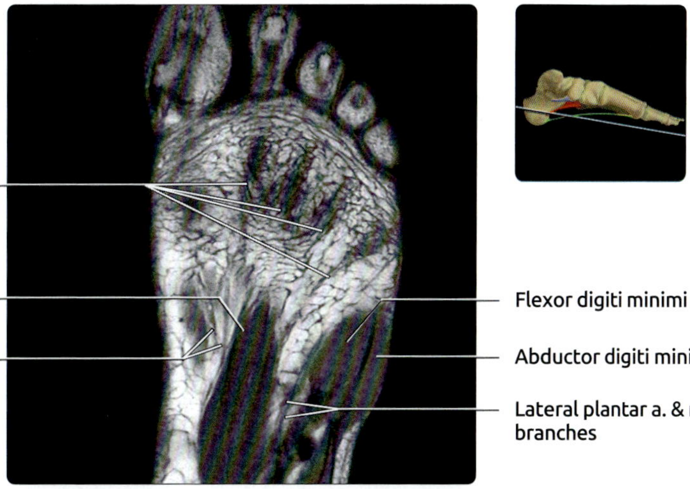

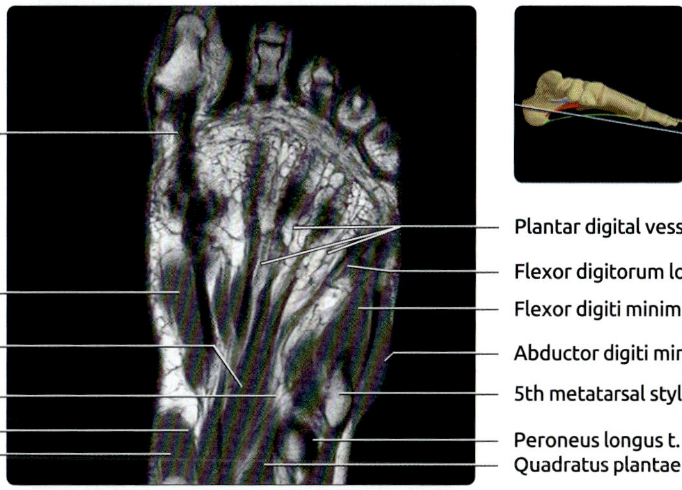

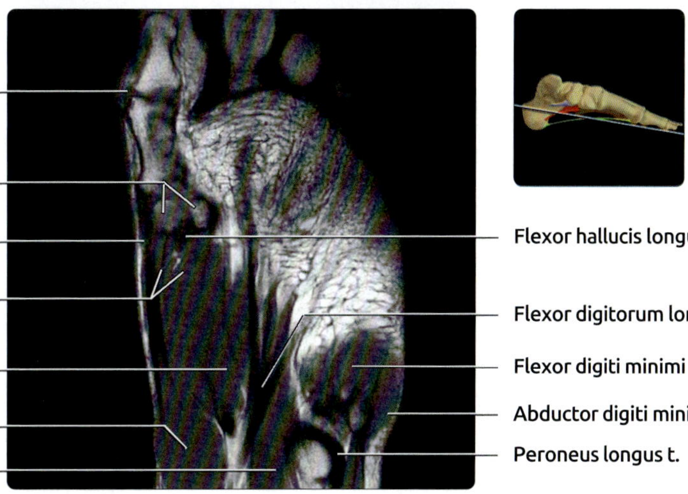

(Top) *First in a series of axial long-axis T1 MR images shows the left foot from plantar to dorsal. Plantar fascia, superficial to the flexor digitorum brevis muscle, is seen dividing into digital bands in the forefoot.* **(Middle)** *The medial plantar nerve courses lateral to the medial plantar artery, between the abductor hallucis and flexor digitorum brevis. The lateral plantar nerve courses between the flexor digitorum brevis muscle and quadratus plantae muscle and continues laterally, dividing into deep and superficial branches at the level of the 5th metatarsal base, between the flexor digitorum brevis muscle and abductor digiti minimi.* **(Bottom)** *The medial and lateral heads of the flexor digitorum brevis muscle are seen attaching to the sesamoids of the 1st toe. Their distal insertion onto base of 1st proximal phalanx is not seen on this image.*

AXIAL LONG-AXIS T1 MR: RIGHT FOOT

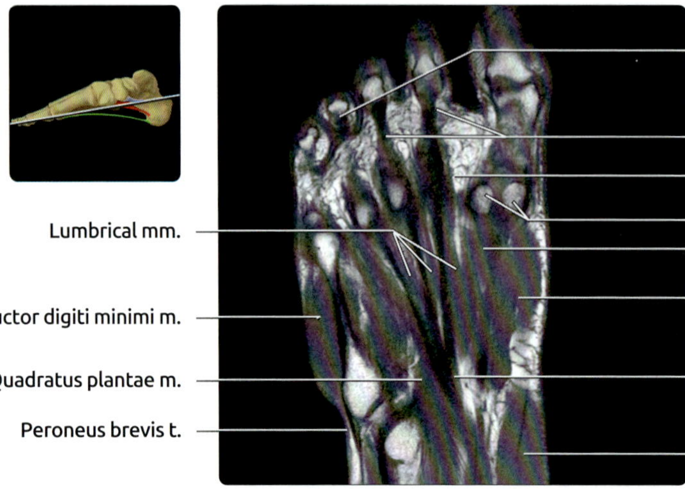

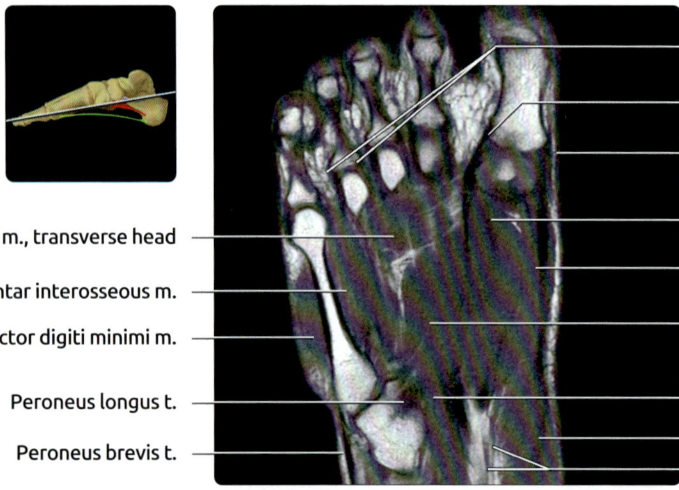

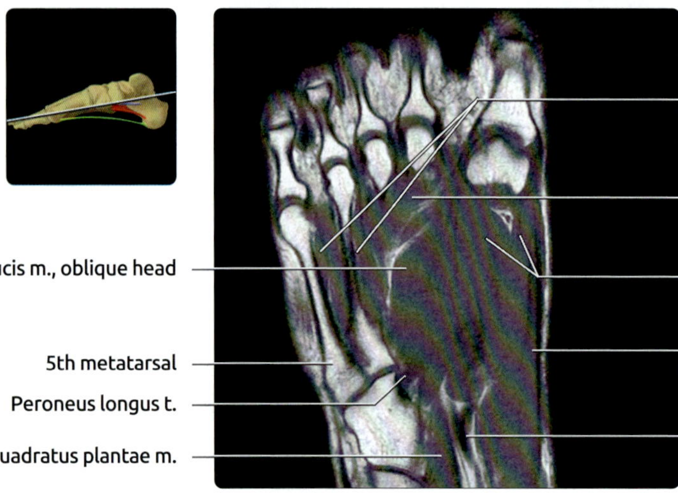

(Top) *Note the insertion of the quadratus plantae muscle into the flexor digitorum longus tendon just proximal to its division into slips to 4 lateral toes. The lumbrical muscles arise from individual slips of the flexor digitorum longus tendon and insert on the medial aspect of the proximal phalanx. A flexor digitorum longus tendon slip to the 5th digit is variably present.* **(Middle)** *Terminology for adductor and abductor hallucis muscles becomes clear once it is remembered that abductor pulls 1st toe away from 2nd toe and adductor pulls it toward 2nd toe (i.e., axis of reference here is the foot, not the entire body).* **(Bottom)** *The oblique head of the adductor hallucis muscle is thick and broad, while the transverse head is thinner and sometimes congenitally absent.*

AXIAL LONG-AXIS T1 MR: LEFT FOOT

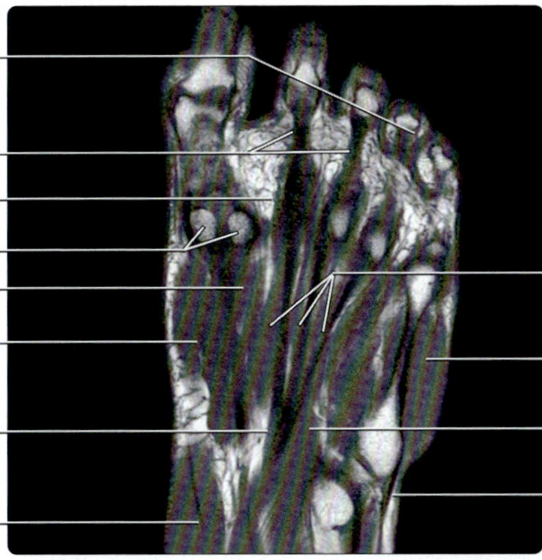

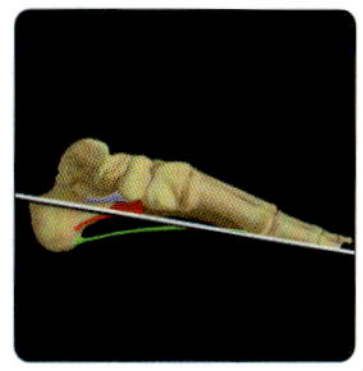

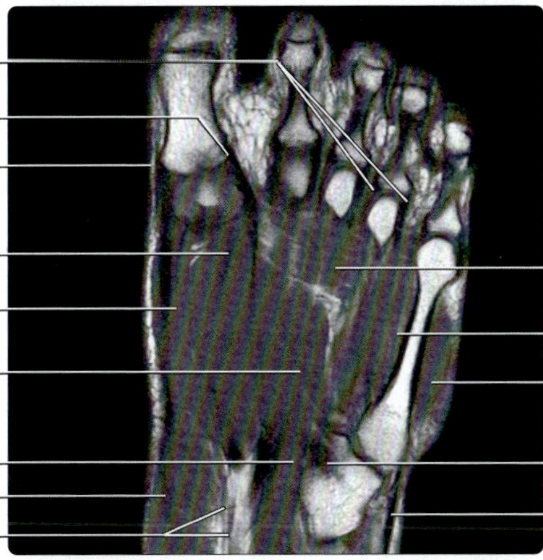

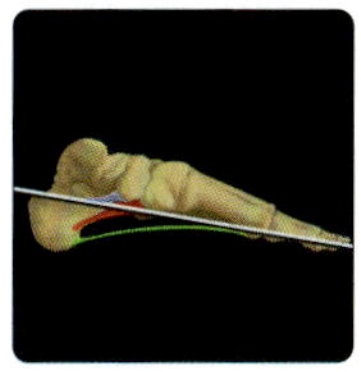

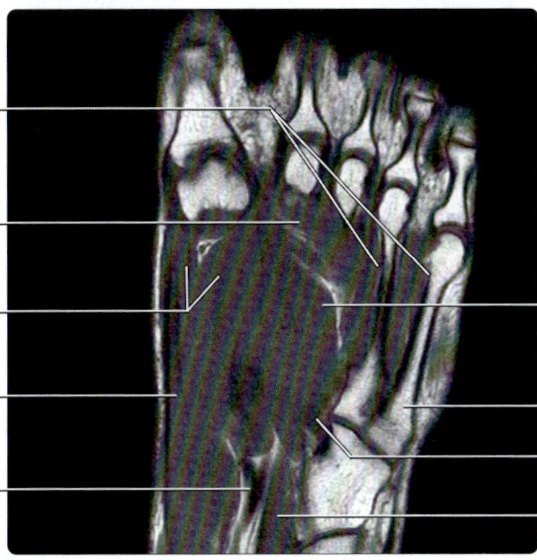

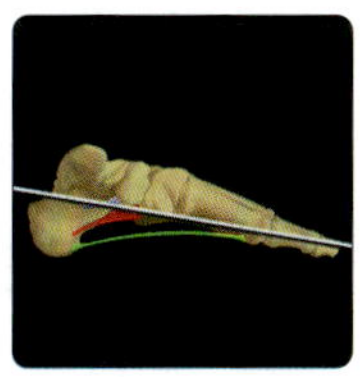

(Top) *Note the insertion of the quadratus plantae muscle into the flexor digitorum longus tendon just proximal to its division into slips to 4 lateral toes. The lumbrical muscles arise from individual slips of the flexor digitorum longus tendon and insert on the medial aspect of the proximal phalanx. A flexor digitorum longus tendon slip to 5th digit is variably present.* **(Middle)** *Terminology for adductor and abductor hallucis muscles becomes clear once it is remembered that the abductor pulls the 1st toe away from the 2nd toe, and the adductor pulls it toward the 2nd toe (i.e., axis of reference here is foot, not entire body).* **(Bottom)** *The oblique head of the adductor hallucis muscle is thick and broad, while the transverse head is thinner and sometimes congenitally absent.*

AXIAL LONG-AXIS T1 MR: RIGHT FOOT

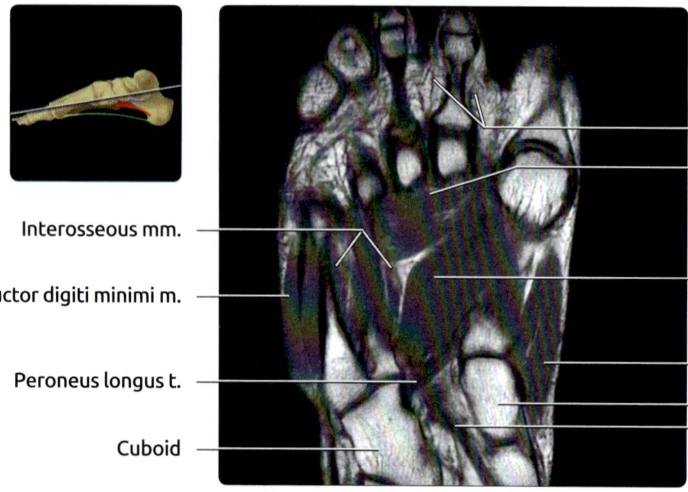

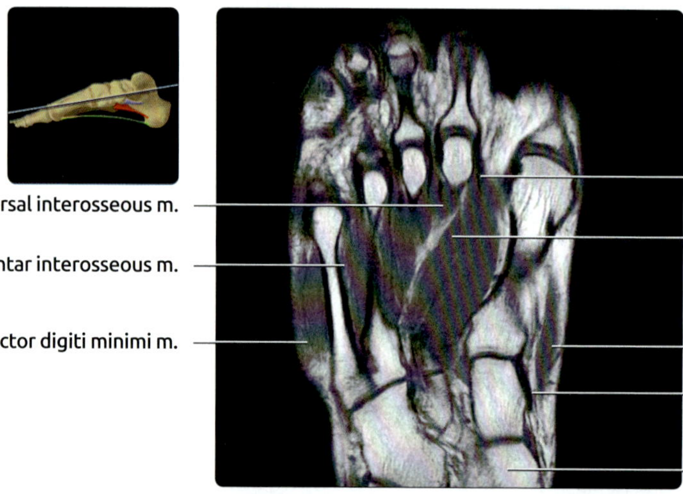

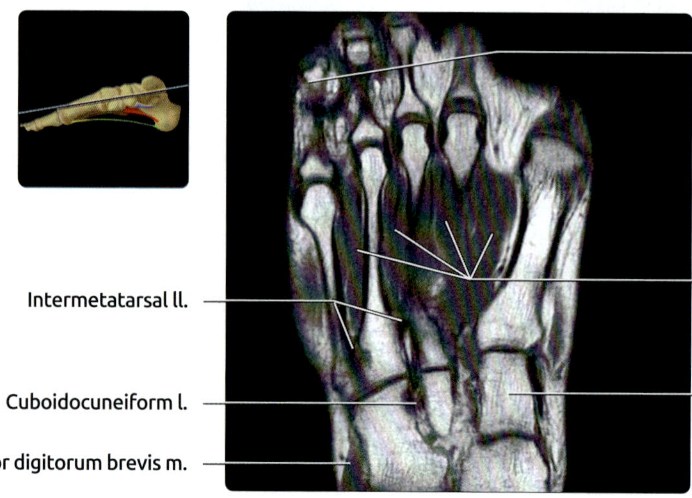

(Top) *The insertion of the peroneus longus tendon on the 1st metatarsal is well seen. Note the thread-like digital vessels at the medial and lateral margins of the 2nd toe.* **(Middle)** *The plantar interossei arise from the medial margin of 3 lateral toes and insert on the medial aspect of the base of their respective proximal phalanges.* **(Bottom)** *There are 4 dorsal interosseous muscles, each with 2 heads ("bipennate") arising from the bases of the adjacent metatarsals. The 1st dorsal interosseous inserts on the medial aspect of the 2nd proximal phalanx base, and the 2nd-4th on to the lateral aspect of the base of the 2nd-4th metatarsals.*

AXIAL LONG-AXIS T1 MR: LEFT FOOT

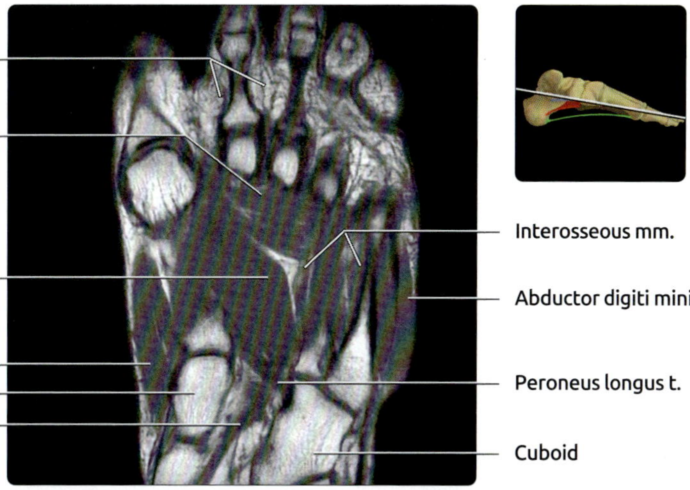

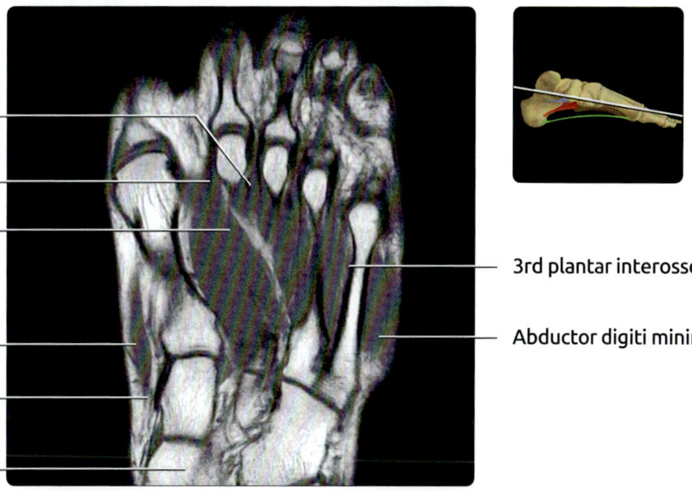

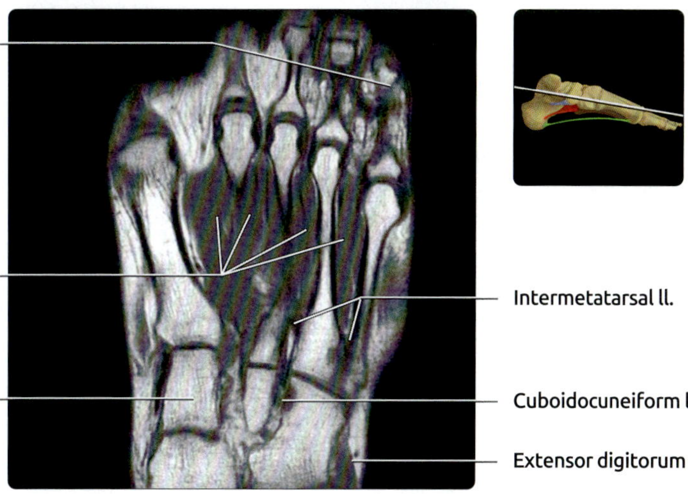

(Top) *The insertion of the peroneus longus tendon on the 1st metatarsal is well seen. Note the thread-like digital vessels at the medial and lateral margins of the 2nd toe.* **(Middle)** *The plantar interossei arise from the medial margin of the 3 lateral toes and insert on the medial aspect of the base of their respective proximal phalanges.* **(Bottom)** *There are 4 dorsal interosseous muscles, each with 2 heads ("bipennate") arising from the bases of the adjacent metatarsals. The 1st dorsal interosseous inserts on the medial aspect of the base of the 2nd proximal phalanx, and the 2nd-4th on to the lateral aspect of the base of the 2nd-4th metatarsals.*

AXIAL LONG-AXIS T1 MR: RIGHT FOOT

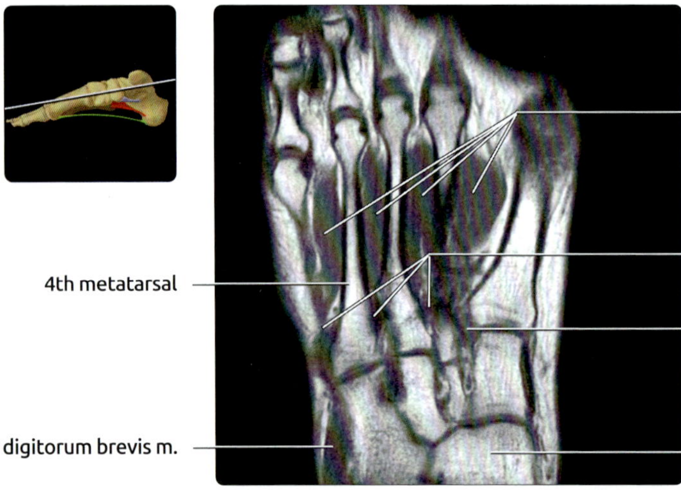

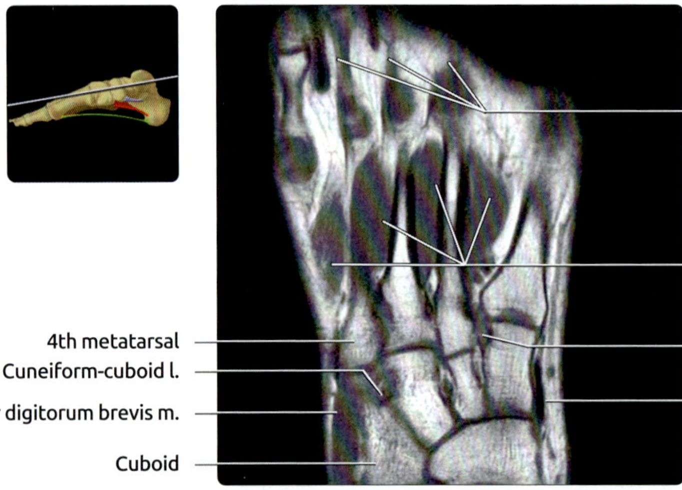

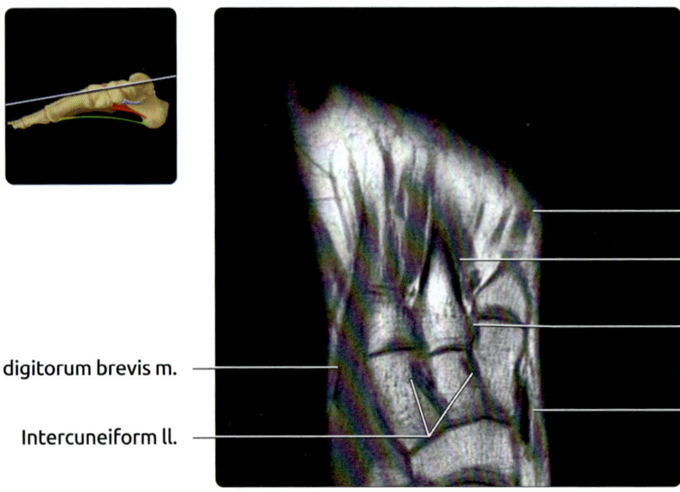

(Top) *The 2nd-5th metatarsal bases are joined by dorsal, interosseous, and plantar intermetatarsal ligaments. Stability between the 1st and 2nd rays is achieved by the 3 ligaments from the 1st cuneiform to the base of the 2nd metatarsal: Dorsal, interosseous, and plantar. The interosseous 1st cuneiform to the 2nd metatarsal ligament is the broadest and strongest and is a true Lisfranc ligament; however, "plantar" and "dorsal Lisfranc ligament" are terms that are commonly and appropriately used.* **(Middle)** *Note the articulations between the metatarsal bases. These are constant at the lateral toes, but variability is seen in the articulations between the 1st and 2nd metatarsals where an articulation is variably present.* **(Bottom)** *Extensor digitorum brevis muscle originates at the lateral margin of the calcaneus and fans out to toes. The tibialis anterior tendon wraps around the 1st cuneiform to insert on its plantar surface as well as on the plantar surface of the 1st metatarsal.*

AXIAL LONG-AXIS T1 MR: LEFT FOOT

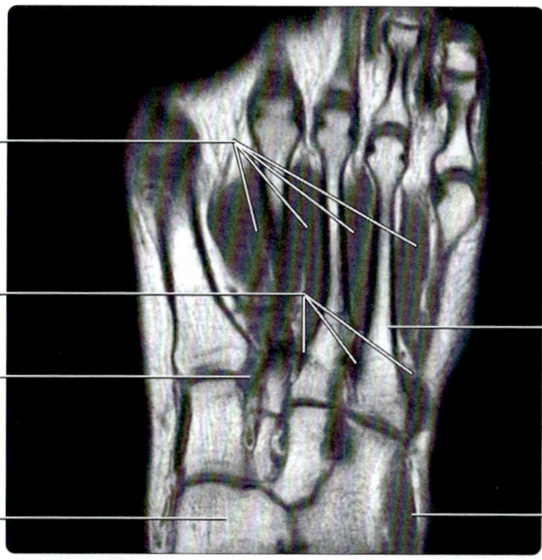

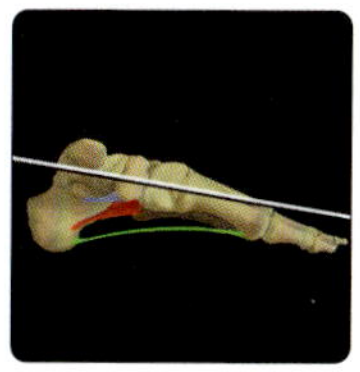

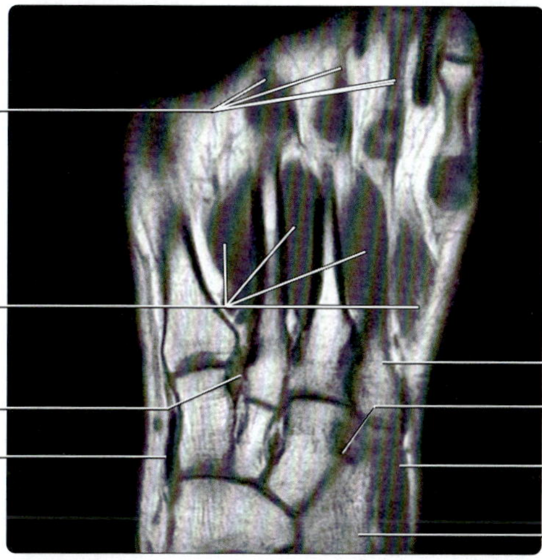

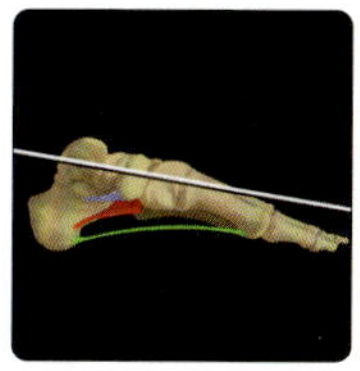

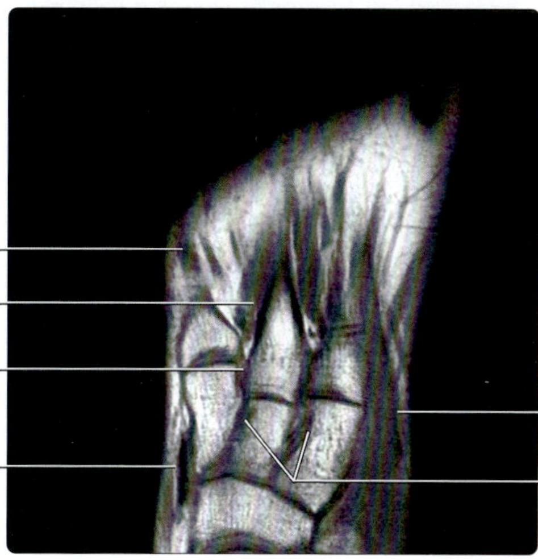

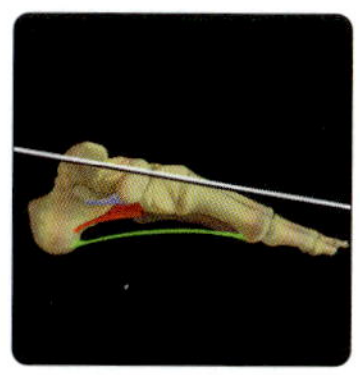

(Top) *The 2nd-5th metatarsal bases are joined by dorsal, interosseous, and plantar intermetatarsal ligaments. Stability between the 1st and 2nd rays is achieved by 3 ligaments from the 1st cuneiform to the base of the 2nd metatarsal: Dorsal, interosseous, and plantar. Interosseous 1st cuneiform to 2nd metatarsal ligament is broadest and strongest and is a true Lisfranc ligament; however, "plantar" and "dorsal Lisfranc ligament" are terms that are commonly and appropriately used.* **(Middle)** *Note the articulations between metatarsal bases. These are constant at the lateral toes, but variability is seen in the articulations between the 1st and 2nd metatarsals, where an articulation is variably present.* **(Bottom)** *The extensor digitorum brevis muscle originates at the lateral margin of the calcaneus and fans out to toes. The tibialis anterior tendon wraps around the 1st cuneiform to insert on its plantar surface as well as on the plantar surface of the 1st metatarsal.*

CORONAL SHORT-AXIS T1 MR: RIGHT FOOT

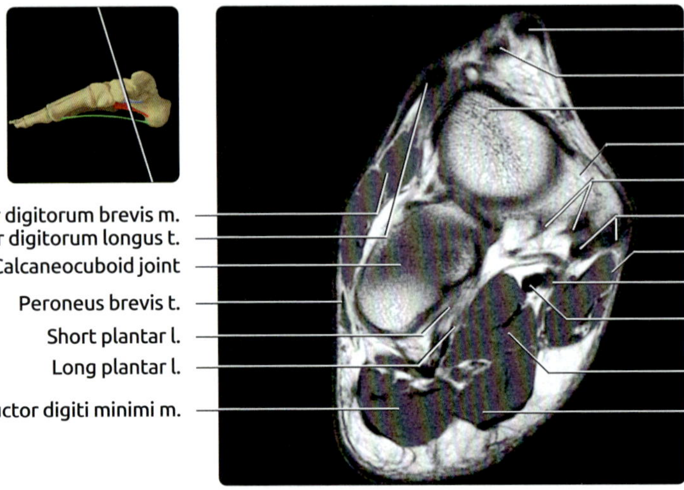

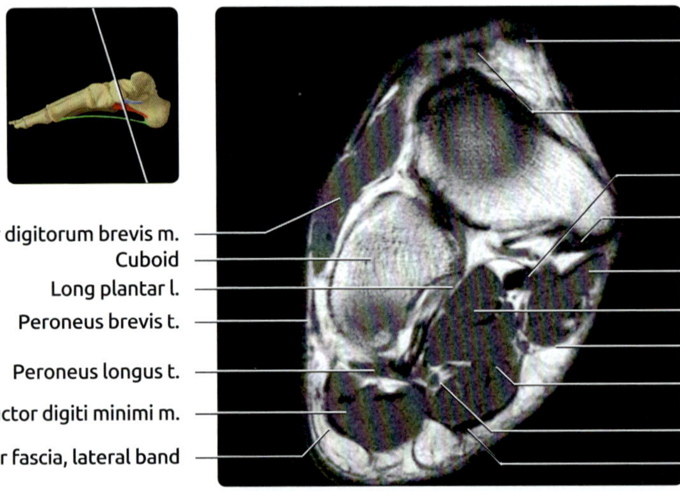

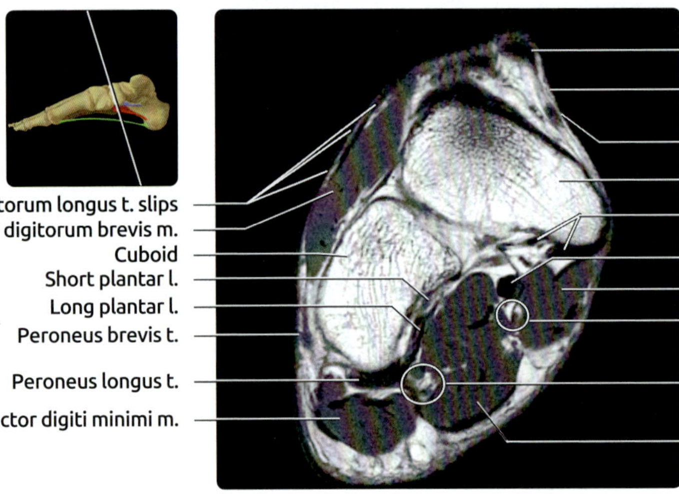

(Top) *First of 24 sequential coronal T1 MR images of the foot, from the Chopart joint to the phalanges, is shown. At the level of the talonavicular and calcaneocuboid joint (together known as the Chopart joint), the flexor digitorum longus and flexor hallucis longus tendons converge, exchanging fibers at the master knot of Henry.* **(Middle)** *Plantar fascia (aponeurosis) has 3 divisions: Medial overlies the abductor hallucis, central overlies the flexor digitorum brevis, and lateral overlies the abductor digiti minimi. The central portion is the strongest and functionally most important.* **(Bottom)** *The posterior tibial neurovascular bundle bifurcates into medial and lateral plantar divisions at the origin of the abductor hallucis muscle. The medial plantar neurovascular bundle courses between the abductor hallucis and quadratus plantae. The lateral plantar neurovascular bundle diverges laterally between the quadratus plantae and flexor digitorum brevis.*

CORONAL SHORT-AXIS T1 MR: LEFT FOOT

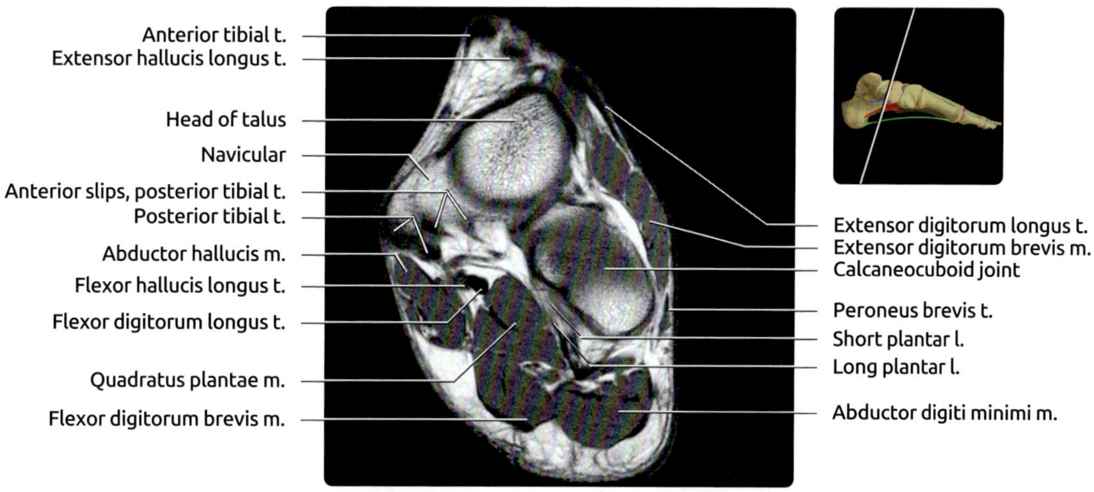

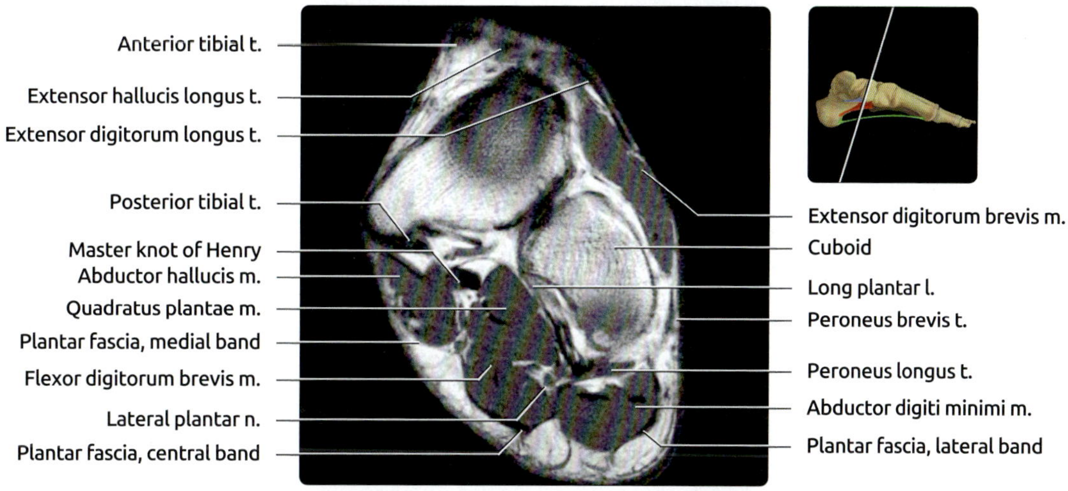

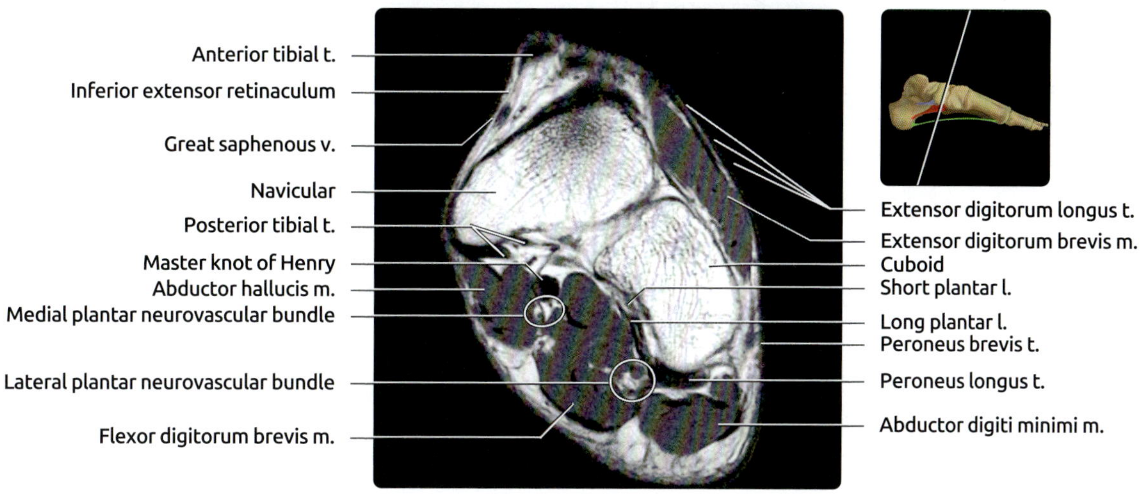

(Top) *At the level of the talonavicular and calcaneocuboid joint (together known as Chopart joint), the flexor digitorum longus and flexor hallucis longus tendons converge, exchanging fibers at the master knot of Henry.* **(Middle)** *Plantar fascia (aponeurosis) has 3 divisions: Medial overlies the abductor hallucis, central overlies the flexor digitorum brevis, and lateral overlies the abductor digiti minimi. The central portion is the strongest and functionally most important.* **(Bottom)** *The posterior tibial neurovascular bundle bifurcates into medial and lateral plantar divisions at the origin of the abductor hallucis muscle. The medial plantar neurovascular bundle courses between the abductor hallucis and quadratus plantae. The lateral plantar neurovascular bundle diverges laterally between the quadratus plantae and flexor digitorum brevis.*

CORONAL SHORT-AXIS T1 MR: RIGHT FOOT

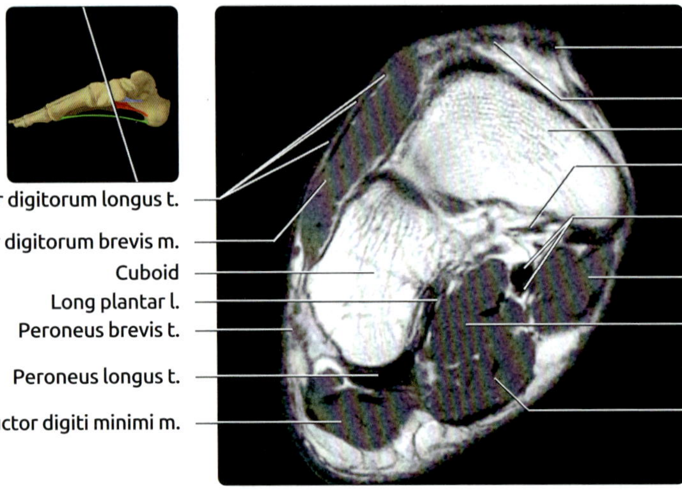

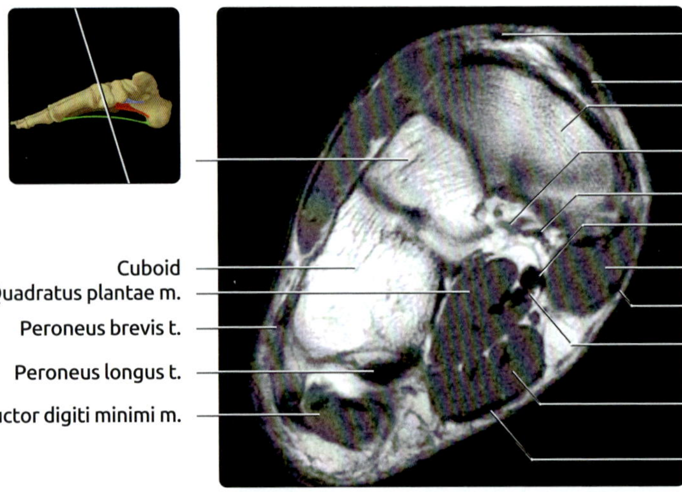

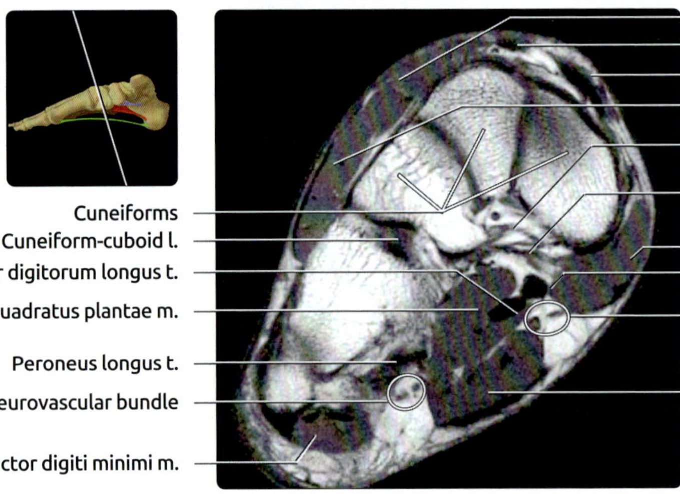

(Top) *The peroneus longus tendon begins to curve medially beneath the plantar aspect of the cuboid. Long plantar ligament superficial fibers form the roof, and deep fibers form the floor of the tunnel through which it passes.* **(Middle)** *The navicular and cuneiforms are bridged by plantar cuneonavicular ligaments, which lie deep to the anterior slips of the posterior tibial tendon.* **(Bottom)** *The quadratus plantae muscle has a broad insertion on the flexor digitorum longus tendon. The anterior tibial tendon is turning medially towards its insertion on the plantar aspect of the 1st cuneiform and 1st metatarsal.*

CORONAL SHORT-AXIS T1 MR: LEFT FOOT

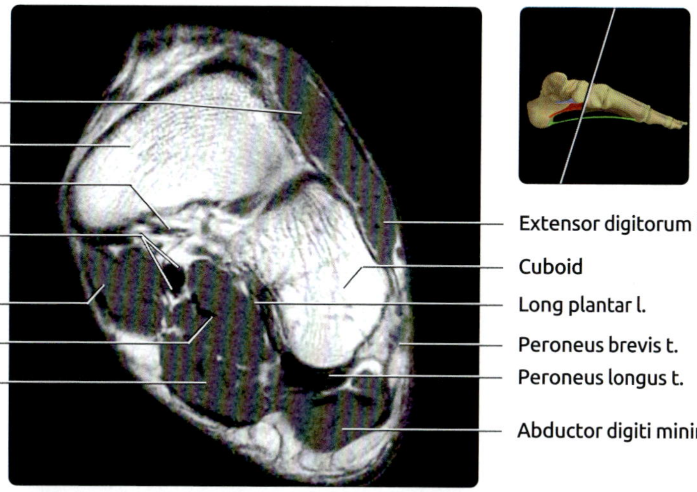

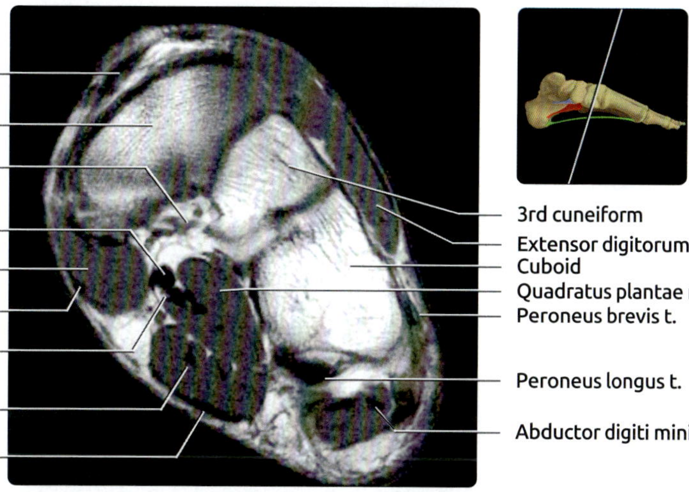

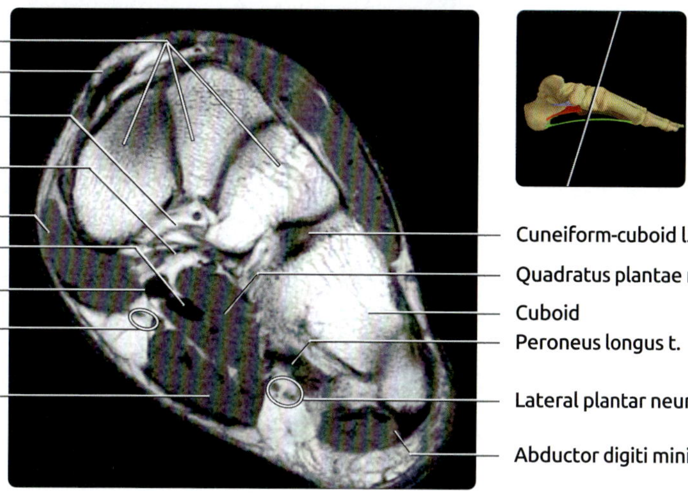

(Top) *The peroneus longus tendon begins to curve medially beneath the plantar aspect of the cuboid. The long plantar ligament superficial fibers form the roof, and deep fibers form the floor of the tunnel through which it passes.* **(Middle)** *The navicular and cuneiforms are bridged by plantar cuneonavicular ligaments, which lie deep to the anterior slips of the tibialis posterior tendon.* **(Bottom)** *The quadratus plantae muscle has a broad insertion on the flexor digitorum longus tendon. The anterior tibial tendon is turning medially towards its insertion on the plantar aspect of the 1st cuneiform and 1st metatarsal.*

CORONAL SHORT-AXIS T1 MR: RIGHT FOOT

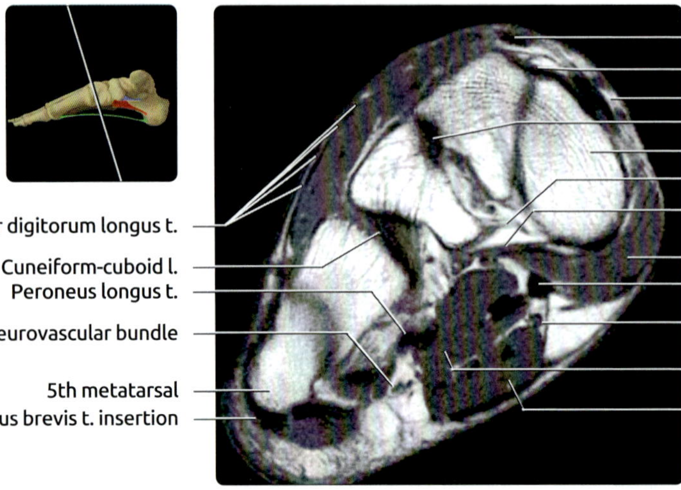

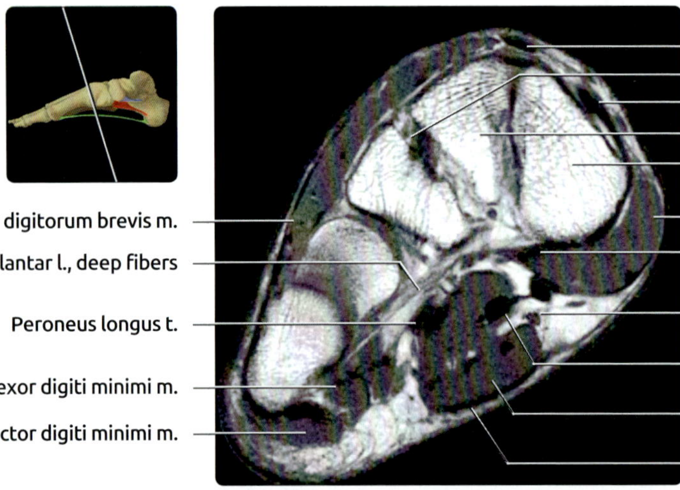

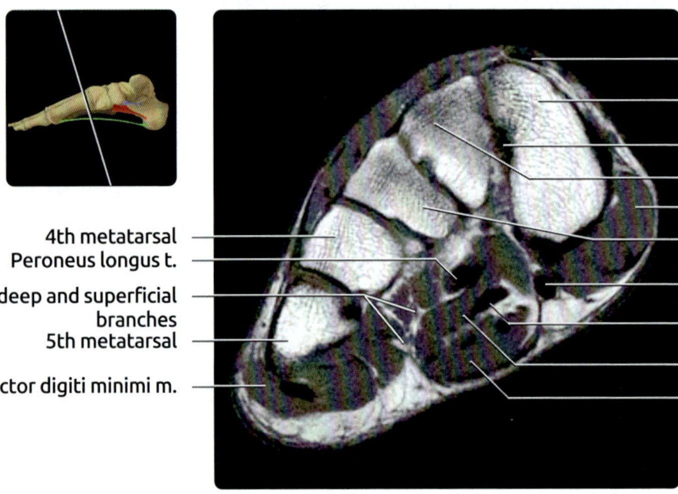

(Top) *The wedge shape of the cuneiform bones create the transverse arch. They are held in position by the dorsal, plantar, and interosseous ligaments.* **(Middle)** *At this level, the 3 major compartmental divisions of the plantar muscles are well seen: The medial compartment beneath the 1st ray, the lateral compartment beneath the 5th ray, and the middle compartment beneath the 2nd-4th rays. The compartments are separated by vertically oriented fascial layers.* **(Bottom)** *The interosseous Lisfranc ligament is seen at its origin from the 1st cuneiform.*

CORONAL SHORT-AXIS T1 MR: LEFT FOOT

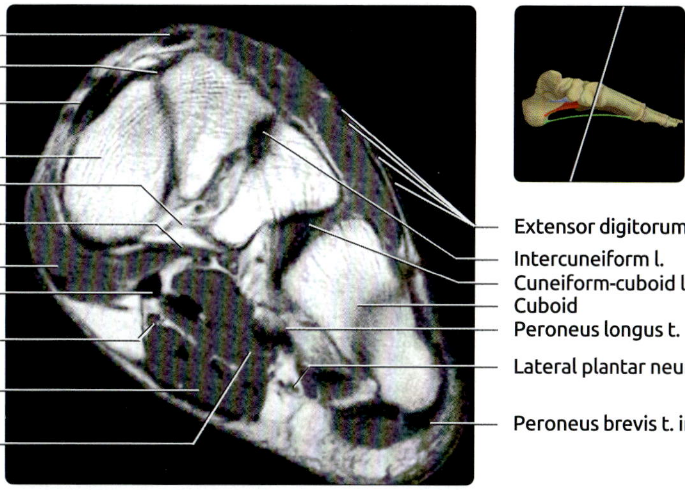

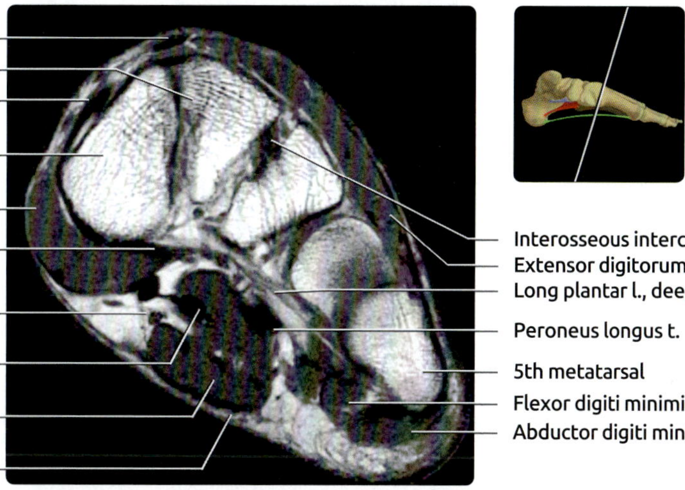

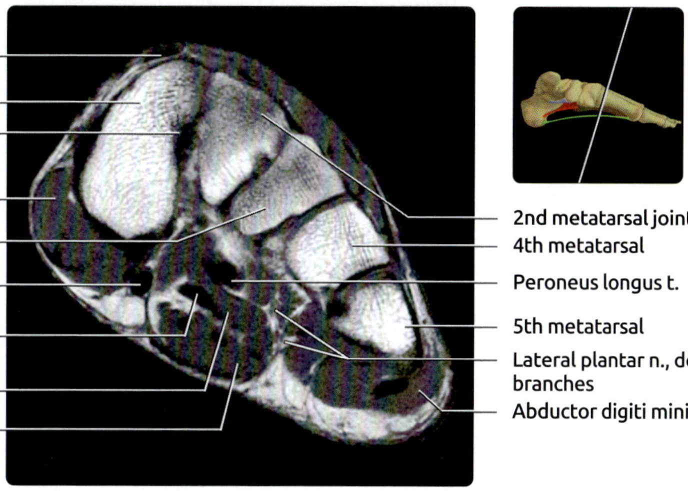

(Top) *The cuneiform bones form the transverse arch by virtue of their wedge shape. They are held in position by the dorsal, plantar, and interosseous ligaments.* **(Middle)** *At this level, the 3 major compartmental divisions of plantar muscles are well seen: The medial compartment beneath the 1st ray, the lateral compartment beneath the 5th ray, and the middle compartment beneath the 2nd-4th rays. The compartments are separated by vertically oriented fascial layers.* **(Bottom)** *The interosseous Lisfranc ligament is seen at its origin from the 1st cuneiform.*

CORONAL SHORT-AXIS T1 MR: RIGHT FOOT

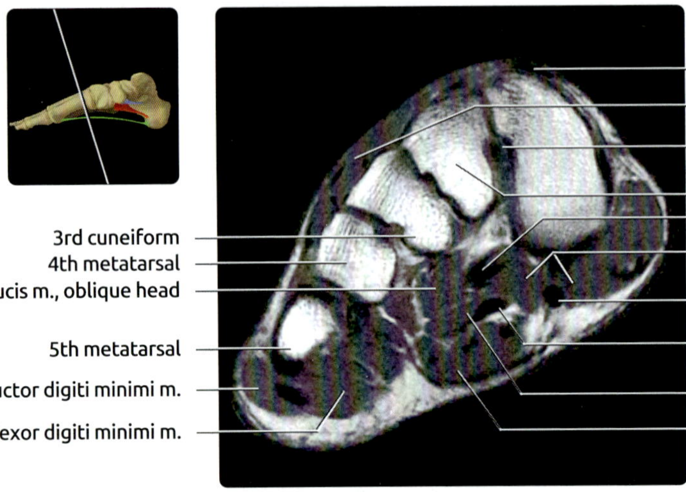

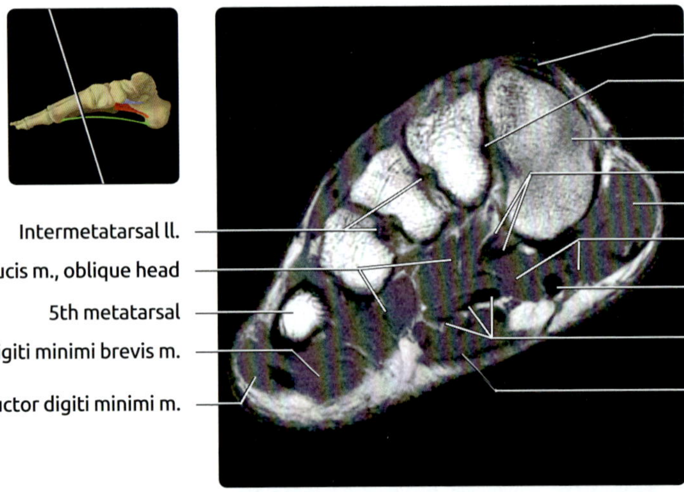

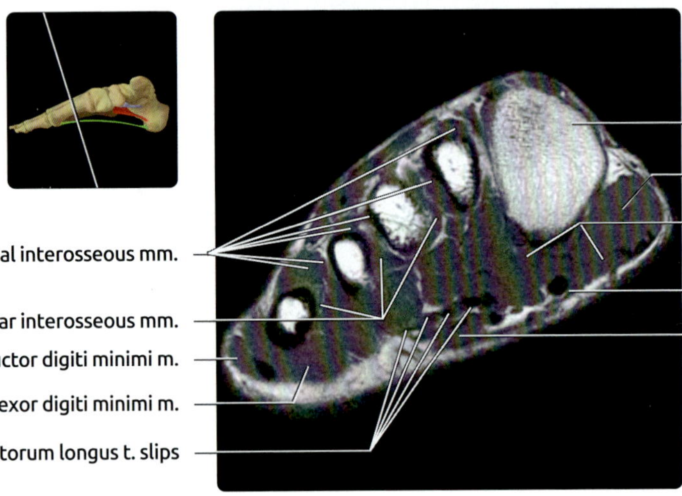

(Top) *The Lisfranc ligament courses distally between the 1st cuneiform and 2nd cuneiform, attaching to the medial margin of the 2nd metatarsal base. It consists of distinct dorsal, interosseous, and plantar bands. The interosseous band is the strongest portion.* **(Middle)** *The peroneus longus tendon ends in slips attaching to the base of the 1st metatarsal, the 1st cuneiform, and sometimes, the base of the 2nd metatarsal. The oblique head of the adductor hallucis muscle originates from the bases of the 3rd and 4th metatarsals and from the tendon sheath of the peroneus longus.* **(Bottom)** *The flexor hallucis brevis muscle has 2 heads, and the flexor hallucis longus tendon is centered between them. The abductor hallucis muscle is closely apposed to the medial head of the flexor hallucis brevis muscle.*

CORONAL SHORT-AXIS T1 MR: LEFT FOOT

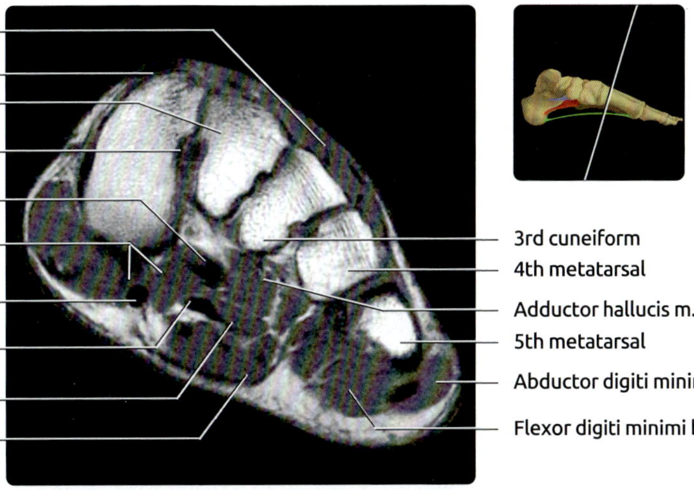

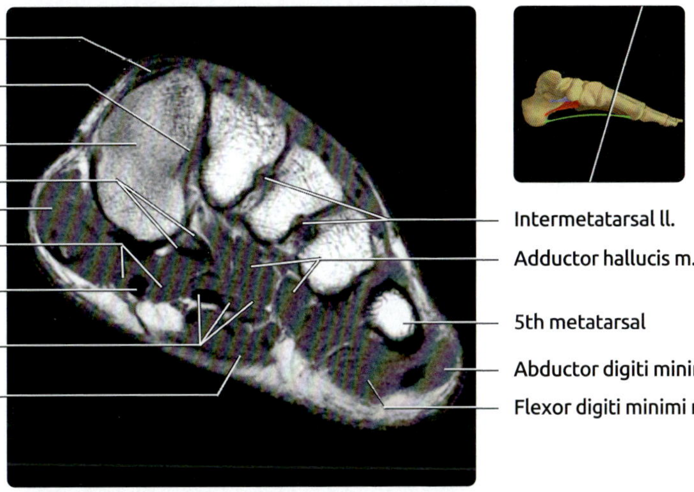

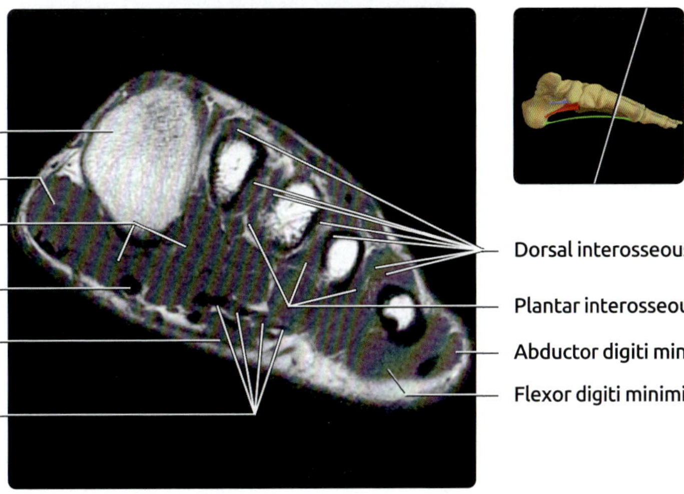

(Top) *The Lisfranc ligament courses distally between the 1st cuneiform and 2nd cuneiform, attaching to the medial margin of the 2nd metatarsal base. It consists of distinct dorsal, interosseous, and plantar bands. The interosseous band is the strongest portion.* **(Middle)** *The peroneus longus tendon ends in slips attaching to the base of the 1st metatarsal, the 1st cuneiform and sometimes, the base of the 2nd metatarsal. The oblique head of the adductor hallucis muscle originates from the bases of the 3rd and 4th metatarsals and from the tendon sheath of the peroneus longus.* **(Bottom)** *The flexor hallucis brevis muscle has 2 heads, and the flexor hallucis longus tendon is centered between them. The abductor hallucis muscle is closely apposed to the medial head of the flexor hallucis brevis muscle.*

CORONAL SHORT-AXIS T1 MR: RIGHT FOOT

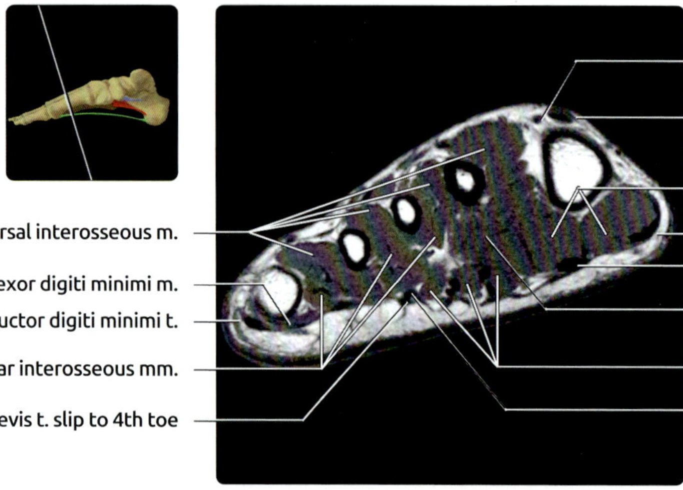

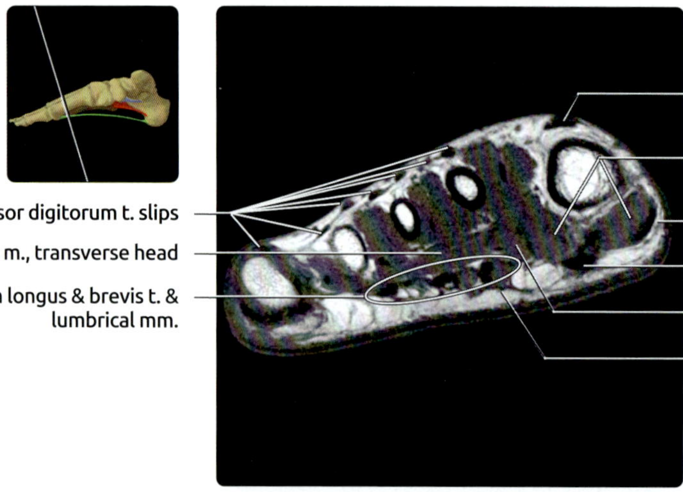

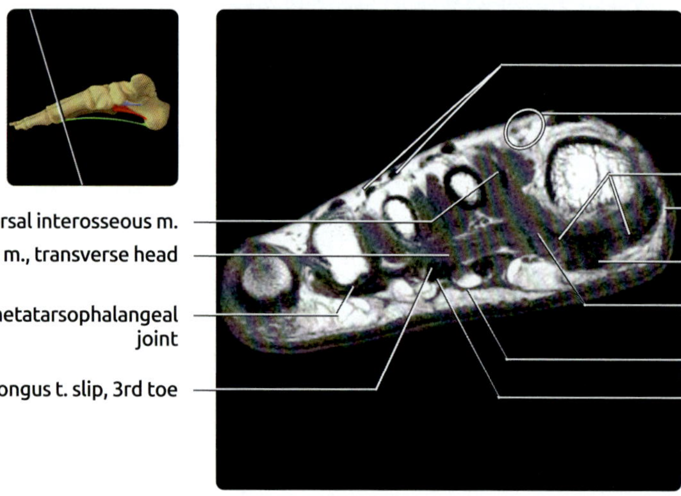

(Top) *The flexor digitorum brevis and longus tendons have divided into individual slips to the toes. The brevis tendon slips are superficial to those of the longus tendon. The lumbrical muscles are seen adjacent to the flexor digitorum longus tendon slips.* **(Middle)** *Transverse head of adductor hallucis muscle supports metatarsal heads. It may be congenitally absent. Transverse and oblique heads are shown converging towards their attachment on the lateral sesamoid of the great toe.* **(Bottom)** *The plantar fascia sends fibers dorsally and superficially in an arborizing pattern.*

CORONAL SHORT-AXIS T1 MR: LEFT FOOT

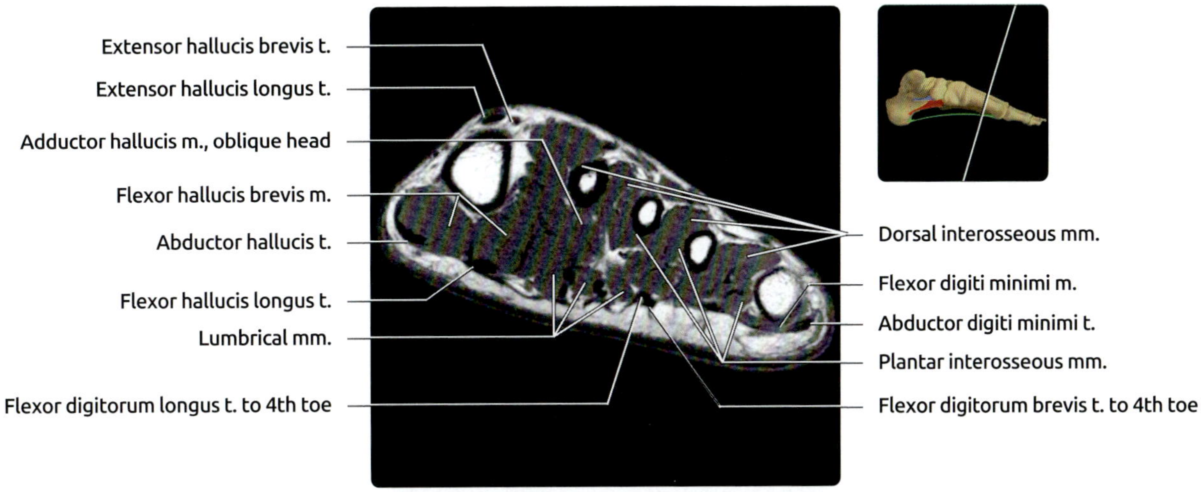

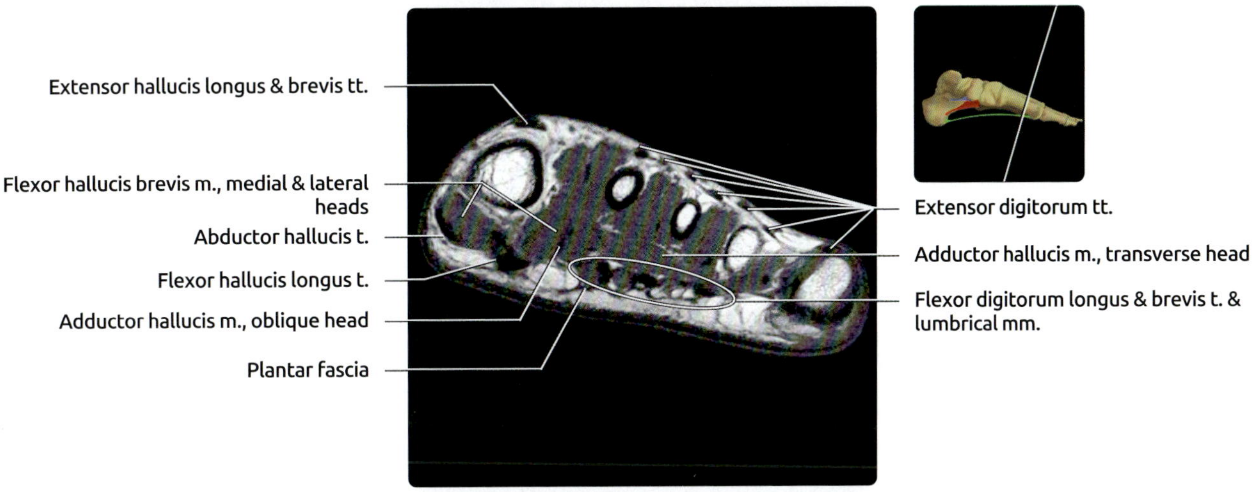

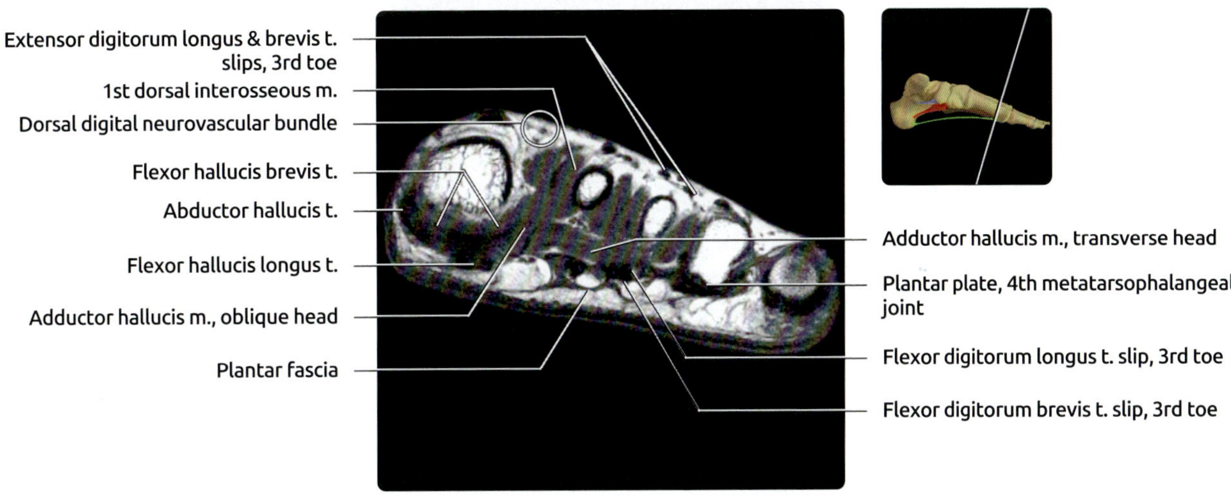

(Top) *The flexor digitorum brevis and longus tendons have divided into individual slips to the toes. The brevis tendon slips are superficial to those of the longus tendon. The lumbrical muscles are seen adjacent to the flexor digitorum longus tendon slips.* **(Middle)** *The transverse head of the adductor hallucis muscle supports the metatarsal heads. It may be congenitally absent. The transverse and oblique heads are shown converging towards their attachment on the lateral sesamoid of the great toe.* **(Bottom)** *The plantar fascia sends fibers dorsally and superficially in an arborizing pattern.*

CORONAL SHORT-AXIS T1 MR: RIGHT FOOT

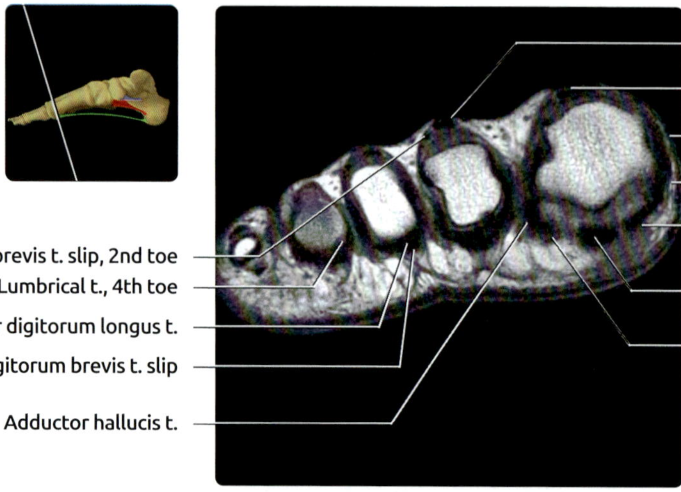

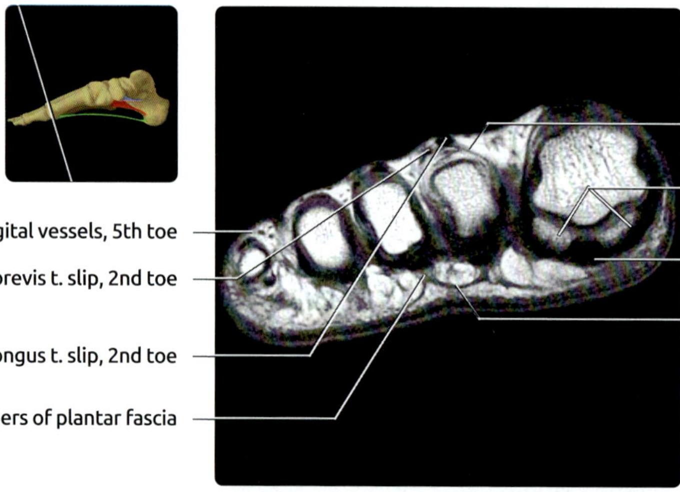

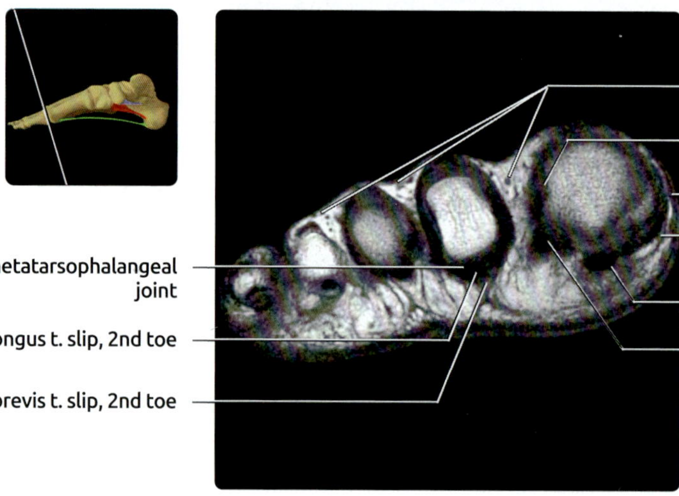

(Top) *The flexor digitorum longus and brevis tendons are centered beneath the metatarsal heads, with the brevis superficial to the longus, in close proximity to the plantar plate of the metatarsophalangeal joints. Lumbrical muscles course medial to the metatarsal heads and will insert on the medial margin of the proximal phalanges.* **(Middle)** *The medial sesamoid of the 1st toe is in the tendon of the medial head of the flexor hallucis brevis tendon and is also attached to the adductor hallucis tendon. The lateral sesamoid is in the lateral head of the flexor hallucis brevis tendon and is also attached to the abductor hallucis tendon. The flexor hallucis longus tendon courses between the sesamoids. Fibrous septa extending from the main portion of plantar fascia to the metatarsophalangeal joints are well seen on this image.* **(Bottom)** *The plantar plate extends from the metatarsal neck to the base of the proximal phalanx and is an important stabilizer of the MTP joints.*

CORONAL SHORT-AXIS T1 MR: LEFT FOOT

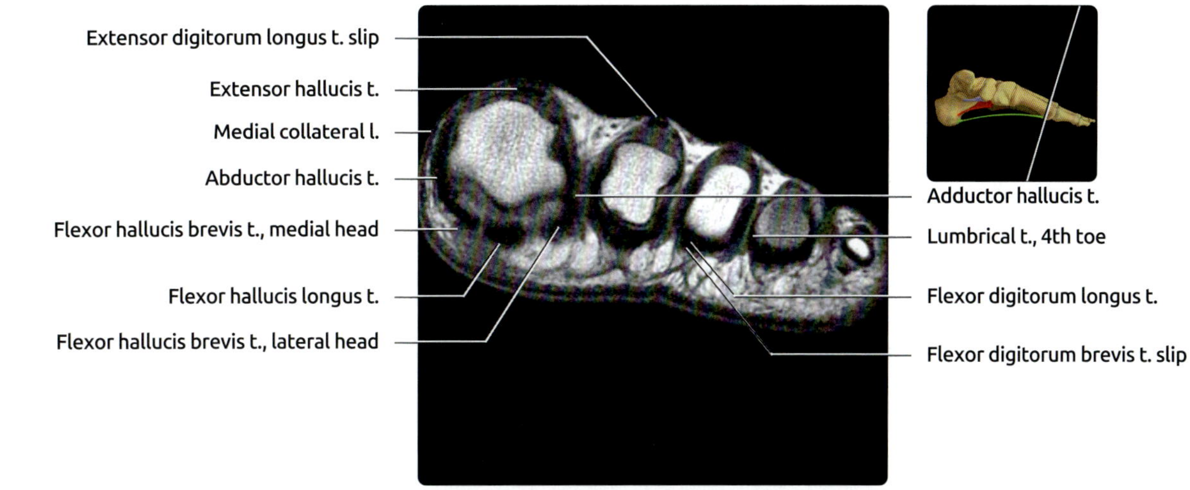

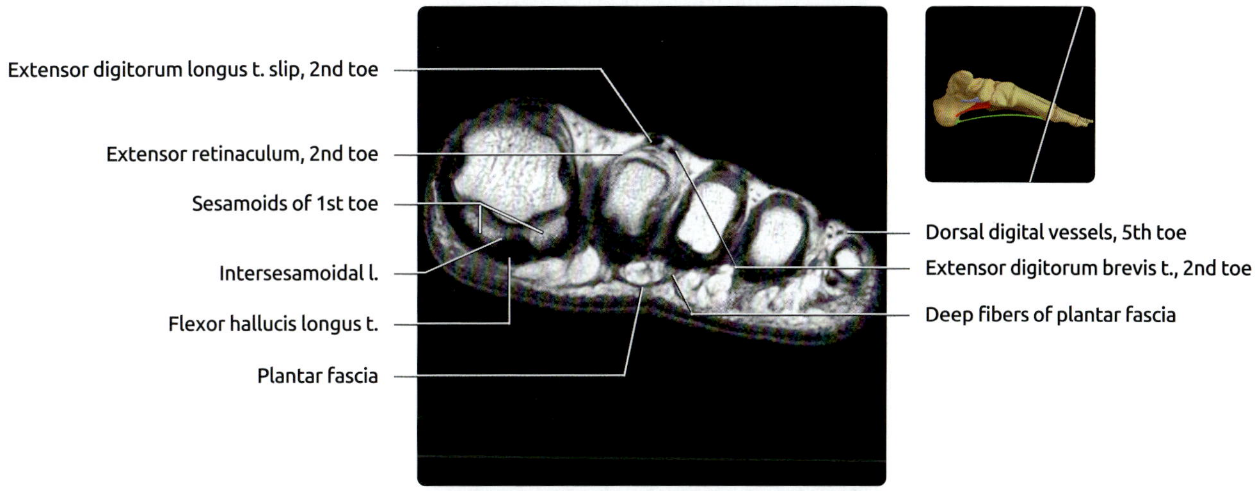

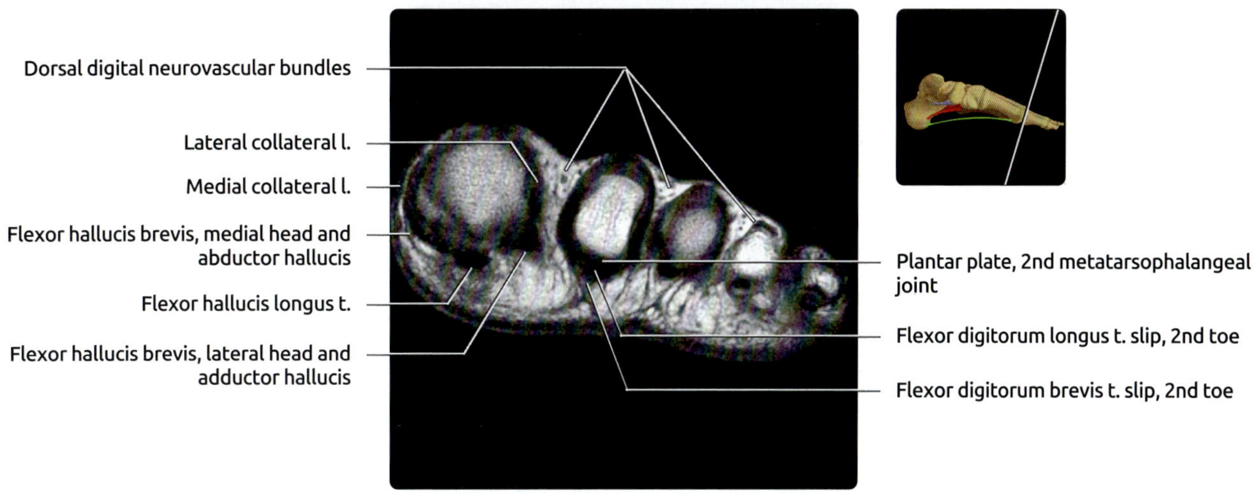

(Top) *The flexor digitorum longus and brevis tendons are centered beneath metatarsal heads, with brevis superficial to longus, in close proximity to the plantar plate of the metatarsophalangeal joints. The lumbrical muscles course medial to the metatarsal heads and will insert on the medial margin of the proximal phalanges.* **(Middle)** *The medial sesamoid of the 1st toe is in the tendon of the medial head flexor hallucis brevis tendon, and is also attached to the adductor hallucis tendon. The lateral sesamoid is in the lateral head flexor hallucis brevis tendon, and is also attached to the abductor hallucis tendon. The flexor hallucis longus tendon courses between the sesamoids. Fibrous septa extending from the main portion of plantar fascia to the MTP joints are well seen on this image.* **(Bottom)** *The plantar plate extends from the metatarsal neck to the base of the proximal phalanx and is an important stabilizer of the MTP joints.*

CORONAL SHORT-AXIS T1 MR: RIGHT FOOT

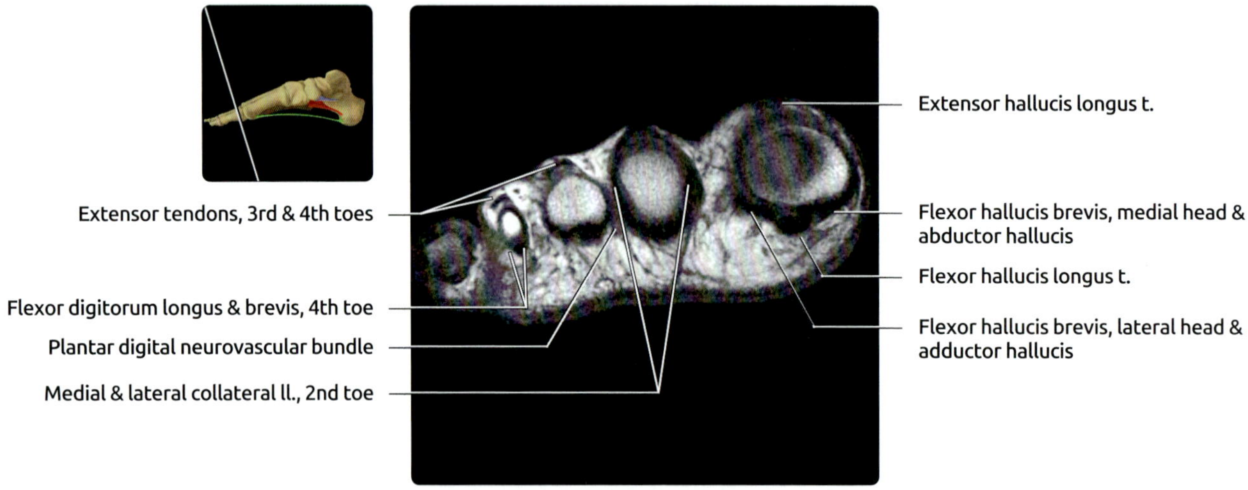

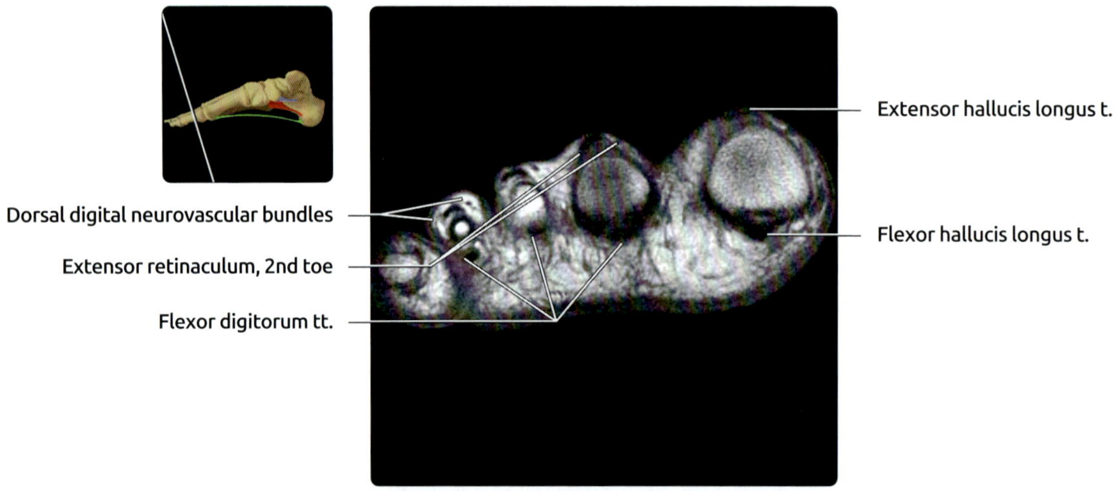

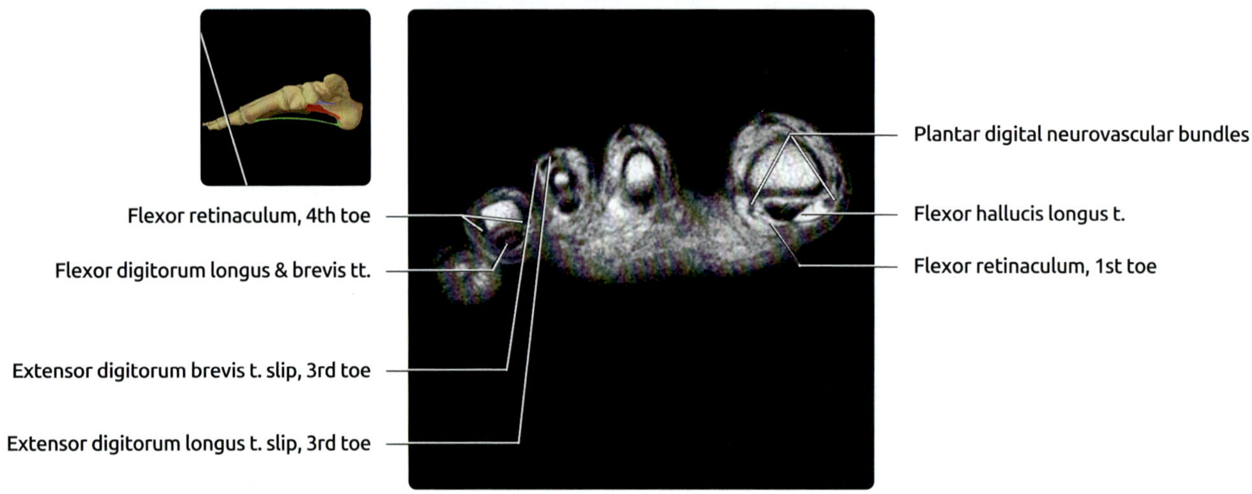

(Top) *The plantar vessels and nerves lie between the metatarsal heads where nerves are susceptible to compression.* **(Middle)** *The extensor retinacula are seen superficial to the extensor tendons and attaching to the dorsolateral margins of the phalanges. The flexor retinacula are not well seen on this image because of their obliquity to the imaging plane. At the level of the proximal phalanges, the flexor digitorum brevis tendons split into medial and lateral slips, which attach to the middle phalanges. The flexor digitorum longus tendon courses between them. The tiny slips are difficult to distinguish on MR. Dorsal digital neurovascular bundles are present at the medial and lateral aspects of the digits.* **(Bottom)** *The flexor digitorum brevis divides into 2 tendon slips to each toe, inserting on the middle phalanx. The flexor digitorum longus has a single slip that passes between them to insert on the distal phalanx.*

CORONAL SHORT-AXIS T1 MR: LEFT FOOT

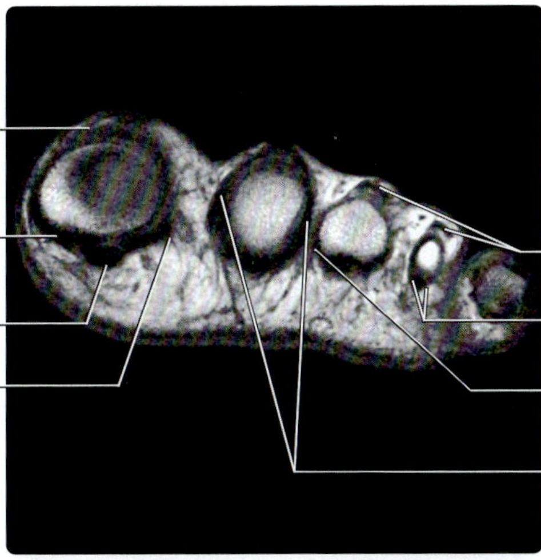

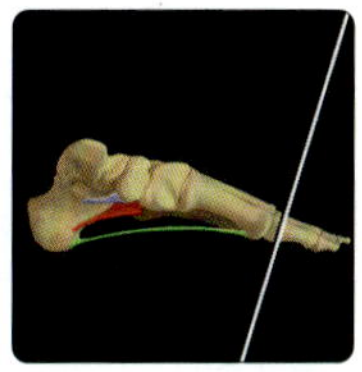

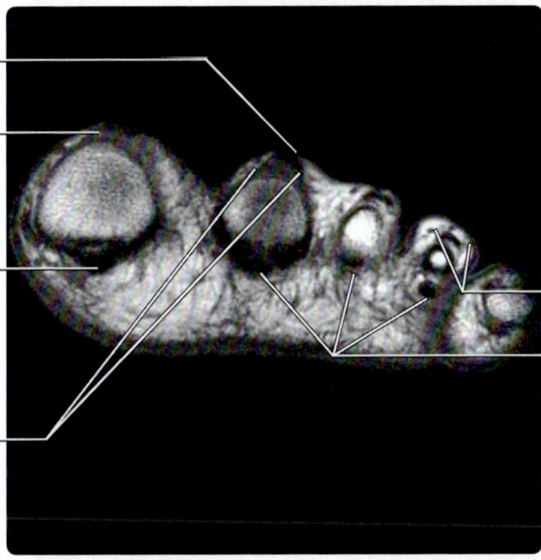

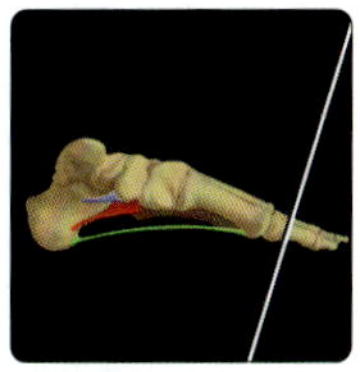

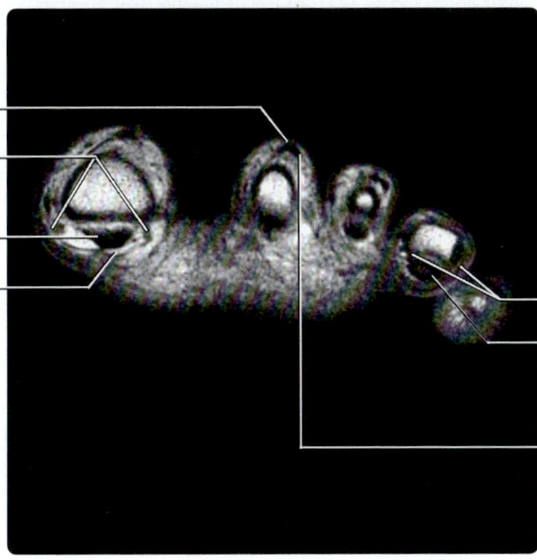

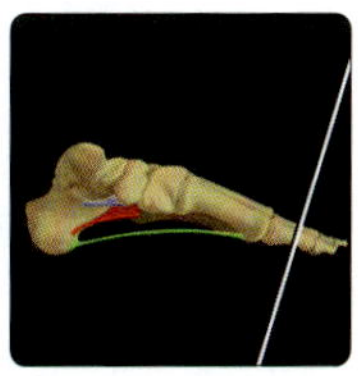

(Top) *The plantar vessels and nerves lie between the metatarsal heads where the nerves are susceptible to compression.* **(Middle)** *The extensor retinacula are seen superficial to the extensor tendons and attaching to the dorsolateral margins of the phalanges. The flexor retinacula are not well seen on this image because of their obliquity to the imaging plane. At the level of the proximal phalanges, the flexor digitorum brevis tendons split into medial and lateral slips, which attach to the middle phalanges. The flexor digitorum longus tendon courses between them. The tiny slips are difficult to distinguish on MR. Dorsal digital neurovascular bundles are present at medial and lateral aspects of digits.* **(Bottom)** *The flexor digitorum brevis divides into 2 tendon slips to each toe, inserting on the middle phalanx. The flexor digitorum longus has a single slip that passes between them to insert on the distal phalanx.*

SAGITTAL T1 MR: FOOT

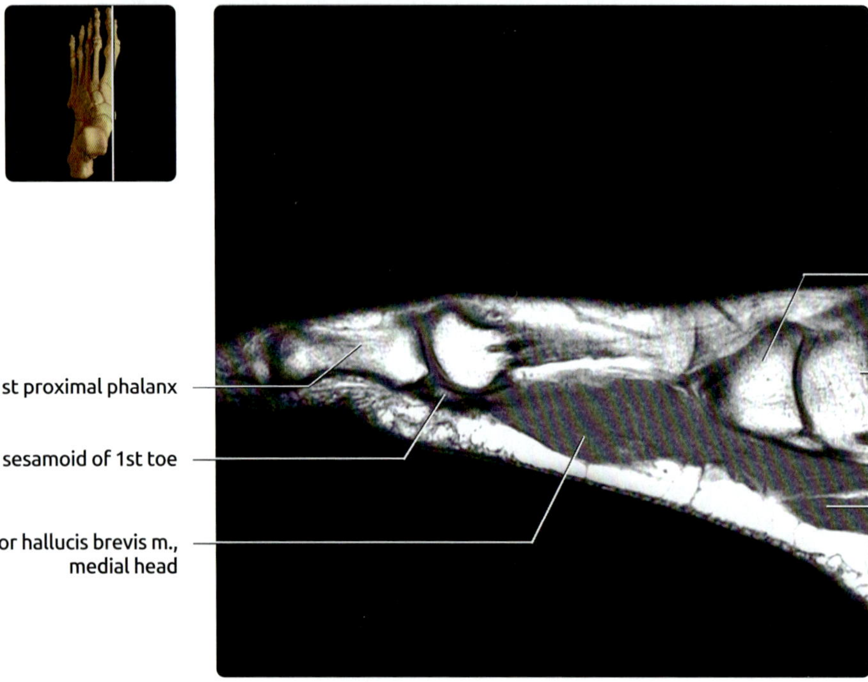

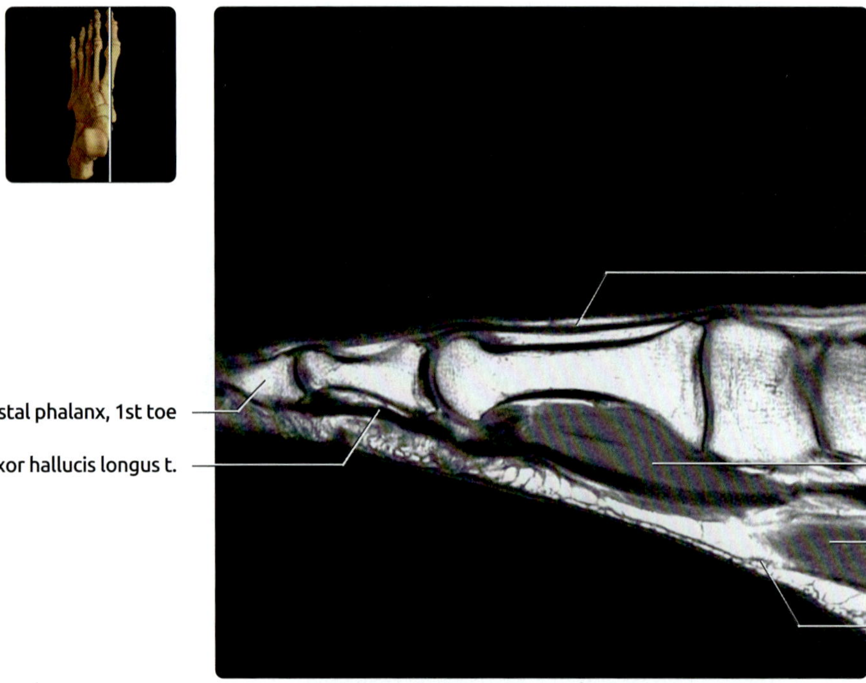

(Top) *First of 16 sagittal MR images shows the forefoot from medial to lateral, aligned along the axis of the 1st metatarsal. The abductor hallucis muscle lies medial to the 1st metatarsal, while the flexor hallucis brevis lies beneath it.* **(Bottom)** *The flexor hallucis longus tendon courses between the sesamoids of the 1st toe and inserts on the distal phalanx of the 1st toe. The extensor hallucis brevis tendon lies lateral to the longus tendon and inserts on the proximal phalanx of the 1st toe.*

SAGITTAL T1 MR: FOOT

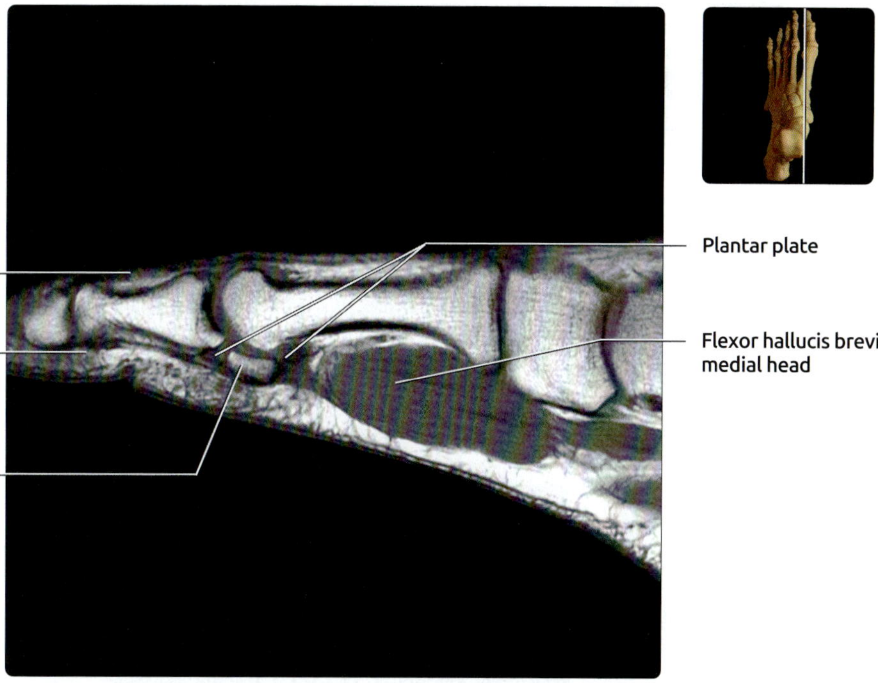

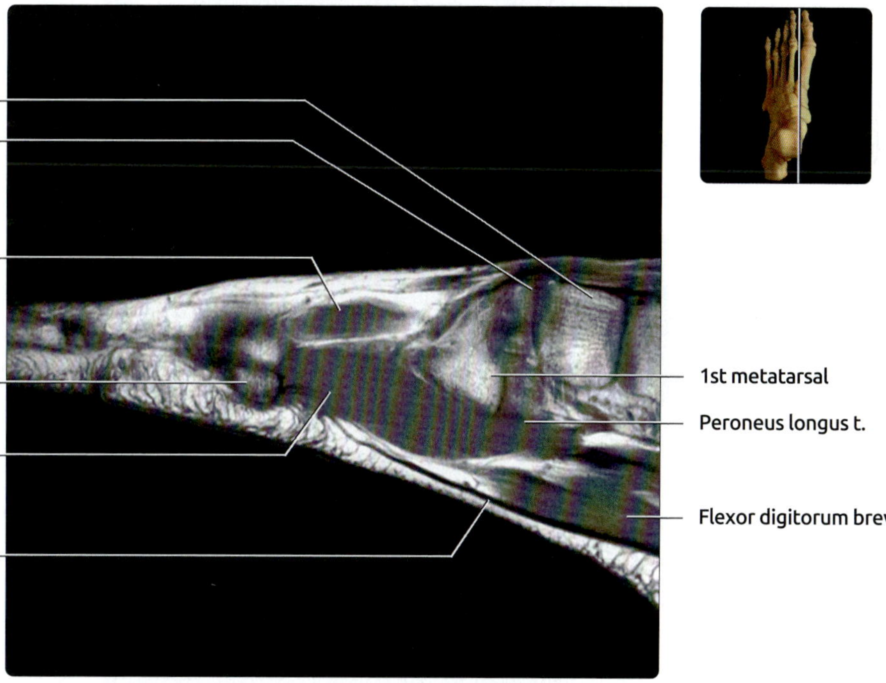

(Top) *The plantar plate of the 1st metatarsophalangeal joint is a strong fibrocartilaginous thickening of the plantar joint capsule. It is attached to both sesamoids, the metatarsal neck, the medial and lateral collateral ligaments, and the base of the proximal phalanx.* **(Bottom)** *The distal portion of the peroneus longus tendon is seen attaching to the 1st metatarsal base.*

SAGITTAL T1 MR: FOOT

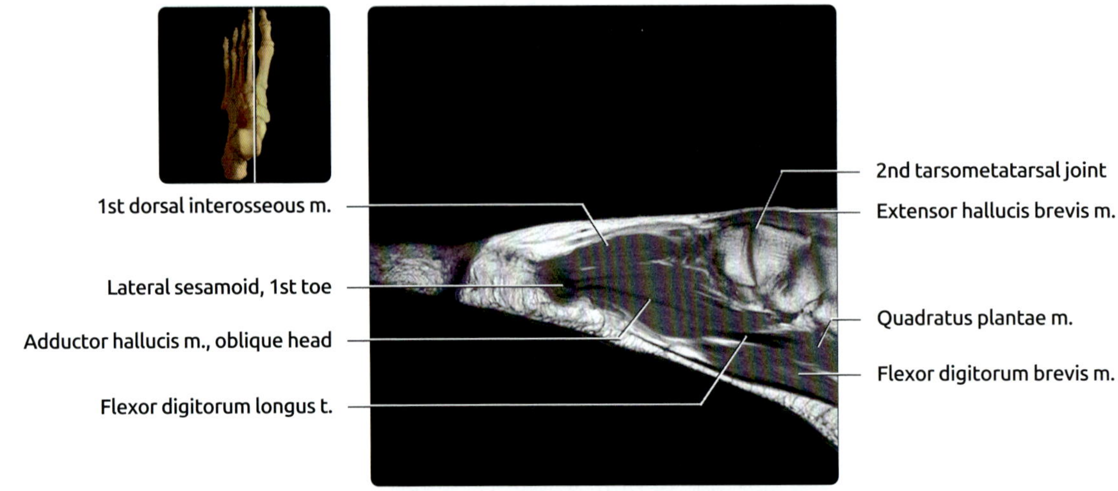

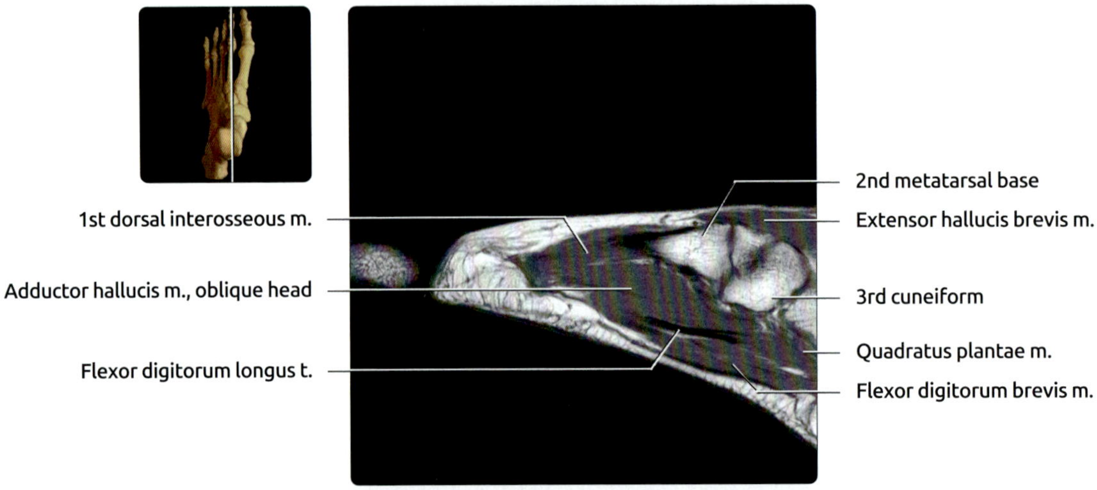

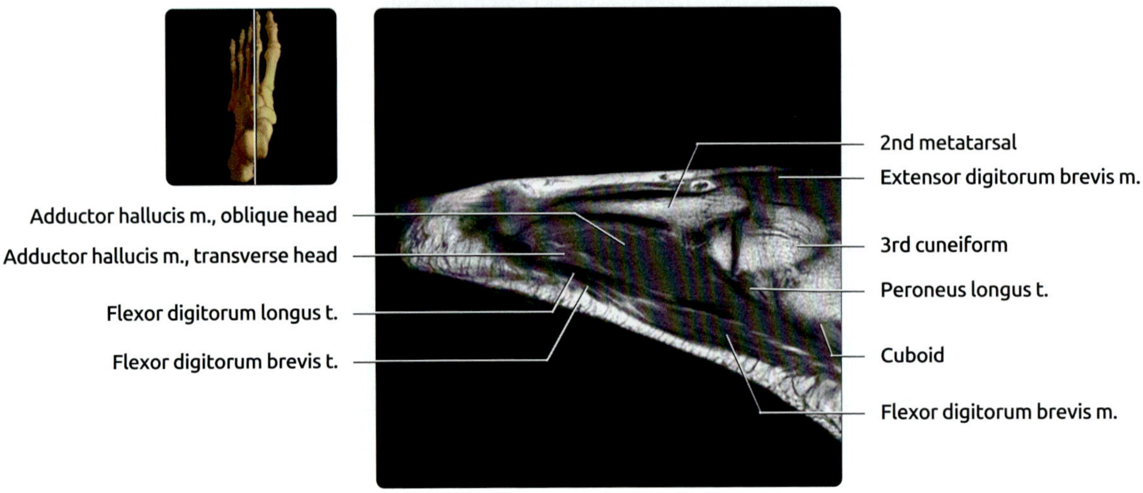

(Top) *The thick, broad adductor hallucis muscle is seen attaching to the lateral sesamoid of the 1st toe. The quadratus plantae muscle is seen attaching to the flexor digitorum longus tendon.* **(Middle)** *Interspace between the 1st and 2nd metatarsals contains only a dorsal interosseous muscle, attaching to the medial aspect of the 2nd proximal phalanx. The remaining intermetatarsal interspaces contain dorsal and plantar interosseous muscles. The dorsal muscles attach to the lateral aspect of proximal phalangeal bases 2-4, and the plantar muscles attach to the medial aspect of proximal phalangeal bases 3-5.* **(Bottom)** *The flexor digitorum brevis muscle divides into slips to toes 2-4, and sometimes 5, at the level of the metatarsal shafts. The tendons are superficial to the flexor digitorum longus tendons.*

SAGITTAL T1 MR: FOOT

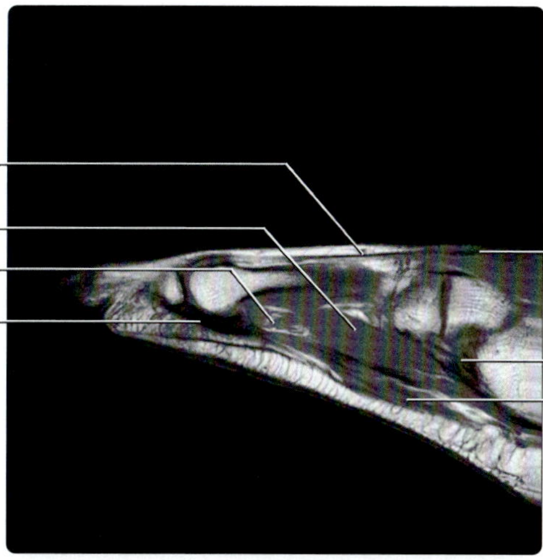

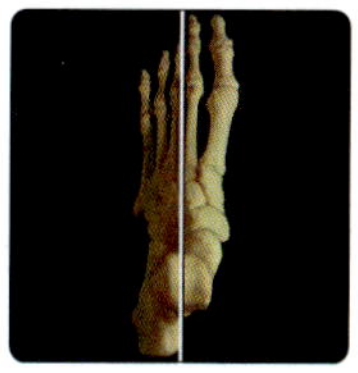

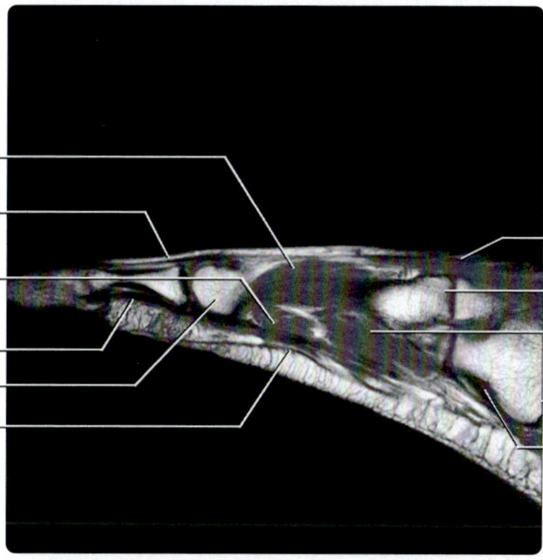

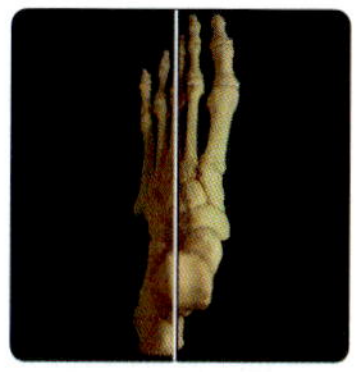

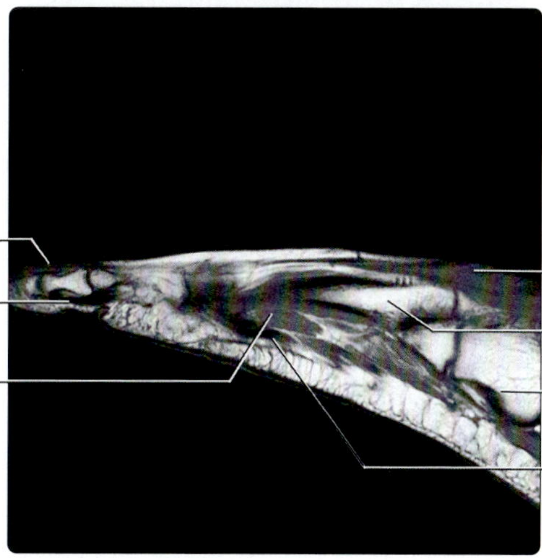

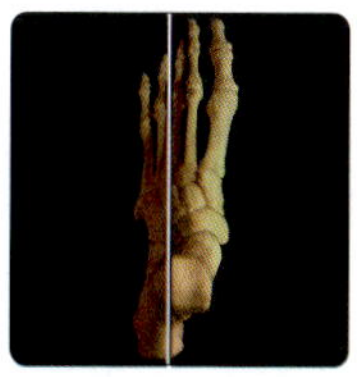

(Top) *The extensor digitorum longus and brevis tendons run side-by-side in the forefoot with the brevis lateral to the corresponding longus tendon. The brevis tendon attaches to the lateral margin of the longus tendon.* **(Middle)** *In the forefoot, the plantar fascia divides into digital bands. At the level of the metatarsal heads, it arborizes into superficial and deep components.* **(Bottom)** *The peroneus longus tendon lies in a groove beneath the cuboid, held in place by the long plantar ligament.*

SAGITTAL T1 MR: FOOT

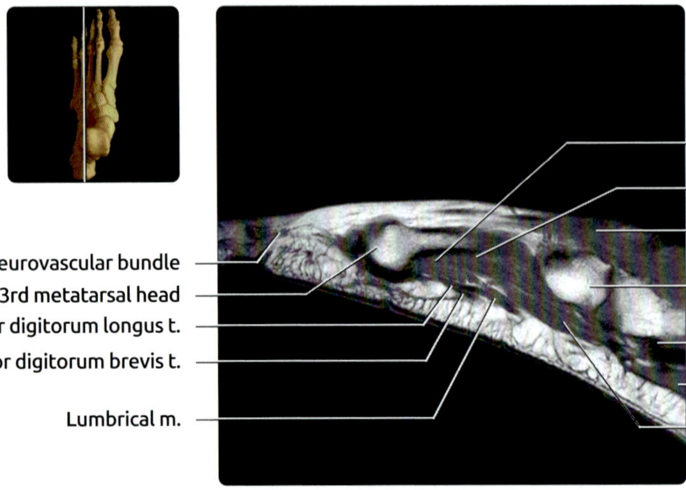

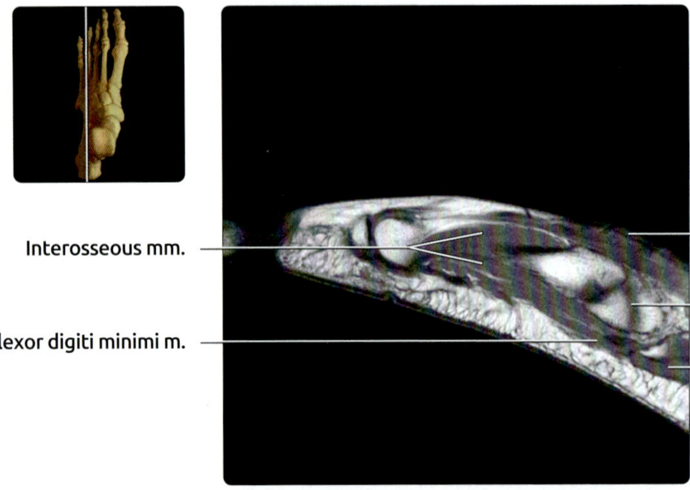

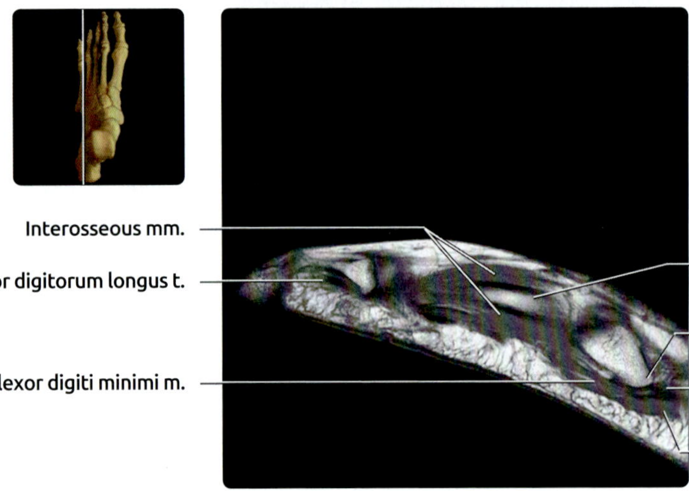

(Top) *The thin lumbrical muscles lie adjacent to the flexor digitorum tendon slips in the 2nd layer of plantar muscles.* **(Middle)** *Because of the normal fanning of toes, sagittal images angled to the 1st metatarsal will become oblique at the lateral aspect of the foot, as shown on this image. The 3rd metatarsophalangeal joint, as well as the 4th metatarsal and 5th metatarsal base are seen here on a single 3-mm thick slice. In clinical practice, the sagittal axis for imaging the forefoot will be chosen for the metatarsal of concern, or as default along the 1st metatarsal axis.* **(Bottom)** *The flexor digiti minimi muscle lies at the plantar aspect of the 5th metatarsal, and the abductor digiti minimi muscle lies at its lateral aspect. The peroneus brevis tendon attaches to the tuberosity (styloid process) at the lateral margin of the metatarsal base.*

SAGITTAL T1 MR: FOOT

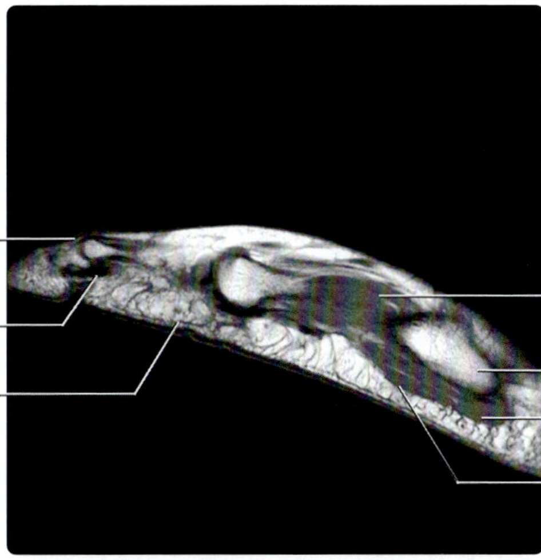

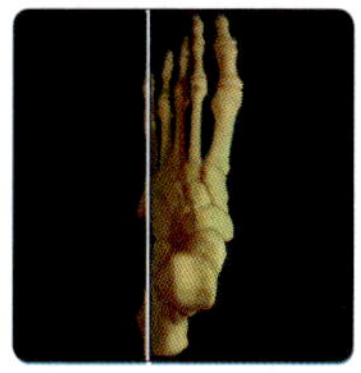

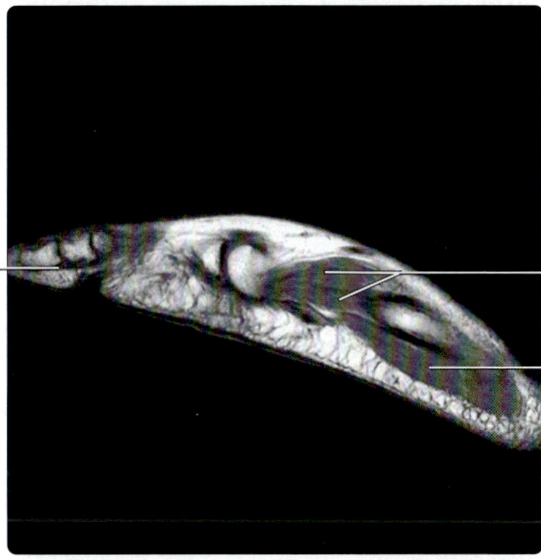

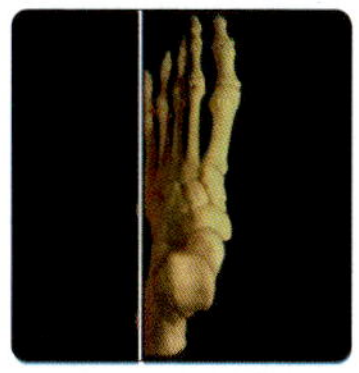

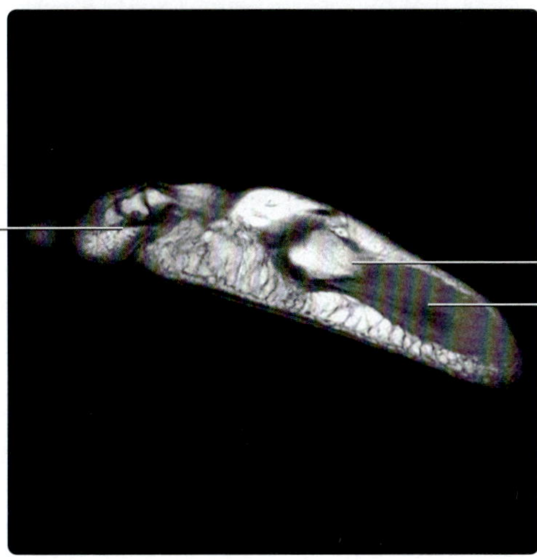

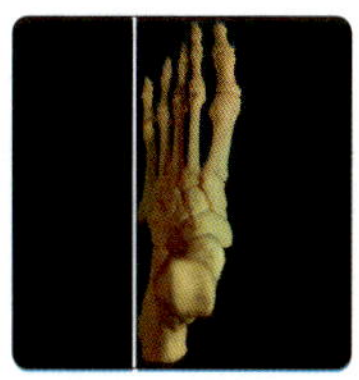

(Top) *The fine digital fascial network, which is the distal termination of the plantar fascia, is well seen.* **(Middle)** *Note that in a resting, non-weight-bearing position, the proximal interphalangeal joint is minimally flexed, and the distal interphalangeal joint is straight.* **(Bottom)** *The abductor digiti minimi is the most lateral muscle of the forefoot.*

GROSS ANATOMY

Plantar Musculature

- 4 layers of muscles deep to plantar aponeurosis
- Peroneus longus tendon crosses all 4 layers
- **Superficial (1st) muscle layer**
  - Abductor hallucis
    - Origin: Medial aspect posterior process calcaneus, flexor retinaculum, plantar fascia, intermuscular septum
    - Insertion: Medial sesamoid of 1st toe and medial aspect 1st proximal phalangeal base
    - Innervation: Medial plantar nerve
    - Function: Moves 1st toe medially
  - Flexor digitorum brevis
    - Origin: Posterior process calcaneus, plantar fascia, intermuscular septum
    - Divisions: 4 tendon slips split into medial and lateral tendons at metatarsophalangeals (MTPs)
    - Insertion: Medial and lateral margins of bases of middle phalanges
    - Innervation: Medial plantar nerve
    - Function: Flexes proximal interphalangeals (PIPs)
  - Abductor digiti minimi
    - Origin: Posterior process calcaneus
    - Insertion: Base 5th proximal phalanx
    - Innervation: Lateral plantar nerve
    - Function: Moves 5th toe laterally
    - Variant: Abductor ossis metatarsi quinti arises tuberosity 5th metatarsal, merges with abductor digiti minimi
  - Tendon of extrinsic muscle: Peroneus brevis
- **Middle (2nd) muscle layer**
  - Quadratus plantae (also called flexor accessorius)
    - Origin: 2 heads arise from posterior process calcaneus and long plantar ligament
    - Insertion: Tendon of flexor digitorum brevis
    - Innervation: Lateral plantar nerve
    - Function: Flexes lateral 4 toes
  - 4 lumbricals
    - Origin: Tendons of flexor digitorum longus
    - Insertion: Medial side of proximal phalanges of 4 lateral toes, into dorsal hood expansion of extensor tendons
    - Innervation: 1st lumbrical from medial plantar nerve, others by deep branch lateral plantar nerve
    - Function: Maintain extension of interphalangeal joints, flex MTP joints
  - Tendons of 2 extrinsic muscles: Flexor digitorum longus and flexor hallucis longus
    - Fibers from these 2 tendons join at master knot of Henry and exchange fibers
- **Deep (3rd) muscle layer**
  - Flexor hallucis brevis
    - Origin: Lateral head originates from plantar surface cuboid; medial head arises lateral division tibialis posterior and medial intermuscular septum
    - Insertion: Medial and lateral heads insert respectively on medial and lateral aspects base 1st proximal phalanx
    - Contains: Medial and lateral sesamoids of 1st toe
    - Innervation: Medial plantar nerve
    - Function: Flexes proximal phalanx of 1st toe
  - Adductor hallucis
    - Origin: Oblique head originates from bases of 2nd, 3rd, and 4th metatarsals, transverse head originates from 3rd, 4th, and sometimes 5th plantar MTP ligaments
    - Insertion: Lateral sesamoid of 1st toe and base of 1st proximal phalanx
    - Innervation: Deep branch lateral plantar nerve
    - Function: Stabilizes metatarsal heads, flexes proximal phalanx of 1st toe
    - Variant: Transverse head may be absent
  - Flexor digiti minimi brevis
    - Origin: Base of 5th metatarsal and sheath of peroneus longus tendon
    - Insertion: Lateral margin, base of 5th proximal phalanx
    - Innervation: Superficial branch of lateral plantar nerve
    - Function: Flexes MTP joint of 5th toe
  - Tendon of extrinsic muscle: posterior tibial
- **Interosseous (4th) layer**
  - Plantar interossei: 3 muscles, to 3rd, 4th, and 5th toes
    - Origin: Medial bases of 3rd, 4th, and 5th metatarsals
    - Insertion: Medial base of proximal phalanges of same toes
    - Innervation: Deep branch lateral plantar nerve
    - Function: Adduct 3rd-5th toes, flex MTP joints, extend PIP joints
  - Dorsal interossei: 4 muscles, to 2nd, 3rd, 4th, 5th toes
    - Origin: Each has 2 heads, from lateral and medial margins of 2 adjacent metatarsals
    - Insertion: 1st to medial margin 2nd proximal phalanx, 2nd-4th to lateral margin of 2nd-4th proximal phalanges
    - Innervation: Deep branch lateral plantar nerve
    - Function: Deviate toes laterally, flex MTP joints, extend PIP joints

Dorsal Muscles

- Extrinsic muscles: Tendons of anterior tibial, extensor hallucis longus, extensor digitorum brevis, peroneus tertius
- Intrinsic muscles
  - Extensor hallucis brevis: Partially joined to extensor digitorum brevis
    - Origin: Anterior aspect calcaneus
    - Insertion: Base proximal phalanx of 1st toe
    - Innervation: Deep peroneal nerve
    - Function: Extends proximal phalanx
  - Extensor digitorum brevis
    - Origin: Anterolateral aspect calcaneus
    - Insertion: Lateral margins of extensor digitorum longus tendons to 2nd-4th digits and bases middle phalanges
    - Innervation: Deep peroneal nerve
    - Function: Extend phalanges of toes
- In hindfoot, extrinsic tendons superficial to intrinsic tendons
- In forefoot, intrinsic (brevis) tendons lateral to extrinsic (longus) tendons

GRAPHICS: MUSCLE ATTACHMENTS OF FOOT

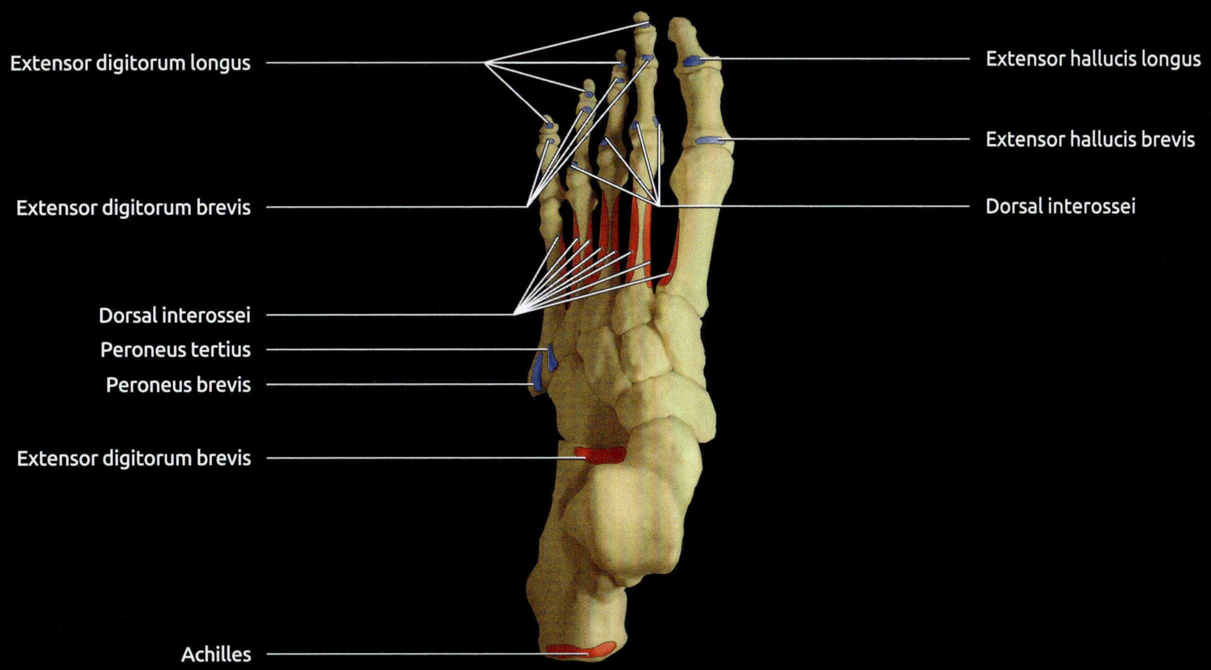

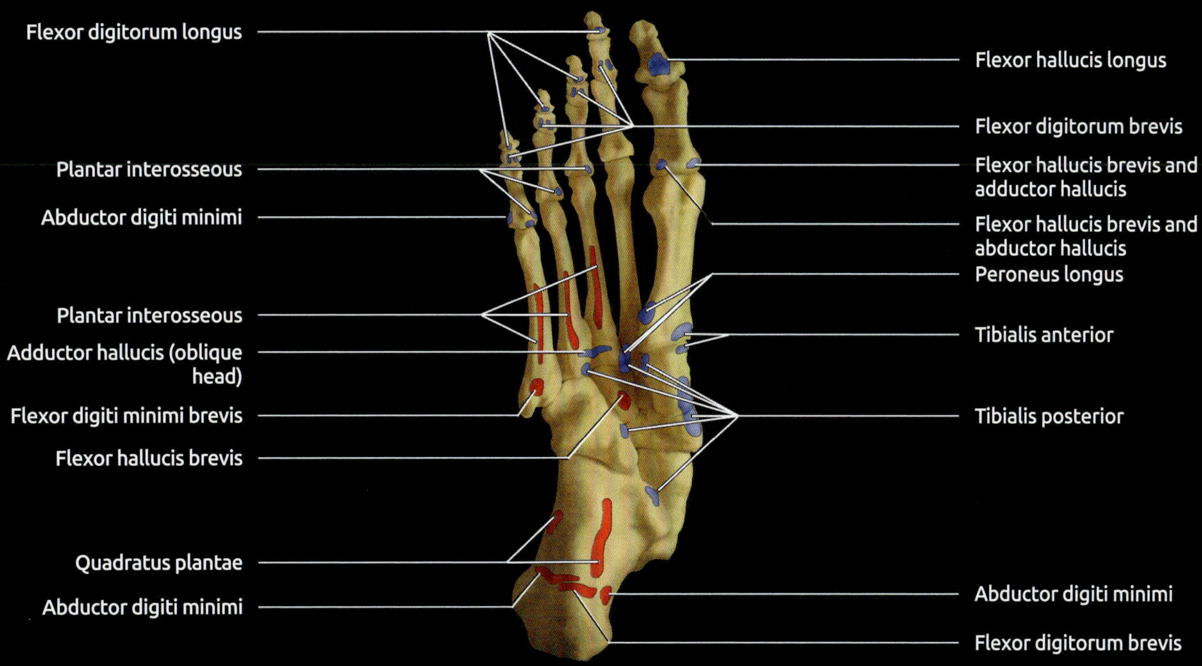

(Top) *Graphic shows muscle origins (red) and insertions (blue) at the dorsal surface of the foot. Note the dorsal interossei insert on the proximal phalangeal bases, extensor digitorum brevis on the middle phalangeal bases, and extensor digitorum longus on the distal interphalangeal bases.* **(Bottom)** *Graphic shows muscle origins (red) and insertions (blue) at the plantar surface of the foot. Note the multiple attachments of the tibialis posterior tendon. Flexor digitorum brevis tendons to each toe split into 2 slips, attaching at the plantar margins of the middle phalanges with the flexor digitorum longus tendon coursing between them to attach at the base of the distal phalanges.*

GRAPHICS: 1ST & 2ND PLANTAR MUSCLE LAYER

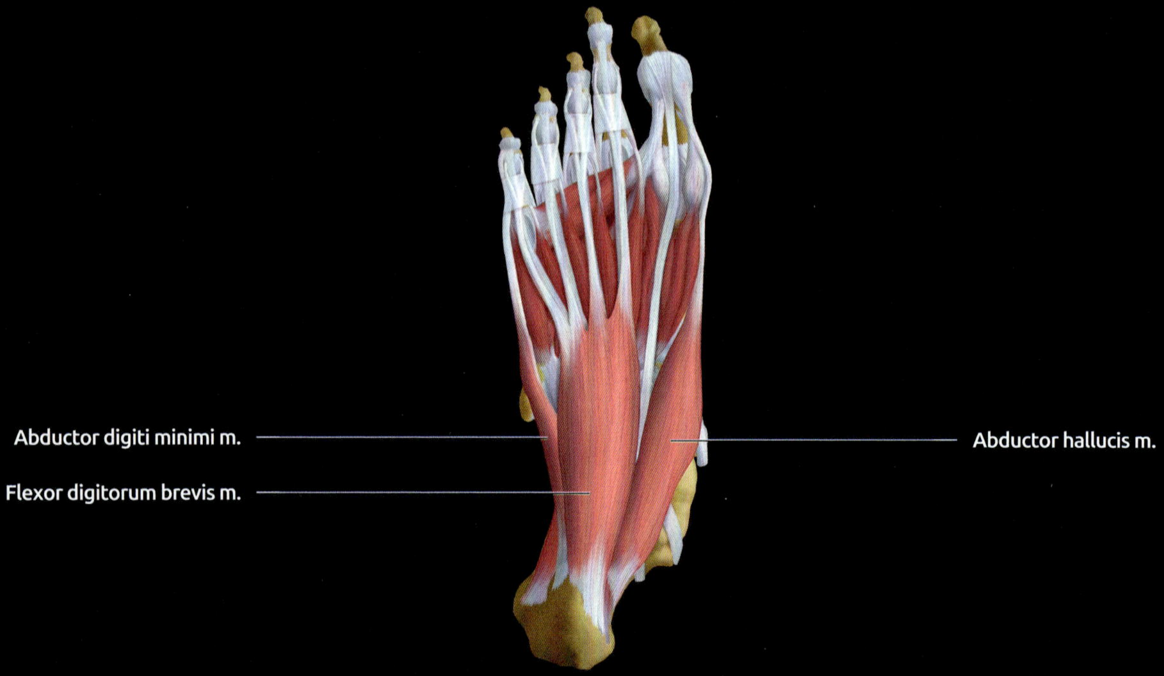

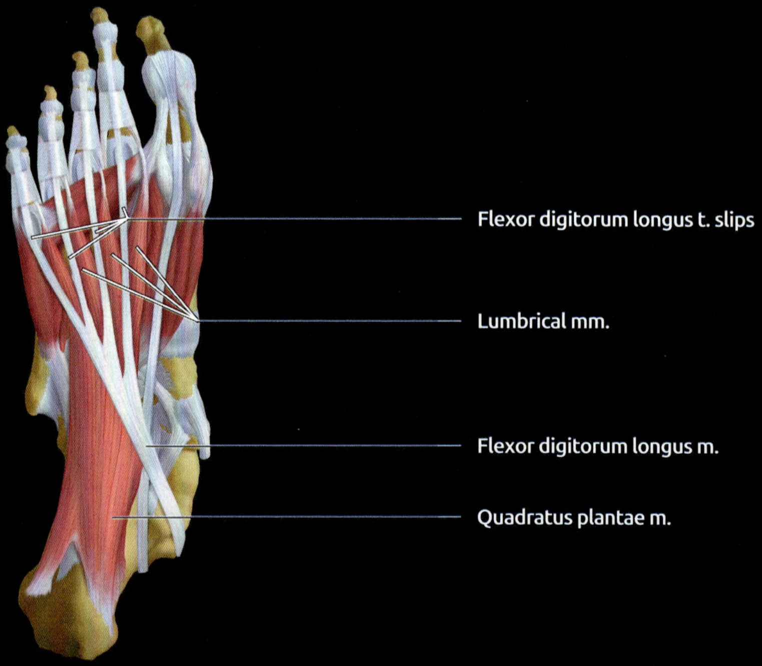

(Top) *The 1st, or superficial, layer of plantar muscles is composed of the abductor hallucis, flexor digitorum brevis, and abductor digiti minimi. Abduction in the foot is motion away from the central axis, the 2nd metatarsal. The peroneus brevis (not shown) is the only extrinsic tendon in this layer.* **(Bottom)** *The 2nd layer of plantar muscles is composed of the intrinsic muscles, quadratus plantae (also called the flexor accessorius) lumbricals, and also the extrinsic tendons of the flexor hallucis longus and flexor digitorum longus. This graphic shows how the lumbricals arise from the tendon slips of the flexor digitorum longus.*

GRAPHICS: 3RD & 4TH PLANTAR MUSCLE LAYER

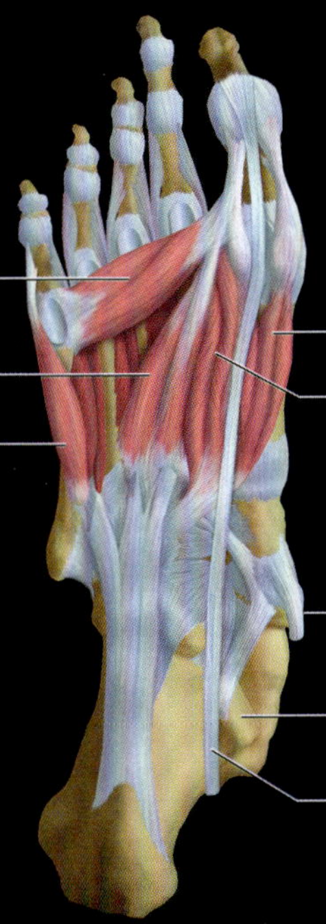

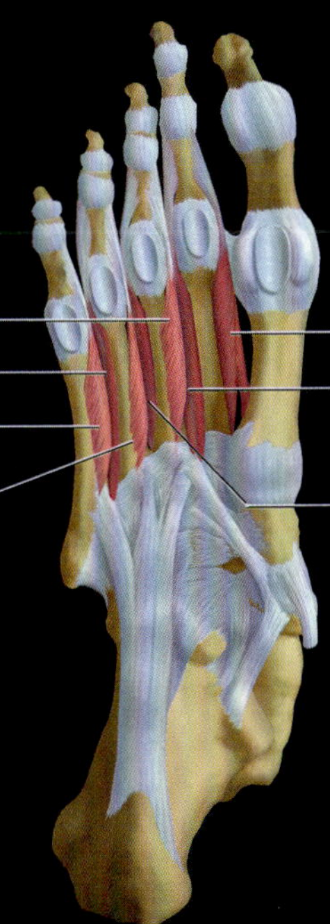

(Top) *The 3rd layer consists of 1 extrinsic tendon, the posterior tibial tendon, and 3 intrinsic muscles: Flexor hallucis brevis (which has medial and lateral heads), the adductor hallucis (which has oblique and transverse heads), and the flexor digiti minimi.* **(Bottom)** *The 4th layer of plantar muscles contains the interossei. There are 4 dorsal interossei, which have bipennate origins from 2 adjacent metatarsals. The 1st dorsal interosseous inserts on medial side of 2nd proximal phalanx, and the remaining dorsal interossei insert on lateral side of the proximal phalanx, corresponding to the metatarsal of origin. There are 3 plantar interossei. They originate from the medial side of the 3rd-5th metatarsals and insert on the medial side of the corresponding proximal phalanges.*

CORONAL T1 MR: INTRINSIC FOOT MUSCLES

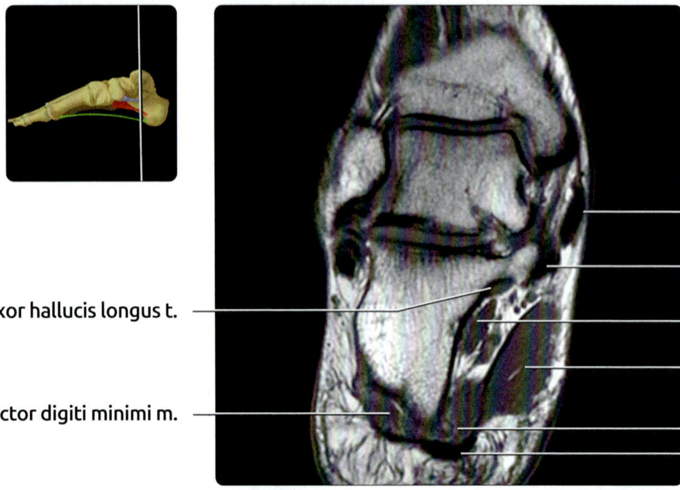

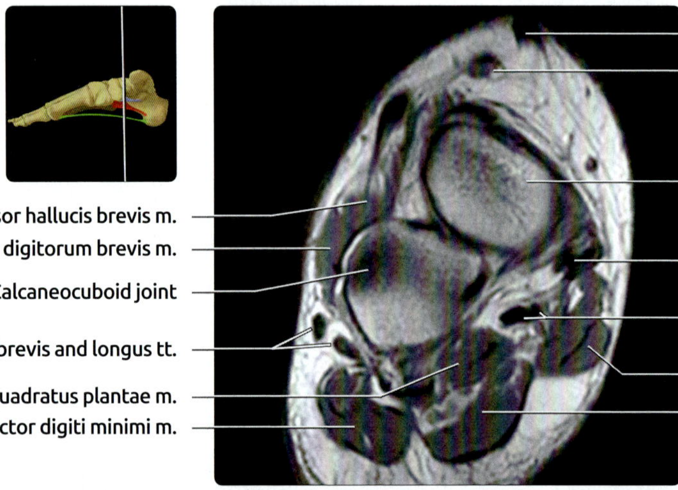

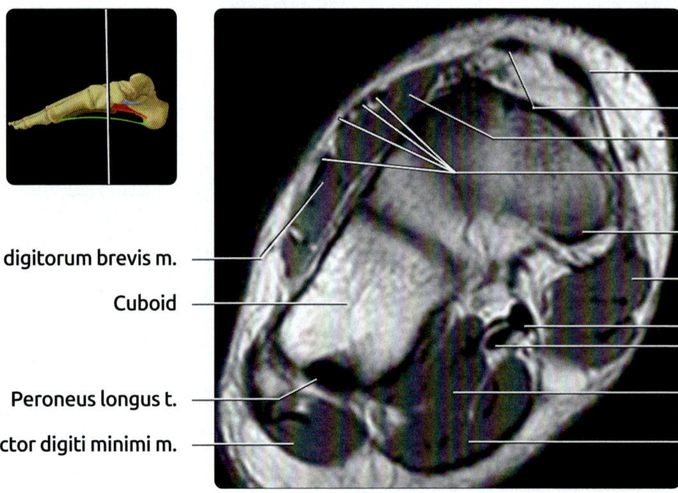

(Top) *First of 6 coronal T1 MR images shows the relationships of the intrinsic muscles. The superficial layer of plantar muscles includes the abductor hallucis, flexor digitorum brevis, and abductor digiti minimi. In the hindfoot, the quadratus plantae shares the 2nd (middle) level with 2 extrinsic tendons, the flexor hallucis longus and flexor digitorum longus.* **(Middle)** *This image is at the level of the calcaneocuboid joint. The extensor digitorum brevis and extensor hallucis brevis arise adjacent to each other on the dorsal surface of the calcaneus.* **(Bottom)** *At the level of the cuboid sulcus, the flexor hallucis and digitorum tendons have crossed. The quadratus plantae muscle is approaching its insertion on the flexor digitorum longus tendon.*

CORONAL T1 MR: INTRINSIC FOOT MUSCLES

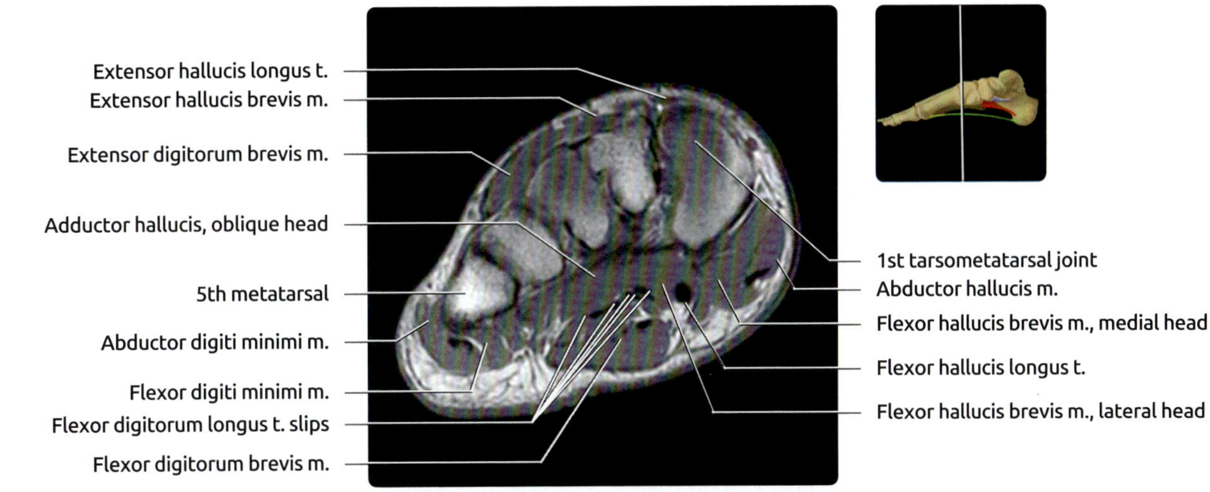

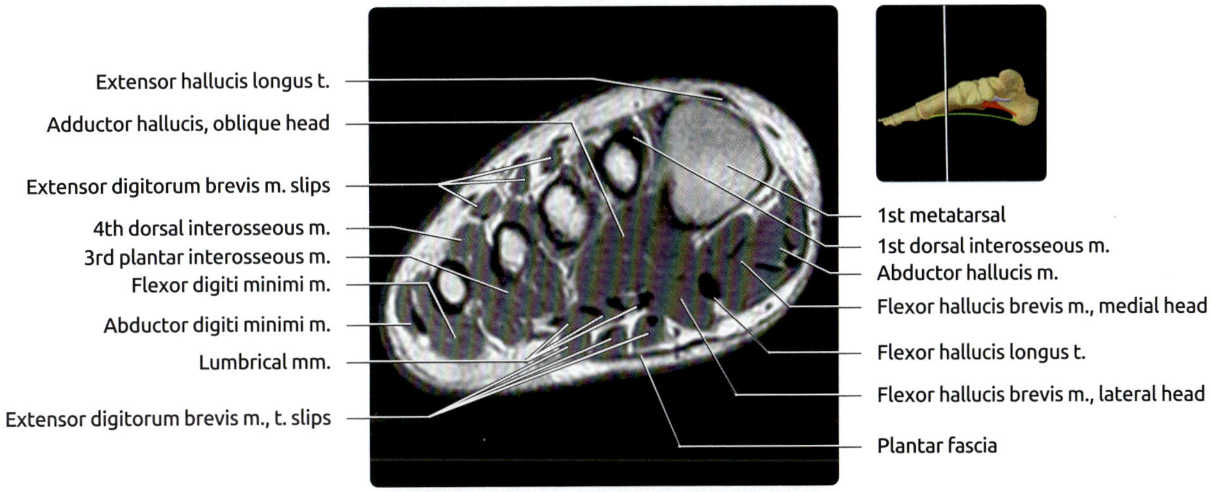

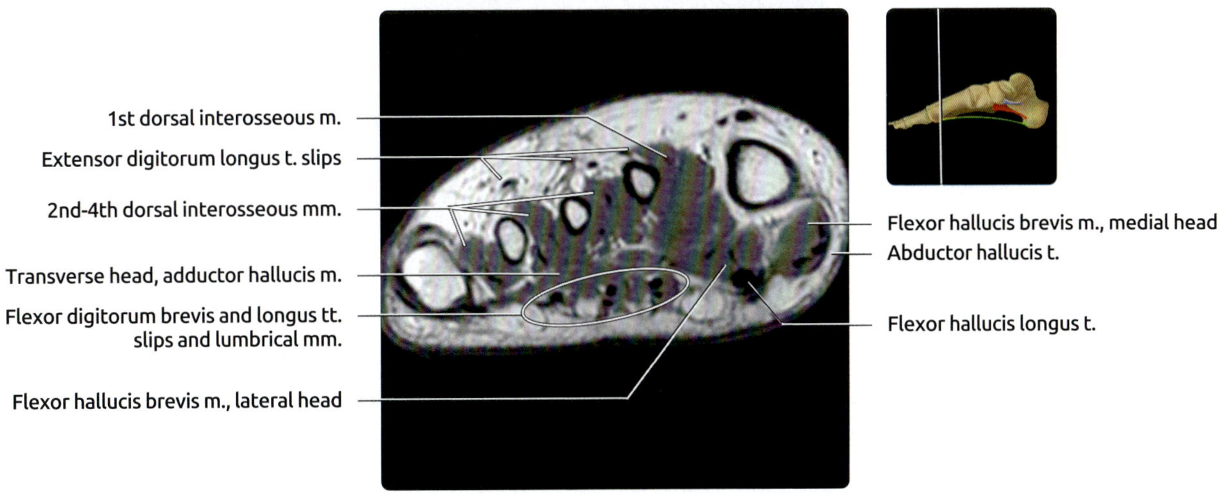

(Top) *At the level of the 1st tarsometatarsal joint, the 2 heads of the flexor hallucis brevis muscle are seen flanking the flexor hallucis longus tendon. They lie in the 3rd layer of intrinsic plantar muscles. The flexor digiti minimi muscle, seen here at its origin from the plantar surface of the 5th metatarsal, and adductor hallucis muscle are also part of the deep layer.* **(Middle)** *This image is through the proximal metatarsals. The interosseous, or 4th layer of plantar muscles, is composed of the plantar and dorsal interossei. Lumbrical muscles are part of the 2nd plantar layer. The slips of the extensor digitorum brevis muscle are deep and lateral to the corresponding slips of extensor digitorum longus tendon.* **(Bottom)** *At the level of the 5th metatarsal head, the abductor digiti minimi and flexor digiti minimi are both tendinous. The transverse head of the adductor hallucis, seen here, is variably present.*

TERMINOLOGY

Synonyms

- Lisfranc joint

IMAGING ANATOMY

Overview

- 1st-5th tarsometatarsal articulations usually considered functionally as 1 joint
- Follows transverse arch configuration established by wedge shape of cuneiforms
  - Bases of 2nd and 3rd metatarsals also have wedge shape
- In coronal plane, joint extends obliquely from anteromedial to posterolateral
  - 2nd metatarsal recessed relative to 1st and 3rd
    - This provides added bony stability (mortise and tenon configuration)
    - Some individuals lack recessed position of 2nd metatarsal; they have higher incidence of dislocation
  - Cuboid slightly recessed relative to 3rd cuneiform
    - Creates mortise and tenon configuration in opposite orientation to 2nd tarsometatarsal joint
- Small intermetatarsal joints are present between metatarsal bases 2-5, sometimes between bases of 1-2

Motion

- 1st tarsometatarsal joint allows abduction, slight flexion, and extension
- 2nd and 3rd tarsometatarsal joints are relatively immobile
- 4th and 5th tarsometatarsal joints have ~ 10° of flexion and extension

Synovial Divisions

- 3 separate synovial joint cavities
  - 1st tarsometatarsal joint
  - 2nd-3rd tarsometatarsal joints
    - Usually continuous with joint between 2nd and 3rd cuneiforms and naviculocuneiform joint
  - 4th-5th tarsometatarsal joints
- Intermetatarsal joints have continuous cavity with tarsometatarsal joints

Ligaments

- **1st tarsometatarsal joint**
  - Dorsal, plantar, and medial and lateral collateral ligaments from 1st cuneiform to 1st metatarsal
- **Tarsometatarsal ligaments 2-5**
  - Dorsal and plantar ligaments at each digit
  - 2nd, 3rd interosseous cuneometatarsal ligaments variably present
- **Lisfranc ligament**
  - Prevents lateral displacement of 2nd cuneiform, helps maintain transverse arch of foot
  - Oblique orientation from 1st cuneiform to 2nd metatarsal
  - 3 separate bands
  - Dorsal bands are most thin
  - Interosseous band is thick, 0.5-1.0 cm; striated appearance, sometimes 2 separate bands
    - Cuneiform origin is slightly dorsal to metatarsal insertion
  - Interosseous band is critical stabilizer of Lisfranc joint
  - Plantar band is 2x thickness of dorsal band
    - Attaches to 3rd as well as 2nd metatarsal base, just dorsal to peroneus longus tendon
- **Intermetatarsal ligaments**
  - Dorsal, interosseous, and plantar ligaments between 2nd-5th metatarsal bases
  - No dorsal or plantar ligaments between 1st and 2nd metatarsal bases
    - Weak interosseous ligaments are present in this region
    - Lack of intermetatarsal ligaments between 1st and 2nd metatarsals increases importance of Lisfranc ligament

Bursae

- Bursa between 1st and 2nd metatarsal bases
- Lateral and plantar bursae at base 5th metatarsal, under abductor and flexor muscle origins
- Bursa at plantar 1st tarsometatarsal joint, under origin flexor hallucis brevis
- Bursae at plantar tarsometatarsal joints, under extensor tendons

ANATOMY IMAGING ISSUES

Imaging Recommendations

- Radiographs must be weight-bearing to evaluate alignment
  - Abduction stress views may elicit instability
- Axial and coronal MR provide best visualization of Lisfranc ligament
  - Optimize with small flex coil centered at Lisfranc joint

Imaging Pitfalls

- Interosseous Lisfranc ligament structurally most important stabilizer of Lisfranc joint
  - Since obliquely oriented, see on sequential coronal MR images
  - See on axial MR images through midportion of cuneiforms and metatarsal bases

CLINICAL IMPLICATIONS

Clinical Importance

- Injuries of Lisfranc joint commonly missed in emergency department setting
- Isolated tears of Lisfranc ligament occur with plantar flexion, axial load
- Even slight lateral displacement of 2nd metatarsal medial margin relative to medial margin of 2nd cuneiform indicates disruption of Lisfranc ligament
- Flattening of transverse and longitudinal arches of foot and osteoarthritis of Lisfranc joint develop rapidly if ligamentous disruption untreated

SELECTED REFERENCES

1. Castro M et al: Lisfranc joint ligamentous complex: MRI with anatomic correlation in cadavers. AJR Am J Roentgenol. 195(6):W447-55, 2010
2. Johnson A et al: Anatomy of the lisfranc ligament. Foot Ankle Spec. 1(1):19-23, 2008

RADIOGRAPHS: LISFRANC JOINT

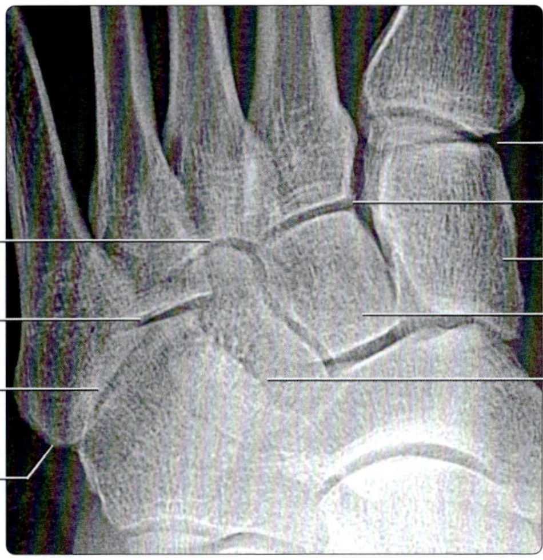

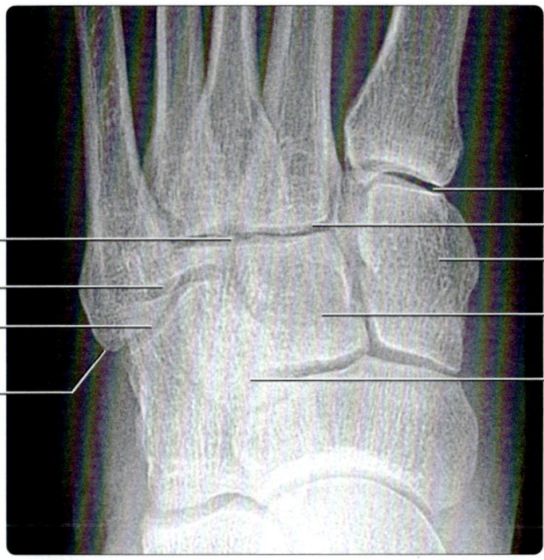

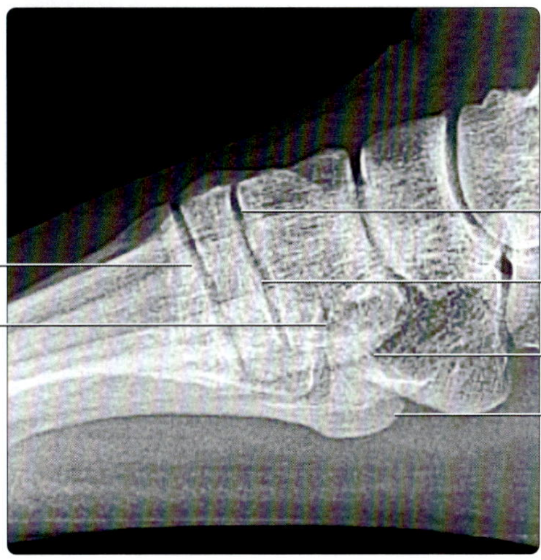

(Top) *Anteroposterior radiograph shows normal relationships: 1st metatarsal (MT) centered on 1st cuneiform, medial margins of 2nd cuneiform and MT aligned, and 5th MT styloid process extending lateral to cuboid.* **(Middle)** *Anteroposterior radiograph shows that 2nd MT base is not recessed relative to the 3rd, a normal variant that predisposes to dislocation.* **(Bottom)** *On lateral radiograph, the 1st and 2nd tarsometatarsal joints are at the dorsum of foot, and the 2nd tarsometatarsal joint is located more proximally.*

SAGITTAL CT: LISFRANC JOINT

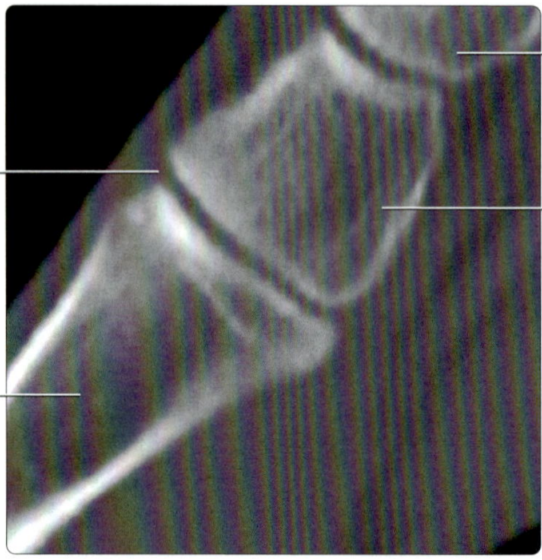

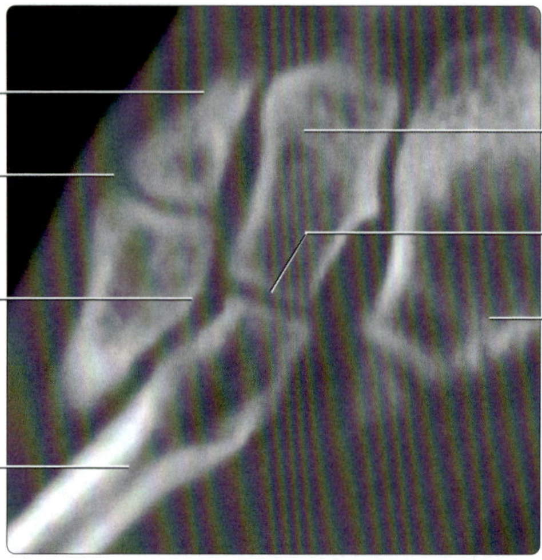

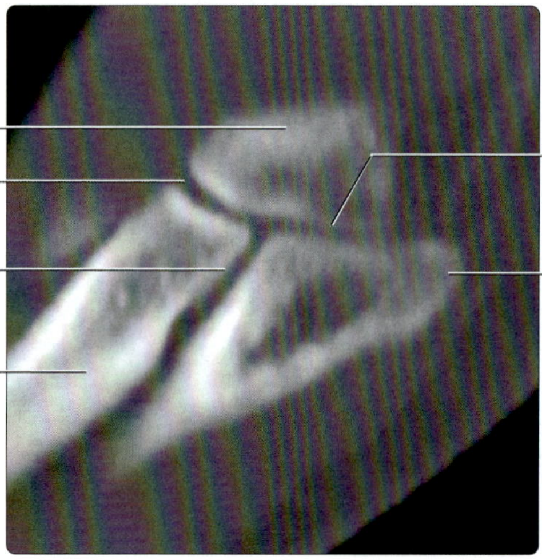

(Top) *First of 3 sagittal CT scans through the Lisfranc joint shows bony anatomy. The 1st cuneiform, MT base, and tarsometatarsal joint are much larger than the corresponding bones of the lateral digits. There should be no plantar or dorsal offset of the 1st MT relative to the 1st cuneiform, even on nonweight-bearing studies.* **(Middle)** *Sagittal CT through the 2nd and 3rd tarsometatarsal joints shows the recessed position of the 2nd MT base relative to the 3rd. The intermetatarsal joint between the bases of the 2nd and 3rd MTs is also well seen.* **(Bottom)** *Sagittal CT through the 4th and 5th tarsometatarsal bases shows the articulation of the cuboid with the 4th and 5th MTs. The tuberosity (styloid process) of the 5th MT extends beyond the lateral margin of the cuboid.*

GRAPHICS: LISFRANC LIGAMENT

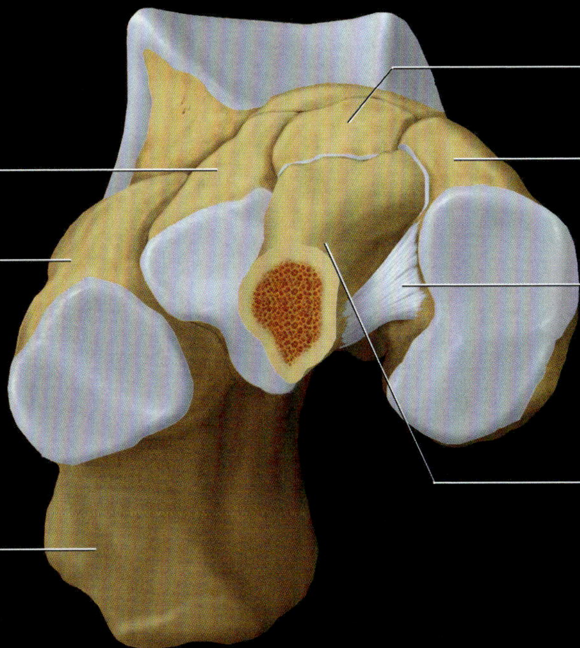

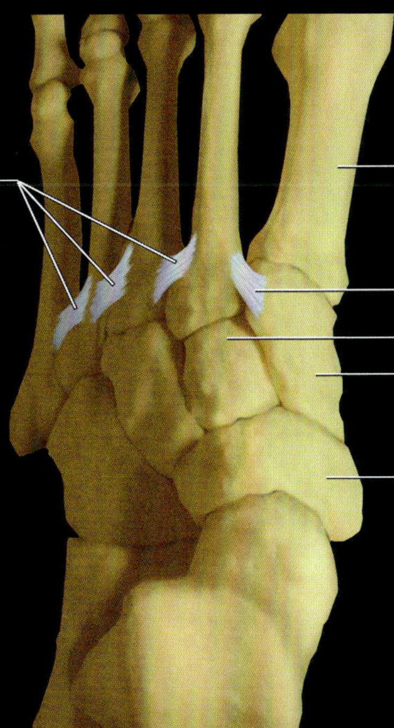

(Top) *Three separate ligaments extend from the lateral aspect of the 1st cuneiform to the medial aspect of the 2nd MT: Dorsal, interosseous, and plantar. The interosseous ligament is the strongest of these. The function of all 3 is to prevent lateral displacement of the 2nd MT.* **(Bottom)** *Dorsally strong intermetatarsal ligaments are seen between the 2nd and 5th MTs but not between the 1st and 2nd MTs. The dorsal Lisfranc ligament extends from the 1st cuneiform to the 2nd MT.*

AXIAL T1 MR: LISFRANC LIGAMENT

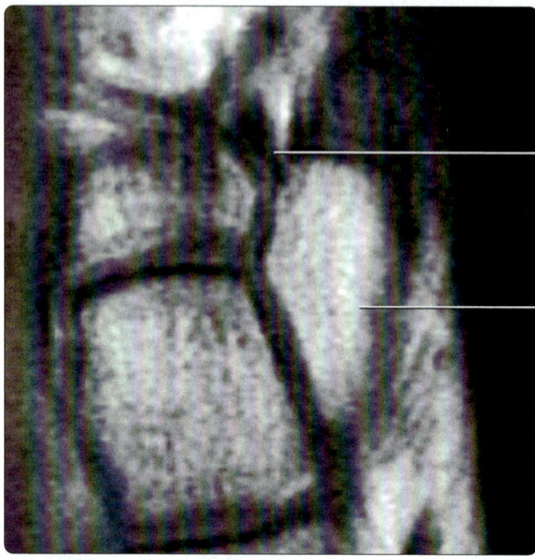

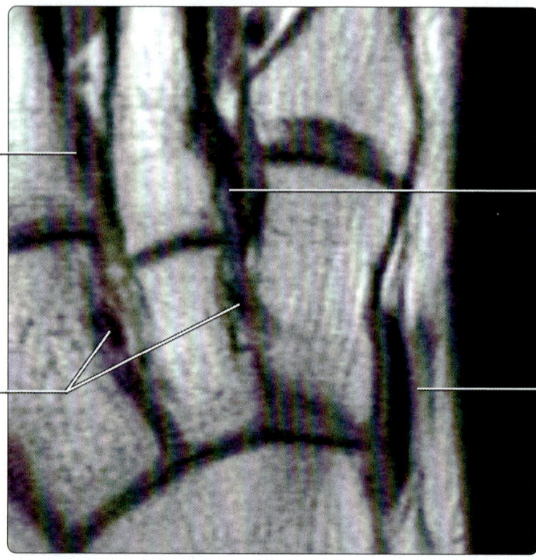

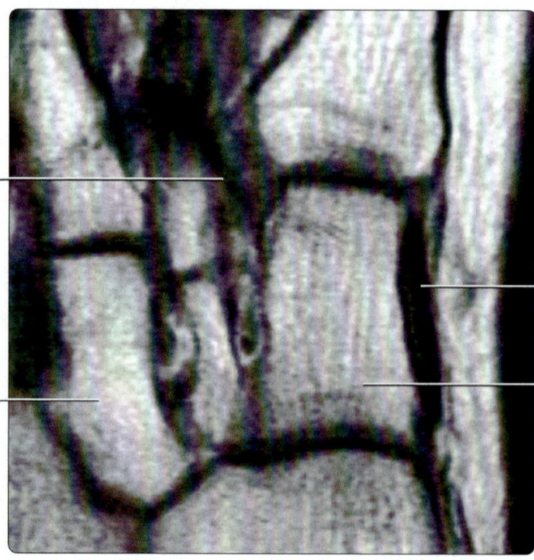

(Top) *First of 3 axial T1 MR images, from dorsal to more plantar positions through the Lisfranc joint, is shown. At the dorsal aspect of the tarsometatarsal joint, a thin ligament extends from the 1st cuneiform to the 2nd MT. Isolated injury to the Lisfranc ligament occurs with plantarflexion of midfoot, so this ligament is 1st to be injured.* **(Middle)** *The interosseous Lisfranc ligament is the primary stabilizer between the 1st and 2nd rays. It is thick and broad when compared to the other interosseous ligaments of the foot.* **(Bottom)** *The plantar Lisfranc ligament is a thin structure paralleling the dorsal and interosseous Lisfranc ligaments.*

CORONAL T2 MR: LISFRANC LIGAMENT

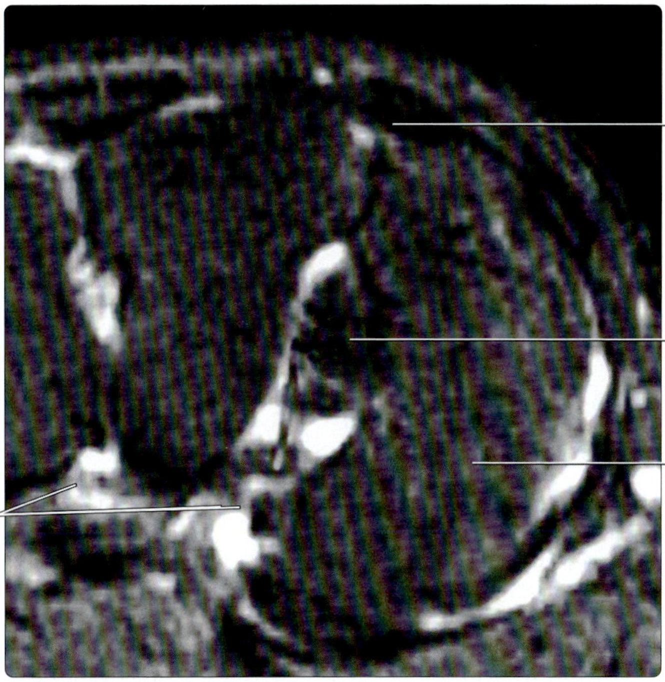

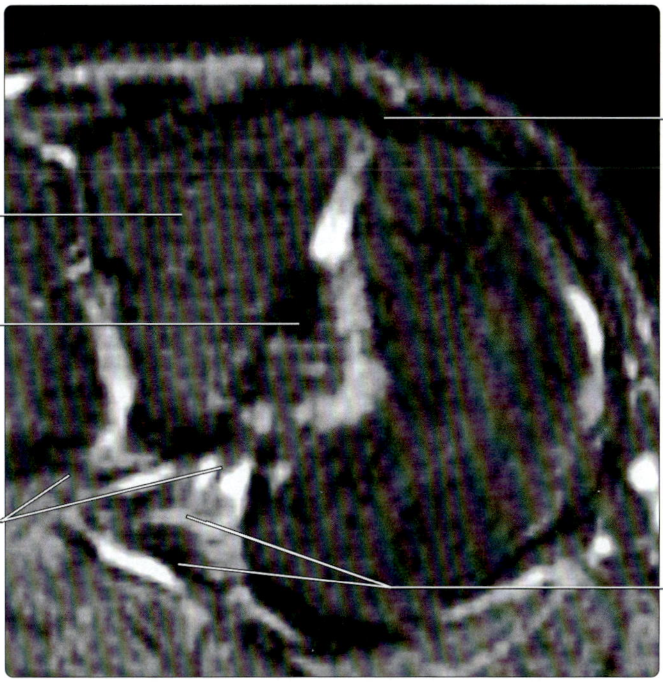

(Top) *First of 2 coronal T2 MR images of the Lisfranc ligaments is shown. Since the ligaments are obliquely oriented, their entire course will not be seen on a single coronal image. This image shows the origin from the 1st cuneiform.* **(Bottom)** *This image, adjacent to the previous image, shows the insertion of the interosseous Lisfranc ligament on the 2nd MT base. Note the striated appearance of ligament.*

IMAGING ANATOMY

Overview

- In normal weight-bearing stance, all of metatarsal heads are at same level, and all are weight-bearing
  - Metatarsophalangeal (MTP) joints are slightly extended in standing position
- Each MTP joint is separate synovial cavity

1st Metatarsophalangeal Joint

- Dorsiflexion of toe important in push-off phase of gait
- Metatarsal head has 2 concave facets at plantar surface, 1 for each sesamoid, separated by ridge (crista)
- Distal articular surface of metatarsal head may be flat, rounded, or have central prominence
- Base of proximal phalanx has concave contour
- **Sesamoids**
  - Either sesamoid may be unipartite or bipartite
  - Medial sesamoid in medial head flexor hallucis brevis and abductor hallucis
  - Lateral sesamoid in lateral head flexor hallucis brevis and adductor hallucis and deep metatarsal ligament
  - Medial and lateral sesamoids joined by intersesamoid ligament
    - Intersesamoid ligament is roof of canal in which flexor hallucis longus tendon runs
  - Both are embedded in plantar plate of joint
- **Plantar plate**
  - Fibrocartilaginous plantar capsular thickening extending from metatarsal neck to base proximal phalanx
  - Incorporates sesamoids + tendons distal to sesamoids
- **Sesamophalangeal apparatus**
  - Consists of sesamoids + tendon attachments + plantar plate
  - Inserts on plantar aspect of 1st proximal phalanx
  - Sesamoids fixed in position relative to 1st proximal phalanx but move relative to 1st metatarsal
  - Therefore displaced laterally in hallux valgus

Lateral Metatarsophalangeal Joints

- Convex metatarsal head articular surface articulates with concave articular surface of proximal phalangeal base
- Plantar aspect of metatarsal head has rounded contour
- Dorsal aspect of metatarsal head is smaller than plantar aspect
  - Has concave or notched contour along medial and lateral margins
- Sesamoids variably present, most commonly at 5th toe
- **Phalangeal apparatus** is combination of plantar plate and proximal phalanx
- **Plantar plate**
  - Fibrocartilaginous plantar capsular thickening extending from metatarsal neck to base proximal phalanx
  - Attached to deep transverse metatarsal ligament, plantar fascia and flexor tendon sheath, medial and lateral collateral ligaments
  - Instability may mimic Morton neuroma symptomatically

Ligaments

- Intermetatarsal ligaments: Between metatarsal heads
- Plantar fascia: Distal attachments to joint capsules
- Medial and lateral collateral ligaments: Well defined at each digit

Bursae

- 1st MTP
  - Dorsal: Variably present separate from tendon sheath of extensor hallucis longus
  - Plantar: Subcutaneous, at plantar and medial aspect of metatarsal head
- Inter-MTP
  - Located between metatarsal heads
  - Dorsal to transverse metatarsal ligament
  - Adjacent to plantar digital neurovascular bundle
    - Bursitis may irritate nerve, mimic Morton neuroma
  - Usually absent between 4th-5th toes
- 5th MTP
  - Plantar: Subcutaneous, at plantar aspect of metatarsal head

Nerves

- Plantar and dorsal nerves course with arterioles along medial and lateral aspects of digits
- Plantar nerves vulnerable to impingement between metatarsal heads

ANATOMY IMAGING ISSUES

Imaging Recommendations

- MTP MR
  - Use wrist or small wrap coil, 10- to 12-cm FOV
  - 3-mm slices allow excellent visualization of ligaments

CLINICAL IMPLICATIONS

Clinical Importance

- Instability of MTP joints results in pain and deformity of forefoot

Stability of 1st Metatarsophalangeal Joint

- Collateral ligaments
- Flexor and extensor hallucis brevis mm
- Flexor and extensor hallucis longus mm have smaller contribution to stability

Stability of Lateral Metatarsophalangeal Joints

- Collateral ligaments
- Plantar plate
  - Rupture of plantar plate results in dorsal subluxation of MTP joint

Short 1st Metatarsal (Morton Foot)

- Normal variant but increases stress on 2nd metatarsal (transfer metatarsalgia)
- Predisposes to
  - Osteonecrosis of 2nd metatarsal head (Freiberg infraction)
  - Stress fracture
  - Dorsal subluxation of 2nd MTP

GRAPHICS: 1ST METATARSOPHALANGEAL JOINT

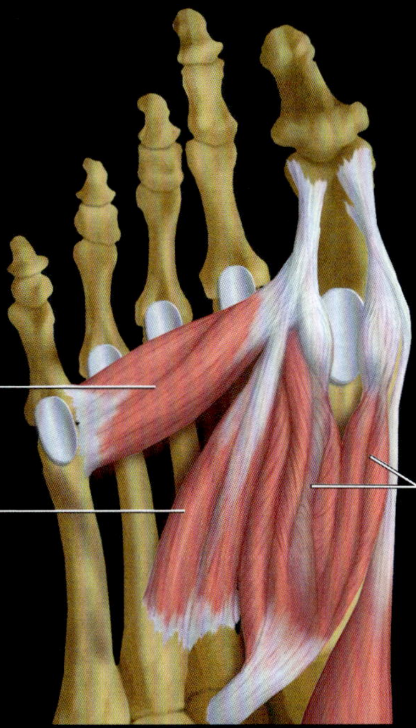

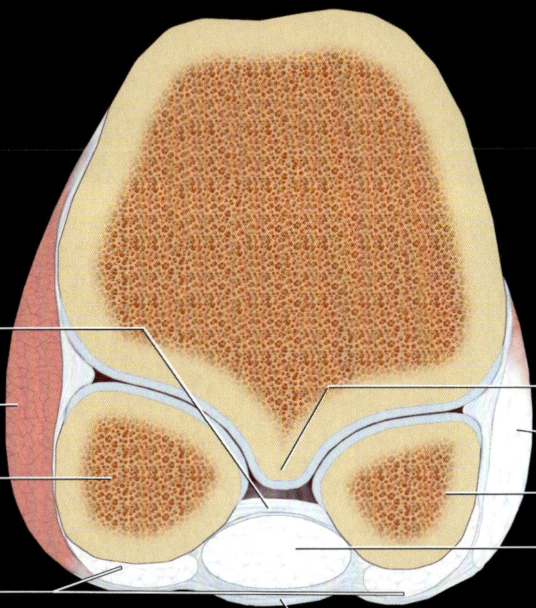

(Top) *Axial graphic shows muscle attachments to the sesamoids of the 1st metatarsophalangeal (MTP) joint. The abductor hallucis and medial head of the flexor hallucis brevis attach to the medial sesamoid. The lateral head of the flexor hallucis brevis and adductor hallucis attach to the lateral sesamoid.* **(Bottom)** *Coronal graphic shows sesamoids positioned at the plantar surface of the 1st metatarsal head, separated by the median crest of the metatarsal. The sesamoids are united by the intersesamoid ligament. The intersesamoid ligament forms the roof of the groove between the sesamoids, and the flexor hallucis longus tendon runs in this groove.*

1ST METATARSOPHALANGEAL JOINT

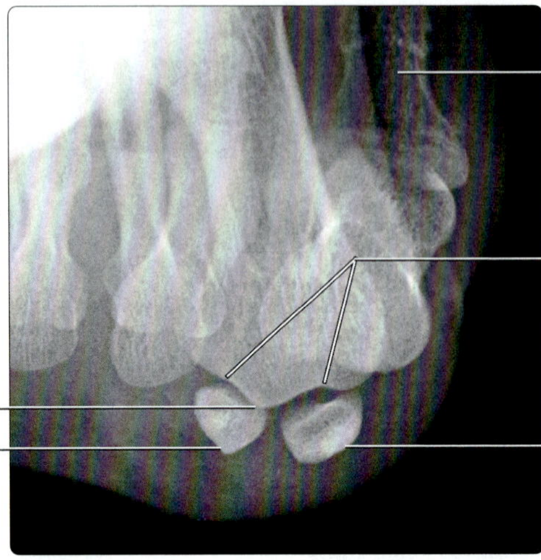

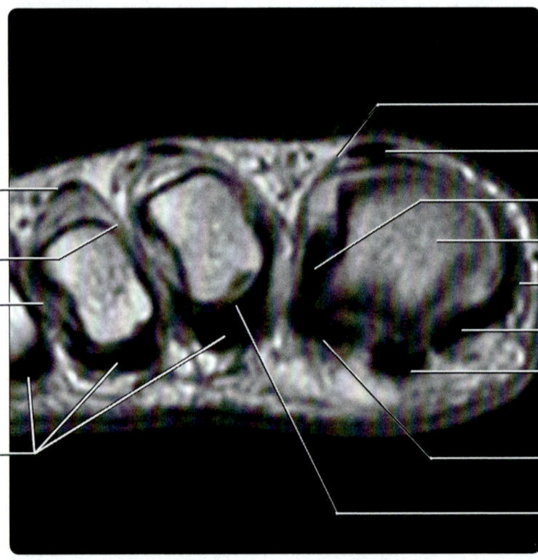

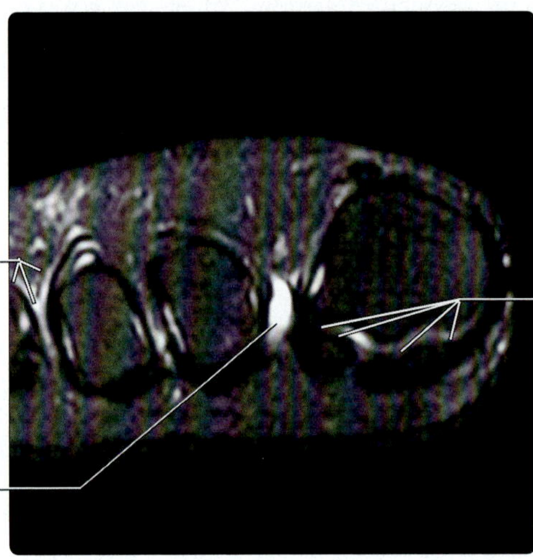

(Top) *Sesamoid radiograph was obtained tangent to the sesamoids, with the toe dorsiflexed. The sesamoids are centered on articular facets of the metatarsal head.* **(Middle)** *Coronal PD MR through the 1st MTP joint and the 2nd and 3rd metatarsal heads shows the stabilizing ligaments. Note the plantar plate is much thicker than the dorsal capsule.* **(Bottom)** *Coronal T2WI FS MR shows the normal intermetatarsal bursa between 1st and 2nd metatarsal heads. The digital vessels are also well seen. Both of these normal structures are sometimes mistaken for Morton neuroma.*

METATARSOPHALANGEAL JOINTS

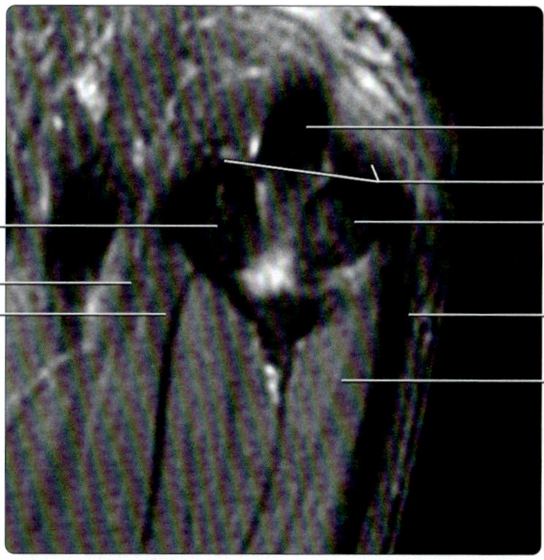

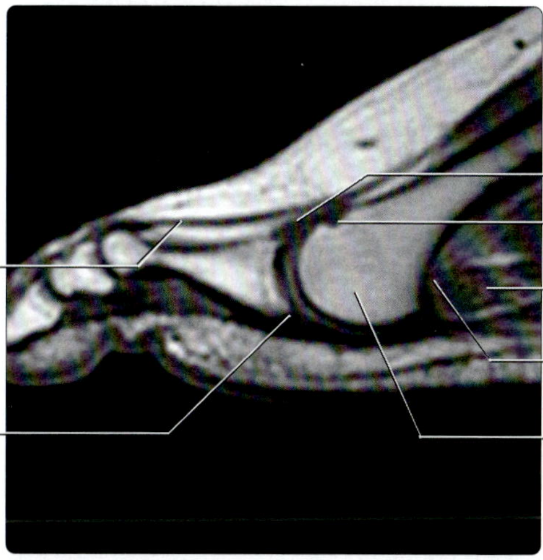

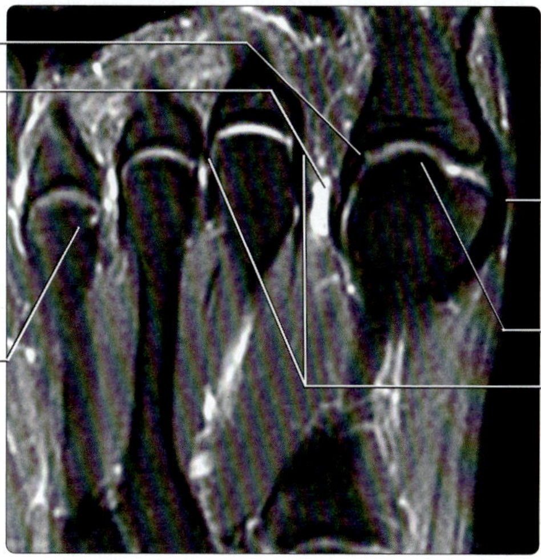

(Top) *Axial PD FS MR through the sesamoids of the 1st metatarsal head shows the tendon attachments to the sesamoids. Distal to their attachment on the sesamoids, the tendons form thickenings in the plantar plate of the 1st MTP joint.* **(Middle)** *Sagittal T1WI MR through the 2nd MTP joint shows the proximal origin of the plantar plate from the metatarsal neck and its insertion on the base of the proximal phalanx.* **(Bottom)** *Axial PD FS MR shows collateral ligaments of the MTP joints. A small bursa is visible between the 1st and 2nd MTP joints.*

TERMINOLOGY

Definitions

- **3 major divisions**
  - Hindfoot: Calcaneus and talus
  - Midfoot: Navicular, cuneiforms, and cuboid
  - Forefoot: Metatarsals and phalanges
- **2 columns**
  - Medial column: Talus, navicular, cuneiforms and digits 1-3
  - Lateral column: Calcaneus, cuboid, digits 4 and 5
- Some authors use 2 columns in hind- and midfoot as above, but divide forefoot into 3 columns
  - Medial column: 1st toe
  - Middle column: 2nd-4th toes
  - Lateral column: 5th toe

IMAGING ANATOMY

Overview

- US useful for evaluation of muscles, tendons, nerves, and blood vessels of foot
- Used to guide selective nerve injections in entrapment syndromes

Musculature

- **Plantar muscles**: 4 muscle layers, numbered from superficial to deep
  - 1st layer: Abductor hallucis, flexor digitorum brevis, abductor digiti minimi
  - 2nd layer: Quadratus plantae (flexor accessorius), flexor digitorum and hallucis longus tendons, lumbricals
  - 3rd layer: Flexor hallucis brevis, adductor hallucis, flexor digiti minimi brevis, tibialis posterior tendon
  - 4th layer: Plantar interossei, dorsal interossei
  - Peroneus longus tendon courses across all layers, from superficial plantar laterally to deep plantar medially
- **Dorsal muscles**: 2 muscle layers
  - Superficial layer: Tibialis anterior tendon, extensor hallucis longus tendon, extensor digitorum longus tendon, peroneus tertius tendon
  - Deep layer: Extensor hallucis brevis, extensor digitorum brevis
  - In forefoot, long and short extensors run side by side in single layer

Compartments

- **Plantar compartments**
  - Muscles are divided by fascial layers into 4 compartments
  - **Medial plantar compartment**
    - Contains abductor hallucis, flexor hallucis longus, and flexor hallucis brevis tendons
  - **Central plantar compartment**
    - Superficial subcompartment: Contains flexor digitorum brevis, distal portion of flexor digitorum longus tendons
    - Intermediary subcompartment: Contains proximal plantar portion of flexor digitorum longus tendon, quadratus plantae, lumbricals
    - Deep subcompartment: Limited to forefoot, contains adductor hallucis
  - **Lateral plantar compartment**
    - Contains abductor and flexor digiti minimi
  - **Interosseous compartment**
    - Contains plantar and dorsal interosseous muscles
- **Dorsal compartment**
  - Superficial layer: Extrinsic extensor tendons
  - Deep layer: Intrinsic extensor muscles

Major Ligaments

- Plantar fascia (aponeurosis): 3 portions extend from tuberosity of calcaneus to transverse metatarsal ligaments of toes
  - Medial band: Thin structure superficial to abductor hallucis muscle
  - Central band: Thick, strong structure superficial to flexor digitorum brevis
    - Divides into separate bands to each toe; these are linked by transverse bands
    - Distally sends septa superficially into subcutaneous fat and deep to metatarsophalangeal (MTP) joints
  - Lateral band: Thin structure superficial to abductor digiti minimi
  - Medial and lateral bands sometimes terminate at level of midmetatarsals
- Long plantar ligament: Originates at calcaneal tuberosity, inserts at cuboid and bases of 2nd-4th metatarsals
  - Forms retinaculum for peroneus longus tendon as it courses medially on plantar aspect of foot
- Short plantar (plantar calcaneocuboid) ligament: Deep to long ligament, inserts more proximally on cuboid
- Plantar calcaneocuboid (spring) ligament: Originates on sustentaculum tali, inserts on plantar aspect navicular
- Bifurcate ligament: Originates on anterior process of calcaneus dorsally, inserts on navicular and cuboid
- Lisfranc ligament: Originates at 1st cuneiform, inserts at base of 2nd metatarsal
- Intermetatarsal ligaments: Dorsal and plantar ligaments between 2nd-5th metatarsal bases
- Transverse metatarsal ligaments: Superficial and deep ligaments between metatarsal heads

Nerves

- **Tibial nerve** divides into medial and lateral plantar branches at level of tarsal tunnel
  - **Medial plantar nerve**
    - Between 1st and 2nd muscle layers, accompanies medial plantar artery
    - Motor branches: Abductor hallucis, flexor digitorum and hallucis brevis, 1st lumbrical
    - Plantar digital nerves to 1st-3rd toes, medial aspect of 4th toe
  - **Lateral plantar nerve**: Has deep and superficial divisions
    - Motor branches: Abductor digiti minimi, flexor digiti minimi brevis, lumbricals, interossei, adductor hallucis
    - Baxter's nerve, to abductor digiti minimi, is first branch of lateral plantar nerve
      - Runs between quadratus plantae & flexor digitorum brevis muscles
    - Superficial lateral plantar nerve: Between 1st and 2nd muscle layers
    - Plantar digital nerves to 5th toe, lateral aspect of 4th toe

  - Deep lateral plantar nerve: Between 3rd and 4th muscle layers; accompanies lateral plantar artery
- **Deep peroneal nerve**: Extends along dorsum of foot, between tibialis anterior and extensor hallucis longus
  - Motor branch: Extensor digitorum brevis
- **Superficial peroneal nerve**: Divides into medial and lateral branches at dorsum of foot
  - Sensory branches to dorsal foot
- **Sural nerve**: Lateral, superficial branch of tibial nerve
  - Extends along lateral margin of foot
  - Sensory branches to lateral foot

Arteries

- Posterior tibial artery divides into medial and lateral plantar arteries at level of tarsal tunnel
  - Plantar arteries accompany medial and deep lateral plantar nerves
- Peroneal artery accompanies superficial peroneal nerve down anterolateral aspect of ankle
  - May join or replace posterior tibial artery
- Anterior tibial artery continues into foot as dorsalis pedis artery, deep to extensor retinaculum
  - Divides into multiple branches in midfoot, forming arcade

Bursae

- Extensor digitorum brevis: Between muscle and 2nd cuneiform and metatarsal bases
- Extensor hallucis longus: Between tendon and 1st cuneiform and metatarsal bases
- Abductor digiti minimi: Between muscle and tuberosity of 5th metatarsal
- MTP joints: Dorsally between metatarsal heads and medial to 1st metatarsal head

Metatarsal Bones

- 1st metatarsal
  - Largest metatarsal
  - Articulates with 1st cuneiform, 1st proximal phalanx, sesamoids
  - Medially receives attachments from tibialis anterior tendon, plantar side receives peroneus longus tendon
  - Origin of medial head of 1st dorsal interosseous muscle on its lateral surface
- 2nd-4th metatarsals
  - Gradually smaller and shorter moving laterally
  - Receive interosseous muscle on medial and lateral sides
- 5th metatarsal
  - Insertion of peroneus tertius and brevis

Phalanges

- Distal phalanx is insertion site for tendons from flexor and extensor digitorum longus
- Middle phalanx is insertion site for tendons from flexor and extensor digitorum brevis
- 2nd-4th proximal phalanges are attachments of interosseous muscles on both sides and lumbricals on medial side

1st Metatarsophalangeal Joint

- Dorsiflexion of toe important in push-off phase of gait
- Metatarsal head has 2 concave facets at plantar surface, 1 for each sesamoid, separated by ridge (crista)
- Distal articular surface of metatarsal head may be flat, rounded, or have central prominence
- Base of proximal phalanx has concave contour
- **Sesamoids**
  - Either sesamoid may be unipartite or bipartite
  - Medial sesamoid in medial head flexor hallucis brevis and abductor hallucis
  - Lateral sesamoid in lateral head flexor hallucis brevis and adductor hallucis and deep metatarsal ligament
  - Medial and lateral sesamoids joined by intersesamoid ligament
    - Intersesamoid ligament is floor of canal in which flexor hallucis longus tendon runs
  - Both are embedded in plantar plate of joint
  - **Sesamophalangeal apparatus**
    - Sesamoids fixed in position relative to 1st proximal phalanx, move relative to 1st metatarsal
    - Therefore, displaced laterally in hallux valgus
- **Plantar plate**
  - Fibrocartilaginous plantar capsular thickening extending from metatarsal neck to base of proximal phalanx
  - Incorporates sesamoids

Lateral Metatarsophalangeal Joints

- Convex articular surface of metatarsal head articulates with concave articular surface of proximal phalangeal base
- Plantar aspect of metatarsal head has rounded contour
- Dorsal aspect of metatarsal head is smaller than plantar aspect
  - Has concave or notched contour along medial and lateral margins
- Sesamoids variably present, most commonly at 5th toe
- **Phalangeal apparatus** is combination of plantar plate and proximal phalanx
- **Plantar plate**
  - Fibrocartilaginous plantar capsular thickening extending from metatarsal neck to base of proximal phalanx
  - Attached to deep transverse metatarsal ligament, plantar fascia and flexor tendon sheath, medial and lateral collateral ligaments
  - Instability may mimic Morton neuroma

Arteries

- **Dorsalis pedis artery**
  - Dorsal artery of foot
  - Direct continuation of anterior tibial artery, changing name at ankle joint
  - Course and relations
    - Crosses superficial to talocrural articular capsule, talus, navicular, and intermediate cuneiform bones
    - Passes deep to inferior extensor retinaculum and distal to extensor hallucis brevis
    - Lies lateral to extensor hallucis longus tendon
    - Passes to proximal end of intermetatarsal space and curves deeply to enter sole between heads of 1st dorsal interosseous muscle
    - Forms part of plantar arch
  - Main branches

- Medial and lateral tarsal arteries: Arise at level of navicular bone
- Lateral tarsal artery runs under extensor digitorum brevis
- 2 or 3 medial tarsal arteries run on medial surface of tarsus
- Arcuate artery: Arises at medial cuneiform level and runs laterally over metatarsal bases, deep to extensor tendons; gives off branches to metatarsals and toes
- 1st dorsal metatarsal artery: Arises just before dorsalis pedis dives deep into sole

- **Posterior tibial artery**
  - Continuation of calf vessel by same name, branch of popliteal artery
  - Runs in tarsal tunnel behind and below medial malleolus accompanied by tibial nerve
  - Divides into medial and lateral plantar arteries in tarsal tunnel
  - Medial plantar artery: Runs in medial aspect of foot medial to medial plantar nerve
    - Then deep to abductor hallucis and flexor digitorum brevis muscles
  - Lateral plantar artery: Runs in lateral aspect of foot lateral to lateral plantar nerve
    - Then deep to abductor hallucis muscle and distally between flexor digitorum brevis and quadratus plantae muscles
    - Runs distally between flexor digitorum brevis and abductor digiti minimi, then runs between base of 1st and 2nd metatarsals, and
    - Joins dorsalis pedis to form plantar arch
- **Plantar arch**
  - Arterial arch at level of metatarsals
  - Formed by dorsalis pedis and lateral plantar arteries
  - Gives off branches to metatarsals and toes
- **Peroneal artery**
  - Accompanies superficial peroneal nerve, sends off perforating branch that joins communicating branch from anterior tibial artery
  - May join or replace posterior tibial artery

Veins

- Superficial veins
  - Great saphenous vein
    - Arises from medial part of dorsal venous arch of foot
    - Runs subcutaneously over muscles and tendons to pass anterior to medial malleolus
    - Passes superiorly on medial aspect of calf and thigh to join common femoral vein at femoral triangle
  - Small saphenous vein
    - Arises from lateral part of dorsal venous arch
    - Runs subcutaneously over muscles and tendons to pass posterior to lateral malleolus
    - Passes superiorly on lateral and posterior side of calf to join popliteal vein in popliteal fossa
- Deep veins
  - Plantar venous arch: Receives venous drainage from dorsal and plantar aspects of toes and metatarsals
  - Medial and lateral plantar veins: Arise from plantar venous arch to accompany same-named arteries
  - Communication exists with great and small saphenous veins
  - Medial and lateral plantar veins form posterior tibial veins in tarsal tunnel and run proximally to calf, accompanying posterior tibial artery

ANATOMY IMAGING ISSUES

Imaging Recommendations

- Diagnostic US
  - As result of transverse arch of foot, interrogation should be performed separately for medial and lateral sides for best visualization
  - Due to complex soft tissue anatomy, panoramic (extended field of view) images provide better depiction of location and extent of lesion and course of different structures
  - Dorsal foot structures tend to be very superficial and thin (tendons) or compressible (vessels)
    - To better visualize these structures, minimal compression and thick layer of coupling gel may help
  - Good for assessing tendon integrity and joint alignment
    - Tendon integrity recognized by morphology (continuity of tendon and densely packed appearance of tendon fibers) and by behavior during passive movement
    - Joints can also be assessed dynamically during flexion and extension
  - Color Doppler scans allow assessment for vessel occlusion and thrombosis
  - Spectral Doppler scans allow quantitative and semiquantitative documentation of flow velocity, resistance, waveform, etc.
  - Augmentation of foot veins usually only requires small degrees of flexion/extension of toes to produce enough venous flow for detection (unlike need to squeeze muscles in calf)
- Therapeutic US
  - Guide therapeutic injection for nerve entrapment syndromes, arthritis, tenosynovitis

Imaging Sweet Spots

- Tendon movement can be easily demonstrated with ultrasound by moving bone onto which it inserts
  - Helps with confirming tendon location and also with establishing tendon integrity
- Tarsal ligaments are usually seen as hypoechoic thickenings on cortices and between bones
  - Orientation of transducer along long axis makes ligament stand out and easier to identify

Imaging Pitfalls

- Superficial veins are easily compressed even with lightest transducer pressure
  - Thick layer of coupling gel helps act as spacer between transducer and skin to minimize pressure and allows for better visualization of vessels

GRAPHICS: DORSAL FOOT

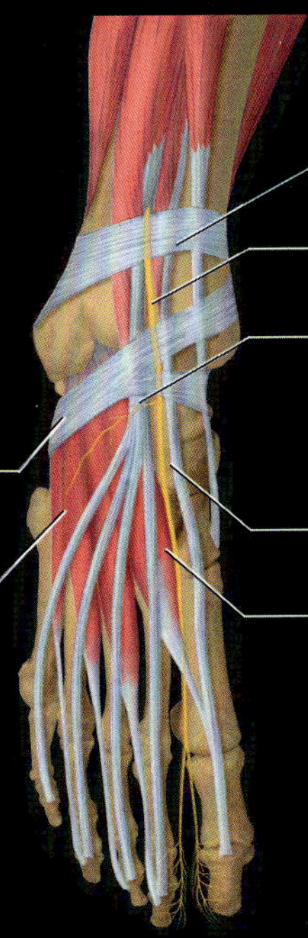

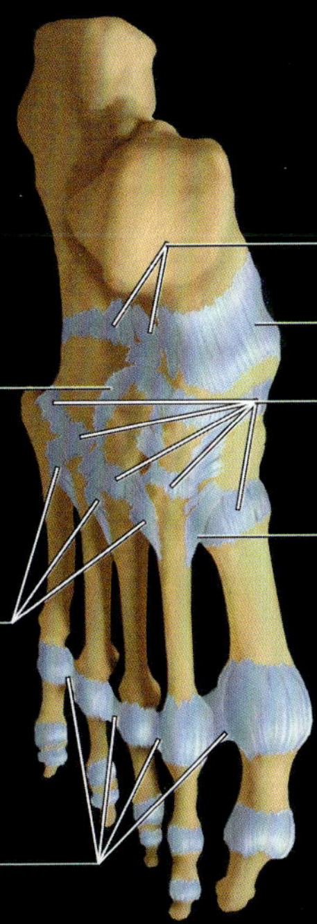

(Top) *The deep peroneal nerve travels deep to the extensor retinacula, in the anterior tarsal tunnel, and gives a lateral motor branch to the extensor digitorum brevis muscle. The medial branch continues dorsal to the talonavicular joint, middle cuneiform, and in between the 1st and 2nd metatarsals to provide mostly sensory but some motor supply to the 1st web space.* **(Bottom)** *Graphic of the dorsal ligaments shows dense ligaments between the tarsal bones and between tarsals and metatarsals. Ligaments are generally named for the bones they bridge. Exceptions are the bifurcate ligament, which extends from the anterior process of the calcaneus to the cuboid and the navicular, and the dorsal Lisfranc ligament, from the 1st cuneiform to the 2nd metatarsal.*

US: DORSAL FOOT

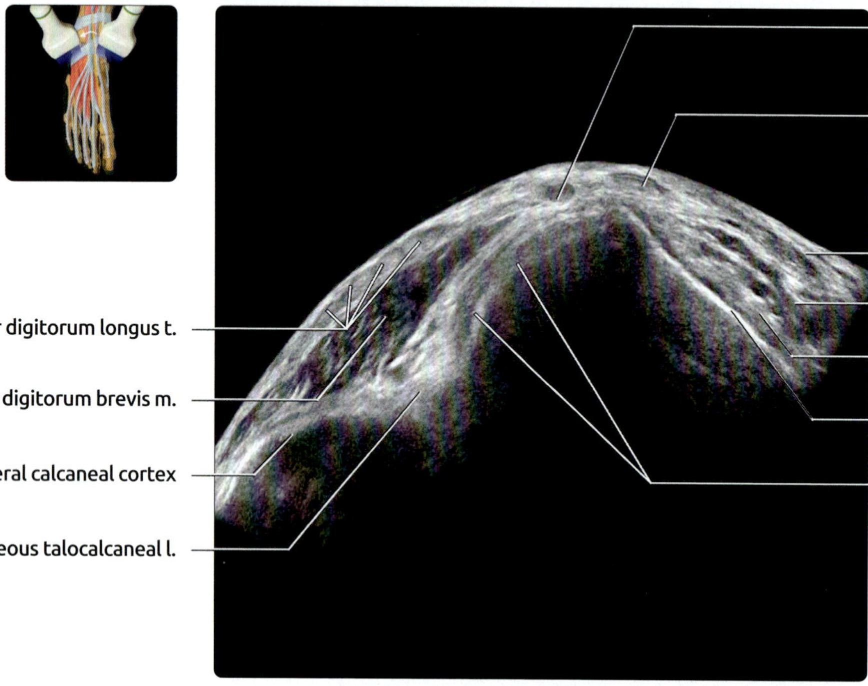

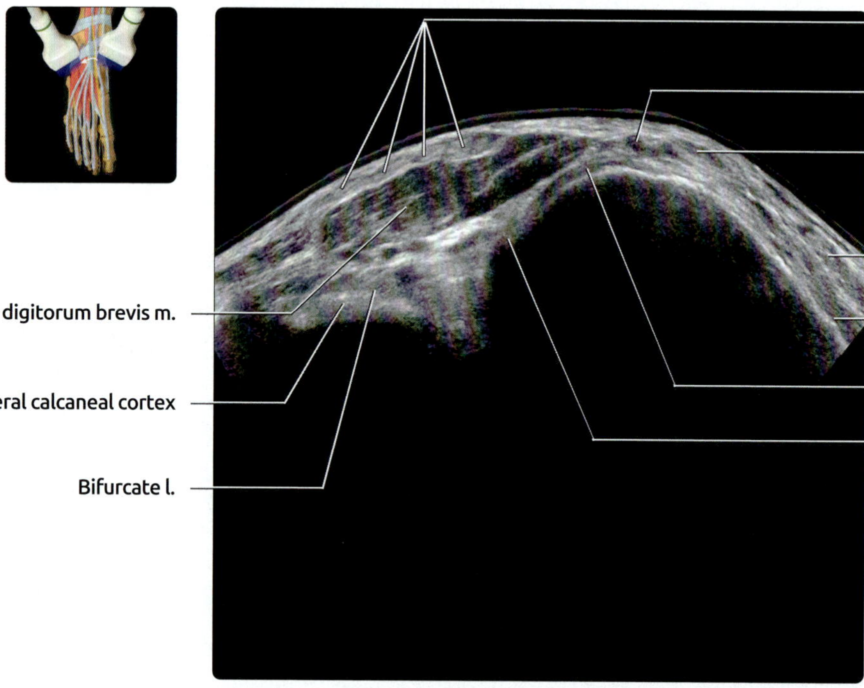

(Top) *Coronal panoramic scan shows the dorsal foot at the level of the talar head The foot can be divided into 2 columns: The medial column (talus, navicular, and cuneiforms) and lateral column (calcaneus and cuboid) form the anteromedial and anterolateral surfaces of the transverse midfoot arch. The dorsalis pedis artery runs at the apex of this arch.* **(Bottom)** *Coronal panoramic scan shows the dorsal foot through the navicular. The transverse arch of the dorsal foot creates 2 surfaces: Anteromedial and anterolateral, over which extensor tendons and small muscles lie. More focal examination of these structures requires scanning along each surface separately. Panoramic scans give an overview of anatomy. However, high-resolution imaging of the site of interest provides more details, and both should be performed as complementary techniques.*

US: DORSAL FOOT

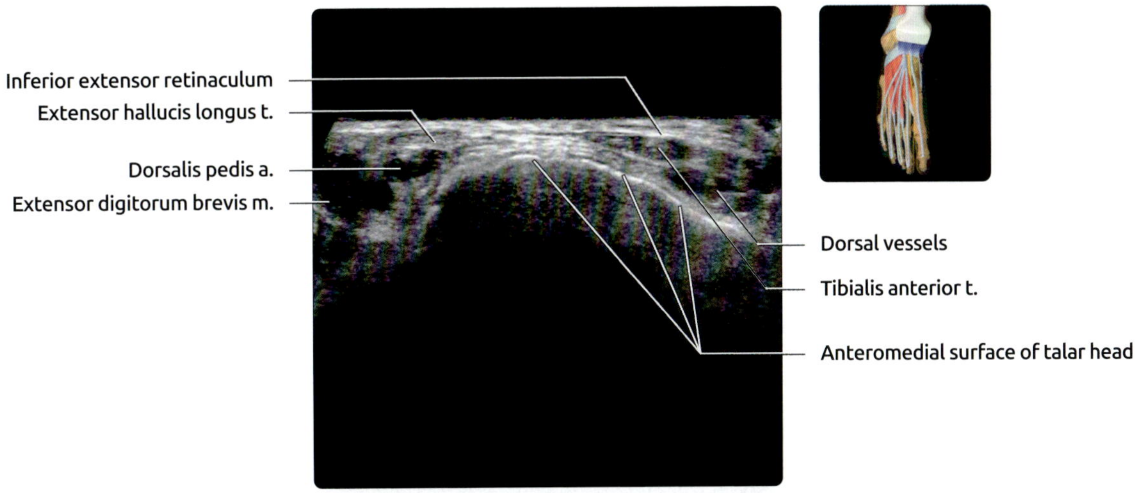

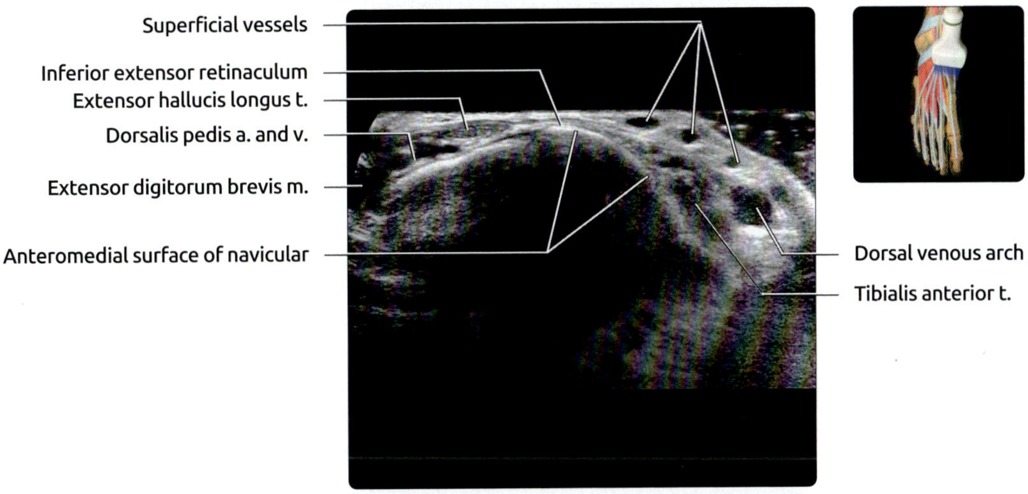

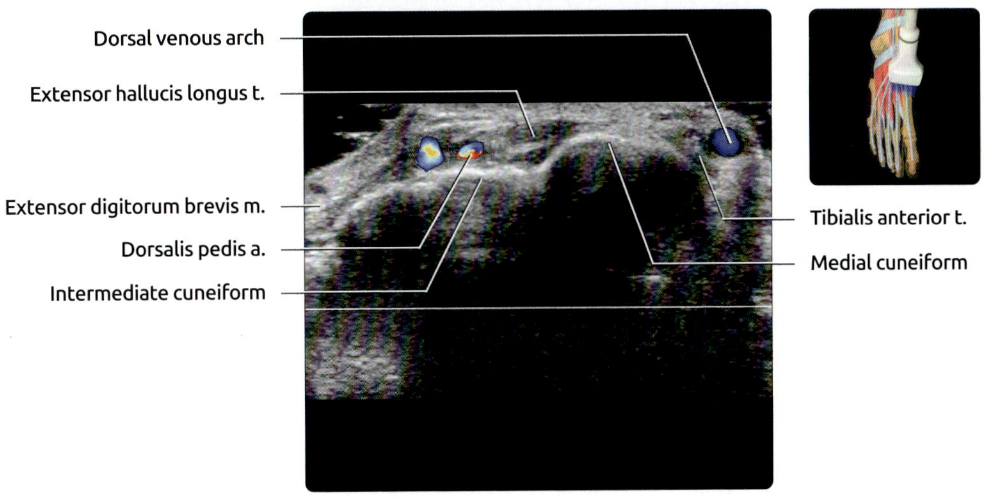

(Top) *Series of 3 coronal scans shows the dorsal medial surface of the foot. At this most proximal level, the talus is the underlying bone. The extensor hallucis can be seen partially covering the dorsalis pedis artery. More medially, the tibialis anterior tendon can be found.* **(Middle)** *At a midtarsal level, this coronal scan shows the anteromedial surface of the navicular. The tibialis anterior tendon begins to turn acutely medially to curve around to the medial edge of the foot, eventually inserting on the medial cuneiform. As seen here, the use of light pressure and copious amounts of gel will allow visualization of small superficial veins, which are numerous on the dorsum of the foot.* **(Bottom)** *Coronal color Doppler scan shows the level of the cuneiforms. The intimate relationship between the dorsalis pedis artery and the extensor hallucis longus tendon continues.*

US: DORSAL FOOT

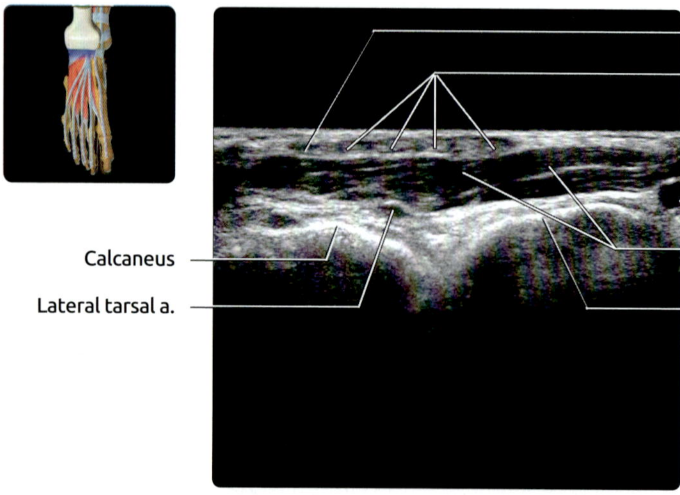

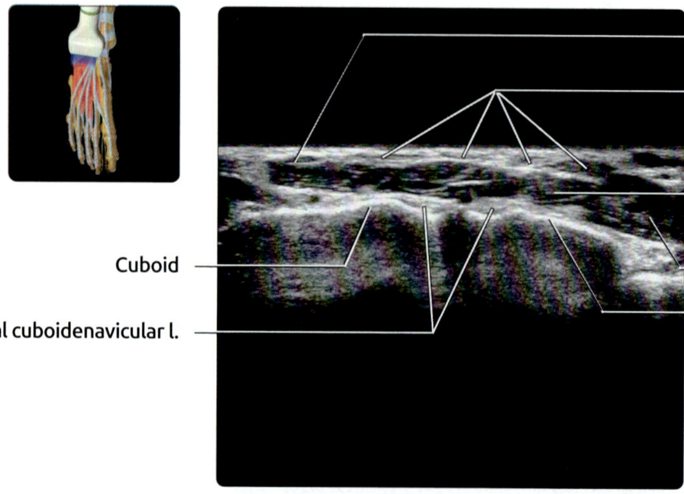

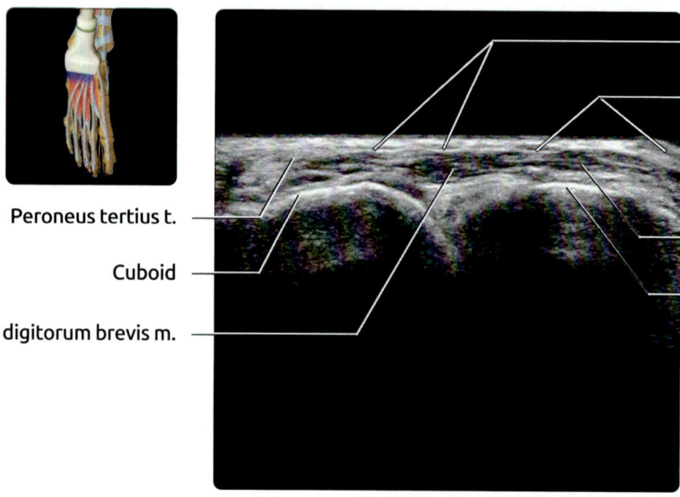

(Top) *Series of 3 coronal scans are shown over the dorsal lateral surface of the tarsus. At this proximal level, the lateral surface of the calcaneus and the talus are the underlying bones. The extensor digitorum longus tendons are close to each other and share a common synovial sheath. The extensor digitorum brevis muscle lies deep to the longus tendons. The lateral tarsal artery runs deeper and is a branch of the dorsalis pedis artery.* **(Middle)** *At the level of the midtarsus, the extensor digitorum longus tendons for individual toes begin to spread out and also flatten (the latter making them just discernible on ultrasound). At this level, the extensor hallucis brevis muscle can also be seen.* **(Bottom)** *At a more distal level, the extensor digitorum brevis muscle and the extensor hallucis brevis muscle are much thinner and will turn into tendons distally.*

US: DORSAL FOOT

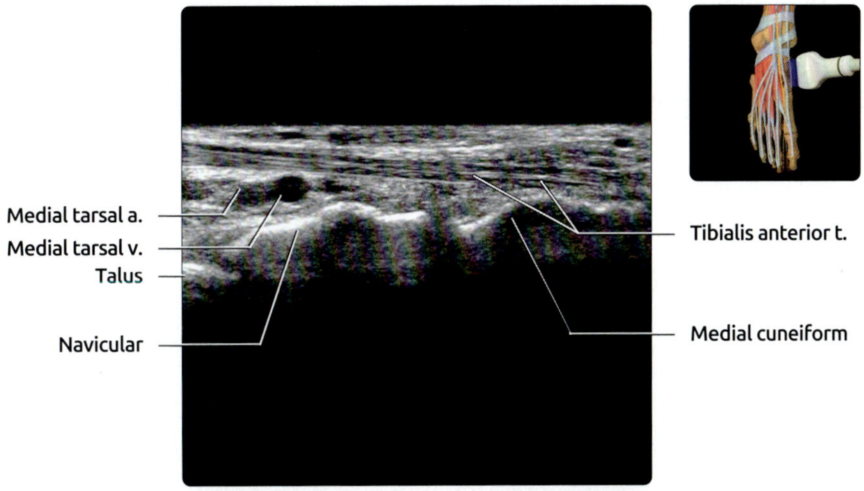

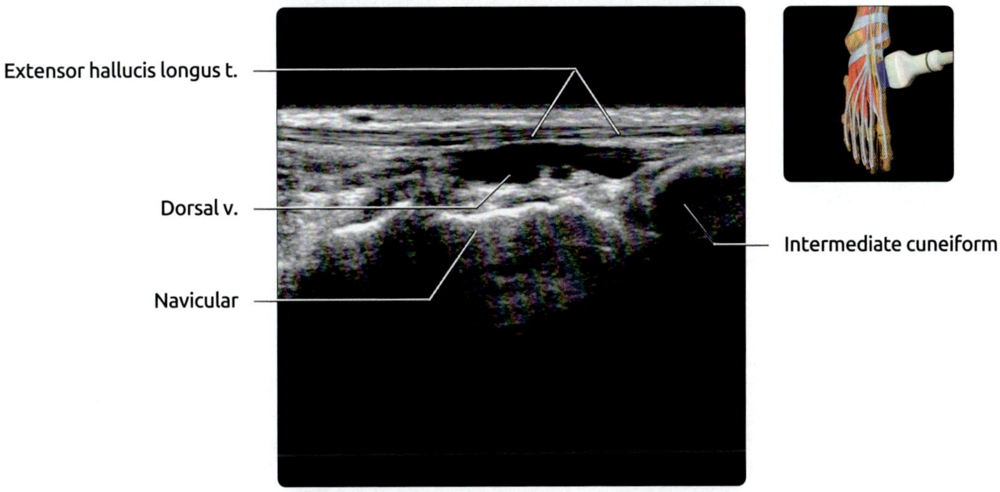

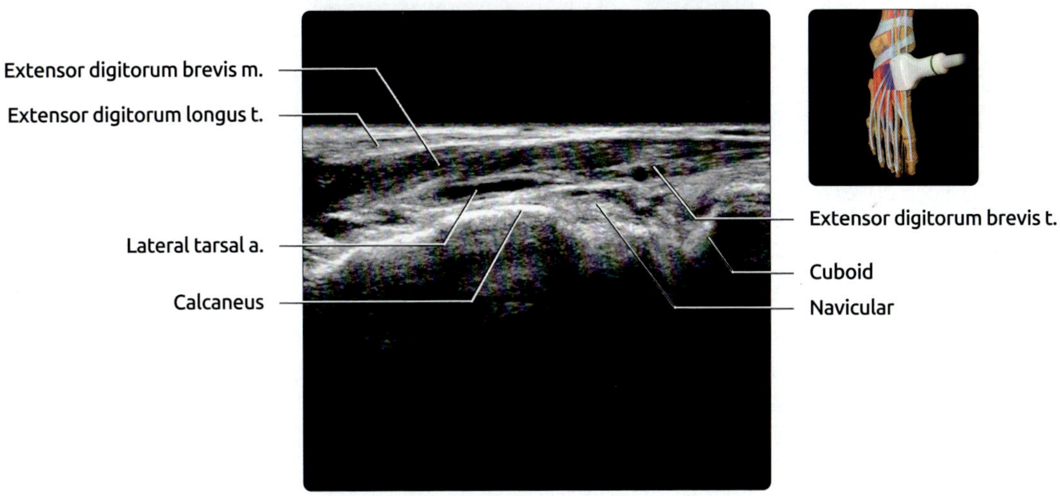

(Top) *Series of sagittal scans are shown through the tarsus. Medially, the tibialis anterior is seen running over the medial tarsal vessels (branch of dorsalis pedis) to insert on the medial and inferior surfaces of the base of the medial cuneiform.* **(Middle)** *Slightly laterally, the extensor hallucis longus tendon runs toward the big toe, passing over the intermediate cuneiform bone.* **(Bottom)** *More laterally, the extensor digitorum longus tendon and the extensor digitorum brevis muscle come into view. They lie on the surface of the calcaneus with the lateral tarsal artery coursing between the muscle and bone. The gradual tapering of the extensor digitorum brevis muscle distally can be appreciated here.*

GRAPHICS: PLANTAR MUSCLES, SUPERFICIAL LAYERS

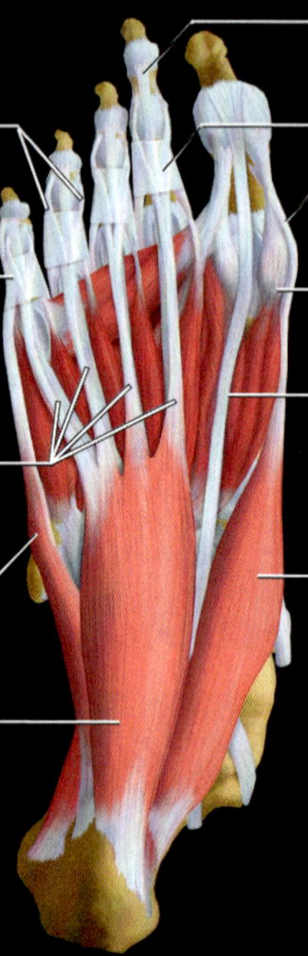

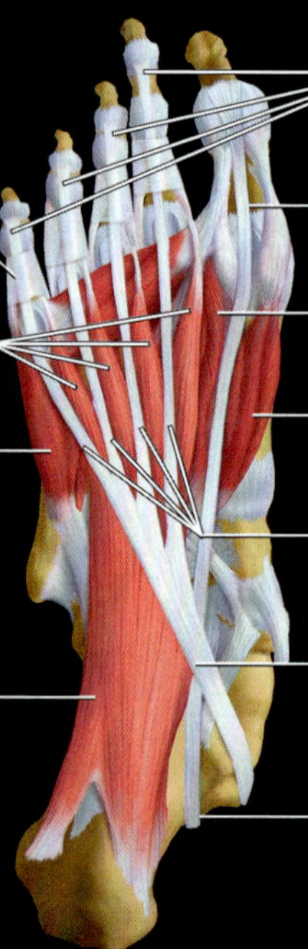

(Top) *Graphic shows the superficial layer of the plantar foot muscles: Abductor digiti minimi, flexor digitorum brevis, and abductor hallucis. The deep muscles are partially visible deep to the superficial layer. The flexor digitorum brevis tendons split in each digit (4th digit labeled), attaching at lateral aspects of the middle phalangeal bases. The flexor tendon sheaths hold the flexor mechanism in close proximity to the phalanges.* **(Bottom)** *Graphic shows the 2nd layer of plantar muscles. The interesting arrangement of interactions between flexors is well seen: Quadratus plantae inserting on flexor digitorum longus tendon and lumbricals arising from individual flexor digitorum longus tendon slips. In the toes, the flexor tendons are contained within fibrous tendon sheaths.*

GRAPHICS: PLANTAR FOOT MUSCLES, DEEP LAYERS

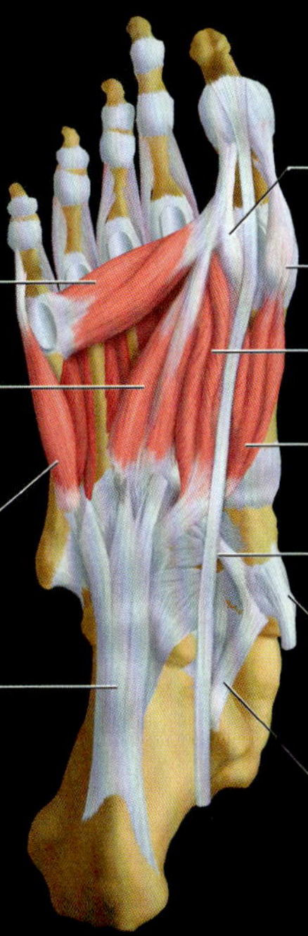

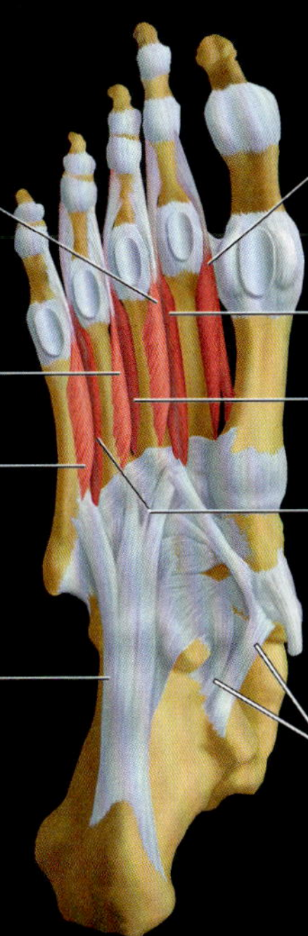

(Top) *Graphic shows the 3rd layer of plantar muscles. This layer contains the flexor hallucis brevis and flexor digiti minimi as well as the adductor hallucis muscle. The oblique head of the adductor hallucis is thick and broad, whereas the transverse head is thin.* **(Bottom)** *Graphic shows the 4th layer of plantar muscles, the interosseous muscles. There are 4 dorsal interossei. They have bipennate origins from 2 adjacent metatarsals. There are 3 plantar interossei. The 1st plantar interosseous muscle originates from the medial side of the 3rd metatarsal and inserts on the medial side of the 3rd proximal phalanx. The 2nd and 3rd plantar interossei originate on the medial sides of the 4th and 5th metatarsals, respectively, and insert on the medial side of the corresponding proximal phalanx.*

US: PLANTAR FASCIA

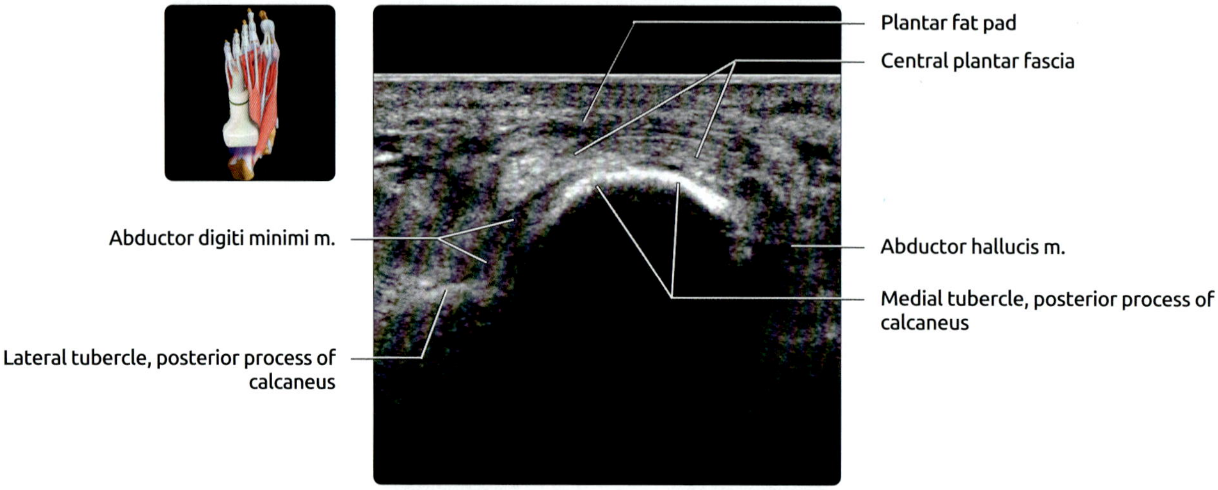

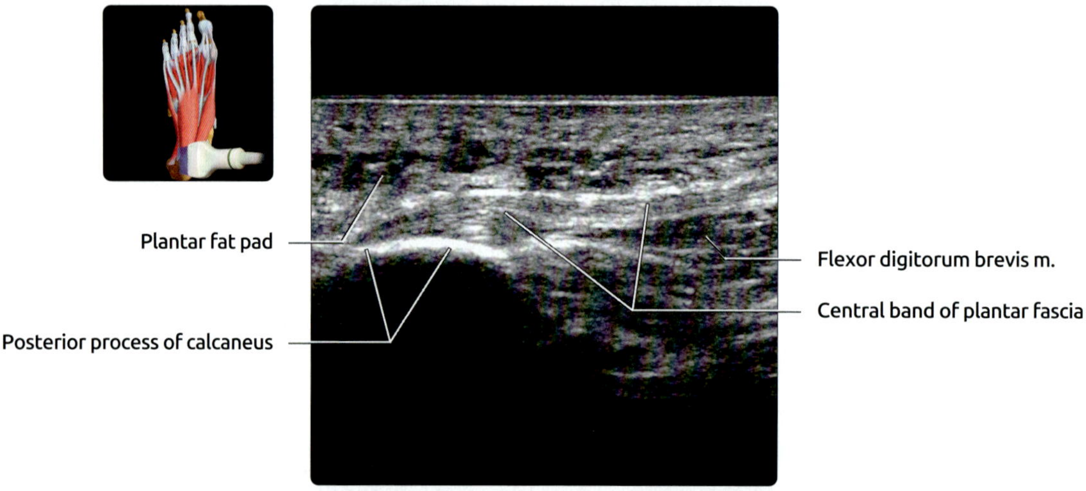

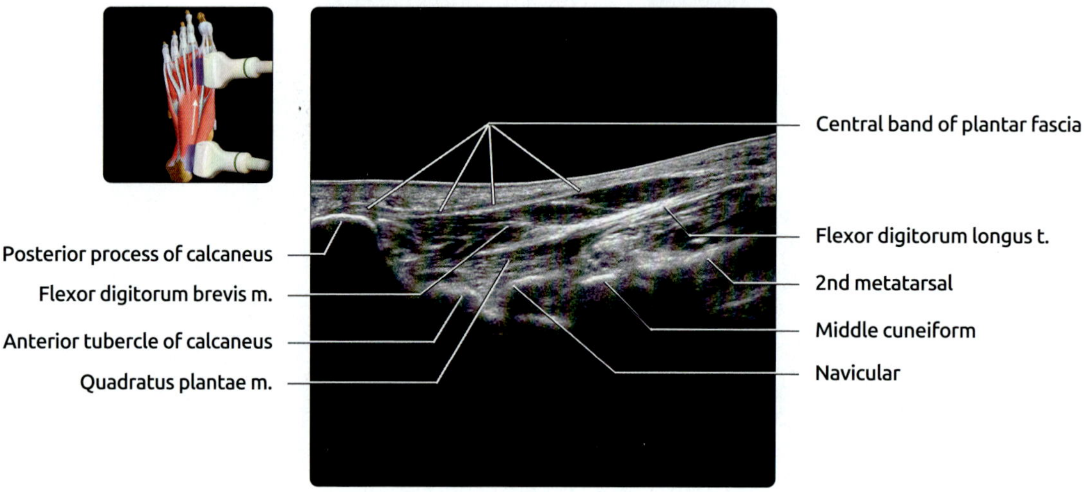

(Top) *Coronal scan of the calcaneus shows the origin of the plantar fascia. The plantar aponeurosis fascia consists of 3 parts: A strong, thick central band over the flexor digitorum brevis muscle; a lateral band over the abductor digiti muscle; and a thin medial band over the abductor hallucis muscle.* **(Middle)** *Sagittal scan shows the origin of the central band of the plantar fascia. This arises from the plantar surface of the posterior process of the calcaneus and arborizes distally with the superficial fascia at the level of the metatarsophalangeal joints.* **(Bottom)** *Sagittal panoramic scan shows the central band of plantar fascia The central is the thickest and most easily identified component of the plantar fascia and the most commonly injured band. Deep to this are the flexor digitorum brevis and quadratus plantae muscles, which form the bulk of the central tarsal plantar compartment.*

US: SAGITTAL FOOT OVERVIEW

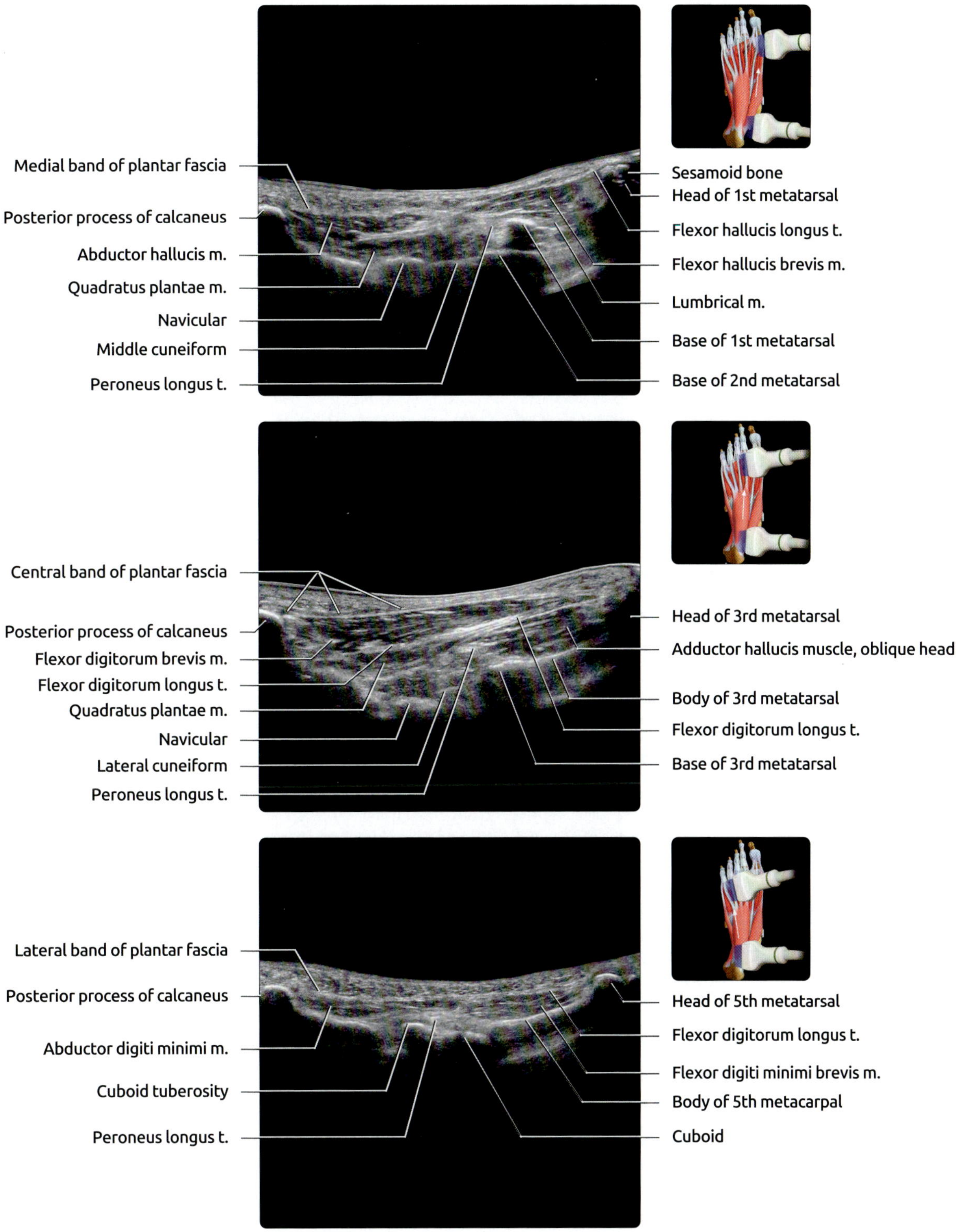

(Top) *Series of 3 panoramic sagittal scans are shown through the plantar aspect of the foot. This scan shows the content of the medial compartment: The abductor hallucis muscle, flexor hallucis longus tendon, and flexor hallucis brevis muscle, together with smaller structures.* **(Middle)** *In the central plantar compartment, the contents can be divided into layers. Superficially, there is the flexor digitorum brevis muscle and the flexor digitorum longus tendon. Deep to this layer are the quadratus plantae muscle, oblique head of the adductor hallucis muscle, and the lumbricals.* **(Bottom)** *A scan through the lateral compartment containing the abductor digiti minimi muscle and the flexor digiti minimi muscle is shown.*

US: MEDIAL TARSUS

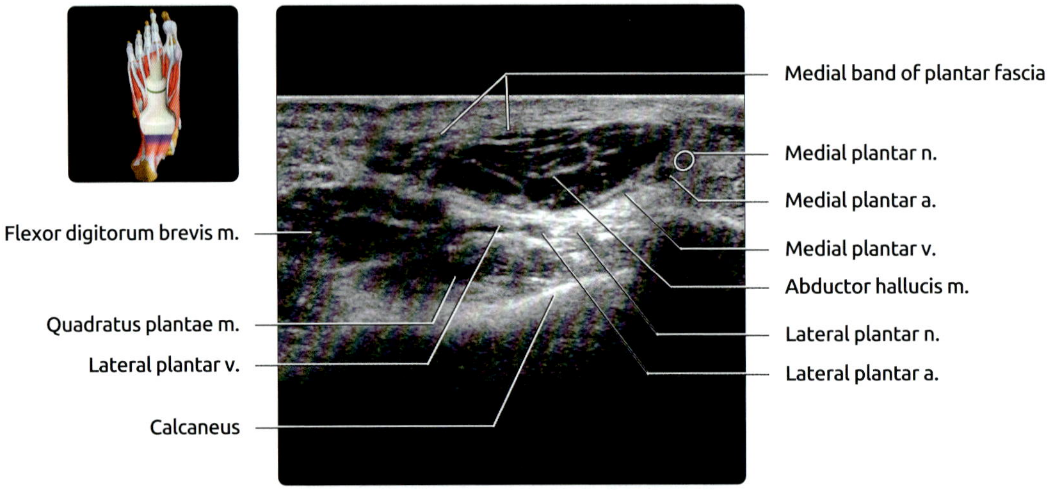

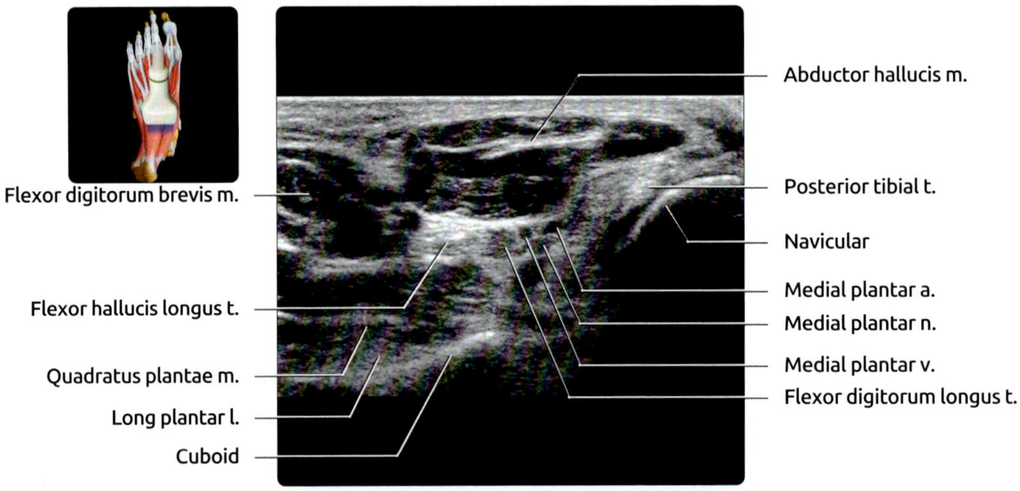

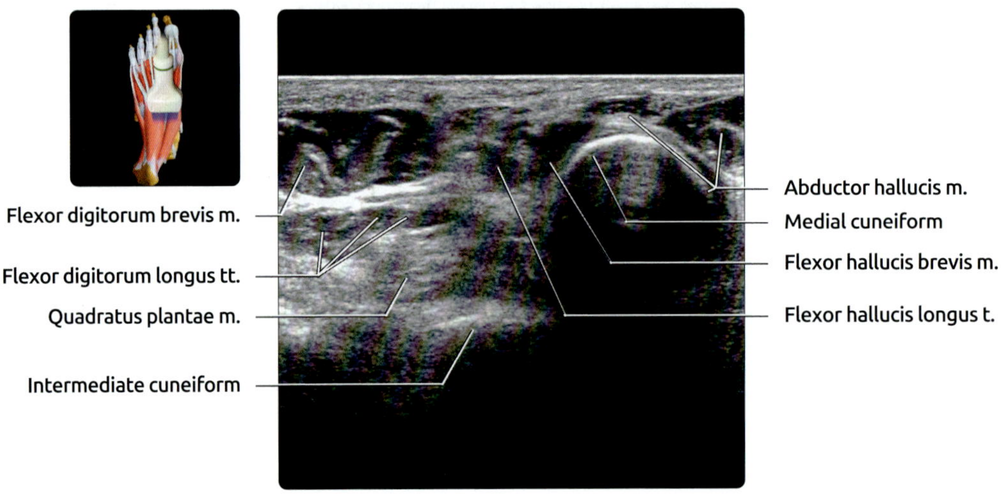

(Top) *Series of 3 coronal scans are shown through the medial 1/2 of the plantar aspect of the foot. At this proximal level, the 2 main muscles (flexor digitorum brevis and quadratus plantae) of the central compartment can be seen lying superficial to the calcaneus. The medial compartment muscle (abductor hallucis) can also be seen medially.* **(Middle)** *At the level of the midtarsus, the knot of Henry can be seen, where the flexor digitorum longus and flexor hallucis longus tendons cross and exchange fibers. The medial plantar neurovascular bundle lies in close proximity to this.* **(Bottom)** *More distally, the flexor hallucis longus and digitorum longus tendons separate and head toward their respective insertions. The flexor hallucis brevis arises at this level and divides into 2 heads, which will flank the flexor hallucis longus more distally.*

US: LATERAL TARSUS

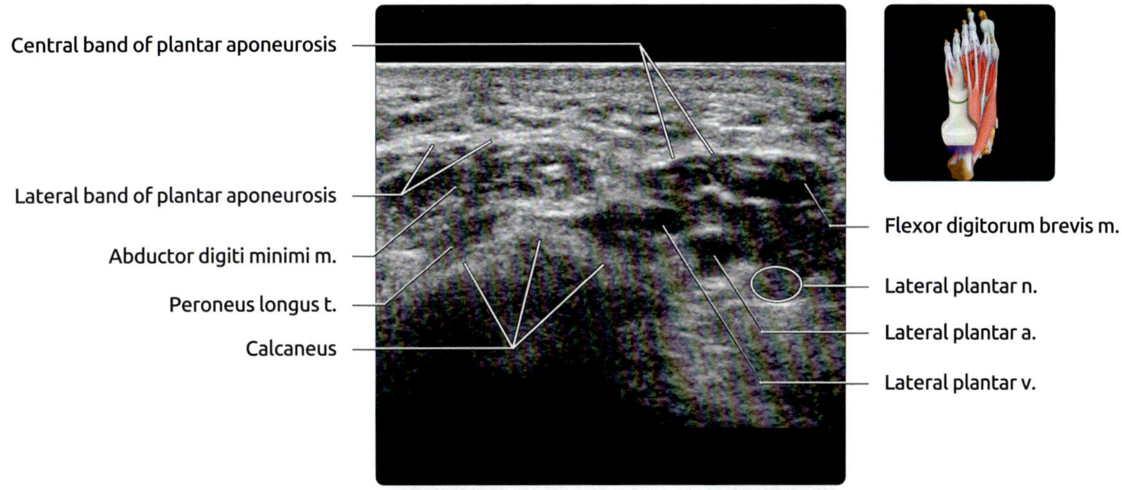

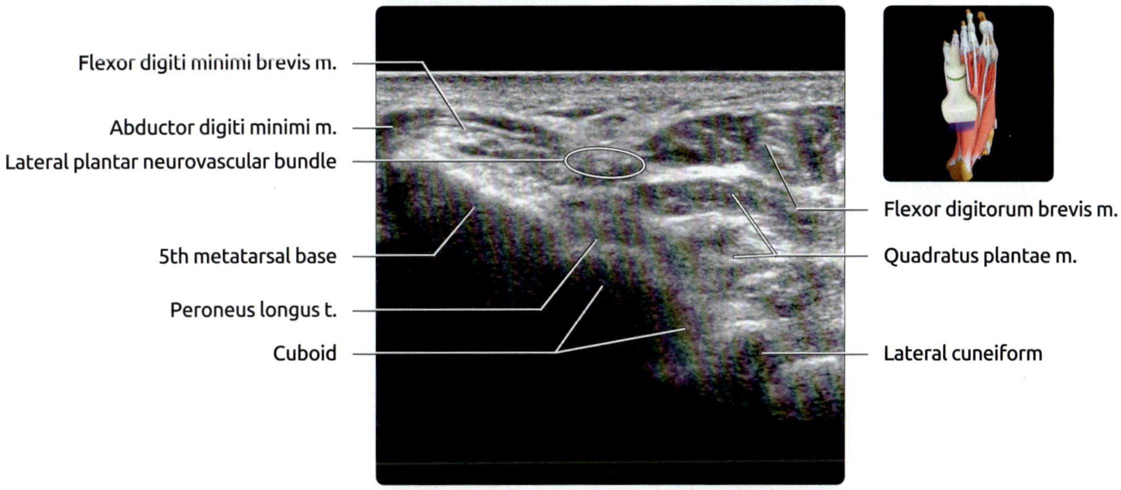

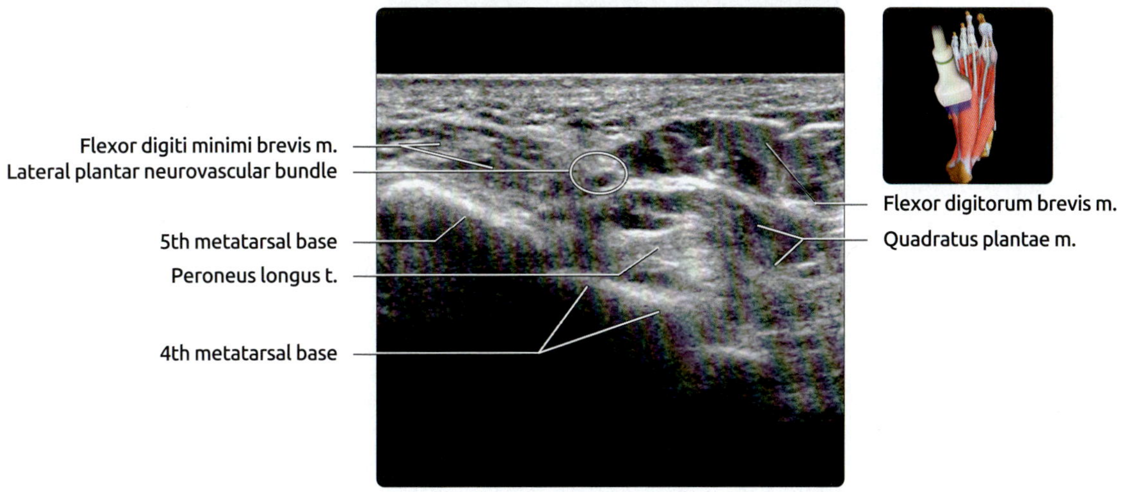

(Top) *Series of 3 coronal scans are shown through the lateral 1/2 of the plantar aspect of the foot. The lateral compartment (abductor digiti minimi) and 1/2 of the central compartment can be seen here, separated by the lateral plantar neurovascular bundle. The calcaneus forms the bony support of all structures at this level.* **(Middle)** *At the level of the midtarsus, the separation between the lateral and the central compartment by the neurovascular bundle continues. Within the lateral compartment, the abductor digiti minimi muscle moves laterally to give way to the other component of the lateral compartment, the flexor digiti minimi brevis muscle.* **(Bottom)** *Most distally, the abductor digiti minimi muscle runs on the lateral border, and only the flexor digiti minimi brevis muscle is seen on the plantar aspect of the foot.*

GRAPHICS: DORSAL AND PLANTAR ARTERIES AND NERVES

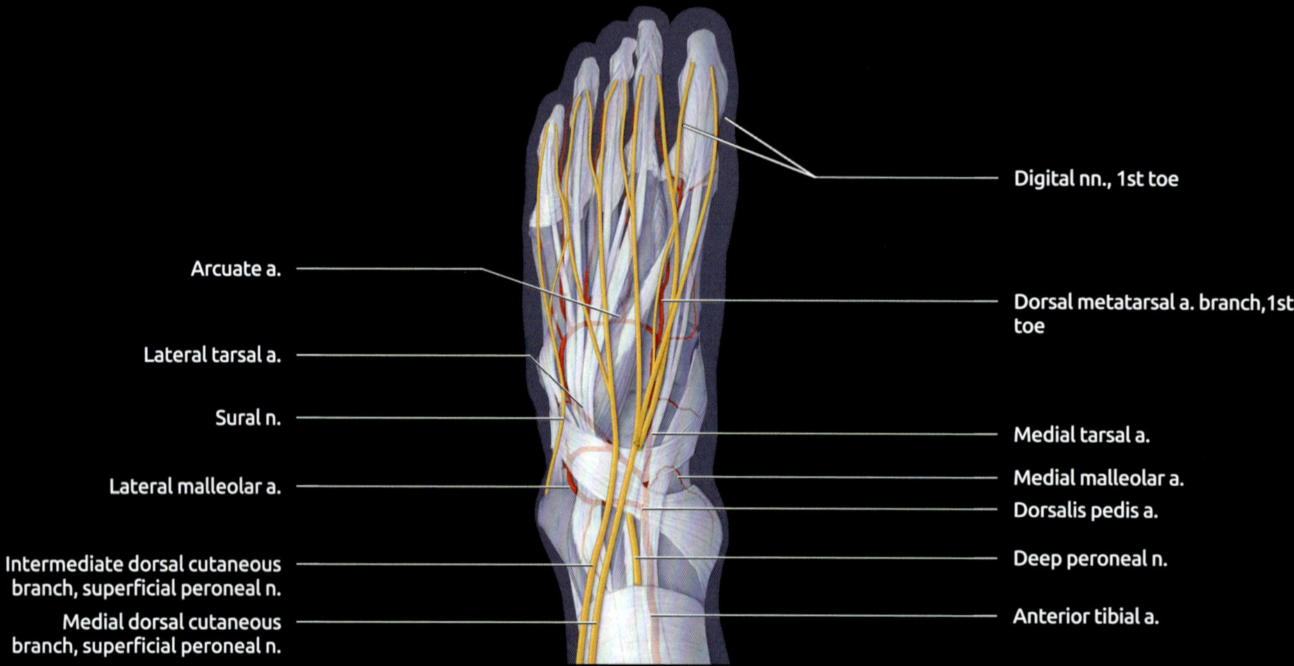

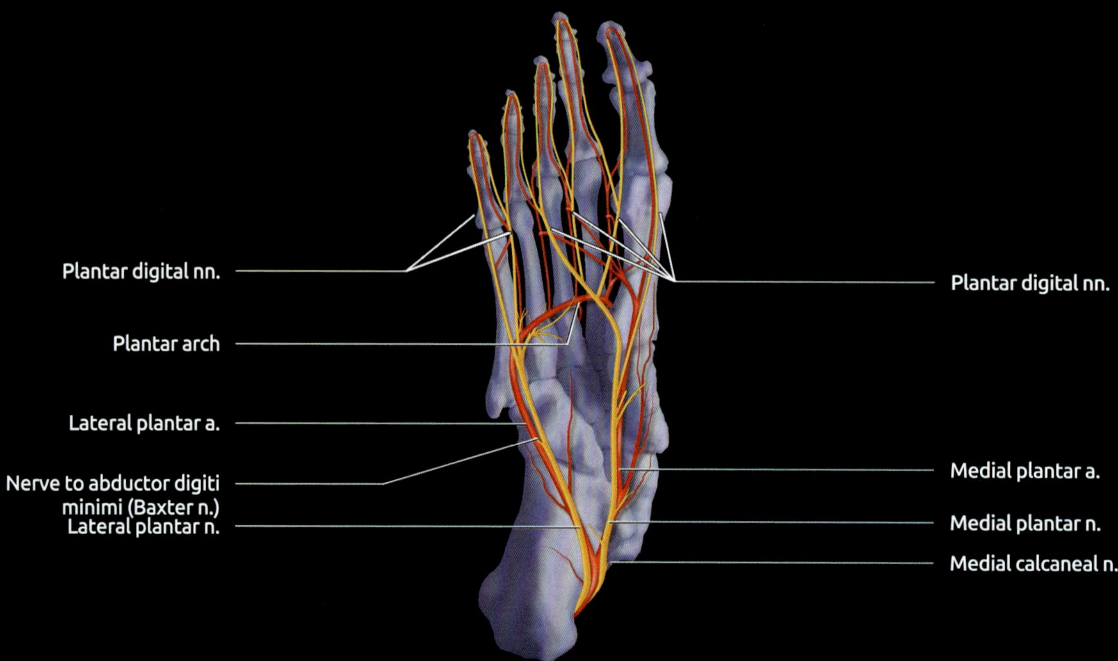

(Top) *Graphic shows the nerves and arteries of the dorsal foot. The deep peroneal nerve accompanies the anterior tibial artery. The superficial peroneal nerve divides in the distal 1/3 of the leg into medial and intermediate cutaneous branches, which provide sensation to the dorsum of the foot except the 1st web space, which is innervated by the deep peroneal nerve. The sural nerve has a number of anatomic variants and is vulnerable to fascial entrapment, which can be treated with ultrasound-guided injection.* **(Bottom)** *Graphic shows the nerves and arteries of the plantar foot. The plantar arch forms from the anastomosis of the lateral plantar artery and the dorsalis pedis artery. Medial calcaneal nerve arises in the proximal portion of the tarsal tunnel and provides cutaneous sensation to the medial heel. Baxter nerve is the 1st branch of the lateral plantar nerve and usually arises more proximally than shown here.*

US: DORSALIS PEDIS ARTERY

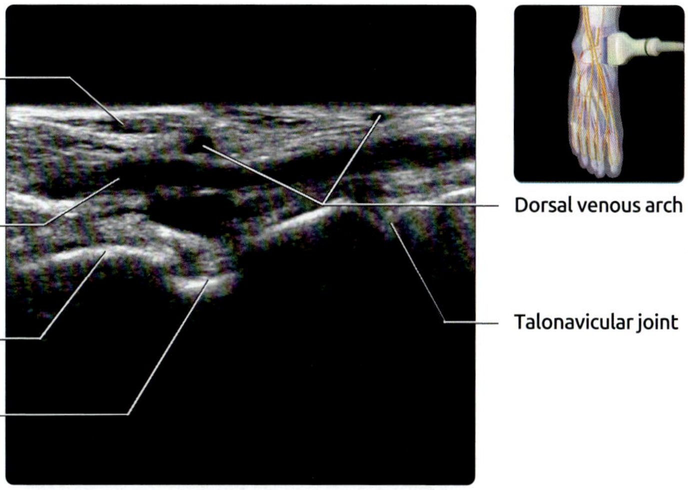

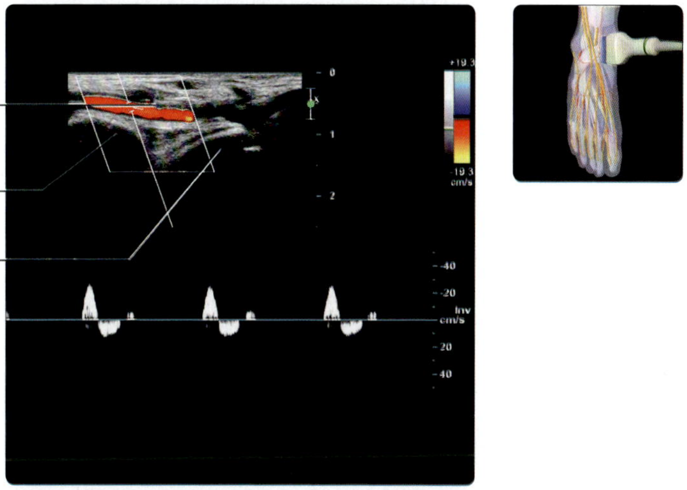

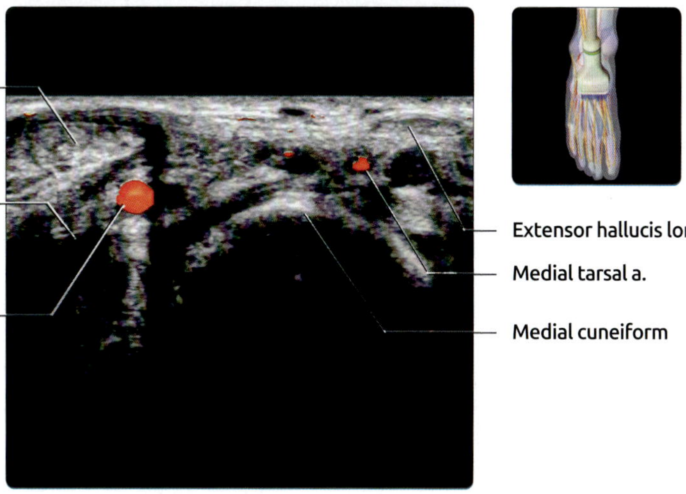

(Top) *Sagittal scan of the dorsum of the foot shows the dorsalis pedis artery, the continuation of the anterior tibial artery. It is lateral to the extensor hallucis longus tendon, a small portion of which is included on this image.* **(Middle)** *Sagittal spectral Doppler exam of the dorsalis pedis artery shows the typical triphasic artery flow.* **(Bottom)** *Coronal color Doppler scan shows the continuation of the dorsalis pedis artery as the medial and lateral tarsal arteries. The lateral tarsal artery runs deep to the extensor digitorum brevis muscle.*

US: METATARSAL AND DIGITAL ARTERIES

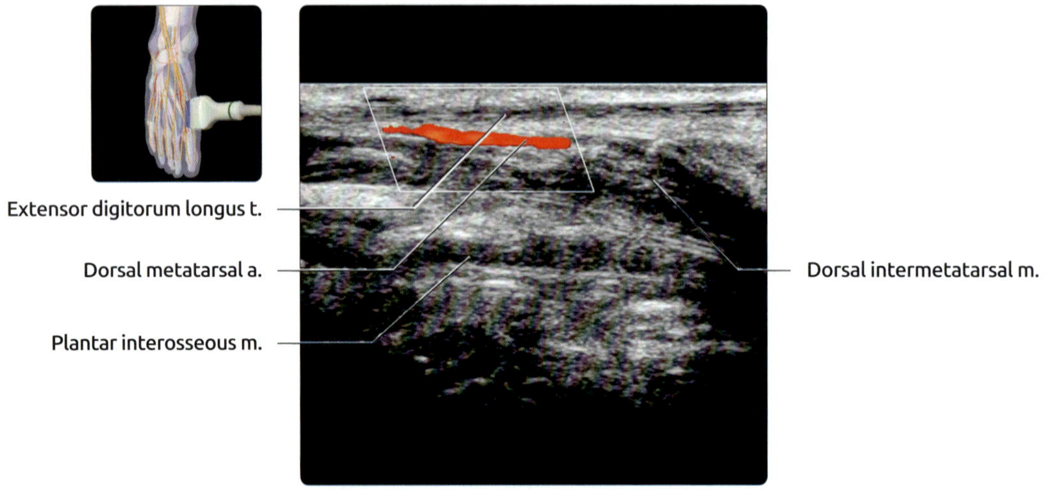

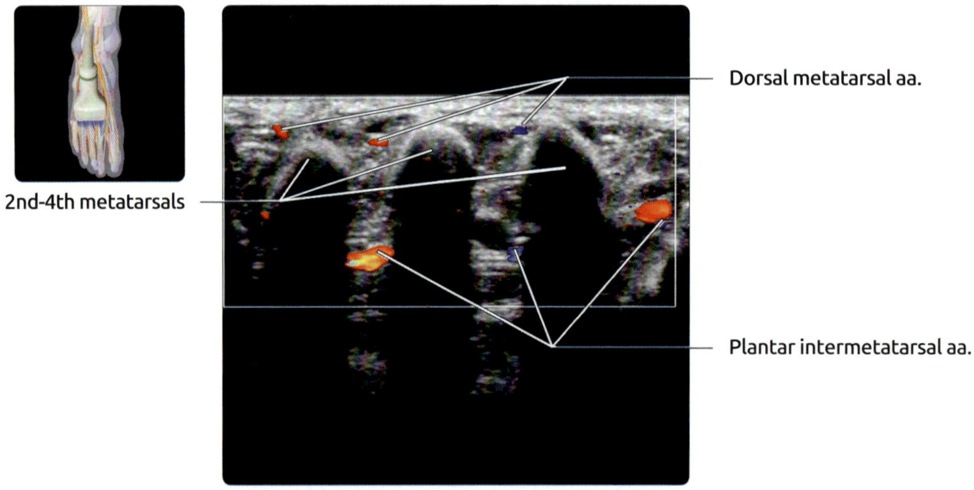

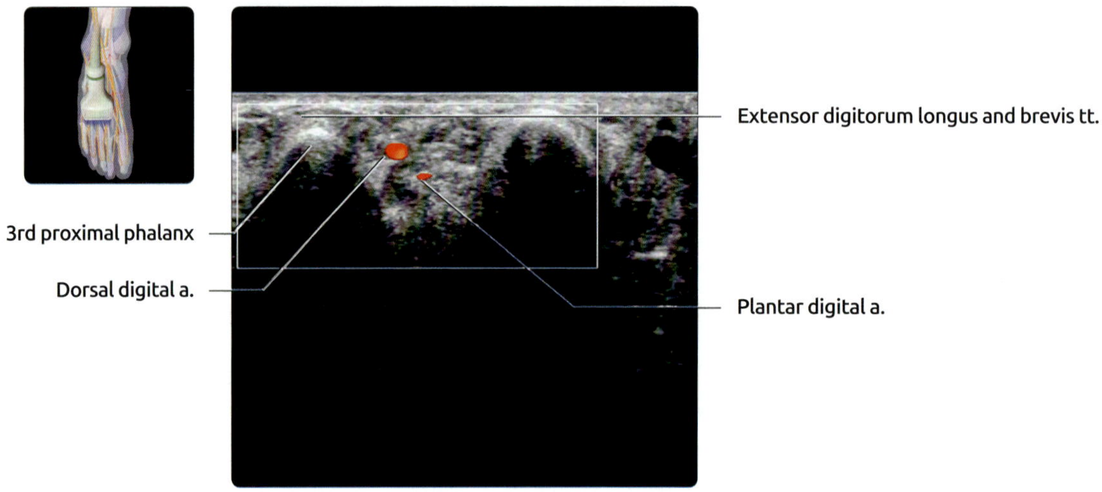

(Top) *Sagittal color Doppler scan shows the 2nd intermetatarsal space. Dorsal metatarsal arteries arise from the arcuate artery and run in the intermetatarsal spaces to supply the metatarsals and toes.* **(Middle)** *Coronal color Doppler scan shows the relationship of the plantar and dorsal metatarsal arteries to the metatarsals.* **(Bottom)** *Coronal color Doppler scan at the level of the proximal phalangeal bases shows the continuation of the intermetatarsal arteries as the digital arteries. The digital arteries each divide into branches along the medial and lateral sides of the phalanges.*

US: PLANTAR ARTERIES

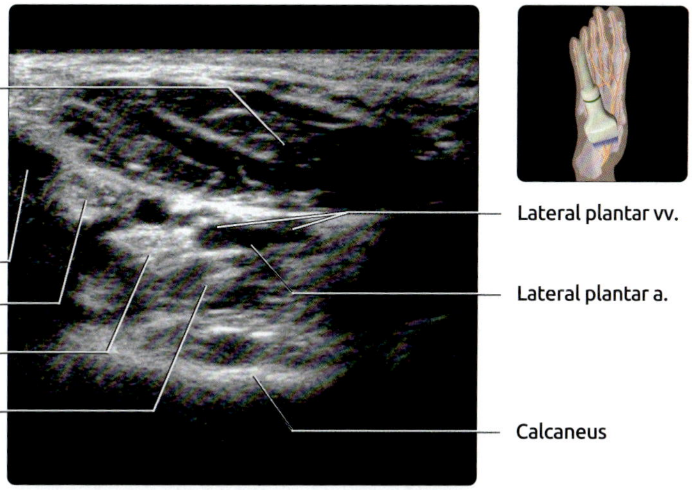

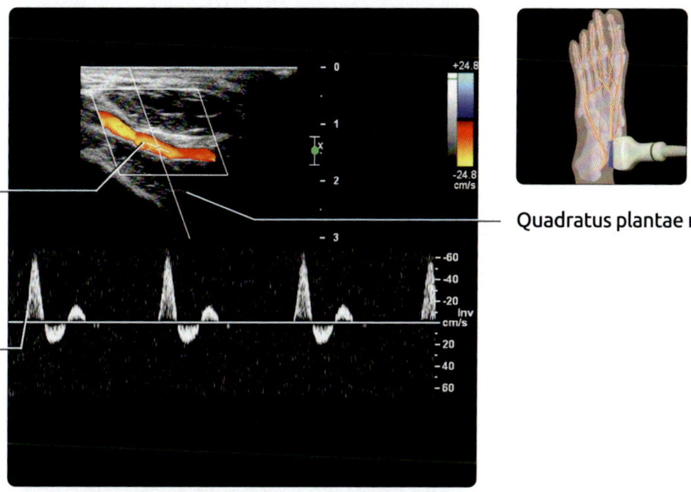

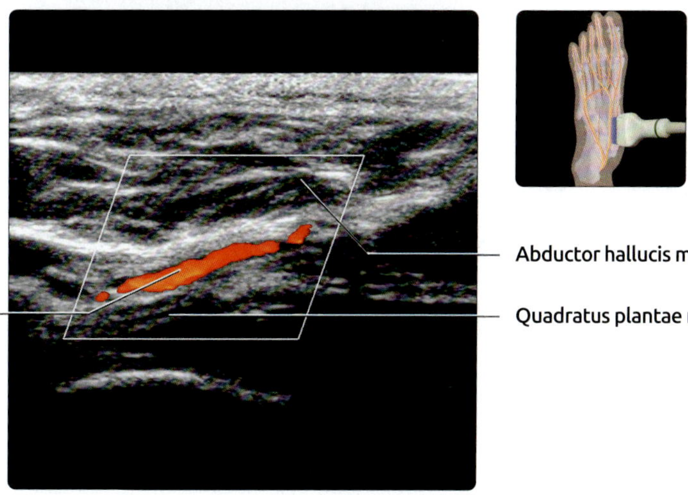

(Top) *Coronal scan shows the medial plantar compartment in the hindfoot. The tibial nerve has divided into medial and lateral plantar nerves, and the posterior tibial artery and veins have also divided into medial and lateral plantar branches.* **(Middle)** *Spectral Doppler scan of the medial plantar artery shows the normal triphasic arterial waveform.* **(Bottom)** *Longitudinal color Doppler scan of the medial compartment shows the medial plantar artery running between the abductor hallucis muscle and the quadratus plantae muscle.*

US: DORSAL METATARSALS

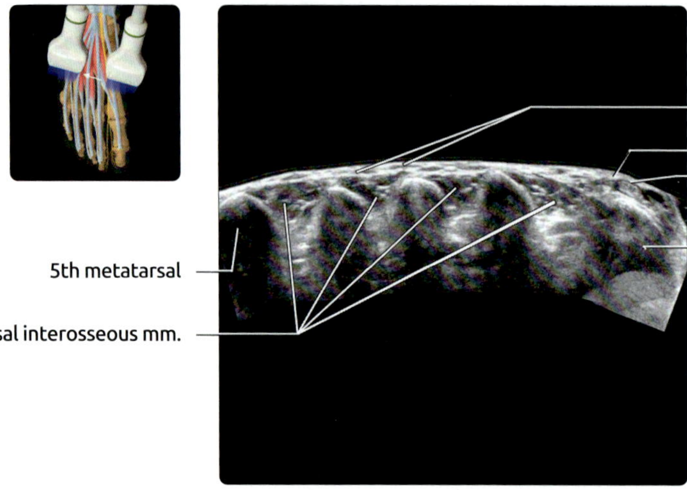

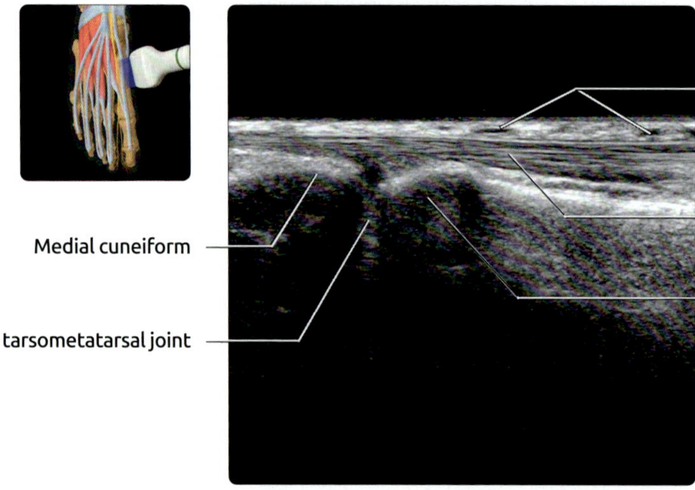

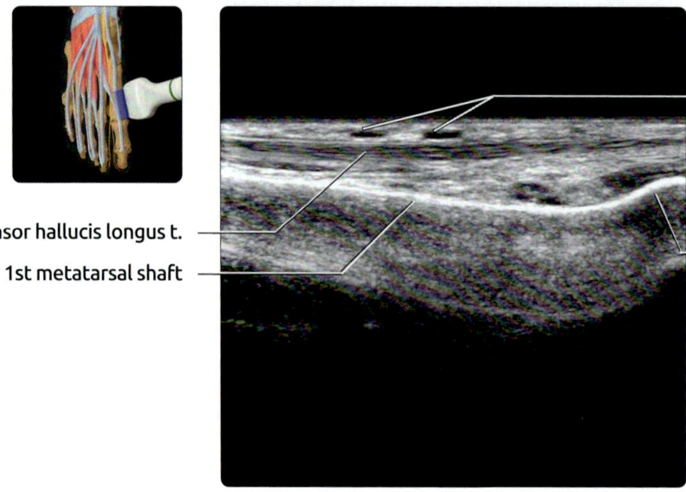

(Top) *Coronal panoramic scan shows the dorsal surface of the metatarsal shafts. The extensor digitorum longus tendon slips lie slightly dorsal and medial to the corresponding slips of the extensor digitorum brevis tendon.* **(Middle)** *Sagittal scan shows the dorsum of the 1st toe at the level of the tarsometatarsal joint. Extensor hallucis longus tendon is closely apposed to the bones; the extensor hallucis brevis is situated slightly more laterally.* **(Bottom)** *Sagittal scan more distally in the 1st metatarsal shows that the extensor hallucis longus is separated from the distal metatarsal shaft by fibrofatty tissue.*

US: PLANTAR METATARSALS

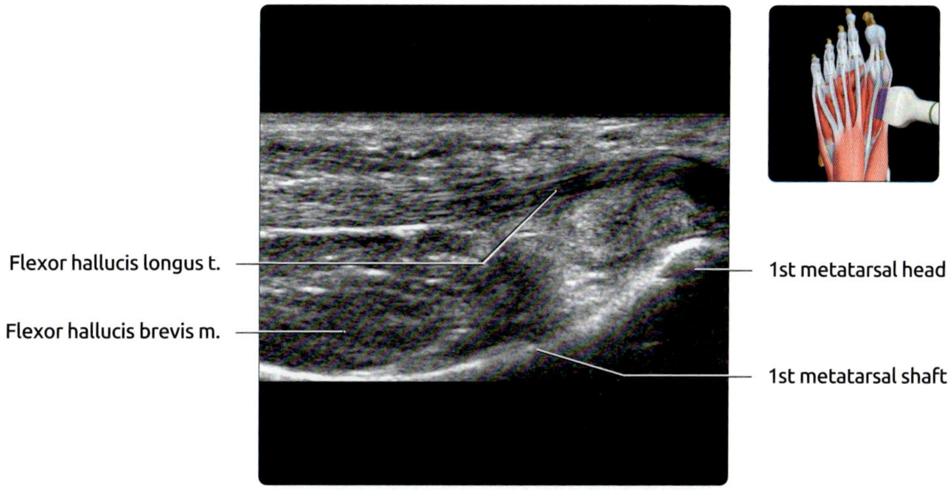

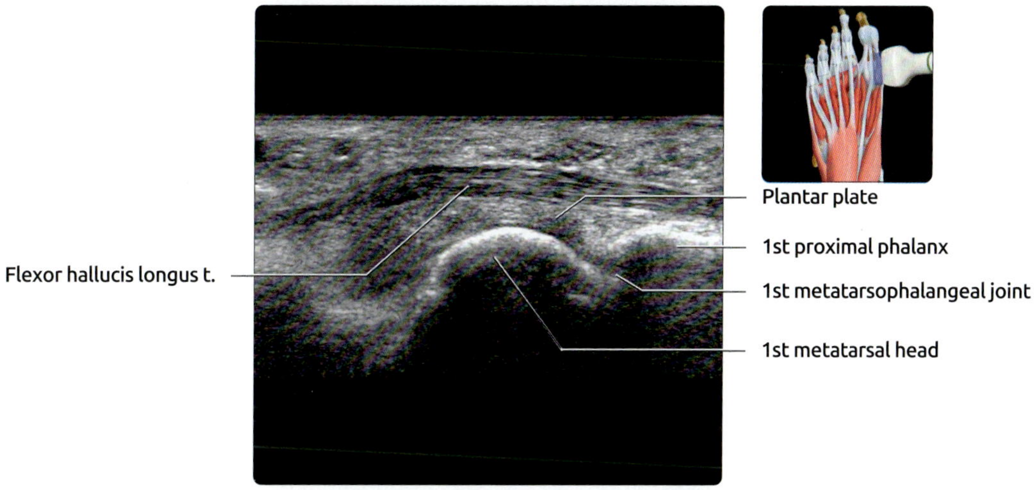

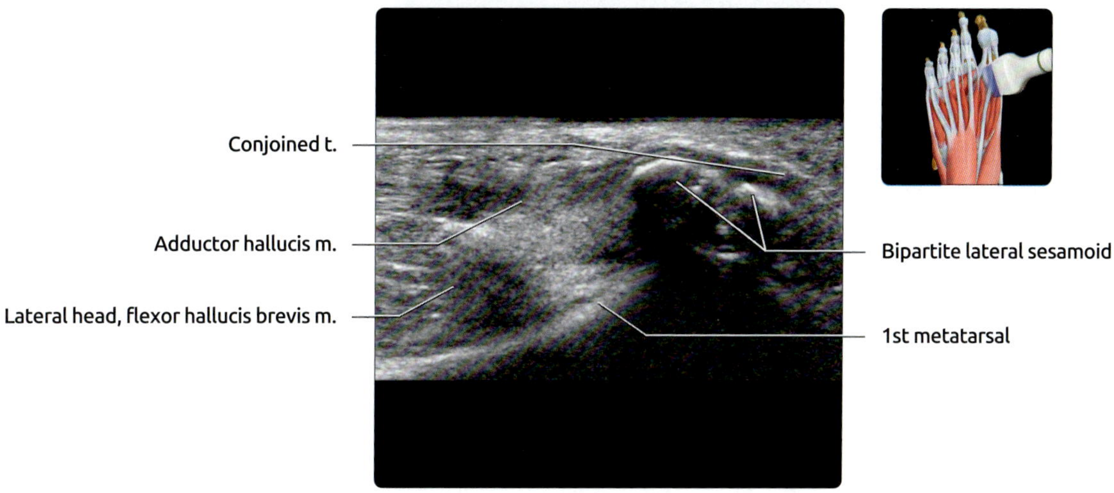

(Top) *Sagittal scan shows the plantar aspect of the distal portion of the 1st metatarsal. The medial and lateral heads of the flexor hallucis brevis muscles diverge to the sides of the flexor hallucis longus tendon to insert on the sesamoids of the 1st metatarsal head.* **(Middle)** *Sagittal scan through the center of the 1st metatarsophalangeal joint shows the plantar plate deep to the flexor hallucis longus tendon. The plantar plate together with the flexor hallucis brevis, abductor hallucis and adductor hallucis muscles, and sesamoids form the sesamophalangeal apparatus, which is important in stabilization of the 1st metatarsophalangeal joint.* **(Bottom)** *Sagittal scan through the lateral sesamoid of the 1st metatarsophalangeal joint shows the lateral head of the flexor hallucis brevis muscle and the adductor hallucis muscle as they converge to attach on the lateral sesamoid. They then form a conjoined tendon that inserts on the base of the proximal phalanx.*

US: PLANTAR METATARSALS

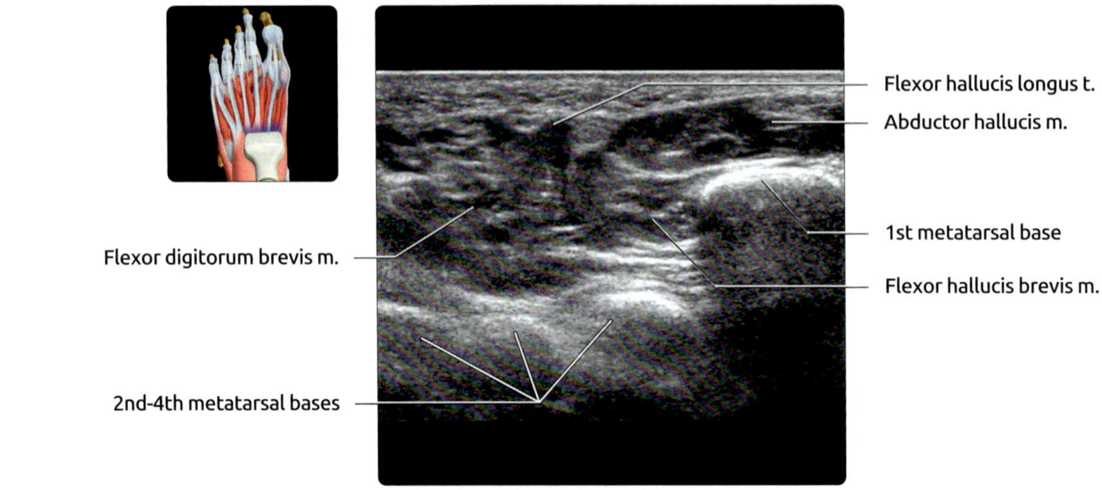

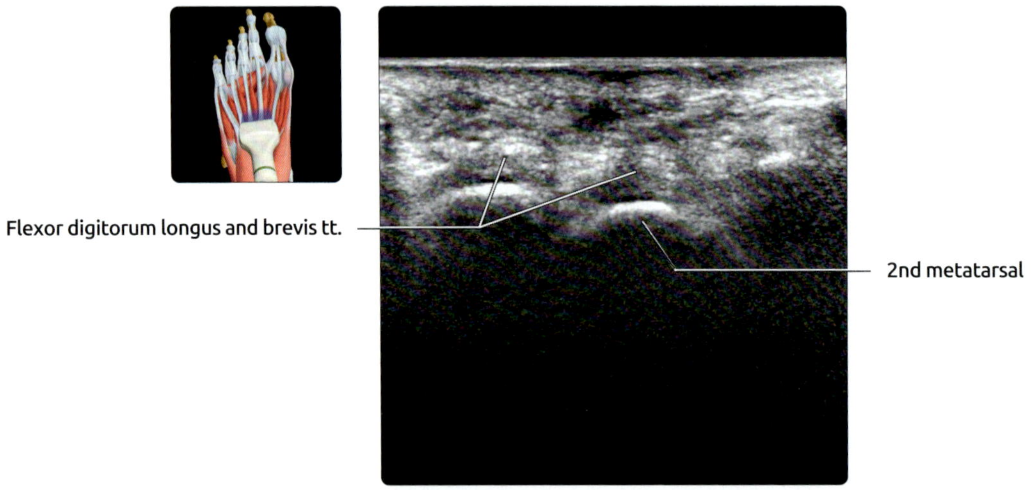

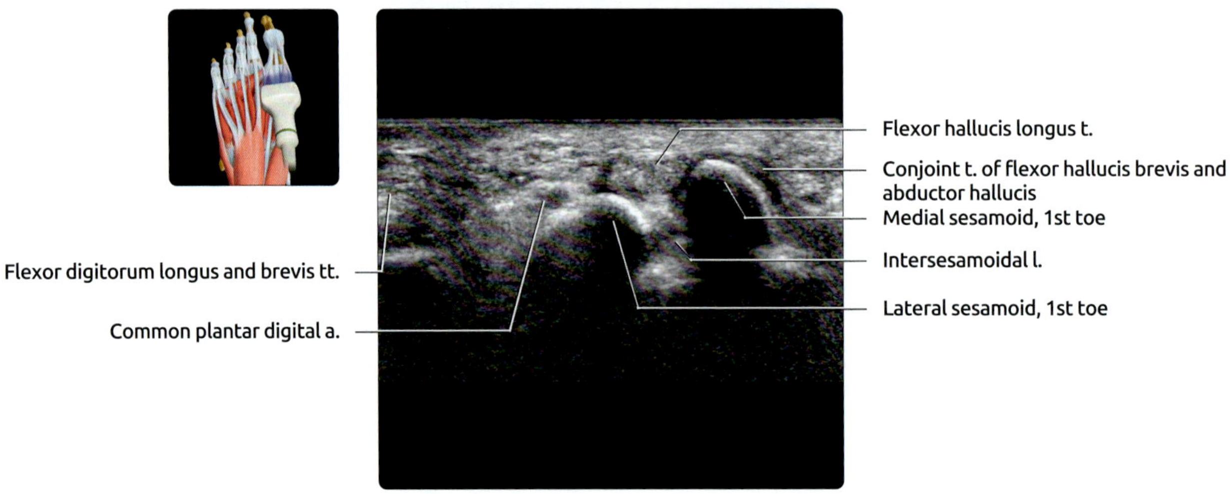

(Top) *Coronal scan shows the plantar structures at the level of the metatarsal bases. The transverse arch of the metatarsals is well seen. Abductor hallucis and flexor digitorum brevis muscles form the superficial layer of plantar muscles together with the abductor digiti minimi (positioned more laterally and not included on this image).* **(Middle)** *Coronal scan shows the plantar structures at the level of the shafts of the 2nd and 3rd metatarsals. The flexor digitorum brevis tendon slips lie superficial to the flexor digitorum longus and split at the level of the proximal phalanx to allow the flexor digitorum tendon slip to pass between them.* **(Bottom)** *Coronal scan shows the sesamoids of the 1st metatarsal head. The medial head of the flexor hallucis brevis and the abductor hallucis attach to the medial sesamoid, and their conjoined tendon attaches to the 1st proximal phalangeal base. Similarly, the lateral head of the flexor hallucis brevis and the adductor hallucis attach to the lateral sesamoid and continue to the 1st proximal phalangeal base.*

US: PLANTAR AND DORSAL TOE

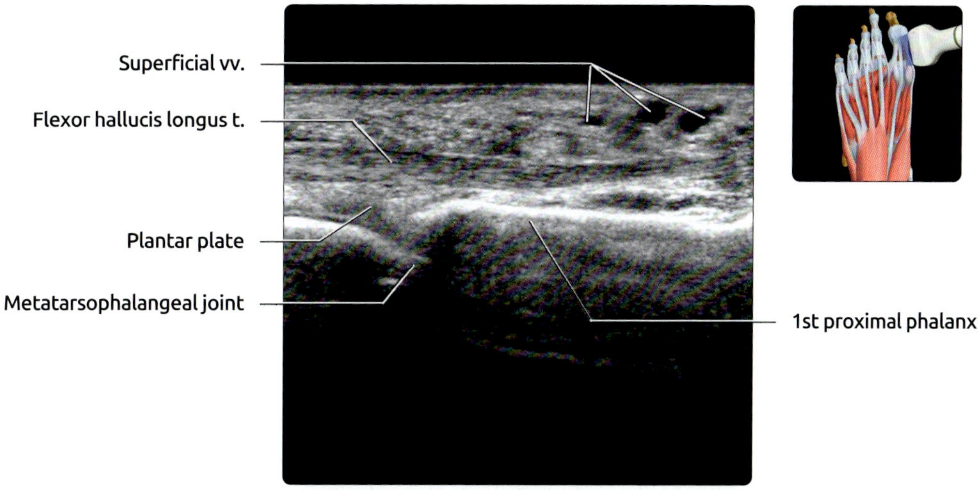

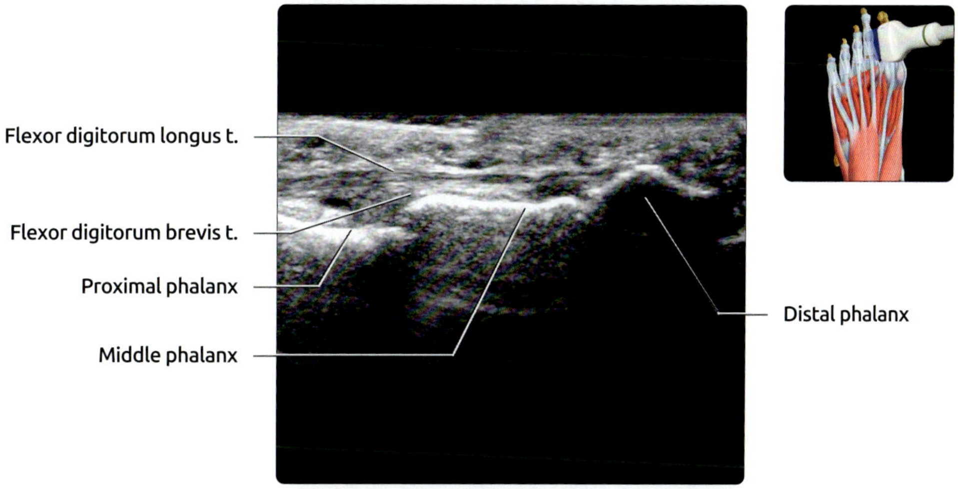

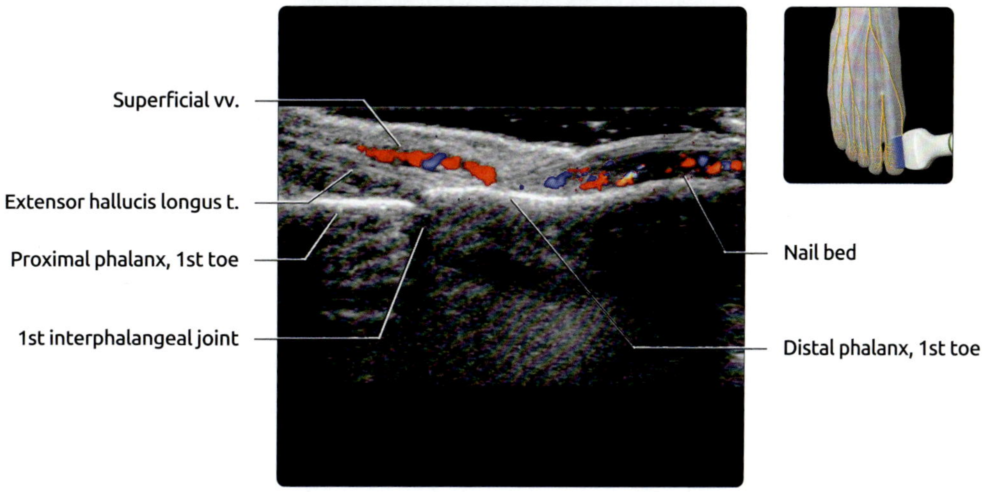

(Top) *Sagittal scan shows the plantar surface of the 1st metatarsophalangeal joint between the sesamoids. Flexor hallucis longus tendon will insert on the base of the distal phalanx.* **(Middle)** *Sagittal scan shows the plantar surface of the 2nd toe. The flexor digitorum brevis tendon has split into bands that insert along the midshaft of the middle phalanx. The flexor digitorum longus tendon inserts on the base of the distal phalanx.* **(Bottom)** *Sagittal color Doppler scan shows the dorsal surface of the distal phalanx of the 1st toe. The extensor digitorum longus tendon inserts on the base of the distal phalanx. The nail bed has a rich vascular supply as demonstrated by the color flow.*

SECTION 5

Angles and Measurements

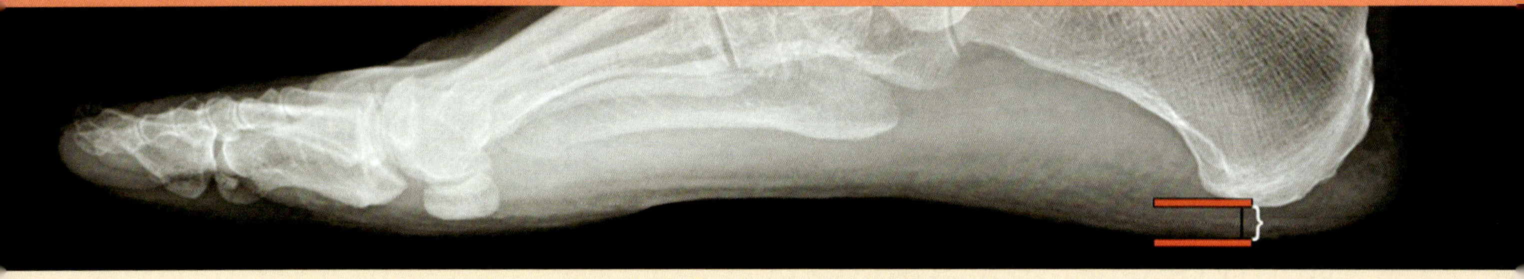

IMAGING ANATOMY

Valgus/Varus on Standing AP View: 2 Methods

- Mechanical axis
  - Line drawn from center of femoral head to center of tibial plafond
  - Should fall through middle of knee
  - Lateral position to center of knee indicates valgus; medial position indicates varus angulation
- Angle described by line bisecting distal femur and line bisecting proximal tibia
  - Normal angle 6° ± 2°

Measurement of Translational Force Exerted on Patella With Contraction of Extensor Mechanism

- Q angle: Standing AP view; angle described by 2 lines
  - One line joins center of patella and anterior superior iliac spine
  - 2nd line joins center of patella and tibial tuberosity
  - Normal angle for males: 14° ± 3°, for females: 17° ± 3°
- Tibial tubercle-trochlear groove method
  - Cross-sectional method (CT or MR) in extension
  - Axial image through apex of intercondylar notch superimposed on axial image through tibial tubercle
  - Horizontal distance between apex of notch and tibial tubercle measured
  - Normal 1.5 ± 0.4 cm; if > 2.0 cm, specific for patellar maltracking

Measurement of Patellar Height

- Insall-Salvati method uses sagittal image in 30° flexion
  - Measure maximum diagonal length of patella (A)
  - Measure shortest length of patellar tendon (B)
  - Ratio B:A = 1.0 ± 0.2
  - If < 0.8, shows patella baja
  - If > 1.2, shows patella alta
- Caton method uses sagittal image in full extension
  - Measure length of patellar cartilage (A)
  - Measure shortest line between patellar articular surface and tibial plateau (B)
  - Ratio B:A = 1.0 ± 0.2
  - If < 0.8, shows patella baja
  - If > 1.2, shows patella alta

Measurement of Trochlear Inclination

- Knee in either flexion or extension, axial image through apex of intercondylar notch
- Reference line: Posterior transcondylar line
- Angle described by posterior transcondylar line and line extending down lateral facet of trochlea
- Normal trochlear inclination: ≥ 11°; if < 11°, describes trochlear dysplasia

Measurement of Trochlear Sulcus Angle

- Knee in either flexion or extension, axial image through apex of intercondylar notch
- Angle described by line along trochlear medial facet and line along trochlear lateral facet
- Normal trochlear angle: 138° ± 6°; if > 145°, describes trochlear dysplasia

Measurement of Patellar Tilt

- Knee in 20° flexion, axial radiographic view
  - Line drawn across tops of medial and lateral trochlea
  - 2nd line drawn along lateral patellar facet
  - Angle should be "open" laterally
- Patellar tilt angle: Knee in flexion or extension, axial image through equator of patella
  - Draw line across posterior condyles, then auxiliary line at level of trochlea parallel to 1st line
  - Draw line through equator of patella; 2 lines form patellar tilt angle; normal 2° ± 2°

Qualitative Assessment of Patellar Subluxation

- Knee in 20° flexion, axial radiographic view
- Draw line across tops of medial and lateral trochlea
- Draw perpendicular line to that, 2 mm lateral to tip of medial trochlea
- That line should intersect patella; if it does not, there is lateral patellar subluxation

Measurement of Patellar Congruence to Trochlea

- Knee in 30° flexion, axial image through patellofemoral joint
- Draw A and B, medial and lateral trochlear facet lines
- Draw line C, bisecting trochlear sulcus (angle formed by A and B)
- Draw line D, from patellar apex to trochlear sulcus
- Congruence angle is formed between lines C and D
- Normal ranges from -6° to +6°

Dynamic Assessment of Patellar Congruence

- 4 axial images through patellofemoral joint taken in extension, 15° flexion, 30° flexion, and 30° flexion with contraction of quadriceps
- Check for changing position of patellar tilt and subluxation in these different positions

Measurement of Femoral and Tibial Torsion

- Femoral torsion
  - Measure degree of hip anteversion by superimposing CT through mid femoral head and femoral shaft at level of lesser trochanter
  - Measure degree of femoral torsion by angle formed by hip anteversion relative to line at posterior femoral condyles
  - Distal femur is normally internally rotated relative to hip (femoral anteversion or antetorsion)
- Tibial torsion
  - Superimpose proximal tibial axial cut on distal tibial axial cut
  - Measured by angle formed by transverse axes of these 2 levels
  - Distal tibia is normally externally rotated relative to proximal tibia (average 30° in adults; range 20-50°)

SELECTED REFERENCES

1. Keats TE et al: Atlas of Radiologic Measurement. 7th ed. Mosby, St. Louis, 2001

MECHANICAL AXIS, KNEE ANGULATION

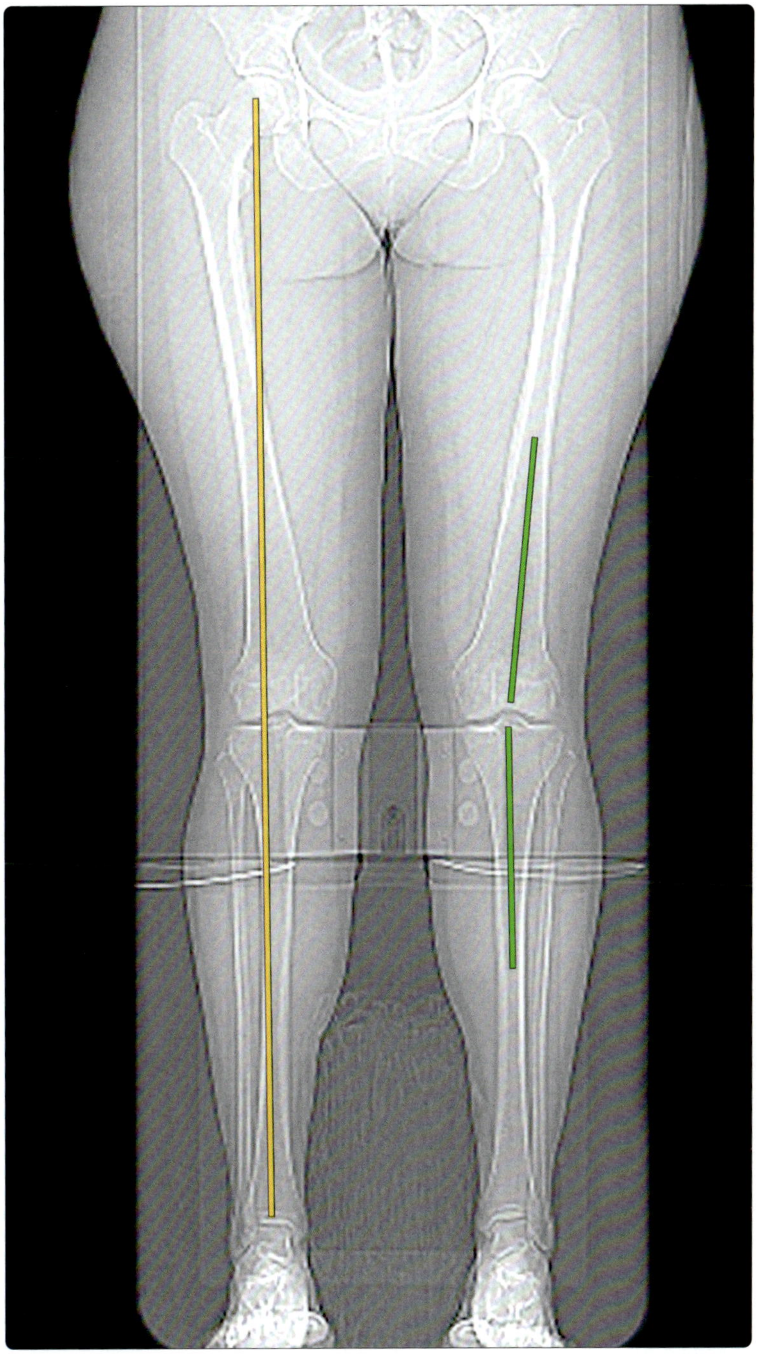

The yellow line drawn on the right lower extremity depicts the mechanical axis, drawn from the center of the femoral head to the center of the tibial plafond. The normal mechanical axis traverses the center of the knee joint. The green lines bisecting the distal femur and proximal tibia shows the normal valgus angulation of the knee (average 6°).

Q ANGLE: TRANSLATIONAL FORCE ON PATELLA

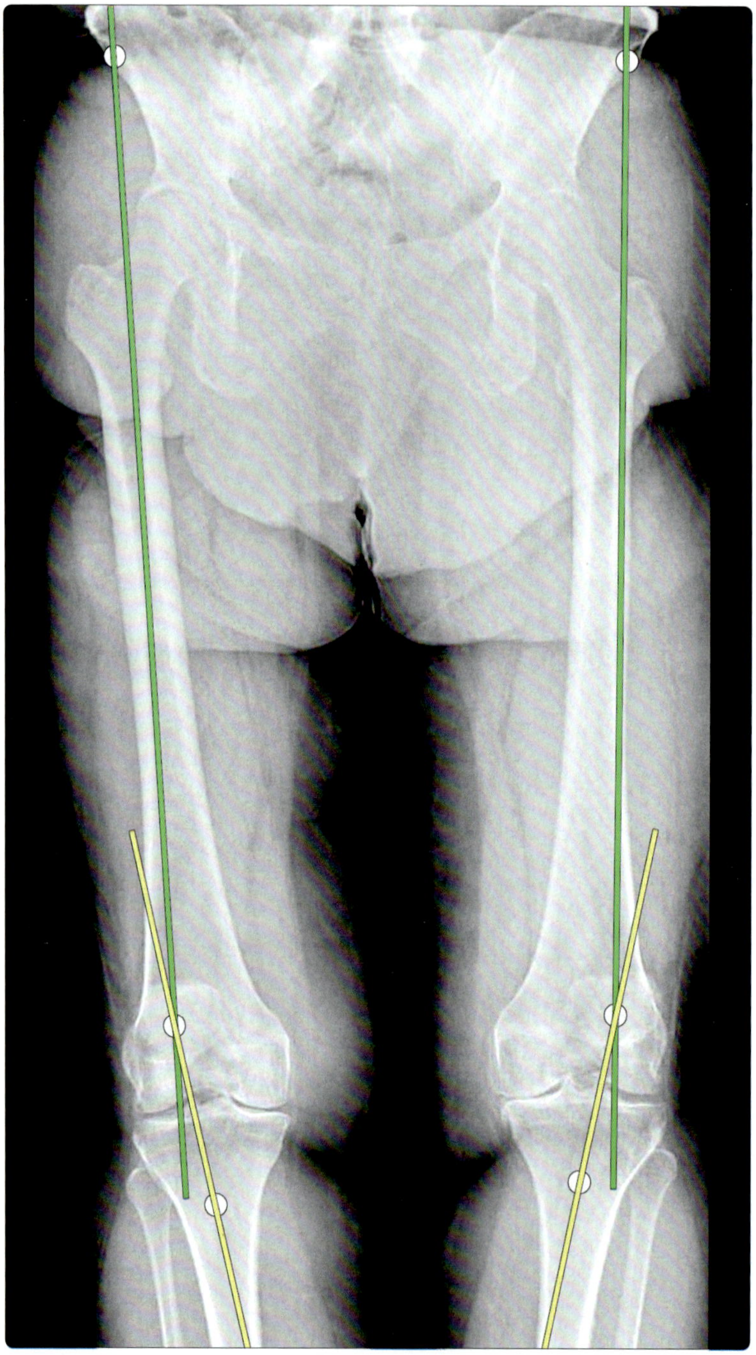

The Q angle measures the translational force exerted on the patella with contraction of the extensor mechanism. A standing AP view is used; the angle is described by 2 lines. The 1st line (green) joins the center of the patella and the anterior superior iliac spine. The 2nd line joins the center of the patella and tibial tuberosity (yellow). The normal angle is 14° ± 3° in males and 17° ± 3° in females. The Q angle in this case is at the upper limits of normal on the right but abnormal on the left.

LATERAL TRANSLATION: TT-TG METHOD

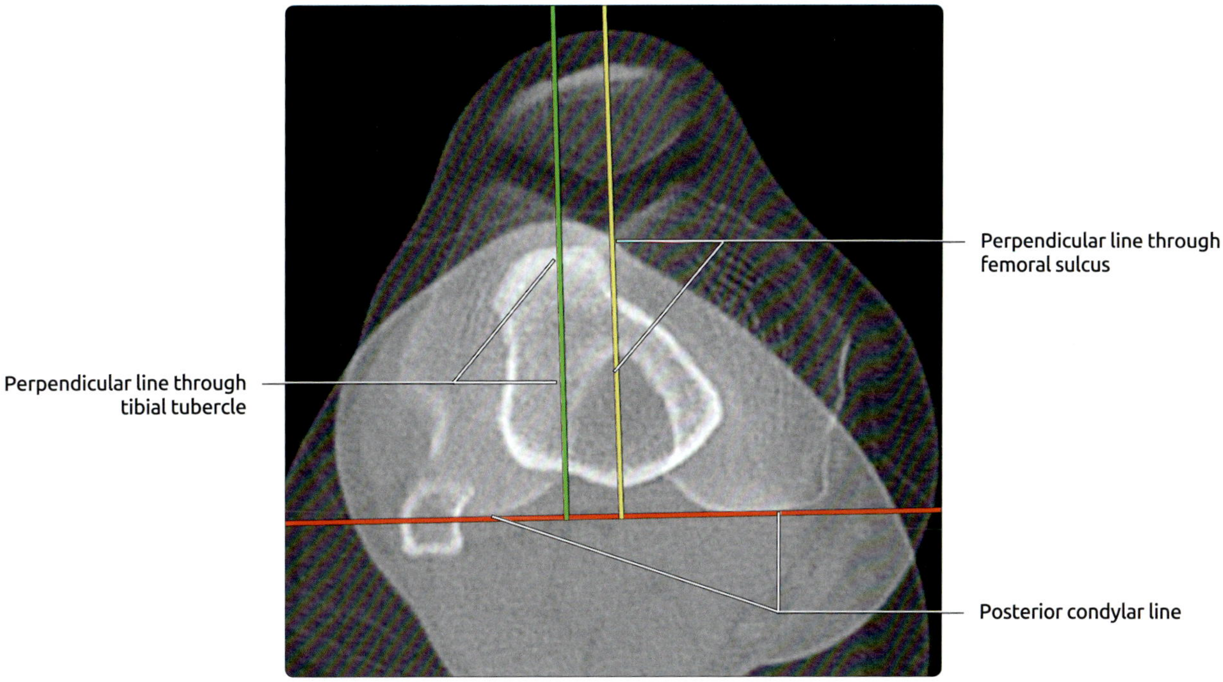

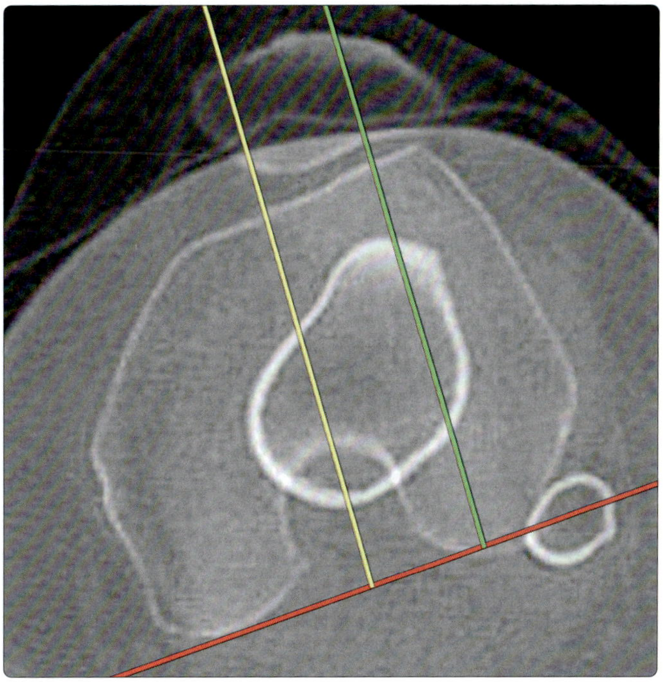

(Top) *Translational force exerted on the patella may be measured by the tibial tubercle-trochlear groove (TT-TG) method. This is performed using cross-sectional images (CT or MR) with the knee in extension. An axial image through the apex of the intercondylar notch is superimposed on an axial image through the tibial tubercle. The horizontal distance between the apex of the notch and tibial tubercle is measured in the following manner: Draw the posterior condylar line (red); draw a perpendicular line to red line, through the tibial tubercle (green; this is the TT line); draw a perpendicular line to red line, through the trochlear groove sulcus (yellow; this is the TG line). The normal TT-TG distance is 1.5 ± 0.4 cm. In this case, the measurement falls within normal limits.* **(Bottom)** *In this case, the TT-TG distance is greater than 2 cm, indicating patellar maltracking.*

MEASUREMENT OF PATELLAR HEIGHT

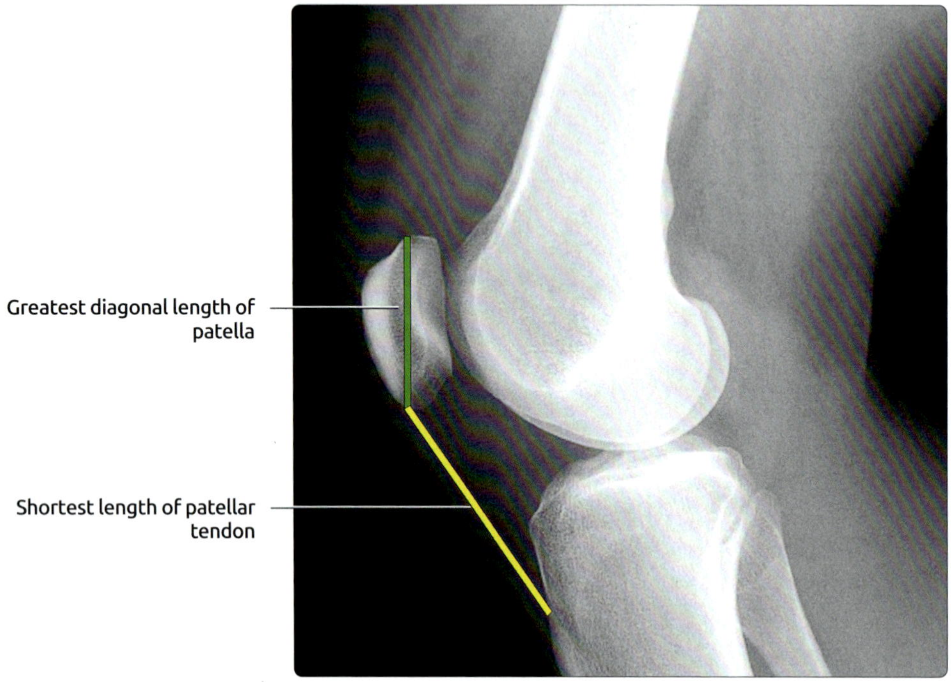

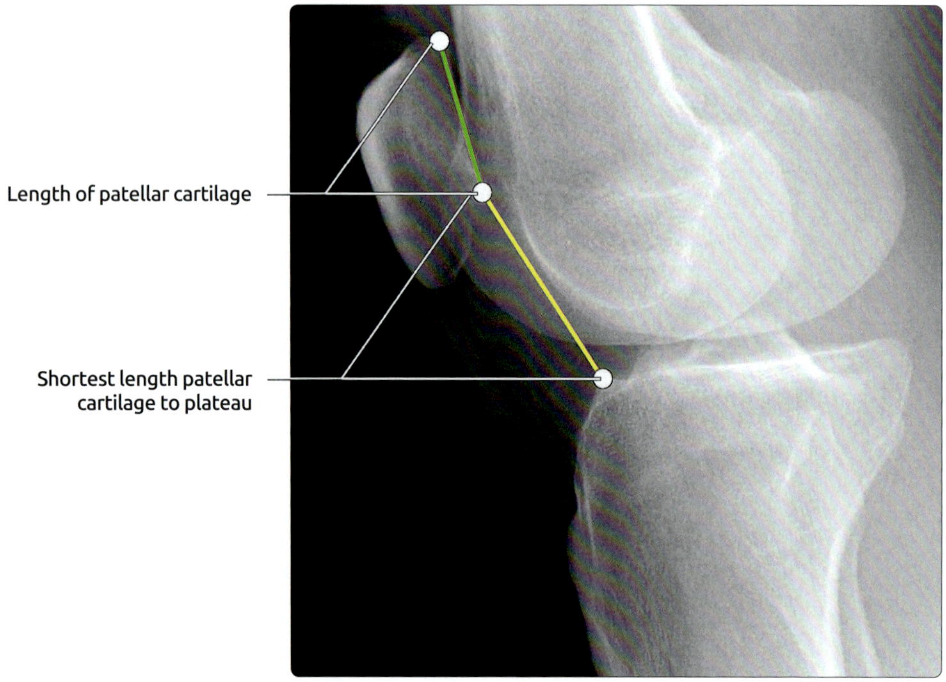

(Top) *Patellar height, by the Insall-Salvati method, is shown. On lateral radiograph, in 30° flexion, the shortest length of the patellar tendon (yellow line), and the greatest diagonal length of the patella (green line), form a ratio that averages 1.0 ± 0.2 (range: 0.8-1.2). If the ratio is less than 0.8, it represents patella baja; if the ratio is greater than 1.2, it is patella alta.* **(Bottom)** *If the landmarks are not clear for the Insall-Salvati method, the Caton method may be used. It requires a lateral image in full extension. The length of the patellar cartilage is measured (A; green line). The shortest line between the patellar articular surface and tibial plateau is measured (B; yellow line). The ratio of B:A is normally 1.0 ± 0.2. A ratio less than 0.8 indicates patella baja, while a ratio greater than 1.2 indicates patella alta.*

MEASUREMENT OF TROCHLEAR INCLINATION

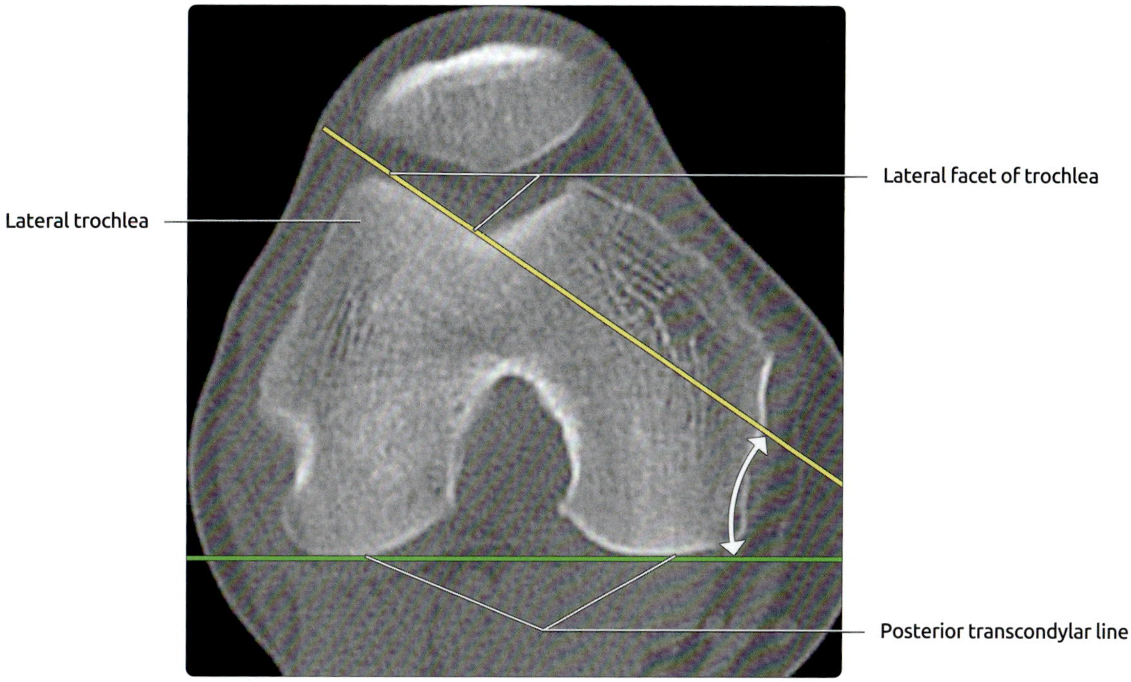

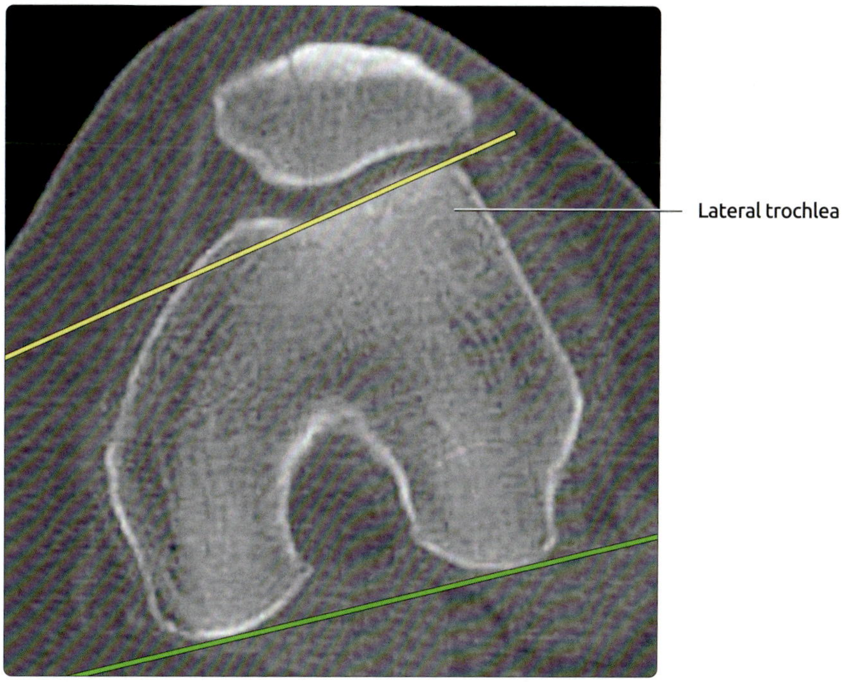

(Top) *The degree of trochlear inclination relates to trochlear dysplasia and consequent patellofemoral disorders. The measurement is obtained on an axial image through the apex of the intercondylar notch, with the knee in either flexion or extension. The posterior transcondylar line is drawn as a reference line (green). The angle is described by the posterior transcondylar line and a line extending along the lateral facet of the trochlea (yellow). The normal trochlear inclination is greater than or equal to 11°. If the angle is less than 11°, it describes trochlear dysplasia. In this example, the angle is greater than 11°, and there is no dysplasia.* **(Bottom)** *This image shows a trochlear inclination angle that measures less than 11°; this is a case of trochlear dysplasia, with a fairly flat trochlear sulcus.*

MEASUREMENT OF TROCHLEAR SULCUS ANGLE

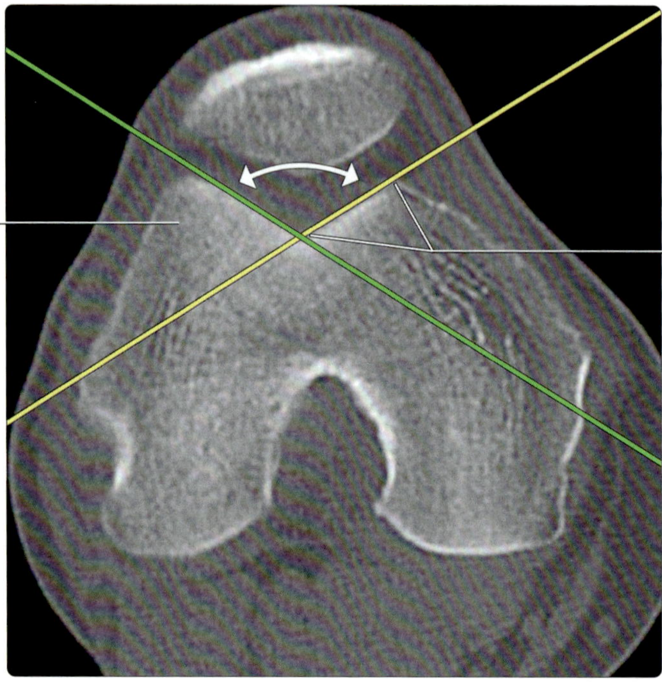

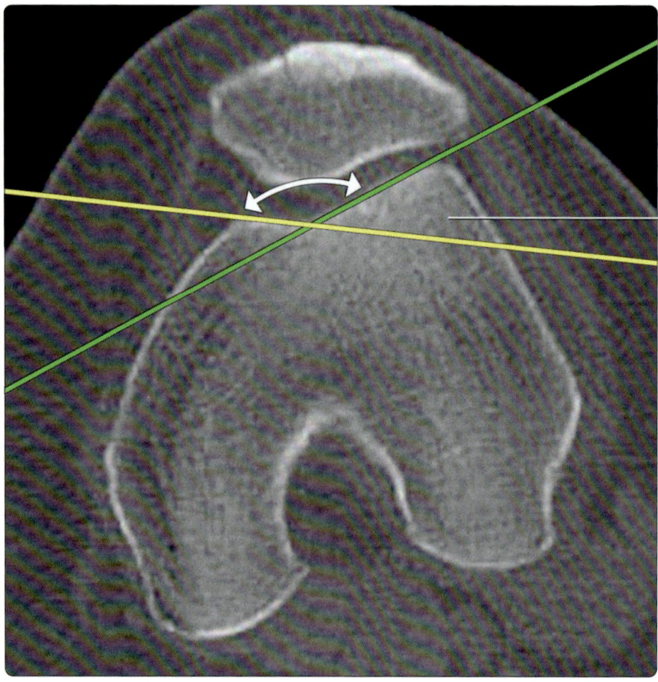

(Top) *This is another measurement that is used to evaluate trochlear dysplasia. The sulcus angle is measured on an axial image through the apex of the intercondylar notch, with the knee in either flexion or extension. The angle is described by a line along the trochlear medial facet (yellow) and another line along the trochlear lateral facet (green). The normal trochlear sulcus angle is 138° ± 6°. If the angle is greater than 145°, it demonstrates trochlear dysplasia. In this case, there is no evidence of dysplasia.* **(Bottom)** *In this patient, the trochlear sulcus angle is much greater than 145°; this demonstrates flattening of the trochlear angle in a patient with dysplasia.*

MEASUREMENT OF PATELLAR TILT

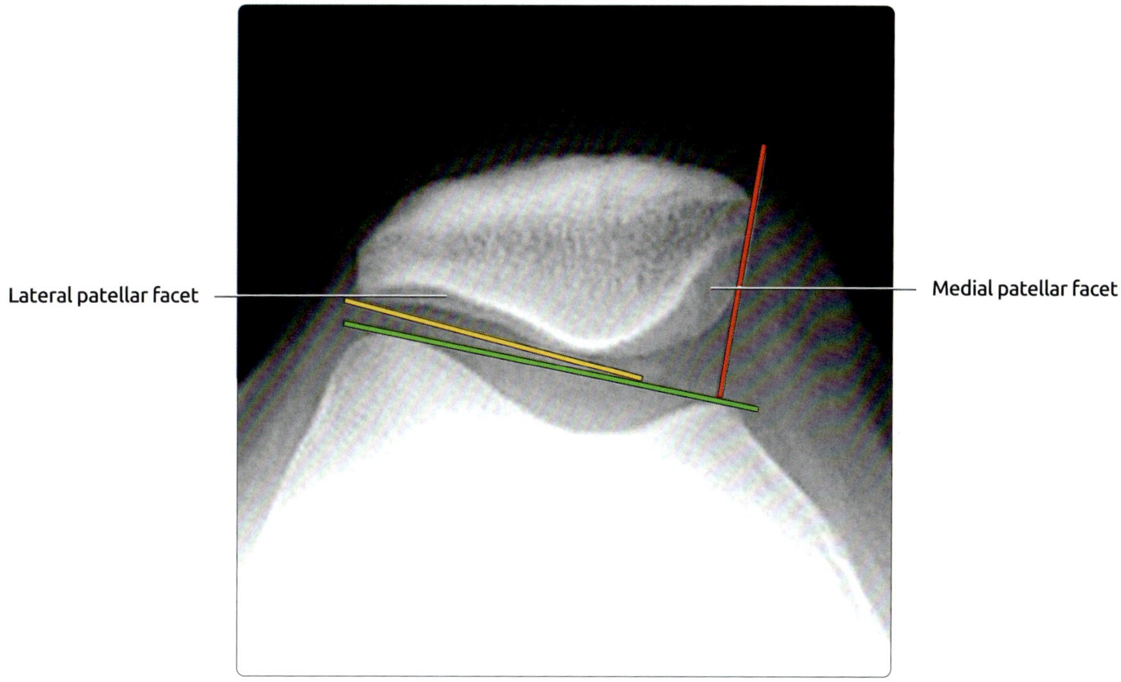

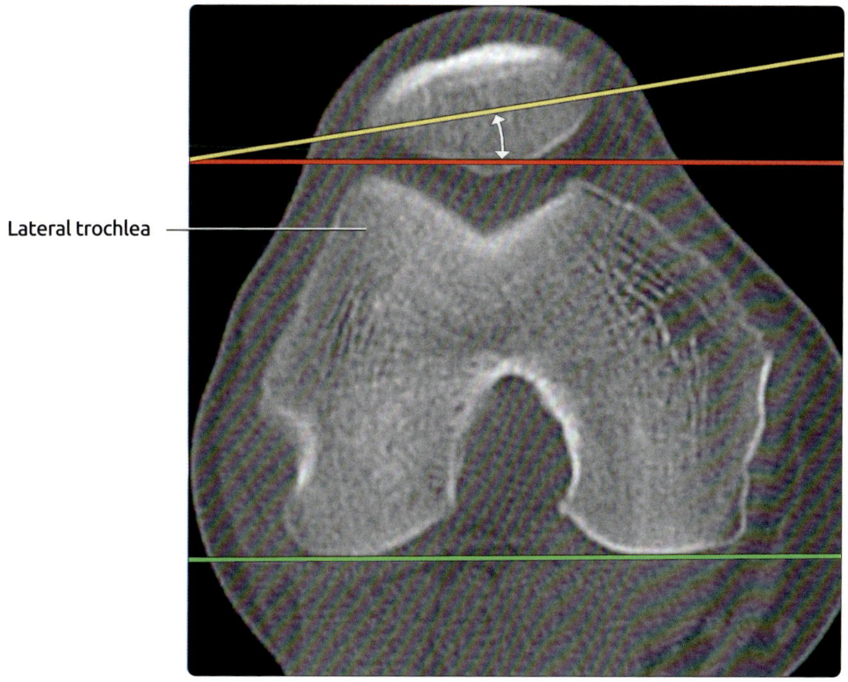

(Top) *Axial radiograph of the knee, obtained with the knee flexed 20°, is shown. The lateral patellar facet is elongated and less sharply angled than the medial. The angle formed by the line through the condylar peaks (green) and lateral patellar facet (yellow) is normally open laterally; reversal of this angle constitutes patellar tilt. A line drawn perpendicular (red) to the condylar peaks line (green), 2 mm lateral to the medial condylar peak, should intersect the patella. If the patella lies lateral to this line, it is laterally subluxed.* **(Bottom)** *Patellar tilt can be measured on an axial image through the equator of the patella. A line is drawn across the posterior condyles (green), then an auxiliary line parallel to it at the level of the trochlea (red). An angle is formed between that and a line drawn through the equator of the patella (yellow). Normal is 2° ± 2°.*

PATELLAR CONGRUENCE TO TROCHLEA

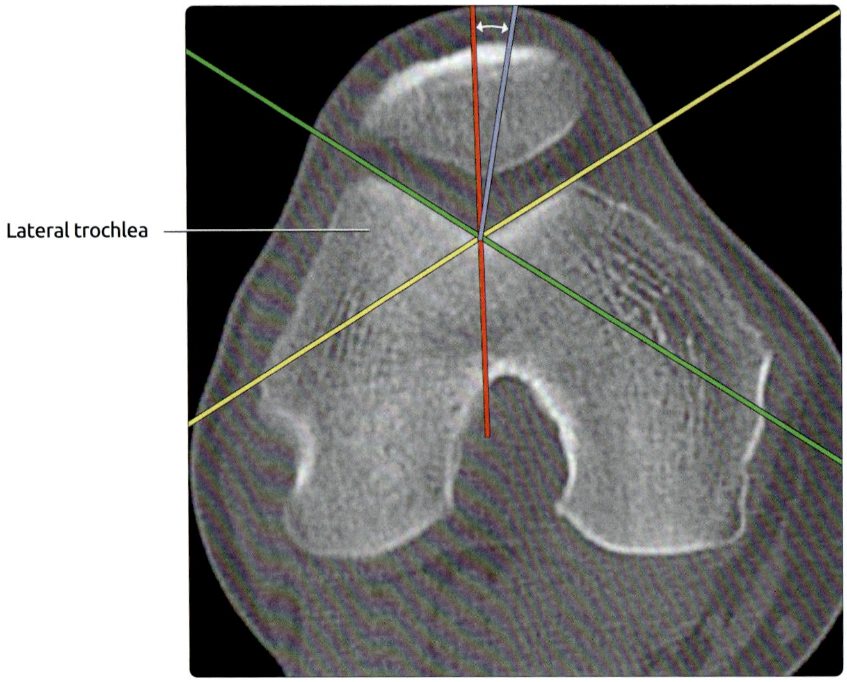

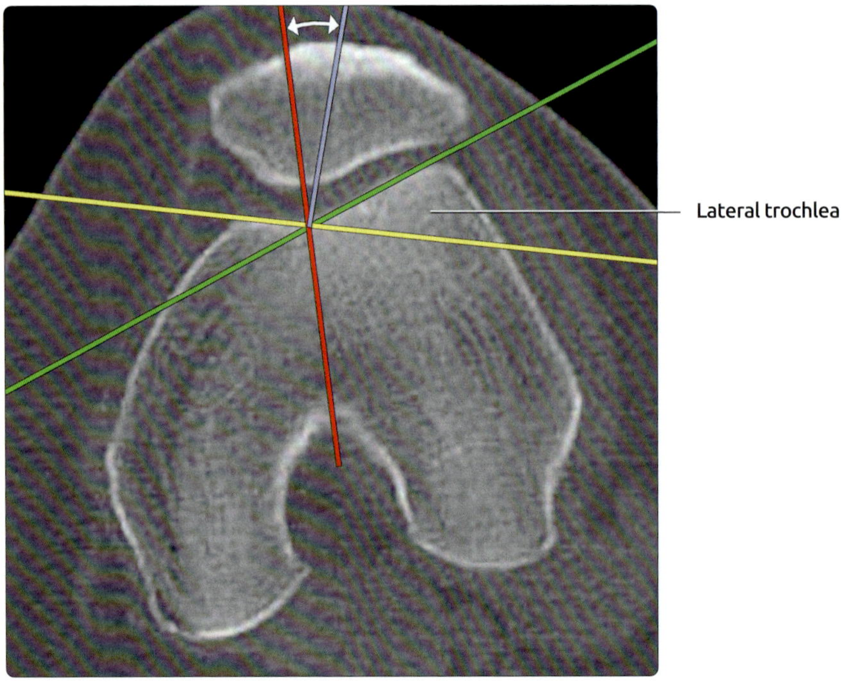

(Top) *Measurement of the patellar congruence to the trochlea is obtained on an axial image through the patellofemoral joint with the knee in 30° flexion. Draw the medial trochlear facet line (yellow) and lateral facet line (green). The angle formed by these 2 lines is then bisected (red line). Next, a line is drawn from the patellar apex to trochlear sulcus (blue; this line is termed the congruence line). The angle formed between the red and blue lines measures the patellar congruence. If the congruence angle is lateral to the bisector of the sulcus, the angle is positive. If the congruence angle is medial to the bisector of the sulcus, the angle is negative. The normal average congruence angle is -6° in males and -10° in females. In this case, the congruence angle is negative and within normal measurements.* **(Bottom)** *In this case, the congruence angle is positive and therefore abnormal.*

DYNAMIC ASSESSMENT PATELLAR CONGRUENCE

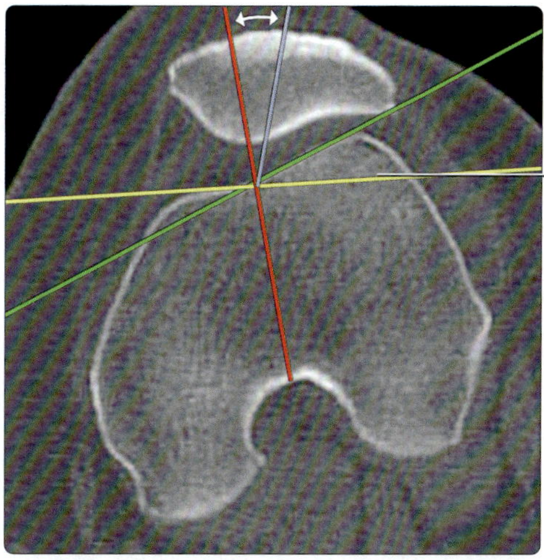

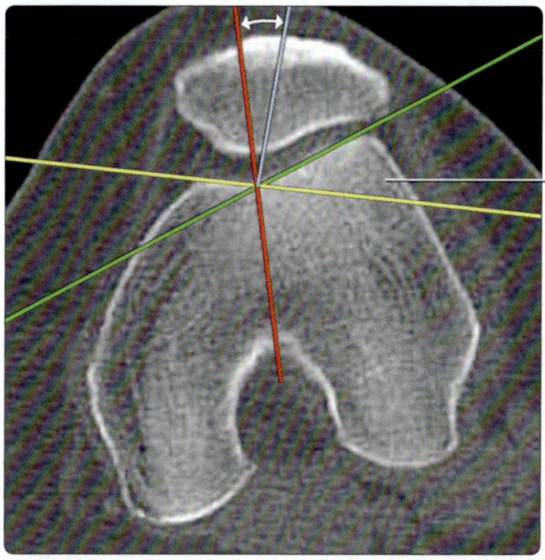

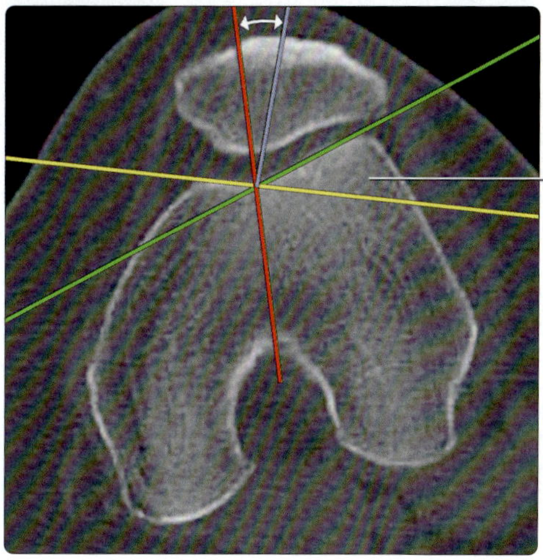

(Top) *Dynamic assessment of patellar congruence is performed either by axial radiographic imaging or by CT or MR axial imaging. Four axial images are obtained through the patellofemoral joint (one each in extension: 15° flexion, 30° flexion, and 30° flexion during contraction of the quadriceps). The congruence angle can be measured on each, and changing position of patellar tilt and subluxation is evaluated in each position. This image is obtained with the knee in extension and shows a positive congruence angle with lateral subluxation of the patella, both of which are abnormal.* **(Middle)** *With flexion of 15°, the lateral subluxation of the patella is reduced, but the congruence angle is still positive.* **(Bottom)** *With 30° flexion, the congruence angle remains slightly positive, though there is no subluxation or patellar tilt. Note the flattened trochlear dysplasia.*

HIP ANTEVERSION & FEMORAL TORSION

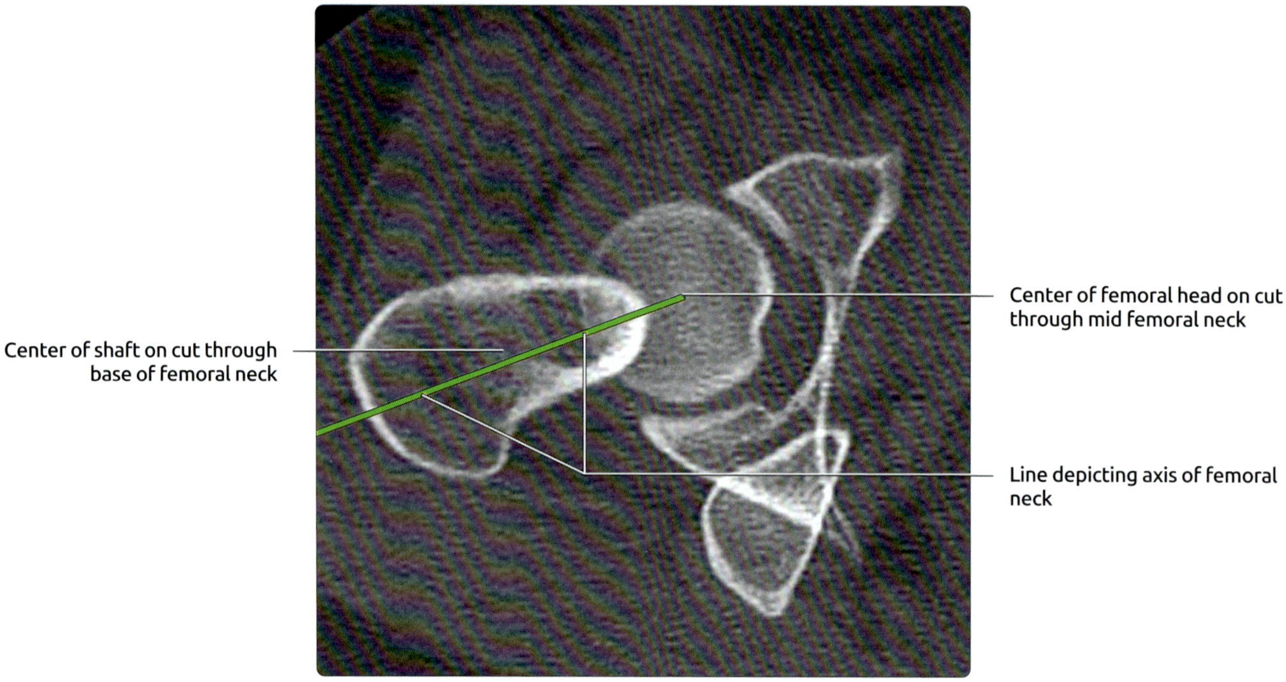

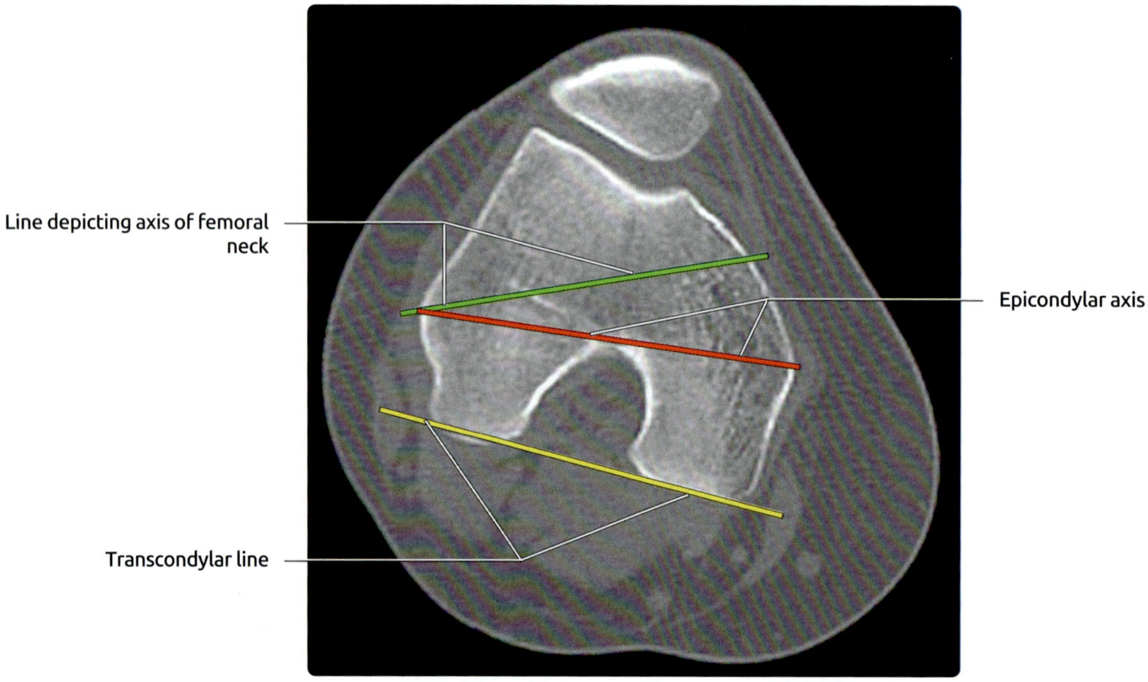

(Top) *Axis of femoral neck, determined by superimposed CT scans through the mid femoral neck and base of femoral neck, is shown. The line connecting the center of the head in the superior cut and the center of shaft in the lower cut determines the femoral neck axis; this line makes an angle with the transischial line (in this case there is 15° femoral neck anteversion).* **(Bottom)** *Femoral torsion, measured by CT, is shown. The angle formed by the axis of the femoral neck (green line from previous image) and transcondylar line (yellow) gives the degree of femoral torsion. Normally, the distal femur is internally rotated relative to the femoral neck, which is termed femoral anteversion or antetorsion; different studies show average anteversion to be 15-24° in adults (range: 3-48°). Epicondylar axis (red line) is another useful landmark. The epicondylar/posterior condylar angle should be 5.7 ± 1.7°.*

TIBIAL TORSION

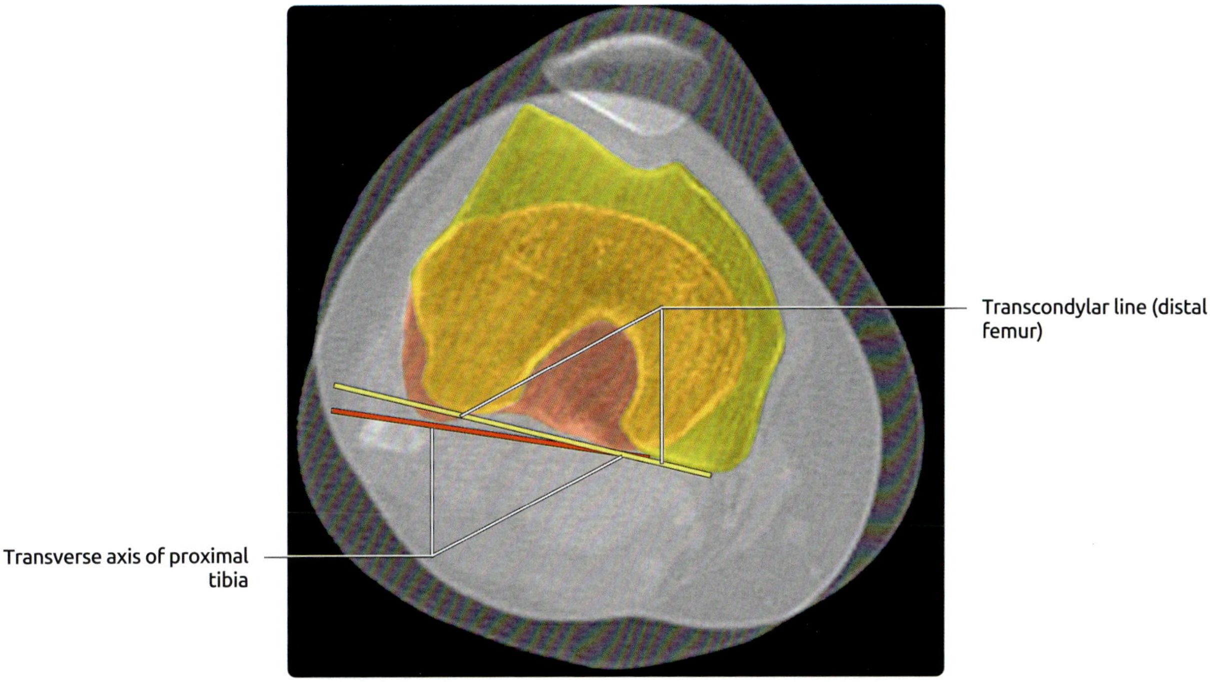

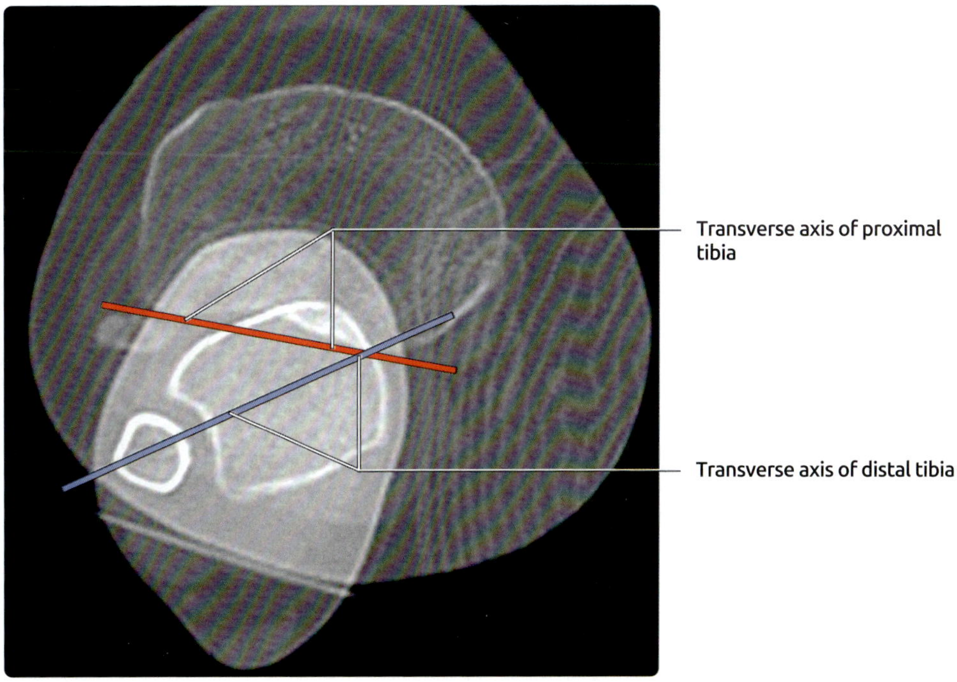

(Top) *Occasionally, one may be required to measure the rotation of the proximal tibia on the distal femur. There is usually slightly external rotation of the tibia relative to the femur; it is measured by the angle formed by the transcondylar line of the distal femur (yellow) and the transverse axis of the proximal tibia (red line).* **(Bottom)** *Tibial torsion is measured by the angle formed by the proximal tibial transverse axis (red line) and distal tibial transverse axis (blue line). There is normally external rotation (torsion) of the distal tibia, measuring 30° in adults (range: 20-50°), as shown by several CT studies. Tibial torsion greater than 40° shows an increased incidence of adverse patellar mechanics and malalignment syndrome.*

PCL RATIO/ANGLE: 2° SIGNS OF ACL TEAR

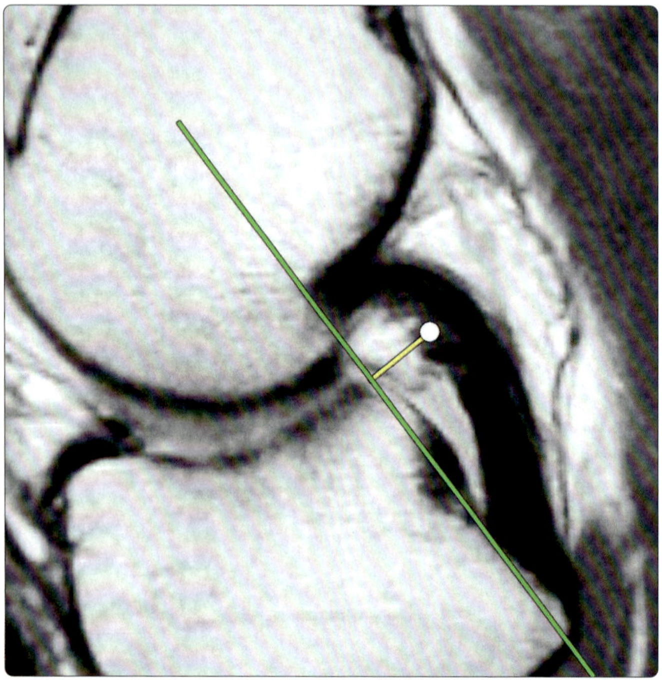

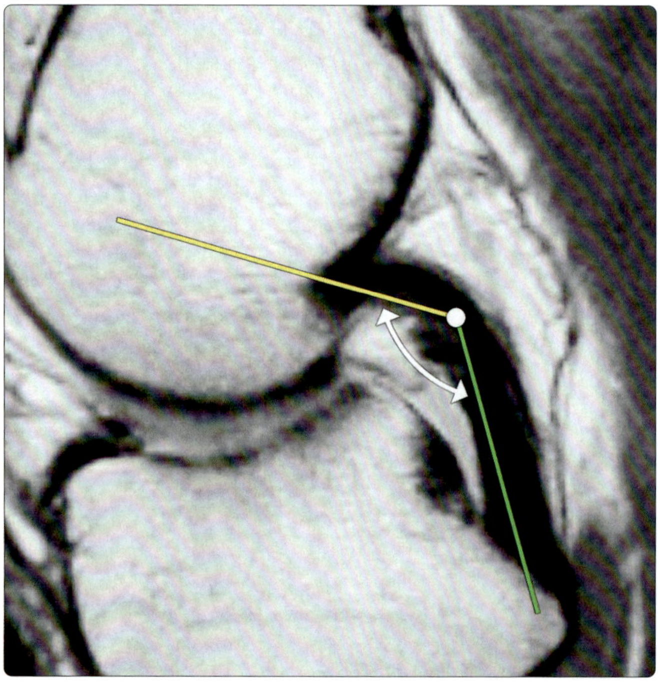

(Top) *The posterior cruciate ligament (PCL) is normally mildly concave in an anterior direction. With anterior cruciate ligament (ACL) tear and anterior subluxation of the tibia, the PCL may become "buckled." This may be measured on a sagittal image through the mid PCL. The PCL index is formed by a line drawn between the anterior portions of the femoral and tibial attachments of the PCL (green line) and a line across the maximum perpendicular distance between the green line and the apex of the PCL (yellow line). The normal ratio of yellow:green is 0.19.* **(Bottom)** *PCL bowing or buckling can also be assessed by the PCL angle. This is measured by a line drawn through the proximal portion of the PCL (yellow) and another through the distal portion of the PCL (green). The normal PCL angle ranges from 114-123°. An increase in either the PCL ratio or angle suggests ACL tear.*

ACL ANGLE RELATIVE TO FEMUR AND TIBIA

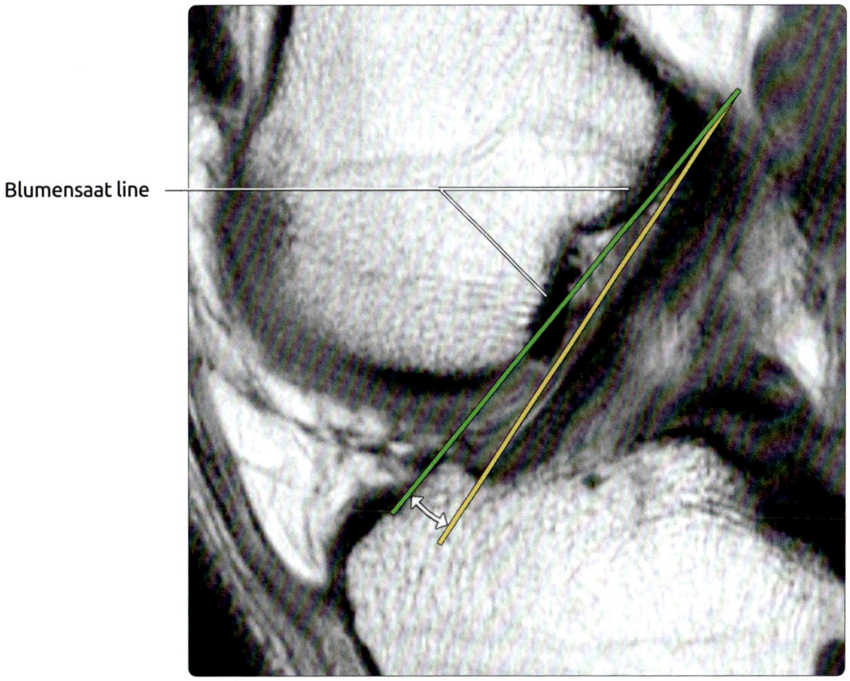

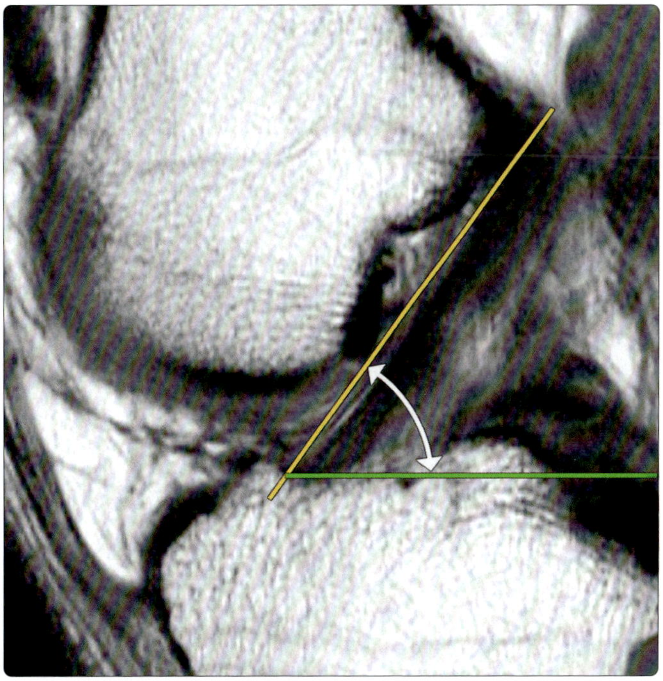

(Top) *The ACL is normally straight, running nearly parallel to Blumensaat line. The ACL angle relative to the femur can be measured by drawing a line along the anterior margin of the ACL (yellow) and another along the Blumensaat line (green). The angle described by these lines averages -1.6°. Abnormal criteria are published ranging from 9-15°.* **(Bottom)** *The ACL can be evaluated relative to the tibial plateau. The angle is described by a line along the anterior margin of the ACL (yellow) and another along the tibial plateau (green). This angle normally averages 56°; abnormal criteria are published ranging from 45-50°.*

LAT. FEMORAL SULCUS/LAT. MENISCAL COVERAGE

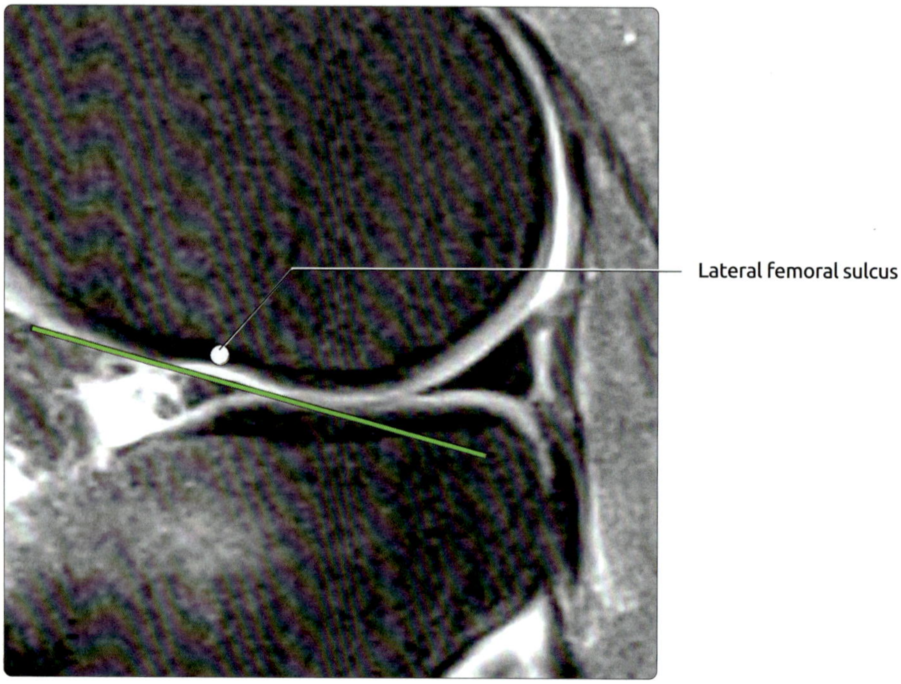

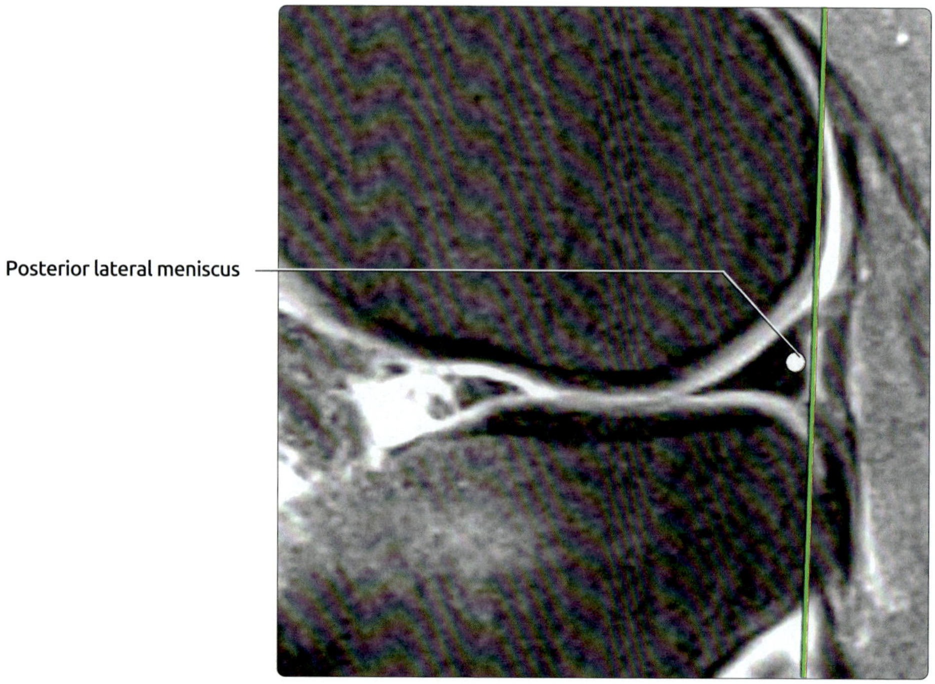

(Top) *The lateral femoral sulcus is a normal slight concavity. This sulcus may be impacted with an injury mechanism that often results in an ACL tear. The depth of the sulcus can be measured on the lateral image, which maximizes it. A line is drawn across the roof of the notch and the maximal depth is measured. Normal depth averages 0.35 mm. Depth greater than 2 mm is considered abnormal.*
(Bottom) *Anterior tibial translation can be measured by evaluation of lateral meniscal "uncovering." This is measured on the sagittal image midway between the tibial insertion of the PCL and the lateralmost portion of the tibial condyle. A line is drawn through the posterior tibia parallel to the long axis of the tibia. The distance of the line from the posterior lateral meniscus is measured (if the meniscus is anterior to the line, it is negative). Average is 2 mm; greater than 5 mm is abnormal.*

ACL/PCL ISOMETRIC TUNNEL LOCATIONS

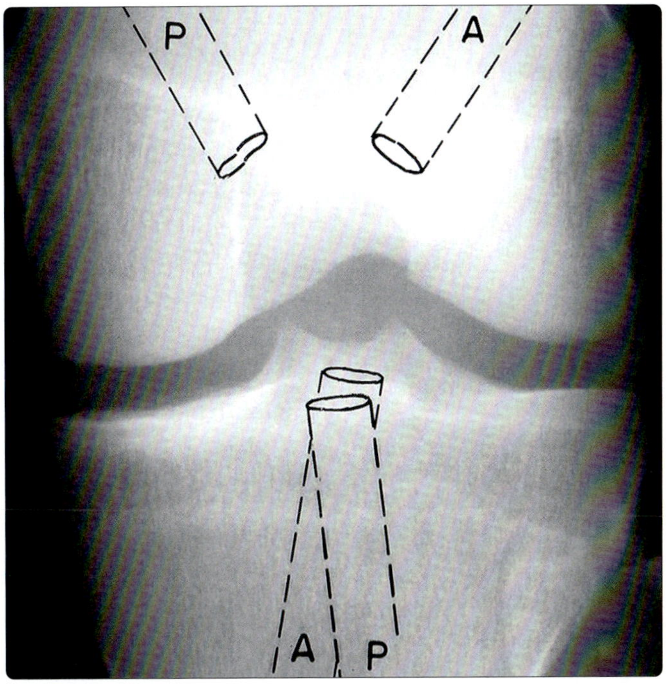

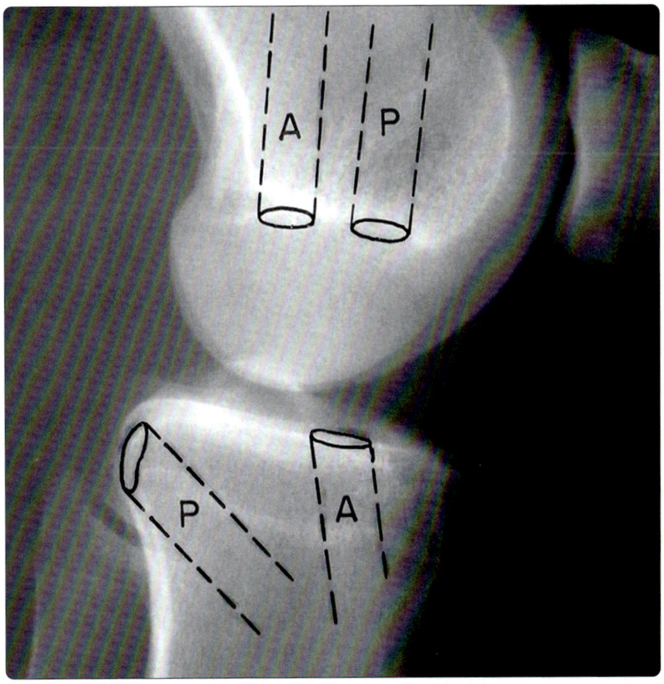

(Top) *AP radiograph demonstrates isometric tunnel positions for ACL and PCL reconstruction grafts. In this projection, both the femoral and tibial tunnel openings appear to be at the normal expected positions of the cruciate ligaments. Note that A stands for ACL, and P stands for PCL.* **(Bottom)** *Lateral radiograph depicts isometric tunnel openings for ACL and PCL reconstructions. The femoral tunnel for the ACL should lie at the intersection of the posterior cortex and Blumensaat line. The tibial tunnel for the ACL should lie 2-3 mm posterior to the normal ACL insertion site; the impingement-free zone has the tunnel centered 22-28 mm posterior to the anterior edge of tibia. The femoral PCL tunnel is at the normal origin of the PCL; note the tibial tunnel opening for the PCL is posterior and distal to the tibial articular surface, matching the normal insertion.*

IMAGING ANATOMY

Overview

- Abnormal alignment leads to foot pain and dysfunction
- All measurements made on weight-bearing radiographs

Anatomy Relationships

- Axes of foot are designated on AP radiograph
  - Anatomic axis
    - Line from center of 2nd metatarsal head to midpoint of posterior tuberosity of calcaneus
  - Mechanical axis
    - Line from center of 1st metatarsal head to midpoint posterior calcaneal tuberosity

Longitudinal Arch of Foot

- Flatfoot normally present at birth
- Arch develops in 1st decade of life
- 20% of normal adults have flatfoot configuration
- Assess with Meary angle or calcaneal pitch

Talometatarsal Angle (Meary Angle)

- Lines drawn along axes of 1st metatarsal and talus on lateral radiograph
- Normally axes are same
- Pes cavus = talar axis > 4° above 1st metatarsal axis
- Pes planus = talar axis > 4° below 1st metatarsal axis

Calcaneal Pitch

- Line 1: Tangential to inferior surface of calcaneus
- Line 2: Horizontal
- Normal: 20-25°, pes planus: < 20°, pes cavus > 25°

Talocalcaneal Angles

- Anteroposterior radiograph (Kite angle)
  - Lines drawn along central axis of talus and lateral margin of calcaneus
  - 27-56° in newborn
  - 25-45° (mean 35°) in adult
  - > 45° = hindfoot valgus
  - < 20° = hindfoot varus
- Lateral radiograph
  - Lines drawn along central axis of talus and inferior margin of calcaneus
  - 23-55° in newborn
  - 30-50° (mean 35°) in adult

Boehler Angle

- Line 1: Anterior process calcaneus to posterior margin posterior facet
- Line 2: Posterior margin posterior facet to superior margin calcaneal tuberosity
- Normal = 20-40°
- Decreased in most central calcaneal fractures

Gissane Angle

- Line 1: Along superior margin anterior process calcaneus
- Line 2: Along lateral border of posterior subtalar facet
- Normal = 100-130°
- Decreased in most central calcaneal fractures

Hindfoot Width (AP Radiograph)

- Distance from medial margin head of talus to lateral margin calcaneus
- Normal = 4-5.5 cm

Talonavicular Relationship (AP Radiograph)

- Distance between midpoint articular surfaces talus and navicular at talonavicular joint
- Normal = < 7 mm, > 7 mm indicates hyperpronation

1st-5th Intermetatarsal Angle (AP Radiograph)

- Normal = 14-35°
- Increased in splayfoot

1st Intermetatarsal Angle (AP Radiograph)

- Normal = < 9°
- Increased in metatarsus primus varus

4th-5th Intermetatarsal Angle (AP Radiograph)

- Normal = < 5°
- Increased in bunionette deformity

Forefoot Width (AP Radiograph)

- Distance from medial margin 1st metatarsal head to lateral margin 5th metatarsal head
- Normal = 7-9 cm

Relative Metatarsal Lengths (AP Radiograph)

- 1st metatarsal may be equal, shorter, or longer than 2nd
  - Abnormally short 1st metatarsal called Morton foot configuration
  - Predisposes to transfer metatarsalgia of 2nd, 3rd metatarsals
- 2nd-5th metatarsals become progressively shorter
- Relative lengths can be assessed by metatarsal break angle of Meschan
  - Line 1: Tangential to 1st and 2nd metatarsal head articular surfaces
  - Line 2: Tangential to 2nd and 5th metatarsal head articular surfaces
  - Normal = 140°; < 135° indicates relatively short 1st metatarsal

Hallux-Metatarsophalangeal Angle (AP Radiograph)

- Normal = < 15°; > 15 indicates hallux valgus

Hallux-Interphalangeal Angle (AP Radiograph)

- Normal = 6-14°

Plantar Soft Tissue Measurements

- Thickness increases with weight, decreases with age
- Increased plantar soft tissue thickness: Acromegaly, infection, myxedema
- Calcaneal fat pad: 4-17 mm
- Metatarsal fat pad
  - 1st metatarsal head: 7-25 mm
  - 5th metatarsal head: 1-16 mm

ANKLE MORTISE ALIGNMENT

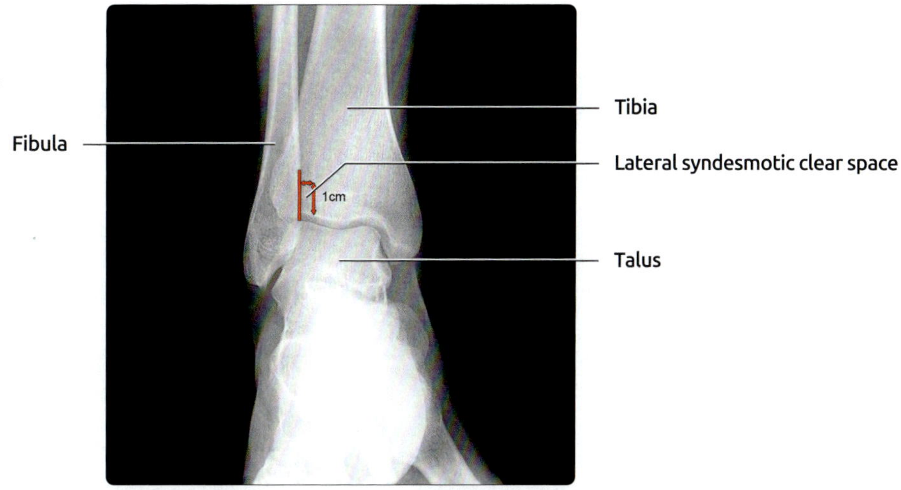

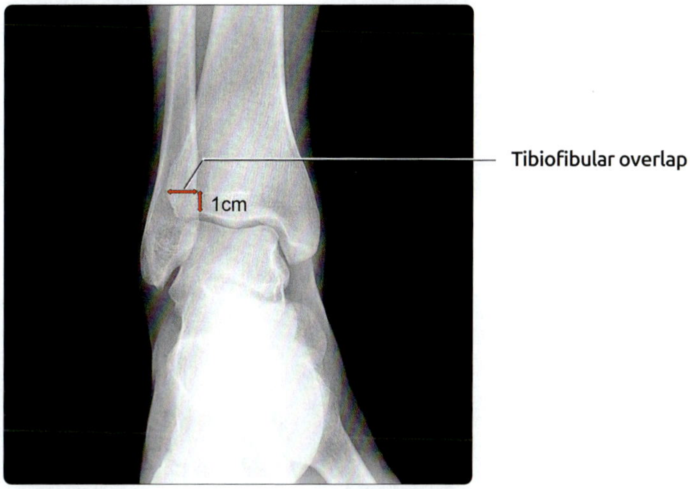

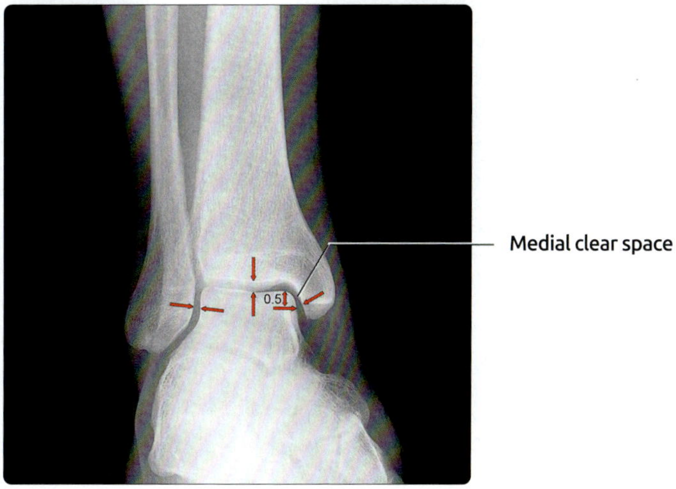

(Top) *The lateral syndesmotic clear space & tibiofibular overlap, indicators of the integrity of the tibiofibular syndesmotic joint, are measured approximately 1 cm above the tibial plafond. The lateral syndesmotic clear space is measured from the posterior tibial margin to the medial fibular margin. Normal measurements vary in the literature and range from 4-6 mm on both the AP ankle and ankle mortise views.* **(Middle)** *The tibiofibular overlap measurements also vary and range from 6-10 mm in the literature. An overlap of 6 mm, however, on the AP view and 1 mm on the ankle mortise view, is considered normal by most.* **(Bottom)** *The talus should be equidistant from the tibial plafond on the AP and ankle mortise views. Minimal tilts are within normal. The normal medial clear space, measured 0.5 cm below the talar articular surface, should be 4 mm in size.*

HINDFOOT ALIGNMENT

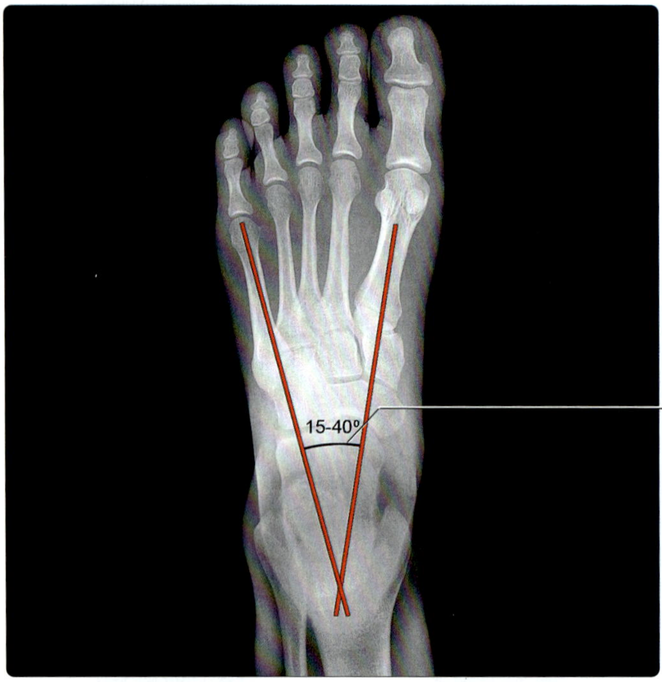

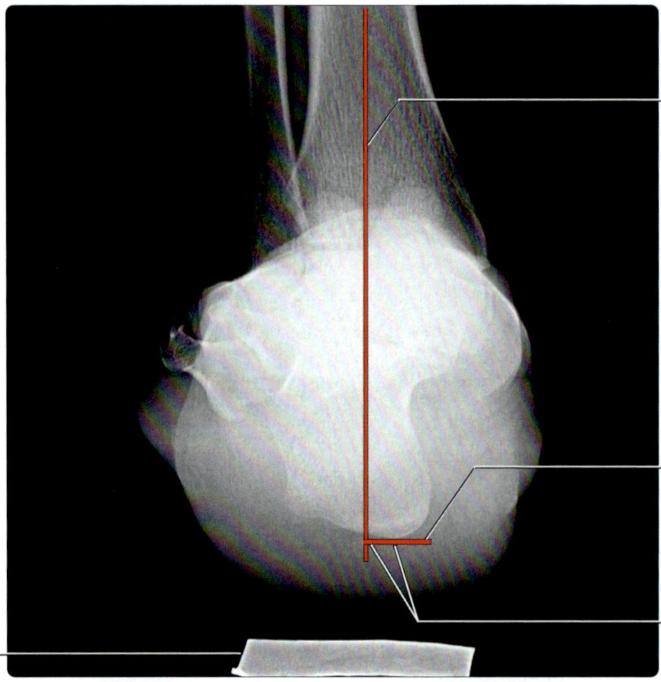

(Top) *Normal AP talocalcaneal angle, measured along longitudinal axes of talus & calcaneus, is 15-40°. Decrease in AP angle is indicative of varus hindfoot deformity & increase is indicative of valgus hindfoot deformity.* **(Bottom)** *Hindfoot alignment view obtained with patient standing is shown. Toes are against radiographic cassette, which is angled 20° from vertical with its top edge tilted away from the foot. X-ray beam angled 20° caudad from heel to toes. Distance from the lowest point of the heel to the line bisecting the tibia (tibial axis) is < 8 mm in normal, asymptomatic subjects. If the distance is > 8 mm, the lateral position of the lowest point of the calcaneus indicates hindfoot valgus, medial position indicates varus.*

HINDFOOT ALIGNMENT

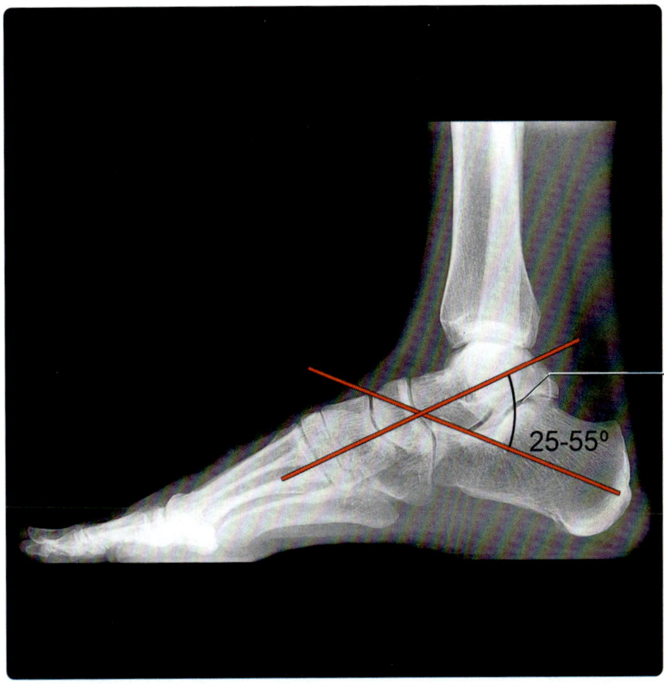

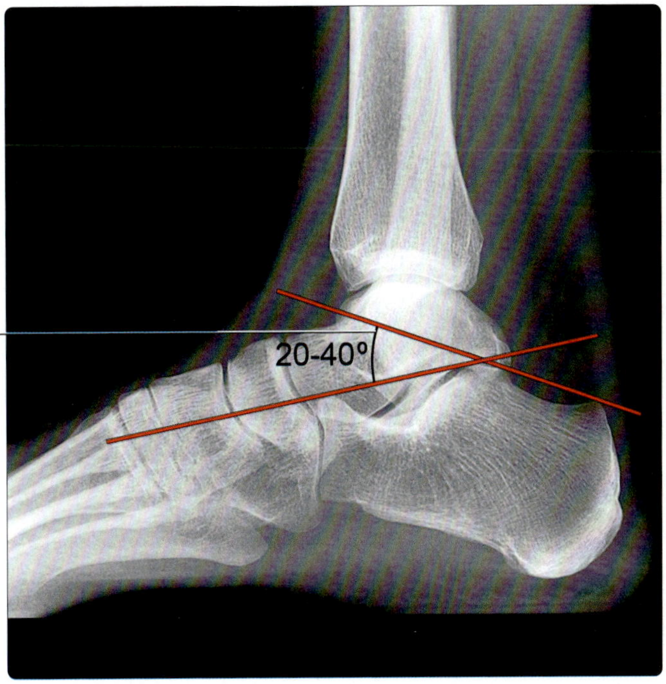

(Top) *Normal lateral talocalcaneal angle (kite angle), formed by intersection of talar & calcaneal longitudinal axes, measures 25-55°. Decrease in lateral angle is indicative of varus hindfoot deformity & increase is indicative of valgus hindfoot deformity.* **(Bottom)** *Boehler angle reflects integrity of the posterior calcaneal facet & calcaneal height. The angle is formed by the intersection of a line drawn along the apices of anterior calcaneal process & posterior calcaneal facet & a line drawn along the apices of posterior calcaneal tuberosity & posterior calcaneal facet. The normal range is 20-40°.*

MIDFOOT ALIGNMENT

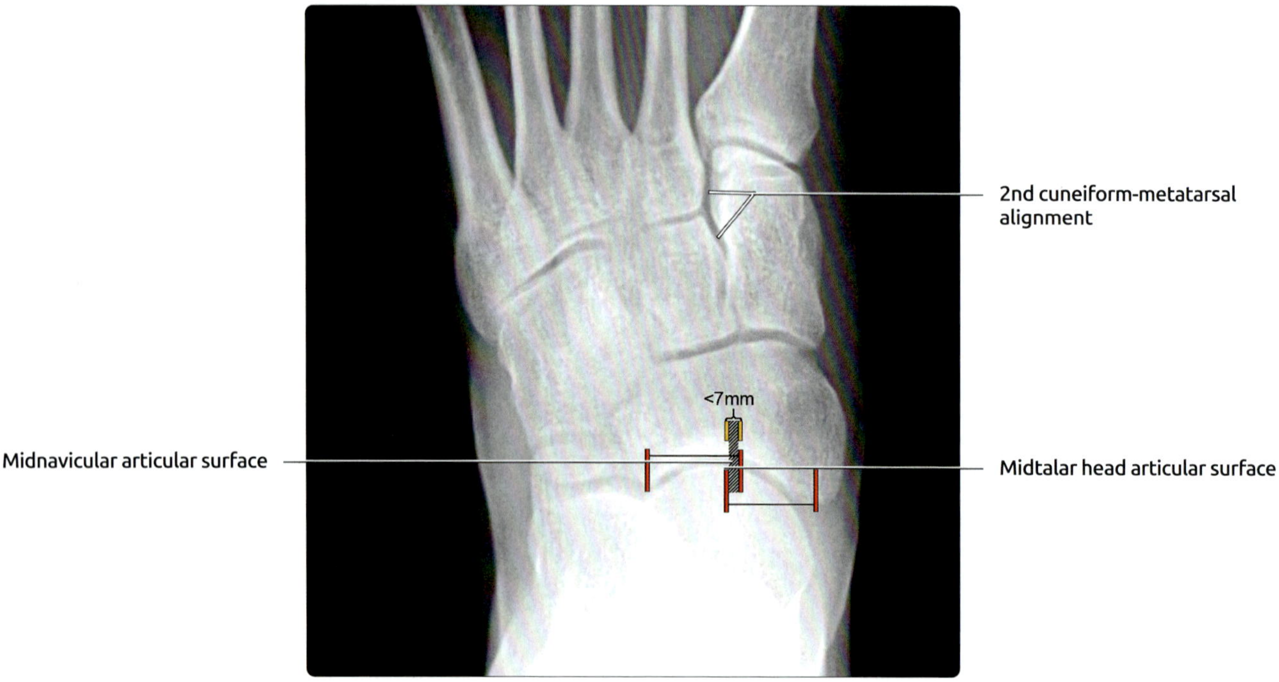

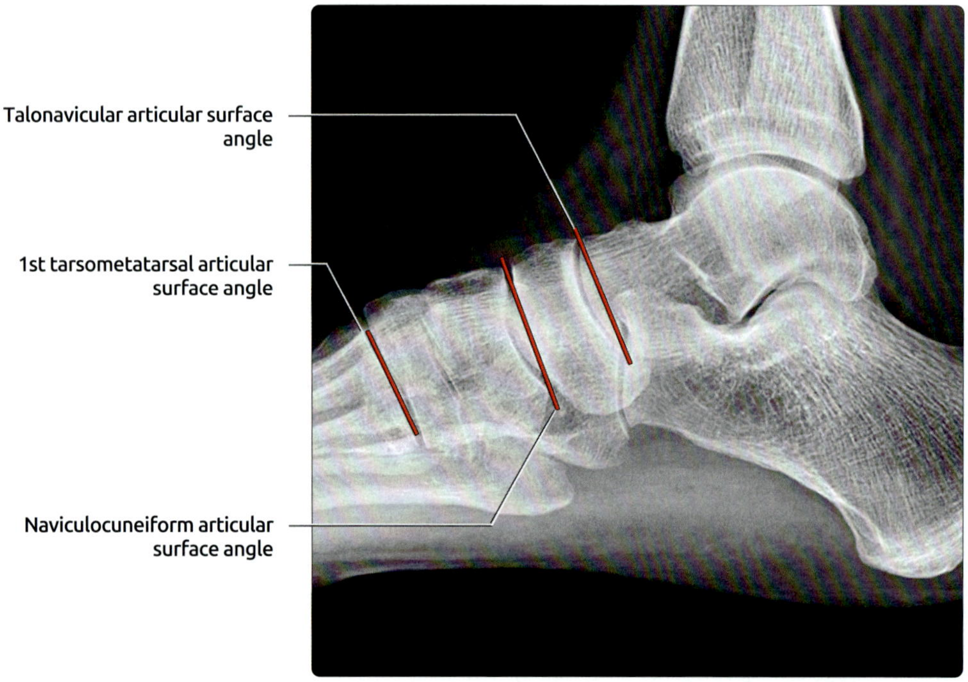

(Top) *Anteroposterior radiograph shows the normal relationship between the talus and navicular. Distance from the midpoint articular surface head of the talus to the midpoint articular surface proximal margin navicular is < 7 mm. The medial margins of 2nd cuneiform and 2nd metatarsal are exactly aligned; lateral displacement indicates Lisfranc ligament rupture.* **(Bottom)** *Lateral radiograph shows the normal relationship of the talus, navicular, and cuneiforms. Lateral articular surface angles of talonavicular, naviculocuneiform, and 1st tarsometatarsal joints are approximately parallel.*

TARSOMETATARSAL JOINT ALIGNMENT

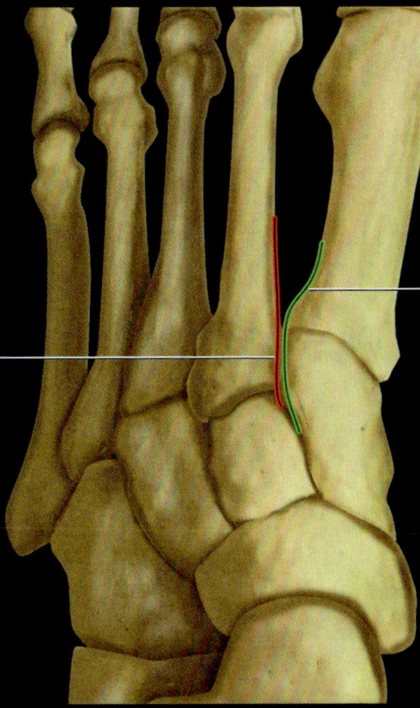

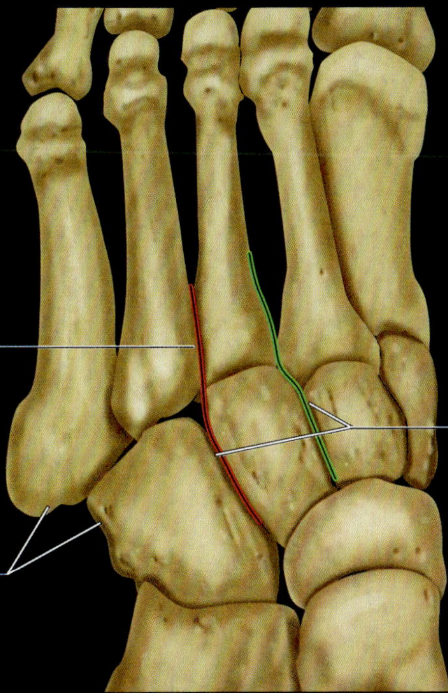

(Top) *Anteroposterior graphic shows that the 1st metatarsal is centered on the 1st cuneiform. The line drawn along the lateral margin of the cuneiform and metatarsal is often curved, and there may be focal offset. In contradistinction, the line along medial margins of the 2nd cuneiform and metatarsal should be straight, and any deviation of the line indicates disruption of the Lisfranc ligament.* **(Bottom)** *Oblique graphic shows the 3rd metatarsal centered on the 3rd cuneiform. The medial margin of the 4th metatarsal is aligned with the medial margin of the cuboid. The 5th metatarsal styloid process extends beyond the lateral margin of the cuboid.*

LONGITUDINAL ARCH OF FOOT

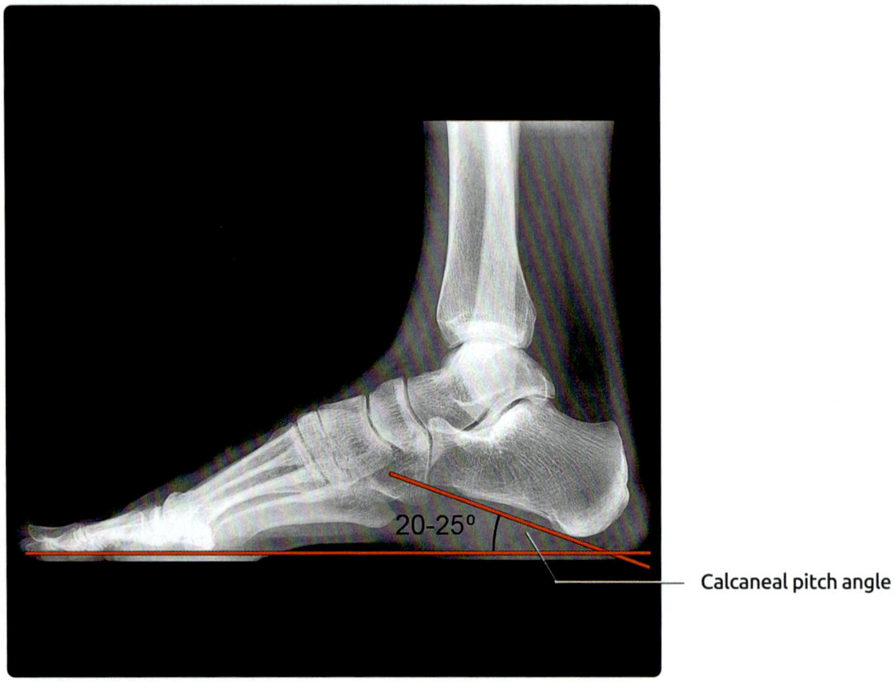

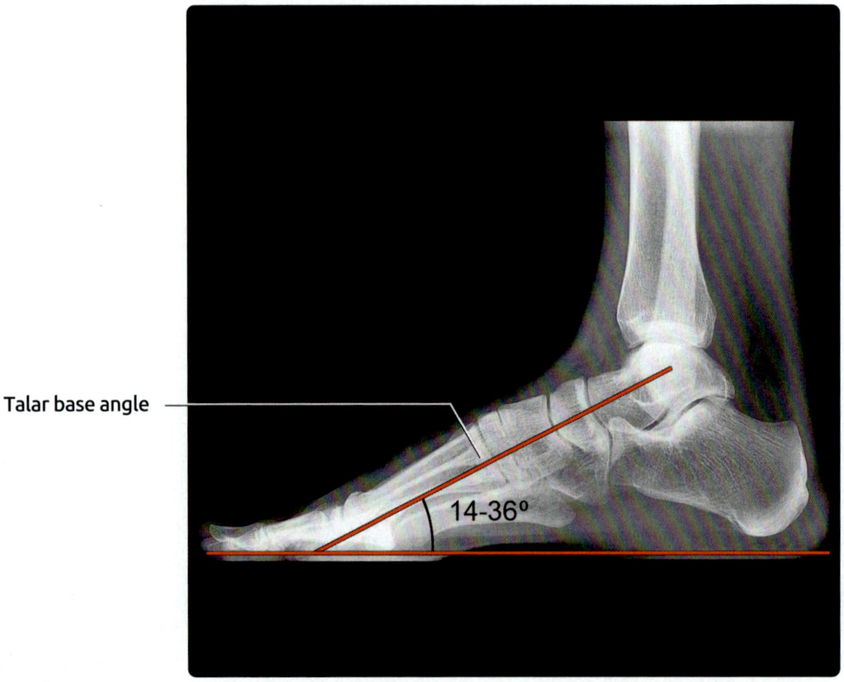

(Top) *Weight-bearing lateral view of the foot provides information on the height of the longitudinal arch. The calcaneal pitch is an angle formed by intersection of a line along the plantar aspect of the calcaneus with a line parallel to floor. It should measure about 20-25°.* **(Bottom)** *The normal talar base angle is formed by the intersection of the longitudinal axis of the talus with a line parallel to the floor. It normally measures 14-36°.*

METATARSAL ALIGNMENT LATERAL

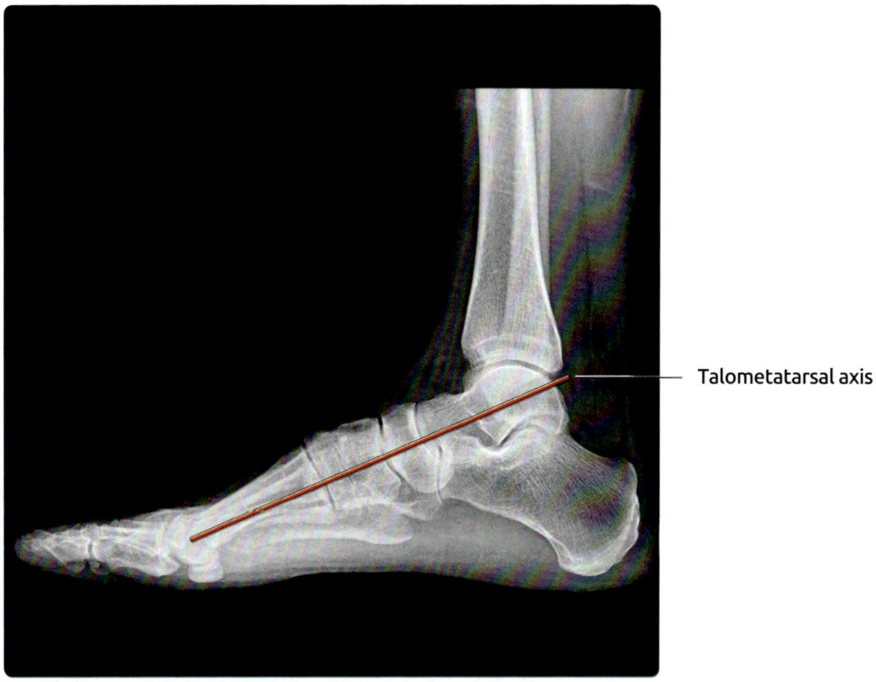

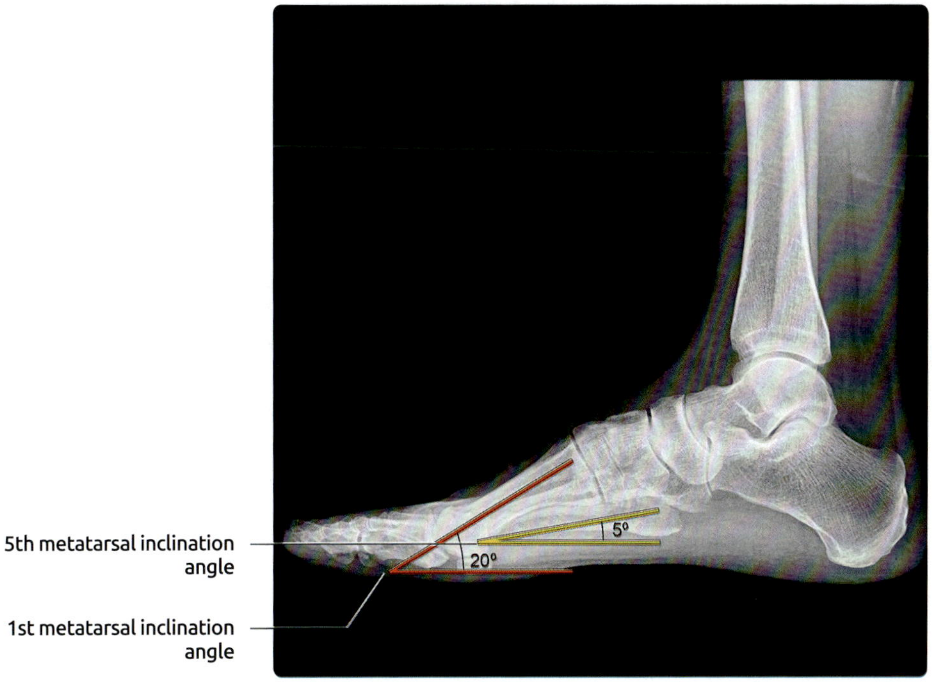

(Top) *Lateral weight-bearing radiograph shows the talometatarsal axis. Meary angle is the angle between the talar angle and the axis of the 1st metatarsal. The line drawn along the center of the talar axis is aligned with the axis of the 1st metatarsal in a normally aligned foot. If the axis of the of the talus extends > 4° above the 1st metatarsal axis, there is pes cavus. If > 4° below the axis of the 1st metatarsal, there is pes planus.* **(Bottom)** *Lateral weight-bearing radiograph shows the plantigrade inclination of the metatarsals. The inclination angle is the angle between the horizontal and the axis of a metatarsal. It decreases from 20° for the 1st metatarsal to 15° for the 2nd, 10° for the 3rd, 8° for the 4th and 5° for the 5th.*

METATARSAL ALIGNMENT AP

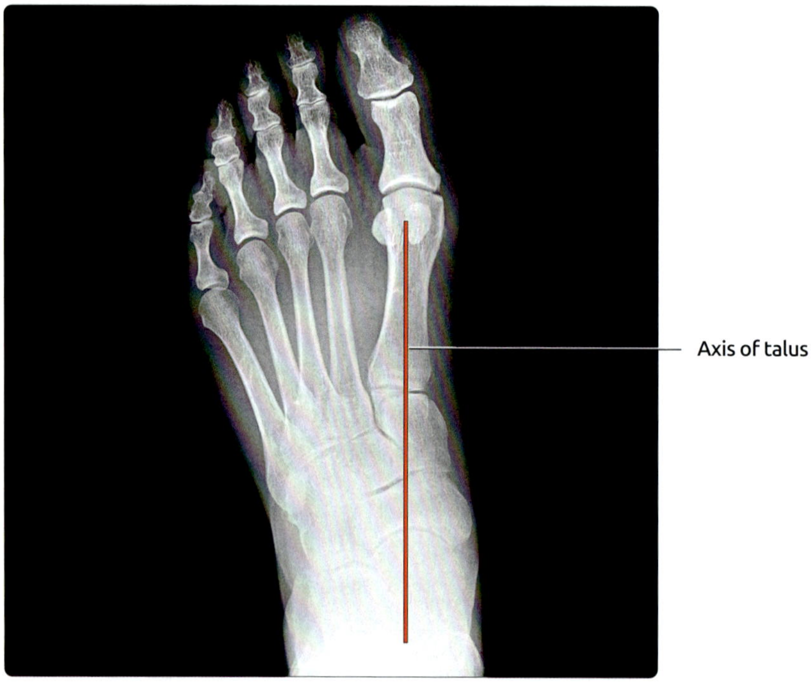

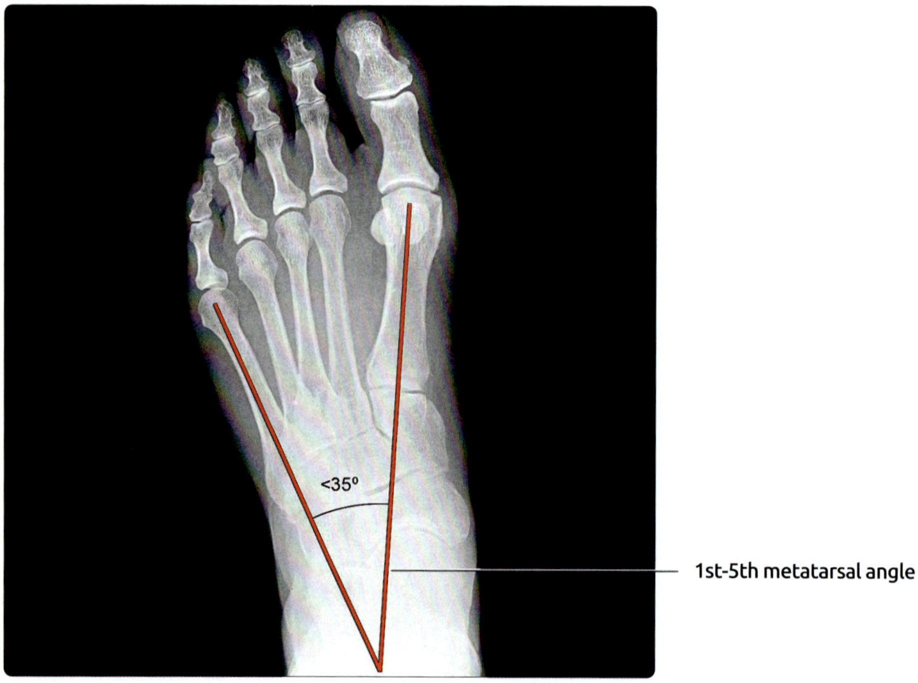

(Top) *Anteroposterior radiograph shows the normal relationship between the axis of the talus and the axis of the 1st metatarsal. The axis of the talus extends along the axis of the 1st metatarsal, or between the 1st and 2nd metatarsal. In the forefoot varus or adductus, the axis of the 1st metatarsal deviates medially from the axis of the talus. In the forefoot valgus or adductus, the 1st metatarsal deviates laterally.* **(Bottom)** *Anteroposterior radiograph shows that metatarsals overlap at the base and fan outward. Splayfoot is present when 1st-5th metatarsal angle is > 35°. The normal angle between the 1st and 2nd metatarsals is < 9°, and between the 4th and 5th metatarsals is < 5°. An increased 1st-2nd metatarsal angle is termed metatarsus primus varus, and an increased 4th-5th metatarsal angle is termed metatarsus quintus valgus.*

METATARSAL LENGTHS

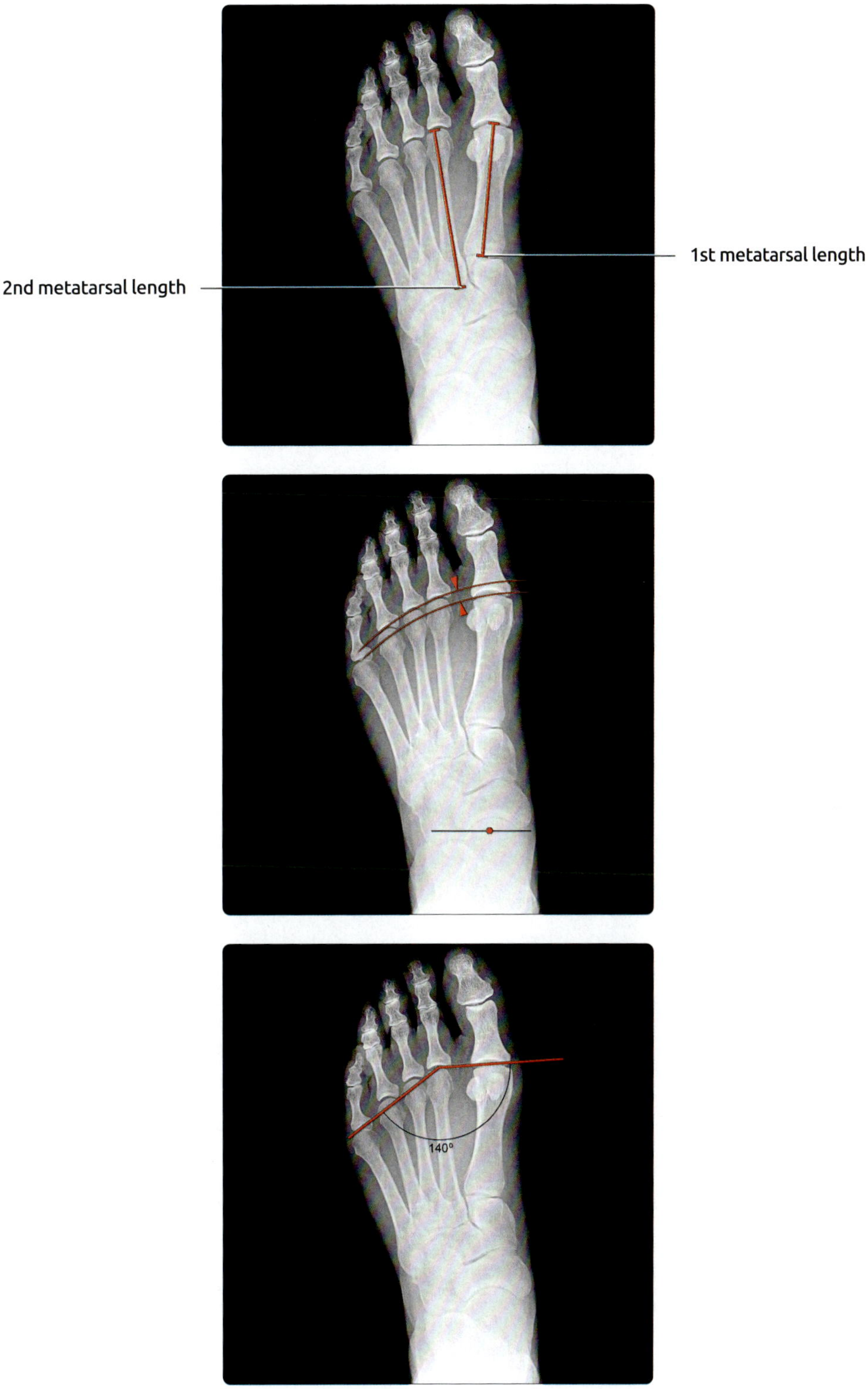

(Top) *Anteroposterior radiograph shows the relative metatarsal lengths measured by the method of Stokes. In this method, absolute metatarsal lengths are measured, but overall alignment is not considered.* **(Middle)** *Anteroposterior radiograph shows relative metatarsal lengths by the method of Hardy and Clapham. An arc is drawn centered on the metatarsal head, with the center of the arc at the center of the talar head. The difference in metatarsal length is measured as the distance between the arcs of the 1st and 2nd metatarsal.* **(Bottom)** *Anteroposterior radiograph shows the metatarsal break angle of Meschan. This is angle formed between the line tangential to the 1st and 2nd metatarsal head articular surfaces and the line tangential to the 2nd and 5th metatarsal head articular surfaces. Normal is 140°; < 135° indicates relatively short 1st metatarsal.*

HALLUX ALIGNMENT

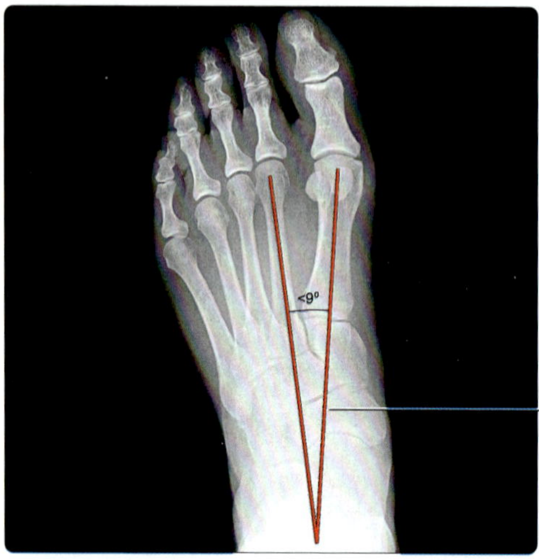

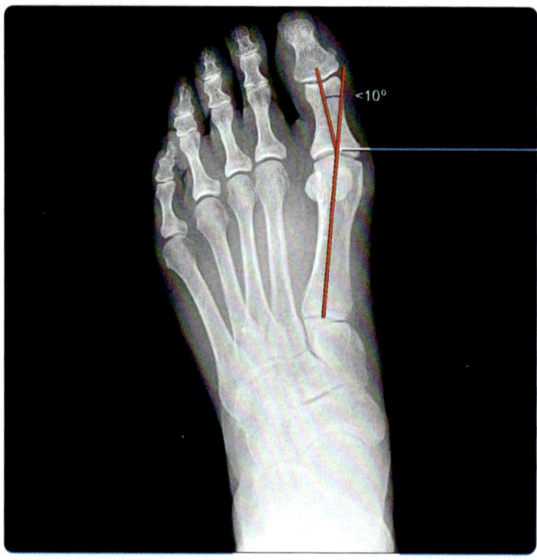

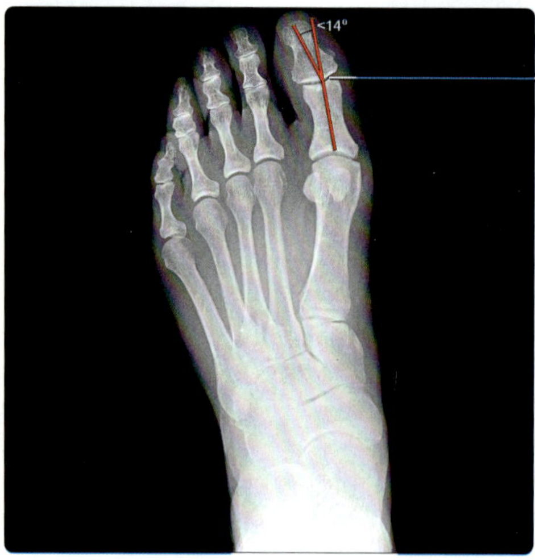

(Top) *Anteroposterior radiograph shows a normal intermetatarsal angle of < 10°.* **(Middle)** *Anteroposterior radiograph shows a normal hallux angle of < 10°. The threshold for definition of hallux valgus varies 15-20°.* **(Bottom)** *Anteroposterior radiograph shows a hallux interphalangeal angle. Lines are drawn along the axes of the 1st proximal and distal phalanges. Normal angle is 6-14°.*

SOFT TISSUE MEASUREMENTS

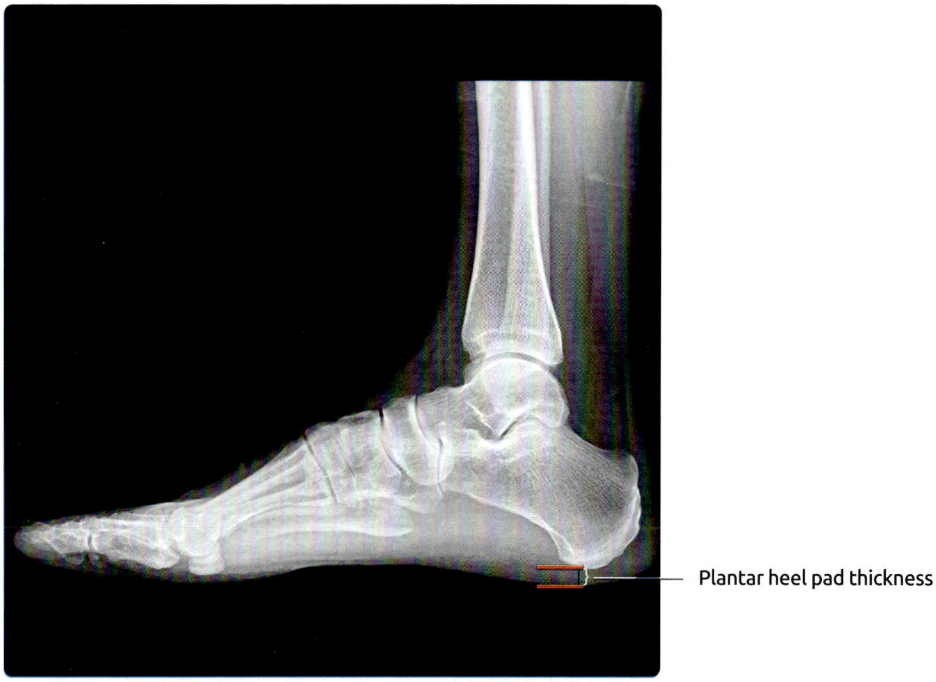

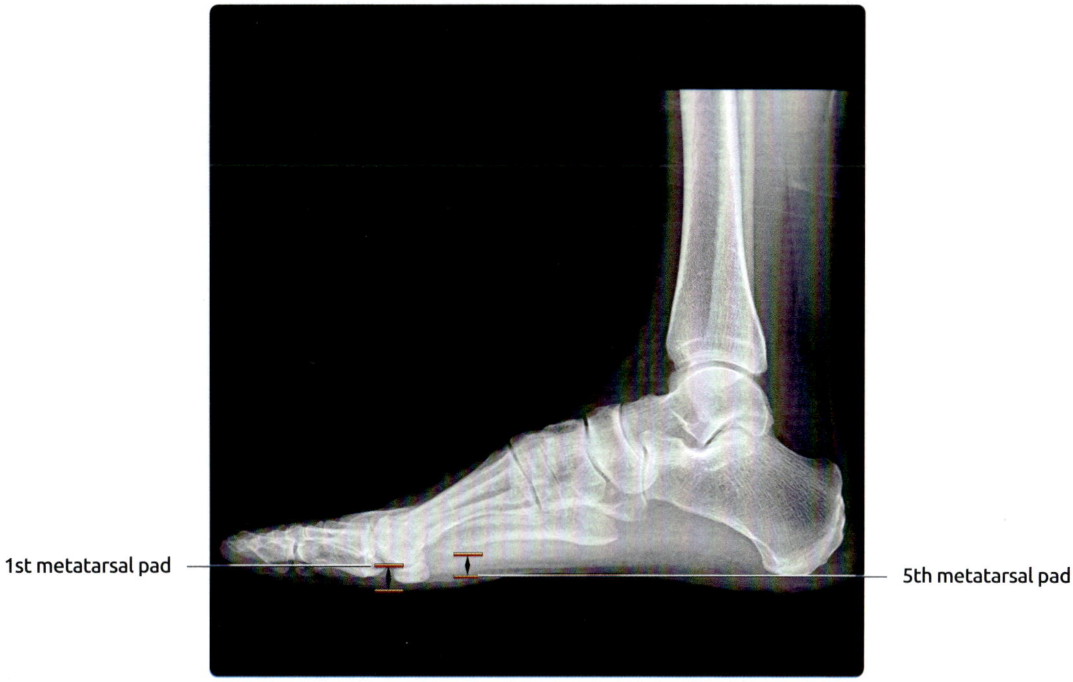

(Top) *Lateral radiograph shows a normal thickness of plantar heel pad, which can range from 4-17 mm.* **(Bottom)** *Lateral weight-bearing radiograph shows a normal thickness of metatarsal soft tissue pads. The 1st measures between 7-25 mm, and the 5th measures between 1-16 mm. Note that it is difficult to discern the soft tissue margin at the lateral aspect of the foot, limiting accuracy of the 5th metatarsal pad measurement.*

SECTION 6

Normal Variants

NORMAL VARIANTS

Muscle Variants

- Many minor variations of muscle size, insertion, and origin exist
  - Most are clinically nonconsequential
  - Absence of plantaris muscle is one of more frequent of these
- Biceps femoris muscle hypertrophy
  - Common peroneal nerve follows biceps femoris to fibular head insertion of muscle
  - If biceps femoris is hypertrophied, it can entrap common peroneal nerve; may be symptomatic
  - Other morphologic abnormalities that may affect nerve at this site: Hypertrophy of lateral head of gastrocnemius or fatty hypertrophy (often secondary to diabetes)
- Gastrocnemius muscle origin variants and popliteal artery entrapment (prevalence estimated at 0.16%)
  - Popliteal artery is normally adjacent and lateral to medial head of gastrocnemius muscle
    - Popliteal artery may take abnormal course medial to attachment of medial gastrocnemius
    - Numerous anomalous popliteal fossa relationships can result in entrapment
  - Several gastrocnemius anomalies described that may entrap popliteal vessels
    - Origin lateral head gastrocnemius from medial femoral condyle
    - Origin medial head gastrocnemius from lateral femoral condyle
    - 3rd head gastrocnemius (seen in 1.9% knee MR exams)
    - Fibrous bands
  - Clinical association
    - Many variants are not symptomatic
    - May produce symptoms of claudication
    - Rarely, repetitive insult can cause arterial aneurysm or thrombosis
    - Anomalous structure usually splits vessels in symptomatic cases
- Accessory muscles at ankle
  - Multiple accessory muscles are described; will be more fully described in ankle section
- Articularis genus muscle
  - Originates distal femur, deep to vastus intermedius, inserts on superior knee joint capsule
  - Pulls suprapatellar recess superiorly during knee extension

Osseous Variants

- Fabella: Sesamoid in lateral head of gastrocnemius
  - To qualify as fabella, rounded ossific density must be located both posteriorly and laterally, at expected site of lateral gastrocnemius
  - Fabella may be absent, then fabellofibular ligament is also absent and arcuate ligament enlarged
  - Fabella may be bipartite or multipartite
- Bipartite patella (prevalence ~ 2%)
  - 40% bilateral; M:F = 9:1
  - Separate ossification site, usually superior and lateral to main patella
  - May be bipartite or multipartite
  - Fragments appear rounded but may not appear to "fit" perfectly together
  - Overlying cartilage is smooth, uniting parts
  - Rarely may be symptomatic
  - Debated whether it is anomaly of ossification or stress related
  - Synchondrosis between parts may be injured
- Dorsal defect of patella (prevalence < 1%)
  - Well-defined lucent lesion, usually in superolateral quadrant of patella
  - Should not be confused with osteochondral defect
  - Defect may become smaller and sclerotic over time
  - Overlying cartilage is normal
  - Debated whether it is anomaly of ossification or stress related
- Posterior femoral condylar irregularity
  - Seen in adolescents (girls < 10 years of age, boys < 12 years of age)
  - Distinctly located in posterior 1/3 of weight-bearing portion of femoral condyle; seen well on lateral view
  - Because of posterior location, better seen on notch view than AP
  - No extension to intercondylar notch
  - Overlying cartilage is normal
  - No significant marrow edema
  - With maturation, ossification becomes smooth and regular
  - Do not confuse with osteochondral defect or injury
  - Does not require reduction of activity or other treatment
- Posteromedial distal femoral metaphyseal cortical defect
  - Variably called cortical desmoid or cortical avulsive tug lesion
  - Seen in adolescents or teenagers
  - Very specific in location, adjacent to insertion of adductor magnus aponeurosis
  - May appear somewhat aggressive: Cortical indistinctness, mild spiculation, scalloping of bone, small soft tissue mass
  - Debated as to whether it is chronic avulsive lesion or normal growth phenomenon
  - Important to not suggest it is more aggressive lesion as long as it precisely fits this description
- FOPE zone
  - FOPE = focal periphyseal edema
  - Occurs in skeletally immature patients approaching age of physeal fusion at knee
  - Edema signal seen surrounding central portion of physis
  - Entire physis is open, and no other abnormality is seen
  - Edema felt to relate to early stages of physiologic physeal closure
  - May be associated with pain when no other MR abnormality is present
  - If characteristic, no further diagnostic procedure or imaging follow-up required
  - No treatment recommended

Ligamentous Variants

- Meniscofemoral ligaments (Wrisberg and Humphrey)

- Both originate at intercondylar notch of medial femoral condyle and insert on posterior horn lateral meniscus, Humphrey anterior to posterior cruciate ligament (PCL), and Wrisberg posterior to PCL
- Variable presence: 1 or both are present in 83% of knees
- Seen in profile as round low signal on sagittal; do not mistake for loose body
- May mimic tear as ligament approaches its attachment on posterior horn lateral meniscus

- Transverse ligament
  - Connects 2 anterior meniscal horns; occasionally, may be absent or hypertrophied
  - May mimic anterior horn tear at anterior horn lateral meniscus as it inserts
  - May be site of origin of meniscomeniscal or meniscocruciate ligament
- Meniscocruciate ligament
  - Extends from anterior horn lateral meniscus to lateral femoral condyle
  - Rarely originates at transverse ligament
  - Parallels anterior cruciate ligament (ACL); distinguish from partial ACL tear
- Oblique meniscomeniscal ligament
  - Anterior horn of one meniscus to posterior horn of other; appears to split ACL
  - May mimic loose body

Plica Variant

- Infrapatellar plica
  - Arises from inferior patella, crosses Hoffa fat pad, and extends along anterior surface ACL
  - Parallels ACL; must distinguish from partial ACL tear

Meniscal Variants

- Discoid meniscus
  - Extra meniscal material extends toward intercondylar notch, making meniscus discoid rather than C shape
    - Generally seen on both coronal and sagittal imaging (occasionally axial)
    - May be partial and seen in only 1 plane
  - Lateral meniscus more commonly discoid than medial
  - Posterolateral knee morphology unusual
    - Posterior horn appears to be drawn in, leaving large popliteal hiatus and elongated superior and inferior fascicles
  - At greater risk for tear, particularly at young age
- Anterior horn medial meniscus origin
  - Usual origin from tibial plateau, far anteriorly
  - Occasionally originates anterior to this, off edge of plateau
  - Location may mimic extrusion, but meniscus itself is normal with normal surrounding tissue
  - On axial, anterior horn tissue mimics bucket handle tear fragment
- Meniscal ossicle
  - Trabeculated osseous tissue formed within meniscus
  - Almost exclusively located in posterior horn medial meniscus
    - Other locations rarely occur
  - Follows osseous signal throughout (fatty signal on T1, saturates out on fat-saturated sequences)
  - Usually associated with meniscal tear, often radial tear at posterior root
  - Uncertain whether it is true normal variant or related to trauma in childhood

IMAGING PITFALLS

Radiographic Positioning

- Axial (tangential) radiographs of patella should be obtained at 20° flexion
  - Over- or under-flexion may reduce subluxating patella, resulting in missed diagnosis

MR Positioning

- Choice of obliquity of sagittal and coronal obliques is crucial
  - Failure to oblique sagittals along ACL results in poor visualization of that structure
  - Over-obliquing sagittals or coronals may give false impression of extrusion of meniscus

Cartilage Thickness

- Posterior weight-bearing femoral cartilage thickness exaggerated
- T2 underestimates cartilage thickness since cortex and cartilage have similar signal
- PD may have similar signal for cartilage and adjacent joint fluid, obscuring defects
  - Fat saturation on PD solves this issue

Partial Voluming Over Convex Surfaces

- Morphology of trochlea, femoral condyles, and patella makes them difficult to evaluate in 3 standard planes

Truncation Artifact

- Occurs due to approximation errors in Fourier transform analysis
- Seen at boundary between high- and low-signal structures
- Menisci with adjacent high-signal effusion particularly subject to this
  - Gives false appearance of horizontal tear in meniscus in fat-saturated images
  - Compare nonfat-saturated PD image to fat-saturated ones; former will not show "tear"

Motion Mimicking Meniscal Tear

- Slight motion of knee during acquisition of images may give false appearance of horizontal meniscal tear with slightly convex line crossing meniscus
- Slightly convex lines through adjacent femoral condyle, exactly paralleling line through meniscus, are best hint of situation; use other planes and sequences to determine integrity of meniscus

Vacuum Phenomenon Mimicking Loose Body

- Full extension of knee may result in vacuum-produced air bubble within joint
  - Round low signal of air bubble may mimic loose body or meniscal tear
  - Particularly prominent on gradient-echo imaging in which air bubble "blooms"

HYPERTROPHIED BICEPS FEMORIS

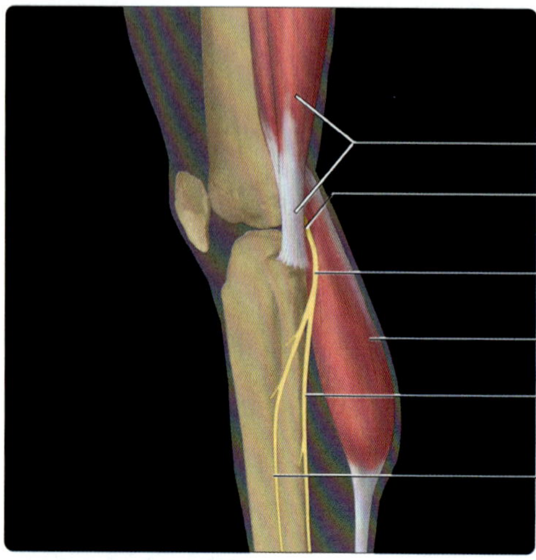

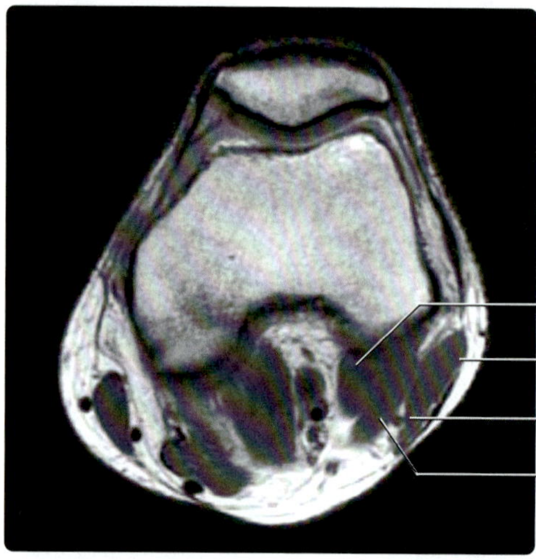

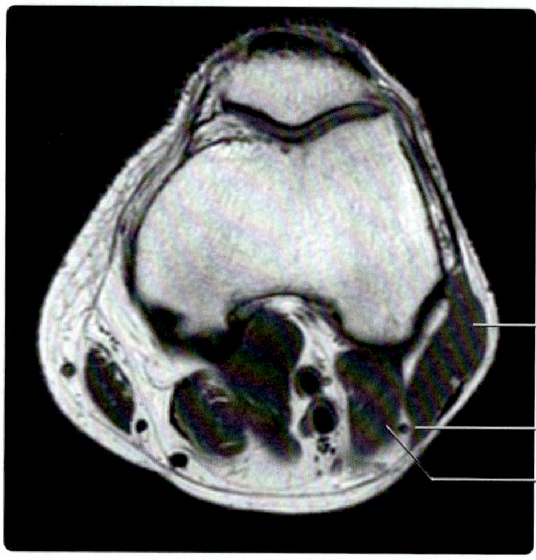

(Top) *Lateral graphic shows the peroneus longus muscle peeled away showing the site at which the common peroneal nerve can be compressed proximal to the fibular head. Compression at this site has been described with hypertrophy of biceps femoris, lateral gastrocnemius, or fat.* **(Middle)** *First of 2 axial T1 MR images shows the top of the intercondylar notch. These images show compression of the common peroneal nerve between a hypertrophied biceps femoris muscle and the lateral gastrocnemius. Normally, the biceps are more gracile in this location with the common peroneal nerve located more posteriorly. This variant may cause nerve compression and may be symptomatic.* **(Bottom)** *Slightly more distal axial T1WI MR shows persistence of the relationship of the hypertrophied biceps, compressing the common peroneal nerve against the gastrocnemius muscle.*

3RD HEAD GASTROCNEMIUS

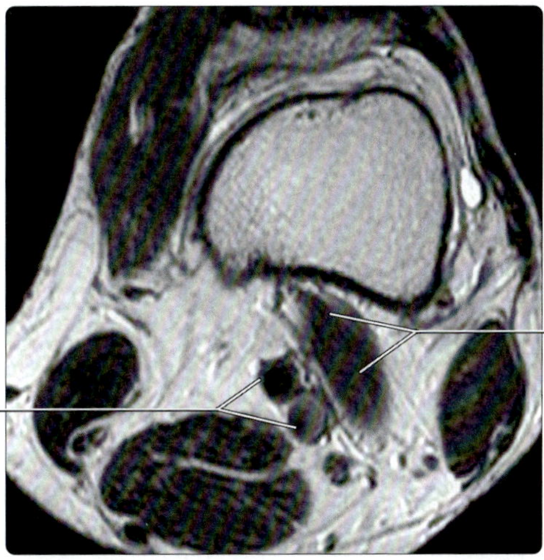

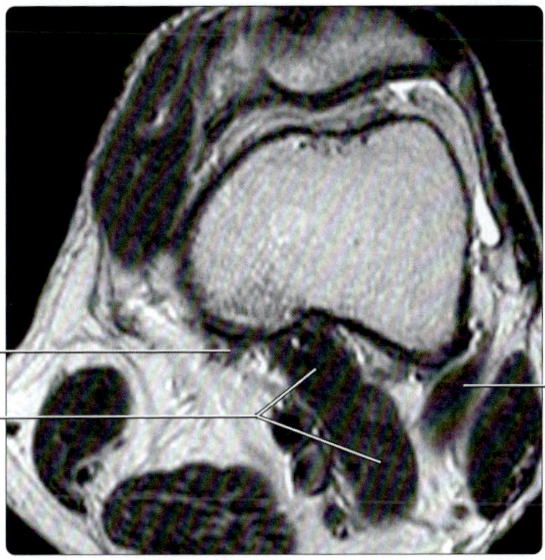

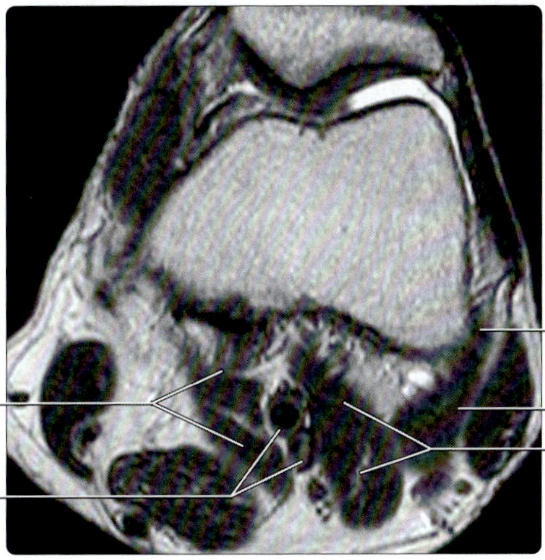

(Top) *First of 3 axial T2 MR images shows a variant 3rd head of gastrocnemius. The aberrant head arises from the medial femoral metaphysis adjacent to the normal medial head gastrocnemius. However, it deviates laterally, forming a muscular sling around the popliteal vessels.* **(Middle)** *Slightly more distal T2WI MR shows the aberrant 3rd head as well as the normal medial head of gastrocnemius and plantaris.* **(Bottom)** *Slightly more distal T2WI MR toward the knee joint shows the popliteal vessels surrounded by the normal medial head and the 3rd head of the gastrocnemius. This may result in symptoms of claudication. However, the variant is more likely to cause symptoms if it splits the popliteal artery and vein.*

ABERRANT ORIGIN LATERAL HEAD GASTROCNEMIUS

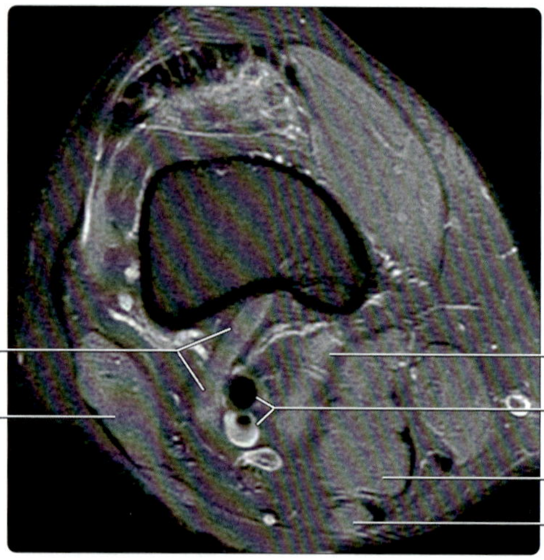

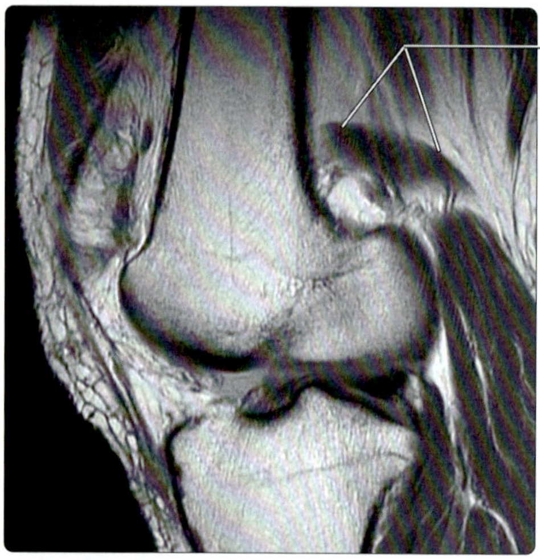

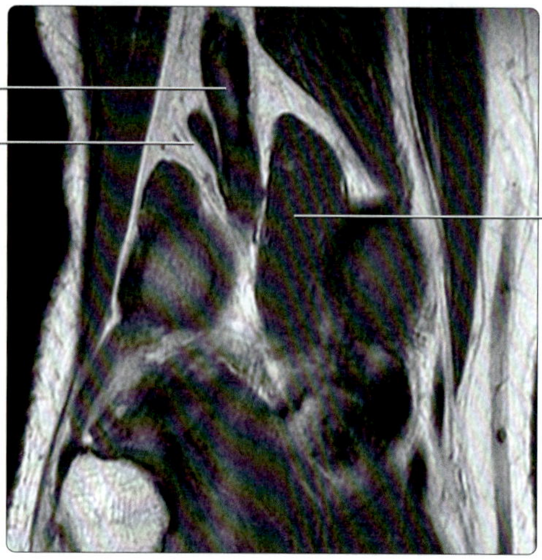

(Top) *Axial PD FS MR demonstrates an aberrant origin of the lateral head of gastrocnemius encircling the popliteal neurovascular bundle. Although patients with this abnormality may be asymptomatic, others present with symptoms of claudication.* **(Middle)** *Sagittal PD MR in the same patient shows the aberrant origin of the lateral head of the gastrocnemius. The course of the muscle is more horizontal than normal, which may be the only hint of the abnormal morphology.* **(Bottom)** *Coronal T1WI MR in the same patient shows the aberrant lateral head of gastrocnemius encircling the popliteal vessels. This static image alone is not diagnostic; however, scrolling through the image stack shows this muscle slip originating more medially, corresponding to the morphology seen on the axial view.*

ABERRANT ORIGIN LATERAL HEAD GASTROCNEMIUS

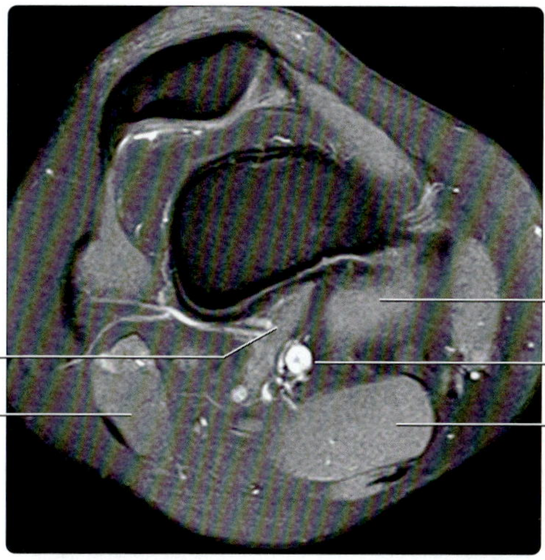

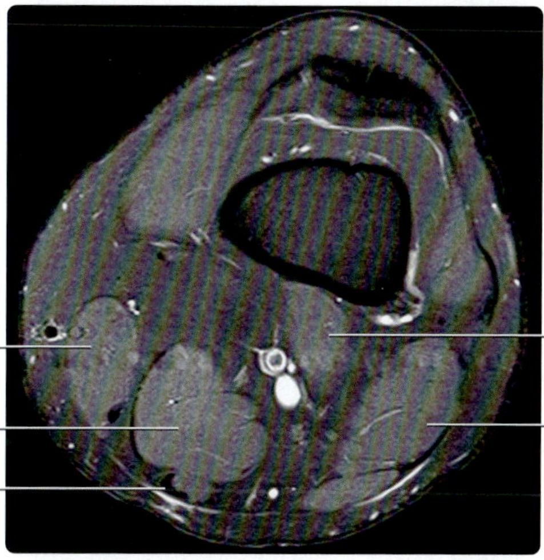

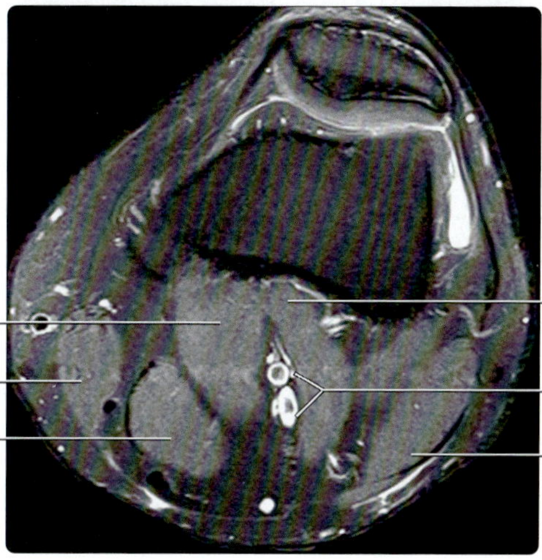

(Top) *Axial PD FS through the supracondylar region of the right distal femur shows an aberrant origin of the lateral head of the gastrocnemius. As it heads toward its normal position posterolaterally, it encircles the popliteal vessels, potentially resulting in claudication symptoms.* **(Middle)** *Axial PD FS MR of the left knee in a different patient shows the lateral head of the gastrocnemius arising from the central/medial portion of the femoral metaphysis.* **(Bottom)** *Axial PD FS MR in the same patient shows the aberrant head of the lateral head of the gastrocnemius and the normal medial head of the gastrocnemius encircling the popliteal vessels. This patient had symptoms of claudication secondary to this morphologic anomaly.*

ARTICULARIS GENU

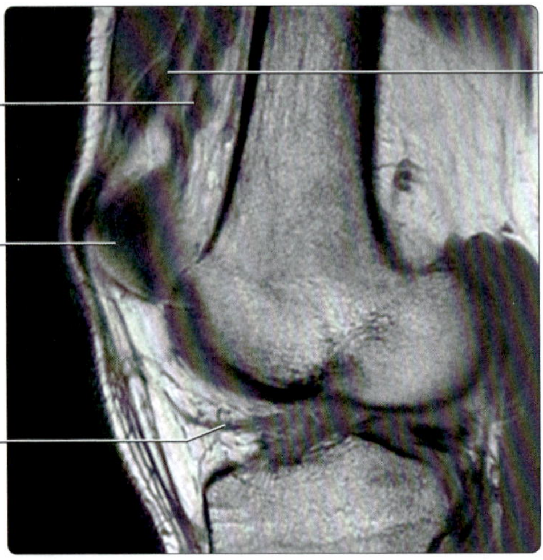

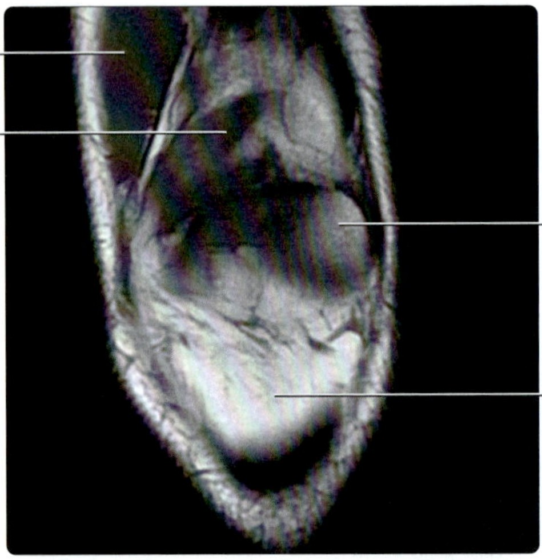

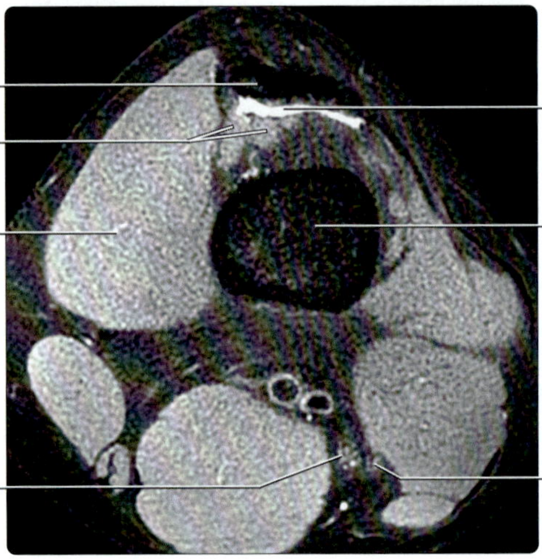

(Top) *Sagittal PD MR shows the articularis genu muscle, which is variably present in the knee. It is sometimes merged with the vastus intermedius muscle. It originates from the distal femur and inserts on the suprapatellar synovium and acts to pull the suprapatellar recess superiorly during knee extension.* **(Middle)** *Coronal T1WI MR immediately posterior to the patella shows the articularis genus as an ellipsoid, wispy structure. Its appearance is quite variable. It is innervated by the femoral nerve.* **(Bottom)** *Axial PD FS MR immediately superior to the patella shows the articularis genu muscle attaching to the synovium of the suprapatellar recess. In this case, 2 separate muscle bundles are seen. The articularis genu may have single or multiple bundles and is variable in appearance.*

ACCESSORY TENSOR FASCIA SURALIS

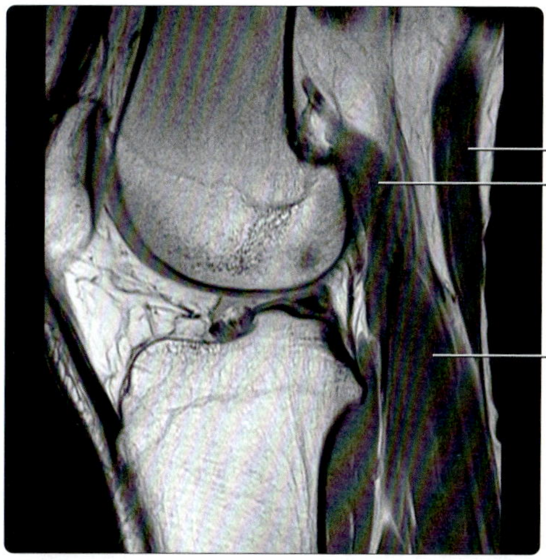

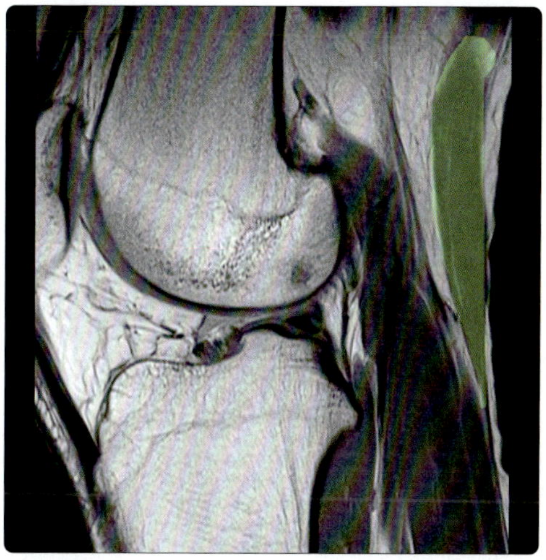

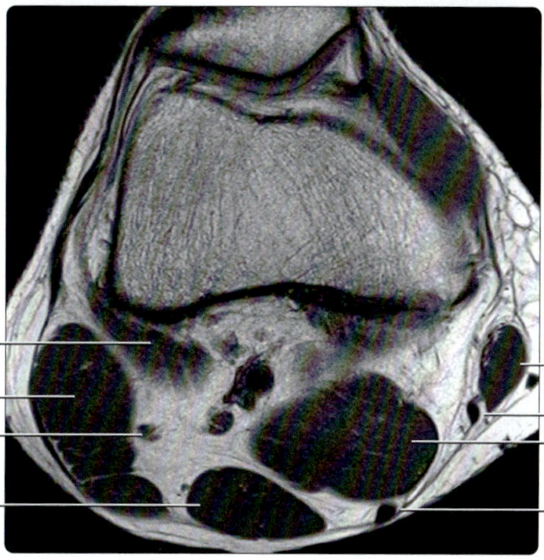

(Top) *Sagittal PD MR of the knee through the lateral condyle demonstrates the expected plantaris and gastrocnemius muscles. However, there is an additional longitudinal structure located posterior to the gastrocnemius that displays signal and texture of muscle.* **(Middle)** *Sagittal PD MR shows the knee through the lateral condyle with accessory muscle shaded green. This accessory muscle is termed the tensor fascia suralis. Such accessory muscles may present clinically as a mass, as in this case.* **(Bottom)** *Axial PD MR in the same patient shows the accessory muscle (tensor fascia suralis) with nearby normal muscles. It is important to note expected muscles and be certain that there are not "extras" since there is no signal abnormality to alert one to the abnormality. (Courtesy A. Kingzett-Taylor, MD.)*

ACCESSORY SOLEUS

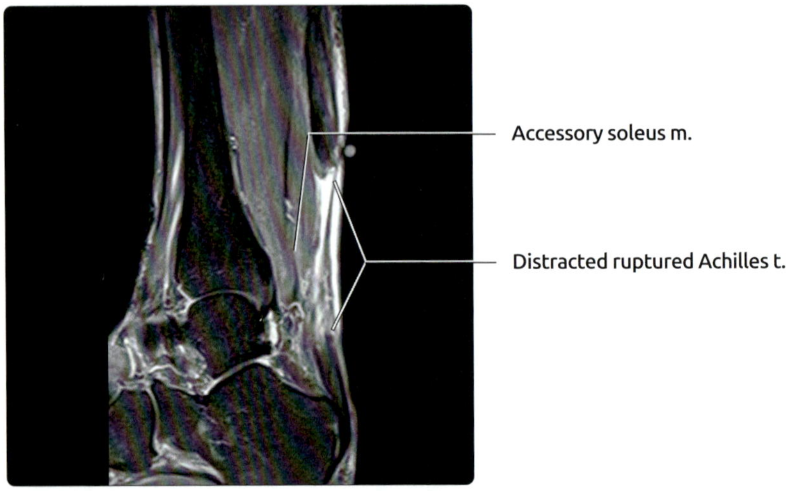

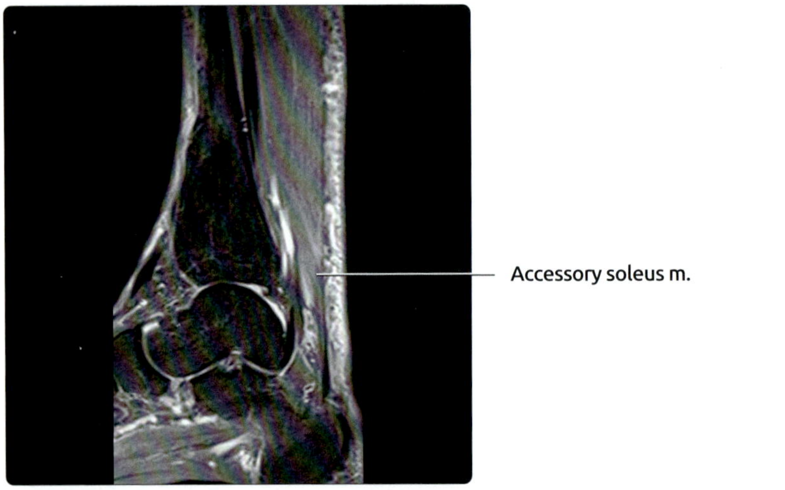

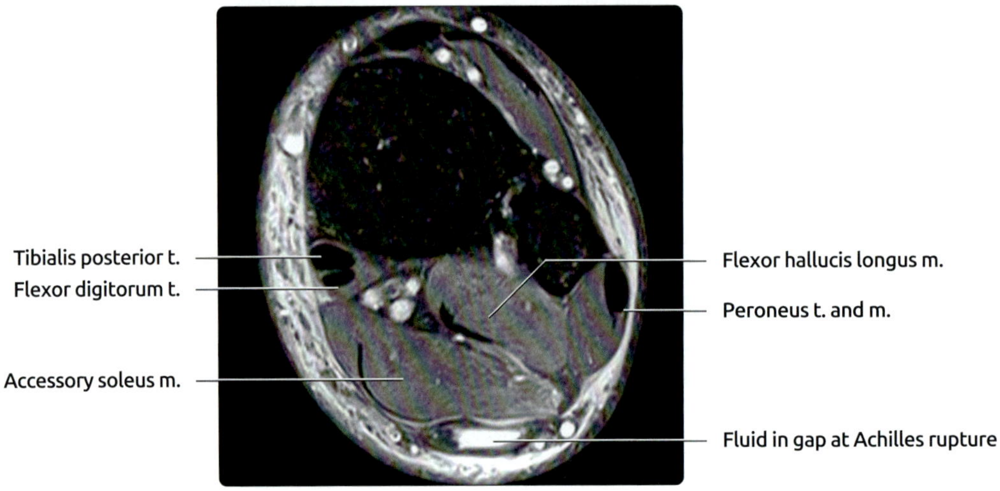

(Top) *Sagittal T2WI FS MR demonstrates not only a widely distracted Achilles tendon tear, but also an accessory soleus muscle. Note the space normally occupied by Kager fat pad.* **(Middle)** *Adjacent sagittal cut shows full bulk of accessory soleus muscle.* **(Bottom)** *Axial PD FS shows fluid at the gap from the Achilles rupture. However, the space normally occupied by Kager fat pad is filled with a large accessory soleus muscle.*

ACCESSORY FLEXOR HALLUCIS LONGUS

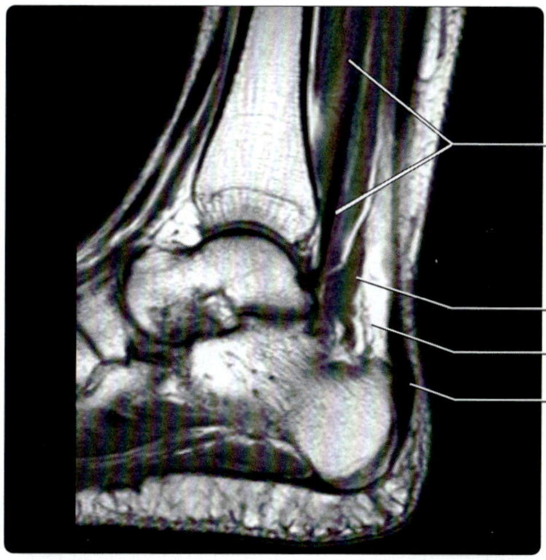

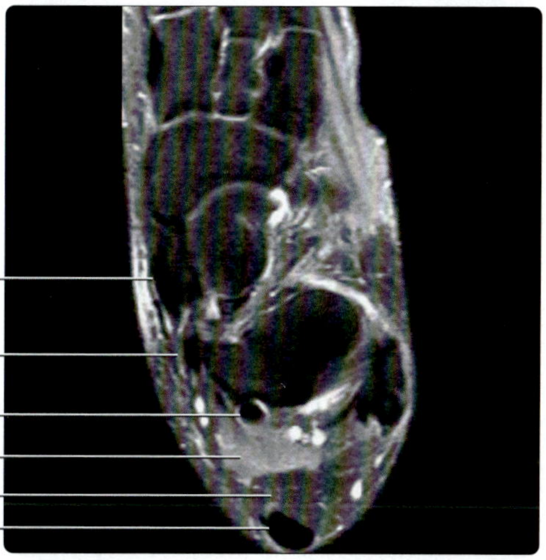

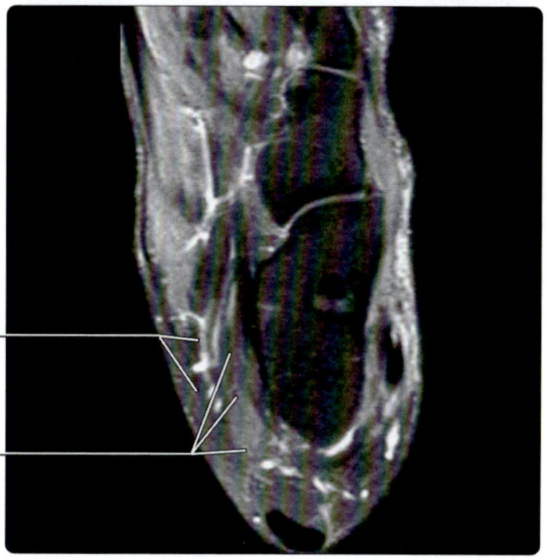

(Top) *Sagittal PD MR demonstrates the flexor hallucis longus muscle and tendon with the muscle fibers extending distally to the level of the tibiotalar joint before becoming entirely tendinous. In addition, there is a structure that has signal intensity of muscle located within the Kager fat pad anterior to the Achilles tendon. In this region, the structure is likely to be an accessory muscle. Axial imaging will prove the origin of this accessory muscle.* **(Middle)** *Long-axis PD FS MR in the same patient shows the expected locations of the tibialis posterior, flexor digitorum, and flexor hallucis longus tendons. In addition, there is a mass located posterior to the flexor hallucis longus tendon that has signal intensity of muscle and encroaches upon Kager fat pad. By location, this muscle is the flexor hallucis longus accessory muscle.* **(Bottom)** *Long-axis PD FS MR located slightly distal to the prior image shows the muscle fibers of the accessory muscle continue medial to the calcaneus. This space-occupying muscle may compress the medial plantar nerve.*

ENLARGED FABELLOFIBULAR LIGAMENT

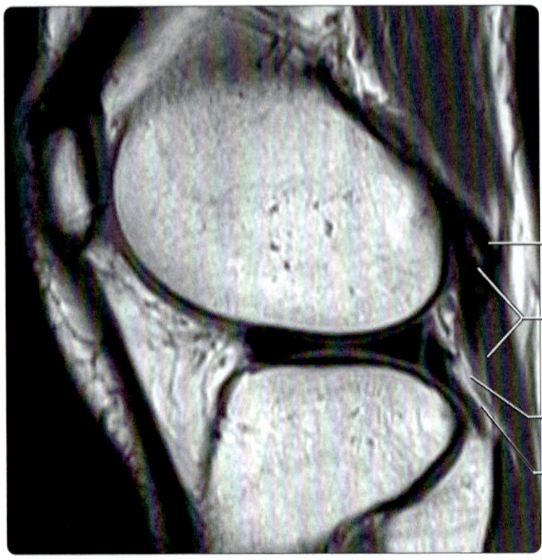

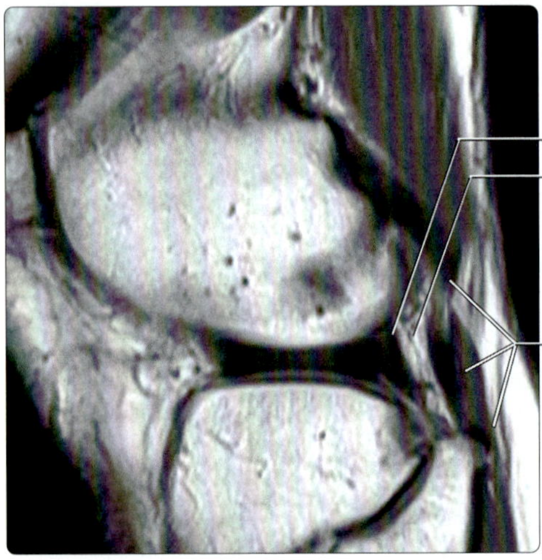

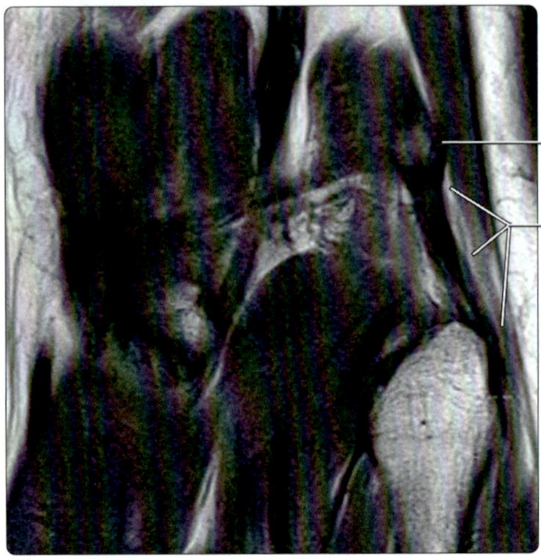

(Top) *Sagittal PD MR shows a fabella with prominent fabellofibular ligament. The size of the fabellofibular and arcuate ligaments tends to be inversely related; if there is no fabella (and therefore no fabellofibular ligament) present, then the arcuate ligament is well seen. In this patient, there is an enlarged fabellofibular ligament, and the arcuate ligament is not visible.* **(Middle)** *A slightly more lateral image shows the enlarged fabellofibular ligament extending to the fibular styloid insertion. The arcuate ligament is extremely thin.* **(Bottom)** *Coronal T1WI MR, far posterior, shows the enlarged fabellofibular ligament extending from the fabella to its insertion on the fibular styloid process.*

MULTIPARTITE PATELLA

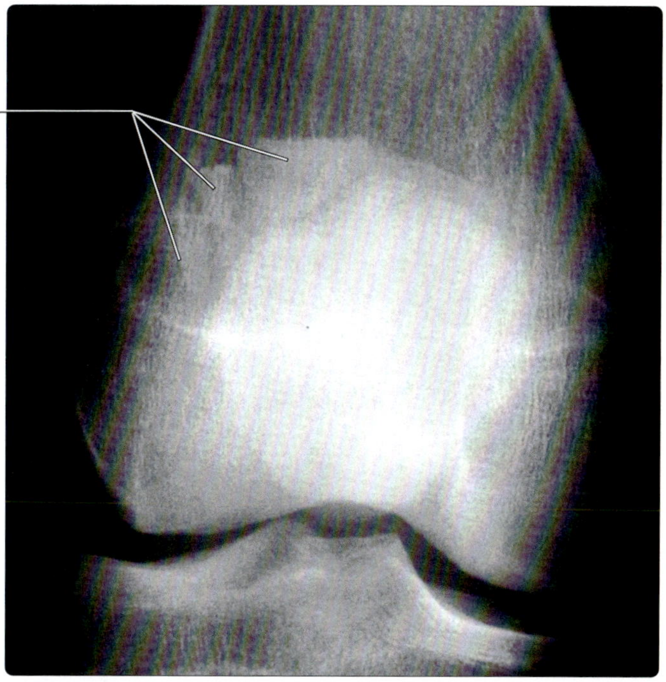

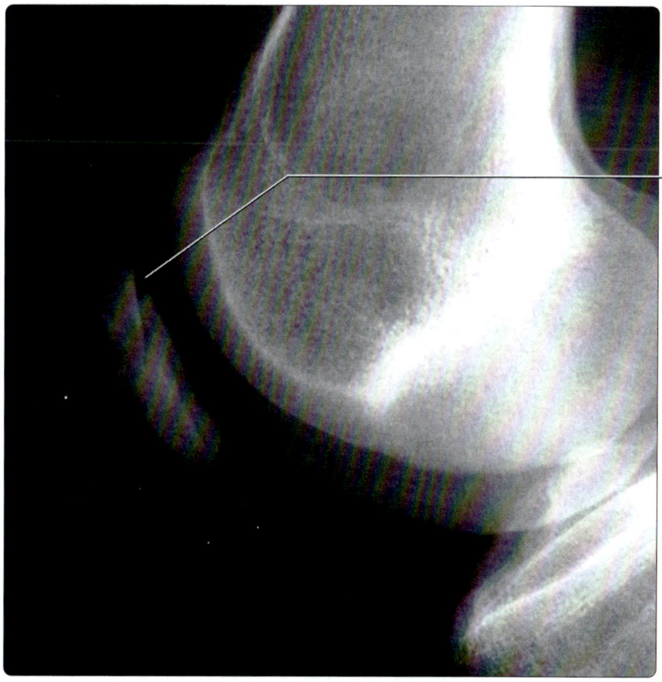

(Top) *The patellar ossification center may be segmented resulting in a bipartite or multipartite structure. The "fragments" may not appear to fit together perfectly (the pieces do not always correspond perfectly with their underlying fossa). The majority of bipartite or multipartite patella have the fragmentation at the superolateral quadrant, as in this case.* **(Bottom)** *The lateral view of this patient demonstrates the common feature of the bipartite fragments not aligning perfectly with the adjacent patellar surfaces. Despite this apparent angulation of ossific structures, the overlying cartilage is intact, and the abnormality is not symptomatic.*

BIPARTITE PATELLA

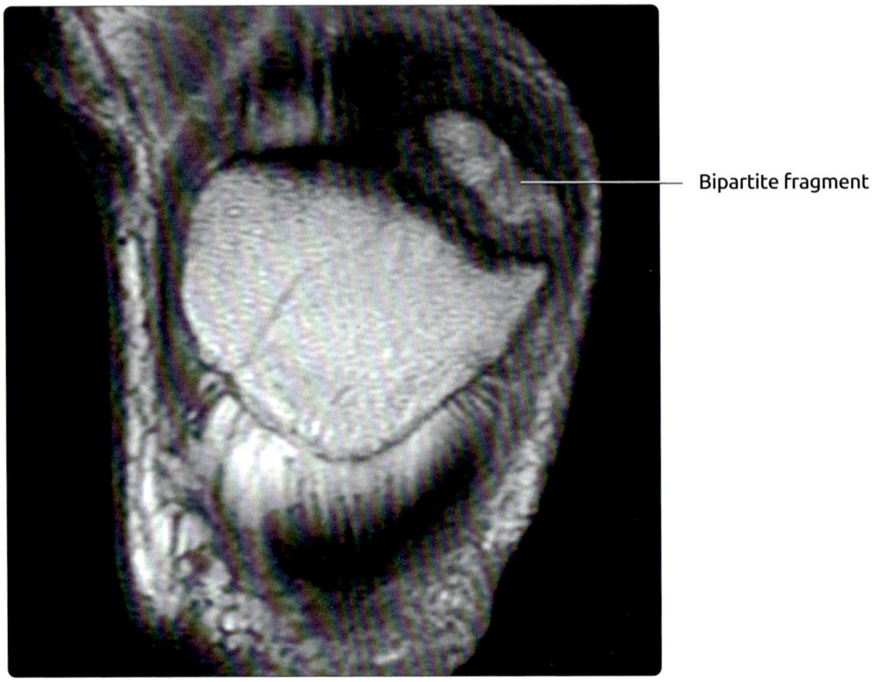

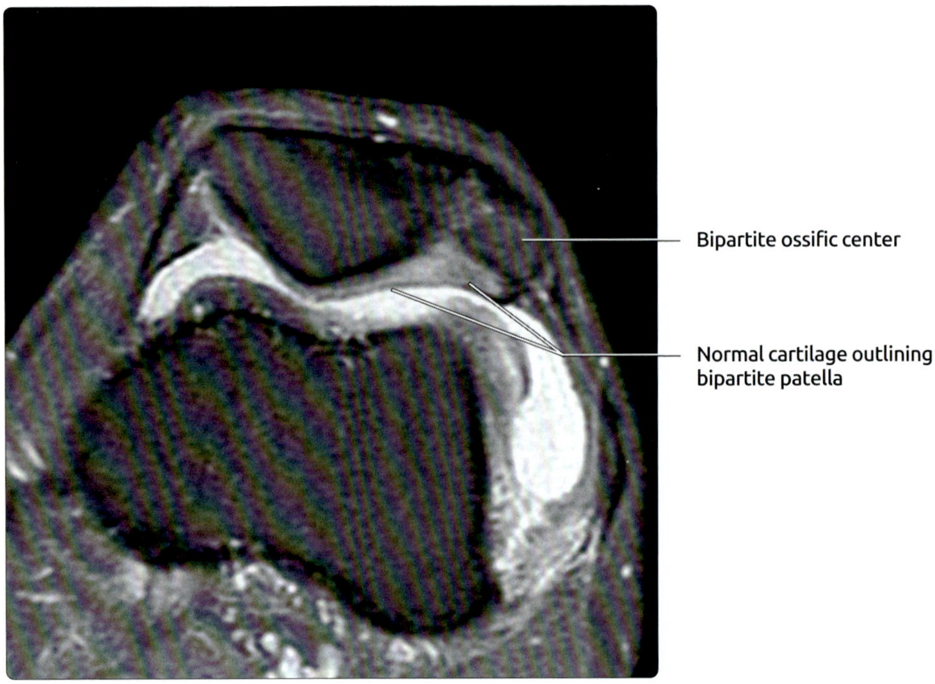

(Top) *Coronal T1WI MR located far anteriorly demonstrates a bipartite patella with the fragment located in the superolateral quadrant. Note the rounded edges of both the fragment and adjacent patella. Additionally, there is no edema present. Both of these findings negate the possibility that this is a fracture.* **(Bottom)** *Axial T2WI FS MR through the superior portion of the patella shows the bipartite ossific center adjacent to the remainder of the patella. The small effusion nicely outlines the patellar cartilage. Note that the cartilage is smooth and completely covers the osseous "defect." Normal cartilage coverage of a bipartite or multipartite patella is standard. (Courtesy A. Sonin, MD.)*

DORSAL DEFECT OF PATELLA

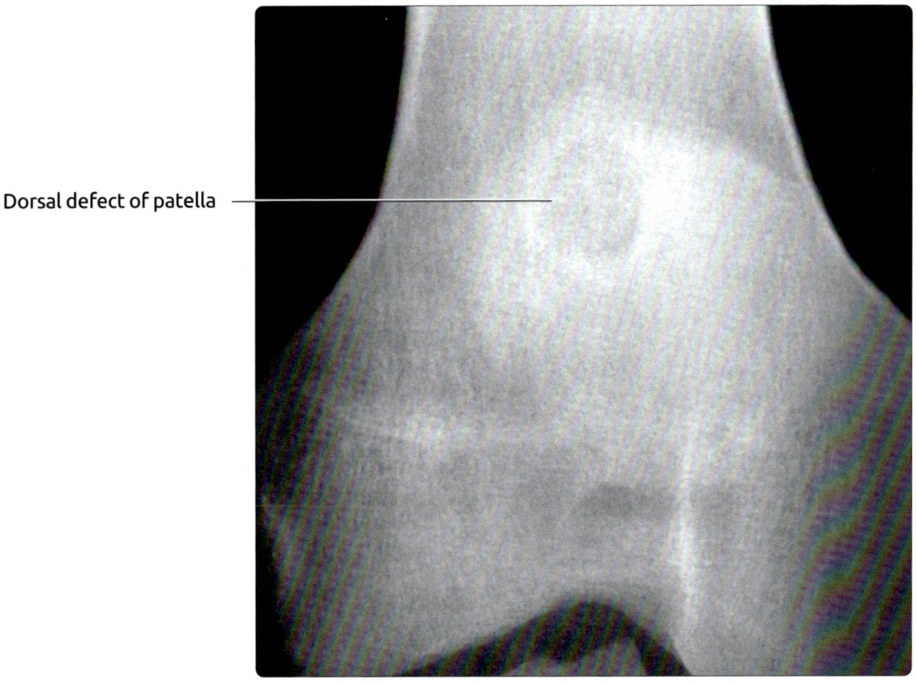

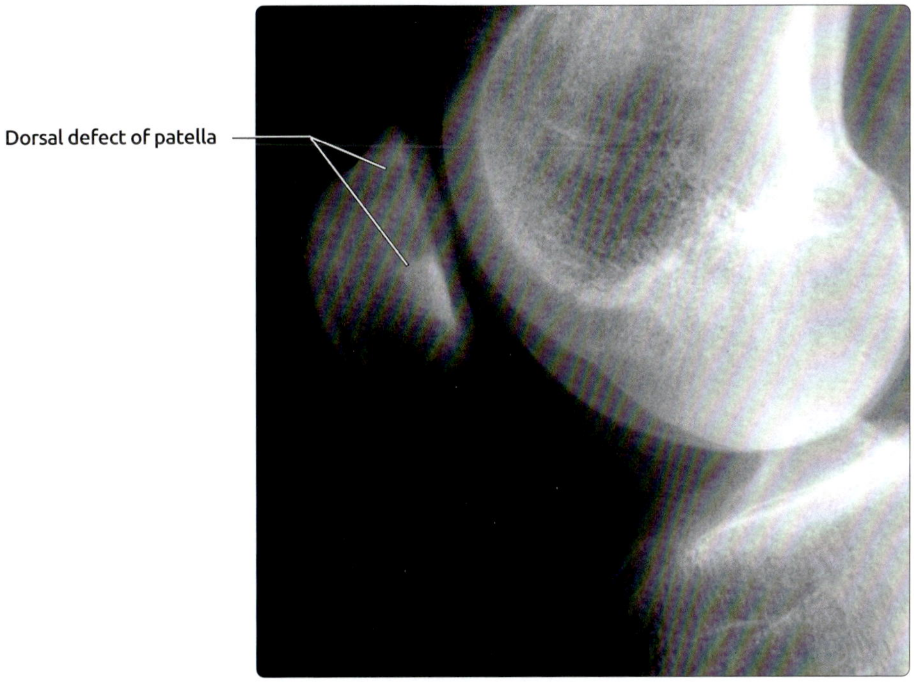

(Top) *Dorsal defect of the patella is considered a normal variant. It is well defined with a sclerotic border. It is usually located within the superolateral quadrant of the patella.* **(Bottom)** *The defect appears less distinct on this lateral view, but the appearance overall is classic for the diagnosis. If a MR was performed, it would show the cartilage to be normal overlying the osseous abnormality. It is important that the abnormality be distinguished from an osteochondral injury.*

DORSAL DEFECT OF PATELLA

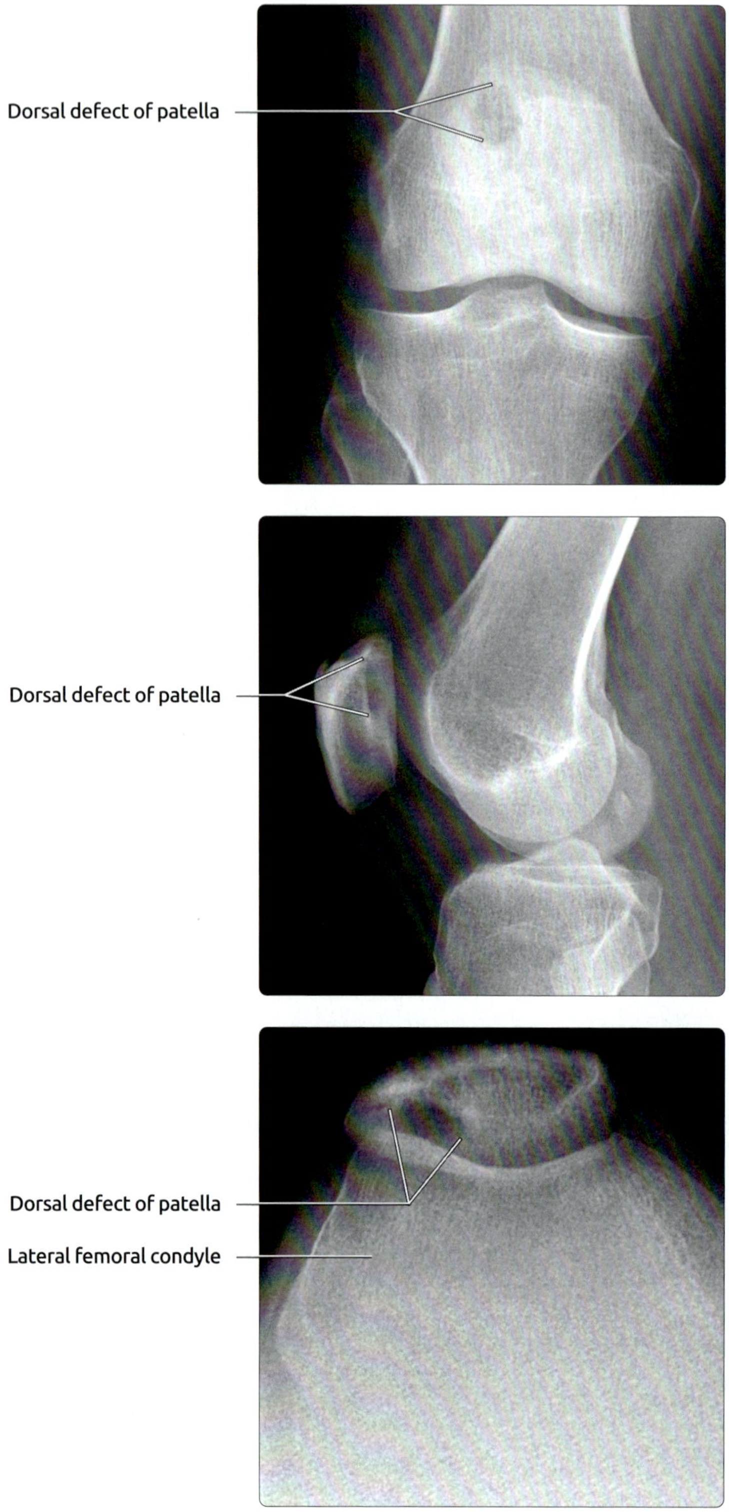

(Top) *AP radiograph shows a rounded lucency superimposed over the upper outer aspect of the patella.* **(Middle)** *Lateral radiograph confirms that the rounded lucency is within the upper aspect of the patella. No other abnormality is seen.* **(Bottom)** *Axial radiograph in the same patient shows the smooth, rounded lucency at the upper outer quadrant of the patella. This is the typical appearance and location of dorsal defect of the patella.*

DORSAL DEFECT OF PATELLA

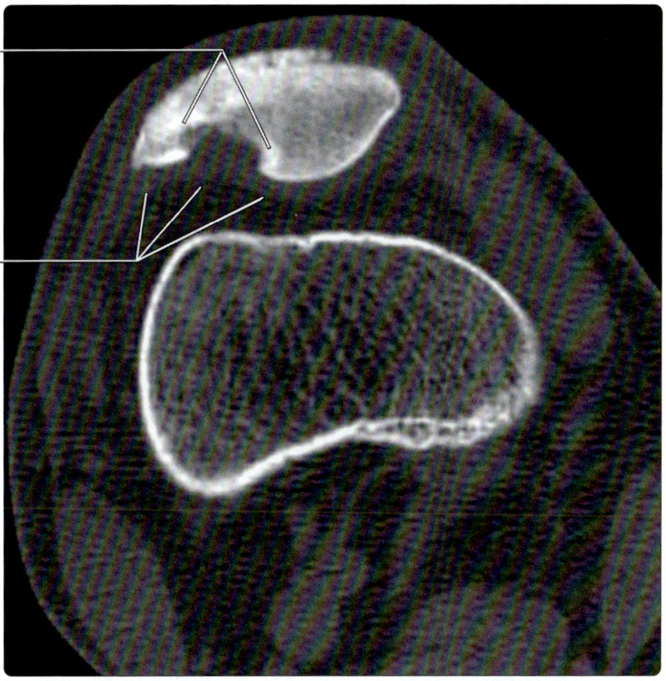

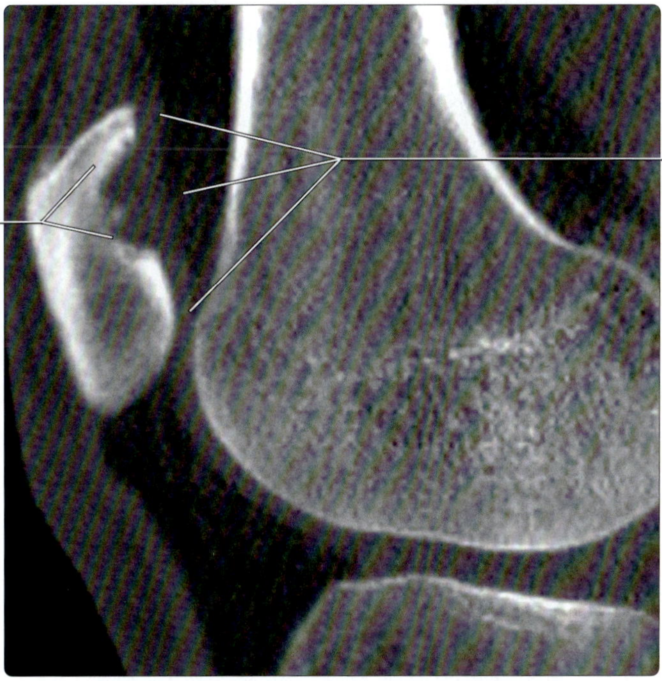

(Top) *Axial CT in the same patient shows the large dorsal defect of the patella. Note the cartilage overlying the defect is completely normal. Given the smooth defect, typical location, and normal overlying cartilage, the diagnosis of dorsal defect is definitive. No further work-up or treatment is needed.* **(Bottom)** *Sagittal CT reconstruction again shows normal cartilage overlying the dorsal defect.*

DEVELOPMENTAL VARIATION LATERAL FEMORAL CONDYLE

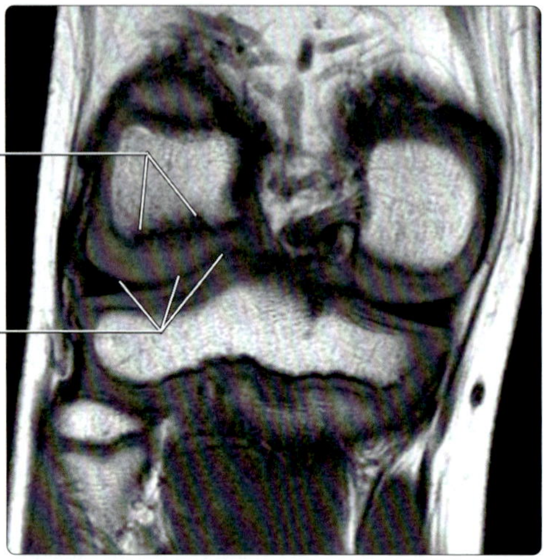

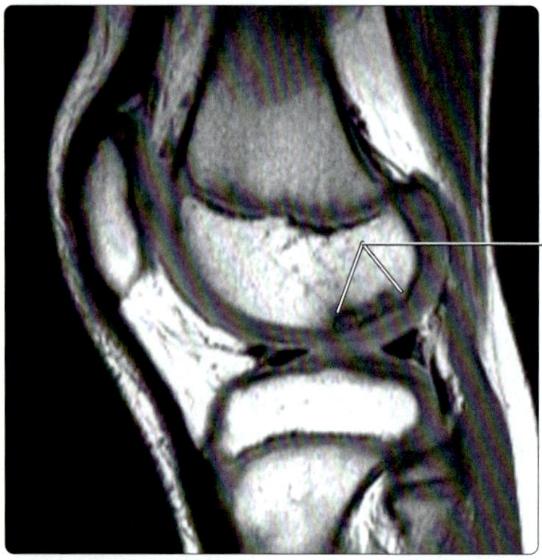

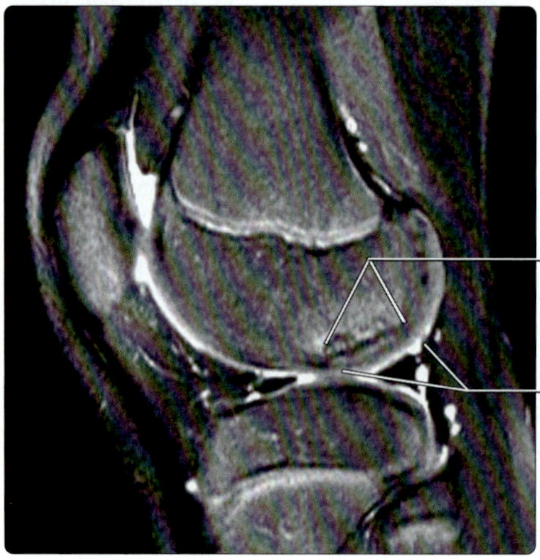

(Top) *Coronal T1WI MR in the posterior aspect of the joint demonstrates irregularity of the lateral femoral condyle in a 9-year-old girl. The overlying cartilage is thick and normal. The location in the posterior 1/3 of the condyle, without extension to the intercondylar notch, helps to differentiate this normal variant from an osteochondral defect.* **(Middle)** *Sagittal T1WI MR in the same patient confirms the irregularity is located in the posterior 1/3 of the femoral condyle.* **(Bottom)** *Sagittal T2WI FS MR in the same patient shows slight hyperintensity at the femoral condylar defect with normal overlying cartilage. This is considered normal in this developmental variant, and the patient was given instructions to continue normal activity.*

DEVELOPMENTAL VARIATION LATERAL FEMORAL CONDYLE

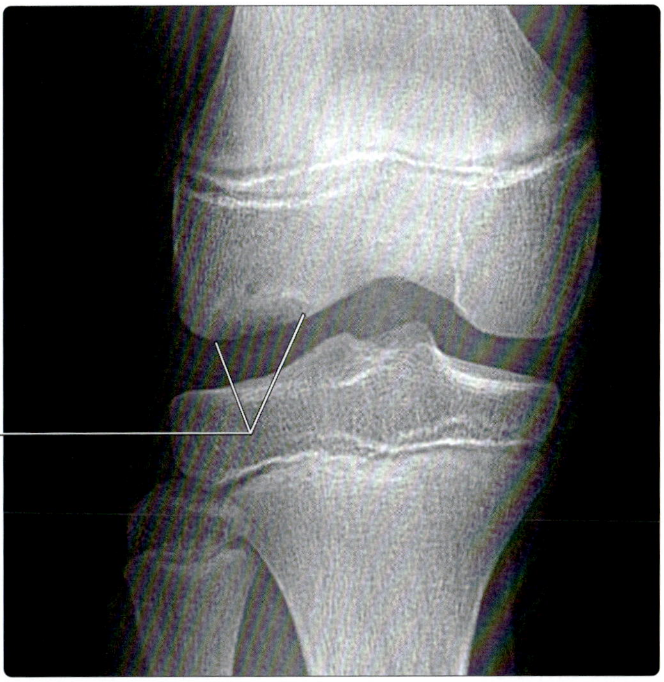

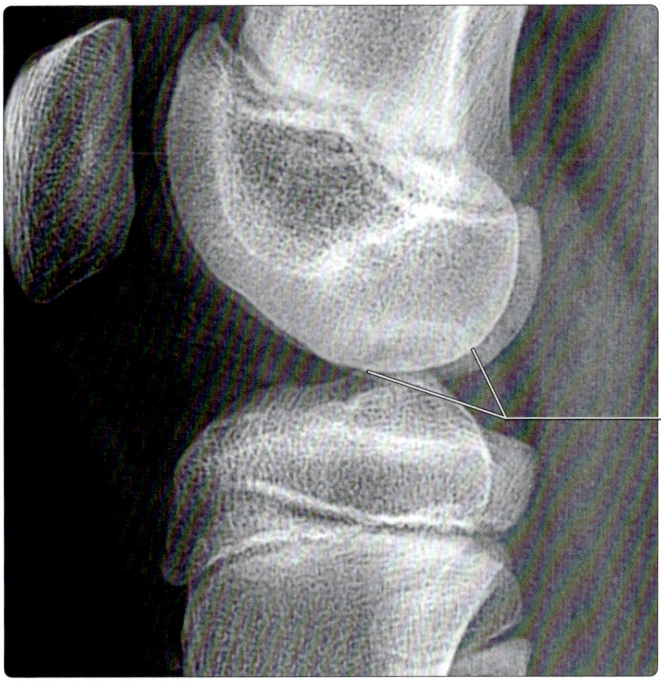

(Top) *AP radiograph obtained 1 year later of the same patient shows apparent "healing in" or normal growth at the site of femoral condylar irregularity.* **(Bottom)** *Lateral radiograph confirms that the developmental irregularity is forming normal bone and that there is no collapse at the site. Remember that the location of the abnormality is restricted to the posterior portion of the condyle and does not extend to the intercondylar notch. The lack of significant marrow edema can help differentiate this normal developmental variant from an osteochondral lesion. Treatment of the 2 is significantly different.*

DEVELOPMENTAL VARIATION LATERAL FEMORAL CONDYLE

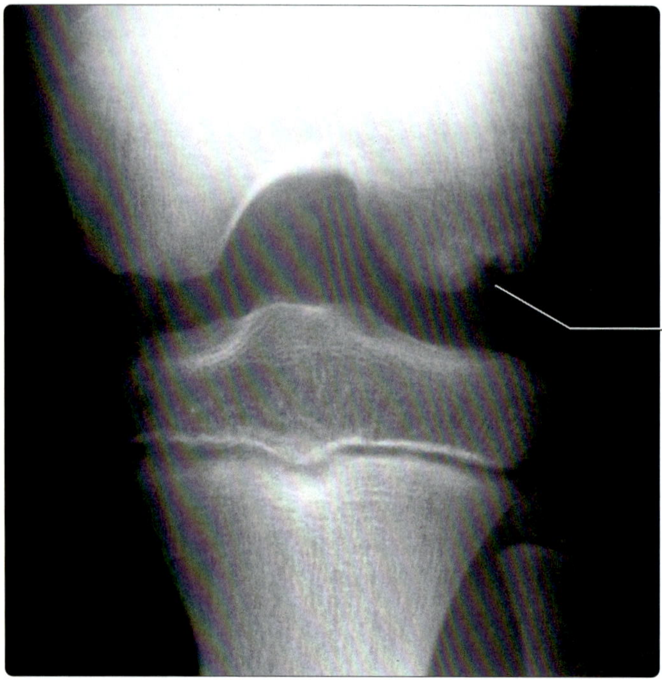

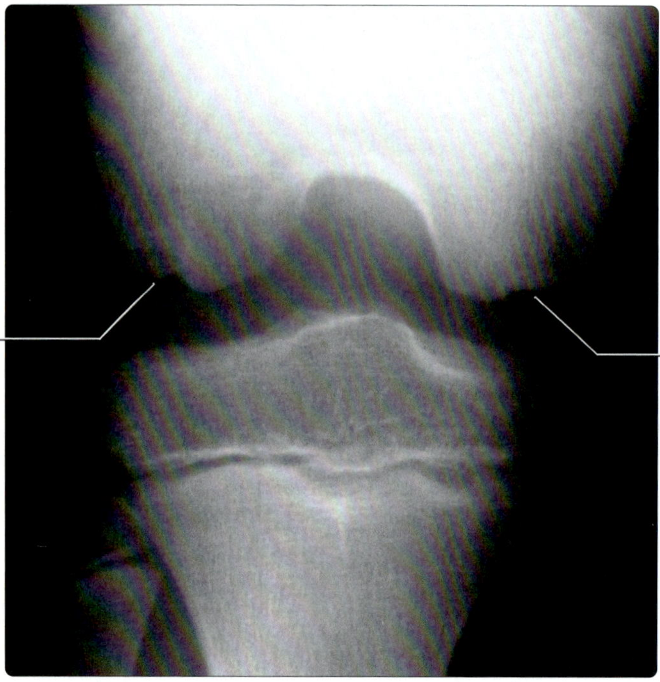

(Top) *This is a notch view of the same patient. Because the notch position brings the posterior portion of the femoral condyle into profile, the cortical irregularity is seen much more distinctly than on either AP or lateral views.* **(Bottom)** *Notch view of the contralateral knee in the same patient shows posterior cortical irregularity on both the medial and lateral femoral condyles. As in this case, the findings may be bilateral, though not necessarily symmetric. The involvement of the lateral femoral condyle is far more common than the medial. This appearance and location is typical in adolescents and must not be mistaken for an osteochondral defect or injury. The overlying cartilage is normal.*

DEVELOPMENTAL VARIATION LATERAL FEMORAL CONDYLE

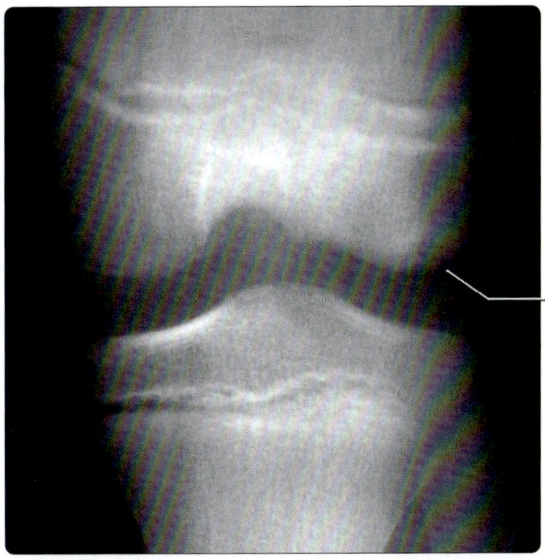

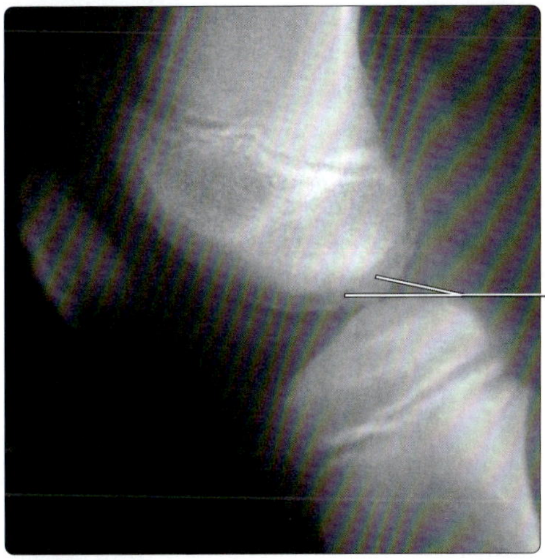

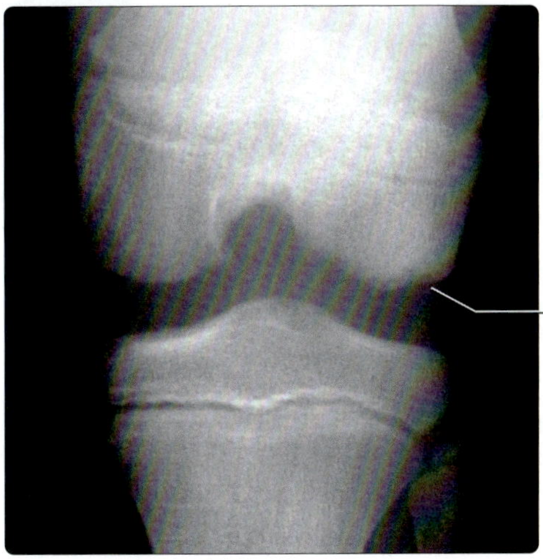

(Top) *AP view shows a mild lateral femoral condylar irregularity in an adolescent patient.* **(Middle)** *Lateral view confirms the location of the irregularity as being typical for the normal variant.* **(Bottom)** *Notch view of the same patient shows the abnormality more clearly and confirms its posterior location. The radiographs are sufficient to make the diagnosis of normal variant. No further imaging should be required, and since it does not represent an osteochondral injury, no treatment need be instituted.*

DEVELOPMENTAL VARIATION LATERAL FEMORAL CONDYLE

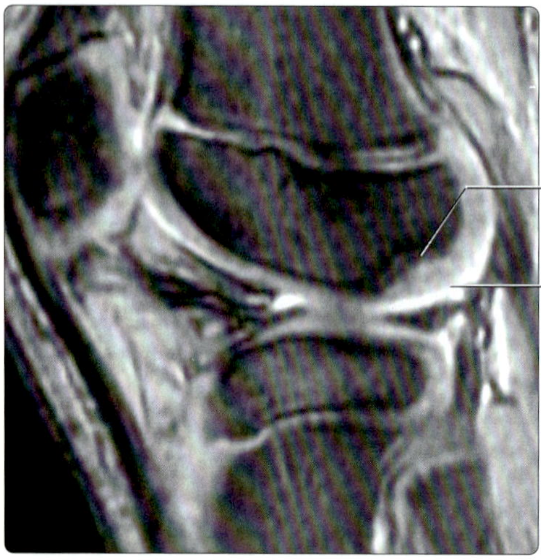

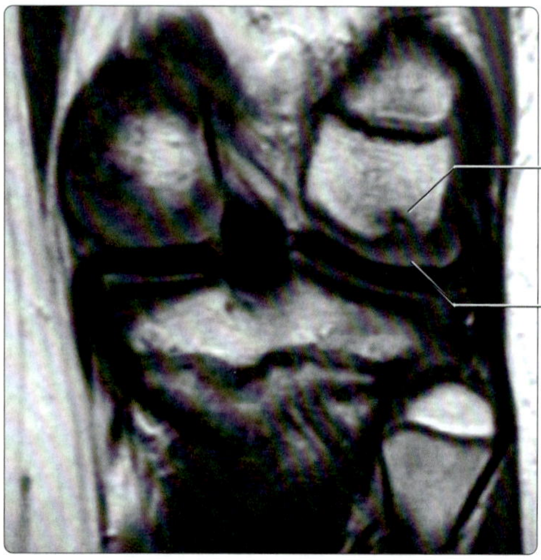

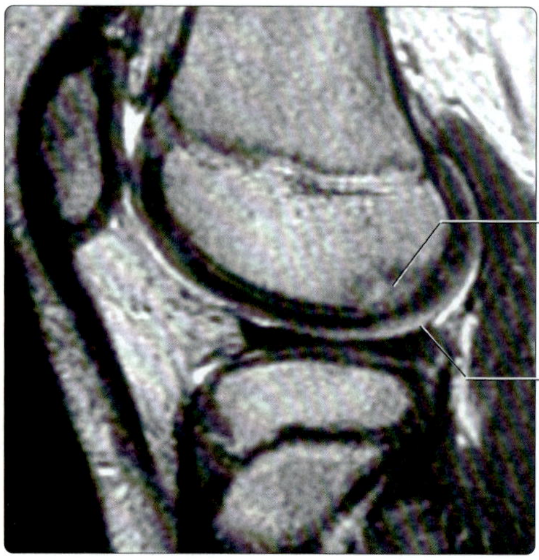

(Top) *Sagittal gradient-echo MR in the same patient shows the osseous defect in the posterior lateral femoral condyle. The overlying cartilage is seen to be normal in thickness and contour, confirming that this is a variant rather than a true osteochondral injury.* **(Middle)** *Coronal PD MR located posteriorly in the joint shows both the femoral condylar defect and the normal overlying cartilage.* **(Bottom)** *Sagittal T2WI MR in the same patient shows both the osseous defect in the typical posterior lateral femoral condylar region and the normal overlying cartilage. There is no marrow edema and no other abnormality. The defect is a normal variant that is seen in adolescents (note the open physes), which routinely ossifies normally. It is not in the usual location to suggest an osteochondral defect.*

POSTEROMEDIAL CORTICAL DEFECT

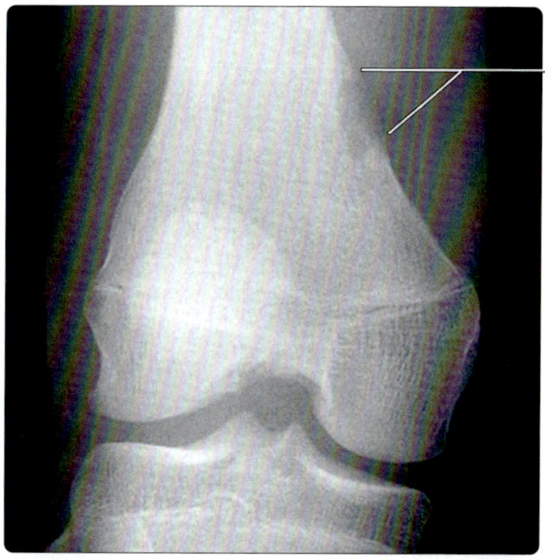

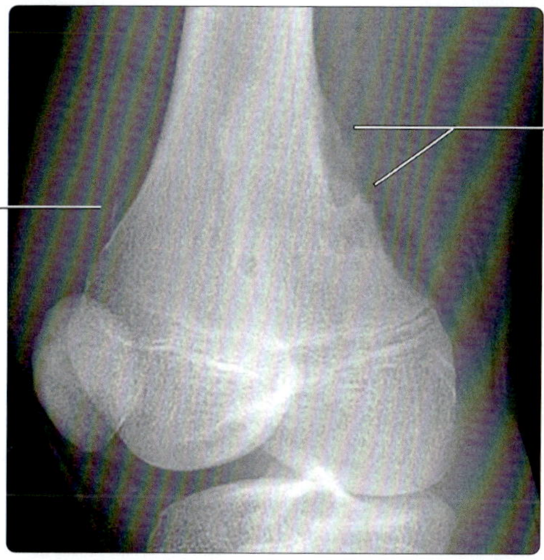

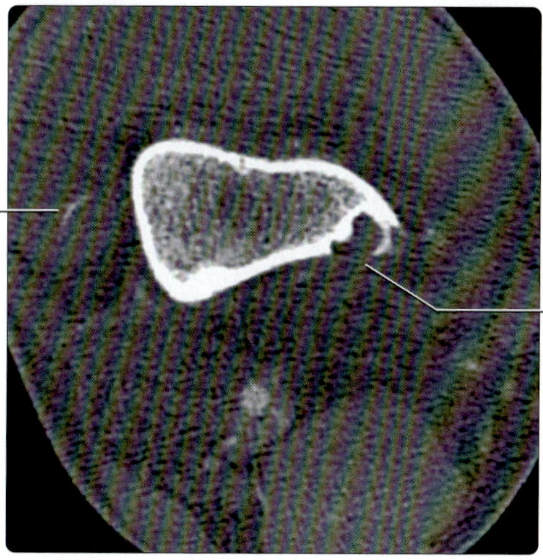

(Top) *This defect seen on the AP radiograph in the posteromedial distal femoral metaphysis has variably been termed "cortical desmoid," "avulsive or tug lesion," or simply a "cortical defect." These authors prefer the latter term. It is site specific at the posteromedial corner and is anatomically related to the adductor magnus aponeurotic insertion. It is debated as to whether it represents a chronic avulsive injury or is a normal growth phenomenon.* **(Middle)** *External oblique view profiles the cortical defect. Note that the defect may not have overlying cortex; it may sometimes even appear slightly spiculated. Despite that appearance, it is judged by location to be a normal variant rather than something more aggressive. This patient also has a large effusion and chip fracture, unrelated to the defect.* **(Bottom)** *CT confirms location and appearance of posteromedial cortical defect.*

POSTEROMEDIAL CORTICAL DEFECT

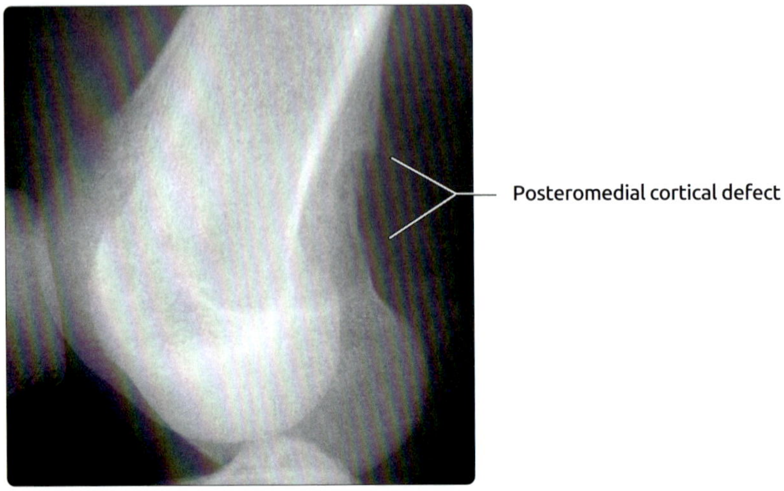

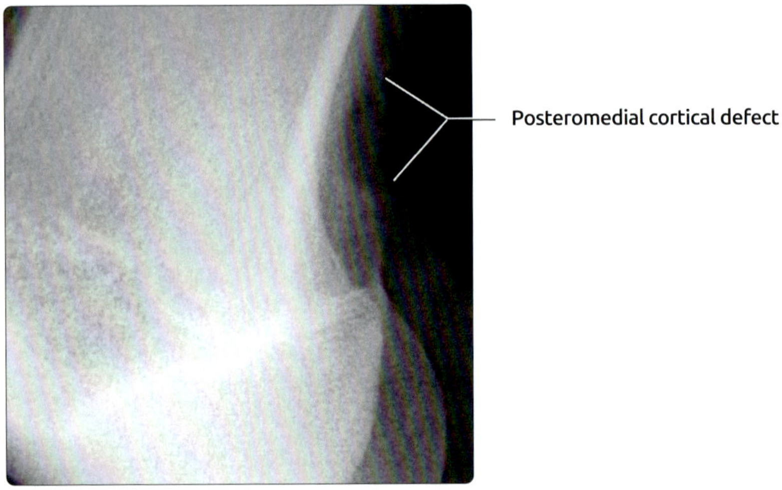

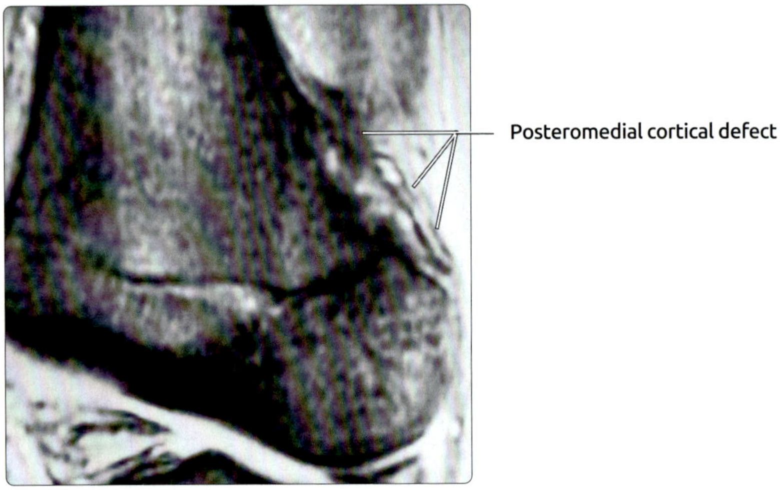

(Top) *Slightly obliqued lateral radiograph shows a posteromedial cortical defect with typically slightly aggressive appearance of scalloping and indistinct cortex.* **(Middle)** *Lateral radiograph shows another posteromedial cortical defect.* **(Bottom)** *Radial gradient-echo MR profiles the posteromedial distal femoral cortical defect. Note how indistinct the cortex and scalloped margin are and the suggestion of soft tissue mass. This is typical of the normal variant cortical defect. As long as the location corresponds to the posteromedial distal femoral metaphysis and appearance shows nothing more aggressive, this can be considered a normal variant.*

FOCAL PERIPHYSEAL EDEMA (FOPE) ZONE

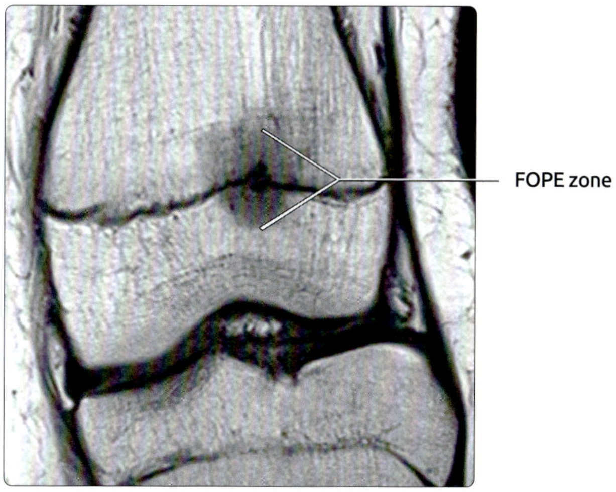

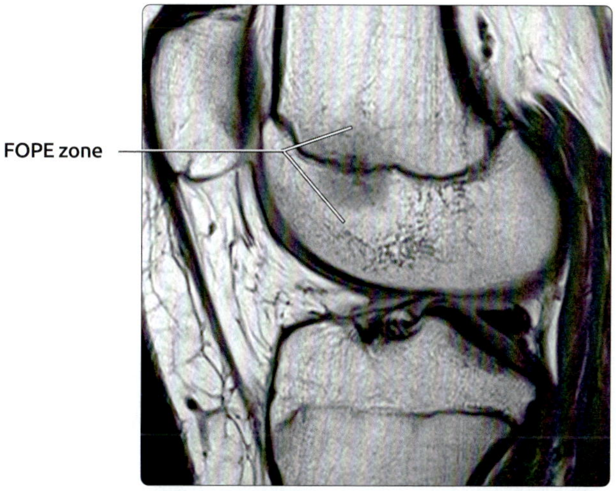

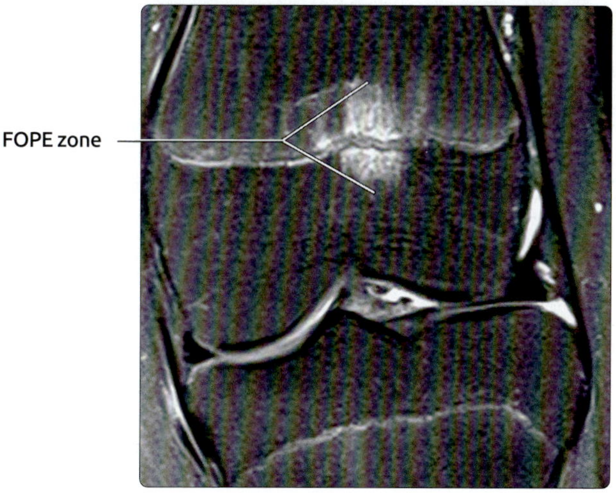

(Top) *Coronal T1WI MR in a skeletally immature patient demonstrates low signal surrounding a central portion of the femoral physis. The entire physis is open and shows no other abnormality.* **(Middle)** *Sagittal PD MR in the same patient confirms that the region of abnormal signal is periphyseal and central. No other abnormality is seen.* **(Bottom)** *Coronal PD FS MR shows edema within the bone surrounding the central physis. This edema is felt to relate to the early stages of physiologic physeal closure. It may be associated with pain, particularly when no other MR abnormalities are present. When the characteristic appearance of a FOPE zone is observed, as in this case, the patient requires no invasive diagnostic procedure and does not need imaging follow-up.*

MENISCOCRUCIATE LIGAMENT ARISING FROM TRANSVERSE LIGAMENT

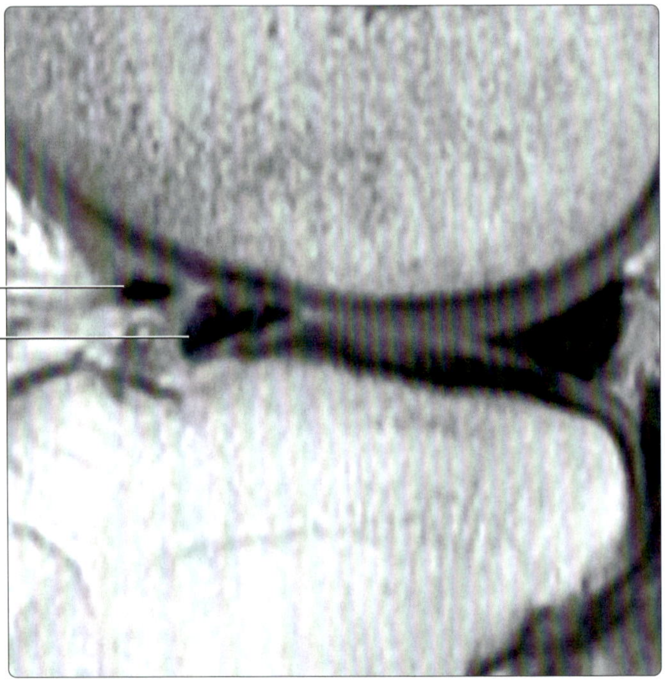

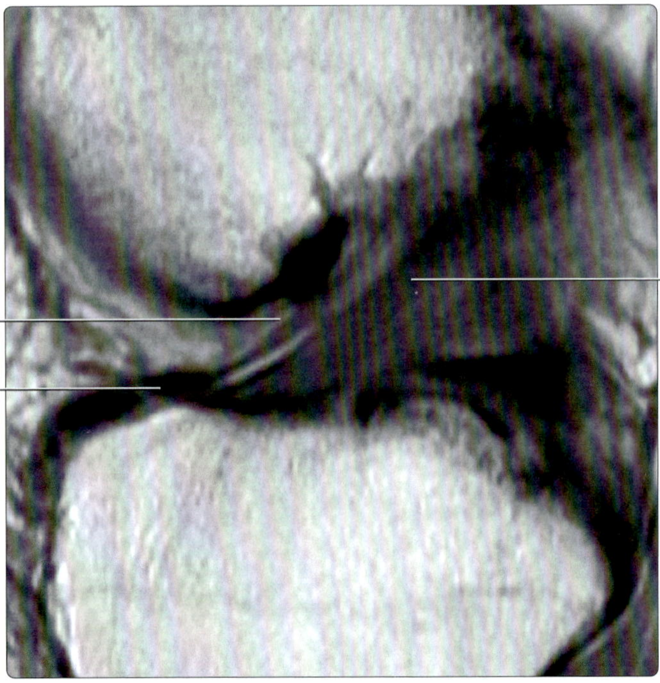

(Top) *Sagittal PD MR near the intercondylar notch, lateral to medial, shows a large transverse ligament. This ligament connects the 2 anterior meniscal horns and is seen in cross section on sagittal images. It could possibly be confused for a meniscal tear as it merges with the lateral meniscus closer to the notch. The ligament is generally smaller than this or may be absent.* **(Bottom)** *Image through the lateral portion of the intercondylar notch shows a discrete structure that parallels the anterior cruciate ligament and extends from the junction of the transverse ligament and root of the anterior horn of the lateral meniscus to the lateral femoral condyle. This represents the normal variant, anterior lateral meniscocruciate ligament. It is distinguished from infrapatellar plica (which can also parallel the anterior cruciate ligament in the same manner) by its site of origin at the meniscus rather than the patella.*

MENISCOCRUCIATE LIGAMENT ARISING FROM TRANSVERSE LIGAMENT

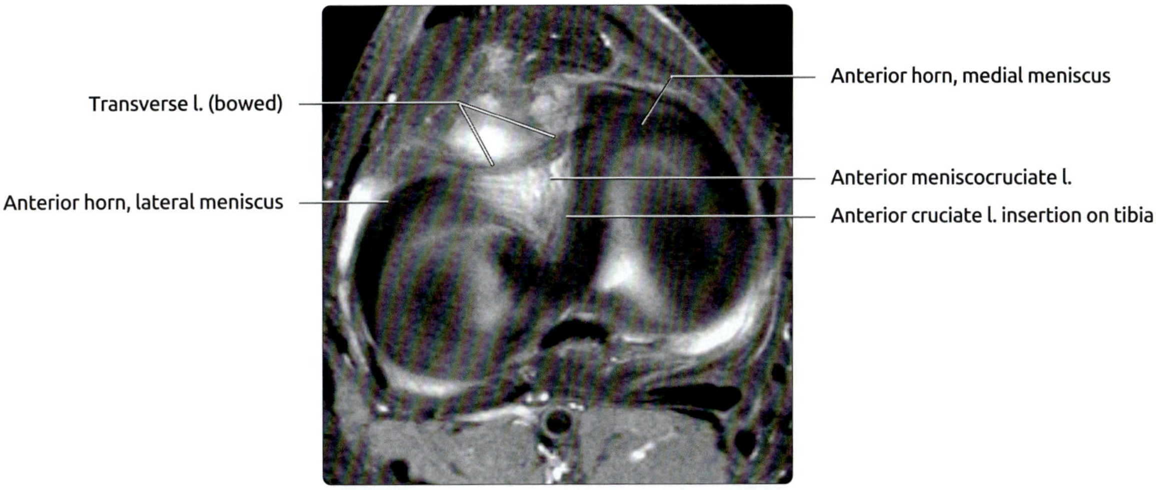

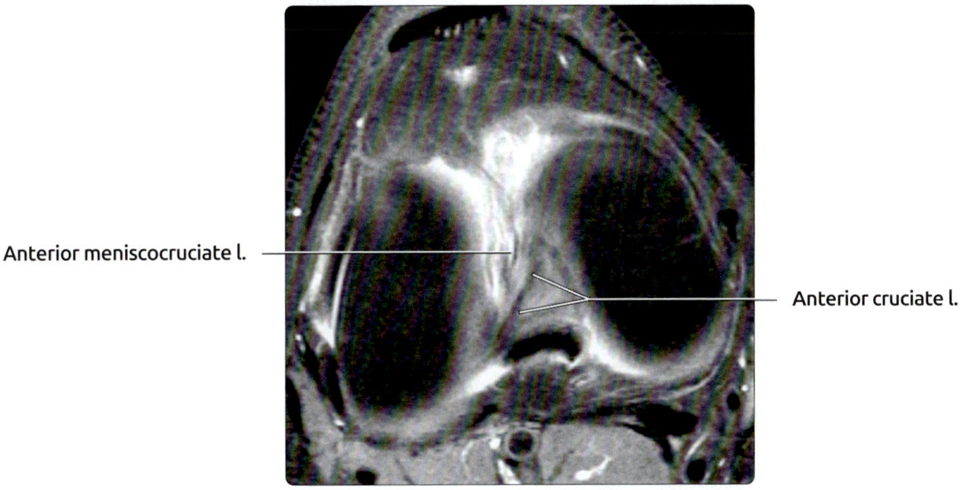

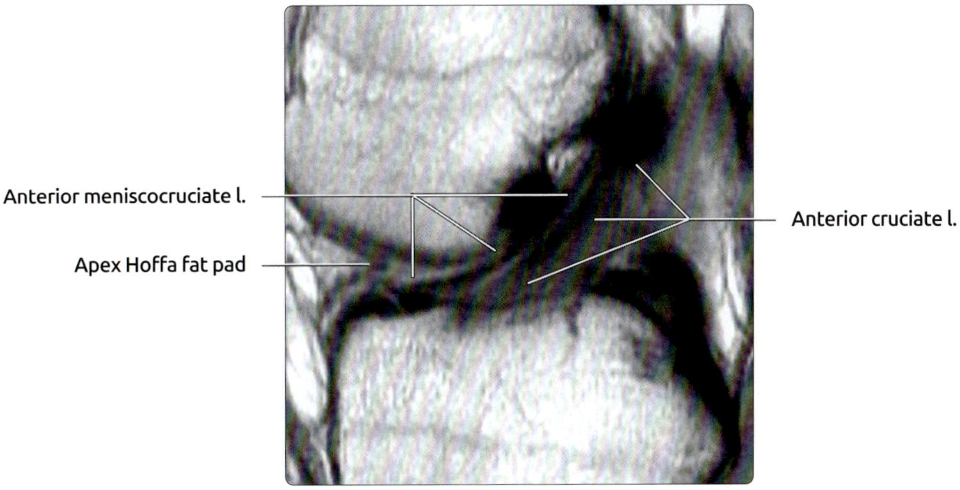

(Top) *Axial PD FS MR at the level of the joint line shows a slightly tethered transverse ligament with an anterior meniscocruciate ligament arising from it. Note that the ligament is anterior to the anterior cruciate ligament.* **(Middle)** *Axial PD FS MR, slightly higher in the intercondylar notch, shows that the anterior meniscocruciate ligament parallels the anterior cruciate ligament throughout the notch.* **(Bottom)** *Sagittal PD MR shows the length of the anterior meniscocruciate ligament paralleling the anterior cruciate ligament. This normal variant should not be mistaken for an intrasubstance tear of the anterior cruciate. Note that the apex of Hoffa fat pad is free of this ligament (not attached as in an infrapatellar plica).*

MENISCOCRUCIATE LIGAMENT

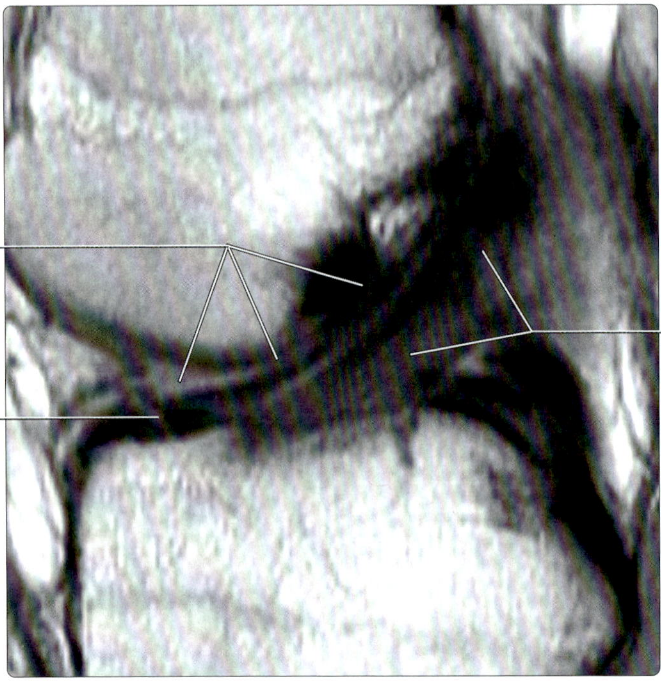

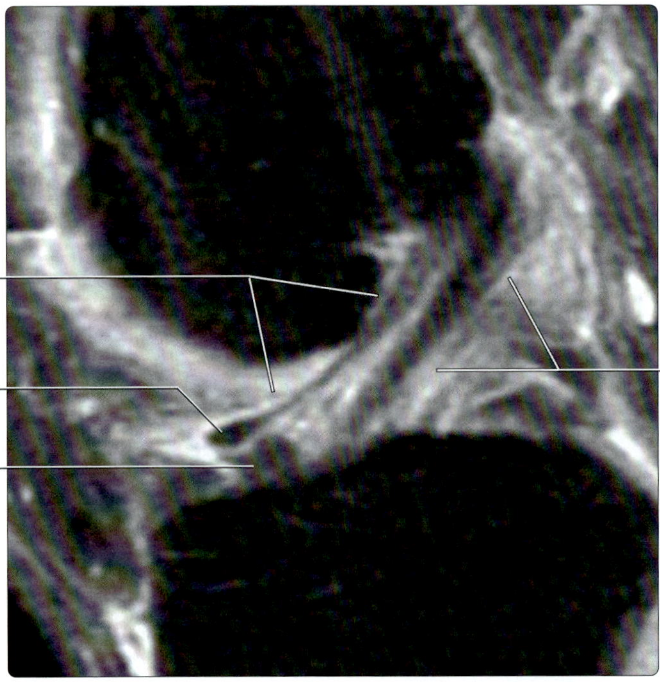

(Top) *Sagittal PD MR through the intercondylar notch shows a meniscocruciate ligament. The ligament arises from the anterior horn of the medial meniscus and extends along the anterior surface of the anterior cruciate ligament to the femoral condyle. It could possibly be mistaken for a longitudinal tear in the anterior cruciate.* **(Bottom)** *Sagittal PD FS MR shows another variant meniscocruciate ligament. This ligament is arising from the transverse ligament; as it extends parallel to and anterior to the anterior cruciate ligament, it could simulate a longitudinal or partial tear in this cruciate.*

LATERAL MENISCAL FASCICLES

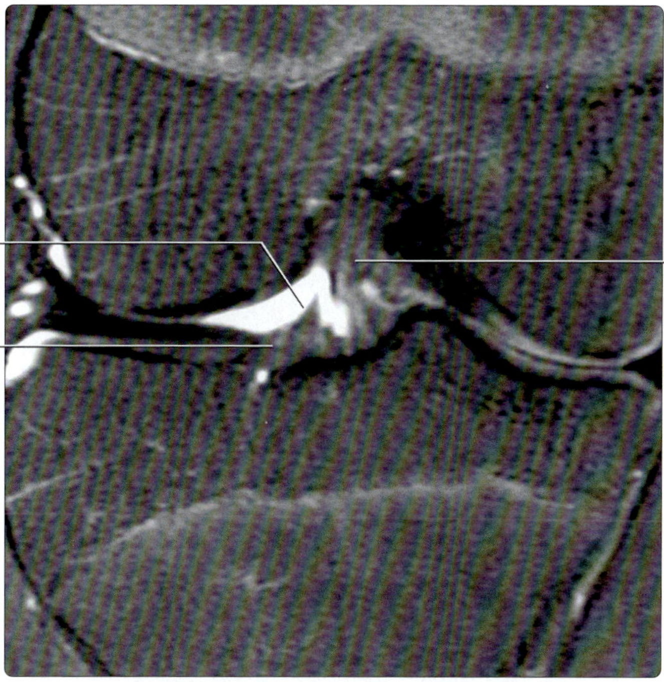

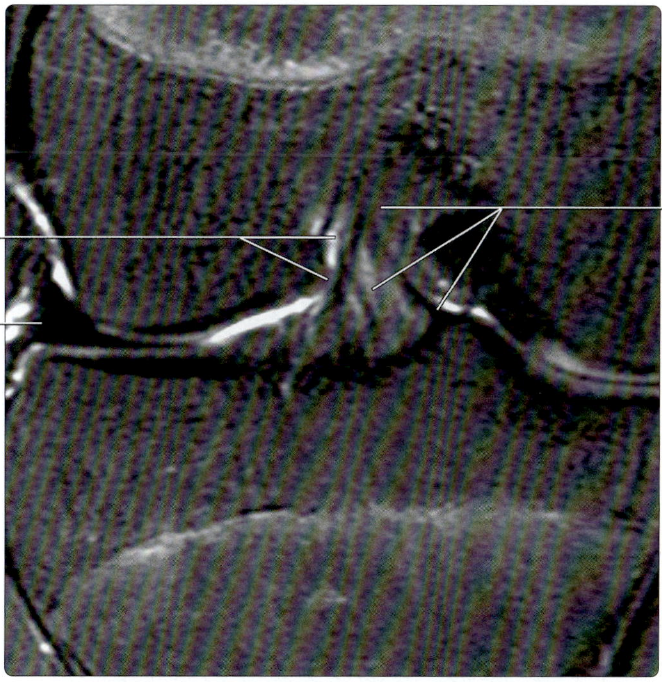

(Top) *Coronal PD FS MR in the anterior portion of the joint shows a patient with an absent transverse ligament (more anterior cut not shown). The fibers of the anterior horn of the lateral meniscus, which normally blend into the transverse ligament, form discrete lateral meniscal fascicles, which ascend toward the anterior cruciate ligament.* **(Bottom)** *Coronal image, slightly posterior, shows the lateral meniscal fascicles ascending to intersect the anterior cruciate ligament. These fibers clearly are not part of the anterior cruciate ligament since they ascend at a different angle. This normal variant should not be mistaken for pathology, such as a disrupted anterior cruciate ligament or a meniscal fragment from a bucket handle tear.*

MENISCOCRUCIATE LIGAMENT MIMICKING MENISCAL TEAR

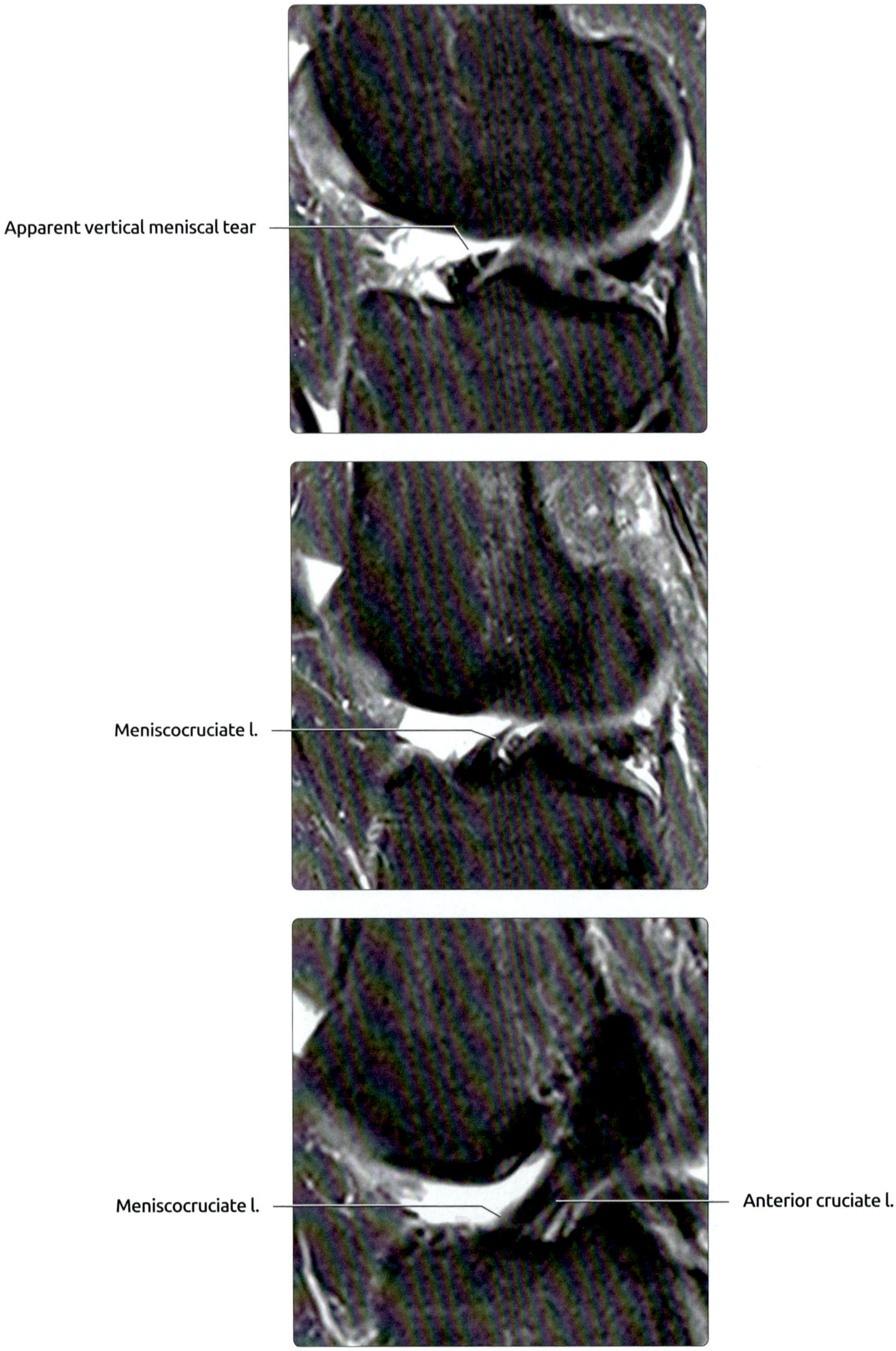

(Top) *Adjacent sagittal PD FS MR, beginning just lateral to the intercondylar notch, shows an apparent vertical tear in the anterior horn of the lateral meniscus.* **(Middle)** *Adjacent sagittal PD FS MR shows that the apparent meniscal fragment in fact is continuous with a ligamentous structure extending in the direction of the anterior cruciate ligament.* **(Bottom)** *Adjacent sagittal PD FS MR, at the level of the intercondylar notch, shows the ligamentous structure to blend into the anterior cruciate ligament. Since the abnormal structure extends from the meniscus to the cruciate ligament, it represents a normal variant meniscocruciate ligament. These may mimic partial cruciate ligament tears or, as in this case, a vertical peripheral meniscal tear.*

MENISCOCRUCIATE LIGAMENT MIMICKING PARTIAL ACL TEAR

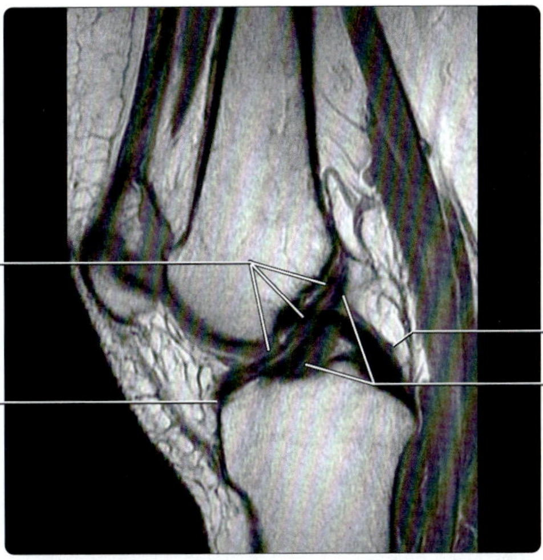

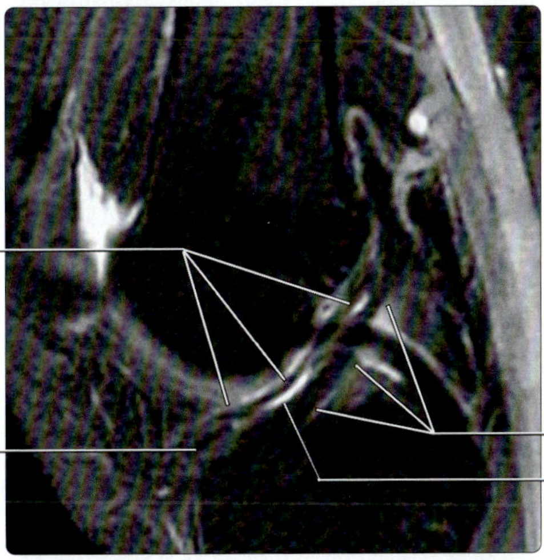

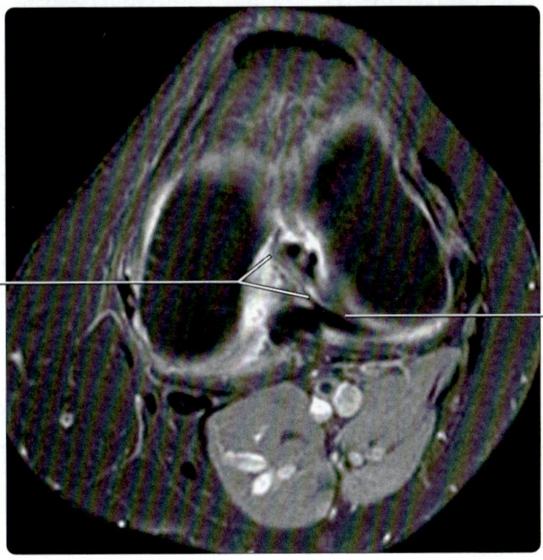

(Top) *Sagittal PD MR demonstrates a low-signal curvilinear structure extending from the anterior horn of the medial meniscus along and immediately anterior to the medial fibers of the anterior cruciate ligament. This is a meniscofemoral ligament seen in its full extent. These normal variants may mimic partial cruciate ligament tears.* **(Middle)** *Sagittal T2WI FS MR in the same patient and same level demonstrates synovial fluid between the meniscocruciate ligament and the anterior cruciate ligament. Since the anterior cruciate ligament is an extrasynovial structure, a tear should not be bathed in synovial fluid. Therefore, the presence of fluid between the 2 structures helps solidify the diagnosis of normal variant meniscocruciate ligament.* **(Bottom)** *Axial PD FS MR in the same patient demonstrates the intercondylar notch course of the meniscocruciate ligament traveling along the course of, and eventually blending in with, proximal fibers of the anterior cruciate ligament.*

OBLIQUE MENISCOMENISCAL LIGAMENT

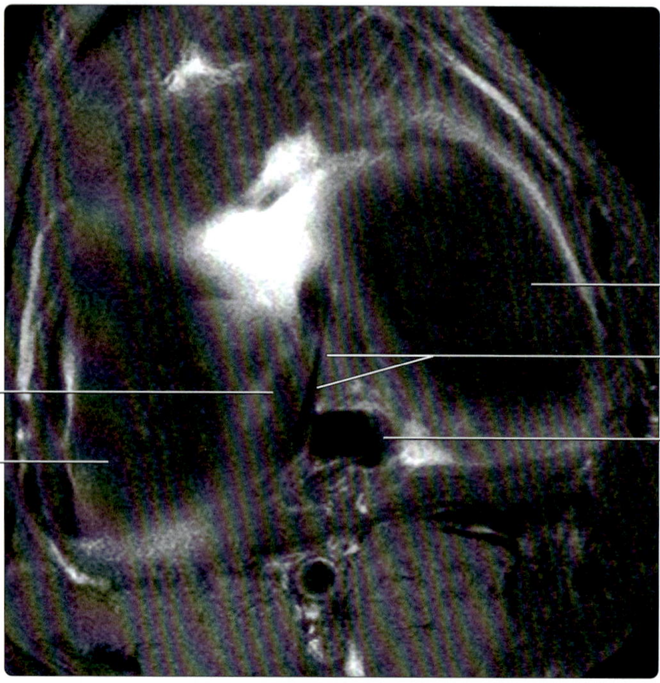

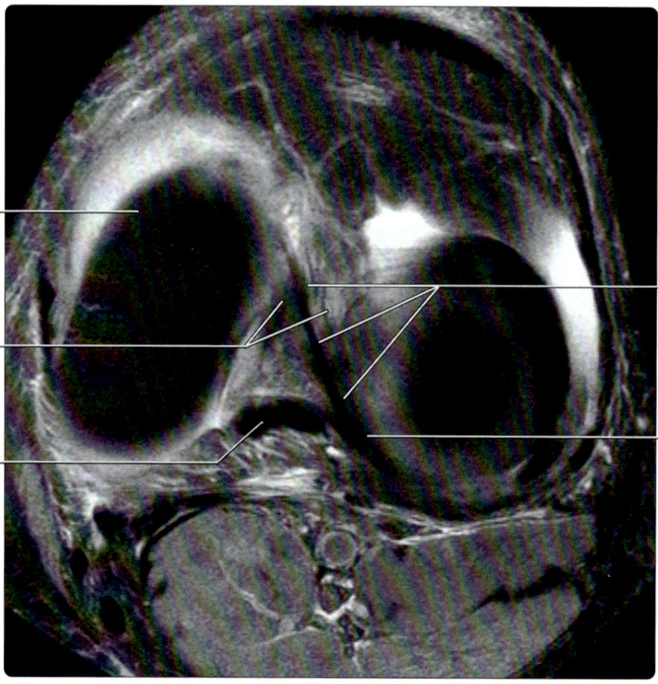

(Top) *Single axial image, just above the joint line, shows the normal variant medial oblique meniscomeniscal ligament. It arises from the anterior horn of the medial meniscus and inserts on the posterior horn of the lateral meniscus, threading its way between the anterior cruciate ligament and posterior cruciate ligament.* **(Bottom)** *Axial PD FS MR through the joint line shows a normal variant, the medial oblique meniscomeniscal ligament. The ligament extends from the anterior horn of the medial meniscus across the intercondylar notch to insert on the posterior horn of the lateral meniscus. At this level of the menisci, the variant ligament appears to split the anterior cruciate ligament at its insertion on the tibia. It normally extends between the anterior cruciate ligament and the posterior cruciate ligament. The mirror image variant, lateral meniscomeniscal ligament, extends from the anterior horn of the lateral meniscus to the posterior horn of the medial meniscus (not shown here).*

OBLIQUE MENISCOMENISCAL LIGAMENT

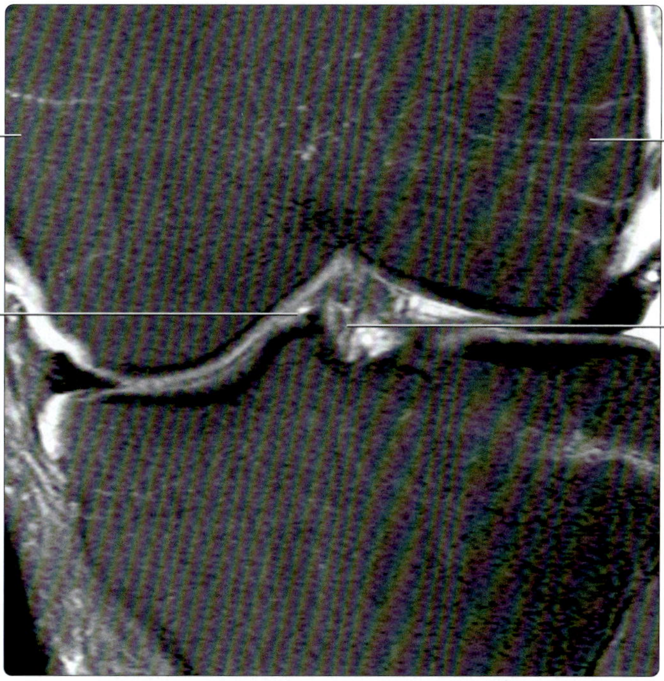

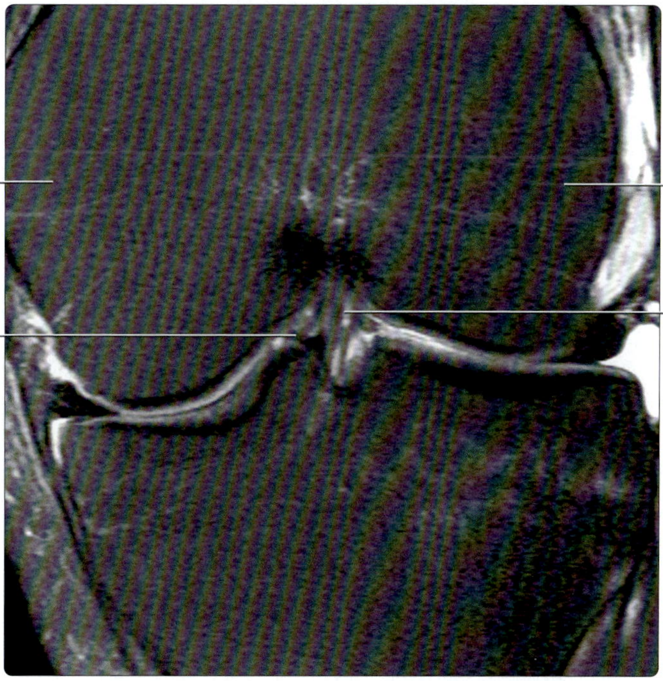

(Top) *Coronal MR, at the anterior portion of midjoint, shows the tiny medial meniscomeniscal ligament in cross section adjacent to the anterior cruciate ligament.* **(Bottom)** *Coronal MR, 3 mm posterior, shows the meniscomeniscal ligament giving the appearance of a loose body or fragment adjacent to the anterior cruciate ligament. The location and low signal of this normal variant ligament may be misdiagnosed as a meniscal fragment or bucket handle fragment. It is important to correlate it with the appearance on either axial or sagittal images, where the ligament will be seen as a longitudinal structure placed between the anterior cruciate ligament and posterior cruciate ligament and angling obliquely across the notch between the 2 menisci.*

OBLIQUE MENISCOMENISCAL LIGAMENT; INFRAPATELLAR PLICA

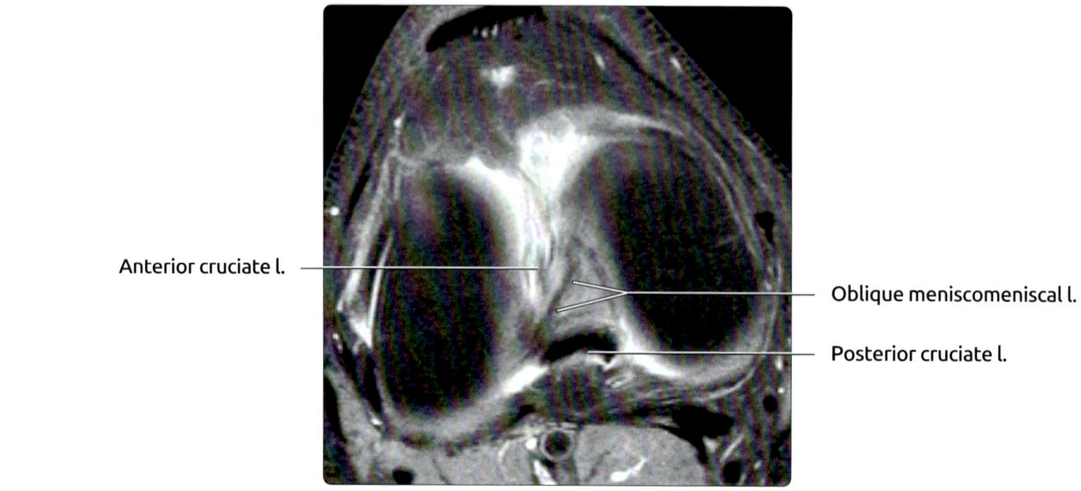

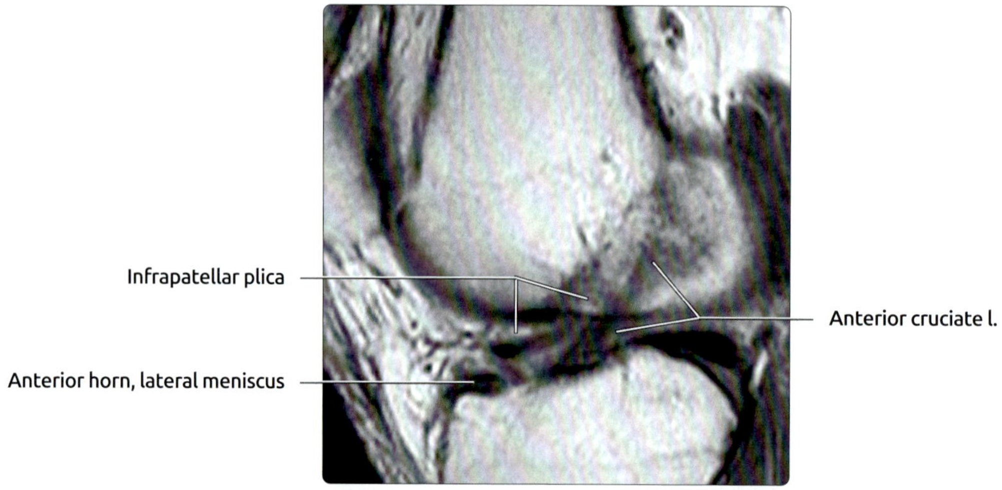

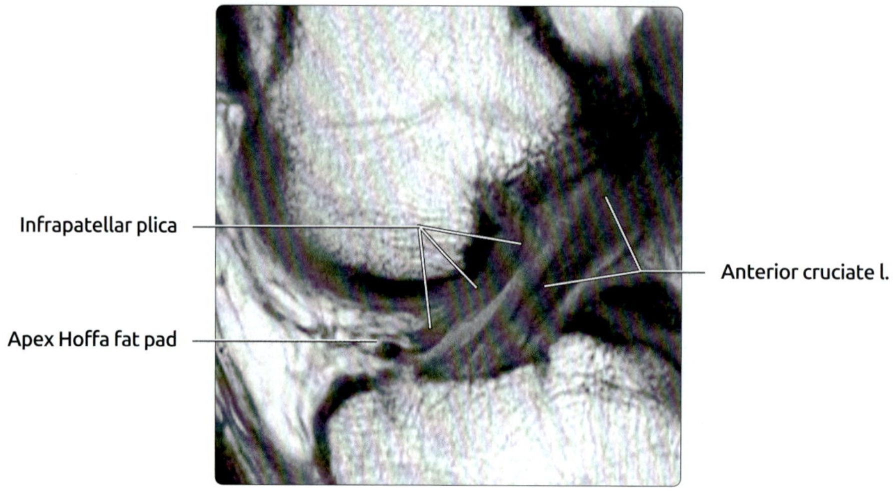

(Top) *Axial PD FS MR through the femoral condyles shows an oblique meniscomeniscal ligament. This uncommon variant connects the anterior horn of one meniscus with the posterior horn of the contralateral meniscus. It runs between the anterior and posterior cruciate ligaments.* **(Middle)** *Sagittal PD MR through the intercondylar notch shows the variant infrapatellar plica. This plica arises from the patella, extends across Hoffa fat pad, and along the anterior surface of the anterior cruciate ligament.* **(Bottom)** *Sagittal PD MR through the intercondylar notch shows an infrapatellar plica. The plica is seen extending through the Hoffa fat pad, paralleling the curvature of the femoral condyle, and then paralleling the anterior cruciate ligament.*

DISCOID MENISCUS

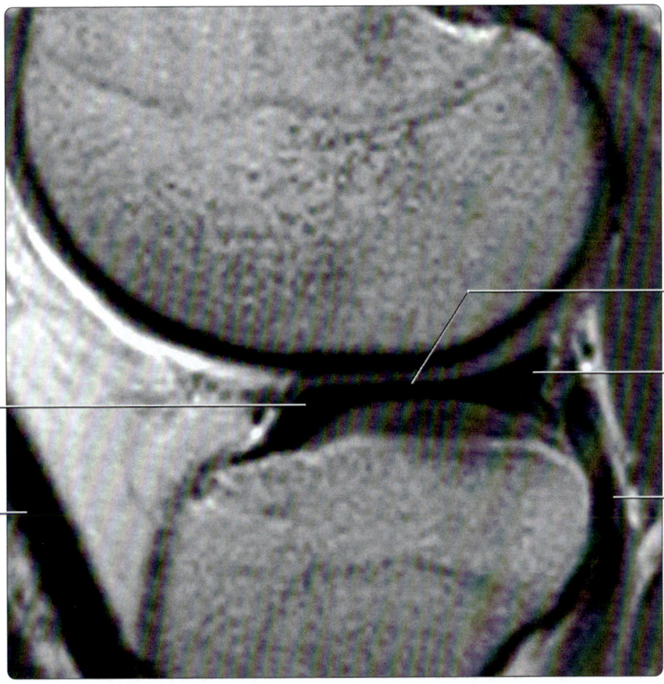

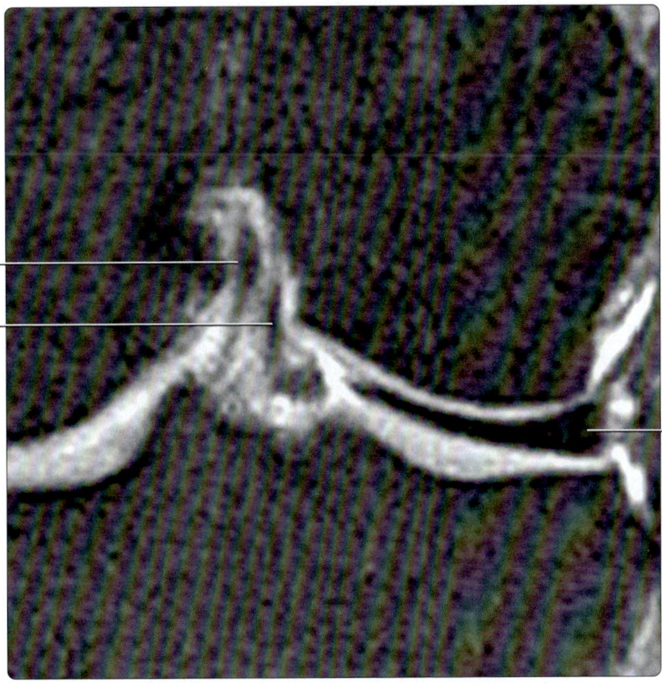

(Top) *Sagittal MR from the midportion of the lateral compartment and shows a discoid lateral meniscus. Note that the meniscus is seen with all 3 portions (anterior horn, body, and posterior horn). This bowtie appearance should be seen only in the outer portion of the joint. The fact that the fibula is not seen, as well as that the popliteus musculotendinous junction (rather than just the popliteus tendon) and patellar tendon are both in this image, indicates that the location is far too interior in the joint for a normal body of meniscus to be seen. Thus, the body of the meniscus is too large, indicating the discoid variant.* **(Bottom)** *Coronal MR through the midportion of the joint (as indicated by the morphology and presence of the anterior cruciate ligament) shows the body of the lateral meniscus to be too large, confirming that it is discoid.*

DISCOID LATERAL MENISCUS MORPHOLOGY

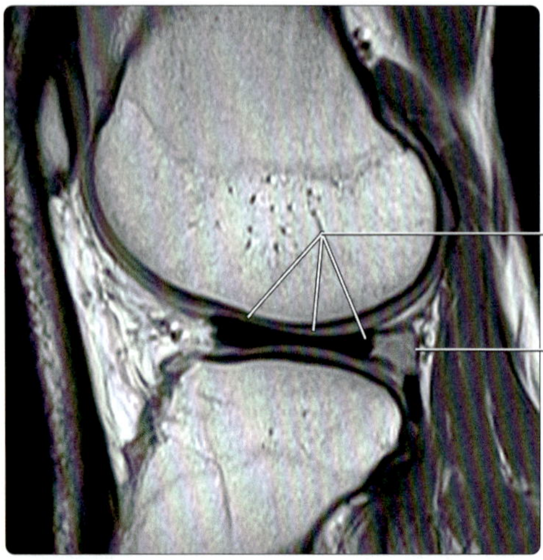

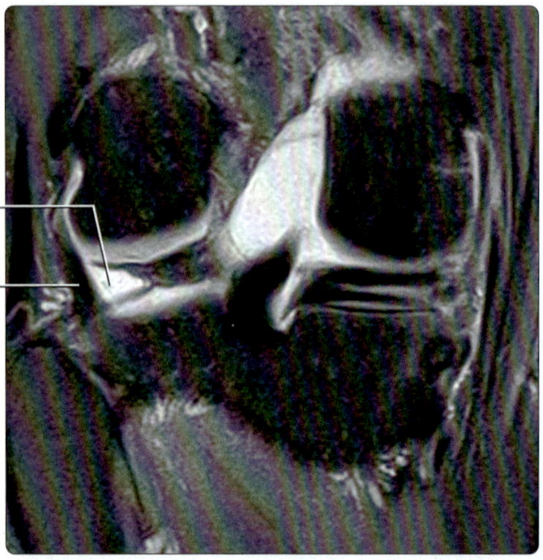

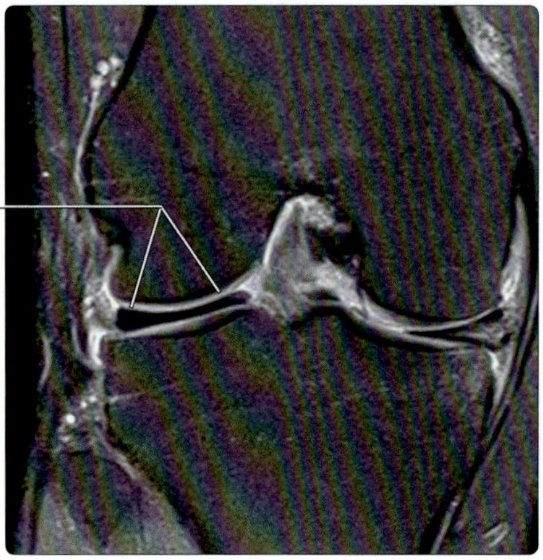

(Top) *Sagittal PD MR in the midlateral compartment demonstrates a discoid lateral meniscus. The lateral meniscus is discoid in morphology far more frequently than is the medial. It is interesting that, with this variant meniscus, the popliteal hiatus is large with prominent fascicles.* **(Middle)** *Coronal PD FS MR located posteriorly in the joint of the same patient again demonstrates the unusual morphology of the popliteal hiatus in the presence of a discoid meniscus. The hiatus becomes enlarged with thickened fascicles.* **(Bottom)** *Coronal PD FS MR in the same patient, midjoint, confirms the discoid morphology of the lateral meniscus.*

DISCOID MENISCUS

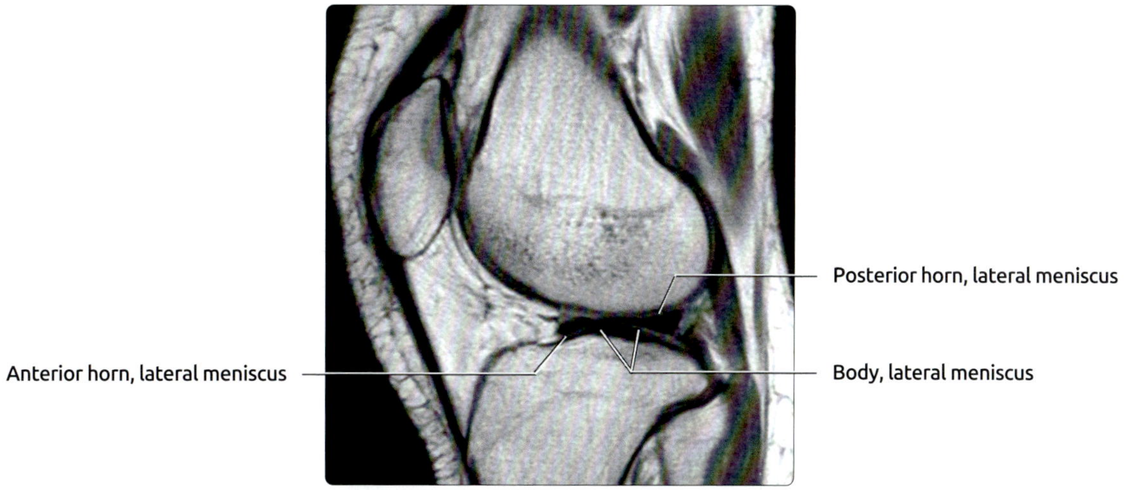

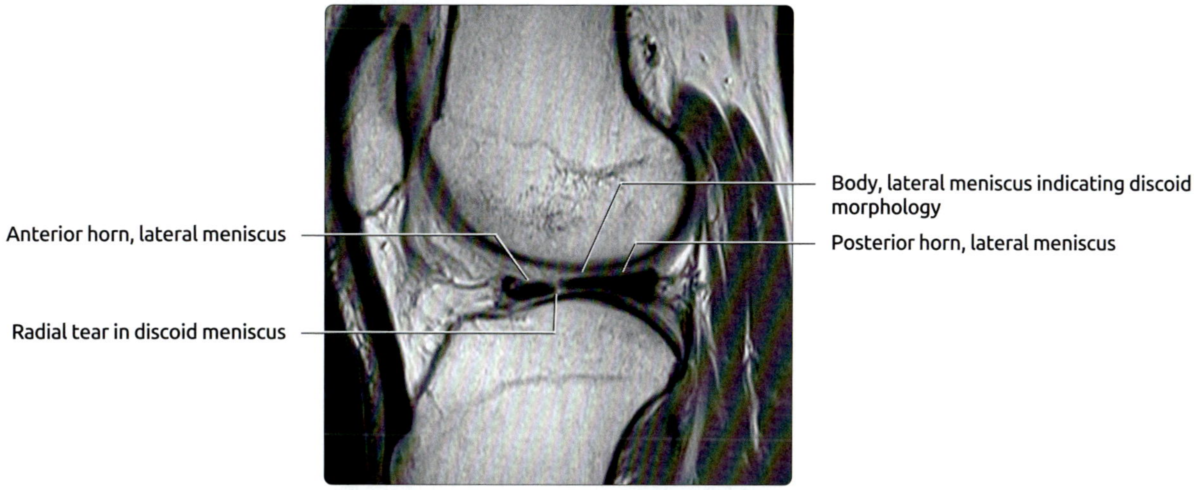

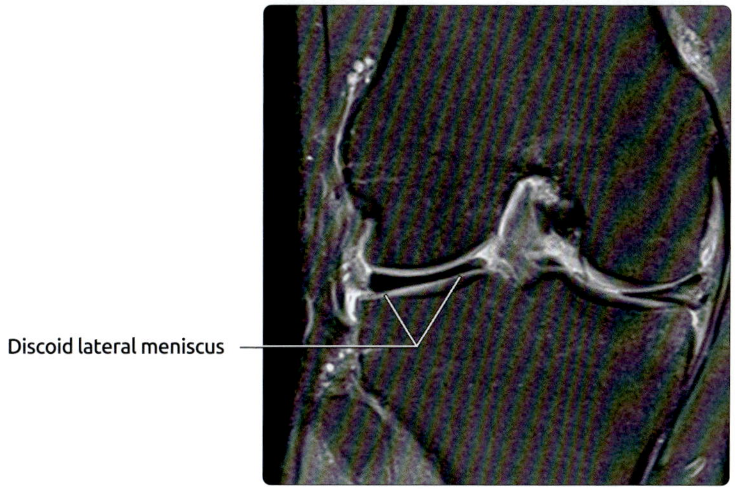

(Top) *Sagittal PD MR in the lateral compartment, near the intercondylar notch, shows the anterior and posterior horns of the lateral meniscus with a thin body of meniscus. This far within the joint, the body of meniscus should not be seen. Therefore, this represents a discoid meniscus.* **(Middle)** *Sagittal PD MR 1 cut closer to the intercondylar notch confirms the discoid meniscus with a radial tear at the junction of the anterior horn and body.* **(Bottom)** *Coronal PD FS MR at midjoint confirms the discoid morphology of the lateral meniscus. The radial tear noted on the sagittal is not seen directly but may be inferred by the blunted edge of the meniscus.*

ANTERIOR HORN MEDIAL MENISCUS ORIGINATING FROM TIBIAL PLATEAU

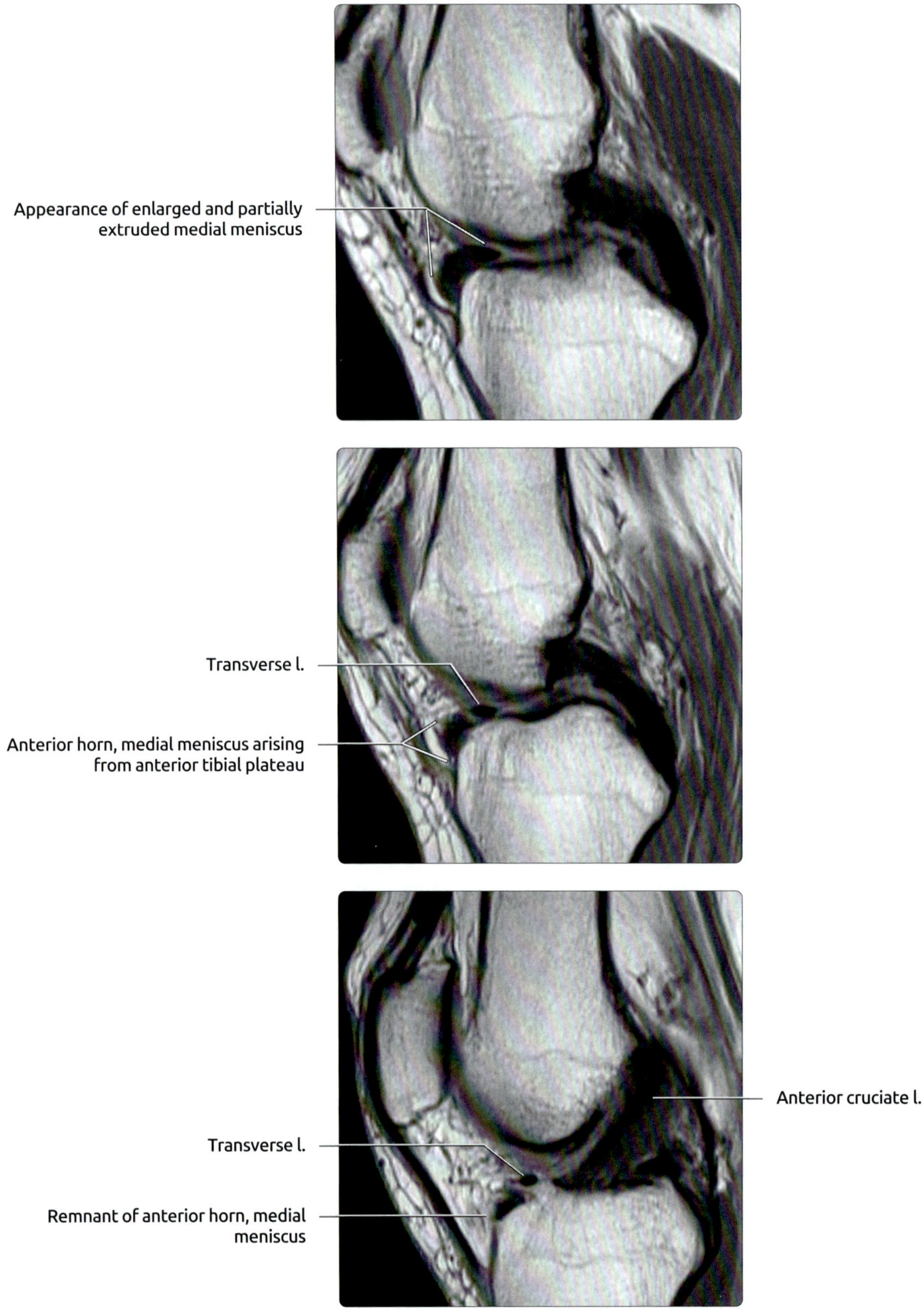

(Top) *First of 3 sagittal PD MR images through the intercondylar notch shows both the posterior cruciate ligament and the anterior horn of the medial meniscus. This image suggests an enlarged and partially extruded medial meniscus. In fact, it is a normal anterior horn that is arising in a slightly variant position of the anterior tibial plateau with the attached transverse ligament that has not yet separated.* **(Middle)** *Second consecutive image, slightly lateral (toward the anterior cruciate ligament), shows an apparent "vertical tear" in the enlarged meniscus. In actuality, this represents the normal anterior horn originating from the anterior tibial plateau with the transverse ligament separating from it.* **(Bottom)** *Third consecutive image, now at the level of the anterior cruciate ligament, shows the remnant of anterior horn medial meniscus, as well as the prominent transverse ligament.*

ANTERIOR HORN MEDIAL MENISCUS ORIGINATING FROM TIBIAL PLATEAU

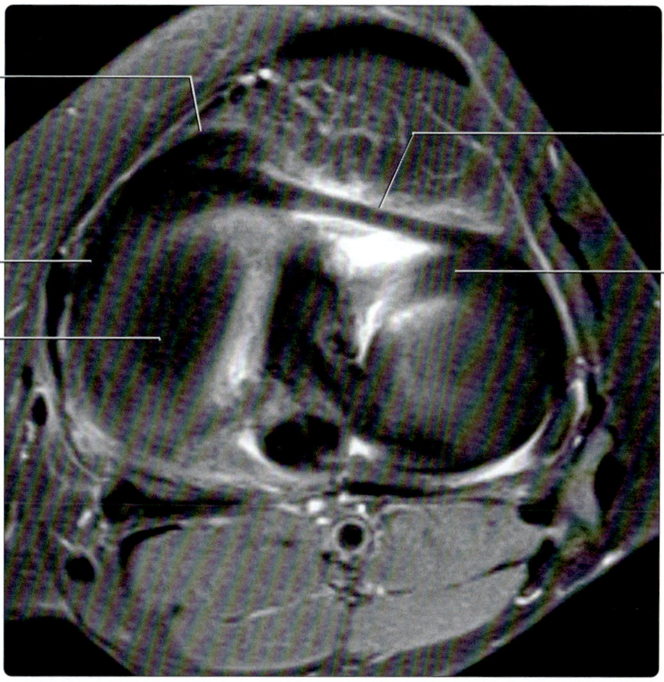

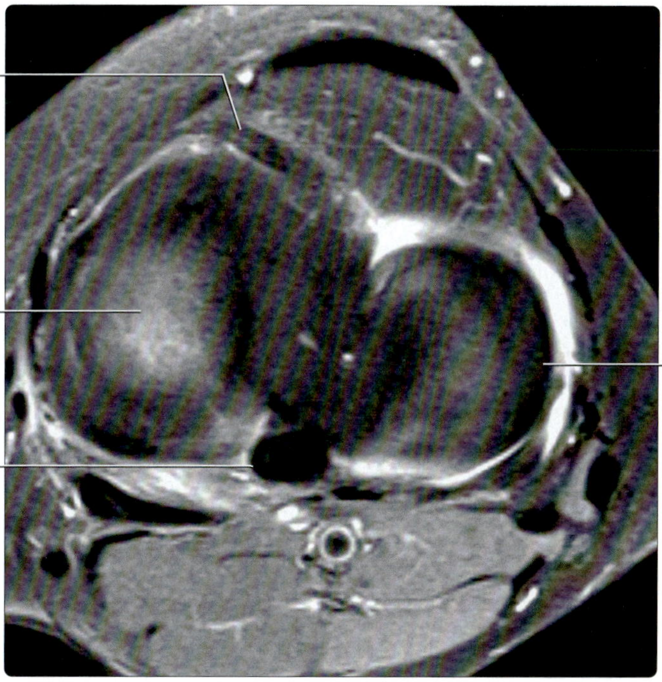

(Top) *First of 2 axial PD FS MR images at the joint line shows both the large transverse ligament and the anterior horn of the medial meniscus that arises anterior to the tibial plateau rather than from on top of the plateau. This is a normal variant origin of the anterior horn of the medial meniscus.* **(Bottom)** *Second axial image, at the level of the joint and tibial plateau, shows the anterior horn of the medial meniscus still as a prominent structure arising anteriorly from the tibia rather than from the top of the plateau. It is important to not misinterpret this appearance as a bucket handle fragment.*

MENISCAL OSSICLE

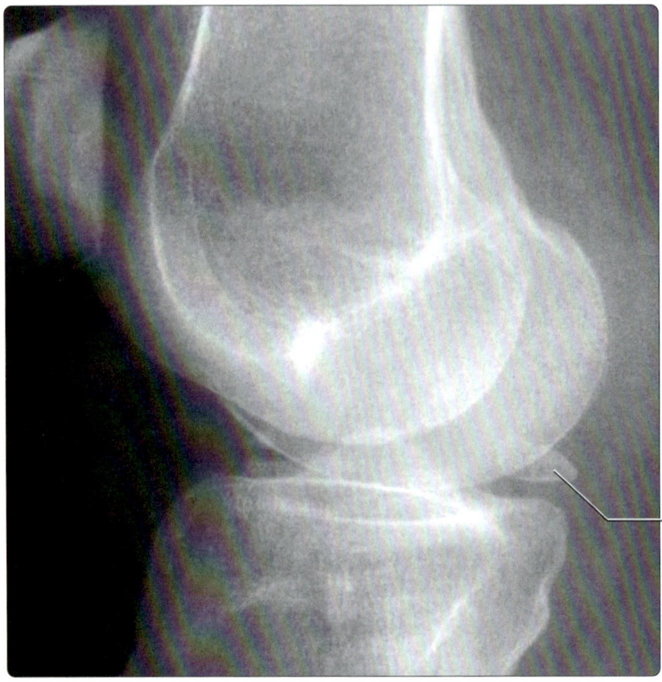

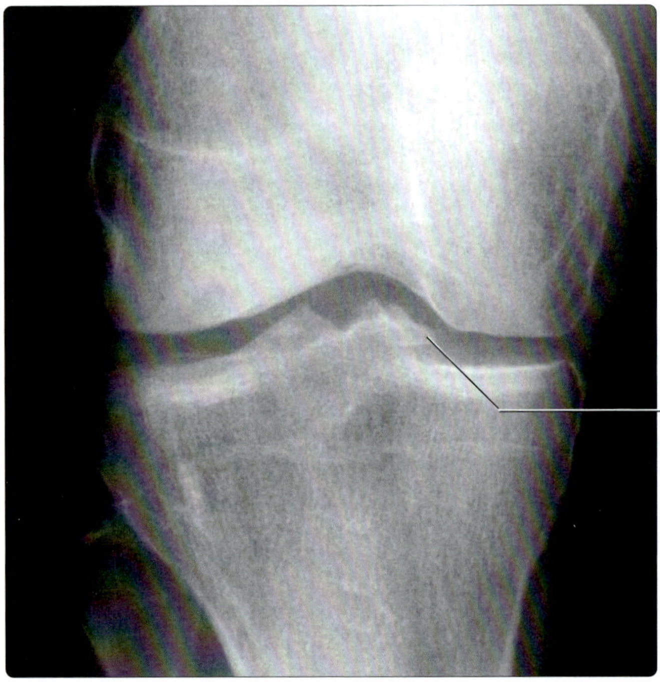

(Top) *Lateral radiograph in a case of meniscal ossicle shows an ossicle located in the region of the posterior horn of the meniscus. It is too low and too horizontally oriented to represent a fabella.* **(Bottom)** *AP radiograph confirms the location of the ossicle to be within the posterior horn of the medial meniscus. It is important to differentiate a meniscal ossicle from a loose body since they are treated differently. Shape and location are both useful parameters in the differentiation. It is also useful to remember that the most common location of a meniscal ossicle is the posterior horn of the medial meniscus, as in this case.*

MENISCAL OSSICLE

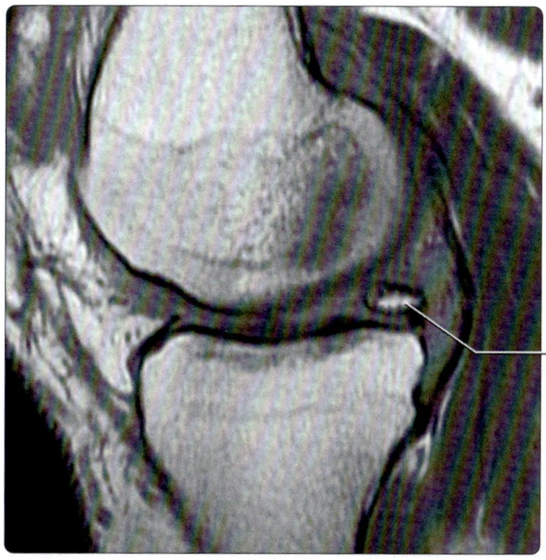

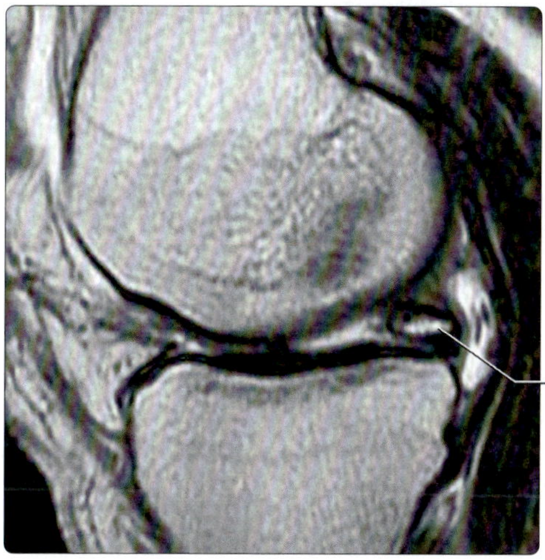

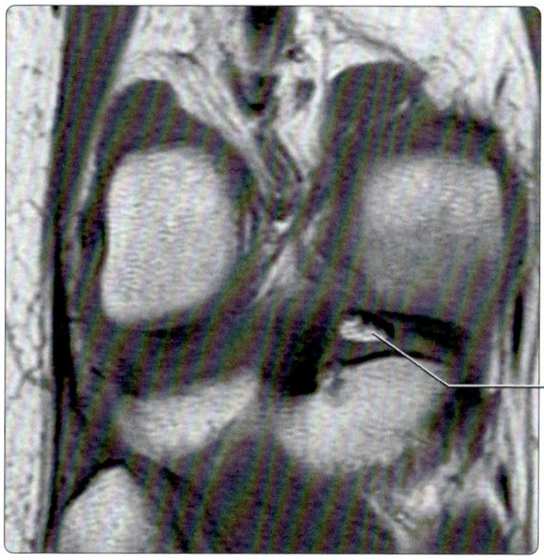

(Top) *Sagittal PD MR shows ossicle (note trabeculae and signal, which matches that of bone) within the posterior horn of the medial meniscus.* **(Middle)** *Sagittal T2WI MR at the same level as the prior image shows the ossicle to occupy the majority of the posterior horn.* **(Bottom)** *Coronal T1WI MR, located posteriorly in the joint, shows the meniscal ossicle within the posterior horn of the medial meniscus. Trabeculae and cortex of the ossicle are seen, and the signal matches that of bone. Meniscal ossicles are uncommon (prevalence 0.15% on one series) and may be symptomatic. (Courtesy A. Sonin, MD.)*

MENISCAL OSSICLE

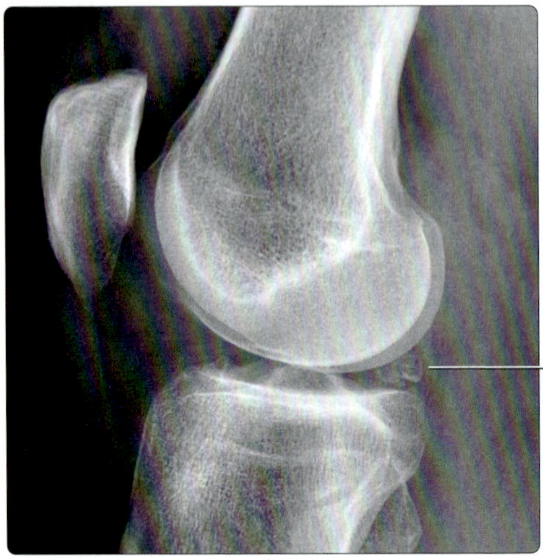

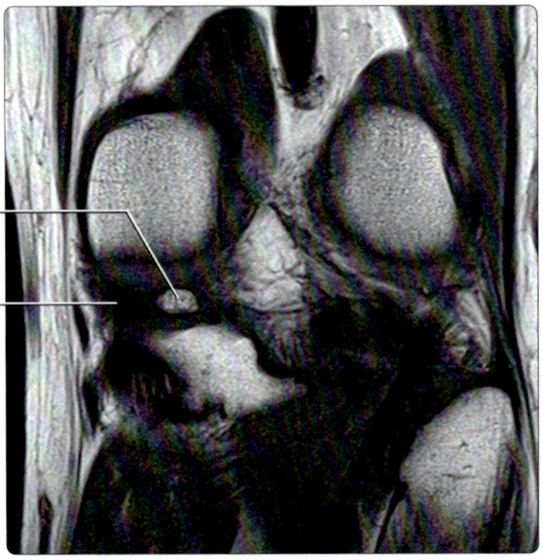

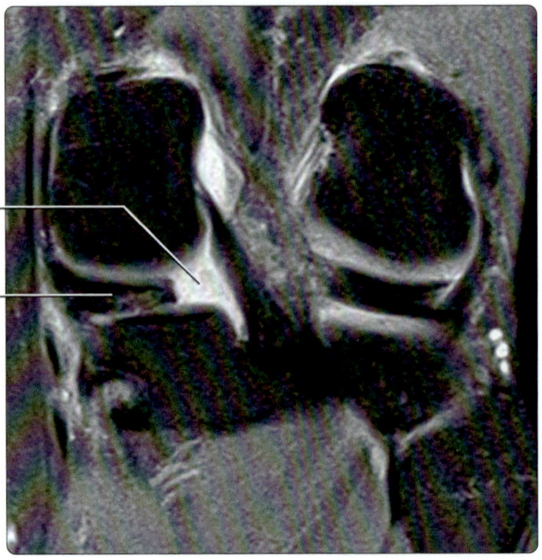

(Top) *Lateral radiograph shows an osseous density superimposed over the posterior knee joint space. It is in a typical position of meniscal ossicle.* **(Middle)** *Coronal T1WI MR, located posteriorly in the joint, shows that there is a rounded structure located within the posterior horn of the medial meniscus that retains the high signal expected of bone. Both the osseous signal and location confirm the diagnosis of meniscal ossicle.* **(Bottom)** *Coronal PD FS MR, located in the posterior portion of the knee joint, shows that there is a radial tear in the root of the posterior horn of the medial meniscus. This is associated with the meniscal ossicle. This cut is slightly anterior to the previous image so that the ossicle is out of the plane.*

MENISCAL OSSICLE

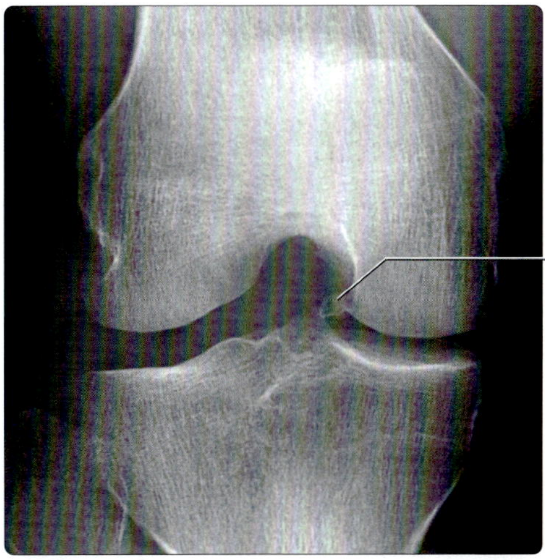

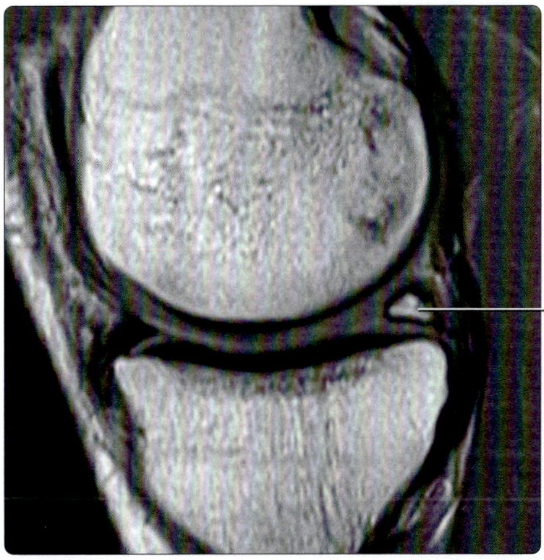

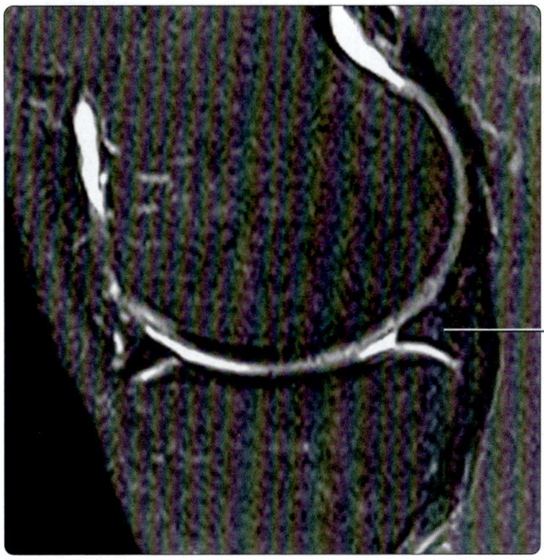

(Top) *AP radiograph shows a rounded osseous density in a location corresponding with the posterior horn of the medial meniscus. This is the typical location of meniscal ossicle. Note that although meniscal ossicle is being treated as a "normal variant" in this discussion, some believe it to be a result of trauma occurring at a young age. Since the posterior horn of the medial meniscus is an area at high risk for meniscal injury at any age, if trauma is indeed the etiology of meniscal ossicle, it is not surprising that the location of an ossicle would most often be within the posterior horn of the medial meniscus.* **(Middle)** *Sagittal PD MR through the medial condyle shows the posterior horn medial meniscus to be replaced by osseous signal. This corresponds to the location of the meniscal ossicle noted on the previous radiograph.* **(Bottom)** *Sagittal T2WI FS MR of the same patient in the same location shows the fat density of the meniscal ossicle to be saturated out.*

MENISCAL OSSICLE

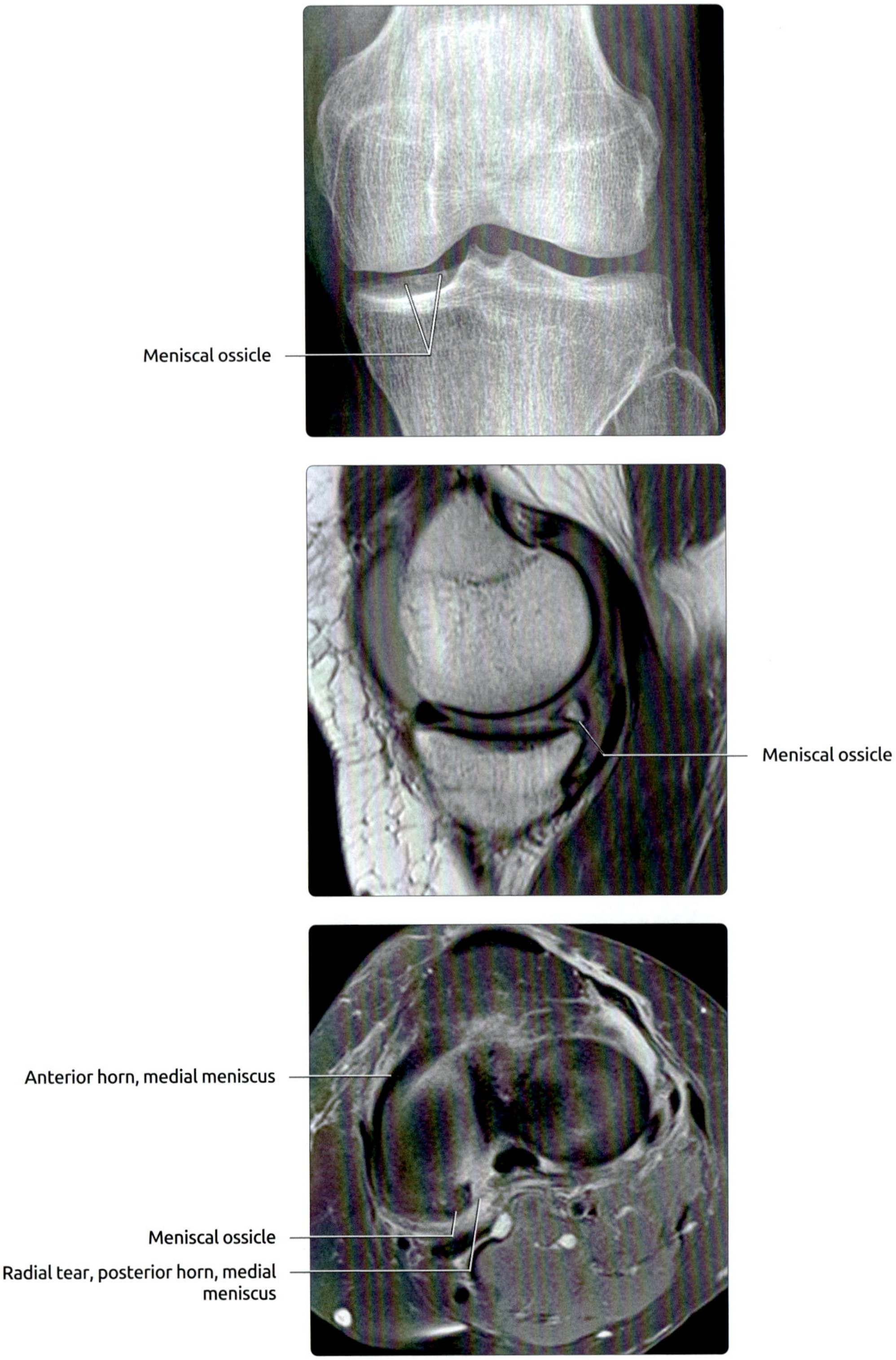

(Top) *AP radiograph shows a trabeculated ossicle located at the posterior horn of the medial meniscus (confirmed on lateral radiograph, not shown). By location, this represents a meniscal ossicle rather than a loose body.* **(Middle)** *Sagittal PD MR in the same patient confirms the bone marrow signal within the ossicle, which itself is located within the posterior horn of the medial meniscus.* **(Bottom)** *Axial PD FS MR in the same patient, at the level of the joint line, shows the meniscal ossicle (low signal since it is fat saturated). The ossicle is, as expected, within the posterior horn of the medial meniscus. Immediately adjacent to the ossicle, there is a gap in the posterior horn representing a large radial tear. It is common to have meniscal tears associated with meniscal ossicle.*

MENISCAL OSSICLE, UNUSUAL LOCATION

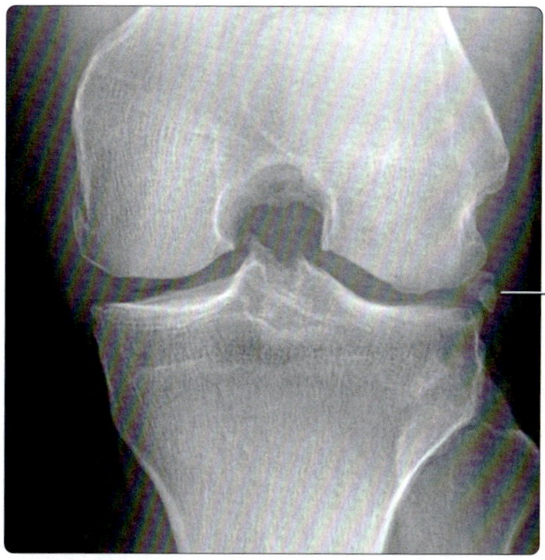

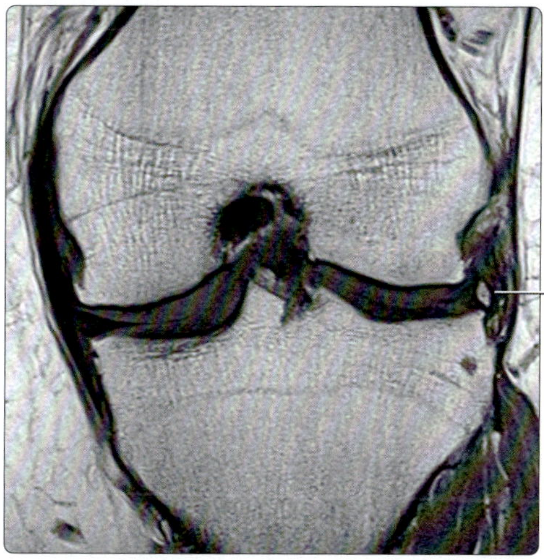

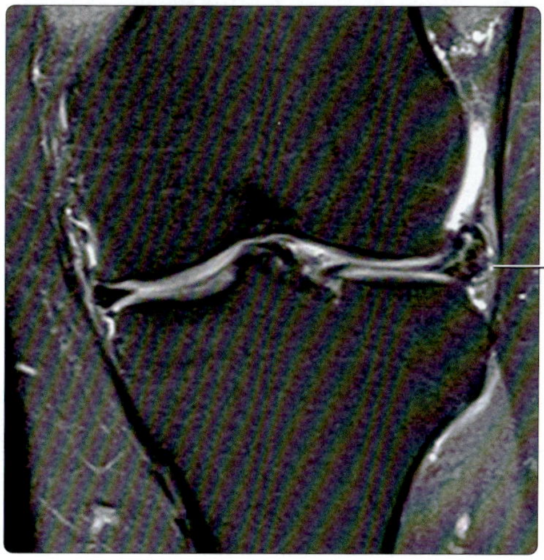

(Top) *AP radiograph demonstrates a meniscal ossicle in an unusual location, the body of the lateral meniscus.* **(Middle)** *Coronal T1WI MR in the midjoint shows the bone-signal meniscal ossicle within the body of the lateral meniscus. It is unusual for a meniscal ossicle to be found either in the lateral rather than medial meniscus or in the body rather than posterior horn of the meniscus.* **(Bottom)** *Coronal PD FS MR at the same level as the prior image shows the ossicle to be fat saturated and an associated tear of the body of the lateral meniscus.*

TRUNCATION ARTIFACT

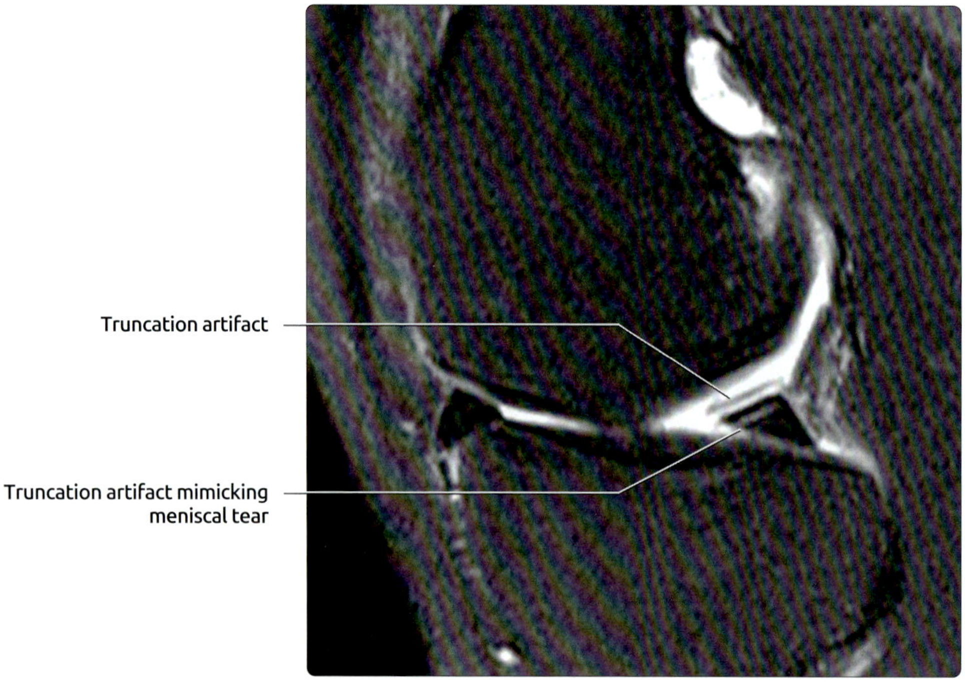

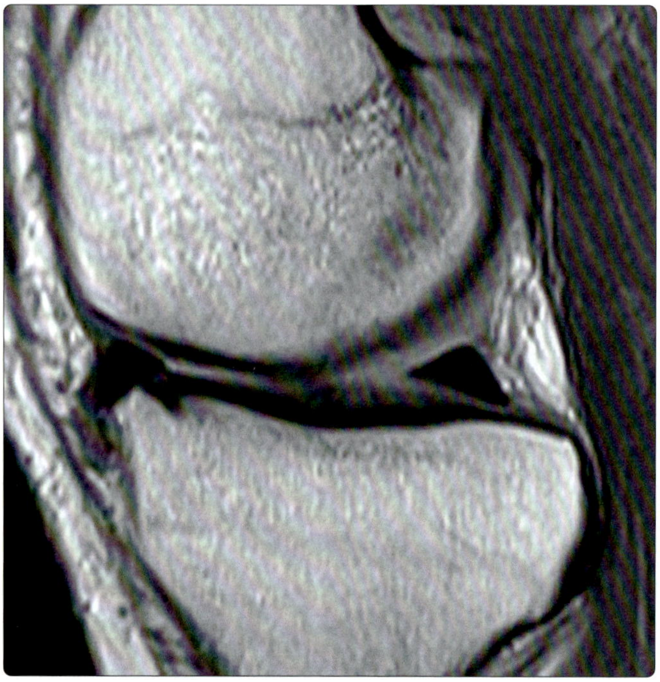

(Top) *Sagittal T2WI FS MR demonstrates posterior horn meniscus with an apparent linear high signal extending to the free edge. Although this gives the appearance of an oblique meniscal tear, there is also a low-signal linear appearance extending along the superior aspect of the meniscus. This parallel linear signal should cause suspicion that the "tear" is due to truncation artifact.* **(Bottom)** *Sagittal PD MR in the same patient, same cut as the previous T2 FS MR, shows a normal posterior horn with no evidence of tear. PD is the most reliable sequence for evaluating menisci; this image proves that the "tear" seen on the T2 FS MR is due to truncation artifact, often seen at the boundary between high- and low-signal structures. These artifacts are caused by approximation errors in Fourier transform analysis.*

MOTION & VACUUM ARTIFACTS

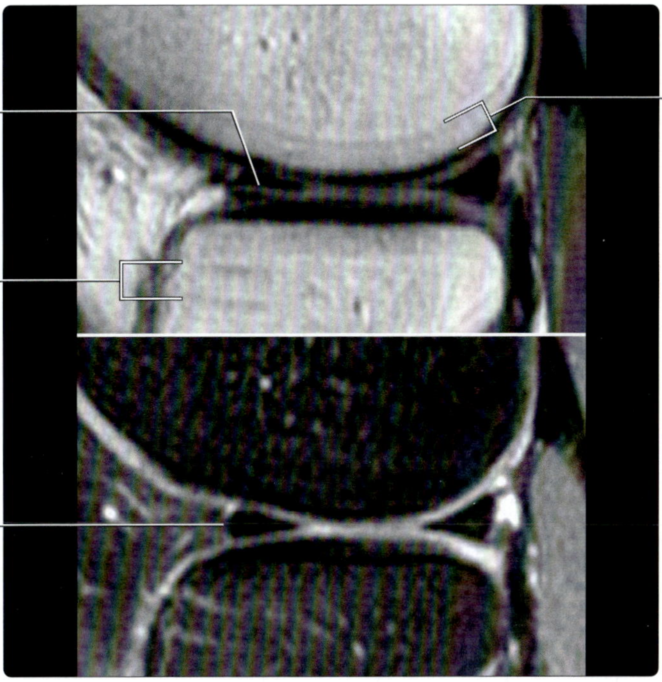

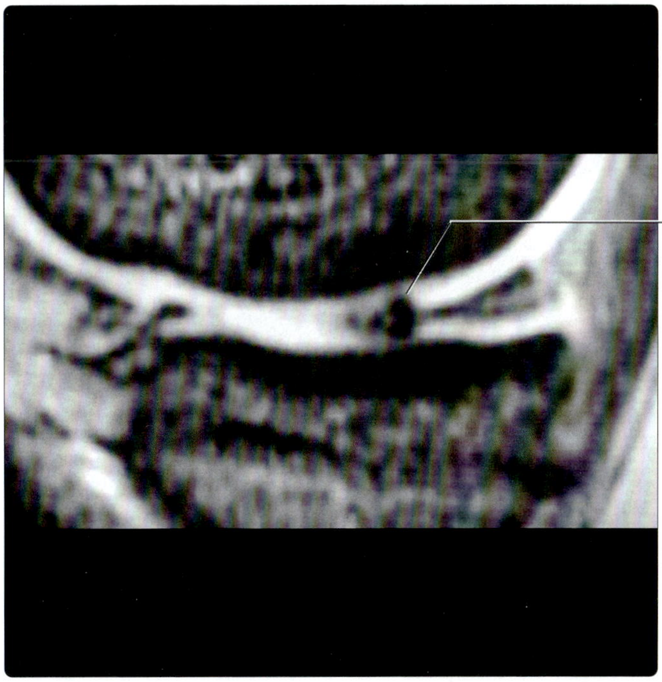

(Top) *Sagittal PD and sagittal PD FS MR images, same cuts at same time, show the effects of slight patient motion. The PD image shows a horizontal high signal through the anterior horn, suggesting a meniscal tear. However, there are also horizontal lines within the tibia paralleling the meniscal line as well as the tibial plateau cortex. There are, in addition, concave lines in the femoral condyle paralleling the concavity of the femoral condylar cortex. These paralleling lines indicate motion and that the meniscal "tear" is artifactual.* **(Bottom)** *Sagittal gradient-echo MR demonstrates a low-signal, round "body" superimposed over the free edge of the posterior horn. This is an air bubble that developed via vacuum phenomenon when the knee was extended in the coil. The air bubble "blooms" on gradient-echo imaging; it would not be as prominent on other sequences, though may be visible.*

IMAGING ANATOMY

Overview

- **Distal fibular variants**
  - Absent retromalleolar fibular groove
    - Predisposes to peroneal retinaculum injury, peroneal tendon subluxation
  - Os subfibulare: Accessory center of ossification, anteroinferior margin of fibula
- **Distal tibial variants**
  - Medial malleolus accessory ossification center for anterior colliculus
- **Ankle capsule variants**
  - 10-15% of population have ankle joint capsule communication with subtalar joint
- **Talus variants**
  - Os trigonum: Accessory center of ossification for posterior process talus
  - Stieda process: Enlarged posterior process of talus
  - Talar ridge: Bony prominence at insertion of anterior ankle joint capsule on talar neck
- **Calcaneal variants**
  - Peroneal tubercle of calcaneus
    - Variably present at lateral margin, separates peroneus longus and brevis
  - Os calcis secondarius: Small ossicle adjacent to anterior process calcaneus
  - Childhood: Sclerotic ossification center of posterior process
    - May be multipartite, may mimic osteonecrosis (Sever disease)
- **Navicular variants**
  - Childhood: May be sclerotic, flat, multipartite
    - Mimics avascular necrosis of navicular (Köhler disease)
  - Accessory navicular (a.k.a. os tibiale externum): Ossicle at median eminence of navicular
    - Type 1: Sesamoid in tibialis posterior tendon
    - Type 2: Accessory center of ossification joined to navicular by synchondrosis
    - Type 3: Enlarged median eminence of navicular
  - Os supranaviculare (a.k.a. os talonaviculare dorsale or Pirie bone)
    - Small ossicle at dorsal, proximal navicular margin
- **Cuboid variant: Cuboides secondarium** (rare)
  - Small ossicle at proximal medial aspect of cuboid, between cuboid and navicular
- **Cuneiform variants**
  - Os intercuneiform: Dorsal aspect foot, between 1st and 2nd cuneiforms
  - Medial cuneiform may arise from 2 ossification centers
- **Metatarsal variants**
  - Accessory centers of ossification
    - Pars peronea metatarsalis primi: Between base of 1st metatarsal and 1st cuneiform
    - Os vesalianum: Base of 5th metatarsal
    - Os intermetatarseum: Dorsal, between 1st and 2nd metatarsals
    - Accessory epiphysis: At opposite end of bone from true epiphysis
  - Intermetatarsal joint of 1st and 2nd digits
    - Articular facet between bases of 1st and 2nd metatarsals variably present
  - Morton foot: 1st metatarsal is short relative to 2nd
    - Results in increased stress on 2nd metatarsal
- **Phalangeal variants**
  - Failure of segmentation of middle and distal phalanges
  - Exostosis of 1st distal phalangeal base

Sesamoids

- **Os peroneale**: Sesamoid within peroneus longus muscle, seen adjacent to lateral margin of cuboid
  - May be bipartite or multipartite
- **Sesamoids of great toe**
  - 30% bipartite or multipartite
  - Medial (tibial) sesamoid rarely congenitally absent
  - Interphalangeal sesamoid: At interphalangeal joint, within flexor hallucis longus tendon
- **Sesamoids of 2nd-5th toes**
  - Variably present at metatarsophalangeal or interphalangeal joints

Pediatric Marrow Variation

- May see islands of low T1, high T2 signal in bone marrow in pediatric population
- Residual hematopoietic bone marrow, resolves by age 15

Muscle Variants

- Accessory soleus
  - Originates anterior margin soleus, inserts on calcaneus
- Accessory flexor muscles
  - Variable origins and insertions, description of course preferred to specific names
- Peroneus quartus
  - Originates distal fibula, peroneus brevis, or peroneus longus
  - Variable insertion lateral foot: 5th toe, calcaneus, cuboid, lateral retinaculum
- Quadratus plantae: May be absent; may send slip to 5th toe, 2nd-4th toes, or 2nd-3rd toes
- Opponens digiti minimi: Variably present muscle slip of flexor digiti minimi, sharing its origin, and inserting on distal 5th metatarsal shaft
- Peroneus tertius: Absent in 10% of population

ANATOMY IMAGING ISSUES

Imaging Recommendations

- Use radiographic CT or MR criteria to distinguish normal variants from fracture
  - Fracture: Jagged margins, acute angular contour
  - Accessory ossicle/bipartite ossicle: Smooth, rounded, corticated margins
- Accessory centers may be symptomatic, due to injury of synchondrosis between ossicle and parent bone
  - If symptomatic, edema will be seen on MR, centered on synchondrosis
- Accessory muscles may be symptomatic, should not be mistaken for mass

ACCESSORY CENTERS & SESAMOIDS

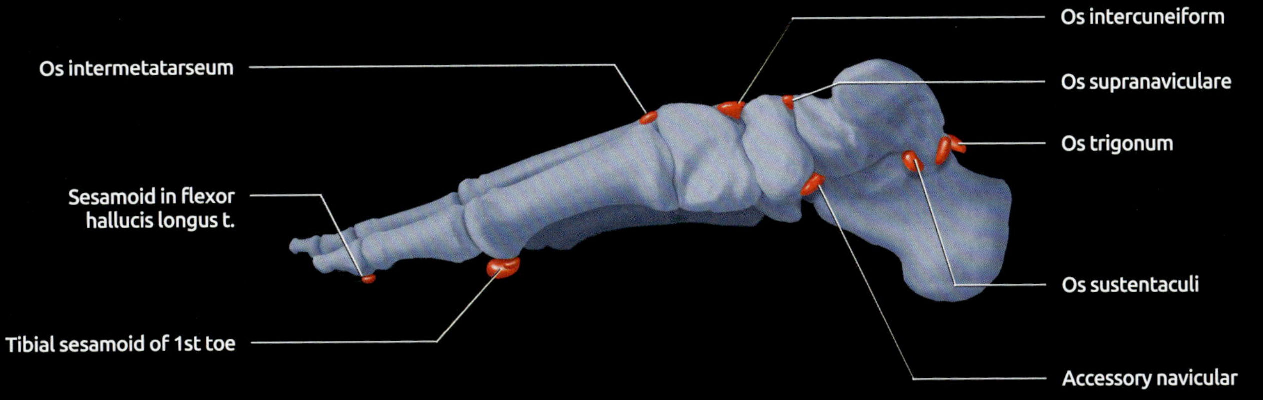

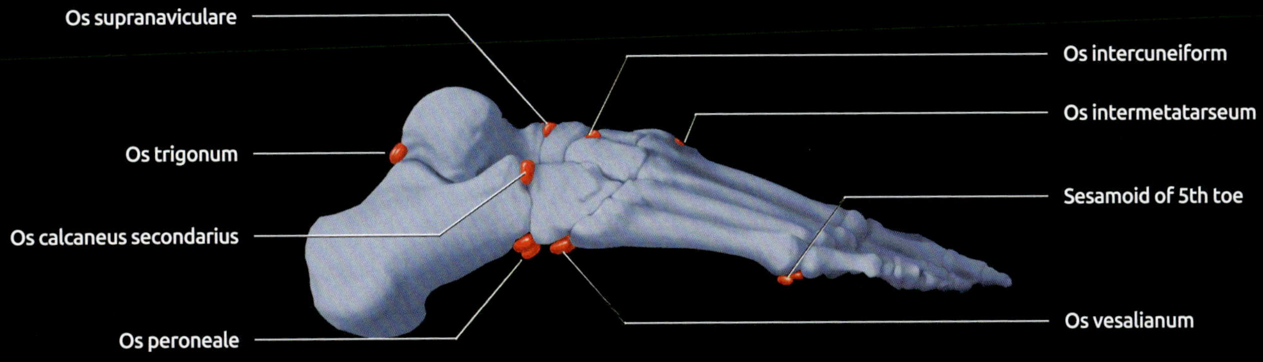

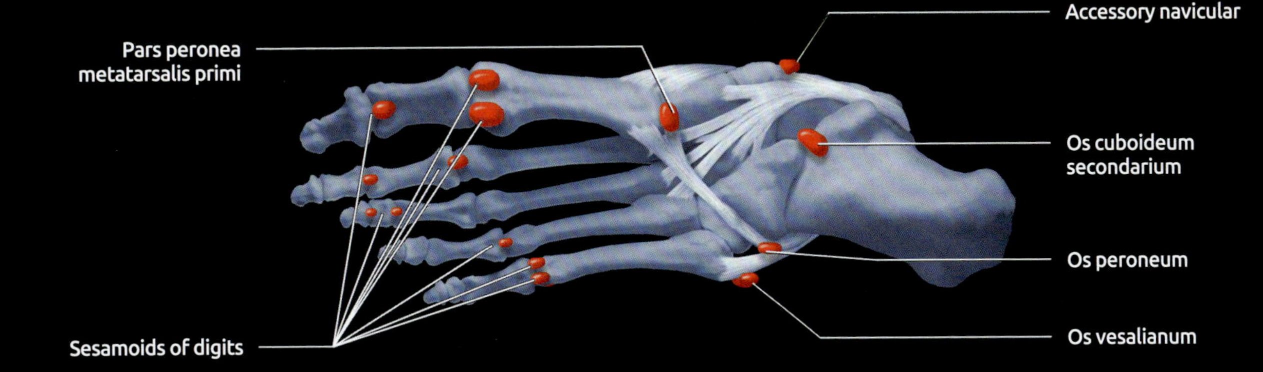

There are multiple, variably present accessory ossicles of the foot. Os sustentaculi and pars peronea metatarsalis primi are quite uncommon, while the others that are shown are frequently seen. Ossicles are frequently called by Latin names. Os tibiale externum, however, is usually called by its simple English name, accessory navicular.

ANKLE JOINT CAPSULE VARIANTS

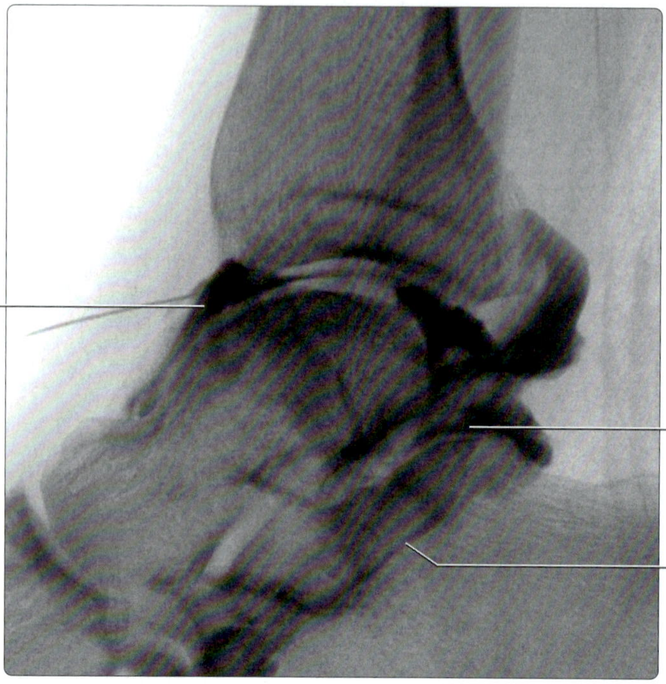

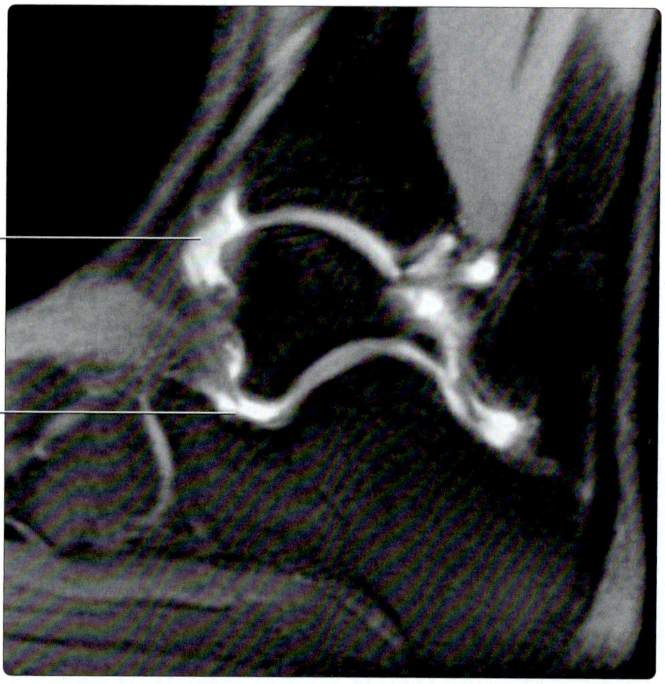

(Top) *Lateral arthrogram shows communication of the ankle joint with the flexor hallucis longus tendon sheath and the posterior subtalar joint. Communication to the flexor hallucis longus tendon sheath is always present, but communication with the posterior subtalar joint happens in only 10-15% of the population.* **(Bottom)** *Sagittal T1WI FS MR arthrogram shows contrast filling ankle and posterior subtalar joints.*

ACCESSORY OSSIFICATION CENTER, MEDIAL MALLEOLUS

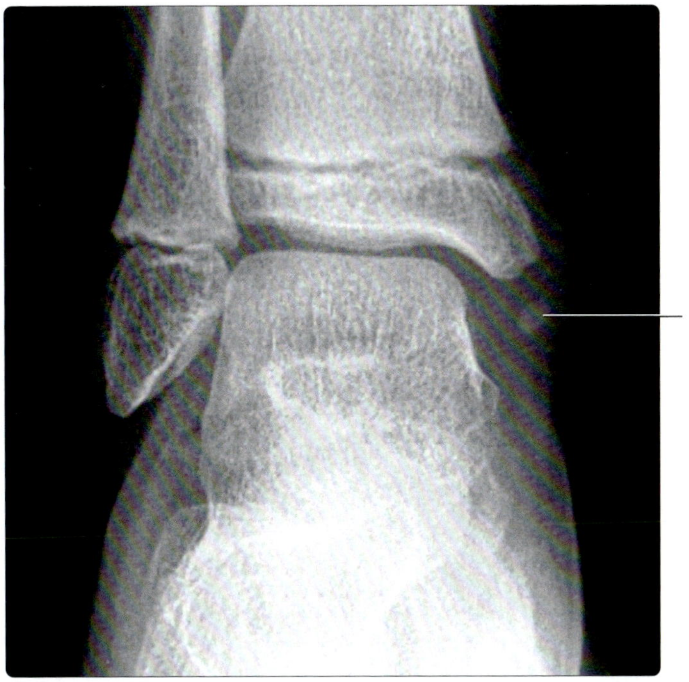

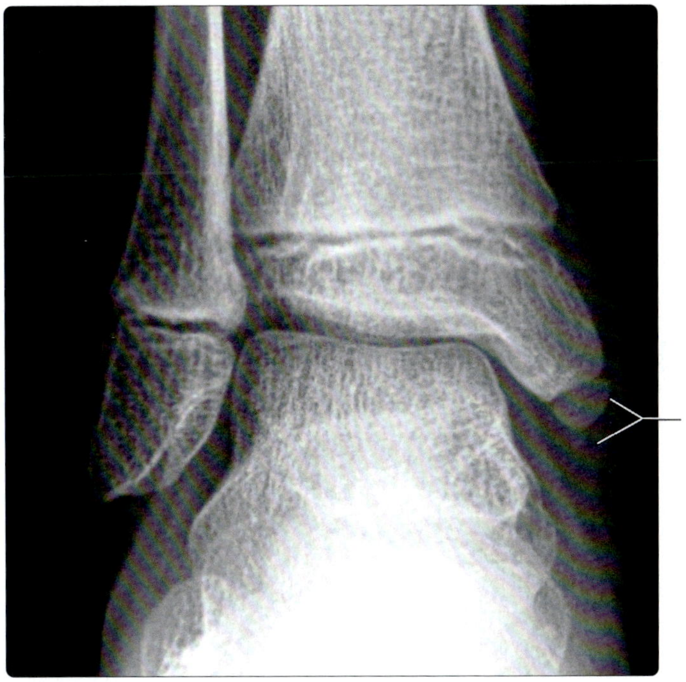

(Top) *Anteroposterior radiograph shows os subtibiale (accessory medial malleolus center of ossification) in a child. This ossicle occurs in ~ 20% of children, becoming radiographically apparent between 7-10 years of age and fusing at skeletal maturity. It may be symptomatic due to injury of synchondrosis, uniting it to the remainder of medial malleolus.* **(Bottom)** *Anteroposterior radiograph in a different child shows bipartite os subtibiale (accessory center of ossification of medial malleolus).*

ACCESSORY OSSIFICATION CENTER, LATERAL MALLEOLUS

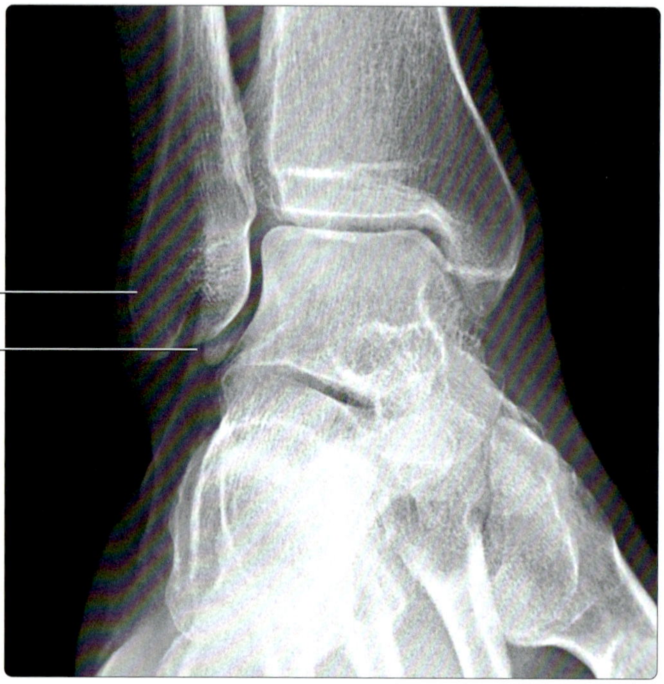

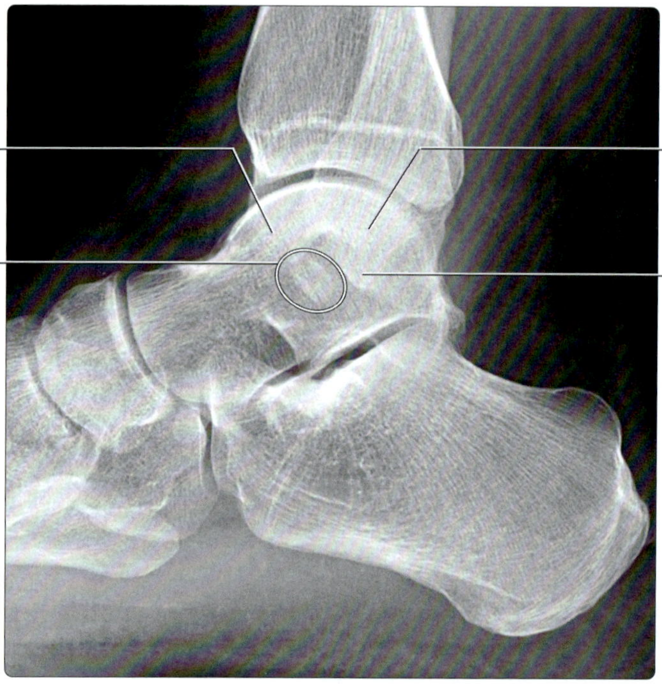

(Top) *Mortise view shows os subfibulare in an adult patient. Os subfibulare occurs in ~ 1% of children but usually fuses by adulthood. Shape of ossicle as well as normal size and configuration of adjacent lateral malleolus help to distinguish ossicle from nonunited fracture.* **(Bottom)** *Lateral radiograph in the same patient shows the characteristic location of os subfibulare at the anteroinferior margin of the fibula. Overlap of malleoli may initially be confusing on lateral radiographs, but malleoli and lateral malleolar accessory center of ossification can reliably be identified.*

OS TRIGONUM AND STIEDA PROCESS

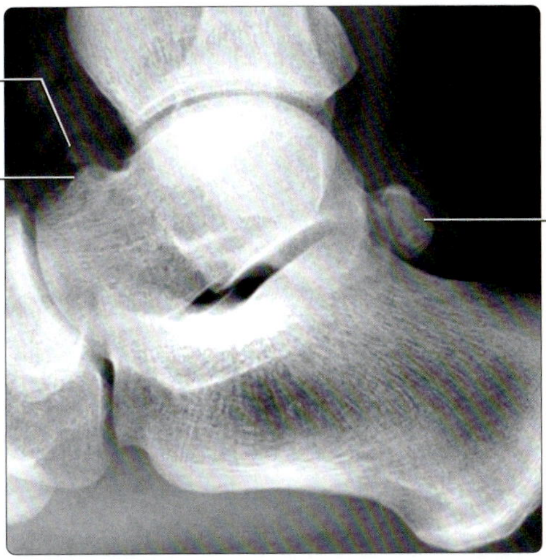

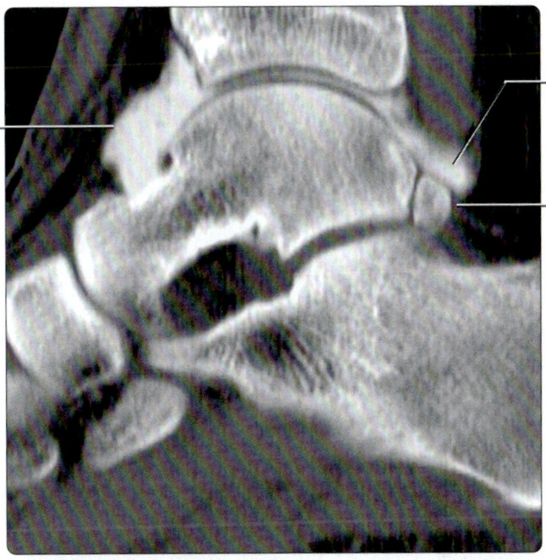

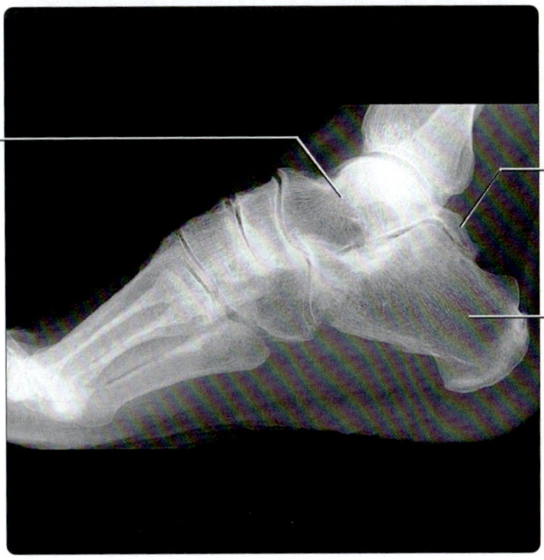

(Top) *Lateral radiograph shows an unusually large os trigonum. Cysts in the ossicle suggest os trigonum syndrome in which there is impingement of the ossicle against talus or flexor hallucis longus. Note that the patient also has a slightly prominent talar ridge, another normal variant. Ossicle adjacent to the talar ridge is an old fracture, not a normal variant.* **(Middle)** *Sagittal CT arthrogram shows contrast in the ankle joint flowing smoothly over the superior margin of a triangular os trigonum.* **(Bottom)** *Lateral radiograph shows a Stieda process, an elongated lateral tubercle of the posterior process of the talus. The Stieda process, while a normal variant, can predispose to posterior impingement of the ankle or flexor hallucis longus tendon, especially in plantar flexion.*

CALCANEAL VARIANTS

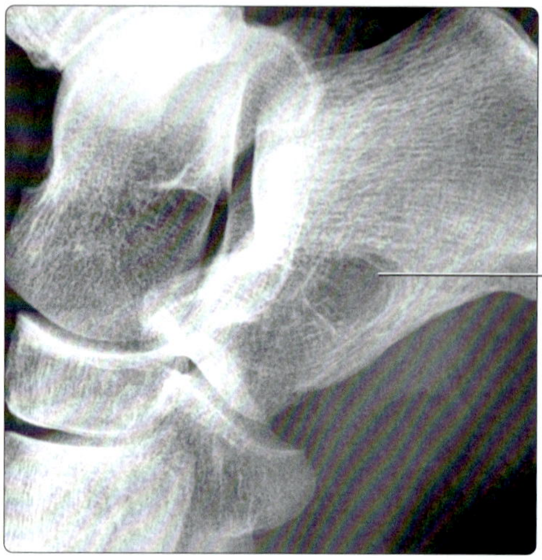

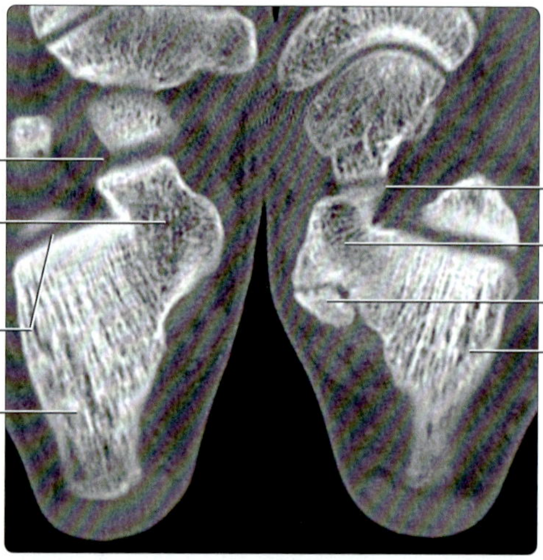

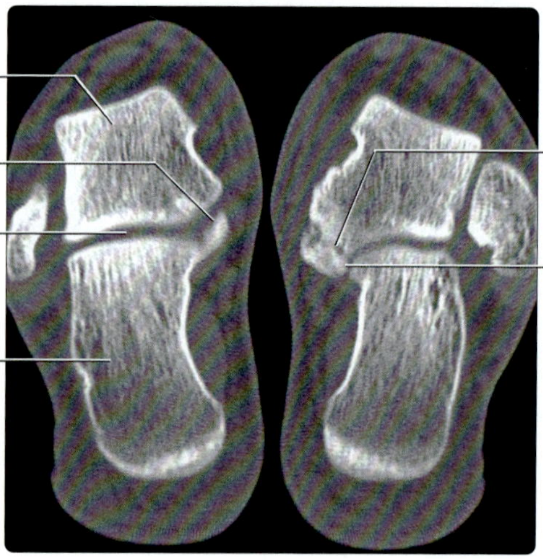

(Top) *Lateral radiograph shows a calcaneal pseudocyst. This area of lucency is seen inferior to the sustentaculum tali and reflects the normal paucity of trabeculae in this region. True cysts and lipomas also occur in this region but will show a more well-defined and continuous border.* **(Middle)** *Axial oblique CT shows left foot os sustentaculi, a rare ossicle arising from the calcaneus at the posterior margin of sustentaculum tali. The right side is normal.* **(Bottom)** *Coronal CT through left-sided os sustentaculi, posterior to sustentaculum tali, shows nonbony coalition between os sustentaculi and talus, a common finding with this ossicle. Right foot is normal.*

CALCANEAL VARIANTS

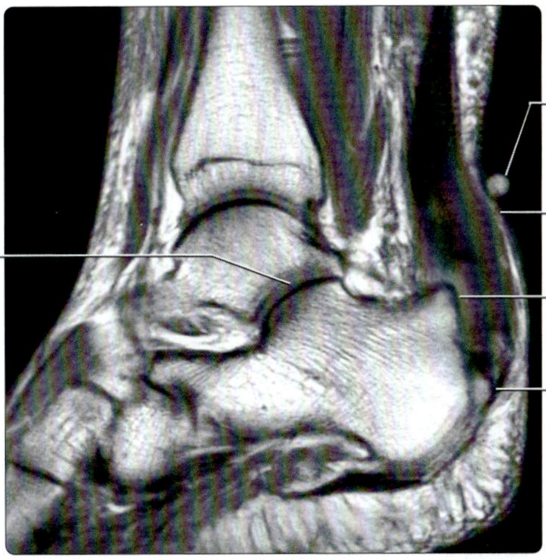

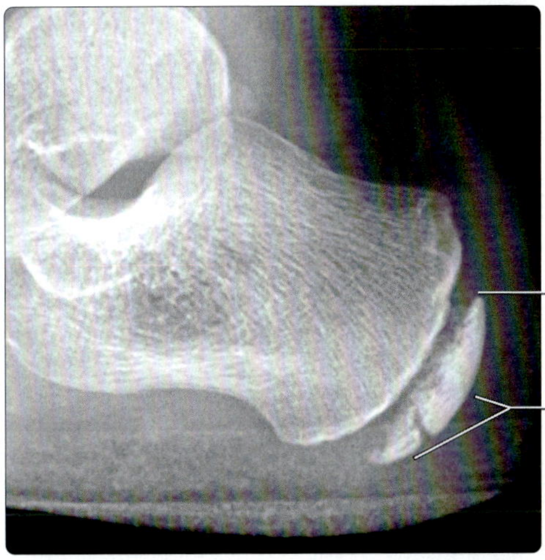

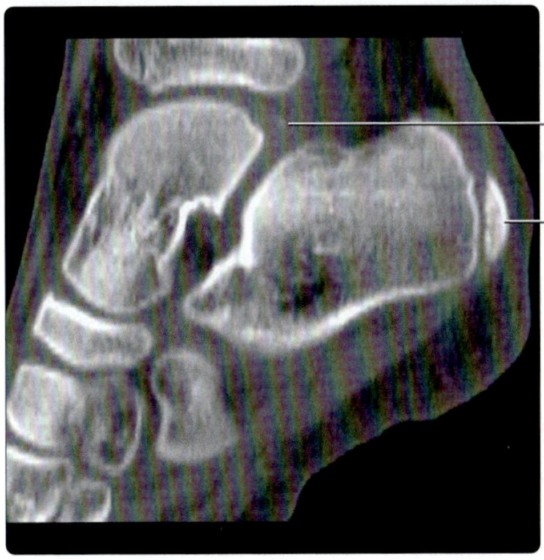

(Top) *Sagittal T1WI MR shows a large Haglund deformity (known as "pump bump"). This is prominence of the superior margin of posterior process of calcaneus. This normal variant often impinges against high backs of shoes and results in retrocalcaneal bursitis as well as Achilles tendinopathy.* **(Middle)** *Lateral radiograph in a child shows bipartite and sclerotic calcaneal apophysis. At the superior margin, apophysis appears to have several tiny fragments, also a normal variant.* **(Bottom)** *Sagittal CT shows the normal sclerotic appearance of calcaneal apophysis in a child. Note the undulating contour of adjacent metaphysis, also a normal variant. This patient has also begun to form an os trigonum.*

CALCANEAL VARIANTS

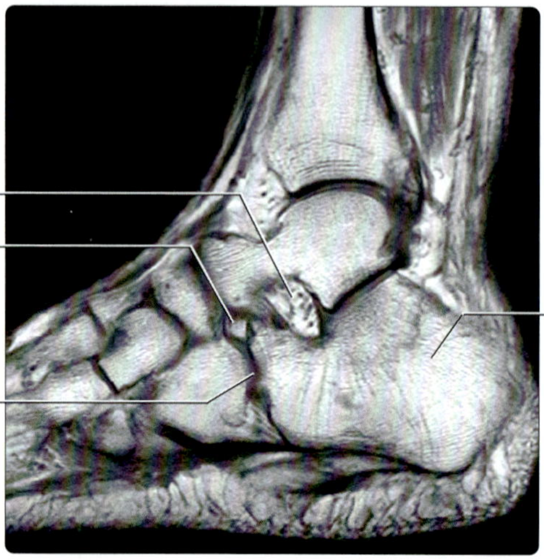

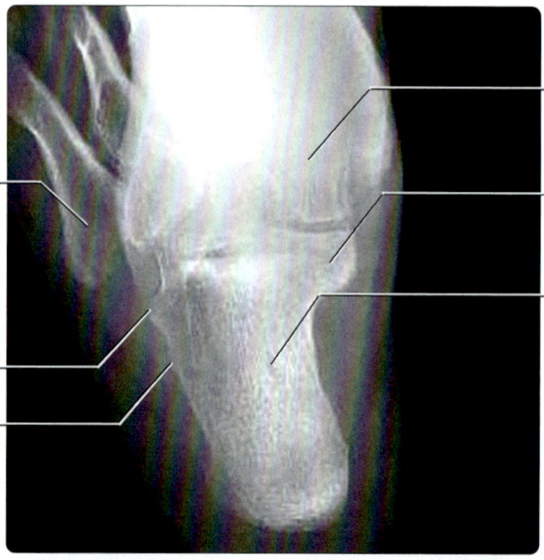

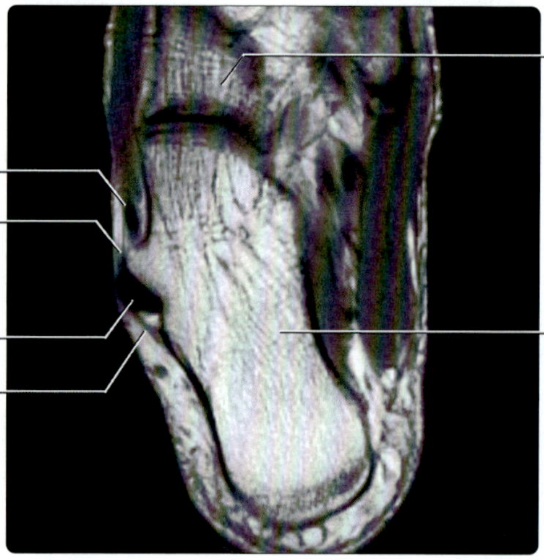

(Top) *Os calcaneus secundarius, with an incidence of 2-7%, is found at the apex of the anterior process of calcaneus between the talar head, navicular, and cuboid. The os may be angular or round and may be confused with an old avulsion fracture at the calcaneal origin of the bifurcate ligament.* **(Middle)** *Calcaneal (a.k.a. axial or Harris) view shows a small peroneal tubercle. The peroneal tubercle, also called trochlear process, is a protuberance of lateral calcaneal wall and is present in ~ 40% of individuals. It separates the peroneus longus and brevis tendons.* **(Bottom)** *Axial MR of the ankle depicts mildly enlarged peroneal tubercle. The peroneus brevis and peroneus longus tendons are anterior and posterior to the tubercle, respectively. Fibers from the inferior peroneal retinaculum insert on the peroneal tubercle, forming 2 fibroosseous tunnels for each peroneal tendon.*

MARROW VARIANT, PEDIATRIC

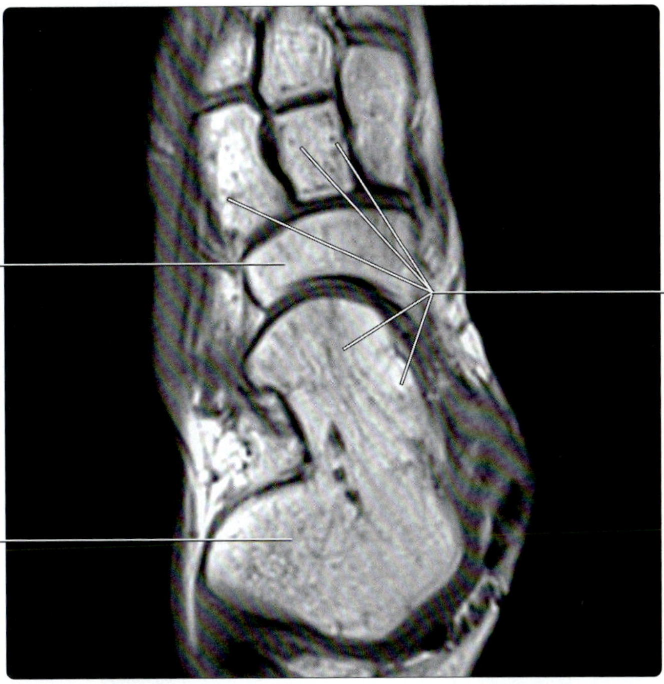

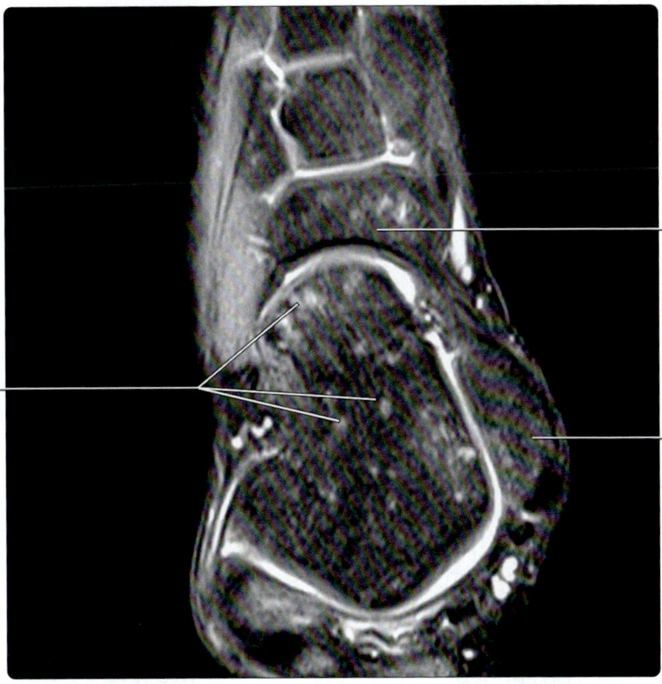

(Top) *Axial T1WI MR in a 12-year-old boy shows multiple islands of low signal intensity in the marrow. These are thought to represent residual erythropoietic marrow and resolve by ~ 13-14 years of age.* **(Bottom)** *Axial PD FS MR in the same patient shows the red marrow foci become bright on fluid-sensitive sequences. A few of the foci are labeled. Patient age, the generalized distribution of small foci, and the absence of localizing findings are helpful in making the correct diagnosis of residual erythropoietic marrow.*

ACCESSORY NAVICULAR BONE

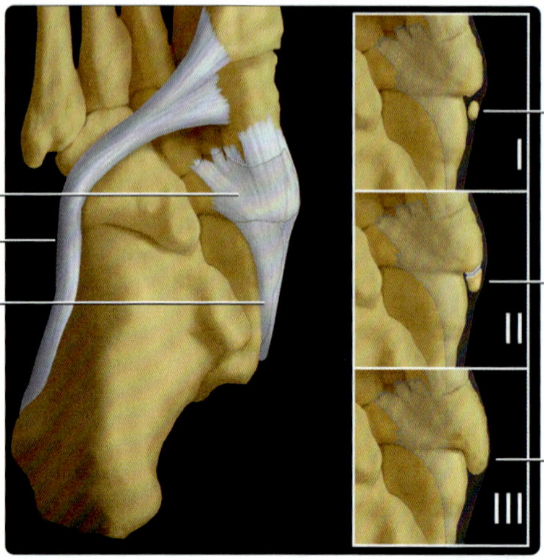

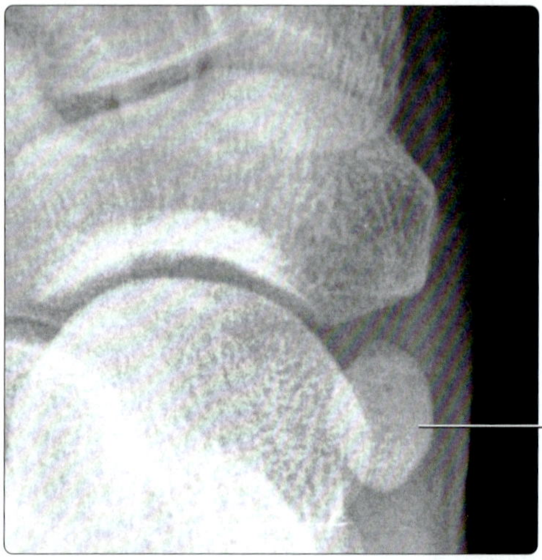

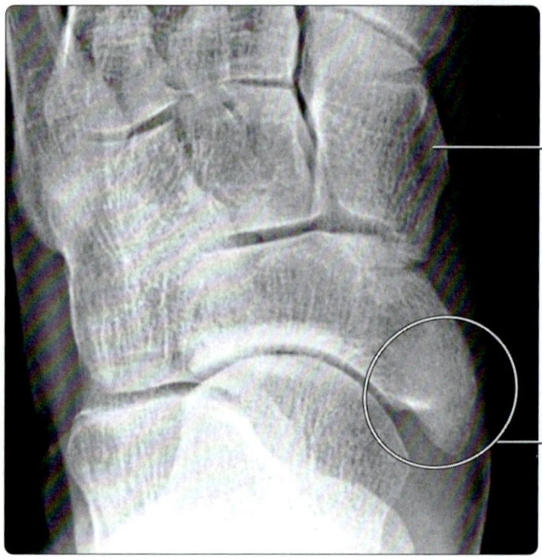

(Top) *Graphic shows plantar view of accessory navicular (os tibiale externum) variants. Normally, tibialis posterior tendon attaches to plantar aspect of median eminence of navicular. A type 1 accessory navicular is a sesamoid in the posterior tibial tendon. Type 2 is an accessory center of ossification. Type 3 is an elongated median eminence ("cornuate navicular").* **(Middle)** *Anteroposterior radiograph shows a large type 1 accessory navicular. This ossicle is larger than most type 1 accessory naviculars. It is distinguished from type 2 by the lack of an articular facet with the main navicular body.* **(Bottom)** *Anteroposterior radiograph shows a type 3 navicular, also called cornuate or gorilloid. This is an assimilated accessory navicular ossicle, which forms a projection at the medial eminence of the navicular. This configuration may cause impingement on shoes, especially on ski boots.*

ACCESSORY NAVICULAR BONE

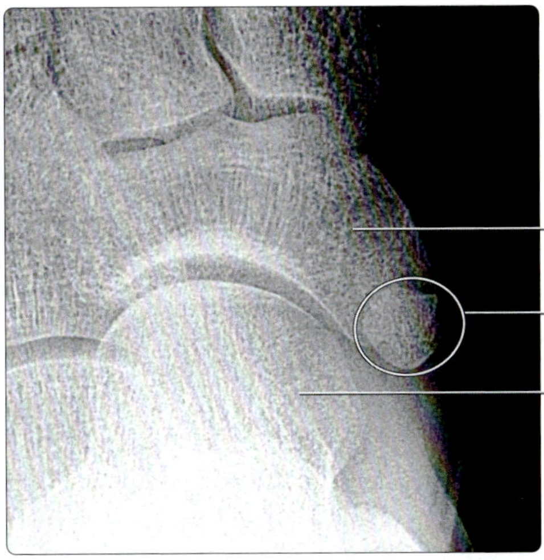

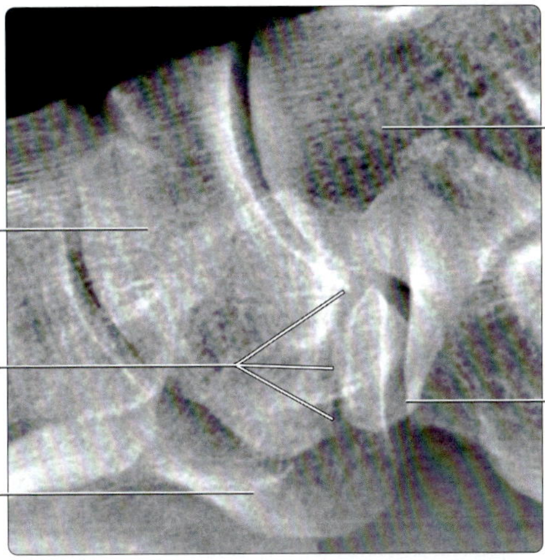

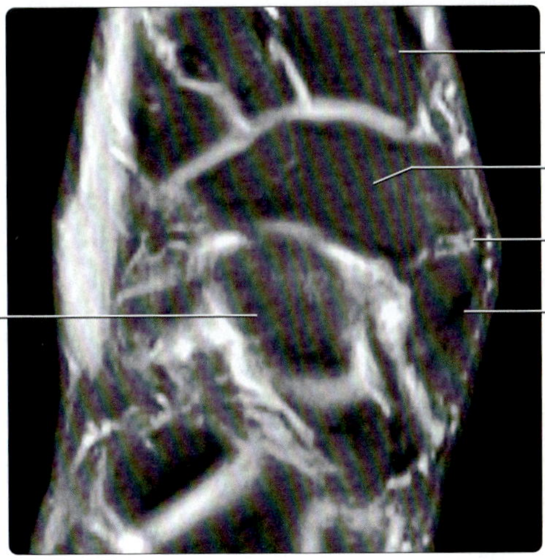

(Top) *Anteroposterior radiograph shows a rounded type 2 accessory navicular overlying the medial eminence of navicular. Synchondrosis with navicular may or may not be seen in the profile on anteroposterior view.* **(Middle)** *Lateral radiograph in the same patient shows the characteristic, relatively plantar position of an accessory navicular. Note its flat anterior facet where it is joined through a synchondrosis to the main navicular.* **(Bottom)** *Axial PD FS MR shows a type 2 accessory navicular having a flat facet joined by a synchondrosis to the parent navicular.*

ACCESSORY NAVICULAR BONE

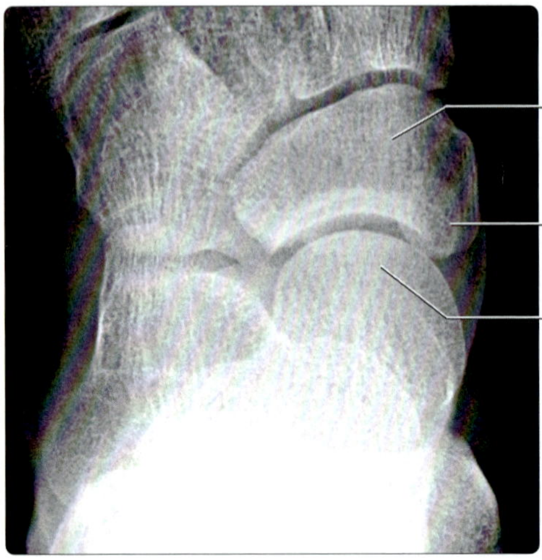

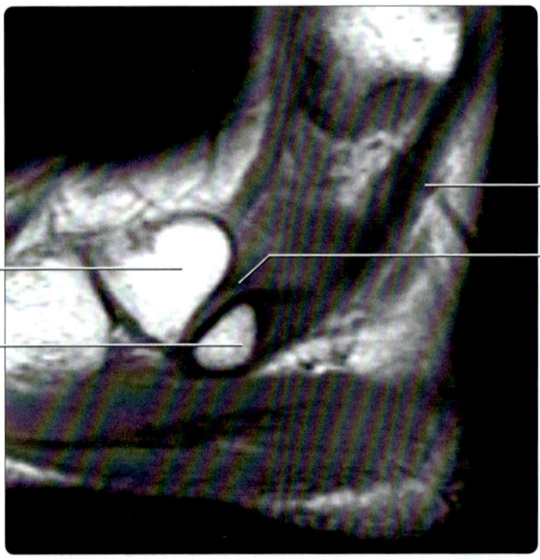

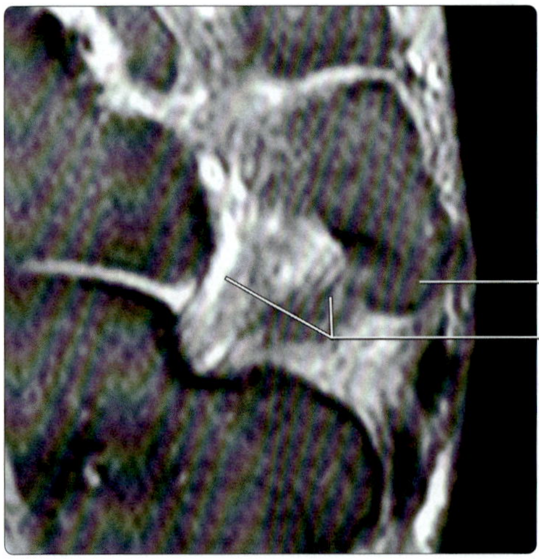

(Top) *Anteroposterior radiograph shows a type 2 accessory navicular. It appears superimposed on the median eminence of the navicular because it is at the plantar margin of navicular.* **(Middle)** *Sagittal PD MR in the same patient shows a plantar position of type 2 accessory navicular relative to the median eminence of navicular. The accessory ossicle has a flat superior facet and articulates with the navicular via a synchondrosis. Note the attachment of the posterior tibial tendon to accessory navicular, stressing the synchondrosis and predisposing to posterior tibial tendon dysfunction.* **(Bottom)** *Axial PD FS MR shows a type 3 accessory navicular. The spring ligament is seen attaching both to the bony prominence and more medially to the main portion of the navicular.*

NAVICULAR VARIANTS

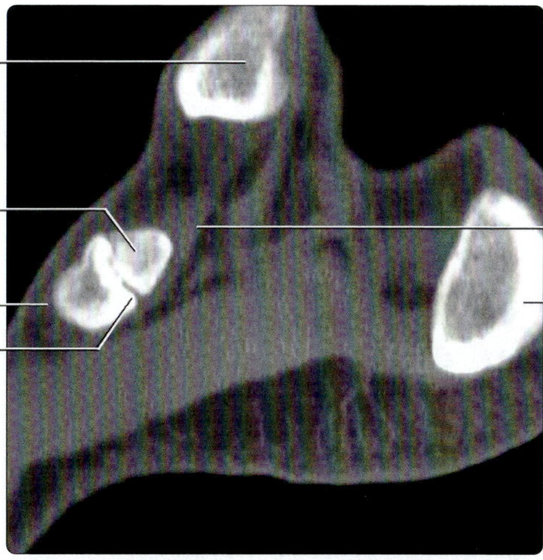

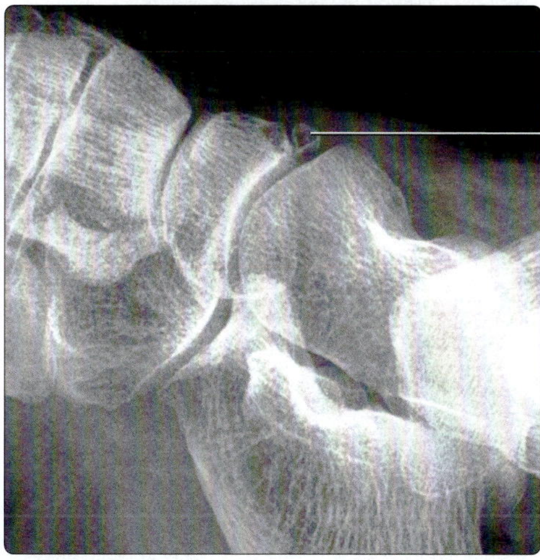

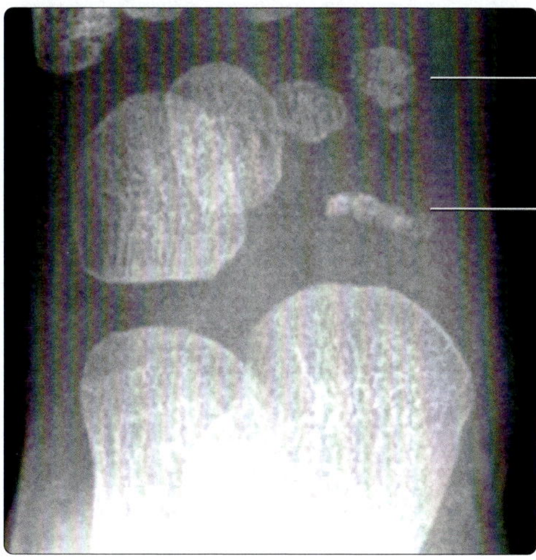

(Top) *Sagittal CT shows a type 2 accessory navicular and a synchondrosis.* **(Middle)** *Lateral radiograph shows a triangular ossicle at the proximal, dorsal margin of the navicular. Os supranaviculare is also known as os talonaviculare dorsale or Pirie bone. Many so-called cases of os supranaviculare probably represent old, nonunited fractures.* **(Bottom)** *Anteroposterior radiograph shows an irregular, flattened, sclerotic but asymptomatic navicular. The appearance resolves as the child grows. Note also the dual ossification centers for the 1st cuneiform, also a normal variant. Köhler disease is avascular necrosis of the navicular in childhood and cannot be distinguished radiographically from the normal variant, so diagnosis is made on clinical findings.*

OS CUBOIDES SECONDARIUM

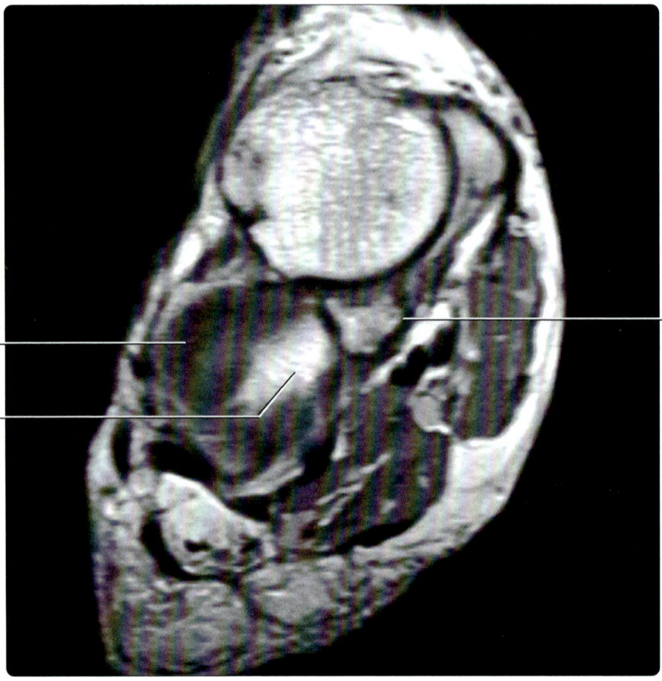

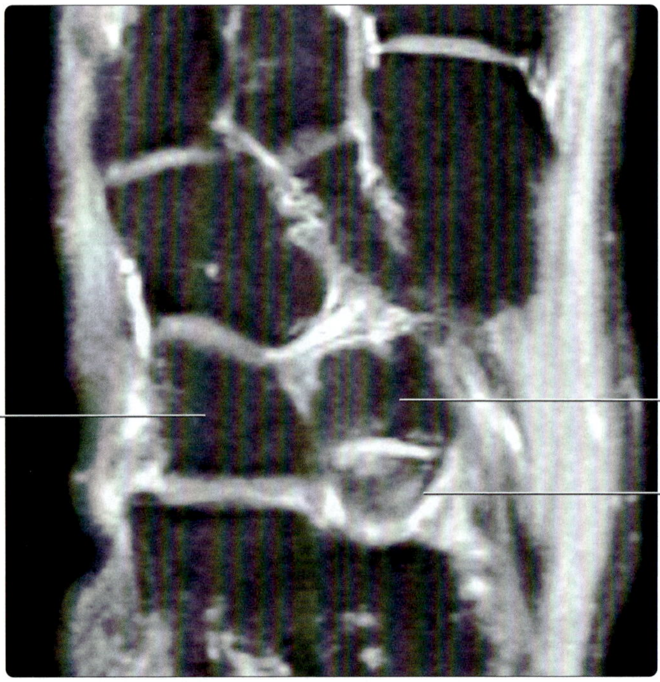

(Top) *Coronal T1WI MR shows cuboides secondarium ossicle at the proximal, medial, and superior margin of the cuboid between the cuboid and the navicular. This ossicle is rare and difficult to see on radiographs.* **(Bottom)** *Axial PD FS MR shows the relationship of the cuboides secondarium ossicle to both the cuboid and navicular.*

OS PERONEUM

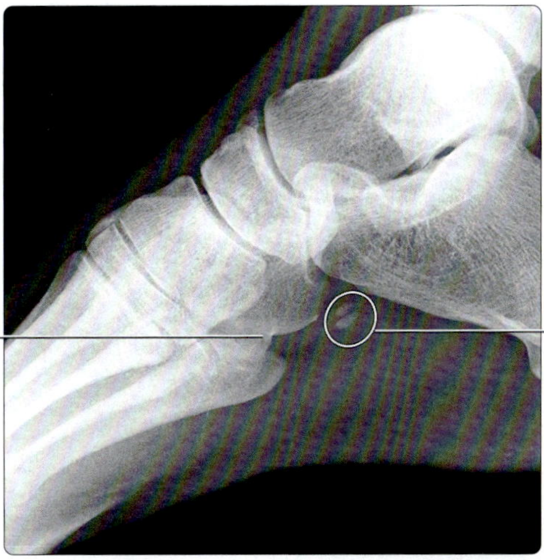

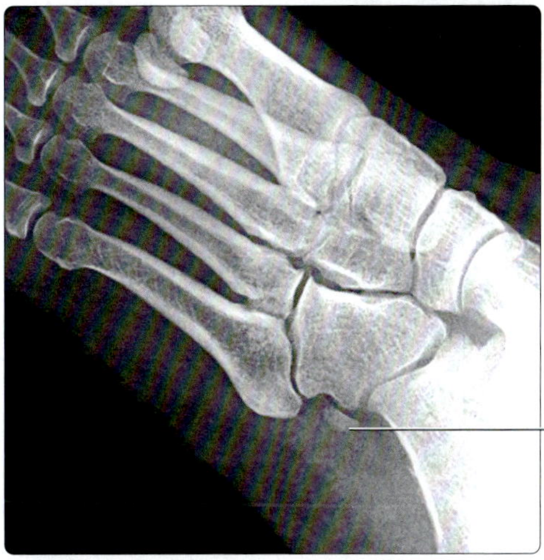

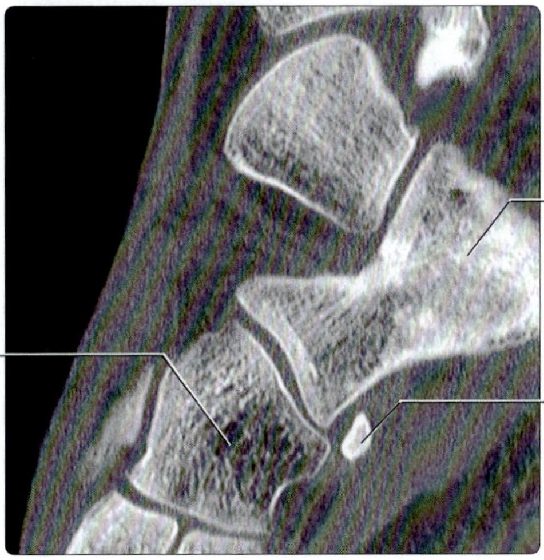

(Top) *Lateral radiograph shows bipartite os peroneum. The os peroneum may be unipartite, bipartite, or multipartite. It lies in the peroneus longus tendon, adjacent to the calcaneocuboid joint or cuboid. Proximal displacement of os peroneum can be seen as a radiographic manifestation of a peroneus longus tendon rupture.* **(Middle)** *Oblique radiograph shows unipartite os peroneum. The ossicle is just proximal to the point where the peroneus longus courses under the cuboid sulcus.* **(Bottom)** *Sagittal CT reformation depicts an os peroneum adjacent to the calcaneocuboid joint.*

OS VESALIANUM

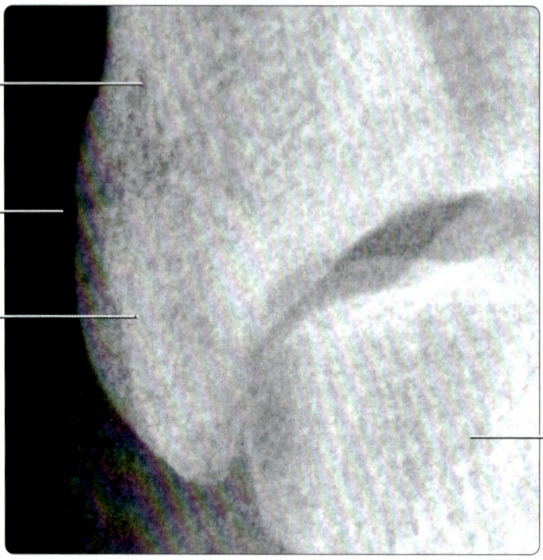

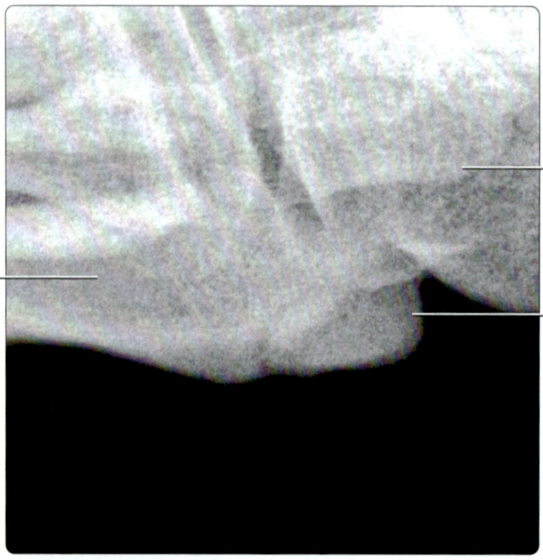

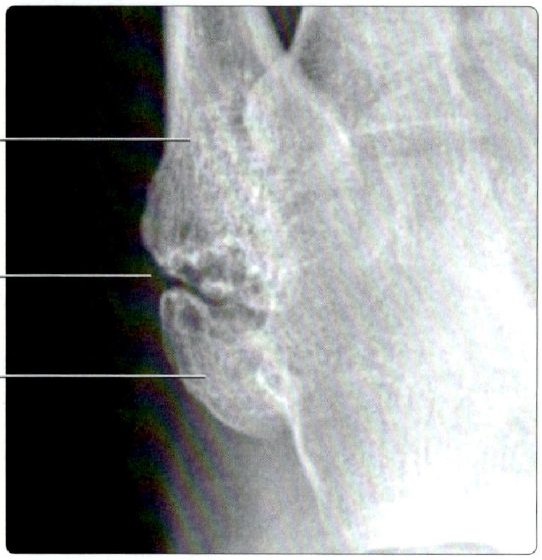

(Top) *On anteroposterior radiograph, the os vesalianum overlies the styloid process of the 5th metatarsal, and a synchondrosis may be mistaken for a fracture.* **(Middle)** *Lateral radiograph in the same patient shows the rounded contour of the ossicle, consistent with accessory center of ossification rather than a fracture.* **(Bottom)** *Anteroposterior radiograph shows a patient with a large os vesalianum and multiple cysts at the synchondrosis between the os and the 5th metatarsal base. Cysts are most likely stress related due to tugging of the peroneus brevis on the os vesalianum and indirectly on the synchondrosis.*

TARSOMETATARSAL JOINT VARIANTS

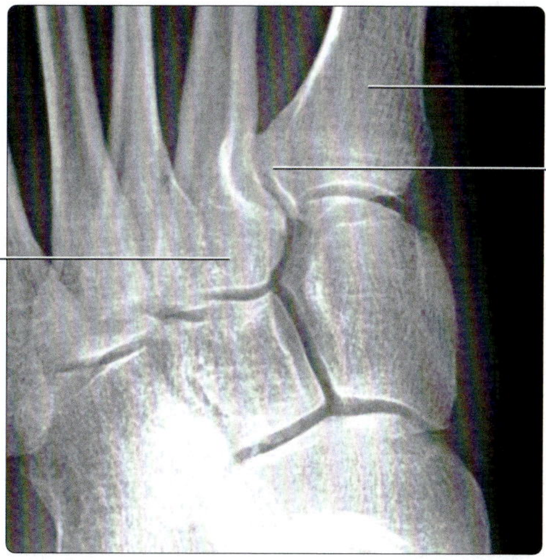

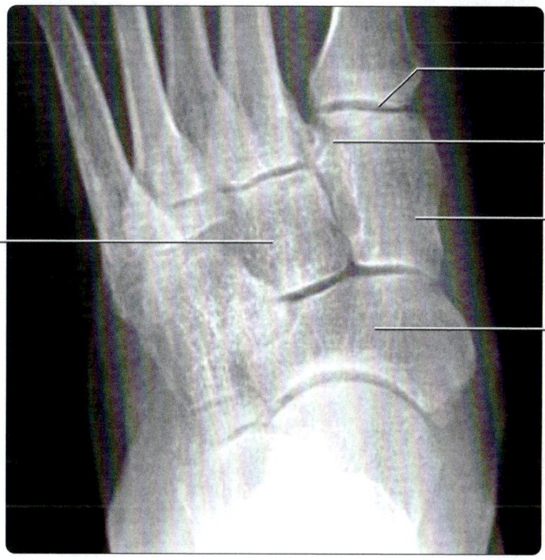

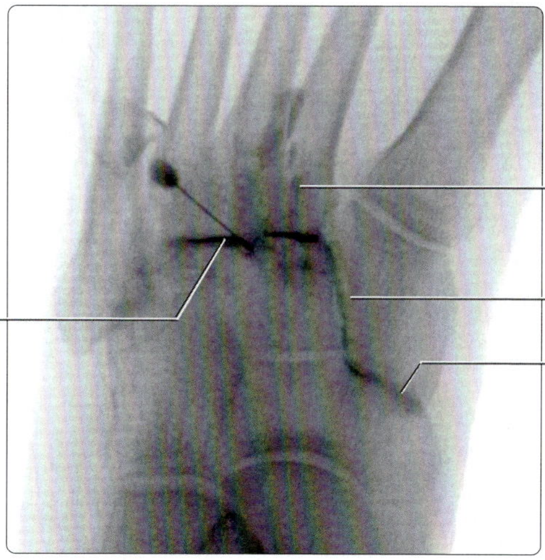

(Top) *Anteroposterior radiograph shows an articulation between the bases of the 1st and 2nd metatarsals. This joint may be absent, small, or fairly large, as in this case.* **(Middle)** *Anteroposterior radiograph shows an uncommon accessory articulation between the 1st cuneiform and the 2nd metatarsal.* **(Bottom)** *Anteroposterior radiograph from the 3rd tarsometatarsal arthrogram shows a normal variant of extension of contrast between the 1st and 2nd cuneiforms as well as into the naviculocuneiform joint. In most feet, the 2nd and 3rd tarsometatarsal joints form a separate cavity. Extension into the 2nd intermetatarsal joint is usually present, as in this case.*

OS INTERMETATARSEUM

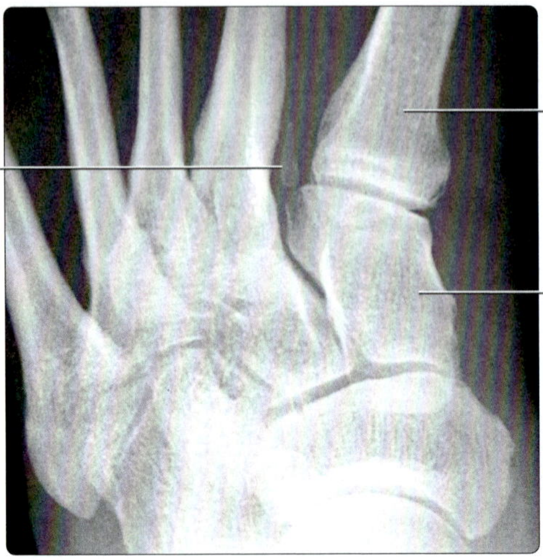

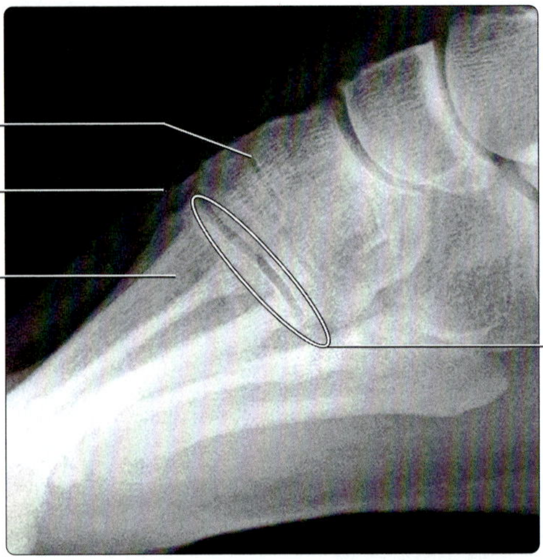

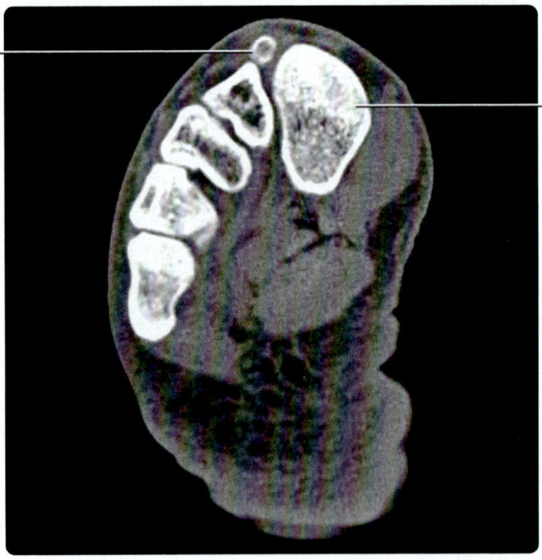

(Top) *Anteroposterior radiograph shows a teardrop-shaped os intermetatarseum arising between the 1st and 2nd metatarsal bases. Occasionally, this ossicle will be partially assimilated to the 1st metatarsal base.* **(Middle)** *On this lateral radiograph, the ossicle is dorsal in position, adjacent to the base of the 1st metatarsal.* **(Bottom)** *On this coronal CT, the os intermetatarseum is rounded in appearance, and no donor site from adjacent bones is visible. These signs help distinguish it from a fracture fragment.*

METATARSAL VARIANTS

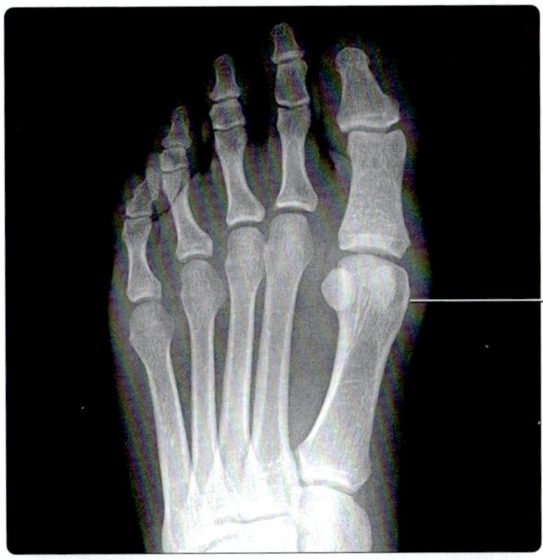

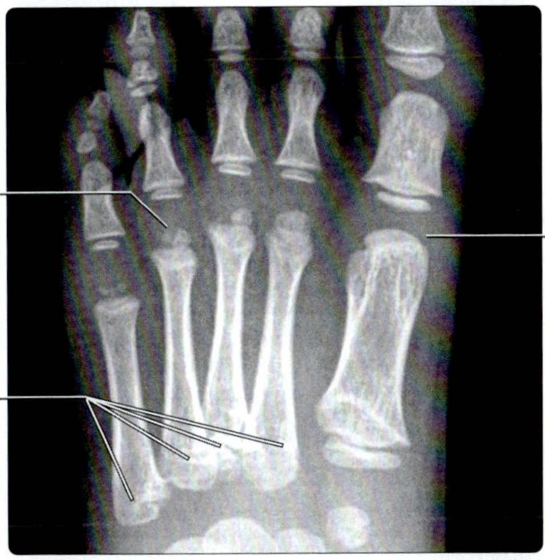

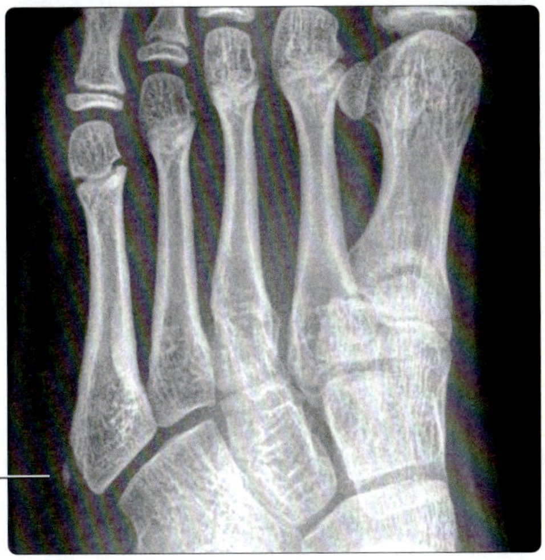

(Top) *Anteroposterior radiograph shows Morton foot configuration. The 1st metatarsal is significantly shorter than the 2nd. This is a very common variant that increases stress on the 2nd metatarsal head.* **(Middle)** *Anteroposterior radiograph shows multiple accessory epiphyses of the metatarsals. The normal ossification center for the 1st metatarsal is at the proximal end of the bone. The normal ossification centers of the remaining metatarsals are distal. Accessory epiphyses may form at the opposite end of the metatarsal from normal epiphysis. Accessory epiphyses may be complete or incomplete.* **(Bottom)** *Normal apophysis at the base of the 5th metatarsal is shown. Fractures in this location tend to be horizontally oriented, while apophysis is longitudinally oriented.*

1ST METATARSOPHALANGEAL SESAMOID VARIANTS

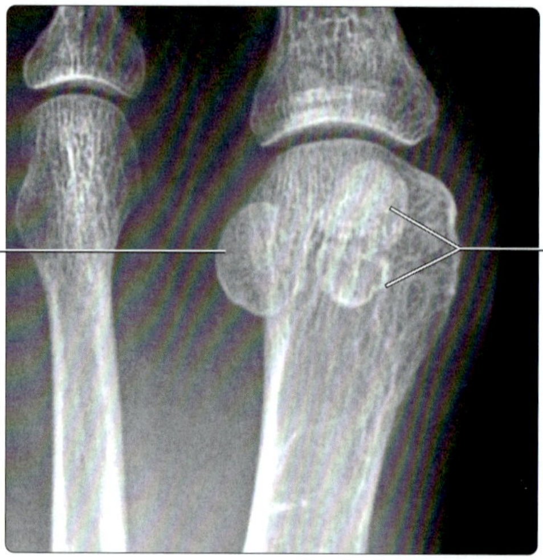

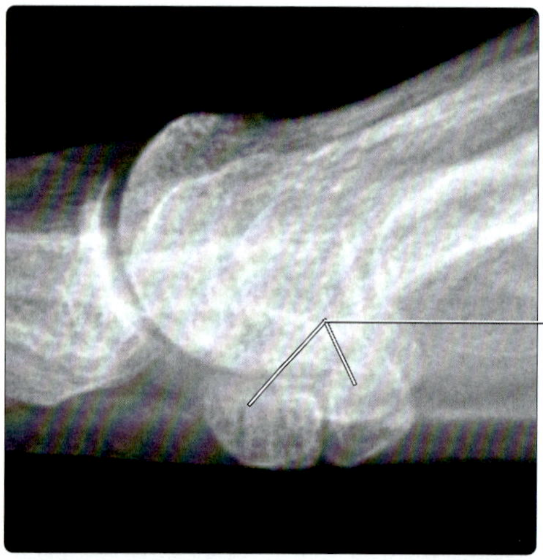

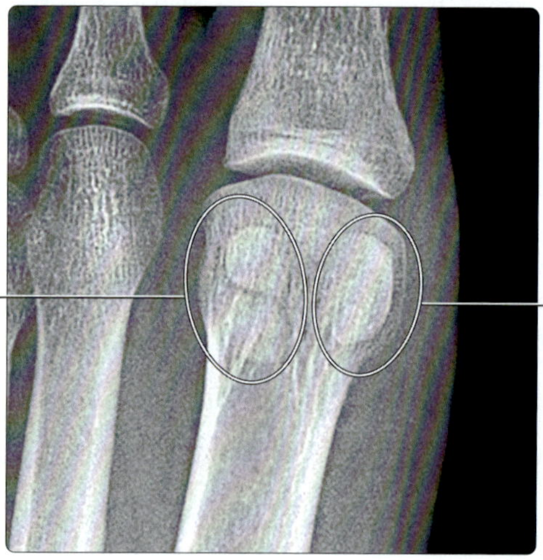

(Top) *Anteroposterior radiograph shows bipartite medial sesamoid of the 1st toe and unipartite lateral sesamoid.* **(Middle)** *Lateral radiograph shows a rounded contour characteristic of bipartite sesamoids. Fracture fragments, in contrast, will show angular margins.* **(Bottom)** *Anteroposterior radiograph shows bipartite lateral sesamoid of the 1st toe and unipartite medial sesamoid. Bipartite sesamoids are usually more rounded in contour than fractured sesamoids. Bipartite sesamoids are usually larger than unipartite sesamoids. Bipartite sesamoids may or may not be present on contralateral foot.*

SESAMOID VARIANTS

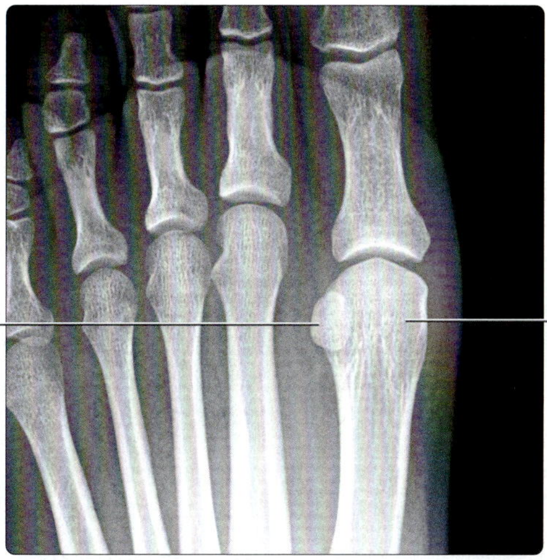

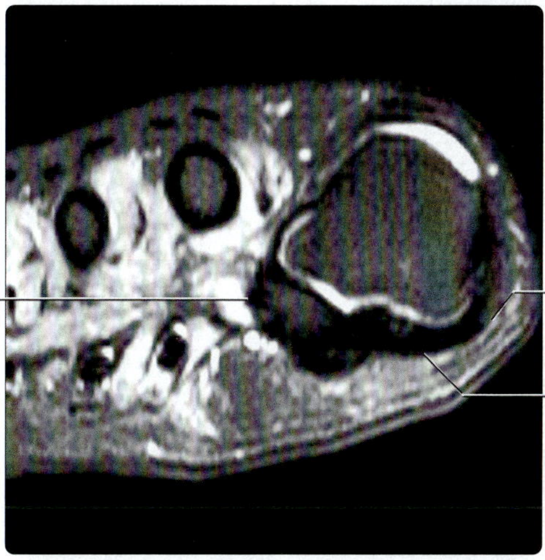

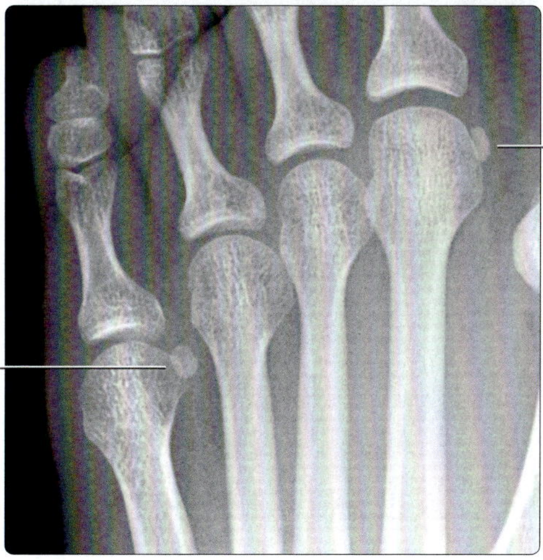

(Top) *Anteroposterior radiograph shows absent medial sesamoid in a patient with no history of trauma. This is a very rare normal variant, and most cases where the sesamoid is not visible probably reflect resorption of the sesamoid after remote trauma.* **(Middle)** *Coronal T2WI FS MR in the same patient confirms absence of the medial sesamoid.* **(Bottom)** *Anteroposterior radiograph shows sesamoids of the 2nd and 5th metatarsal heads. Sesamoids of the lateral toes are variably present. They are always small and may be round or oval. The 5th toe may have medial and lateral sesamoids.*

TOE VARIANTS

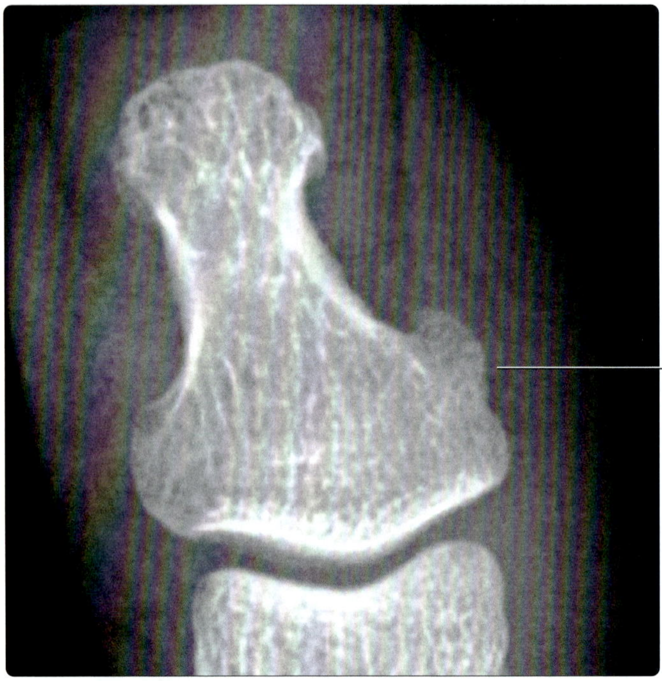

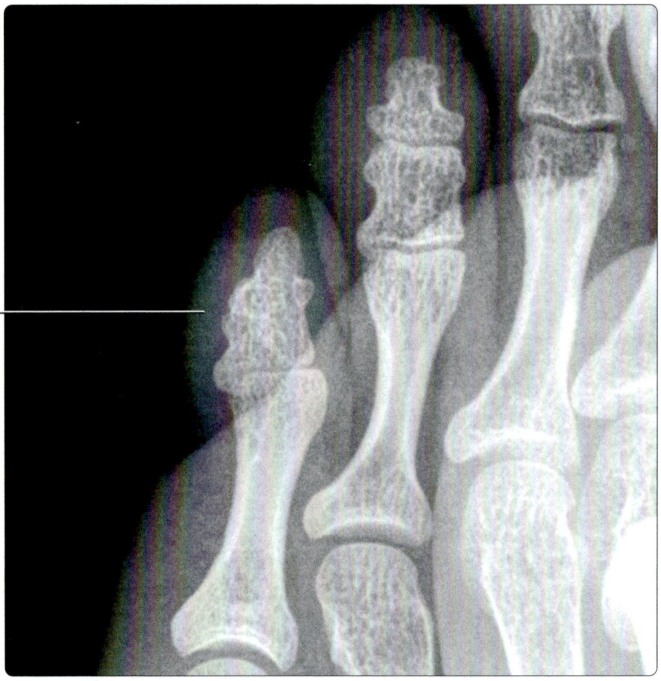

(Top) *Anteroposterior radiograph shows an exostosis from the medial margin, the base of the 1st distal phalanx. This is commonly seen, often large and asymptomatic.* **(Bottom)** *Anteroposterior radiograph shows failure of segmentation of the middle and distal phalanges of the 5th toe. This is a very common normal variant.*

SOLEUS VARIANTS

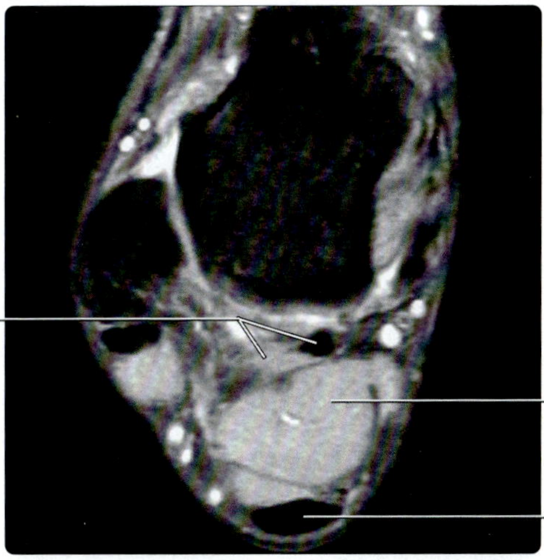

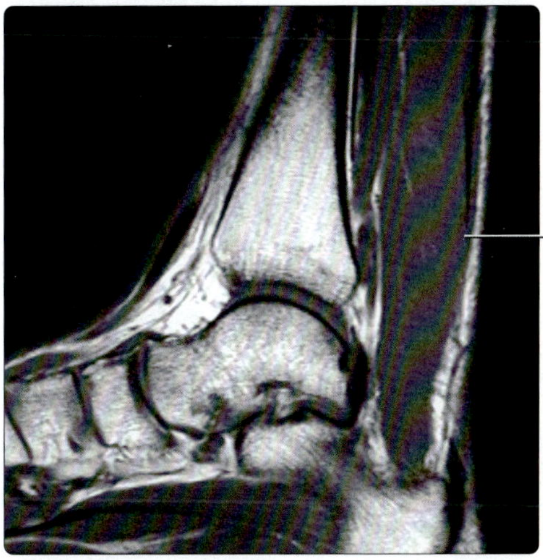

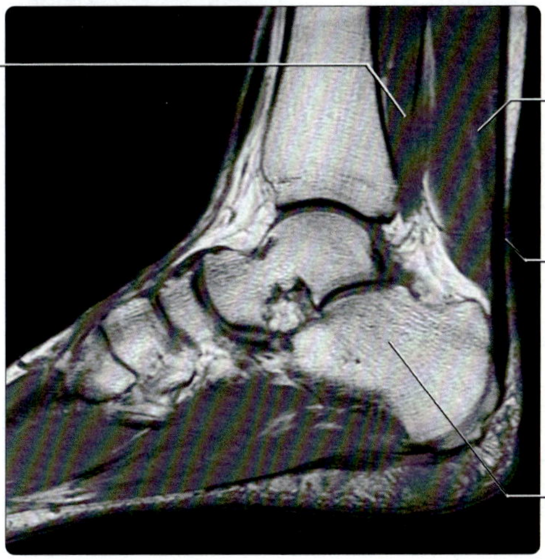

(Top) *Axial PD FS MR shows a bulky accessory soleus muscle anterior to the Achilles tendon. The muscle arises from the anterior margin of soleus and inserts on the medial margin of calcaneus.* **(Middle)** *Sagittal T1WI MR shows a bulky accessory soleus muscle extending to the medial margin of the posterior process of calcaneus. This anomalous muscle may present clinically as a mass or may cause impingement.* **(Bottom)** *Sagittal MR of the low-lying soleus muscle in an asymptomatic patient is shown. In most individuals, the soleus muscle ends between 2.5-7.5 cm above the calcaneus. In ~ 12.5% of individuals, however, the musculotendinous unit is 0.0-2.5 cm above the calcaneus. A low-lying soleus muscle may present clinically as calf fullness. (Courtesy J. Bencardino, MD.)*

ACCESSORY FLEXOR MUSCLES

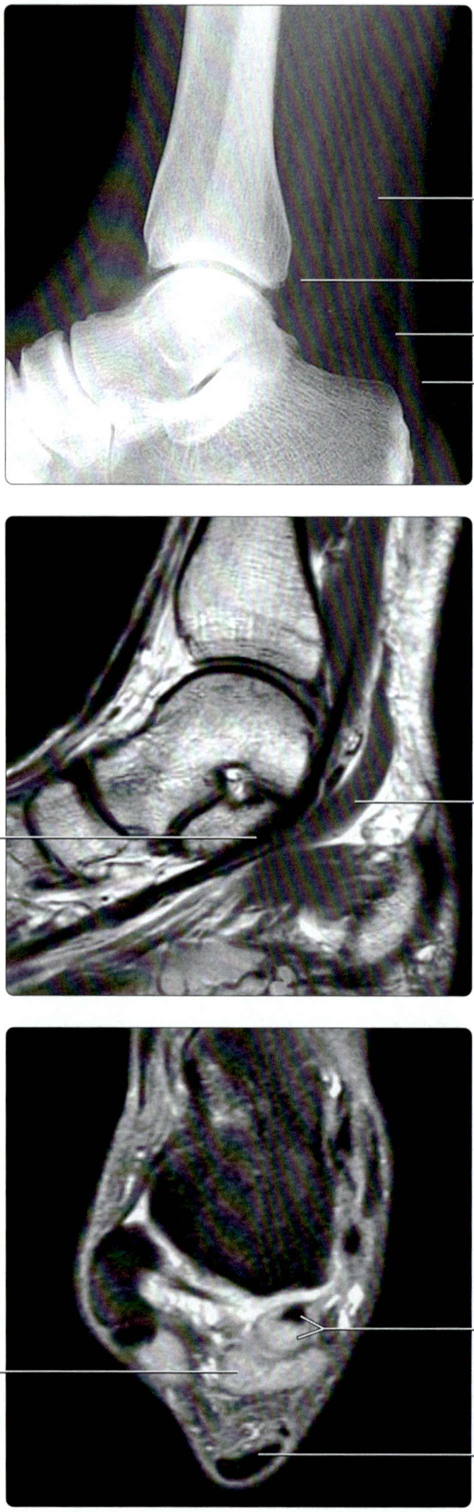

(Top) *Lateral radiograph shows fusiform soft tissue density posterior to the flexor hallucis longus muscle, consistent with an accessory muscle.* **(Middle)** *Sagittal T2WI MR in the same patient shows that the muscle travels with and attaches to the flexor hallucis longus tendon. Due to mass effect from the anomalous muscle, patients may present with tarsal tunnel syndrome or with impingement when the foot is plantar flexed. This patient, a ballerina, had limited plantar flexion, which resolved after excision of accessory muscle.* **(Bottom)** *Axial PD MR in the same patient shows the accessory flexor hallucis longus muscle posterior to the flexor hallucis longus.*

ACCESSORY FLEXOR MUSCLES

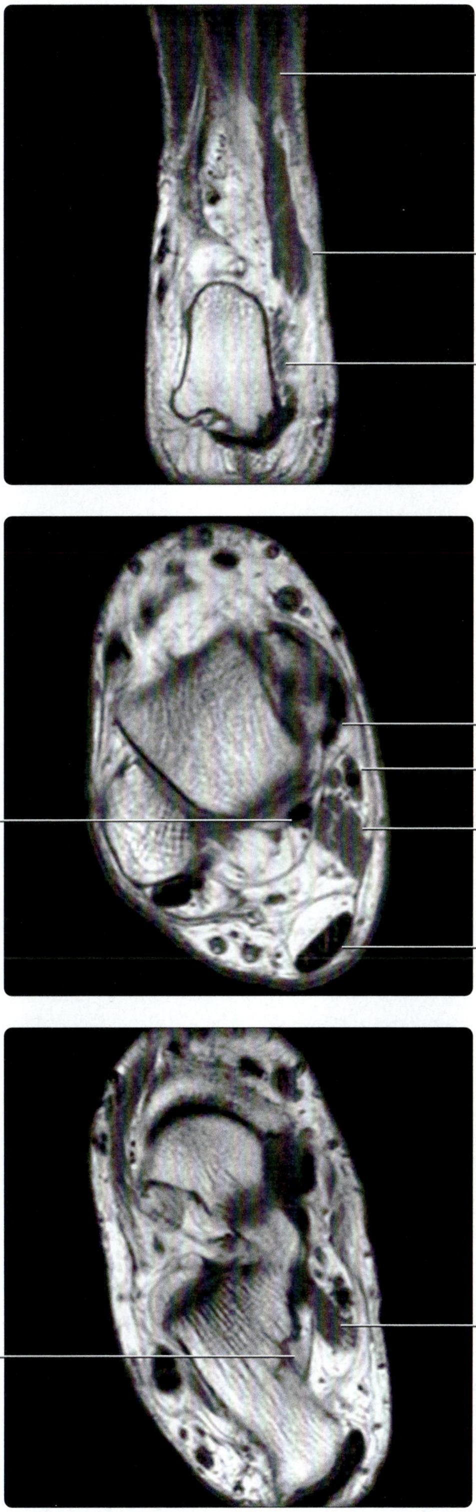

(Top) *Coronal T1WI MR shows the accessory flexor digitorum longus muscle arising from the belly of the flexor digitorum longus muscle and inserting on the quadratus plantae muscle.* **(Middle)** *Axial PD MR shows the position of the accessory flexor digitorum longus muscle immediately posterior to the flexor digitorum longus tendon and neurovascular bundle.* **(Bottom)** *Axial PD MR shows the muscle near its attachment to the atrophic quadratus plantae muscle.*

FLEXOR MUSCLE VARIANTS

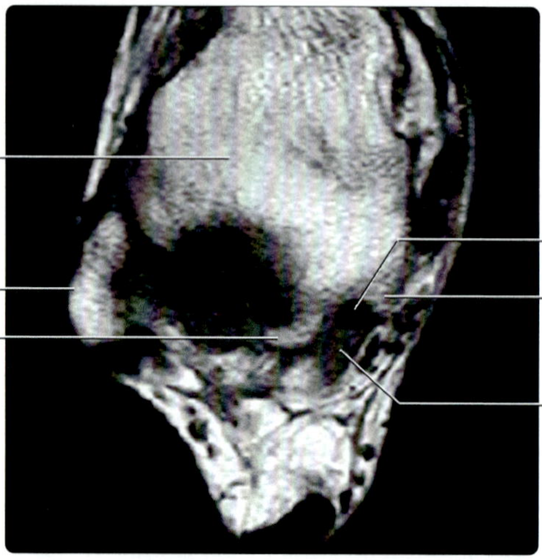

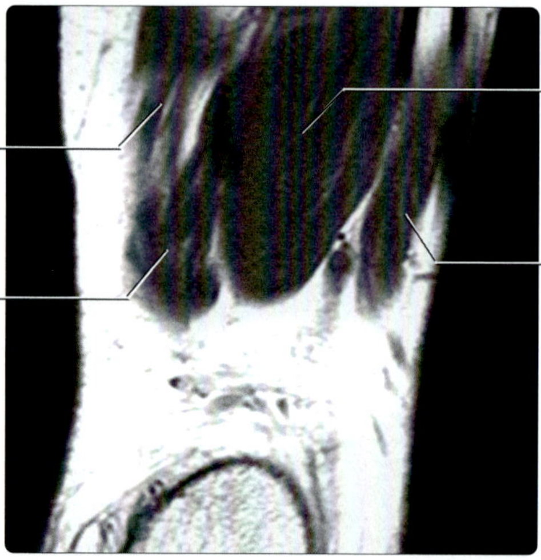

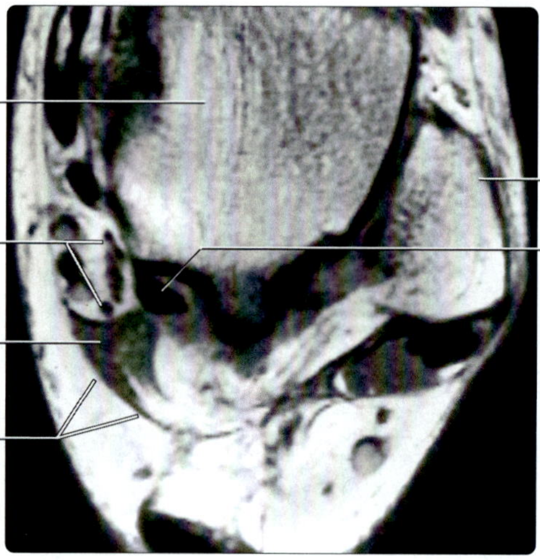

(Top) *Axial T1WI MR depicts low-lying flexor hallucis longus muscle fibers in the talar fibroosseous tunnel between medial and lateral talar tubercles of the posterior talar process. This variant can produce crowding and limit smooth gliding of the tendon in the talar tunnel during foot plantar and dorsiflexion.* **(Middle)** *The accessory flexor digitorum longus muscle is optimally visualized on axial images but may be detected on coronal and sagittal images as well.* **(Bottom)** *The accessory flexor digitorum longus muscle frequently originates directly from the flexor retinaculum in the ankle region. In those instances, it is typically triangular in shape with the apex pointing toward the talus or tibia and base, abutting against the flexor retinaculum. Because of variable origins and insertions of the accessory flexor digitorum longus and accessory flexor hallucis longus muscles, they are lumped by some authors under the category of "long accessory of long flexors," or "quadratus plantae."*

PERONEUS QUARTUS

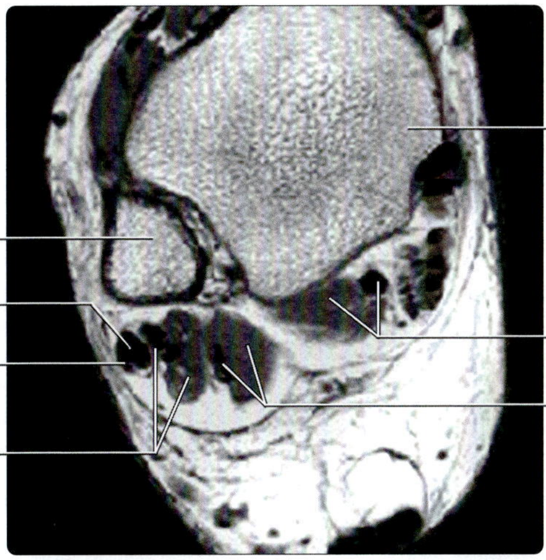

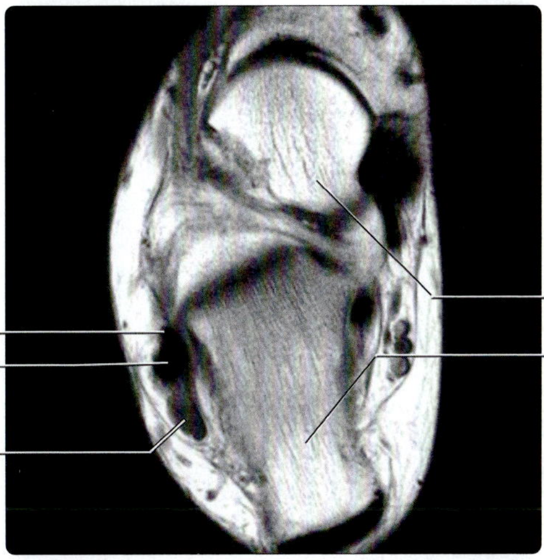

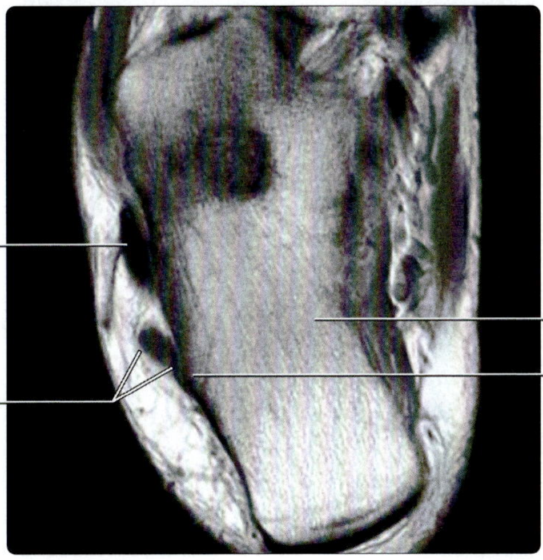

(Top) *The peroneus quartus is frequently seen on axial MR images as an accessory muscle/tendon distinct and medial to the peroneus brevis muscle. The presence of the peroneus quartus muscle on ankle MR study should prompt the radiologist to search for peroneal tendon tears or dislocation. Note the incidental finding of an accessory slip of the peroneus longus tendon.* **(Middle)** *The normal peroneus brevis is tendinous by the level of the retromalleolar groove, although significant variations in its distal extent have been described. In this case, a separate peroneus quartus is visible posterior to the peroneus longus and brevis tendons.* **(Bottom)** *The peroneus quartus inserts into the retrotrochlear eminence and not into the peroneal tubercle (as stated in many reports). The retrotrochlear eminence is seen in 98% of normal individuals posterior and slightly inferior to the peroneal tubercle. The eminence is typically seen on axial MR images and can be quite small, as seen in this patient.*

SECTION 7
Needle Placement for Procedures

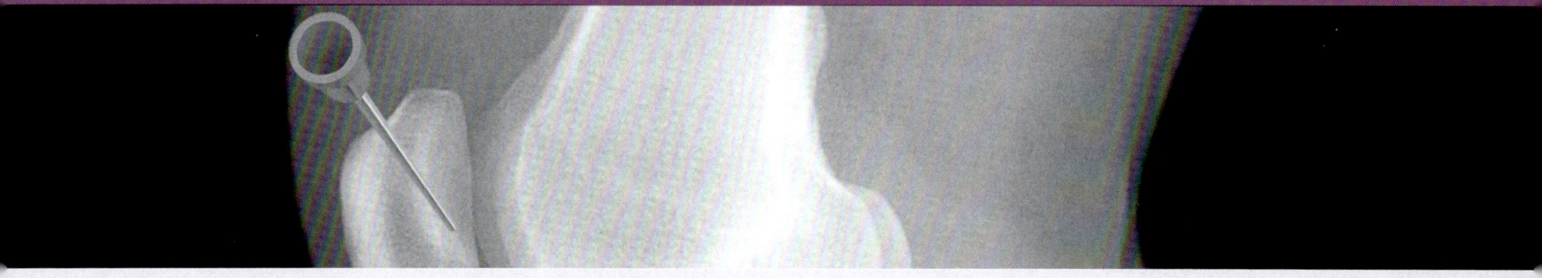

ANATOMY IMAGING ISSUES

Imaging Recommendations

- **Choice of imaging guidance**
  - May perform under fluoroscopy or ultrasound
    - Matter of operator preference
- **Therapeutic injection**: To alleviate pain, decrease inflammation
  - Medication: Anesthetic, steroid, hyaluronic acid preparations, platelet rich plasma (PRP)
    - Steroid choices include betamethasone, triamcinolone, or methylprednisolone acetate
    - 1 mg betamethasone or equivalent in small joints, 2 mg in large joints
  - Confirm position of needle
    - Fluoroscopy: Inject air or iodinated contrast to confirm position
    - Ultrasound: Inject anesthetic under direct visualization to confirm position
- **Diagnostic injection**: Evaluate internal derangement of joint
  - Usually in conjunction with CT or MR
  - Monitor joint distension under fluoroscopy
  - Inject until joint recesses filled, or patient complains of pain
  - Overdistention may cause extravasation
- **Diagnostic aspiration**
  - To evaluate for infection, inflammatory arthritis, or crystal-induced arthropathy
  - Use shortest needle possible, as length of needle increases resistance to aspiration
- **Choice of needle size**
  - Knee: 18- or 20-gauge needle
    - Synovial fluid drips out when needle intraarticular
  - Ankle, foot: 25-gauge needle
    - Except 18 gauge for aspiration of infected joint
- **Tendon sheath injection**
  - Used for therapy of tenosynovitis

Imaging Pitfalls

- **Complications of injection**
  - Allergy rare in arthrography but include risk in consent
    - May present with persistent pain and effusion, treat with Benadryl 25-50 mg orally
  - Infection exceedingly rare, estimated between 1:10,000 and 1:20,000
    - May have delayed presentation up to 1 month
    - Avoid with careful technique, single-use vials: **Never** reuse materials
  - Nerve anesthesia
    - Transient, avoid with consideration of nerve anatomy
  - Bleeding
    - Largely avoided with use of small needles
    - Arthrography can be done on patients on anticoagulation therapy
    - Apply pressure after procedure
- **Unusual communications between joints**
  - Important to document when performing therapeutic injections
  - Response to therapy may not be from targeted joint but from communicating joints

JOINT INJECTION

Basic Approach to Fluoroscopic-Guided Injection

- Picture 3D anatomy prior to needle placement
- Position patient so joint in profile
- Always palpate for arteries in area
- Advance needle to bone, withdraw minimally
  - Slight curve to needle tip often seen and indicates intraarticular location
- If needle tip in joint or tendon sheath, fluid easily injected with minimal force
  - Can do test injection with anesthetic
  - Confirm intraarticular position with air or iodinated contrast
- Use connector tubing between needle and syringe to avoid radiation to hands
  - Stabilize needle with side of hand against skin while attaching tubing
    - Prevents inadvertently moving needle
- For MR arthrography, fill needle hub with fluid prior to injection
  - Prevents air bubbles
- Always document any injection, preferably with 2 views

Basic Approach to Ultrasound-Guided Injection

- Basics of ultrasound joint access
  - Picture 3D anatomy prior to needle placement
  - Choose approach to avoid vessels and nerves
  - Place transducer to see both sides of joint
  - Needle approach as parallel to transducer as possible
  - Inject under direct visualization, confirm joint distends with anesthetic
  - Inject therapeutic agent(s)

Knee Joint Injection

- Position patient supine, with knee flexed about 30° over rolled pillow
- Patient must relax quadriceps
- Needle should be placed between patella and femur distal to superior-inferior midpoint of patella
  - More superior placement may bury tip of needle in prefemoral fat pad
- Needle approach may be either medially or laterally beneath patella
  - Medial approach slightly easier because of tilt of medial patellar facet
  - To "open" patellofemoral joint for needle placement, push from opposite side of patella while advancing needle
- Once needle is intraarticular, effusion should be aspirated
  - Maximize fluid aspiration by "milking" effusion from suprapatellar bursa with one hand while aspirating with other
- Knee joint may communicate with proximal tibiofibular joint in up to 20% of cases

Proximal Tibiofibular Joint Injection

- Patient in lateral position, affected side up
- Rotate joint until in profile
- Entry point center of joint

Ankle Joint Injection

- Patient supine, anterior needle approach, avoid dorsalis pedis artery
- Usual point of entry between extensor tendons
  - If severe arthritis present, easier to enter medial or lateral gutters
- Joint normally communicates with flexor hallucis longus tendon sheath
- **Fluoroscopy**
  - On AP image, needle enters below visualized joint and angles superiorly
  - Often easiest to place with lateral fluoroscopy
- **Ultrasound**
  - Transducer vertically positioned along anterior tibia, needle entry from below

Posterior Subtalar Joint Injection

- Patient lateral decubitus position, affected foot lateral side up
- Point of entry lateral, at anterior margin of joint
- Normal recess extends anterior to articular surfaces, into posterior aspect of tarsal sinus
- May communicate with ankle joint: Important to document for therapeutic injections

Talocalaneonavicular Joint Injection

- Middle & anterior subtalar joints & talonavicular joint communicate
  - Easiest to access them all via talonavicular injection
- Patient supine, knee flexed, foot flat on table
- Enter through center of talonavicular joint

Calcaneocuboid Joint Injection

- Patient in lateral decubitus position, affected side up

Tarsometatarsal Joint Injection

- Patient supine, knee flexed, foot flat on table
- 3 separate joint cavities: 1st tarsometatarsal, 2nd-3rd tarsometatarsal, 4th-5th tarsometatarsal
- Fluoroscopy: Angle needle along joint inclination
- Ultrasound: Transducer in longitudinal plane, needle entry from distal approach
  - Allows more space for needle entry

Metatarsophalangeal or Interphalangeal Joint Injection

- Patient supine, knee flexed, foot flat on table
- Fluoroscopy: Slight angle of needle with curve of metatarsal head
- Ultrasound: Transducer distal to joint, needle entry from proximal approach

TENDON SHEATH INJECTION

Approach to Fluoroscopic-Guided Tendon Sheath Access

- Method 1
  - Palpate tendon in position where overlying bone
  - Advance needle to bone through tendon
  - Withdraw needle tip, injecting lidocaine slowly
  - When injectate flows easily, should be in tendon sheath
  - Confirm position with injection of nonionic iodinated contrast
    - Can "push" contrast along tendon sheath with injected steroid/anesthetic
    - Technique allows visualization of adhesions in tendon sheath
    - Ability to deliver adequate amount of steroid not compromised
  - Inject therapeutic agent(s)
- Method 2
  - Palpate tendon, place needle in tendon
  - Confirm position by having patient contract muscle
    - Needle will move with muscle contraction if needle tip in tendon
  - Then withdraw needle tip slightly while injecting anesthetic
  - Injectate flows freely if needle tip in sheath but not if in tendon
  - Inject small amount of nonionic contrast for confirmation
  - Inject therapeutic agent(s)

Approach to Ultrasound-Guided Tendon Sheath Access

- Visualize tendon in short and long axis, assess for tendon tear
  - Document presence of tendinosis, tenosynovitis
- Advance 25-gauge needle into tendon sheath
  - Often best to go through tendon to stabilize needle, inject on deep side of tendon sheath
  - Usually easiest to accurately localize needle in short axis of tendon
- Inject lidocaine to slightly distend tendon sheath, confirm position
- Inject therapeutic agent(s) under ultrasound visualization

Posterior Tibial Tendon Sheath Injection

- Can inject posterior to medial malleolus or along horizontal portion of tendon
- Do not inject at tendon insertion because no tendon sheath in this location

Flexor Hallucis Longus Tendon Sheath Injection

- Inject inferior to sustentaculum tali or adjacent to medial margin of posterior process talus
  - Aim for superior margin of tendon sheath to avoid tibial nerve

Peroneal Tendon Sheath Injection

- Inject either posterior to lateral malleolus or along horizontal portion of tendon
- Fluoroscopy: Palpate peroneus brevis and longus tendons in horizontal portion

KNEE NEEDLE PLACEMENT

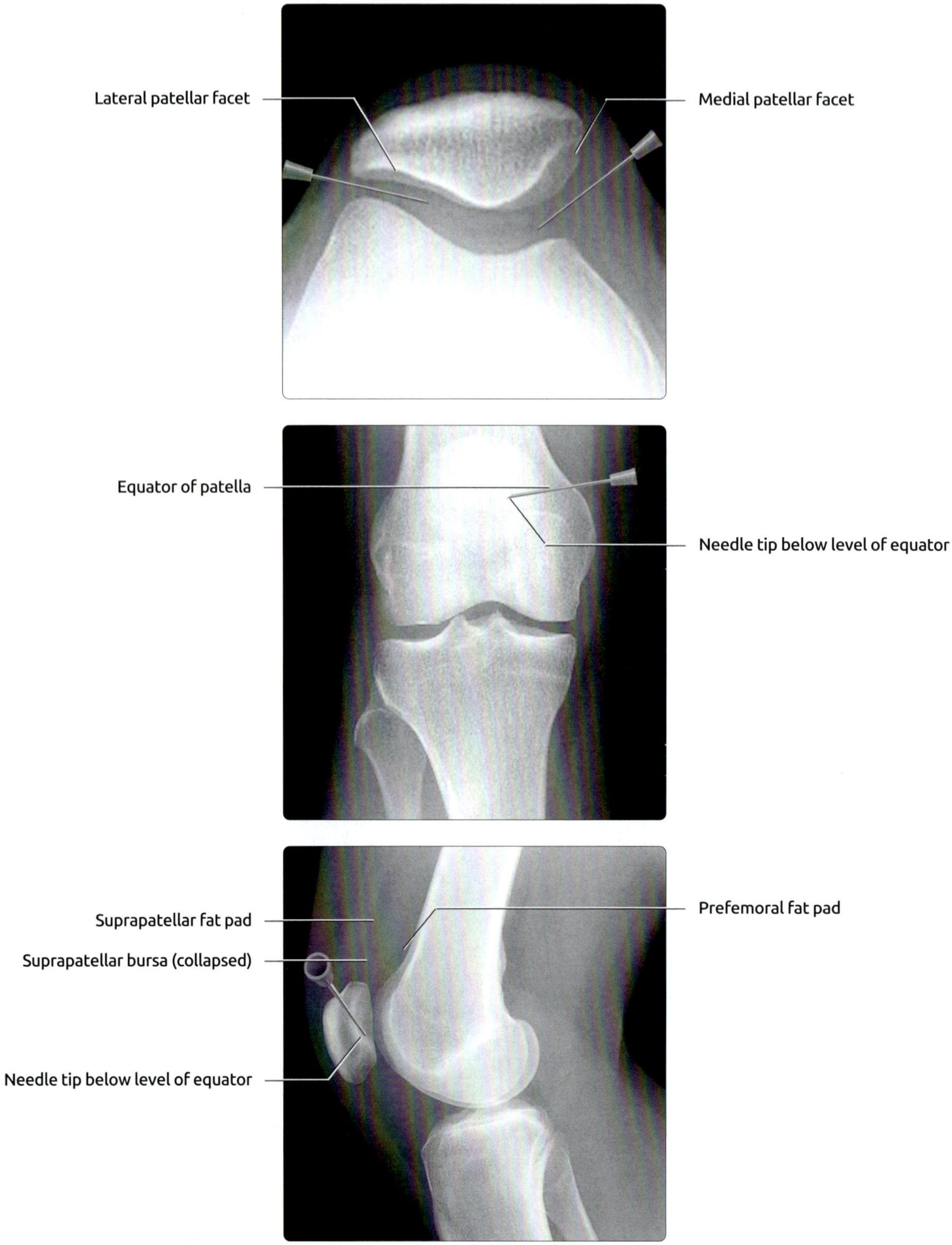

(Top) *Sunrise view shows 2 possible needle approaches to the knee joint. The medial approach is more steeply angulated than the lateral; either is relatively easy since the space between the patella and femoral condyle is easily palpated.* **(Middle)** *AP radiograph of the knee demonstrates that the needle placement should be just below the equator of the patella.* **(Bottom)** *Lateral radiograph of the knee shows a nondistended suprapatellar bursa surrounded by the suprapatellar fat pad anteriorly and the prefemoral fat pad posteriorly. The needle placement should be just below the equator of the patella to avoid inadvertent placement within the prefemoral fat pad.*

ULTRASOUND-GUIDED KNEE ASPIRATION

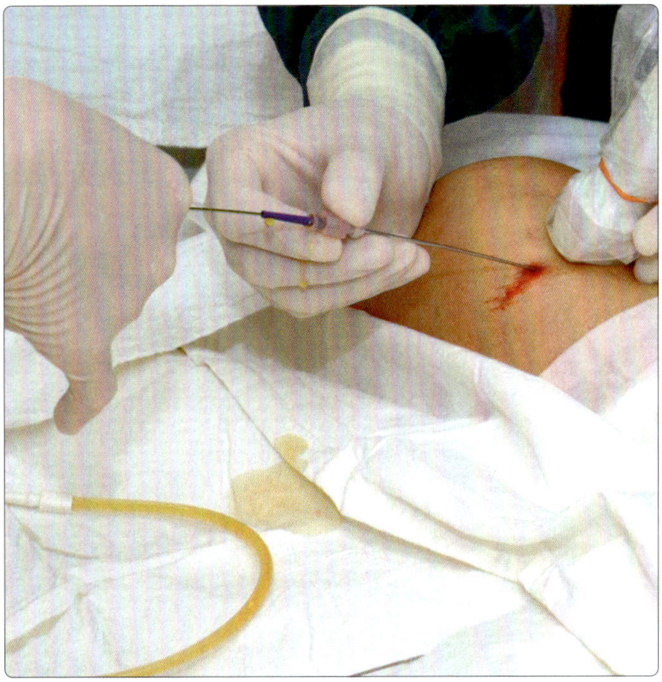

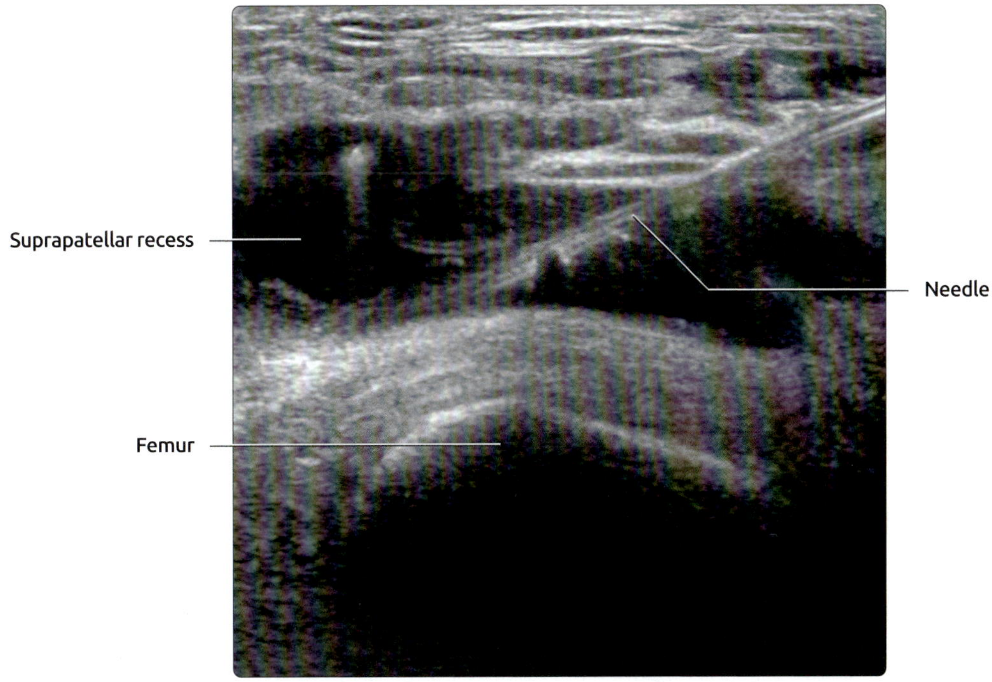

(Top) *Photograph shows puncture of knee joint under ultrasound guidance using the Seldinger technique. The transducer is held in the nondominant hand and the needle in the dominant hand, with direct visualization of the needle under ultrasound.* **(Bottom)** *Transverse ultrasound in the same patient shows needle placement in the suprapatellar recess.*

PROXIMAL TIBIOFIBULAR JOINT ARTHROGRAM

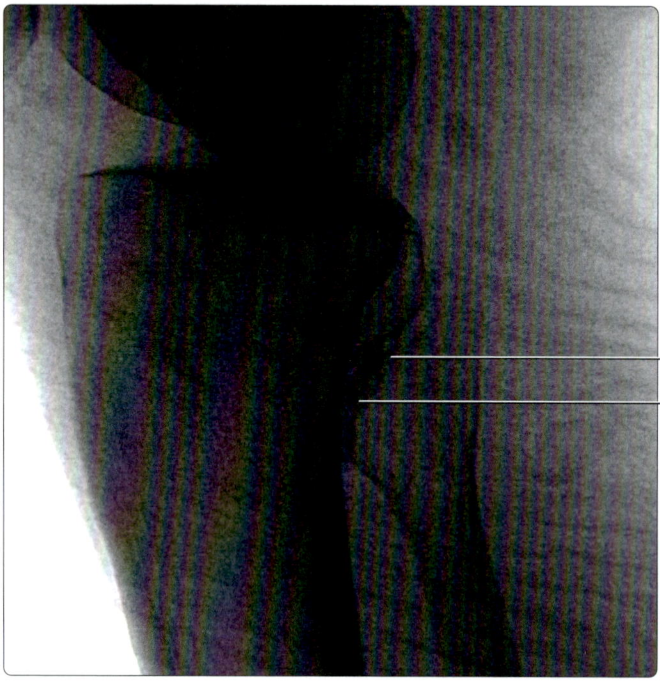

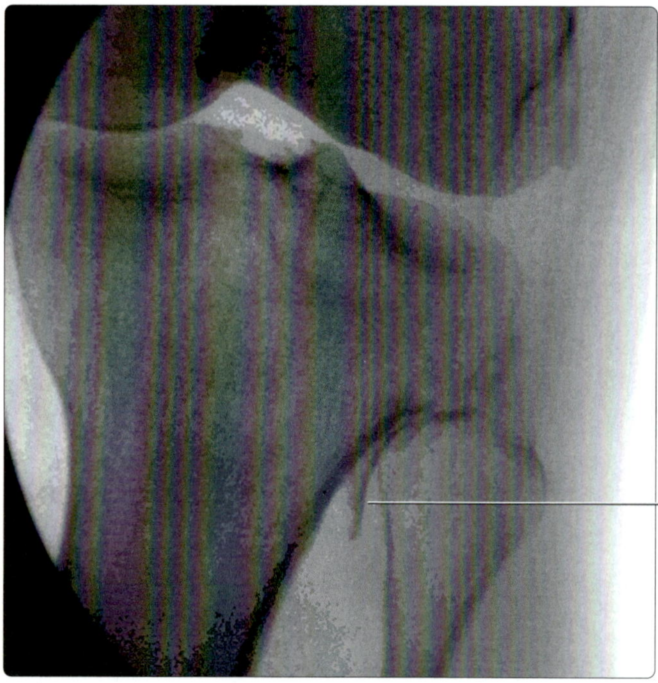

(Top) *Lateral view shows contrast within the proximal tibiofemoral joint. The knee is rotated so that the tibiofibular joint is projected posterior to the tibia.* **(Bottom)** *Anteroposterior view shows freely flowing contrast in the proximal tibiofemoral joint. The joint is not distended since contrast was placed simply to verify intraarticular positioning prior to injection of anesthetic and steroids.*

ANKLE INJECTION/ASPIRATION

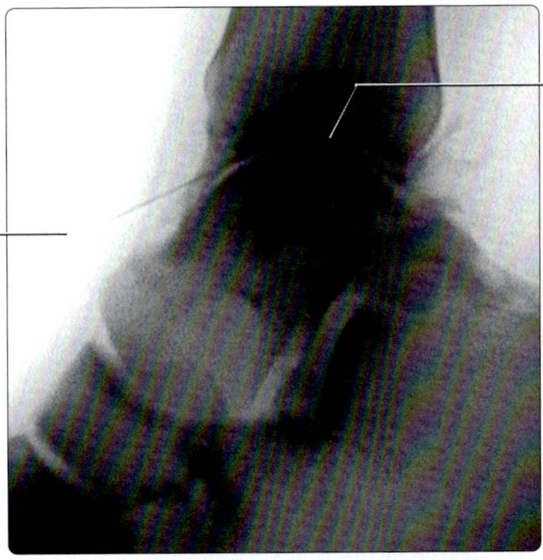

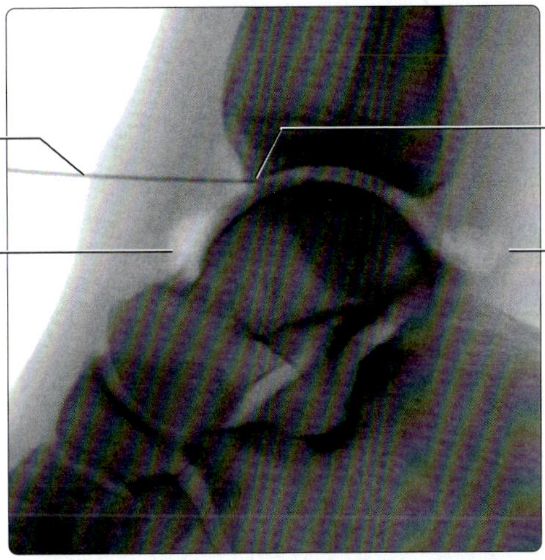

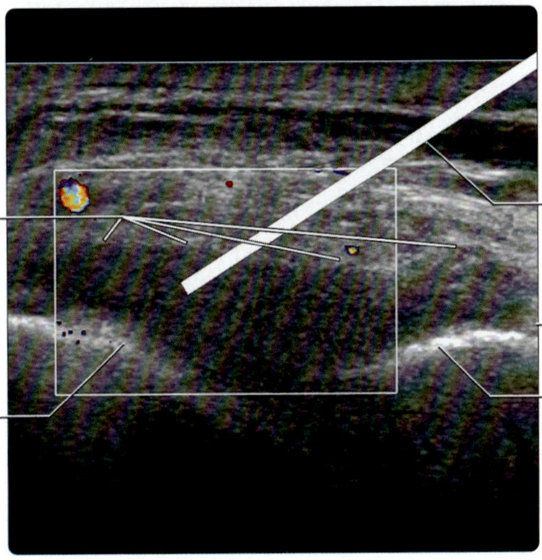

(Top) *Lateral iodine-contrast arthrogram shows cephalad needle angle, with the needle tip under the anterior margin of the tibia. Contrast must always flow away from the needle tip immediately on injection; if contrast puddles around the needle tip, then the needle is not intraarticular.* **(Middle)** *Lateral ankle injection shows the use of air as a contrast agent to verify intraarticular location of the needle.* **(Bottom)** *Sagittal ultrasound through the anterior ankle shows trajectory for needle placement in a patient with septic arthritis of the ankle.*

HINDFOOT AND MIDFOOT INJECTIONS

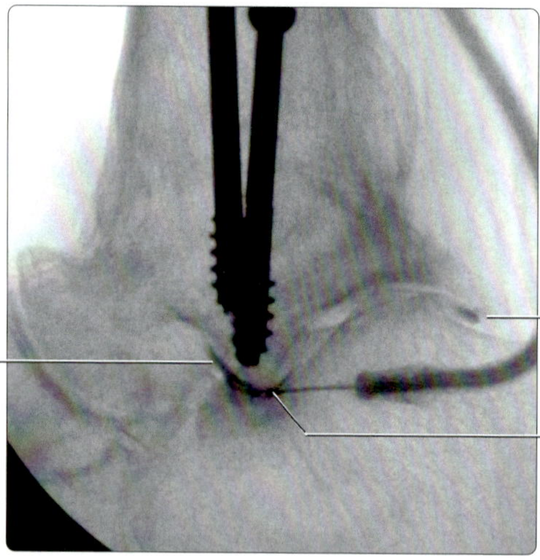

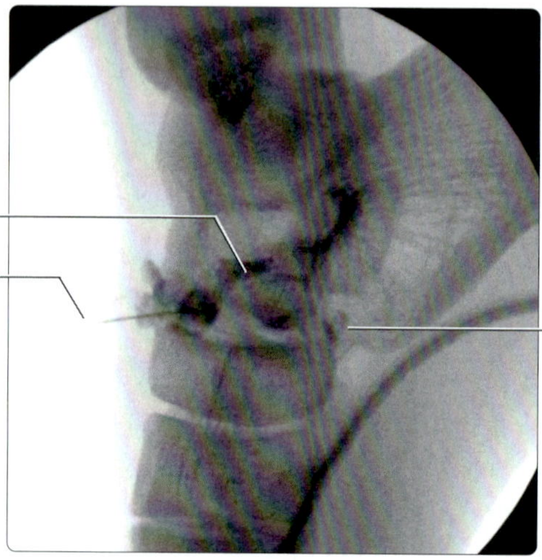

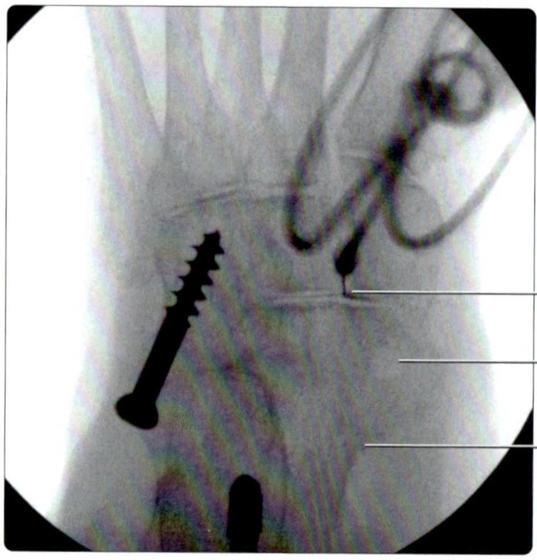

(Top) *Lateral posterior subtalar arthrogram shows point of entry at the anterior margin of the joint, between the lateral process of talus and the angle of Gissane. Contrast normally fills the recess anterior to the lateral process, at the posterior portion of the tarsal sinus.* **(Middle)** *Lateral arthrogram shows the needle in the talonavicular joint. Note the inferior recess of the joint. Contrast also extends into the anterior subtalar joint.* **(Bottom)** *Anteroposterior arthrogram shows needle placement in the midportion of the naviculocuneiform joint. The patient is status post triple arthrodesis (fusion of talonavicular, subtalar, and calcaneocuboid joints).*

TARSOMETATARSAL INJECTIONS

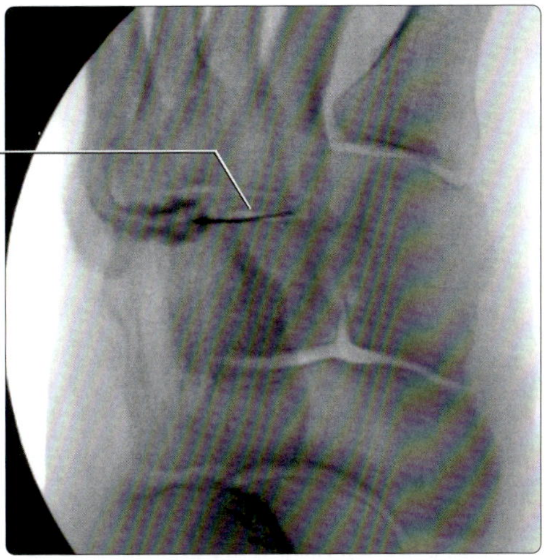

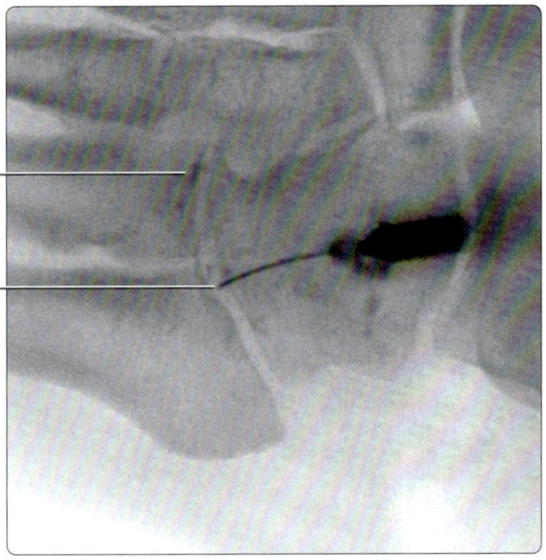

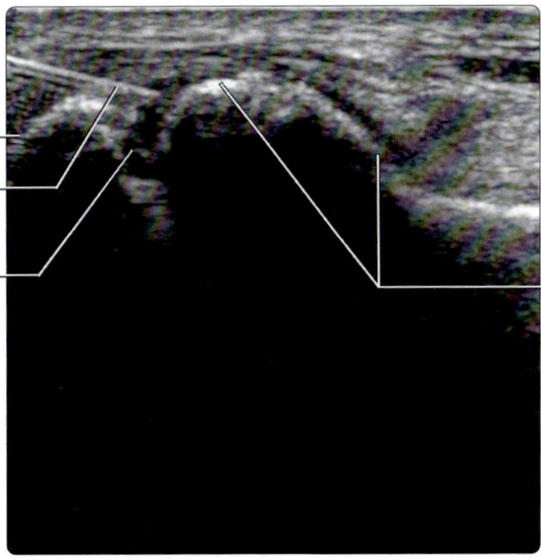

(Top) *Anteroposterior arthrogram of the 2nd tarsometatarsal shows needle placement and flow of contrast away from the needle tip, confirming intraarticular placement.* **(Middle)** *Oblique arthrogram shows needle entry into the 5th tarsometatarsal joint. Contrast flows into the 4th tarsometatarsal joint, which normally communicates with the 5th. A slightly oblique position for the foot helps to avoid overlapping of the joint surfaces in this region and makes arthrography easier.* **(Bottom)** *Longitudinal ultrasound shows placement of a 25-gauge needle in the 4th tarsometatarsal joint. A hockey stick probe is placed centered just proximal to the joint, and the needle enters the joint from a distal approach.*

METATARSOPHALANGEAL JOINT INJECTIONS

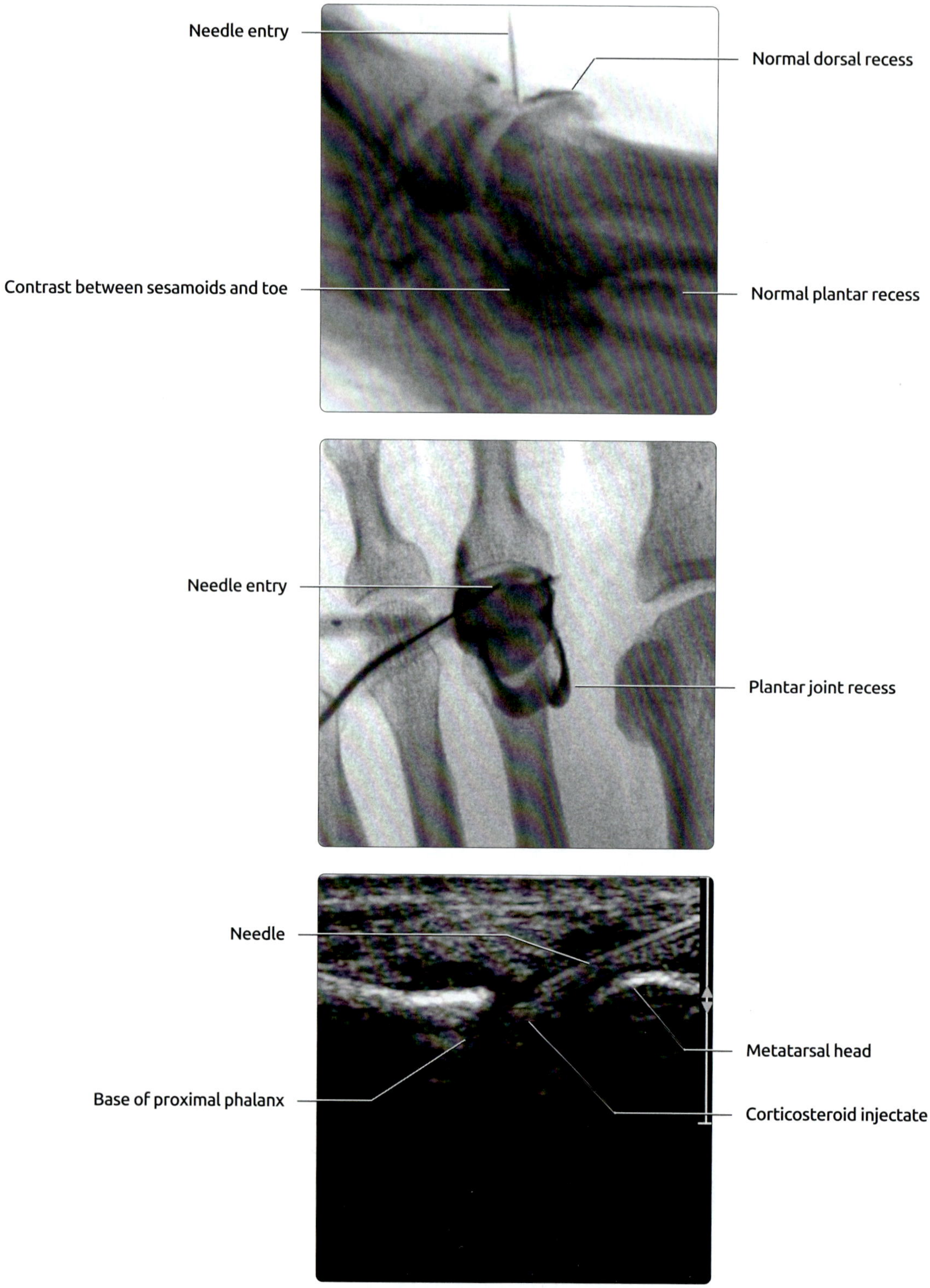

(Top) *Lateral arthrogram shows needle placement from the dorsal approach. Note normal extent of the dorsal and plantar recesses.* **(Middle)** *Anteroposterior arthrogram shows needle placement over the dorsal margin of the 2nd metatarsal head with a slight distal angulation. This angulation parallels the articular surface of the metatarsal head, and aids precise placement.* **(Bottom)** *Sagittal ultrasound shows needle entry into the 2nd metatarsophalangeal joint. A hockey stick transducer has been placed along the long axis of the joint, centered at its distal portion. The needle enters from proximal to distal, following the curve of the metatarsal head. Corticosteroid injectate is visualized in real time as hyperechoic bubbles flowing away from the needle tip.*

TENDON SHEATH INJECTIONS

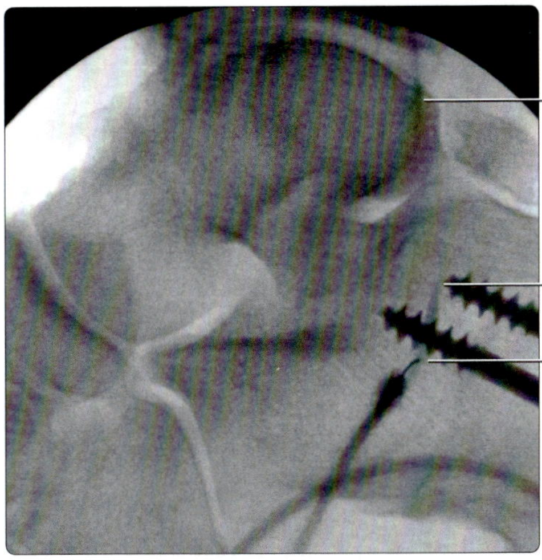

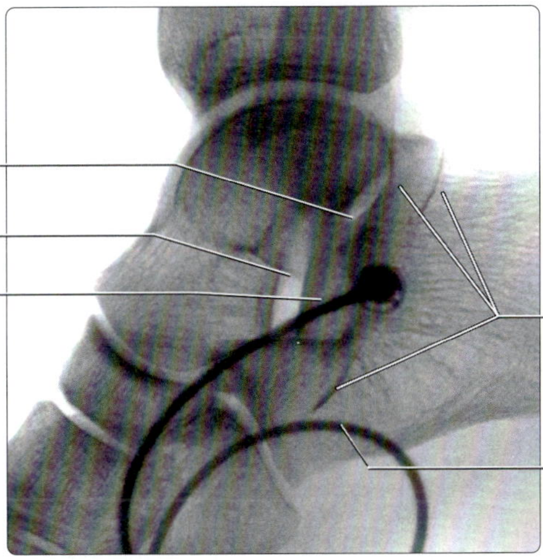

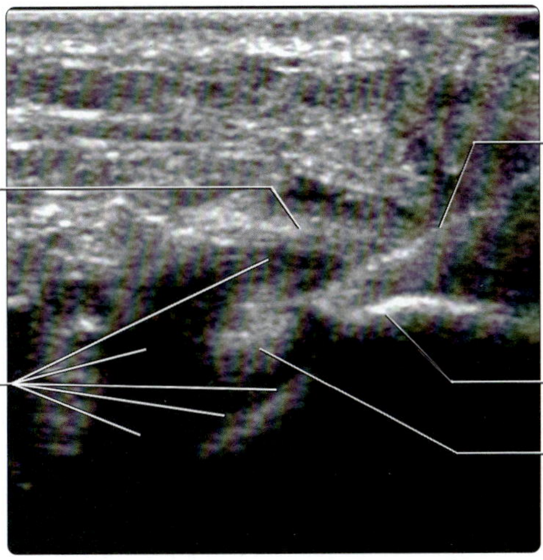

(Top) *Lateral fluoroscopic peroneal tendon sheath injection shows needle entry below the lateral malleolus. The tendons are palpated. The needle is advanced to the bone between the tendons, then withdrawn slightly as lidocaine is injected. When fluid flows freely, the needle tip is in the tendon sheath. Contrast is then injected and flows away from the needle tip along the tendon sheath.* **(Middle)** *Lateral fluoroscopic tendon sheath injection shows placement of a 25-gauge needle in the flexor hallucis longus tendon sheath. The needle was placed along the inferior margin of the sustentaculum tali and advanced to bone. The needle was then withdrawn slowly as lidocaine was injected. When lidocaine flows freely, contrast is injected to confirm flow of contrast along the tendon sheath.* **(Bottom)** *Axial ultrasound-guided posterior tibial tendon sheath injection shows needle tip in tendon sheath and injected fluid surrounding the tendon.*

INDEX

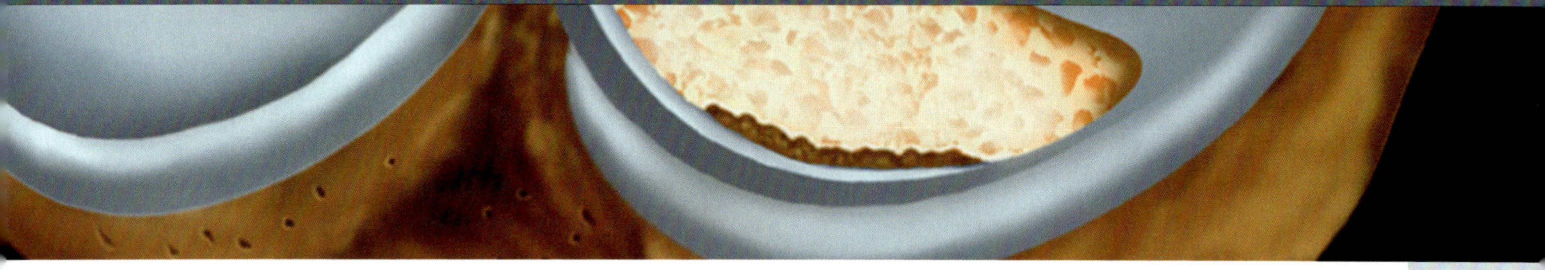

A

INDEX

INDEX

B

C

INDEX

D

E

F

G

H

I

INDEX

J

K

L

INDEX

M

INDEX

INDEX

N

INDEX

O

P

INDEX

INDEX

INDEX

T

INDEX

INDEX

U

V